INFECTION AND AUTOIMMUNITY

INFECTION AND AUTOIMMUNITY

Second Edition

Edited by

YEHUDA SHOENFELD
Zabludowicz Center for Autoimmune Diseases, Sheba Medical Center, Tel Hashomer, affiliated with Sackler Faculty of Medicine, Tel Aviv University, and Laura Schwarz-Kip Chair for Research of Autoimmune Diseases, Sackler Faculty of Medicine, Tel-Aviv University, Ramat Aviv, Israel

NANCY AGMON-LEVIN
Zabludowicz Center for Autoimmune Diseases, Sheba Medical Center, Tel Hashomer, affiliated with Sackler Faculty of Medicine, Tel Aviv University, Ramat Aviv, Israel

NOEL R. ROSE
Department of Pathology, Department of Molecular Microbiology and Immunology, the Center for Autoimmune Disease Research, The Johns Hopkins Schools of Medicine and Public Health, Baltimore, Maryland, USA

AMSTERDAM • BOSTON • HEIDELBERG • LONDON
NEW YORK • OXFORD • PARIS • SAN DIEGO
SAN FRANCISCO • SINGAPORE • SYDNEY • TOKYO
Academic Press is an imprint of Elsevier

Academic Press is an imprint of Elsevier
32 Jamestown Road, London NW1 7BY, UK
525 B Street, Suite 1800, San Diego, CA 92101-4495, USA
225 Wyman Street, Waltham, MA 02451, USA
The Boulevard, Langford Lane, Kidlington, Oxford OX5 1GB, UK

First published 2004

Notices

Knowledge and best practice in this field are constantly changing. As new research and experience broaden our understanding, changes in research methods, professional practices, or medical treatment may become necessary.

Practitioners and researchers must always rely on their own experience and knowledge in evaluating and using any information, methods, compounds, or experiments described herein. In using such information or methods they should be mindful of their own safety and the safety of others, including parties for whom they have a professional responsibility.

To the fullest extent of the law, neither the Publisher nor the authors, contributors, or editors, assume any liability for any injury and/or damage to persons or property as a matter of products liability, negligence or otherwise, or from any use or operation of any methods, products, instructions, or ideas contained in the material herein.

British Library Cataloguing in Publication Data
A catalogue record for this book is available from the British Library

Library of Congress Cataloging-in-Publication Data
A catalog record for this book is available from the Library of Congress

ISBN: 978-0-444-63269-2

For information on all Academic Press publications visit our website at **store.elsevier.com**

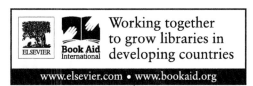

Working together
to grow libraries in
developing countries

www.elsevier.com • www.bookaid.org

CONTENTS

CONTRIBUTORS

Alexander Abdurakhmanov
Department of Medicine, C Wolfson Medical Center, Sackler Faculty of Medicine, Tel Aviv University, Tel Aviv, Israel

Mahmoud Abu-Shakra
Rheumatic Diseases Unit, Soroka Medical Center and Ben-Gurion University, Beer-Sheva, Israel

Marina Afanasyeva
Department of Epidemiology and Community Medicine, Faculty of Medicine, University of Ottawa, Ottawa, Ontario, Canada

Nancy Agmon-Levin
Zabludowicz Center for Autoimmune Diseases, Sheba Medical Center, Tel-Hashomer, Sackler Medical School, and Sackler Faculty of Medicine, Tel Aviv University, Tel Aviv, Israel

Paul J. Albert
Weill Cornell Medical College, New York, USA

Isabel Almeida
Medicine Service and Clinical Immunology Unit—Centro Hospitalar do Porto and Unit for Multidisciplinary Research in Biomedicine (UMIB/ICBAS)—Porto University, Portugal

Rute Alves
Medicine Service—Centro Hospitalar do Porto, Portugal

Howard Amital
Zabludowicz Center for Autoimmune Diseases, Sheba Medical Center, Tel Hashomer, Sackler Faculty of Medicine, Tel Aviv University, Ramat Aviv, and Internal Medicine Department B, Sheba Medical Center, Tel Hashomer, Israel

Paulo Andrade
Infectious Diseases Department Hospital São João, Porto, Portugal

Alessandro Antonelli
Department of Clinical and Experimental Medicine, University of Pisa, Pisa, Italy

Antonio Puccetti
Department of Immunology, Institute G. Gaslini, and Department of Experimental Medicine, Unit of Histology, University of Genoa, Genoa, Italy

María-Teresa Arango
Zabludowicz Center for Autoimmune Diseases, Sheba Medical Center, Tel-Hashomer, Sackler Medical School, Tel Aviv University, Tel Aviv, Israel; Center for Autoimmune Diseases Research, and Doctoral Program in Biomedical Sciences, Universidad del Rosario, Bogotá, Colombia

Fabiola Atzeni
Rheumatology Unit, L. Sacco University Hospital, Milan, Italy

Alison E. Baird
Division of Cerebrovascular Disease and Stroke, Department of Neurology, State University of New York, Downstate Medical Center, Brooklyn, New York, USA

Alexandra Balbir-Gurman
B. Shine Rheumatology Unit, Rambam Health Care Campus, and Bruce and Ruth Rappoport Faculty of Medicine, Technion-Israel Institute of Technology, Haifa, Israel

Tomer Bashi
Zabludowicz Center for Autoimmune Diseases, Sheba Medical Center, Tel Aviv University, Ramat Gan, Israel

Alberto Batticciotto
Rheumatology Unit, L. Sacco University Hospital, Milan, Italy

Maurizio Benucci
Unit of Rheumatology, Ospedale San Giovanni di Dio, Florence, Italy

Miri Blank
Zabludowicz Center for Autoimmune Diseases, Sheba Medical Center, Tel Aviv University, Ramat Gan, Israel

Dimitrios P. Bogdanos
Division of Transplantation Immunology and Mucosal Biology, King's College London School of Medicine at King's College Hospital, Denmark Hill Campus, London, UK, and Department of Rheumatology, School of Health Sciences, University of Thessaly, Larissa, Greece

S. Bombardieri
Dipartimento di Malattie Muscoloscheletriche e Cutanee, U.O. Reumatologia, Pisa, Italy

E. Borella
Division of Rheumatology, Department of Medicine, University of Padova, Padova, Italy

Samantha Bosis
Department of Pathophysiology and Transplantation, Pediatric Highly Intensive Care Unit, Università degli Studi di Milano, Fondazione IRCCS Ca' Granda Ospedale Maggiore Policlinico, Milan, Italy

Vasiliki Kalliopi Bournia
First Department of Propeudeutic and Internal Medicine, Laikon General Hospital, Athens, Greece

Mariana Brandão
Centro Hospitalar do Porto and Unit for Multidisciplinary Research in Biomedicine (UMIB/ICBAS)—Porto University, Portugal

Yolanda Braun-Moscovici
B. Shine Rheumatology Unit, Rambam Health Care Campus, and Bruce and Ruth Rappoport Faculty of Medicine, Technion-Israel Institute of Technology, Haifa, Israel

Neta Brender-Gotlieb
Department of Internal Medicine F, Sheba Medical Center, Tel Hashomer, Israel

Francesca Cainelli
Department of Internal Medicine, Faculty of Medicine, University of Botswana, Gaborone, Botswana

Cezar Augusto Muniz Caldas
Department of Internal Medicine, Universidade Federal do Pará, and Curso de Medicina do Centro Universitário do Estado do Pará—CESUPA, Belém, Pará, Brazil

A. Campar
Clinical Medicine Department, Cento Hospitalar do Porto, Portugal

Graziela Carvalheiras
Centro Hospitalar do Porto and Unit for Multidisciplinary Research in Biomedicine (UMIB/ICBAS)—Porto University, Portugal

R. Cervera
Department of Autoimmune Diseases, Hospital Clínic, Barcelona, Catalonia, Spain

Joab Chapman
Zabludowicz Center for Autoimmune Diseases, Sheba Medical Center, Tel-Hashomer, Sackler Medical School, Tel Aviv University, Tel Aviv, and Department of Neurology and Sagol Center for Neurosciences, Sheba Medical Center, Tel-Hashomer, Israel

Emily M.L. Chastain
Department of Microbiology-Immunology and Interdepartmental Immunobiology Center, Feinberg School of Medicine, Northwestern University, Chicago, Illinois, USA

Lunardi Claudio
Department of Medicine, Unit of Internal Medicine, University of Verona, Verona, Italy

Eytan Cohen
Department of Medicine F, Rabin Medical Center, Beilinson Campus, Sackler Faculty of Medicine, Tel Aviv University, Tel Aviv, Israel

Fabrizio Conti
Reumatologia, Dipartimento di Medicina Interna e Specialità Mediche, Sapienza Università Roma, Roma, Italy

J. Correia
Clinical Immunology Unit, Cento Hospitalar do Porto, Portugal

Jozélio Freire de Carvalho
Rheumatology Division, Aliança Medical Center, Salvador, Bahia, Brazil

A. Della Rossa
Dipartimento di Malattie Muscoloscheletriche e Cutanee, U.O. Reumatologia, Pisa, Italy

Barbara Detrick
Department of Pathology, School of Medicine, The Johns Hopkins University, Baltimore, Maryland, USA

Melanie Deutsch
2nd Department of Medicine and Laboratory, University of Athens Medical School, Hippokration General Hospital, Athens, Greece

Andrea Di Domenicantonio
Department of Clinical and Experimental Medicine, University of Pisa, Pisa, Italy

M. Domeneghetti
Division of Rheumatology, Department of Medicine, University of Padova, Padova, Italy

Vital Domingues
Centro Hospitalar do Porto, Portugal

A. Doria
Division of Rheumatology, Department of Medicine, University of Padova, Padova, Italy

Coad Thomas Dow
McPherson Eye Research Institute, University of Wisconsin-Madison, Madison, United States and Chippewa Valley Eye Clinic, Eau Claire, United States

David H. Dreyfus
Associate Clinical Professor, Department of Pediatrics, Yale SOM, New Haven, Connecticut, USA

Elise E. Drouin
The Center for Immunology and Inflammatory Diseases, Massachusetts General Hospital, Harvard Medical School, Boston, Massachusetts, USA

Anna Dubaniewicz
Department of Pneumology, Medical University of Gdansk, Gdansk, Poland

Malarvizhi Durai
Department of Microbiology and Immunology, University of Maryland School of Medicine, Baltimore, Maryland, USA

Alan Ebringer
Analytical Sciences Group, King's College London, London, UK

Michael Ehrenfeld
Rheumatic Disease Unit, Zabludowicz Center for Autoimmune Diseases, Chaim Sheba Medical Center, Tel Hashomer, Israel

Tinazzi Elisa
Department of Medicine, Unit of Internal Medicine, University of Verona, Verona, Italy

Susanna Esposito
Department of Pathophysiology and Transplantation, Pediatric Highly Intensive Care Unit, Università degli Studi di Milano, Fondazione IRCCS Ca' Granda Ospedale Maggiore Policlinico, Milan, Italy

Poupak Fallahi
Department of Clinical and Experimental Medicine, University of Pisa, Pisa, Italy

Raquel Faria
Medicine Service and Clinical Immunology Unit—Centro Hospitalar do Porto and Unit for Multidisciplinary Research in Biomedicine (UMIB/ICBAS)—Porto University, Portugal

Fátima Farinha
Medicine Service and Clinical Immunology Unit—Centro Hospitalar do Porto and Unit for Multidisciplinary Research in Biomedicine (UMIB/ICBAS)—Porto University, Portugal

Ele Ferrannini
Department of Clinical and Experimental Medicine, University of Pisa, Pisa, Italy

Silvia Martina Ferrari
Department of Clinical and Experimental Medicine, University of Pisa, Pisa, Italy

Alvaro Ferreira
Unidade de Imunologia Clínica, Centro Hospitalar do Porto, and UMIB/ICBAS, Universidade do Porto, Porto, Portugal

C. Ferrão
Clinical Medicine Department, Centro Hospitalar do Porto, Portugal

Ravindra Kumar Garg
Department of Neurology, King George Medical University, Lucknow, Uttar Pradesh, India

M. Gatto
Division of Rheumatology, Department of Medicine, University of Padova, Padova, Italy

A. Ghirardello
Division of Rheumatology, Department of Medicine, University of Padova, Padova, Italy

Zanoni Giovanna
Department of Pathology and Diagnostics, Unit of Immunology, University of Verona, Verona, Italy

Patuzzo Giuseppe
Department of Medicine, Unit of Internal Medicine, University of Verona, Verona, Italy

Gili Givaty
Zabludowicz Center for Autoimmune Diseases, Sheba Medical Center, Tel-Hashomer, Sackler Medical School, Tel Aviv University, Tel Aviv, and Neurology Department and Sagol Neuroscience Center, Sheba Medical Center, Tel-Hashomer, Israel

Luiza Guilherme
Heart Institute—InCor, University of São Paulo, School of Medicine, and Institute for Immunology Investigation, National Institute for Science and Technology, São Paulo, Brazil

Sara Salehi Hammerstad
Division of Endocrinology, Diabetes, and Bone Disease, Department of Medicine, Mount Sinai School of Medicine, New York, New York, USA, and Division of Pediatric Endocrinology and Diabetes, Oslo University Hospital, Oslo, Norway

Emillia Hodak
Department of Dermatology, Rabin Medical Center, Petach Tikva, and Sackler Faculty of Medicine, Tel Aviv University, Tel Aviv, Israel

John J. Hooks
Laboratory of Immunology, National Eye Institute, National Institutes of Health, Bethesda, Maryland, USA

L. Iaccarino
Division of Rheumatology, Department of Medicine, University of Padova, Padova, Italy

Pietro Invernizzi
Liver Unit and Center for Autoimmune Liver Diseases, Humanitas Clinical and Research Center, Rozanno, Milan, Italy

Eitan Israeli
Center for Autoimmune Diseases, Sheba Medical Center, Tel-Hashomer, Israel

Christophe Jamin
Immunologie et Pathologie, LabEx IGO, SFR ScInBioS, Université de Brest et Université Européenne de Bretagne, and Laboratory of Immunology and Immunotherapy, CHRU Brest, Brest, France

Sok-Ja Janket
Department of General Dentistry, Boston University, Henry M. Goldman School of Dental Medicine, Boston, Massachusetts, USA

Peter Jarčuška
1st Department of Internal Medicine, Medical Faculty of P. J. Šafárik University Košice, Slovakia

Rodney P. Jones
Healthcare Analysis & Forecasting, Camberley, UK

Jorge Kalil
Heart Institute—InCor, University of São Paulo, School of Medicine; Institute for Immunology Investigation, National Institute for Science and Technology, and Clinical Immunology and Allergy, Department of Clinical Medicine University of São Paulo, School of Medicine, São Paulo, Brazil

Eleni Kanasi
Department of General Dentistry, Boston University, Henry M. Goldman School of Dental Medicine, Boston, Massachusetts, USA

Shaye Kivity
Zabludowicz Center for Autoimmune Diseases, Sheba Medical Center, Tel-Hashomer, Sackler Medical School, Tel Aviv University, Tel Aviv; Rheumatic Disease Unit, and The Dr. Pinchas Borenstein Talpiot Medical Leadership Program 2013, Sheba Medical Center, Tel-Hashomer, Israel

Tom Konikoff
Zabludowicz Center for Autoimmune Diseases, Sheba Medical Center, Tel Aviv University, Ramat Gan, Israel

D. Kozáková
National Institute of Rheumatic Disease, Piešťany, Slovakia

Ilan Krause
Department of Medicine F, Rabin Medical Center, Beilinson Campus, Sackler Faculty of Medicine, Tel Aviv University, Tel Aviv, Israel

Aaron Lerner
Pediatric Gastroenterology and Nutrition Unit, Carmel Medical Center, B. Rappaport School of Medicine, Technion-Israel Institute of Technology, Haifa, Israel

Merav Lidar
Rheumatology Unit, Sheba Medical Center, Tel Hashomer, Israel and Sackler Faculty of Medicine, Tel Aviv University, Tel Aviv, Israel

Eduard Ling
Pediatric Rheumatic Diseases Unit, Soroka Medical Center and Ben-Gurion University, Beer-Sheva, Israel

Hussein Mahajna
Department of Medicine 'B', Sheba Medical Center, Tel-Hashomer, Sackler Faculty of Medicine, Tel Aviv University, Tel Aviv, Israel

Naim Mahroum
Department of Medicine 'B', Sheba Medical Center, Tel-Hashomer, Sackler Faculty of Medicine, Tel Aviv University, Tel Aviv, Israel

Ramit Maoz-Segal
Zabludowicz Center for Autoimmune Diseases, Sheba Medical Center, Tel-Hashomer, Israel

António Marinho
Unidade de Imunologia Clínica, Centro Hospitalar do Porto, and UMIB/ICBAS, Universidade do Porto, Portugal

Trevor G. Marshall
Autoimmunity Research Foundation, Thousand Oaks, California, USA

Maria Martinelli
Zabludowicz Center for Autoimmune Diseases, Sheba Medical Center, Tel Hashomer, Sackler Faculty of Medicine, Tel Aviv University, Ramat Aviv, Israel, and Division of Rheumatology, Department of Medicine, University of Brescia, Brescia, Italy

Dolcino Marzia
Department of Immunology, Institute G. Gaslini, Genoa, Italy

Clio P. Mavragani
Department of Physiology, School of Medicine, University of Athens, Athens, Greece

Teresa Mendonça
Medicine Service and Clinical Immunology Unit—Centro Hospitalar do Porto and Unit for Multidisciplinary Research in Biomedicine (UMIB/ICBAS)—Porto University, Portugal

Stephen D. Miller
Department of Microbiology-Immunology and Interdepartmental Immunobiology Center, Feinberg School of Medicine, Northwestern University, Chicago, Illinois, USA

Daniel Mimouni
Department of Dermatology, Rabin Medical Center, Petach Tikva, and Sackler Faculty of Medicine, Tel Aviv University, Tel Aviv, Israel

Marta Monteiro
Unidade de Imunologia Clínica, Centro Hospitalar do Porto, and UMIB/ICBAS, Universidade do Porto, Portugal

Kamal D. Moudgil
Department of Microbiology and Immunology, University of Maryland School of Medicine, Baltimore, Maryland, USA

Vaishali R. Moulton
Division of Rheumatology, Department of Medicine, Beth Israel Deaconess Medical Center, Harvard Medical School, Boston, Massachusetts, USA

Haralampos M. Moutsopoulos
Department of Pathophysiology, School of Medicine, University of Athens, Athens, Greece

Kamalpreet Nagpal
Division of Rheumatology, Department of Medicine, Beth Israel Deaconess Medical Center, Harvard Medical School, Boston, Massachusetts, USA

Esmeralda Neves
Centro Hospitalar do Porto and Unit for Multidisciplinary Research in Biomedicine (UMIB/ICBAS)—Porto University, Portugal

Robert Nussenblatt
Laboratory of Immunology, National Eye Institute, National Institutes of Health, Bethesda, Maryland, USA

Ayelet Ollech
Department of Dermatology, Rabin Medical Center, Petach Tikva, Israel

L. Palma
Division of Rheumatology, Department of Medicine-DIMED, University of Padova, Padova, Italy

Sandra Gofinet Pasoto
Rheumatology Division, Hospital das Clínicas da Universidade de São Paulo, São Paulo, Brazil

Daniel Pella
1st Department of Internal Medicine, Medical Faculty of P. J. Šafárik University Košice, Slovakia

Cláudia Pereira
Medicine Service—Centro Hospitalar do Porto, Portugal

Carlo Perricone
Reumatologia, Dipartimento di Medicina Interna e Specialità Mediche, Sapienza Università di Roma, Roma, Italy

Jana Petríková
1st Department of Internal Medicine, Medical Faculty of P. J. Šafárik University Košice, Slovakia

Amy D. Proal
Autoimmunity Research Foundation, Thousand Oaks, California, USA

Taha Rashid
Analytical Sciences Group, King's College London, London, UK

Shimon Reif
Pediatric Department, Hadassah Medical Center, Hebrew University of Jerusalem, Jerusalem, Israel

Yves Renaudineau
Immunologie et Pathologie, LabEx IGO, SFR ScInBioS, Université de Brest et Université Européenne de Bretagne, and Laboratory of Immunology and Immunotherapy, CHRU Brest, Brest, France

Francinne Machado Ribeiro
Rheumatologist; Department of Rheumatology. Universidade do Estado do Rio de Janeiro, RJ, Brazil

Donato Rigante
Institute of Pediatrics, Università Cattolica Sacro Cuore, Rome, Italy

Eirini I. Rigopoulou
Department of Medicine, School of Health Sciences, University of Thessaly, Larissa, Greece

Noel R. Rose
Departments of Pathology and of Molecular Microbiology and Immunology, The Johns Hopkins Schools of Medicine and Public Health, Baltimore, Maryland, USA

Cristina Rosário
Internal Medicine Department, Hospital Pedro Hispano, Matosinhos, Portugal

J. Rovenský
National Institute of Rheumatic Disease, Piešťany, Slovakia

Lazaros I. Sakkas
Department of Rheumatology, School of Health Sciences, University of Thessaly, Larissa, Greece

Piercarlo Sarzi-Puttini
Rheumatology Unit, L. Sacco University Hospital, Milan, Italy

Luciana Parente Costa Seguro
Rheumatology Division, Hospital das Clínicas da Universidade de São Paulo, São Paulo, Brazil

Margherita Semino
Department of Pathophysiology and Transplantation, Pediatric Highly Intensive Care Unit, Università degli Studi di Milano, Fondazione IRCCS Ca' Granda Ospedale Maggiore Policlinico, Milan, Italy

Yehuda Shoenfeld
Zabludowicz Center for Autoimmune Diseases, Sheba Medical Center, Research of Autoimmune Diseases, and Sackler Faculty of Medicine, Tel-Aviv University, Tel-Hashomer, Israel

S. Silva
Clinical Medicine Department, Cento Hospitalar do Porto, Portugal

Laurent Simonin
Laboratory of Immunology and Immunotherapy, CHRU Brest, Brest, France

Daniel S. Smyk
Institute of Liver Studies, King's College London School of Medicine at King's College Hospital, and Division of Transplantation Immunology and Musosal Biology, King's College London School of Medicine at King's College Hospital, Denmark Hill Campus, London, UK

Rita Catarina Medeiros Sousa
Núcleo de Medicina Tropical, Universidade Federal do Pará, Belém, Pará, Brazil

C. Stagnaro
Dipartimento di Malattie Muscoloscheletriche e Cutanee, U.O. Reumatologia, Pisa, Italy

Allen C. Steere
The Center for Immunology and Inflammatory Diseases, Massachusetts General Hospital, Harvard Medical School, Boston, Massachusetts, USA

Klemen Strle
The Center for Immunology and Inflammatory Diseases, Massachusetts General Hospital, Harvard Medical School, Boston, Massachusetts, USA

Maria G. Tektonidou
First Department of Internal Medicine, Medical School, University of Athens, Laikon General Hospital, Athens, Greece

Moshe Tishler
Department of Medicine B, Asaf Harofe Medical Center, Zrifin, and Tel Aviv University, Sackler School of Medicine, Tel Aviv, Israel

Yaron Tomer
Division of Endocrinology, Diabetes, and Bone Disease, Department of Medicine, Mount Sinai School of Medicine, New York, New York, USA

Elias Toubi
Division of Allergy and Clinical Immunology, Bnai-Zion Medical Center, Faculty of Medicine, Technion, Haifa, Israel

George C. Tsokos
Division of Rheumatology, Department of Medicine, Beth Israel Deaconess Medical Center, Harvard Medical School, Boston, Massachusetts, USA

Zahava Vadasz
Division of Allergy and Clinical Immunology, Bnai-Zion Medical Center, Faculty of Medicine, Technion, Haifa, Israel

Guido Valesini
Reumatologia, Dipartimento di Medicina Interna e Specialità Mediche, Sapienza Universitàdi Roma, Roma, Italy

Carlos Vasconcelos
Unidade de Imunologia Clínica, Centro Hospitalar do Porto, and UMIB/ICBAS, Universidade do Porto, Portugal

Júlia Vasconcelos
Centro Hospitalar do Porto and Unit for Multidisciplinary Research in Biomedicine (UMIB/ICBAS) - Porto University, Portugal

Dimitrios Vassilopoulos
2nd Department of Medicine and Laboratory, University of Athens Medical School, Hippokration General Hospital, Athens, Greece

Shivaprasad H. Venkatesha
Department of Microbiology and Immunology, University of Maryland School of Medicine, Baltimore, Maryland, USA

Sandro Vento
Department of Internal Medicine, Faculty of Medicine, University of Botswana, Gaborone, Botswana

Christophe Viale
Laboratory of Immunology and Immunotherapy, CHRU Brest, Brest, France

Ronald Villanueva
Division of Endocrinology, Diabetes, and Bone Disease, Department of Medicine, Mount Sinai School of Medicine, New York, New York, USA

Pedro Vita
Unidade de Imunologia Clínica, Centro Hospitalar do Porto, and UMIB/ICBAS, Universidade do Porto, Porto, Portugal

Clyde Wilson
Departments of Microbiology and Pathology, King Edward VII Memorial Hospital, Hamilton, Bermuda

Pierre Youinou
Immunologie et Pathologie, LabEx IGO, SFR ScInBioS, Université de Brest et Université Européenne de Bretagne, Brest, France

E. Záňová
National Institute of Rheumatic Disease, Piešťany, Slovakia

Gisele Zandman-Goddard
Department of Medicine, C Wolfson Medical Center, Sackler Faculty of Medicine, Tel Aviv University, Tel Aviv, Israel

M. Zen
Division of Rheumatology, Department of Medicine, University of Padova, Padova, Italy

Opinions expressed by the chapter authors are not necessarily those of the editors.

CHAPTER 1

Introduction

Noel R. Rose[1]
Department of Pathology, Center for Autoimmune Disease Research, The Johns Hopkins Schools of Medicine and Public Health, Baltimore, Maryland, USA and
Department of Molecular Microbiology and Immunology, and the Center for Autoimmune Disease Research, The Johns Hopkins Schools of Medicine and Public Health, Baltimore, Maryland, USA
[1]Corresponding Author: nrrose@jhmi.edu

1 INTRODUCTION

Humans and microorganisms have lived together in reasonable harmony for many millennia. Coevolution for so long has resulted in a commensal relationship of mutual benefit. Humans accommodate vast numbers of microorganisms of many descriptions on virtually all exposed body surfaces, especially the skin, mucosal linings and gastrointestinal tract. Evolution produced a wide variety of microorganisms well adapted to living harmoniously with their human partners. These microbes learned to avoid or sometimes even actively suppress immune responses that might interfere with their survival. Humans, for their part, have adapted mechanisms to evade the harmful activities of microorganisms that threaten the host's life and impair their reproduction. The life-long delicate balance between these two essential requirements dictated by coevolution produced a generally stable microbial population – the microbiota – which actually exceeds by 10-fold the number of cells that comprise the human body.

On a day-to-day basis, this balance not only avoids injury to either party, microbial or human, but frequently results in a homeostatic equilibrium advantageous to both. Members of the microbiome have found a congenial environmental niche. The microbial population, in turn, benefits the human host by performing valuable physiologic reactions and generating needed nutrients. Equally important, the resident microbial population itself retards infection or overgrowth by potentially harmful microorganisms.

At times, the symbiotic relationship established between the microbial population and its human counterpart become unbalanced because both parties are constantly subject to change. Aggressive microorganisms with overwhelming disease-inducing properties may gain the upper hand within

Infection and Autoimmunity
http://dx.doi.org/10.1016/B978-0-444-63269-2.09987-6

1

the microbial population. Alternatively, the ability of the human immune system to cope with the microbial population may falter because of changing age, hormonal status, nutrition and lifestyle. An example of a dysfunctional interrelationship between the host and its microbiome is the promotion of autoimmune disease as a consequence of infection. The conditions under which microbes can induce immune-mediated disease in the host remains an overarching topic of discussion today.

2 RHEUMATIC FEVER, A PRIME EXAMPLE

In medicine, the concept that pathogenic microorganisms can induce disease, not only by their direct pathogenic effects but also by affecting the host response, goes back centuries. In the eighteenth century, Edward Jenner, better known for his development of vaccination, noticed that an illness approximating rheumatic fever was sometimes a consequence of pharyngitis.[1] William Osler, arguably the keenest clinical observer, pointed out more than 100 years ago that some patients may die not from infection but from the body's response to it.[2] Paroxysmal cold hemoglobinuria, the first well-established example of an autoimmune disease in humans, was originally considered a sequela of syphilis.[3] Little progress could be made in verifying these clinical impressions, however, until more was learned about the fundamentals of infection and immunity.

Before 1940, the consensus opinion regarding rheumatic fever, a disease relatively well defined by generally accepted (Jones) criteria, was that it was a genetic disease but its expression was affected in some way by poverty and poor living conditions (see chapter 27). A few forward-looking investigators, such as A. F. Coburn in the United States, suggested that a dysregulated immune response was caused by a beta-hemolytic streptococcus infection of the throat.[4] Firm evidence to support this notion was lacking until World War II.

The 1940s brought together large numbers of young men from different parts of the United States in training camps to prepare them for military service. One such institution was the Great Lakes Naval Training Center near Chicago. As one of the major centers for the study of the spread of rheumatic fever among these young recruits, the availability of such a large population for research made it possible to show convincingly that rheumatic fever is associated with previous streptococcal pharyngitis. An entire generation of young American immunologists and microbiologists took up these studies in the years during and after the war and, in the process, received basic training that enabled them to establish many of the fundamental principals upon which are based our present understanding of the interaction of infection and immunity. They included such future stars as Lewis Thomas, Chandler Stetson, Robert Good, and Jonathan Uhr.

In the decades after World War II, studies of the immunologic basis of rheumatic fever were greatly enhanced by the introduction of new immunologic methods. For example, the application of immunofluorescence permitted M. H. Kaplan and his colleagues to show directly a cross-reaction between the beta-hemolytic streptococcus (*Streptococcus pyogenes*) and an antigen in the heart.[5] The introduction of gels for separating antigens in immune reactions allowed Halbert to define the precise cardiac antigens responsible for the association with streptococci.[6] Molecular methods used by Dale and Beachey and by Fischetti and colleagues enabled the delineation of the precise antigens of the streptococcus that are responsible for cross-reactions with human cardiac tissue.[7,8] These studies culminated in work by Beachey's student, Madeleine Cunningham,[9] who showed clearly that antibodies and T lymphocytes specific for epitopes on the streptococcal M protein cross-reacted with cardiac-specific proteins such as cardiac myosin. Furthermore, her investigations indicated that purified streptococcal antigens could actively induce myocarditis in experimental animals. Although heart muscle inflammation is one of the cardinal signs of rheumatic fever, the ultimate course of the disease is determined more often by endocarditis and its effect on the heart valves. Cunningham found that antibodies induced by streptococcal pharyngitis could cross-react with N-acetyl-β-D-glucosamine residues on the cardiac mitral valve endothelium. These classic studies provide the strongest evidence to date that a particular infection can actually induce an autoimmune disease in humans.

3 GUILLAIN–BARRÉ SYNDROME, A SECOND EXAMPLE

Another convincing example of a particular infection as the cause of human autoimmune disease is found in an acute motor axonal form of Guillain–Barré syndrome (GBS) originally encountered in northern China (see chapter 59). *Campylobacter jejuni*, a common intestinal inhabitant, has a constituent ganglioside, GM1, that cross-reacts with a similar antigen in human peripheral nerve axons.[10,11] The antigen has been isolated, defined and used to produce monoclonal antibodies. With these highly specific antiganglioside antibodies, J. W. Griffin and his team were able to induce a GBS-like response in experimental animals.[12] Thus, we now have two excellent examples of a defined microbial antigen mimicking its counterpart in the human host and inducing an immune response capable of reproducing in experimental animals the core features of the autoimmune disease in humans.

4 UNDERLYING MECHANISMS

The paradigm of rheumatic fever has brought to the fore the concept that molecular or epitope mimicry between a microorganism and a host constituent may explain the production of pathogenic autoimmunity following resolution of the infectious process. Multiple studies demonstrate that a microbial antigen very similar to, but perhaps slightly different from, its human equivalent induces an autoantibody response. In some investigations, T cells cross-react with the human counterpart of its cognate antigen. Molecular mimicry is a compelling theory to explain the association of infections with autoimmune disease.

At this time, however, there are few other examples of a human disease with this high level of evidence that mimicry is the cause.[13] Certainly, there are many well-described instances of molecular mimicry where antibodies (and, in some experiments, T cells) induced by exposure to a microbial antigen can cross-react with a human antigen.[14–16] Sometimes the microorganisms involved have little or no clinical or epidemiologic association with the particular human disease. Moreover, the microbial antigen has not been shown to be capable of inducing a reasonable replica of the human disease, even under experimental conditions.

Molecular mimicry is not the only possible explanation for infection-induced autoimmune disease, although it remains the mechanism most often cited. A number of other possibilities have been put forth to explain the induction of autoimmune disease as the result of microbial infection. One reasonable possibility, first suggested by Charles Gauntt, is that, when damaging cells, the invading microorganism may cause the expression of otherwise unavailable autoantigens, providing both a trigger and a vulnerable target for a pathogenic autoimmune response.[17] Cell damage or "spillage" inflicted by the microorganism overcomes "immunologic ignorance" of a previously ignored antigen.

This mechanism has been invoked in a number of instances, including type 1 diabetes mellitus and post-viral myocarditis, where molecular mimicry was not found.[18,19] The finding that coxsackievirus B3, the instigating virus, must actually infect the heart, where the cardiac form of myosin is exclusively produced, is supportive evidence that the host rather than the viral antigen is responsible for autoimmune myocarditis. The same virus that fails to localize in the heart, even though it is plentiful elsewhere in the host, does not induce subsequent myocarditis.[20] Moreover, many unrelated viruses such as cytomegalovirus are capable of producing the same autoimmune disease in the same genetically susceptible strains of mice.[21]

A number of other plausible explanations for the relationship between infection and the initiation of pathogenic autoimmunity have been suggested.[22] The host antigen sometimes becomes incorporated into an infecting virion and can induce an autoimmune response in a manner recalling the classical hapten–carrier relationship. Infecting microorganisms may alter a host protein to the point where it is initially perceived by the host as foreign. These and other possibilities have been suggested as ways that an infecting microorganism can instigate a specific autoimmune response to a human antigen, but the question remains whether the autoimmune response leads to disease.

5 AUTOIMMUNITY VS. AUTOIMMUNE DISEASE: THE ADJUVANT EFFECT

The mechanisms cited in the previous section relate to the possibility that a microorganism provides the cognate antigen-specific first signal in inducing an autoimmune response, as envisioned in the Bretscher–Cohn two-step hypothesis.[23] Infection also has the ability to induce differing non-antigen-specific associative second signals. Many such associative signals that enhance immune responses are produced during the initial innate immune and inflammatory responses to infecting microorganisms. Without appropriate second signals in the form of the requisite cytokine profile or inflammasome, the antigen-specific signal leads to unresponsiveness; autoimmunity would not progress to autoimmune disease. In fact, complete Freund adjuvant, the substance most commonly used to induce experimental pathologic autoimmune responses, probably acts by stimulating an immune response to the mycobacterial component. Bacterial lipopolysaccharide is another potent adjuvant effective in inducing autoimmune disease in experimental animals – sometimes even in mouse strains considered genetically resistant to infection-induced autoimmune disease.[24,25] Genetic resistance and susceptibility to autoimmune disease are relative, not absolute, varying with the type and strength of the stimulus as well as the genetics of the host. Infection is an ideal adjuvant for initiating a pathogenic autoimmune response, providing both a potent antigen-specific first signal and an appropriate second signal.

6 THE PROBLEMS AND THE PROMISE

With mounting interest in the role of infection in inducing autoimmune responses, it is somewhat surprising that there are so few human diseases that so far have been clearly linked to a particular previous microbial infection. The potential value of establishing such a connection cannot be overstated. Knowledge that a beta-hemolytic streptococcus infection is required for the onset of rheumatic fever has provided the critical clue for almost eliminating the disease in the industrialized world. Finding a specific microbial agent for a particular autoimmune disease promises to be the most cost-effective way of preventing autoimmune disease.

A number of major problems have impeded progress to the goal of replicating the success achieved with rheumatic fever. The first problem is that many different microorganisms seem able to produce the same, or virtually the same, disease picture. A long list of diverse microorganisms has been associated in clinical studies of lupus, type 1 diabetes mellitus, myocarditis, and multiple sclerosis.[26] Some of the microbes may simply be passengers, proliferating as a consequence of tissue damage. Yet because the particular immunopathic outcome of an infection is probably dictated by the genetics of the host, the same or virtually the same clinical picture may result from a number of quite different microbial stimuli.

There are also examples where the same microorganism can induce a number of clinically different autoimmune diseases. This suggests some impairment of a regulatory pathway that normally controls different autoimmune responses. A possible example of such an organism is the Epstein–Barr virus (EBV), considered primarily a B cell pathogen.[27] It is seriously considered to be an important initiator of such different autoimmune disorders as rheumatoid arthritis, lupus, type 1 diabetes mellitus and multiple sclerosis (see chapter 29). EBV infection can be thought of as a broadly active adjuvant supplying the necessary associative signals for a number of autoimmune diseases.

Finally, is the problem of timing. A large body of circumstantial evidence suggests that autoimmune diseases may follow environmental exposures by many months or even years. Population studies, for example, have suggested that multiple sclerosis is associated with some (perhaps infectious) exposure during early childhood.[28] The imprint stays with the subject even though the disease does not become clinically evident until the patient is 20 years old. Such a long latent period between the time of infection and its clinical appearance makes establishing a firm connection between a particular infectious agent and a particular autoimmune disease outcome especially daunting.

7 LESSONS OF MOLECULAR (EPITOPE) MIMICRY

Novel lessons can be gleaned from the many studies of molecular or epitope mimicry. Although it has been difficult to identify specific microbial antigens that induce specific autoimmune disorders, studies have consistently implied that epitope mimicry is an extremely common phenomenon.[29] The broad range of responses by a host to microbial invasion inevitably evokes recognition (on both the B cell and T cell levels) of similar epitope patterns found in the tissue of the host. It testifies to the randomness built into the adaptive immune response. Given that the central task of adaptive immunity is to provide a sufficiently diverse population of lymphocytes capable of reacting with virtually any existing or future pathogen, specialized recombination and genetic mechanisms together provide a fulsome range of possible recognition structures. That degree of randomness ensures that many epitopes represented within an infecting microorganism are also present in the host. The host must minimize these cross-reacting lymphocytes using an array of regulatory devices so that they do not cause harmful autoimmunity.

Negative selection of T cells in the thymus is the best established example of such a regulatory measure. Negative selection depends upon a spectrum of binding affinities of T cell receptor, antigen peptide, and major histocompatibility complex product on the thymic medullary antigen-presenting cell. A large proportion of T lymphocytes that recognize a self antigen presented in the thymus with a high affinity are condemned to suicide.[30,31] Experimental studies suggest, however, that they are rarely completely eliminated. Some cross-reactive T lymphocytes and probably B cells remain. The B cell products may be represented in the low affinity of natural autoantibodies usually shunned by immunologists as background noise.

At one end of the negative selection spectrum are a few major antigens (often with carbohydrate moieties) such as the major blood group (ABO) antigens and the Forssman antigen, which are examples of complete clonal deletion.[32] These antigens are well represented in the body, and autoantibodies are never produced. Interestingly, animals that do not express these critical self-epitopes produce prominent natural antibodies against them. At the other end of the spectrum of negative selection are tissue-specific antigens that are strictly limited in their expression to a particular organ, such as the lens of the eye, sperm in the testes and, to some extent, the brain. Because organ- or tissue-specific antigens are poorly presented in the thymus, a relatively large number of self-reactive T lymphocytes can make their way into the periphery. As a consequence they require a large array of regulatory measures to prevent them from progressing to a pathogenic outcome. It was relatively easy experimentally to induce autoimmune disease to a tissue-specific organ antigen like thyroglobulin.[33] Moreover, the tissue-specific antigens are most likely to spontaneously induce disease when immunoregulatory cells are depleted.[34] If the tissue-specific antigen is not expressed by the thymic-presenting cells because of a mutation in the gene *AIRE*, organ-specific autoimmune disease often occurs spontaneously. Thus, self-antigens are distributed along a broad spectrum of clonal deletion ranging from complete to very little.

The common presence of natural autoantibodies in serum or the production of specific natural autoantibodies by B cell hybridomas supports the view that, like T cells, negative selection and receptor editing of B cells are incomplete. Generated in the absence of deliberate immunization, natural autoantibodies make up about two-thirds of the total immunoglobulins in healthy individuals. They characteristically bind with low affinity and thus may react with many apparently unrelated antigens. Because of their polyreactivity they may make up an important part of the initial innate immune response to a wide variety of pathogens. Natural autoantibodies differ markedly from the autoantibodies produced to the incredibly specific antigens that mark tissue-limited autoimmune diseases.[35] Disease-associated autoantibodies are products of processes that differ from those producing natural autoantibodies.

If clonal deletion were complete, the results could be disastrous. Microorganisms bearing key epitopes mimicking self-antigens would inevitably encounter hosts incapable of mounting an effective protective immune response against them. This view recalls the original concept of Damian[36] that antigen sharing by host and parasite permits persistence of the relevant microorganism. If epitope mimicry is so common and clonal dilution were complete, immune deficits would appear. The result would be many "black holes" in the repertoire of the host's protective immunity. Such black holes must be strongly selected against during evolution because they may well render the host vulnerable to multiple infectious (or even malignant) diseases.

Thus, molecular mimicry may explain the evolutionary basis for incomplete negative selection. We can now understand why autoimmunity in the form of natural autoantibodies and self-reactive T cells are common features of a normal, well-regulated immune response. Only when autoimmunity escapes the bounds of normal regulation (or perhaps overcomes them with a powerful stimulus such as infection) that benign, natural autoimmunity progresses to autoimmune disease.

This line of reasoning may be useful in understanding one of the enduring mysteries in the study of infection and autoimmunity. Certain autoantibodies are characteristically elevated in particular infections even if the antibodies play no causative role in the disease itself. A classical example is seen in the consistent production of antibody to cardiolipin in patients with syphilis. There is no evidence that antibody to cardiolipin plays any pathogenic (or even protective) role in the disease. Yet for more than a century it has proven to be of enormous diagnostic value. Such autoantibodies must be the consequence of the activation of particular clones of self-reactive B cells by an ongoing host response to the pathogen. The presence of such antibodies is a diagnostic signal that the pathogenic process is underway. Such an autoantibody represents an empirically useful biomarker of a disease even though it is not completely specific for the disease or the causative agent. Although antibodies reactive to cardiolipin are elevated in cases of antiphospholipid syndrome, their precise specificity differs from those found in syphilis and some other infectious processes. Reflecting on the autoantibodies that have proved to be of value in the diagnosis of autoimmune disease, it seems that the great majority are, in fact, not the cause but the secondary result of a particular disease process.

These considerations have practical consequences. Specifically inhibiting a characteristic, diagnostically valuable autoantibody such as cardiolipin will not benefit patients with syphilis because these autoantibodies are not causative. Of course, we cannot exclude the possibility that some secondary antibodies or T cells that arise in the course of disease may contribute to the final disease picture. In cases of chronic lymphocytic thyroiditis, antibodies to thyroperoxidase are often a relatively late addition to the autoimmune process initiated by thyroglobulin, but their increasing titer may be taken as a sign that the disease is reaching a clinically evident level.[37]

8 VIEWS OF THE FUTURE

Further detailed study of the interrelationship between infection and autoimmune disease holds great promise for improved, more focused therapies and possibly even preventive measures for the disease. The pathways leading from infection to benign autoimmunity to pathologic autoimmune disease most often are based on the changing patterns of inflammatory cells and their cytokine products. From the knowledge gathered from such studies, new tools for blocking the most critical mediators of a particular disease are coming to hand almost daily in the form of monoclonal antibodies and low-molecular-weight receptor inhibitors. There is now hope that one can skillfully disable key steps of the inflammatory response without suppressing the entire immune system. Inhibition of TNFα or its receptor for the treatment of rheumatoid arthritis is the "poster child" of later developments. The next step is to identify the particular antigen initiating the pathogenic phase of the autoimmune response. It may or may not be the antigen identified in the most predictive antibody response. The long-range goal remains avoiding pathogenic autoimmunity without impeding protective immunity. In addition, if a particular infectious agent can be identified as the initiating cause and can be promptly eliminated, it may very well be possible to prevent the disease. Here, rheumatic fever is our guiding light.

As a final thought, we are becoming aware of the unexpected, unpredictable consequences of altering our microbial partners. Through evolutionary time we developed precise mechanisms for tolerating them as they tolerate us. As the human internal condition or external environment change, the microbial population shifts. Sometimes these changes may be beneficial; other times, detrimental. Eliminating helminthic worms from our intestinal environment may be an example where a shift in the consequent microbiome has increased susceptibility to inflammatory bowel disease.[38] Exposures that tend to increase the relative numbers of *C. jejuni* in the intestine, such as raising poultry or swine, increases the likelihood of a Guillain–Barré-like syndrome.[39] We must learn the rules governing the microbiome. A new world of investigation of the interrelationship between infection and autoimmunity is waiting to be explored.

ACKNOWLEDGMENTS

The author's research on infection and autoimmunity was supported by National Institutes of Health Grants HL077611, HL067290, and HL113008. The expert editorial assistance of Starlene Murray is greatly appreciated.

REFERENCES

1. Rose NR. Immune-mediated heart disease: in the footsteps of Jenner. *Autoimmunity* 2001;**34**:159–60.
2. Silverman ME, Murray TJ, Bruam CS. *The quotable Osler.* Philadelphia: American College of Physicians; 2003.

3. Donath J, Landsteiner K. Ueber paroxysmale hamoglobinurie. *Z Klin Med* 1906;**58**:173–89.
4. Coburn AF, Pauli RH. Studies on the relationship of streptococcus hemolyticus to the rheumatic process: III. Observations on the immunological responses of rheumatic subjects to hemolytic streptococcus. *J Exp Med* 1932;**56**(5):651–76.
5. Kaplan MH. The cross-reaction of group A streptococci with heart tissue and its relation to induced autoimmunity in rheumatic fever. *Bull Rheum Dis* 1969;**19**(9):560–7.
6. Halbert SP, Keatinge SL. The analysis of streptococcal infections. VI. Immunoelectrophoretic observations on extracellular antigens detectable with human antibodies. *J Exp Med* 1961;**113**:1013–28.
7. Dale JB, Beachey EH. Epitopes of streptococcal M proteins shared with cardiac myosin. *J Exp Med* 1985;**162**(2):583–91.
8. Martins TB, Hoffman JL, Augustine NH, Phansalkar AR, Fischetti VA, Zabriskie JB, et al. Comprehensive analysis of antibody responses to streptococcal and tissue antigens in patients with acute rheumatic fever. *Int Immunol* 2008;**20**(30):445–52.
9. Cunningham MW. Streptococcus and rheumatic fever. *Curr Opin Rheumatol* 2012;**24**(4):408–16.
10. Kuwabara S, Yuki N. Axonal Guillain–Barre syndrome: concepts and controversies. *Lancet Neurol* 2013;**12**(12):118–1188.
11. Sheikh KA, Nachamkin I, Ho TW, Willison HJ, Veitch J, Ung H, et al. *Campylobacter jejuni* lipopolysaccharides in Guillain–Barre syndrome. *Neurology* 1998;**51**:371–8.
12. Sheikh KA, Zhang G, Gong Y, Schnaar RL, Griffin JW. An anti-ganglioside antibody-secreting hybridoma induces neuropathy in mice. *Ann Neurol* 2004;**56**:228–39.
13. Rose NR, Mackay LR. Molecular mimicry: a critical look at exemplary instances in human diseases. *Cell Mol Life Sci* 2000;**57**:542–51.
14. Bachmaier K, Neu N, de la Maza LM, Pal S, Hessel A, Penninger JM. *Chlamydia* infections and heart disease linked through antigenic mimicry. *Science* 1999;**283**:1335–9.
15. Bachmaier K, Penninger JM. Chlamydia and antigenic mimicry. *Curr Top Microbiol Immunol* 2005;**296**:153–63.
16. Massilamany C, Huber SA, Cunningham MW, Reddy J. Relevance of molecular mimicry in the mediation of infectious myocarditis. *J Cardiovasc Trans Res* 2013;**7**(2):165–71; http://dx.doi.org/10.1007/s12265-013-9519-3, Pub online: Nov.
17. Gauntt CJ, Trousdale MD, LaBadie DLR, Paque RE, Nealon T. Properties of coxsackievirus B3 variants which are amyocarditic or myocarditic for mice. *J Med Virol* 1979;**3**(3):207–20.
18. Rose NR. Viral damage or 'molecular mimicry'—placing the blame in myocarditis. *Nature Med* 2000;**6**(6):693–7.
19. Rose NR, Hill SL. The pathogenesis of postinfectious myocarditis. *Clin Immunol Immunopathol* 1996;**80**:S92–9.
20. Horwitz MS, LaCava A, Fine C, Rodriguez E, Ilic A, Sarvetnick N. Pancreatic expression of interferon-γ protects mice from lethal coxsackievirus B3 infection and subsequent myocarditis. *Nature Med* 2000;**6**(6):693–7.
21. Fairweather D, Kaya Z, Shellam GR, Lawson CM, Rose NR. From infection to autoimmunity. *J Autoimmunity* 2001;**16**:175–86.
22. Rose NR, Griffin DE. Virus-induced autoimmunity. In: Talal N, editor. *Molecular autoimmunity*. San Diego: Academic Press, Inc.; 1991. p. 247–72.
23. Bretscher P, Cohn M. A theory of self-nonself discrimination. *Science* 1970;**169**:1042–9.
24. Rose NR. The role of infection in the pathogenesis of autoimmune disease. *Seminars Immunol* 1998;**10**:5–13.
25. Rose NR. The adjuvant effect in infection and autoimmunity. *Clinic Rev Allerg Immunol* 2008;**34**:279–82.

26. Rose NR. Infection and autoimmunity: theme and variations. *Curr Opin Rheumatol* 2012;**24**:380–2.
27. Draborg AH, Duus K, Houen G. Epstein-Barr virus in systemic autoimmune diseases. *Clin Dev Immunol* 2013:535738; http://dx.doi.org/10.1155/2013/535738, Epub Aug 24, 2013.
28. Djelilovic-Vranic J, Alajbegovic A. Role of early viral infections in development of multiple sclerosis. *Med Arh* 2012;**66**(3S1):37–40.
29. Wucherpfennig KW, Strominger JL. Molecular mimicry in T cell-mediated autoimmunity: viral peptides activate human T cell clones specific for myelin basic protein. *Cell* 1995;**80**:695–705.
30. Kappler JW, Staerz U, White J, Marrack PC. Self-tolerance eliminates T cells specific for Mls-modified products of the major histocompatibility complex. *Nature* 1988;**332**(3):35–40.
31. MacDonald HR, Schneider R, Lees RK, Howe RC, Acha-Orbea H, Festenstein H, et al. T-cell receptor V$_\beta$ use predicts reactivity and tolerance to Mls$^\alpha$-encoded antigens. *Nature* 1988;**332**(3):40–5.
32. Dighiero G, Rose NR. Critical self-epitopes are key to the understanding of self-tolerance and autoimmunity. *Immunol Today* 1999;**20**:423–8.
33. Rose NR, Witebsky E. Studies on organ specificity. V. Changes in the thyroid glands of rabbits following active immunization with rabbit thyroid extracts. *J Immunol* 1956;**76**:417–27.
34. Sakaguchi S, Rose NR. Immune mechanisms in autoimmune disease of endocrine organs. In: Mendelsohn G, editor. *Diagnosis and pathology of endocrine diseases.* Philadelphia: J.B. Lippincott Company; 1988. p. 619–40 [chapter 19].
35. Caturegli P, Mariotti S, Kuppers RC, Burek CL, Pinchera A, Rose NR. Epitopes on thyroglobulin: a study of patients with thyroid disease. *Autoimmunity* 1994;**18**:41–9.
36. Damian RT. Molecular mimicry revisited. *Parasitol Today* 1987;**3**(9):263–6.
37. Hutfless S, Matos P, Talor MV, Caturegli P, Rose NR. Significance of prediagnostic thyroid antibodies in women with autoimmune thyroid disease. *J Clin Endocrinol Metab* 2011;**96**(9):E1466–71.
38. Elliott DE, Weinstock JV. Where are we on worms? *Curr Opin Gastroenterol* 2012;**28**(6):551–6.
39. Davis MF, Kamel F, Hoppin JA, Alavanja MC, Freeman LB, Gray GC, et al. Neurologic symptoms associated with raising poultry and swine among participants in the agricultural health study. *J Occup Environ Med* 2011;**53**(2):190–5.

CHAPTER 2

Infections and Autoimmune Diseases: An Interplay of Pathogenic and Protective Links

Maria Martinelli[*,†,1], **Nancy Agmon-Levin**[*], **Howard Amital**[*,‡], **Yehuda Shoenfeld**[*,§]

[*]Zabludowicz Center for Autoimmune Diseases, Sheba Medical Center, Tel Hashomer, affiliated with Sackler Faculty of Medicine, Tel Aviv University, Ramat Aviv, Israel
[†]Division of Rheumatology, Department of Medicine, University of Brescia, Brescia, Italy
[‡]Internal Medicine Department B, Sheba Medical Center, Tel Hashomer, Israel
[§]Incumbent of the Laura Schwarz-Kip Chair for Research of Autoimmune Diseases, Sackler Faculty of Medicine, Tel-Aviv University, Israel
[1]Corresponding Author: maria.martinelli.ul@gmail.com

1 INTRODUCTION

Autoimmune diseases have considerable incidence and prevalence worldwide, especially in industrialized countries, where their prevalence is increasing steadily.[1] Autoimmunity was found to be induced by a variety of genetic, hormonal, immune and environmental factors that are complementary pebbles of a mosaic, the "mosaic of autoimmunity". These factors interact in complex ways; hence, a particular combination of these elements with a certain balance and timing is required for a specific autoimmune disease to develop. Remarkable progress in understanding the multiplicity of these contributors to autoimmunity, of which infectious agents probably constitute the most important and most studied role, has been achieved.[2] There is a dual association between infections and autoimmunity: infectious agents have, in fact, been proved to be potential triggers of autoimmunity (and this is true for most autoimmune diseases), whereas in different conditions some infections may provide protection from autoimmunity, as was suggested by the "hygiene hypothesis".

This discrepancy represents a challenge in the attempt to develop a predictive model for autoimmunity onset. Facts are even more complex because the same infectious agent can induce or trigger one AD while providing protection from another. For example, hepatitis B virus can contribute to the induction of anti-phospholipid syndrome (APS) and

Infection and Autoimmunity
http://dx.doi.org/10.1016/B978-0-444-63269-2.00001-5

13

polyarteritis nodosa while protecting from the development of systemic lupus erythematosus (SLE).[3] Another example of this compound interrelationship was documented among a unique population of Kitavans from Papua New Guinea,[4] among whom a high prevalence of treponemal infections was linked to the presence of cardioprotective antibodies, namely immunoglobulin M (IgM)-anti-phosphoryl choline antibodies, and the low prevalence of cardiovascular disease. On the other hand, a significantly increased prevalence of anti-double stranded DNA antibodies was documented in the same population, probably originating from cross-reactivity between anti-phosphoryl choline and anti-double stranded DNA antibodies.

This puzzle of genetic and environmental influences differ among both healthy and diseased ethno-geographically distinct populations.[5,6] Moreover, the various mechanisms by which infections induce autoimmunity are not mutually exclusive. Their interrelations are compound, and each mechanism plays a role in different stages of the developing disease. The most studied mechanisms are molecular mimicry, bystander activation,[7] epitope spreading[8] and polyclonal activation.[9] Some of these mechanisms, as well as others such as antigenic competition, bystander suppression and the action of non-antigenic ligands, increase T regulatory cytokines, as IL10, TGF beta which could induce regulatory cells and cytokines, and may induce protection from autoimmunity.[10] This review focuses on the dichotomy between infections and autoimmunity.

2 PATHOGENIC ROLES OF INFECTIONS

Infectious agents are among the many environmental factors that play a major role in triggering autoimmunity. The historical concept of one infectious agent inducing one autoimmune disease (e.g., *Streptococcus* and rheumatic fever) has dramatically changed in the past several decades. This "one-on-one" view has given way to the well-accepted knowledge that several agents are sometimes involved in the pathogenesis of a single AD, while the same pathogen may also play a role in the induction of other ADs. Moreover, autoimmunity is mostly the result of the "burden of infections" during life rather than a single infectious disease; thus infections during childhood may be implicated in the development of ADs during adulthood. Infectious pathogens interact with genetic and epigenetic factors that determine an individual's susceptability for developing autoimmunity. The connections between infections and autoimmunity are diverse and include the ability of pathogens to trigger or aggravate ADs as well as their effect on the predominant clinical manifestations of an AD. For instance, in SLE exposure to the Epstein-Barr virus (EBV) seems to correlate with manifestations in the skin and joints, whereas exposure to rubella correlates with depression or psychosis. The higher prevalence of exposure to infections among patients with autoimmunity may be due to therapy with immunosuppressant agents or the primary immune dysregulations that are involved in the basis of the autoimmune disease. For some ADs such as bullous ADs,[11] the correlation with infections has been posed only in terms of association of the former with different markers of the latter (e.g., bacterial DNA, antibodies against infectious agents). For other ADs, however, specific mechanisms have been proposed and investigated, such as the importance of molecular mimicry between pathogens and β2-glycoprotein I in the pathogenesis of APS[12] or EBV with autoantibodies and AD manifestations in various animal models.[2]

2.1 Viruses

Many viruses have been associated with ADs. One of the most studied pathogens is EBV. This ubiquitous human γ-herpes virus predominantly infects B-lymphocytes and possesses the ability to transform cell growth. It has been associated with many ADs, particularly rheumatoid arthritis (RA), SLE and multiple sclerosis (MS). In the case of MS, even if it is impossible to unequivocally associate the AD with a specific pathogen, EBV is considered to be the most likely candidate, serving both as a trigger and a direct causative agent of central nervous system immunopathology.[13] The plausible mechanisms by which EBV is linked to autoimmunity have recently been reviewed under an interesting unifying hypothesis.[14] A general feature of chronic autoimmune diseases is CD8 + T-cell deficiency; this seems to be genetically determined because it also occurs in healthy blood relatives of patients with ADs. This deficiency has been proposed to impair CD8 + T-cell control of EBV, resulting in the accumulation of autoreactive B cells in target organs, where they provide costimulatory survival signals to autoreactive T cells, and thus facilitating the development of ADs.

Vitamin D has attracted more and more consideration as a fundamental mediator of the immune system. It is widely accepted that its deficiency is linked to autoimmunity.[15] One of the mechanisms by which a lack of vitamin D facilitates the development of autoimmune diseases is the aggravation of the CD8 + T-cell deficiency, thereby constituting a possible enhancing background In which EBV-induced autoimmunity can occur.

Another virus closely linked with autoimmunity is the hepatitis C virus (HCV). The latter can induce autoimmune manifestations ranging from the appearance of autoantibodies to the development of full-blown autoimmune disease. In fact, autoimmunity is a well-recognized part of the extrahepatic manifestations of HCV-induced chronic liver disease. Moreover, the prevalence of anti-HCV antibody was found to be higher in patients with different ADs, whereas a myriad of different autoantibodies can be found in the serum of patients chronically infected with HCV. Notably, the best established association is between HCV and mixed cryoglobulinemia (MC),[16] an immune-mediated vasculitis characterized by the triad of purpura, weakness and arthralgias. The role of HCV in the pathogenesis of MC was firmly established in the 1990s, and an association between viral and clinical status has been confirmed.[17] The link between HCV and MC led to a dramatic change in the treatment of patients with concomitant diseases. Antiviral therapy and additional immunosuppressive drugs, if required, are currently the primary treatment for MC related to HCV. HCV is unequivocally the main culprit in the development of MC, but an association between *Toxoplasma gondii* and cytomegalovirus as an additional contributor to the pathogenesis of MC or, at least, to the flare-up of the vasculitic process upon acquisition of a superimposed infection has also been suggested. This agrees with the "infectious burden" hypothesis. Another piece to the "mosaic of MC" is the importance of the interaction between HCV infections and genetic factors; for example, HLA-DR11 confers a higher risk/protection is referred to the development of MC, whereas other alleles such as HLA-DR7 seem to be protective. Myocarditis is one more autoimmune disease related to viral infections. Direct viral damage plays an important role in this disease, but most of the injury to cardiac muscles derives from an autoimmune response against myocardial antigens that cross-react with infectious microorganisms. In the mid and late 1990s enteroviruses were related to outbreaks of acute myocarditis, but now parvovirus-B19 and adenoviruses are emerging as the most prevalent viral pathogens.[18]

2.2 Bacteria

The best recognized association between an infectious agent and an autoimmune disease is the one linking *Sreptococcus pyogenes* to rheumatic fever. Further associations between bacterial agents and ADs are numerous, such as *Hemophilus influenzae* and *Neisseria gonorrhoeae* as possible triggers of the APS. Heat shock protein 60 (Hsp60), an antigenic peptide of the chaperonins family, seems to play an important role in bacterial-driven autoimmune responses. The possibility that atherosclerosis, diabetes mellitus, and RA follow periodontal infection with *Porphyromonas gingivalis* was recently highlighted, and seroreactivity to *P. gingivalis* Hsp60 was found to be predominant in patients with ADs with ongoing periodontal disease. Moreover, *P. gingivalis* proved to orchestrate chronic inflammatory reactions, enhancing a T helper 17 cell polarization in the immune response.[19] The bacterium *Chlamydia trachomatis* is one of the most common causes of reproductive tract diseases and infertility. It also has been proved to be a possible trigger for different autoimmune diseases by means of overexpression of Hsp60, resulting in the elicitation of autoantibody production.[20] *Helicobacter pylori*, a gram-negative microaerophilic bacterium, is gaining more and more attention because of its complex interactions with and modulatory activities in the immune system. *H. pylori* is implicated as a key agent in the pathogenesis of autoimmune gastritis, able to induce both gastritis and atrophy. This bacterium was also linked with the pathogenesis of atherosclerosis, again with an immune response at Hsp60 as a major target. *H. pylori* shows a strong link with idiopathic thrombocytopenic purpura, and high-quality studies show the improvement of idiopathic thrombocytopenic purpura after the eradication of *H. pylori*, supporting its causative role.[21] A recent prospective cohort study concluded for the first time that *H. pylori* also is associated with an increased incidence of diabetes.[22]

Guillain-Barré syndrome (GBS) is a rare AD characterized by damage to gangliosides in the peripheral nervous system. The first clinical manifestations of the disease normally consist of weakness and tingling sensations in the legs, which can later spread to the arms and the upper body and often occur a few days or weeks after the patient has suffered from a respiratory or gastrointestinal infection. *Campylobacter jejuni* infection precedes about a third of cases of GBS, and molecular mimicry between a lipooligosaccharide of *C. jejuni* strains and peripheral nerves was demonstrated in animal models of human GBS.[23]

Atypical hemolytic uremic syndrome (HUS) has been associated with some non-enteric infectious agents. Compared to the classical HUS caused by verotoxin-producing *Escherichia coli*, atypical HUS has a less favorable prognosis and is particularly prone to recurrence. Among causal agents, *Bordetella pertussis* deserves particular attention, especially in patients who are genetically predisposed to the disease.[24]

2.3 Fungi

Saccharomyces cerevisiae is a commensal yeast that can trigger autoimmunity when fine regulation of immune tolerance does not work properly.[25]

A growing number of studies have detected high levels of anti-*S. cerevisiae* autoantibodies in patients with ADs and especially in patients with inflammatory bowel diseases. A possible role of fungal agents acting by means of molecular mimicry also has been proposed for SLE and other disorders.[26]

2.4 Parasites

Parasites interact in complex ways with the immune system.[27] Some of them can induce autoimmune phenomena, such as *Trypanosoma cruzi* inducing Chagas disease, which may result in severe autoimmune cardiomyopathy.[28] *T. gondii* also was linked with autoimmunity: the prevalence of anti-toxoplasma antibodies was found to be higher in patients with ADs.[29] A particular link with RA was found in several studies.[29,30]

Considering all of this information, the role of infectious agents in the mosaic of autoimmunity seems to be well established, and although the puzzle remains complex—involving exposure to various infections at certain sequences and timing throughout a person's life—it seems that these environmental factors are linked not only with the presence of autoimmunity but also with the manifestation and exacerbations of diseases.

3 PROTECTIVE ROLE OF INFECTIONS

For many years infectious agents were considered to be solemnly pathogenic, both as the cause of infectious diseases as well as triggers of autoimmunity. As mentioned earlier, however, it seems that in some cases infections may protect individuals from the emergence of AD and allergic diseases. In the second half of the 20th century, a dramatic increase in the incidence of some allergic diseases and ADs was observed in Western countries, such as type I diabetes mellitus (T1D), inflammatory bowel disease (IBD) and MS.[31] The idea that this was connected to the decline in infectious diseases and improved hygiene underlies what has been termed the "hygiene hypothesis": the higher frequency of allergy and autoimmunity in economically developed countries might be due to lower rates of childhood infections, which is referred to the lower rate of infections. Demonstrating a protective role of infections is even more challenging than displaying a pathogenic one, but it is an issue of importance because these plausible effects may be harnessed to treat or prevent ADs.

The hygiene hypothesis is strongly supported by evidence from studies of both humans and animals. Studies of helminth-infected cohorts did highlight a lower propensity to allergic diseases. Stronger support for the actual protective role of parasites stems from evidence that anthelmintic therapy in children increases their reactivity to skin tests. This kind of evidence is parallel to the increase of autoantibodies in *Schistosoma*-infected individuals when treated with anti-schistosome therapy. Infected people have been proven to normally have fewer autoantibodies compared to infection-free subjects.[32] Furthermore, epidemiological data showed a remarkable increase in MS incidence in Sardinia after malaria was eradicated.[33] In general there is a clear negative relationship between the incidence of MS and the prevalence of helminthic infections in different countries. The actual protective effect of some pathogens has been demonstrated in animal models, which are ideal for testing the mechanistic relationship between infection, pathology and the immune system. Models of allergic diseases proved the ability of helminths to induce T-regulatory cells capable of suppressing allergic pathology. *Heligmosomoides polygyrus* is an intestinal nematode that has been demonstrated to suppress anaphylaxis in a dietary peanut allergy model, as well as airway hyperresponsiveness, lung histopathology, eosinophil recruitment and T helper 2 (Th2) cytokines in an alum-sensitized model of airway allergy. Similar allergy-suppressing ability in animal models has been demonstrated for other parasites.[34] The protective effect derives from a complex interaction of many different factors such as the parasite load, the sex of the parasite and the stage of infection. There are also multiple rodent models of ADs that underline parasites' capability to suppress T helper 1/T helper 17 cell-mediated immunopathologies, probably skewing the inflammatory response toward Th2 cells. Exposure to *Schistosoma mansoni* prevents non-obese diabetic mice from developing T1D, and helminths proved to be protective in models of IBD and in a mouse model of experimental autoimmune encephalomyelitis. The development of pathology can be abated by many parasites; thus similar to the pathogenic burden, we can expect to have a "protective infectious burden" in which several pathogens contribute to the production of protective antibodies. There are multiple plausible protective mechanisms that probably arise from the reciprocal fine adaptation of humans to coexist with some pathogens. The mutual advantage of not being eradicated for the latter and not developing excessive proinflammatory responses for the former. The most well-recognized protective agents are parasites. There is extensive evidence of their influence on various pathways of the immune system: they are capable of inducing an attenuated regulatory immune network that allows them to survive and cause chronic infestation by skewing the immune reaction toward both a Th2-type response and regulatory responses.[27] Both mice and humans infected with helminths might also have minor susceptibility to Th2/allergic-type diseases, proving that the benefits of a helminths infestation would not stem just from a Th2 polarization of the immune response. The different effects of parasite infections also derive from characteristics of the host, e.g., the genetic background and whether the host is definitive or accidental.

Parasites mostly provide protective effects against pathogens; however, among bacterial agents it is noteworthy to highlight the possible protective role of *H. pylori* from some autoimmune states. A negative association between seropositivity to this infectious agent and specific ADs has been proved for IBD, SLE and, more recently, MC,[16] confirming once more that the same pathogen can be protective against some ADs and a predisposing factor of others.

Animal models provide proof-of-concept data for the use of a "therapeutic helminth". Nevertheless, it is necessary to keep in mind the fundamental principle "first do no harm" and thus to investigate further the potential adverse effects of infection with parasites that were observed in animal models. Patients with Crohn's disease actually achieved symptomatic relief and/or objective improvement of the disease following treatment with *Trichuris suis* ova.[35] Other clinical trials of treatment with live parasites have been performed,[36] contributing to developing immunological insights and therapeutic possibilities. One of these has come from the intuition that parasites had to share the expression of some pathogen–associated molecular patterns that could be used to induce protection against autoimmunity as a therapeutic tool.[37,38] This led to the identification of phosphorylcholine (PC), a component shared by parasites that plays a fundamental role in diverting the immune system towards an anti–inflammatory phenotype.[38] PC is the head group of many phospholipids. *Streptococcus pneumoniae* bears PC on its cell wall as an immunodeterminant. Active immunization with *S. Pneumoniae* reduced atherosclerosis in hypercholesterolemic mice; this was attributed to an immune response to phosphoryl choline. Therefore, the hypothesis of an athero–protective activity of passive immunization with a monoclonal anti–PC IgM antibody was tested in a murine model of native aortic and vein graft atherosclerosis. The hypothesis was actually confirmed because passive immunization with anti–PC IgM reduced vein graft plaque size and neointimal thickness, and it also reduced the inflammatory cell content of the plaques. The role of phosphoryl choline as the main epitope recognized by both anti–pneumococcus and anti–oxidized low–density lipoprotein antibodies was further confirmed when PC immunization of apolipoprotein E knockout mice was proven to drive a specific humoral immune response that reduced foam cell formation *in vitro* and was athero-protective *in vivo*.

The role of the intestinal microbiota in maintaining the healthy status of an individual can be discussed here because it supports the idea that some microbial agents are actually beneficial for the host. A recent article showed the occurrence of dysbiosis in patients affected by chronic fatigue syndrome; the meaning of this correlation requires further investigation to understand any possible causal link between an alteration in the gut flora and the development of a syndrome in the spectrum of autoimmune phenomena.[39] It is becoming established that patients with recurrent *Clostridium difficile* infection may benefit from infusion of donor feces through a nasoduodenal tube in comparison to a vancomycin regimen.[40]

All the data reported here support the idea of a fine-tuning of immune homeostasis by different microorganisms, either naturally present as endogenous or exogenous flora, that is essential to protect the organism from autoimmune/inflammatory diseases.

REFERENCES

1. Shapira Y, Agmon-Levin N, Shoenfeld Y. Defining and analyzing geoepidemiology and human autoimmunity. *J Autoimmun* 2010;**34**:J168–77.
2. Kivity S, Agmon-Levin N, Blank M, Shoenfeld Y. Infections and autoimmunity—friends or foes? *Trends Immunol* 2009;**30**:409–14.
3. Ram M, Anaya JM, Barzilai O, et al. The putative protective role of hepatitis B virus (HBV) infection from autoimmune disorders. *Autoimmun Rev* 2008;**7**:621–25.
4. Agmon-Levin N, Bat-sheva PK, Barzilai O, et al. Antitreponemal antibodies leading to autoantibody production and protection from atherosclerosis in Kitavans from Papua New Guinea. *Ann N Y Acad Sci* 2009;**1173**:675–82.
5. Shapira Y, Poratkatz BS, Gilburd B, et al. Geographical differences in autoantibodies and anti-infectious agents antibodies among healthy adults. *Clin Rev Allergy Immunol* 2012;**42**:154–63.
6. Baldovino S, Montin D, Martino S, Sciascia S, Menegatti E, Roccatello D. Common variable immunodeficiency: crossroads between infections, inflammation and autoimmunity. *Autoimmun Rev* 2013;**12**:796–801.
7. Boyman O. Bystander activation of CD4+ T cells. *Eur J Immunol* 2010;**40**:936–39.
8. Ji Q, Castelli L, Goverman JM. MHC class I-restricted myelin epitopes are cross-presented by Tip-DCs that promote determinant spreading to CD8(+) T cells. *Nat Immunol* 2013;**14**:254–61.
9. Dar SA, Das S, Bhattacharya SN, et al. Possible role of superantigens in inducing autoimmunity in pemphigus patients. *J Dermatol* 2011;**38**:980–87.
10. Okada H, Kuhn C, Feillet H, Bach JF. The 'hygiene hypothesis' for autoimmune and allergic diseases: an update. *Clin Exp Immunol* 2010;**160**:1–9.
11. Sagi L, Baum S, Agmon-Levin N, et al. Autoimmune bullous diseases the spectrum of infectious agent antibodies and review of the literature. *Autoimmun Rev* 2011;**10**:527–35.
12. Cruz-Tapias P, Blank M, Anaya JM, Shoenfeld Y. Infections and vaccines in the etiology of antiphospholipid syndrome. *Curr Opin Rheumatol* 2012;**24**:389–93.

13. Owens GP, Bennett JL. Trigger, pathogen, or bystander: the complex nexus linking Epstein- Barr virus and multiple sclerosis. *Mult Scler* 2012;**18**:1204–8.
14. Pender MP. CD8+ T-cell deficiency, Epstein-Barr virus infection, vitamin D deficiency, and steps to autoimmunity: a unifying hypothesis. *Autoimmune Dis* 2012;**2012**:189096.
15. Agmon-Levin N, Theodor E, Segal RM, Shoenfeld Y. Vitamin D in systemic and organ-specific autoimmune diseases. *Clin Rev Allergy Immunol* 2013;**45**:256–66.
16. Lidar M, Lipschitz N, Agmon-Levin N, et al. Infectious serologies and autoantibodies in hepatitis C and autoimmune disease-associated mixed cryoglobulinemia. *Clin Rev Allergy Immunol* 2012;**42**:238–46.
17. Fabrizi F, Dixit V, Messa P. Antiviral therapy of symptomatic HCV-associated mixed cryoglobulinemia: meta-analysis of clinical studies. *J Med Virol* 2013;**85**:1019–27.
18. Shauer A, Gotsman I, Keren A, et al. Acute viral myocarditis: current concepts in diagnosis and treatment. *Isr Med Assoc J* 2013;**15**:180–85.
19. Moutsopoulos NM, Kling HM, Angelov N, et al. Porphyromonas gingivalis promotes Th17 inducing pathways in chronic periodontitis. *J Autoimmun* 2012;**39**:294–303.
20. Cappello F, Conway de Macario E, Di Felice V, Zummo G, Macario AJ. Chlamydia trachomatis infection and anti-Hsp60 immunity: the two sides of the coin. *PLoS Pathog* 2009;**5**:e1000552.
21. Tan HJ, Goh KL. Extragastrointestinal manifestations of *Helicobacter pylori* infection: facts or myth? A critical review. *J Dig Dis* 2012;**13**:342–49.
22. Jeon CY, Haan MN, Cheng C, et al. *Helicobacter pylori* infection is associated with an increased rate of diabetes. *Diabetes Care* 2012;**35**:520–25.
23. Israeli E, Agmon-Levin N, Blank M, Chapman J, Shoenfeld Y. Guillain-Barre syndrome—a classical autoimmune disease triggered by infection or vaccination. *Clin Rev Allergy Immunol* 2012;**42**:121–30.
24. Cohen-Ganelin E, Davidovits M, Amir J, Prais D. Severe *Bordetella pertussis* infection associated with hemolytic uremic syndrome. *Isr Med Assoc J* 2012;**14**:456–58.
25. Rinaldi M, Perricone R, Blank M, Perricone C, Shoenfeld Y. Anti-Saccharomyces cerevisiae autoantibodies in autoimmune diseases: from bread baking to autoimmunity. *Clin Rev Allergy Immunol* 2013;**45**(2):152–61.
26. Guarneri F, Guarneri B, Vaccaro M, Guarneri C. The human Ku autoantigen shares amino acid sequence homology with fungal, but not bacterial and viral, proteins. *Immunopharmacol Immunotoxicol* 2011;**33**:329–33.
27. Zandman-Goddard G, Shoenfeld Y. Parasitic infection and autoimmunity. *Lupus* 2009;**18**:1144–48.
28. Nunes DF, Guedes PM, de Mesquita Andrade C, Camara AC, Chiari E, Galvao LM. Troponin T autoantibodies correlate with chronic cardiomyopathy in human Chagas disease. *Trop Med Int Health* 2013;**18**:1180–92.
29. Shapira Y, Agmon-Levin N, Selmi C, et al. Prevalence of anti-toxoplasma antibodies in patients with autoimmune diseases. *J Autoimmun* 2012;**39**:112–16.
30. Fischer S, Agmon-Levin N, Shapira Y, et al. *Toxoplasma gondii*: bystander or cofactor in rheumatoid arthritis. *Immunol Res* 2013;**56**:287–92.
31. Cooper PJ. Interactions between helminth parasites and allergy. *Curr Opin Allergy Clin Immunol* 2009;**9**:29–37.
32. Mutapi F, Imai N, Nausch N, et al. Schistosome infection intensity is inversely related to auto-reactive antibody levels. *PloS one* 2011;**6**:e19149.
33. Sotgiu S, Angius A, Embry A, Rosati G, Musumeci S. Hygiene hypothesis: innate immunity, malaria and multiple sclerosis. *Med Hypotheses* 2008;**70**:819–25.
34. Dittrich AM, Erbacher A, Specht S, et al. Helminth infection with Litomosoides sigmodontis induces regulatory T cells and inhibits allergic sensitization, airway inflammation, and hyperreactivity in a murine asthma model. *J Immunol* 2008;**180**:1792–99.

35. Sandborn WJ, Elliott DE, Weinstock J, et al. Randomised clinical trial: the safety and tolerability of Trichuris suis ova in patients with Crohn's disease. *Aliment Pharmacol Ther* 2013;**38**:255–63.
36. McSorley HJ, Maizels RM. Helminth infections and host immune regulation. *Clin Microbiol Rev* 2012;**25**:585–608.
37. Finkelman FD. Worming their way into the pharmacy: use of worms and worm products to treat inflammatory diseases. *Arthritis and rheumatism* 2012;**64**:3068–71.
38. Ben-Ami Shor D, Harel M, Eliakim R, Shoenfeld Y. The hygiene theory harnessing helminths and their ova to treat autoimmunity. *Clin Rev Allergy Immunol* 2013;**45** (2):211–16.
39. Fremont M, Coomans D, Massart S, De Meirleir K. High-throughput 16S rRNA gene sequencing reveals alterations of intestinal microbiota in myalgic encephalomyelitis/ chronic fatigue syndrome patients. *Anaerobe* 2013;**22**:50–56.
40. van Nood E, Vrieze A, Nieuwdorp M, et al. Duodenal infusion of donor feces for recurrent *Clostridium difficile*. *New Engl J Med* 2013;**368**:407–15.

PART 1

Mechanisms of Autoimmunity induction by infectious agents and vaccination

CHAPTER 3

Molecular Mimicry and Autoimmunity

Ramit Maoz-Segal[*,1], **Paulo Andrade**[†]
[*]The Zabludowicz Center for Autoimmune Diseases, Sheba Medical Center, Tel-Hashomer 52621, Israel
[†]Infectious Diseases Department Hospital São João, Porto, Portugal
[1]Corresponding Author: ramitsegal@gmail.com

1 INTRODUCTION

The term *molecular mimicry* was originally defined by Damian as "the sharing of antigens between parasite and host".[1] The sequence similarity between foreign (a microorganism's peptides) and self-peptides (the host's antigen) enable pathogens that mimic self-epitopes to evade the immune system and lead to an immunological tolerance; in this way they gain an evolutionary advantage.[2–4] The mechanism by which pathogens have evolved or obtained by chance similar amino acid sequences or the homologous three-dimensional crystal structure of immune-dominant epitopes remains a mystery, yet there are many examples of common microorganisms that 'use' this mechanism: the *Vaccinia* virus protein A49 mimics nuclear factor κB inhibitor; *Neisseria meningitidis* recruits complement-soluble plasma regulatory protein factor H by mimicking host carbohydrates; and group B *Streptococcus* (GBS) mimics host sialoglycan, resulting in impaired neutrophil function.[5–7]

The phenomenon of molecular mimicry has, however, been just recently discovered as one of several ways in which autoimmunity can be evoked. Under certain circumstances, these infectious 'mimickers' can activate the immune system, initiate an immune response and lead to a breakdown in self-tolerance and autoimmunity.[8] Structural homology – meaning that a single antibody or T-cell receptor can only be activated by a few residues – is crucial for this immune system activation. Following the encounter with the pathogen, activated autoreactive B or T cells can cross-react with self-epitopes, thus leading to autoimmunity.[9] Autoimmunity is the result of a loss of immunological tolerance, the ability of the immunologic system to discriminate between self and nonself. Recent data show that autoimmune diseases affect approximately 1 in 31 people within the general population.[10] Growth also has led to a greater characterisation of what autoimmunity is and how it

Infection and Autoimmunity
http://dx.doi.org/10.1016/B978-0-444-63269-2.00054-4

can be studied and treated. With the increased amount of research, there has been tremendous growth in the study of several different ways in which autoimmunity can occur, one of which is molecular mimicry. Thus, nowadays the term *molecular mimicry* has been transformed and is used to define an autoimmune response elicited by a microorganism's antigenic determinants.[11]

Here we provide some examples of common infectious agents and their roll in creating autoimmune disorders. Later, we present the opposite, describing autoimmune disorders in which there was found a relation to infectious agents via a molecular mimicry mechanism. At the end of each paragraph, the data are summarized in two tables.

2 COMMON INFECTIOUS AGENTS AND THEIR ROLL IN SETTING AUTOIMMUNE DISORDERS

2.1 Viruses

Epstein-Barr virus (EBV), a member of the *herpesviridae* family, is estimated to infect more than 90% of the human population.[12] There is consistent evidence supporting the role of EBV in triggering many autoimmune diseases, particularly systemic lupus erythematosus (SLE).[13–15] The most relevant mechanism by which EBV has been suggested to induce autoimmunity is molecular mimicry. Epstein-Barr nuclear antigen-1 (EBNA-1) has regions bearing homology to SLE-associated antigens such as ribonucleoprotein Smith antigen (Sm) and Ro self-protein.[8,16–18] By tracing autoantibody response in SLE back in time, cross-reactivity was found between the Ro self-protein, the initial SLE autoantigen and EBNA-1, suggesting it is triggered by molecular mimicry.[19] Furthermore, in mice, expression of EBNA-1 may elicit antibodies to Sm and double-stranded DNA (dsDNA), and antibodies elicited in response to EBNA-1 were shown to cross-react with dsDNA.[20,21] Finally, in rabbits, immunization with EBNA-1 fragments containing the PPPGRRP sequence led to the development of antibodies with cross-reactivity to Sm and nuclear ribonucleoproteins; after immunization, most of the rabbits developed leucopenia or lymphopenia (or both), the features of which resemble those of SLE.[22]

Cytomegalovirus (CMV), also a member of the *herpesviridae* family, is an extremely common human pathogen worldwide.[23] Its role in triggering autoimmunity trough molecular mimicry has been pointed out in different autoimmune disorders. Immunoglobulin G antibodies from the sera of patients with systemic sclerosis where found to recognize both autoantigens and human CMV late protein UL94 and to induce endothelial cell apoptosis.[24] Cross-reactivity also was found between glutamic acid decarboxylase (a major autoantigen in diabetes mellitus type 1 and stiff-man syndrome) and CMV major DNA-binding protein pUL57, which supports the role of CMV in triggering those two pathologies.[25] Regarding Guillain-Barré syndrome (GBS), it has been demonstrated that anti-GM2 antibodies cross-react with CMV-infected fibroblasts.[26] Finally, Hsieh et al.[27] demonstrated that most patients with SLE have antibodies to CMV phosphoprotein 65 when compared with controls and that immunization with CMV phosphoprotein 65 in mice elicited the production of antichromatin, anticentriole, antimitotic spindle type I/II and anti-dsDNA antibody, as well as deposition of glomerular immunoglobulin.

Parvovirus B19 (PB19), a single-stranded DNA (ssDNA) virus and ubiquitous human pathogen, is the etiologic agent of erythema infectiosum (the fifth disease) and is responsible for such diverse pathologies as transient aplastic crisis, hydrops fetalis and arthropathy.[28,29] Clinical resemblance of PB19 infection and some autoimmune disorders has raised the possibility of a linkage between the two.[30,31] Loizou et al.[32] compared sera of three groups of patients with acute PB19 infection, patients with other acute viral infections and patients with syphilis. He specified the antiphospholipid antibodies and further compared sera from those three groups with sera from patients with SLE trying to investigate the dependence of anticardiolipin binding on the presence of β2-glycoprotein I as a cofactor. Sera from patients with PB19 was found to have different antiphospholipid specificity when compared with sera from patients with other infections; like sera from patients with SLE trying but unlike sera from patients with other acute viral infections or syphilis, anticardiolipin antibodies of patients with PB19 were found to increase their binding ability in the presence of β2-glycoprotein I.[32] After synthesizing a PB19 viral peptide, Lunardi et al.[33] demonstrated that purified anti-PB19 antibodies cross-reacted with autoantigens such as keratin, collagen type II, ssDNA and cardiolipin. Afterwards, 8 mice were immunised with that same viral peptide, eliciting autoantibody production against keratin, collagen II, cardiolipin and ssDNA in 6 of them.[33]

2.2 Bacteria

Streptococcus pyogenes, a Gram-positive cocci, is the main etiologic agent of bacterial pharyngitis. One of the first and best established linkages between a human pathogen and an autoimmune disorder was that of *S. pyogenes* and rheumatic fever (RF); molecular mimicry was proposed as trigger early on.[34] Evidence of antibody cross-reactivity between the streptococcal M protein and cardiac myosin has been presented in different publications.[35–37] Guilherme et al.[38] demonstrated that T-cell clones from hearts of patients with RF recognized both streptococcal M protein and heart proteins. Regarding Sydenham chorea, cross-reactivity between mammalian lysoganglioside and *S. pyogenes* N-acetyl-beta-D-glucosamine was observed.[39] Finally, Quinn et al.[40] reported that 3 of 6 Lewis rats immunized with recombinant streptococcal M protein developed valvulitis and focal lesions of myocarditis, whereas Bronze and Dale[41] showed that immunization of rabbits with streptococcal protein M elicited the production of antibodies with cross-reactivity to brain proteins, thus establishing a possible etiology for Sydenham chorea in patients with RF.

Helicobacter pylori, a Gram-negative bacillus estimated to infect about 50% of the world's population, is linked with disorders such as atrophic gastritis, peptic ulcer disease and gastric carcinoma.[42] Different autoimmune disorders have been associated with *H. pylori* infection, and molecular mimicry was proposed as a triggering mechanism in some of them. Appelmelk et al.[43] observed that immunization of mice and rabbits with *H. pylori* lipopolysaccharide elicited production of antibodies to Lewis blood group antigens, which recognized human and murine gastric glandular tissue. Amedei et al.[44] showed that cell clones of gastric T cells recovered from *H. pylori*–infected patients with autoimmune gastritis recognized both pathogen antigens and H^+, K^+ ATPase. Finally, Takahashi et al.[45] demonstrated that platelet-associated immunoglobulin G from the sera of patients with idiopathic thrombocytopenic purpura recognized *H. pylori* CagA protein.

Campylobacter jejuni, a Gram-negative, spiral-shaped bacillus, is one of the most common agents of bacterial gastroenteritis in the world.[46] Postinfectious GBS is one of the best examples of autoimmune disease triggered by bacterial infection; up to a third of cases are preceded by *C. jejuni* infection.[47] Structural homology between *C. jejuni* lipo-oligosaccharide (LOS) and human ganglioside GM1 was first demonstrated by Yuki et al.[48] and Willison and Yuki;[49] later, cross-reactivity between *C. jejuni* LOS and human antiganglioside antibodies was observed. Furthermore, animal studies have shown anti-GM1 antibody development and neurologic disorders resembling GBS upon immunization with *C. jejuni* LOS, thus supporting the role of molecular mimicry in this disease.[50]

2.3 Parasites

Trypanosoma cruzi, a flagellated protozoan parasite, is the etiologic agent of Chagas' disease, a disorder with protean clinical manifestations including digestive, nervous and cardiac involvement; the latter is the most important because of its frequency and clinical implications.[51–55] The contribution of molecular mimicry in triggering Chagas' disease cardiopathy has been suggested by a number of publications.[56,57] Immunization of mice with cruzipain, a parasitic antigen, elicited anticruzipain and antimyosin antibody production and was associated with heart conduction disturbances.[58] Cunha-Neto et al.[59,60] demonstrated cross-reactivity between a heart-specific epitope of myosin and *T. cruzi* antigen B13 and further identified simultaneous responsiveness of heart-infiltrating T-cell clones from patients with Chagas' disease cardiopathy to cardiac myosin heavy chain and *T. cruzi* antigen B13. Leon et al.[61,62] showed that mice immunized with *T. cruzi* protein extract emulsified in complete Freund's adjuvant developed antibodies and delayed-type hypersensitivity to cardiac myosin, whereas mice immunized with cardiac myosin developed antibodies and delayed-type hypersensitivity to *T. cruzi*. Induction of peripheral immune tolerance to *T. cruzi* or myosin led to a decrease in cellular immunity to myosin and *T. cruzi*, respectively. Finally, mice immunized with R13 synthetic peptide, corresponding to sequences in the *T. cruzi* ribosomal P1 and P2 proteins, generated antibodies to R13 as well as to H3, an autoantigen, followed by cardiac structure abnormalities[63] (Table 1).

Autoimmunity is believed to be the consequence of a breakdown in self-tolerance that induces an attack of the immune system on different organs and tissues. A combination of genetic, immunologic and environmental factors is required, comprising what is nowadays called 'the mosaic of autoimmunity'.[79]

Microbial antigens have the potential to initiate autoreactivity through molecular mimicry and other mechanisms such as polyclonal activation or the release of previously sequestered antigens.[80] Although the triggering event in most autoimmune diseases is unknown, the process of molecular mimicry between microbial and self-components (e.g., proteins, carbohydrates or DNA epitopes) is postulated to be the most likely mechanism of postinfectious autoimmunity.

Molecular mimicry is one mechanism by which infectious agents (or other exogenous substances) may trigger an immune response against auto-antigens. According to this hypothesis, a susceptible host acquires an

Table 1 Examples of molecular mimicry mechanisms of infectious pathogens in autoimmune disorders

	Pathogen	Associated autoimmune disorder	Mimicking pathogenic antigen	References
Virus	CMV	DM1	pUL94	24
		SS	pUL57	25
		APS	TIFI	64
	EBV	MS	LMP-1	65
		SLE	EBNA-1	16–22
		RA	BZLF-1, BMLF-1	66
	Enterovirus	DM1	Several viral peptides	67
	HBV	MS	HBV DNA polymerase	68
	HCV	AH	Core protein	69
		CryG	Core protein	70
		AT	HCV polyprotein	71
	HIV	SjS	p24 Capsid antigen	72
		SLE	p24 Capsid antigen	72
	HSV	MG	Glycoprotein D	73
	PB19	APS	VP1u	74
	Rubella	DM1	Several viral peptides	75
Bacteria	Campylobacter jejuni	GBS	LOS	48–50
	Clostridium tetani (toxoid)	APS	TLRVYK hexapeptide	76
	Chlamydia trachomatis	AS	DNA primase	77
	Hemophilus influenzae	MS	Protease IV	73
		APS	TLRVYK hexapeptide	76
	Helicobacter pylori	AG	LPS	43
		ITP	CagA	45
	Neisseria gonorrhoeae	APS	TLRVYK hexapeptide	76
	Streptococcus pyogenes	RF	M protein	35–38,40,41
			N-acetyl-β-D-glucosamine	39
Parasites	Trypanosoma cruzi	CD	Cruzipain	58
			B13	59,60
			R13 synthetic peptid	63
			F1-160	78

AG, autoimmune gastritis; AH, autoimmune hepatitis; APS, antiphospolipid syndrome; AS, ankylosing spondylitis; AT, autoimmune thyroiditis; CD, Chagas disease; CMV, cytomegalovirus; CryG, cryoglobulinemia; DM1, type 1 diabetes mellitus; EBV, Epstein–Barr virus; GBS, Guilain–Barré syndrome; HBV, hepatitis B virus; HCV, hepatitis C virus; HIV, human immunodeficiency virus; HSV, herpes simplex virus; ITP, idiopathic thrombocytopenic purpura; LOS, lipo-oligosaccharide; LPS, lipopolysaccharide; MG, myasthenia gravis; MS, multiple sclerosis; PB19, parvovirus B19; RA, rheumatoid arthritis; RF, rheumatic fever; SLE, systemic lupus infection with an agent that has antigens that are immunologically similar to the host antigens but differ sufficiently to induce an immune response when presented to T cells. As a result, the tolerance to autoantigens breaks down, and the pathogen-specific immune response that is generated cross-reacts with host structures to cause tissue damage and disease. This model has persisted for more than three decades because it offers an attractive conceptual link between physiologic responses (defence against infection) and a pathologic process (autoimmunity).

Cross-reactivity between foreign (i.e., infectious) and self-antigens can be determined by different methods. One approach is to enable the detection of cross-reactive self-antigens and humoral response by identifying a suspected causative organism and its antigenic epitopes. Another method, when the causative organism is unknown, is identifying T-cell determinants capable of inducing autoimmunity and then searching for homologous microbial sequences that might activate the immune system in a major histocompatibility complex–dependent way.[81]

In recent years, the role of different infectious agents has been extensively studied, and several mechanisms were found to be associated with postinfectious autoimmunity pathogenesis, of which molecular mimicry is the dominant mechanism.[82] For example, it was found that several human monoclonal antibodies can react specifically with infectious agents as well as with human antigens.[83] These antibodies are believed to be at least partially responsible for initiating a pathogenic process that eventually results in autoimmunity. Those studies led to the suggested criteria for 'diagnosing' the role of molecular mimicry in autoimmune diseases.[50] The first requirement is that the suspected pathogen must be associated with the presence, onset or exacerbation of the autoimmune disease in a convincing number of patients. Second, the infectious agent must provoke either a T-cell-dependent or T-cell-independent immune response (i.e., autoantibodies) that cross-reacts with host antigens and is clinically relevant to the autoimmune disease. The proof of the causality between the mimic epitope and the autoimmune disease can be achieved by active immunization with the shared epitope in animal models and induction of the autoimmune disease or by passive transfer of the disease using autoreactive T cells or autoantibodies.

In conclusion, molecular mimicry has been linked to the pathogenesis of many autoimmune diseases. Here we review a few major examples of different autoimmune diseases that have been linked to this mechanism. The data of these examples as well as other autoimmune diseases and related infectious agents that were found to be escaping the immune system through the roll of molecular mimicry are summarized in Table 2.

3 NEURO-AUTOIMMUNE DISEASE

Multiple sclerosis is a chronic human autoimmune disease characterized by mononuclear cell infiltration and demyelization within the central nervous system (CNS) and neurological dysfunction. In the case of multiple sclerosis, it has been hypothesized that the disease is initiated by an infection early in life by a virus that shares antigenic structures with the host's CNS tissue. The host immune response against EBV, influenza virus type A and human papillomavirus peptides cross-reacts with CNS self-antigens, such as myelin basic protein, leading to demyelization. Subsequent viral infections are thought to cause exacerbations of the disease by reactivating the immune response against viral antigens and autoantigens.[99]

4 ENDOCRINOLOGICAL AUTOIMMUNE DISEASE

Insulin-dependent diabetes mellitus (IDDM), or type I diabetes, is an auto-immune disease involving mononuclear cell infiltration of the pancreatic islets (insulitis), destruction of the beta islet cells and insulin deficiency. In autoimmune diabetes, T cells recognize both a peptide derived from the autoantigen glutamic-acid decarboxylase and a highly analogous peptide from the coxsackievirus P2-C protein (see Table 2).

5 INFLAMMATORY ARTICULAR DISEASE

Rheumatoid arthritis (RA) is a human autoimmune disease with an unknown etiology and is characterized by symmetrical persistent inflamma-tory synovitis of the peripheral joints. Rheumatic fever (RF) is the classical example of molecular mimicry resulting in postinfectious autoimmunity. A timely association between streptococcal infection and RF had been dem-onstrated in the majority of patients. Streptococcal epitopes such as N-acetylglucosamine or M-protein mimic cardiac myosin and a-helical proteins present in the valve, whereas N-acetyl glucosamine also mimics neuronal ganglioside. T-cell clones originating from human RF heart lesions recognize bacterial M-protein peptides and heart-derived peptides. These mimic peptides are clearly associated with major manifestations of RF that affect the heart valves and neuronal elements, among other organs.[100,39]

Table 2 Molecular mimicry mechanism in different autoimmune disorders

Autoimmune Disorder	Self-antigen	Pathogen	References
Rheumatic fever	Cardiac myosin, tropomyosin, laminin, vimentin, actin, keratin, N-acetyl-glucosamine	*Streptococcus pyogens* M protein and N-acetyl-glucosamine	84–86
Chagas cardiomyopathy	Humen β1-adrenergic receptor, cardiac myosin, Cha antigen, common glycolipid antigenson nervous tissue	*Trypanosoma cruzi* ribosomal PO, B13 protein, shed acute-phase antigen (SAPA); 160-kDa flagellum; trypomastigote stage specific glycoprotein	58
Rheumatoid arthritis	BZLF1, BMLF1	EBV	13,66
Ankylosing spondylitis	HLA B27 Type I, II, IV collagen	Klebsiella pneumonia, chlamydia	87
Systemic lupus erythematosus	Ro 60 kD, Sm, MDA, dsDNA	Mycobacteria, Klebsiella pneumonia Pneumococcal polysaccharide EBV, HERV, Coxsackie virus 2B, parvovirus, retroviruses	13,88–93
Sjögren's syndrome	Ro 60 kD	Coxsackie virus 2B	94
Antiphospholipid syndrome	β2 Glycoprotein I	*Hemophilus influenza, Niesseria gonorrhoeae,* tetanus toxin, parvovirus B12, CMV	64,76
Autoimmune liver diseases	Core protein	HCV	69,70
Inflammatory bowel diseases	Cruzipain	*Trypanosoma cruzi*	58
Type I diabetes mellitus	pUL94, viral peptides	CMV, enterovirus, rubella	67,75
Autoimmune thyroid diseases	HCV polyprotein	HCV	71

Continued

Table 2 Molecular mimicry mechanism in different autoimmune disorders—cont'd

Autoimmune Disorder	Self-antigen	Pathogen	References
Multiple sclerosis	Myelin basic protein Myelin oligodendrocyte glycoprotein 18–32	Corona virus, measles, mumps, EBV, human herpes Semliki Forest virus E2 peptide 115–129, *Acanthamoeba castellanii*, influenza virus type A, human papillomavirus	95,88,96,13
Myasthenia gravis	Acetylcholine receptor neurofilaments	Herpes virus, hemophilus influenza	97
Guillain-Barré syndrome	Gangliosides	*Campylobacter jejuni* lipo-oligosaccharide	98

CMV, cytomegalovirus; dsDNA, double-stranded DNA; EBV, Epstein-Barr virus; HCV, hepatitis C virus; HERV, human endogenous retrovirus; HLA, human leukocyte antigen; MDA, malondialdehyde; Sm, Smith.

Moreover, active immunization with these cross-reactive peptides induces myocarditis in mice, and passive transfer of purified antibodies from rats immunised with cardiac myosin resulted in immunoglobulin G deposition and apoptosis, leading to cardiomyopathy.[101,102]

6 VASCULITIDES

SLE is a multisystem human autoimmune disease characterized by multiple autoantibodies: anti-dsDNA, anti-Ro/La, antiribonucleoprotein complex, antihistone and other nuclear components. Among autoimmune diseases, SLE was linked to several viral and bacterial agents, especially the EBV, which is a ubiquitous pathogen associated with many autoimmune diseases. The interaction between EBV and SLE is not unidirectional. EBV may trigger autoimmunity (the appearance of SLE-associated autoantibodies and clinical manifestations), but it can also affect the immunologic system in patients with SLE, who seem to have an impaired anti-EBV immune response and dysregulation of the viral latency period compared with controls.[103,104] In recent years, several other viruses have been linked to SLE as well, and molecular mimicry was suggested as the responsible mechanism. For the majority of them, however, only antigenic cross-reactivity had been demonstrated so far. The first example for cross-reactivity is the peptide derivative from Coxsackie virus 2B protein (pepCoxs), which has 87% amino acid homology with the 222–229 region of the major linear antibody binding site of the Ro 60-kD autoantigen. The Coxsackie virus was suggested to have a potential role in the autoimmune response against Ro/SSA and La/SSB as well.[94] The second example of cross-reactivity is the PB19, which has been implicated as a causative agent of several autoimmune disorders, including SLE. A peptide that shares homology with the parvovirus VP1 protein and with human cytokeratin (the transcription factor GATA1) and that plays an essential role in megakaryopoiesis and erythropoiesis was identified and was suggested to have a role in the induction of cross-reactive autoantibodies.[88] Furthermore, endogenous retrovirus elements and nonendogenous elements were found to be linked with autoimmunity, and molecular mimicry between those retroviruses and a host antigen was proposed.[89] The complex interplay between infections, genetics and autoimmunity regarding retroviruses in SLE patients is reviewed elsewhere.[90]

A molecular mimicry mechanism in lupus was studied in bacterial infections as well (i.e., mycobacteria, Klebsiella pneumonia), mainly with anti-dsDNA antibodies, and has been documented in animal models and in humans.[91,105] For example, in healthy individuals, elevated titers of anti-dsDNA antibodies can be detected following different bacterial infections.[92] Furthermore, sera from patients infected with the Gram-negative pathogen *Klebsiella pneumoniae* were found to have high titers of a common anti-DNA idiotype (16/6ID). Another example is the similarity found between the B 561 peptides from *Burkholderia* bacteria and anti-dsDNA antibodies.[106] The cross-reactivity between anti-dsDNA and *Burkholderia* peptides points to the possible role of bacterial infection in inducing the production of autoantibodies.

6.1 Summary and Suggestions for the Future: 'Control' of Molecular mimicry

The complex causes of autoimmune diseases not only present a challenge to the development and testing of new therapies but also offer a framework that allows the identification of subgroups of patients who might benefit from particular approaches. Molecular mimicry is one of the most logical explanations for the linkage between infection and autoimmunity, and its concept is a useful tool in understanding the etiology and pathogenesis of autoimmune disorders. The examples detailed in this chapter supply evidence for the role of specific pathogens in triggering particular autoimmune disorders by molecular mimicry. However, a definite direct causality between this mechanism and autoimmunity is yet to be established.

Understanding the mechanism of molecular mimicry in autoimmune disorders, one cannot avoid thinking that autoimmunity caused by molecular mimicry can be avoided. Control of the initiating factor (pathogen) via vaccination seems to be the most common method of avoiding autoimmunity. Inducing tolerance to the host autoantigen in this way may also be the most stable factor. The development of a downregulating immune response to the epitopes shared between the pathogen and the host may be the best way of treating an autoimmune disease caused by molecular mimicry.[107] Unfortunately, this method is not straightforward. Recently, a large number of published case reports of immunologic late reactions to vaccines raised the hypothesis that specific vaccines containing adjuvants are responsible for autoimmune diseases, especially in genetically susceptible patients. The entity autoimmune/auto-inflammatory syndrome induced by adjuvants describes the role of various environmental factors in the pathogenesis of immune-mediated diseases. Of these factors, those entailing immune adjuvant activity, such as infectious agents, silicone, aluminium salts and others, were associated with defined and nondefined immune-mediated diseases both in animal models and in humans.[108]

Understanding the mechanisms of molecular mimicry may allow future research to be directed towards uncovering the initiating infectious agent as well as recognizing the self-determinant. Willingly, future research may be able to design strategies for the treatment and prevention of autoimmunity.

REFERENCES

1. Damian RT. Molecular mimicry: antigen sharing by parasite and host and its consequences. *Am Nat* 1964;**98**(900):129–49.
2. Damian RT. Parasite immune evasion and exploitation: reflections and projections. *Parasitology* 1997;**115**(Suppl):S169–75.
3. Würzner R. Evasion of pathogens by avoiding recognition or eradication by complement, in part via molecular mimicry. *Mol Immunol* 1999;**36**(4-5):249–60.
4. Elde NC, Malik HS. The evolutionary conundrum of pathogen mimicry. *Nat Rev Microbiol* 2009;**7**(11):787–97.
5. Mansur DS, Maluquer de Motes C, Unterholzner L, Sumner RP, Ferguson BJ, Ren H, et al. Poxvirus targeting of E3 ligase β-TrCP by molecular mimicry: a mechanism to inhibit NF-κB activation and promote immune evasion and virulence. *PLoS Pathog* 2013;**9**(2):e1003183.
6. Schneider MC, Prosser BE, Caesar JJ, Kugelberg E, Li S, Zhang Q, et al. Neisseria meningitidis recruits factor H using protein mimicry of host carbohydrates. *Nature* 2009;**458**(7240):890–3.
7. Carlin AF, Uchiyama S, Chang YC, Lewis AL, Nizet V, Varki A. Molecular mimicry of host sialylated glycans allows a bacterial pathogen to engage neutrophil Siglec-9 and dampen the innate immune response. *Blood* 2009;**113**(14):3333–6.
8. Agmon-Levin N, Blank M, Paz Z, Shoenfeld Y. Molecular mimicry in systemic lupus erythematosus. *Lupus* 2009;**18**(13):1181–5.
9. Kohm AP, Fuller KG, Miller SD. Mimicking the way to autoimmunity: an evolving theory of sequence and structural homology. *Trends Microbiol* 2003;**11**(3):101–5.
10. Shoenfeld Y, Gershwin ME. Autoimmunity at a glance. *Autoimmun Rev* 2002;**1**.
11. Blank M, Barzilai O, Shoenfeld Y. Molecular mimicry and auto-immunity. *Clin Rev Allergy Immunol* 2007;**32**(1):111–18.
12. Cohen JI. Epstein-Barr virus infection. *N Engl J Med* 2000;**343**(7):481–92.
13. Barzilai O, Sherer Y, Ram M, Izhaky D, Anaya JM, Shoenfeld Y. Epstein-Barr virus and cytomegalovirus in autoimmune diseases: are they truly notorious? A preliminary report. *Ann N Y Acad Sci* 2007;**1108**:567–77.
14. Berkun Y, Zandman-Goddard G, Barzilai O, Boaz M, Sherer Y, Larida B, et al. Infectious antibodies in systemic lupus erythematosus patients. *Lupus* 2009;**18**(13):1129–35.
15. Zandman-Goddard G, Berkun Y, Barzilai O, Boaz M, Blank M, Ram M, et al. Exposure to Epstein-Barr virus infection is associated with mild systemic lupus erythematosus disease. *Ann N Y Acad Sci* 2009;**1173**:658–63.
16. Sabbatini A, Bombardieri S, Migliorini P. Autoantibodies from patients with systemic lupus erythematosus bind a shared sequence of SmD and Epstein–Barr virus-encoded nuclear antigen EBNA I. *Eur J Immunol* 1993;**23**:1146–52.
17. McClain MT, Ramsland PA, Kaufman KM, James JA. Anti-Sm autoantibodies in systemic lupus target highly basic surface structures of complexed spliceosomal autoantigens. *J Immunol* 2002;**168**:2054–62.

18. James JA, Scofield RH, Harley JB. Lupus humoral autoimmunity after short peptide immunization. *Ann N Y Acad Sci* 1997;**815**:124–7.
19. McClain MT, Heinlen LD, Dennis GJ, Roebuck J, Harley JB, James JA. Early events in lupus humoral autoimmunity suggest initiation through molecular mimicry. *Nat Med* 2005;**11**(1):85–9.
20. Sundar K, Jacques S, Gottlieb P, Villars R, Benito ME, Taylor DK, et al. Expression of the Epstein-Barr virus nuclear antigen-1 (EBNA-1) in the mouse can elicit the production of anti-dsDNA and anti-Sm antibodies. *J Autoimmun* 2004;**23**(2):127–40.
21. Yadav P, Tran H, Ebegbe R, Gottlieb P, Wei H, Lewis RH, et al. Antibodies elicited in response to EBNA-1 may cross-react with dsDNA. *PLoS One* 2011;**6**(1):e14488.
22. Poole BD, Gross T, Maier S, Harley JB, James JA. Lupus-like autoantibody development in rabbits and mice after immunization with EBNA-1 fragments. *J Autoimmun* 2008;**31**(4):362–71.
23. Cannon MJ, Schmid DS, Hyde TB. Review of cytomegalovirus seroprevalence and demographic characteristics associated with infection. *Rev Med Virol* 2010;**20**(4):202–13.
24. Lunardi C, Bason C, Navone R, Millo E, Damonte G, Corrocher R, et al. Systemic sclerosis immunoglobulin G autoantibodies bind the human cytomegalovirus late protein UL94 and induce apoptosis in human endothelial cells. *Nat Med* 2000;**6**(10):1183–6.
25. Hiemstra HS, Schloot NC, van Veelen PA, Willemen SJ, Franken KL, van Rood JJ, et al. Cytomegalovirus in autoimmunity: T cell crossreactivity to viral antigen and autoantigen glutamic acid decarboxylase. *Proc Natl Acad Sci U S A* 2001;**98**(7):3988–91.
26. Ang CW, Jacobs BC, Brandenburg AH, Laman JD, van der Meché FG, Osterhaus AD, et al. Cross-reactive antibodies against GM2 and CMV-infected fibroblasts in Guillain-Barré syndrome. *Neurology* 2000;**54**(7):1453–8.
27. Hsieh AH, Jhou YJ, Liang CT, Chang M, Wang SL. Fragment of tegument protein pp 65 of human cytomegalovirus induces autoantibodies in BALB/c mice. *Arthritis Res Ther* 2011;**13**(5):R162.
28. Mossong J, Hens N, Friederichs V, Davidkin I, Broman M, Litwinska B, et al. Parvovirus B19 infection in five European countries: seroepidemiology, force of infection and maternal risk of infection. *Epidemiol Infect* 2008;**136**(8):1059–68.
29. Sabella C, Goldfarb J. Parvovirus B19 infections. *Am Fam Physician* 1999;**60**(5):1455–60.
30. Lehmann HW, Von Landenberg P, Modrow S. Parvovirus B19 infection and autoimmune disease. *Autoimmun Rev* 2003;**2**(4):218–23.
31. Pavlovic M, Kats A, Cavallo M, Shoenfeld Y. Clinical and molecular evidence for association of SLE with parvovirus B19. *Lupus* 2010;**19**(7):783–92.
32. Loizou S, Cazabon JK, Walport MJ, Tait D, So AK. Similarities of specificity and cofactor dependence in serum antiphospholipid antibodies from patients with human parvovirus B19 infection and from those with systemic lupus erythematosus. *Arthritis Rheum* 1997;**40**(1):103–8.
33. Lunardi C, Tiso M, Borgato L, Nanni L, Millo R, De Sandre G, et al. Chronic parvovirus B19 infection induces the production of anti-virus antibodies with autoantigen binding properties. *Eur J Immunol* 1998;**28**(3):936–48.
34. Zabriskie JB. Mimetic relationships between group A streptococci and mammalian tissues. *Adv Immunol* 1967;**7**:147–88.
35. Dale JB, Beachey EH. Epitopes of streptococcal M proteins shared with cardiac myosin. *J Exp Med* 1985;**162**(2):583–91.
36. Cunningham MW, McCormack JM, Fenderson PG, Ho MK, Beachey EH, Dale JB. Human and murine antibodies cross-reactive with streptococcal M protein and myosin recognize the sequence GLN-LYS-SER-LYS-GLN in M protein. *J Immunol* 1989;**143**(8):2677–83.

37. Quinn A, Ward K, Fischetti VA, Hemric M, Cunningham MW. Immunological relationship between the class I epitope of streptococcal M protein and myosin. *Infect Immun* 1998;**66**(9):4418–24.

38. Guilherme L, Cunha-Neto E, Coelho V, Snitcowsky R, Pomerantzeff PM, Assis RV, et al. Human heart-infiltrating T-cell clones from rheumatic heart disease patients recognize both streptococcal and cardiac proteins. *Circulation* 1995;**92** (3):415–20.

39. Kirvan CA, Swedo SE, Heuser JS, Cunningham MW. Mimicry and autoantibody-mediated neuronal cell signaling in Sydenham chorea. *Nat Med* 2003;**9**(7):914–20.

40. Quinn A, Kosanke S, Fischetti VA, Factor SM, Cunningham MW. Induction of autoimmune valvular heart disease by recombinant streptococcal m protein. *Infect Immun* 2001;**69**(6):4072–8.

41. Bronze MS, Dale JB. Epitopes of streptococcal M proteins that evoke antibodies that cross-react with human brain. *J Immunol* 1993;**151**(5):2820–8.

42. Go MF. Review article: natural history and epidemiology of Helicobacter pylori infection. *Aliment Pharmacol Ther* 2002;**16**(Suppl 1):3–15.

43. Appelmelk BJ, Simoons-Smit I, Negrini R, Moran AP, Aspinall GO, Forte JG, et al. Potential role of molecular mimicry between Helicobacter pylori lipopolysaccharide and host Lewis blood group antigens in autoimmunity. *Infect Immun* 1996;**64** (6):2031–40.

44. Amedei A, Bergman MP, Appelmelk BJ, Azzurri A, Benagiano M, Tamburini C, et al. Molecular mimicry between Helicobacter pylori antigens and H+, K+ –adenosine triphosphatase in human gastric autoimmunity. *J Exp Med* 2003;**198**(8):1147–56.

45. Takahashi T, Yujiri T, Shinohara K, Inoue Y, Sato Y, Fujii Y, et al. Molecular mimicry by Helicobacter pylori CagA protein may be involved in the pathogenesis of H. pylori-associated chronic idiopathic thrombocytopenic purpura. *Br J Haematol* 2004;**124** (1):91–6.

46. Allos BM. Campylobacter jejuni Infections: update on emerging issues and trends. *Clin Infect Dis* 2001;**32**(8):1201–6.

47. Israeli E, Agmon-Levin N, Blank M, Chapman J, Shoenfeld Y. Guillain-Barré syndrome–a classical autoimmune disease triggered by infection or vaccination. *Clin Rev Allergy Immunol* 2012;**42**(2):121–30.

48. Yuki N, Taki T, Inagaki F, Kasama T, Takahashi M, Saito K, et al. A bacterium lipopolysaccharide that elicits Guillain-Barré syndrome has a GM1 ganglioside-like structure. *J Exp Med* 1993;**178**(5):1771–5.

49. Willison HJ, Yuki N. Peripheral neuropathies and anti-glycolipid antibodies. *Brain* 2002;**125**(Pt 12):2591–625.

50. Yuki N, Susuki K, Koga M, Nishimoto Y, Odaka M, Hirata K, et al. Carbohydrate mimicry between human ganglioside GM1 and Campylobacter jejuni lipooligosaccharide causes Guillain-Barre syndrome. *Proc Natl Acad Sci U S A* 2004;**101**(31):11404–9.

51. Chagas C. Nova tripanozomiase humana. Estudos sobre a morfolojia e o ciclo evolutivo do *Schizotrypanum cruzi* n. gen. n. sp., ajente etiológico de uma nova entidade morbida do homem. *Mem Inst Oswaldo Cruz* 1909;**1**:159–218.

52. Chagas C. Tripanosomiase americana. Forma aguda da moléstia. *Mem Inst Oswaldo Cruz* 1916;**8**:37–60.

53. Chagas C. Processos patojénicos da Tripanozomiase Americana. *Mem Inst Oswaldo Cruz* 1916;**8**:5–36.

54. Chagas C, Villela E. Forma cardíaca da Trypanosomiase Americana. *Mem Inst Oswaldo Cruz* 1922;**14**:5–61.

55. Prata A. Clinical and epidemiological aspects of Chagas disease. *Lancet Infect Dis* 2001;**1** (2):92–100.

56. Cunha-Neto E, Bilate AM, Hyland KV, Fonseca SG, Kalil J, Engman DM. Induction of cardiac autoimmunity in Chagas heart disease: a case for molecular mimicry. *Autoimmunity* 2006;**39**(1):41–54.
57. Bonney KM, Engman DM. Chagas heart disease pathogenesis: one mechanism or many? *Curr Mol Med* 2008;**8**(6):510–18.
58. Giordanengo L, Maldonado C, Rivarola HW, Iosa D, Girones N, Fresno M, et al. Induction of antibodies reactive to cardiac myosin and development of heart alterations in cruzipain-immunized mice and their offspring. *Eur J Immunol* 2000;**30**(11):3181–9.
59. Cunha-Neto E, Duranti M, Gruber A, Zingales B, De Messias I, Stolf N, et al. Autoimmunity in Chagas disease cardiopathy: biological relevance of a cardiac myosin-specific epitope crossreactive to an immunodominant Trypanosoma cruzi antigen. *Proc Natl Acad Sci U S A* 1995;**92**(8):3541–5.
60. Cunha-Neto E, Coelho V, Guilherme L, Fiorelli A, Stolf N, Kalil J. Autoimmunity in Chagas' disease. Identification of cardiac myosin-B13 Trypanosoma cruzi protein cross-reactive T cell clones in heart lesions of a chronic Chagas' cardiomyopathy patient. *J Clin Invest* 1996;**98**(8):1709–12.
61. Leon JS, Daniels MD, Toriello KM, Wang K, Engman DM. A cardiac myosin-specific autoimmune response is induced by immunization with Trypanosoma cruzi proteins. *Infect Immun* 2004;**72**(6):3410–17.
62. Leon JS, Wang K, Engman DM. Myosin autoimmunity is not essential for cardiac inflammation in acute Chagas' disease. *J Immunol* 2003;**171**(8):4271–7.
63. Motrán CC, Fretes RE, Cerbán FM, Rivarola HW. Vottero de Cima E. Immunization with the C-terminal region of Trypanosoma cruzi ribosomal P1 and P2 proteins induces long-term duration cross-reactive antibodies with heart functional and structural alterations in young and aged mice. *Clin Immunol* 2000;**97**(2):89–94.
64. Gharavi AE, Pierangeli SS, Espinola RG, Liu X, Colden-Stanfield M, Harris EN. Anti-phospholipid antibodies induced in mice by immunization with a cytomegalovirus-derived peptide cause thrombosis and activation of endothelial cells in vivo. *Arthritis Rheum* 2002;**46**(2):545–52.
65. Gabibov AG, Belogurov Jr AA, Lomakin YA, Zakharova MY, Avakyan ME, Dubrovskaya VV, et al. Combinatorial antibody library from multiple sclerosis patients reveals antibodies that cross-react with myelin basic protein and EBV antigen. *FASEB J* 2011;**25**(12):4211–21.
66. Scotet E, David-Ameline J, Peyrat MA, Moreau-Aubry A, Pinczon D, Lim A, et al. T cell response to Epstein-Barr virus transactivators in chronic rheumatoid arthritis. *J Exp Med* 1996;**184**(5):1791–800.
67. Härkönen T, Lankinen H, Davydova B, Hovi T, Roivainen M. Enterovirus infection can induce immune responses that cross-react with beta-cell autoantigen tyrosine phosphatase IA-2/IAR. *J Med Virol* 2002;**66**(3):340–50.
68. Fujinami RS, Oldstone MB. Amino acid homology between the encephalitogenic site of myelin basic protein and virus: mechanism for autoimmunity. *Science* 1985;**230** (4729):1043–5.
69. Kammer AR, van der Burg SH, Grabscheid B, Hunziker IP, Kwappenberg KM, Reichen J, et al. Molecular mimicry of human cytochrome P450 by hepatitis C virus at the level of cytotoxic T cell recognition. *J Exp Med* 1999;**190**(2):169–76.
70. Hartmann H, Schott P, Polzien F, Mihm S, Uy A, Kaboth U, et al. Cryoglobulinemia in chronic hepatitis C virus infection: prevalence, clinical manifestations, response to interferon treatment and analysis of cryoprecipitates. *Z Gastroenterol* 1995;**33**(11):643–50.
71. Muratori L, Bogdanos DP, Muratori P, Lenzi M, Granito A, Ma Y, et al. Susceptibility to thyroid disorders in hepatitis C. *Clin Gastroenterol Hepatol* 2005;**3**(6):595–603.
72. Deas JE, Liu LG, Thompson JJ, Sander DM, Soble SS, Garry RF, et al. Reactivity of sera from systemic lupus erythematosus and Sjögren's syndrome patients with peptides

derived from human immunodeficiency virus p24 capsid antigen. *Clin Diagn Lab Immunol* 1998;**5**(2):181–5.

73. Schwimmbeck PL, Dyrberg T, Drachman DB, Oldstone MB. Molecular mimicry and myasthenia gravis An autoantigenic site of the acetylcholine receptor alpha-subunit that has biologic activity and reacts immunochemically with herpes simplex virus. *J Clin Invest* 1989;**84**(4):1174–80.

74. Tzang BS, Lee YJ, Yang TP, Tsay GJ, Shi JY, Tsai CC, et al. Induction of antiphospholipid antibodies and antiphospholipid syndrome-like autoimmunity in naive mice with antibody against human parvovirus B19 VP1 unique region protein. *Clin Chim Acta* 2007;**382**(1–2):31–6.

75. Ou D, Mitchell LA, Metzger DL, Gillam S, Tingle AJ. Cross-reactive rubella virus and glutamic acid decarboxylase (65 and 67) protein determinants recognised by T cells of patients with type I diabetes mellitus. *Diabetologia* 2000;**43**(6):750–62.

76. Blank M, Krause I, Fridkin M, Keller N, Kopolovic J, Goldberg I, et al. Bacterial induction of autoantibodies to beta2-glycoprotein-I accounts for the infectious etiology of antiphospholipid syndrome. *J Clin Invest* 2002;**109**(6):797–804.

77. Ramos M, Alvarez I, Sesma L, Logean A, Rognan D. López de Castro JA. Molecular mimicry of an HLA-B27-derived ligand of arthritis-linked subtypes with chlamydial proteins. *J Biol Chem* 2002;**277**(40):37573–81.

78. Van Voorhis WC, Schlekewy L, Trong HL. Molecular mimicry by Trypanosoma cruzi: the F1-160 epitope that mimics mammalian nerve can be mapped to a 12-amino acid peptide. *Proc Natl Acad Sci U S A* 1991;**88**(14):5993–7.

79. Shoenfeld Y, Zandman-Goddard G, Stojanovich L, et al. The mosaic of autoimmunity: hormonal and environmental factors involved in autoimmune disease—2008. *Isr Med Assoc J* 2008;**10**:8–12.

80. Macray Ian R, Rosen Fred S. autoimmune disease. *N Engl J Med* 2001;**345**(5):340–50.

81. Lim DG, Haffler DA. Molecular mimicry in multiple sclerosis: role of MHC altered peptide Ligands. In: *Infections and autoimmunity*. 1st ed. Amsterdam: Elsevier; 2004. p. 45–55.

82. Oldstone MB. Molecular mimicry and immune-mediated diseases. *FASEB J* 1998;**12**:1255–65.

83. Srinivasappa J, Saegusa J, Prabhakar BS, et al. Molecular mimicry: frequency of reactivity of monoclonal antiviral Abs with normal tissues. *J Virol* 1986;**57**:397–401.

84. Galvin JE, Hemric ME, Ward K. Cunningham MW; Cytotoxic mAb from rheumatic carditis recognizes hert va;ves and laminin. *J Clin Invest* 2000;**106**:217–24.

85. Guilhrme I, Cunha-Neto E. Coelho V et el; Human heart –infiltrating T cells clones from rheumatic heart disease patients recognize both streptococcal and cardiac proteins. *Circulation* 1995;**92**:415–20.

86. Malkiel S, Liao L, Cunningham MW, Diamond B. T–cell dependant ride, N-acetyl-glucosamines, is cross-reactive with cardiac myosin. *Infect Immun* 2000;**68**:5803–8.

87. Ramos M, Alvarez I, Sesma L, Logean A, Rognan D, de Castro JA López. Molecular mimicry of an HLA-B27-derived ligand of arthritis-linked subtypes with chlamydial proteins. *J Biol Chem* 2002;**277**(40):37573–81.

88. Lunardi C, Tinazzi E, Bason C, Dolcino M, Corrocher R, Puccetti A. Human parvovirus B19 infection and autoimmunity. *Autoimmun Rev* 2008;**8**:116–20.

89. Perl A, Nagy G, Koncz A, et al. Molecular mimicry and immunomodulation by the HRES-1 endogenous retrovirus in SLE. *Autoimmunity* 2008;**41**:287–97.

90. Blank M, Shoenfeld Y, Perl A. Cross-talk of the environment with the host genome and the immune system through endogenous retroviruses in systemic lupus erythematosus. *Lupus* 2009;**18**(13):1136–43.

91. Shoenfeld Y, Vilner Y, Coates AR, et al. Monoclonal anti-tuberculosis Abs react with DNA, and monoclonal anti-DNA autoantibodies react with Mycobacterium tuberculosis. *Clin Exp Immunol* 1986;**66**:255–61.

92. Zandman-Goddard G, Shoenfeld Y. SLE and infections. In: *Infections and autoimmunity*. 1st ed. Amsterdam: Elsevier; 2004. p. 491–503.
93. Zhang W, Reichlin M. A possible link between infection with burkholderia bacteria and systemic lupus erythematosus based on epitope mimicry. *Clin Dev Immunol* 2008;**1–7**.
94. Stathopoulou EA, Routsias JG, Stea EA, Moutsopoulos HM, Tzioufas AG. Cross-reaction between Abs to the major epitope of Ro60 kD autoantigen and a homologous peptide of Coxsackie virus 2B protein. *Clin Exp Immunol* 2005;**141**:148–54.
95. Wucherpfennig KW, Strominger JL. Molecular mimicry in T cellmediated autoimmunity: viral peptides activate human T cell clones specific for myelin basic protein. *Cell* 1995;**80**:695–705.
96. Lang HLE, Jacobsen H, Ikemizu S, et al. A functional and structural basis for TCR cross-reactivity in multiple sclerosis. *Nat Immunol* 2002;**3**:940–3.
97. Peter LS, Thomas D, Daniel BD, Michael BA, Oldstone MB. Molecular Mimicry and Myasthenia Gravis, An Autoantigenic Site of the Acetylcholine Receptor a-Subunit That Has Biologic Activity and Reacts Immunochemically with Herpes Simplex Virus. *J Clin Invest* 1989;**84**(4):1174–80.
98. Yuki N. Pathogenesis of Guillan Barre and Miller Fisher syndromes subsequent to campylobacter jejuni enteritis. *Jpn J Infect Dis* 1999;**52**:99–105.
99. Lori JA, Iman Robert D. Molecular mimicry and autoimmunity. *NEJM* 1999;**341**(27):2068–74.
100. Guilherme L, Kalil J, Cunningham MW. Molecular mimicry in the autoimmune pathogenesis of rheumatic heart disease. *Autoimmunity* 2006;**39**:31–9.
101. Cunningham MW. Streptococcus-induced myocarditis in mice. *Autoimmunity* 2001;**34**:193–7.
102. Li Y, Heuser JS, Cunningham LC, et al. Mimicry and antibodymediated cell signaling in autoimmune myocarditis. *J Immunol* 2006;**177**:8234–40.
103. Niller HH, Wolf H, Minarovits J. Regulation and dysregulation of Epstein–Barr virus latency: implications for the development of autoimmune diseases. *Autoimmunity* 2008;**41**:298–328.
104. Gross AJ, Hochberg D, Rand WM, Thorley-Lawson DA. EBV and systemic lupus erythematosus: a new perspective. *J Immunol* 2005;**174**:6599–607.
105. George J, Shoenfeld Y. Infections, idiotypes and SLE. *Lupus* 1995;**4**:333–5.
106. Zhang W, Reichlin M. A possible link between infection with burkholderia bacteria and systemic lupus erythematosus based on epitope mimicry. *Clin Dev Immunol* 2008;**2008**(683489):1–7.
107. Barnett LA, Fujinami RS. Molecular mimicry: a mechanism for autoimmunity. *FASEB J* 1992;**6**:840–4.
108. Shoenfeld Y, Agmon-Levin N. 'ASIA'–autoimmune/inflammatory syndrome induced by adjuvants. *J Autoimmun* 2011;**36**(1):4–8.

CHAPTER 4

Epitope Spreading in Autoimmune Diseases

Shivaprasad H. Venkatesha, Malarvizhi Durai, Kamal D. Moudgil[1]
Department of Microbiology and Immunology, University of Maryland School of Medicine, Baltimore, Maryland, USA
[1]Corresponding Author: kmoud001@umaryland.edu

1 INTRODUCTION

The phenomenon of "epitope spreading" (or "determinant spreading") is characterized by broadening or diversification of the initial immune response induced by immunization with a single peptide antigen or a multi-determinant antigen.[1-3] The new T cell and/or antibody responses are directed to different epitopes either within the same antigen (intramolecular spreading) or another antigen (intermolecular spreading). The spreading of initial immune reactivity has been shown to occur during the course of a variety of experimentally induced and spontaneously arising autoimmune diseases in animal models (Tables 1 and 2).[2,3] Studies of patients with certain autoimmune diseases (Table 1) have further validated the significance of epitope spreading in disease pathogenesis. Depending on the disease process, epitope spreading can contribute to either the progression or the control of an autoimmune disease (Figure 1).[1,3,10] The timing of epitope spreading during the course of an autoimmune disease and its functional attributes are of significance in designing appropriate immunotherapeutic approaches.

2 EXAMPLES OF EPITOPE SPREADING IN AUTOIMMUNE DISEASES

2.1 Multiple Sclerosis and Experimental Autoimmune Encephalomyelitis

Multiple sclerosis (MS) is a human autoimmune disease characterized by mononuclear cell infiltration and discrete areas of demyelination (plaques) within the central nervous system (CNS) and neurological dysfunction. Experimental autoimmune encephalomyelitis (EAE) is an experimental

Infection and Autoimmunity
http://dx.doi.org/10.1016/B978-0-444-63269-2.00003-9

Table 1 Examples of Epitope Spreading in Animal Models and Human Autoimmune Diseases

Diseases	References
(a) Animal models of autoimmune diseases	
Experimental autoimmune encephalomyelitis (EAE)	1,4–7
Diabetes in the non-obese diabetic (NOD) mouse	8,9
Adjuvant-induced arthritis (AA)	10–15
Lupus or systemic lupus erythematosus (SLE)	16–20
Experimental autoimmune myasthenia gravis (EAMG)	21
Experimental autoimmune neuritis (EAN)	22
Equine recurrent uveitis (ERU)	23
Experimental autoimmune gastritis (EAG)	24
Autoimmune oophoritis	25
Experimental autoimmune thyroiditis (EAT)	26
(b) Human autoimmune diseases	
Multiple sclerosis (MS)	27–29
Insulin-dependent diabetes mellitus (IDDM) or type I diabetes	30–33
Rheumatoid arthritis (RA)	34–37
Systemic lupus erythematosus (SLE) or lupus	38–41
Myasthenia gravis (MG)	21

model of MS, and it can be induced in different mouse/rat strains by immunization (in adjuvant) with myelin antigens such as myelin basic protein (MBP), proteolipid protein (PLP), or myelin oligodendrocyte glycoprotein (MOG) (Table 2).[3,43,44] Epitope spreading was first demonstrated by Lehmann et al. in an EAE model using (SJL × B10.PL) F1 mice.[1] It was shown that the initial T cell response of mice with acute EAE was directed to MBP Ac1-11, but spreading of the T cell response to new determinants of MBP, namely, 35–47, 81–100, and 121–140, subsequently, occurred during the chronic stage of EAE.[1,45] This broadening of the T cell response was attributed to the priming of new T cells by determinants within endogenous MBP following initial CNS damage.

Miller's group established the role of epitope spreading in the pathogenesis of relapsing EAE (R-EAE) and defined the mechanisms underlying epitope spreading. R-EAE can be induced in SJL mice by immunization with PLP 139–151.[4,46] Using this model, it was observed that the T cell response to the disease-initiating epitope, PLP 139–151, was maintained in SJL mice throughout the course of EAE. However, spreading of the T cell response to non-cross-reactive PLP 178–191 and MBP 84–104 epitopes occurred after the first and second relapses, respectively. Furthermore, the T cells against

Table 2 The Antigen Specificity of Epitope Spreading in Experimental Models of Autoimmune Diseases

Disease Model	Animals Tested	Disease-Inducing Antigen/Agent	Antigen/Epitopes Targeted During Epitope Spreading[a]	References
Experimental autoimmune encephalomyelitis (EAE)	(SJL × B10.PL)F1 mice	MBP Ac1–11	MBP 35–47, MBP 81–100, and MBP 121–140	1
	SJL/J mice	PLP 139–151	PLP 178–191 and MBP 84–104	4
	(SWR × SJL)F1 mice	PLP 139–151	PLP 249–273, MBP 87–99, and PLP 137–198	5
	Lewis rats	MBP	Multiple T cell epitopes within MBP	6
	Callithrix jacchus (the common marmoset)	MP4 fusion protein (PLP–MBP)	Anti-MOG antibodies	7
Diabetes in the non-obese diabetic (NOD) mouse	NOD mice	Spontaneous	T cell response to GAD65, carboxypeptidase-H, insulin, and HSP65	8
	NOD mice	Spontaneous	T cell and antibody response to GAD65/67, peripherin, carboxypeptidase-H, and HSP60	9
Adjuvant-induced arthritis (AA)	Lewis rats	Mtb (H37Ra)	417–431, 441–455, 465–479, 513–527, 521–535 of Bhsp65	10
	Lewis rats	Mtb (H37Ra)	Multiple B cell epitopes within Bhsp65 after recovery from acute AA	12,13
Lupus or systemic lupus erythematosus (SLE)	NZW rabbits	Sm B/B' peptide	Antibody response to other epitopes of Sm B/B' antigen and other spliceosomal proteins	16
	Mice	La (or Ro) antigen	Antibody response to both La and Ro proteins	17

(Continued)

Table 2 The Antigen Specificity of Epitope Spreading in Experimental Models of Autoimmune Diseases—cont'd

Disease Model	Animals Tested	Disease-Inducing Antigen/Agent	Antigen/Epitopes Targeted During Epitope Spreading	References
	(SWR × NZB)F1 mice	Spontaneous	Antibody response to nucleosomal components	18
	(NZB/NZW)F1 mice	Spontaneous	Response to epitopes in V_H region of anti-DNA antibody	19
Experimental autoimmune myasthenia gravis (EAMG)	NZW rabbits	Human AChR α-subunit peptides	Antibodies to rabbit AChR	42
Experimental autoimmune neuritis (EAN)	Lewis rats	Peptides 56–71 and 180–199 of P0 protein	T cell response to other epitopes of P0 protein	22
Equine recurrent uveitis (ERU)	Horse	IRBP	Multiple T cell epitopes within IRBP and S-Ag	23
Experimental autoimmune gastritis (EAG)	Mice	H/K ATPase β-subunit	T cell and antibody response to α-subunit of H/K ATPase	24

MBP, myelin basic protein; PLP, proteolipid protein; TMEV, Theiler's murine encephalomyelitis virus; MOG, myelin oligodendrocyte glycoprotein; GAD65/67, glutamic acid decarboxylase 65/67; HSP65, heat shock protein 65; Mtb, heat-killed *Mycobacterium tuberculosis* H37Ra; Bhsp65, mycobacterial hsp65; AA, adjuvant-induced arthritis; Sm B/B′; La & Ro, antigens within ribonucleoprotein complex; AChR, acetylcholine receptor; P0, peripheral nervous system myelin glycoprotein; IRBP, interphotoreceptor retinoid binding protein; S-Ag, retinal S-antigen.
[a]Unless specified, all epitopes mentioned in the table refer to T cell responses.

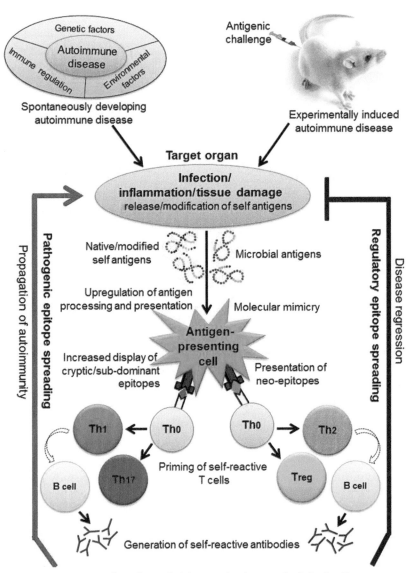

Figure 1 Epitope spreading: the underlying mechanisms and role in the disease process. Initiation of an autoimmune disease, either spontaneously or following an antigenic challenge, creates a local inflammatory milieu that is conducive to the upregulation of antigen processing and presentation. In addition, the tissue damage associated with inflammation and infection may lead to the release of self antigens. Under these circumstances, self antigens are processed efficiently by the antigen-presenting cells, revealing previously cryptic/subdominant epitopes to potentially self-reactive T cells available in the mature T cell repertoire. In addition, the post-translational modification of antigens following inflammation and other stimuli generates neo-epitopes. The outcome of the priming of self-reactive T cells depends on multiple factors, including the balance between Th1/Th17 versus Th2/Treg cells. In parallel, the activated T cells may provide help to autoreactive B cells, leading to the spread of antibody responses. Antibodies and B cells in turn may influence T cell responses as well as disease severity. Accordingly, epitope spreading could either perpetuate (pathogenic epitope spreading) or attenuate (protective epitope spreading) the ongoing disease process.

the spreading epitope (PLP 178–191) could transfer disease to naïve synge-neic recipients.[4] Interestingly, inducing tolerance against relapse-associated epitopes after the acute episode in SJL mice blocked disease progression and decreased the frequency of subsequent relapses.[4] In addition, short-term blockade of either CD28–CD80 (B7.1) interaction by anti-CD80 F(ab) fragment[47] or CD40–CD154 (CD40L) interaction using monoclonal anti-CD154 antibody[48] during remission from acute disease significantly reduced both the incidence of disease relapse and the T cell response to relapse-associated epitopes. Epitope spreading also has been implicated in the induction of autoimmunity in Theiler's murine encephalomyelitis virus (TMEV)-induced demyelinating disease in SJL/J mice.[49]

Tuohy and colleagues studied the specificity of determinants and the functional significance of epitope spreading in R-EAE inducible in (SWR × SJL) F1 mice by injection with PLP 139–151.[5] Interestingly, the T cells specific for the spreading determinant could passively transfer EAE to naïve syngeneic recipients, whereas induction of peptide-specific toler-ance to spreading epitopes after the onset of EAE could prevent the progres-sion of EAE.[5] Furthermore, interferon-β treatment of mice not only reduced the frequency/severity of disease relapses but also suppressed epitope spreading.[50] The diversification of response to MBP epitopes also has been observed during the course of EAE in Lewis rats.[6] The dominant encephalitogenic T cells in the induction phase of the disease were directed to epitope 71–90, whereas T cell responses to new epitopes within MBP appeared during the recovery phase of the disease.[6] Another study revealed that Wistar Kyoto (WKY) rats having the same MHC haplotype as the Lewis rat were resistant to EAE despite raising potent T cell responses to the dom-inant encephalitogenic T cell epitope within MBP.[51] However, the antigen-specific T cell response in WKY rats was skewed towards a predominantly T helper (Th) 2 type compared to a predominantly Th1 type in Lewis rats.

Epitope spreading to MBP and additional MOG epitopes has been reported in the course of MOG peptide-induced EAE in humanized mice expressing DR4, which represents one of the disease susceptibility MHC alleles for patients with MS.[52] In another study, autoantibody responses of mice with EAE were measured using a large set of autoantigens in a protein microarray.[53] Chronic EAE was characterized by both intra- and intermolecular epitope spreading, and attenuation of EAE by a tolerizing DNA vaccination was associated with reduced epitope spreading of auto-antibody responses. Similarly, the treatment of mice with EAE using a variety of other modalities (e.g., tolerance induction using antigen-decorated micro-particles,[54] multi-peptide-coupled splenocyte-induced tolerance,[55] multivalent bifunctional peptide inhibitor,[56] poly(ADP-ribose) polymerase-1 inhibitor,[57] anti-IL-23 antibody therapy[58] and suppressive oligodeoxynucleotide therapy)[59] resulted in the inhibition of epitope spreading and protection against disease, including relapses.

As in rodent EAE, epitope spreading also has been observed during the course of EAE in the common marmoset, *Callithrix jacchus*, and in patients with MS. The *C. jacchus* marmoset develops a chronic relapsing-remitting form of EAE following challenge with myelin antigens, and both the T cells and antibodies serve as immune effector mechanisms in the disease process.[7,60] Interestingly, the treatment of these non-human primates with anti-CD40 antibody prevented intramolecular spreading and afforded protection against EAE.[61,62] In a study of patients with isolated monosymptomatic demyelinating syndrome (IMDS), the T cell reactivity to PLP epitopes was found to decrease over time. However, spreading of T cell responses to other PLP epitopes was observed in those patients with IMDS who progressed to clinically definite MS.[27–29]

2.2 Insulin-Dependent Diabetes Mellitus or Type I Diabetes

Insulin-dependent diabetes mellitus (IDDM) is an autoimmune disease involving mononuclear cell infiltration of the pancreatic islets (insulitis), destruction of β-islet cells, and insulin deficiency. Spontaneously developing diabetes in the non-obese diabetic (NOD) mouse serves as a model for human IDDM. Glutamic acid decarboxylase (GAD65) has been invoked as one of the early target antigens in the pathogenesis of autoimmune diabetes in the NOD mouse.[8,9] With the progression of disease, the T cell responses spread to additional epitopes within GAD65 and to other β-cell antigens (e.g., to carboxypeptidase-H, insulin, and heat shock protein 65 (Hsp65) in one study[8] and to GAD67, carboxypeptidase-H, peripherin, and Hsp60 in another study[9]) (Table 2). Furthermore, tolerization of GAD65-reactive T cells suppressed the development of insulitis, disease progression, and the spreading of T cell responses.[8,9] Further, Th1 cell spreading leads to disease progression, whereas Th2 cell spreading is associated with protection from disease in NOD mice. In another study, new potential target epitopes within GAD65 and GAD67 were described in NOD mice,[63] and mice given a disease-protective regimen (e.g. adjuvant challenge) revealed a different pattern of response to GAD65/67 compared to control mice.

Studies of epitope spreading in human IDDM have revealed a pattern of autoantibody responses to β-cell antigens in children of diabetic patients.[30]

The anti-islet autoantibody response in these subjects was characterized by the appearance of an early immunoglobulin G1 response to one or more islet antigens, particularly insulin. Thereafter, coupled with a decline in the titer of these antibodies, antibodies against other β-cell antigens sequentially appeared over a period of several years.[30] In other studies of pre-clinical childhood type I diabetes, the initial antibody response to GAD of offspring of diabetic patients was directed primarily to epitopes within the middle portion of GAD65 but later spread to epitopes in other regions of GAD65 and GAD67.[31,32] Similarly, intermolecular spreading of the T cell reactivity and antibody responses to islet antigens occurred during the pre-clinical phase of type I diabetes in subjects at risk (as defined by positivity for autoantibodies to β-islet antigens) of developing clinical diabetes.[33]

2.3 Arthritis

Rheumatoid arthritis (RA) is a human autoimmune disease characterized by persistent inflammatory synovitis. Adjuvant-induced arthritis (AA) is an experimental model of human RA, and it can be induced in Lewis rats by immunization with heat-killed *Mycobacterium tuberculosis* H37Ra (Mtb) in mineral oil. The T cell response to the 65-kDa mycobacterial heat shock protein (Bhsp65) has been implicated in the pathogenesis of AA as well as RA.[64–67] We showed that there is a shift in the epitope specificity of the T cell response to Bhsp65 during the course of AA in Lewis rats. In the acute phase of AA, the T cell response of arthritic Lewis rats was focused on peptide 177–191 (which contains the arthritogenic determinant 180–188) and other epitopes in the middle and N-terminal regions of Bhsp65. During the recovery phase of AA, however, new T cell responses directed to the five C-terminal epitopes of Bhsp65 (namely, 417–431, 441–455, 465–479, 513–527, and 521–535) appeared (Table 2). Interestingly, pre-treatment of naïve Lewis rats with the synthetic peptides representing these five Bhsp65 C-terminal determinants (BCTDs) significantly reduced the severity of subsequently induced AA.[10,68] Furthermore, T cell responses to BCTDs were observed early following Mtb challenge in WKY rats that possess the same MHC haplotype as the AA-susceptible Lewis rat but are resistant to the induction of AA. The simultaneous emergence of T cell responses to the pathogenic (180–188/177–191 determinant) and regulatory (BCTD) epitopes could explain, in part, the AA resistance of WKY rats. The results of one of our other studies showed that the C-terminal epitopes of self hsp65 also are disease-regulating in nature.[69,70] The above-mentioned results suggest that spreading of the T cell responses to BCTDs during the course of AA might be involved in natural recovery from acute AA in the Lewis rat. Furthermore, these findings demonstrate that epitope spreading in the course of an autoimmune disease is not always pathogenic; instead, it can regulate disease in another situation. This is the first study[10] reporting the disease-regulating aspect of epitope spreading in the course of an autoimmune disease.

Another aspect of spontaneous emergence and spreading of T cell responses was revealed in a study of the Fischer F344 (F344) rat.[11] We observed that F344 rats kept in a barrier facility (BF-F344) were susceptible to AA, whereas those maintained in a conventional facility (CV-F344) spontaneously acquired protection (or resistance) against AA. CV-F344 but not BF-F344 rats showed an increased T cell response to multiple epitopes of Bhsp65, including BCTD, and the level of these spontaneously arising T cell responses gradually increased with the duration and extent of exposure of F344 rats to the conventional environment. Adoptive transfer of BCTD-restimulated (*in vitro*) splenic cells of naïve CV-F344 rats to naïve BF-F344 recipients offered protection against AA. The role of a conventional environment in facilitating the induction of an autoimmune disease has been observed in various models of autoimmunity. By contrast, our study described above[11] along with others of diabetes[71] reflect on the protective effect of environment on autoimmunity.

As for the T cell-mediated epitope spreading in AA, a couple studies have highlighted the role of spreading of antibody response to Bhsp65 in the regulation of AA. Lewis rats develop antibodies against Bhsp65 during the course of AA, and the number of epitopes within Bhsp65 recognized by these antibodies gradually increases during the recovery phase of the disease.[12,13] Similarly, passive immunization with the antibodies directed against one of these epitopes (peptide 31–46), or the adoptive transfer of serum from late-phase arthritic rats, suppressed subsequent AA.[12,13] Furthermore, the resistance of Brown Norway or WKY rats to AA correlates with natural antibody response to the same B cell epitopes as those involved in epitope spreading in the susceptible Lewis rats.

Spreading of the tolerogenic effect of the disease-related epitope of Bhsp65, p180–188, and that of the suppressive effect of antigen-specific anergic T cells have been invoked in the downmodulation of the course of avridine-induced arthritis and/or AA.[14,15] It was observed that induction of nasal tolerance against p180–188 provided protection against subsequent AA as well as avridine-induced arthritis.[14] It was proposed that tolerization of T cells recognizing p180–188 or its mimic spread to T cells of other specificities that are involved in arthritis induction. Similarly, it was suggested that a subset of anergic T cells, in the presence of the specific antigen recognized by these cells, exerted a suppressive activity on the spreading of T cells of other antigen specificities.[15] Furthermore, this amplification of suppressive effect was attributed to modulation of the activity of antigen-presenting cells (APCs) by anergic T cells.

A study of the T cell repertoire in patients with RA showed that several dominant T cell clones were found in the synovial membrane but not in the peripheral blood.[34] Analysis of the complementarity-determining region 3, following sequencing of the T cell receptor (TCR) Vβ V-D-J junctional regions, showed evidence for antigen-driven selection of the TCR, which was attributed to determinant spreading during the course of RA. Additional similar studies of RA would help define the fine characteristics of the pathogenic T cell repertoire in this disease. Further, epitope spreading involving antibodies to post-translationally modified antigens has been reported in the pre-clinical phase of the disease in patients with RA.[35–37]

2.4 Systemic Lupus Erythematosus

Systemic lupus erythematosus (SLE) is a multi-system human autoimmune disease characterized by the development of autoantibodies against a variety of autoantigens.[72–74] Both intermolecular and intramolecular epitope spreading involving the above-mentioned autoantigens have been observed in SLE and an animal model of lupus (Table 2). For example, James et al.[16] demonstrated that New Zealand white rabbits immunized with an Sm B/B′ peptide (representing a C-terminal epitope) developed antibodies directed against the immunogen and other epitopes within the middle and amino-terminal regions of the Sm B/B′ antigen, along with antibodies against other spliceosomal proteins (e.g., D, 70K, A, and C). In another study, mice immunized with La protein developed autoantibodies not only to the immunogen but also to 60-kDa Ro, whereas mice immunized with 60-kDa Ro produced anti-Ro antibodies as well as anti-La antibodies.[17] The results of another study[75] validated the development of antibodies to multiple components of the La/Ro ribonucleoprotein complex after a challenge with a single component of the antigenic complex. The spreading of the Th and antibody responses to components of the nucleosome[18] and intramolecular spreading of the T cell response to Th epitopes within the V_H region of a pathogenic anti-DNA antibody[19] represent cases of epitope spreading during spontaneously arising disease. Antibodies to post-translationally modified antigens in lupus also are reported.[76] Interestingly, tolerization of lupus-prone mice against either autoantibody-derived peptides or the protein/peptides (e.g., nucleosomal peptides) representing antigenic determinants involved in epitope spreading can successfully halt the progression of epitope spreading as well as the disease process.[20,77]

Patients with SLE also develop autoantibodies to the variety of autoantigens described above. Studies of the antigen reactivity of the sera of patients with lupus have demonstrated temporal shifts in both the recognition of another antigen (e.g., intermolecular spreading from Sm antigen to RNP reactivity) as well as in the reactivity to different epitopes within the same antigen (e.g., intramolecular spreading within a given antigen depending on the model system: Sm B/B', Sm D, ribosomal protein L7, caspase-8, etc.).[38–41]

2.5 Other Autoimmune Diseases

Myasthenia gravis (MG) is an autoimmune disease resulting from antibody-mediated autoimmune attack against the nicotinic acetylcholine receptor (AChR). Epitope spreading has been reported in experimental autoimmune MG,[21] and there is some evidence suggesting epitope spreading in patients with MG as well.[21] Epitope spreading also has been observed in animal models of thyroiditis,[26] neuritis,[22] uveitis,[23] gastritis,[24] and oophoritis[25] (Tables 1 and 2). Progression of myocarditis to dilated cardiomyopathy also has been linked with epitope spreading.[78]

3 MECHANISMS UNDERLYING EPITOPE SPREADING DURING THE COURSE OF AN AUTOIMMUNE DISEASE

Considering the diverse experimental models of autoimmune diseases involving different target organs and predominantly either T cells (CD4+/CD8+) or antibodies as the pathogenic effector mediators (Table 2), various mechanisms have been proposed to explain the phenomenon of epitope spreading (Figure 1 and Table 3). These are described below.

3.1 Upregulation of the Display of Cryptic/Subdominant Epitopes Within a Self Antigen Under Inflammatory Conditions

Native (whole) self and foreign antigens possess potential T cell epitopes that are processed and presented either efficiently (dominant determinants) or poorly (cryptic/subdominant determinants) by APCs.[79] However, both sets of determinants are immunogenic in the peptide form. In the case of a self

Table 3 Proposed Mechanisms Underlying the Phenomenon of Epitope Spreading

1. Upregulation of the display of cryptic/subdominant epitopes within a self antigen
2. Release of self antigens and their processing and presentation following tissue damage in the course of a microbial infection or an autoimmune disease
3. Post-translational modification of antigens generates neo-epitopes
4. The frequency and avidity of epitope-specific precursor T cells within the mature T cell repertoire favoring responsiveness to certain antigenic determinants over others
5. Presentation of neo-epitopes within a particular self antigen by the B cells specific for that antigen
6. The influence of antigen-bound antibodies on the processing and presentation of T cell epitopes within that antigen
7. Antigen cross-presentation and epitope spreading
8. Site of initiation of epitope spreading: target organ versus periphery

antigen, tolerance is readily induced to its dominant but not cryptic/subdominant epitopes.[80–83] For this reason, unlike a foreign dominant epitope that is generally immunogenic, a self-dominant determinant often fails to induce a response because of self-tolerance. However, the T cells against cryptic/subdominant self epitopes escape the induction of tolerance in the thymus and therefore are available in the mature T cell repertoire. These T cells can be activated provided the otherwise poorly processed cryptic/subdominant epitopes within the native self antigen are efficiently presented to the T cells by professional APCs. This could happen under conditions of upregulated antigen processing and presentation events, as in the case of inflammation and/or infection.[3,84–87] The T cells specific for cryptic/subdominant epitopes of an endogenous self antigen thus activated (constituting epitope spreading) can participate in further propagation of the ongoing disease process. This also applies to self antigens released following tissue damage (described below), which can contribute to epitope spreading. Similarly, quantitatively enhanced display of foreign antigenic epitopes that are cross-reactive with self epitopes can further expand the pool of self-reactive T cells via molecular mimicry (see below).

3.2 Release of Self Antigens and Their Processing and Presentation Following Tissue Damage in the Course of a Microbial Infection or an Autoimmune Disease

The etiology of most human autoimmune diseases is not known. However, one trigger or precipitating factor for the induction of autoimmunity is microbial infection. Some of the mechanisms proposed to explain this association include (a) *molecular mimicry*: a microbial antigen/epitope structurally mimics a self antigen/epitope such that the T cells primed following microbial infection can be re-stimulated by the endogenous self antigen and can thereby target cells/tissue expressing that self antigen, leading to tissue damage;[42,88–90] (b) *bystander activation*: inadvertent stimulation of potentially self-reactive T cells under the immune environment where priming of microbial antigen-specific T cells is taking place; the autoreactive T cells can then cause tissue damage[3]; and (c) *tissue injury leading to induction of autoimmune response*: the tissue damage caused by microbial infection results in the release of endogenous self antigens that can then be processed and presented by local as well as distant APCs, leading to the priming of self-reactive T cells.[3,91,92] The role of virus-mediated tissue damage in the induction of autoimmunity has been demonstrated by Miller and colleagues in the TMEV-induced EAE model[49] and by Rose and colleagues in the model of autoimmune myocarditis.[93,94] In TMEV-induced EAE, the induction of autoimmunity also has been linked to epitope spreading resulting from the release of self antigens.[49] Autoimmune myocarditis induced by coxsackievirus B3 has been shown to be a biphasic disease: an early "infection" phase and a subsequent "autoimmune" phase characterized by T cell and antibody response to cardiac myosin.[94] (d) *Apoptotic cells as the source of released antigen* has been proposed by Rosen and colleagues[95,96] as another mechanism for the release of intracellular self antigens; in this process, apoptotic cells serve as an important source of self antigens, and the novel antigenic fragments produced in apoptotic surface blebs are implicated in the reversal of self-tolerance, leading to the induction of autoimmunity.

3.3 Post-Translational Modification of Antigens

Post-translational modification of naturally occurring proteins may lead to the generation of neo-epitopes, which might induce anti-self immune responses. In the face of a susceptible combination of genetic and environmental factors, such an immune response can initiate autoimmunity. In addition, the generation of neo-epitopes and subsequent immune response to them may perpetuate (via epitope spreading) the diversification of ongoing autoimmune response. The conversion of arginine to citrulline, the conversion of aspartate to isoaspartic acid, and the oxidation of amino acids by reactive oxygen species and reactive nitrogen species represent examples of modifications of proteins leading to the generation of neo-epitopes and their relationship with autoimmunity.[97–99] RA and SLE are two of the major autoimmune diseases whose pathogenesis involves the generation of the above-mentioned neo-epitopes, leading to initiation of auto-immunity and epitope spreading.[35,100]

3.4 The Frequency and Avidity of Epitope-Specific Precursor T Cells Within the Mature T Cell Repertoire Favoring Responsiveness to Certain Antigenic Determinants over Others

The T cell responses to various epitopes within a native antigen, or to individual antigens within a mixture of antigens, are hierarchical and are influenced by multiple factors operating at the level of the APC (described above) as well as those relating to the size (frequency) and the composition (e.g. the relative levels of high avidity vs. low avidity T cells) of the mature T cell repertoire.[44,101] These characteristics have been invoked, in part, to explain the hierarchy as well as the ordered sequential appearance of response to different antigens/epitopes involved in inter- or intramolecular epitope spreading.[3–5,46]

3.5 Presentation of Neo-Epitopes Within a Particular Self Antigen by the B Cells Specific for That Antigen

Activated B cells serving as potent APCs also can participate in the induction and propagation of epitope spreading. Mamula and Janeway proposed an interesting model based on the role of B cells as APCs in the diversification of the T cell and antibody response.[102] The initial T cell priming to self epitopes is done by APC-like dendritic cells (DCs); these activated T cells then provide help to the appropriate B cells. The activated B cells in turn can take up, process, and then present that antigen to the T cells. The new subsets of activated T cells then can provide help to a new population of B cells. These T–B interactions thus lead to the diversification of both T cell and antibody responses. These processes in the setting of epitope spreading have been demonstrated in experimental models of lupus.[3,44] However, there also is evidence from studies of PLP-induced EAE in BALB/c mice that B cells can limit epitope spreading.[103] Further, IL-10-producing regulatory B (B10) cells may play an important role in controlling autoreactive responses[104] and thereby contribute to regulating epitope spreading as well.

3.6 The Influence of Antigen-Bound Antibodies on the Processing and Presentation of T Cell Epitopes Within That Antigen

Studies have demonstrated that antigen-bound antibodies can significantly influence the processing and presentation of T cell epitopes within that antigen.[84,105] Depending on the nature and the site (in the context of antigenic structure) of the interaction between the antigenic determinant and the antibody, antibodies bound to specific epitopes of an antigen can either enhance or suppress the T cell response to the epitope involved. This in turn can lead to a shift in the epitope specificity of the T cell response (as observed in epitope spreading) during the course of an immune response directed towards a microbial or self antigen.

3.7 Antigen Cross-Presentation and Epitope Spreading

It has recently been reported that during the course of disease induced by CD4+ T cells, naive, MBP-reactive CD8+ T cells in the CNS were activated.[106] These CD8+ T cells could directly recognize oligodendrocytes, which presented MHC class I-restricted epitopes of MBP. Interestingly, the cross-presentation of MBP leading to the activation of naive CD8+ T cells occurred by a subset of DCs, namely, tumor necrosis factor-α/inducible nitric oxide synthase-producing DCs.[106] Thus, this example illustrates determinant spreading to antigen-specific CD8+ T cells during the course of CD4+ T cell-induced EAE.

3.8 Site of Initiation of Epitope Spreading: Target Organ Versus the Periphery

The CNS has traditionally been viewed as being immune privileged. However, studies of PLP-induced R-EAE and TMEV-induced demyelination revealed that epitope spreading is initiated within the CNS.[107] During the course of disease, naïve T cells enter the inflamed CNS and are activated there by local APCs to initiate epitope spreading. A recent study showing determinant spreading to CD8+ T cell epitopes in CD4+ T cell-induced EAE also emphasized the CNS as the site of epitope spreading.[106] However, there also is evidence to suggest an alternative viewpoint emphasizing that the CNS-draining lymph nodes are important for the induction of immune response during relapses in chronic R-EAE.[108] Surgical removal of these lymph nodes reduced the severity of relapses of EAE. This proposition is supported by the observation that myelin antigens are expressed in the lymph node, spleen, and thymus of SJL mice.[109]

4 PHYSIOLOGICAL SIGNIFICANCE OF EPITOPE SPREADING: INVOLVEMENT OF EPITOPE SPREADING IN THE PATHOGENESIS OF AUTOIMMUNE DISEASE

Experimental evidence from studies of different models of autoimmune diseases supports the role of epitope spreading in the pathogenesis of the disease process. The results of these studies can be categorized into three functional outcomes: (1) *pathogenic epitope spreading*: most of the studies summarized earlier (Table 2) describe that the new T cell responses emerging via epitope spreading are involved in the perpetuation of the initial autoimmune process and thereby the progression and chronicity of the disease process; (2) *protective epitope spreading*: other studies provide evidence favoring a regulatory or protective role for T cell/antibody responses comprising diversification of the initial immune response;[10,12,13] and (3) *epitope spreading unrelated to the disease process or no spreading at all*: in a couple studies of EAE, epitope spreading either was evident but had no functional relationship with the disease process[110] or did not occur at all.[111] In another study, clinically relapsing disease was observed in transgenic mice with a single TCR that lack all T cell specificities except the one required for initiation of the disease process,[112] suggesting that relapses were not dependent on other T cell specificities. Thus, there is no single functional outcome that can a priori be assigned to epitope spreading; therefore, each disease and the antigenic response associated with it needs to be examined objectively and without any pre-formed notion or bias. In this regard, any prediction regarding the contribution of epitope spreading to the disease process in a vastly heterogeneous human population poses an important challenge for both clinical prognosis and the custom designing of therapeutic regimens.

5 IMPLICATIONS OF EPITOPE SPREADING IN IMMUNOTHERAPY OF AUTOIMMUNE DISEASES: HINDERING VS. FACILITATING THE CONTROL OF THE AUTOIMMUNE PROCESS

A great deal of the effort invested in developing immunotherapeutic approaches for autoimmune diseases has centered on the inactivation/tolerization of potentially pathogenic T cells. It is evident from extensive studies of animal models that it is relatively easier to modulate the antigen-specific immune response for preventing the development of autoimmunity than for controlling the ongoing disease process. Epitope spreading that is disease-propagating in nature (Figure 1) may pose a major hurdle in the treatment of ongoing disease. For successful treatment, the patient would have to be treated very early in the course of disease before the occurrence of epitope spreading. However, it is not an easy task to correctly predict the timing of epitope spreading during the natural course of disease in individual members of a patient population. On the other hand, epitope spreading that is disease-regulating in nature (Figure 1) can readily be exploited for therapeutic purposes by developing therapeutic regimens aimed at priming and expanding the regulatory T cells specific for the new epitopes arising during the course of disease. Here, the precise timing of the onset of epitope spreading might not be much of a concern. However, in either situation, carefully planned clinical trials are warranted to insure that the programmed modulation of the immune response delivers the expected outcome. Otherwise, strategies aimed at suppressing the disease might unexpectedly exacerbate the disease or have no effect at all. In this regard, identification of the "window" of therapeutic opportunity, in terms of selecting the right target antigen and the timing of intervention in animal models offers hope for developing better approaches for the treatment of human autoimmune diseases.[3,113]

6 CONCLUDING REMARKS

Epitope spreading represents a dynamic quantitative/qualitative change in the T cell and/or antibody specificities during the course of an immune response that is generally initiated by a dominant antigen/epitope associated with a pathological condition. The primary event may either be triggered experimentally or arise spontaneously. The subsequently developing new T cell and/or antibody responses then participate in perpetuation of the initial pathological changes, leading to chronic disease. Depending on the disease process, however, the spreading of response to potentially disease-regulating antigens/epitopes can be protective in nature; therefore, epitope spreading also represents a mechanism by which initial pathological immune responses can be controlled to effect natural recovery from the acute phase of the disease. We suggest that epitope spreading, like many other physiological processes in the body, represents a snapshot of the dynamic events attempting to strike a balance between the pathogenic and regulatory components of antigen-specific T cell responses and that the "picture" obtained would vary depending on the time when the responses are sampled and tested during the disease process.

Further studies facilitated by the application of new tools such as MHC-peptide tetramers, MHC-Ig dimers, and autoantibody profiling using protein microarrays[53] would help advance our understanding of the role of epitope spreading of antigen-specific T cell/antibody responses in the pathogenesis of autoimmune diseases. In addition, advances in the areas of immune regulation, modulation of adaptive immunity by components of the innate immune response, and interplay between the host and environment are expected to unravel additional mechanisms underlying epitope spreading. At this time there is far more information regarding pathogenic immune responses in epitope spreading than there is for the regulatory aspects of the process. Further integration of the mechanisms involving Foxp3-expressing CD4+CD25+ T cells and other regulatory T cells in the control of disease-propagating epitope spreading would advance our understanding of the pathogenesis of autoimmune diseases. In addition, the regulatory aspects of epitope spreading could be exploited for therapeutic advantage.

ACKNOWLEDGMENT

The authors gratefully acknowledge grant support from the National Institutes of Health (Bethesda, MD).

REFERENCES

1. Lehmann PV, Forsthuber T, Miller A, Sercarz EE. Spreading of T-cell autoimmunity to cryptic determinants of an autoantigen. *Nature* 1992;**358**(6382):155–7.
2. Sercarz EE. Immune focusing vs diversification and their connection to immune regulation. *Immunol Rev* 1998;**164**:5–10.
3. Vanderlugt CL, Miller SD. Epitope spreading in immune-mediated diseases: implications for immunotherapy. *Nat Rev Immunol* 2002;**2**(2):85–95.
4. McRae BL, Vanderlugt CL, Dal Canto MC, Miller SD. Functional evidence for epitope spreading in the relapsing pathology of experimental autoimmune encephalomyelitis. *J Exp Med* 1995;**182**(1):75–85.
5. Yu M, Johnson JM, Tuohy VK. A predictable sequential determinant spreading cascade invariably accompanies progression of experimental autoimmune encephalomyelitis: a basis for peptide-specific therapy after onset of clinical disease. *J Exp Med* 1996;**183** (4):1777–88.
6. Mor F, Cohen IR. Shifts in the epitopes of myelin basic protein recognized by Lewis rat T cells before, during, and after the induction of experimental autoimmune encephalomyelitis. *J Clin Invest* 1993;**92**(5):2199–206.
7. McFarland HI, Lobito AA, Johnson MM, Nyswaner JT, Frank JA, Palardy GR, et al. Determinant spreading associated with demyelination in a nonhuman primate model of multiple sclerosis. *J Immunol* 1999;**162**(4):2384–90.
8. Kaufman DL, Clare-Salzler M, Tian J, Forsthuber T, Ting GS, Robinson P, et al. Spontaneous loss of T-cell tolerance to glutamic acid decarboxylase in murine insulin-dependent diabetes. *Nature* 1993;**366**(6450):69–72.
9. Tisch R, Yang XD, Singer SM, Liblau RS, Fugger L, McDevitt HO. Immune response to glutamic acid decarboxylase correlates with insulitis in non-obese diabetic mice. *Nature* 1993;**366**(6450):72–5.
10. Moudgil KD, Chang TT, Eradat H, Chen AM, Gupta RS, Brahn E, et al. Diversification of T cell responses to carboxy-terminal determinants within the 65-kD heat-shock protein is involved in regulation of autoimmune arthritis. *J Exp Med* 1997;**185**(7):1307–16.

11. Moudgil KD, Kim E, Yun OJ, Chi HH, Brahn E, Sercarz EE. Environmental modulation of autoimmune arthritis involves the spontaneous microbial induction of T cell responses to regulatory determinants within heat shock protein 65. *J Immunol* 2001;**166**(6):4237–43.

12. Ulmansky R, Cohen CJ, Szafer F, Moallem E, Fridlender ZG, Kashi Y, et al. Resistance to adjuvant arthritis is due to protective antibodies against heat shock protein surface epitopes and the induction of IL-10 secretion. *J Immunol* 2002;**168**(12):6463–9.

13. Kim HR, Kim EY, Cerny J, Moudgil KD. Antibody responses to mycobacterial and self heat shock protein 65 in autoimmune arthritis: epitope specificity and implication in pathogenesis. *J Immunol* 2006;**177**(10):6634–41.

14. Prakken BJ, van der Zee R, Anderton SM, van Kooten PJ, Kuis W, van Eden W. Peptide-induced nasal tolerance for a mycobacterial heat shock protein 60 T cell epitope in rats suppresses both adjuvant arthritis and nonmicrobially induced experimental arthritis. *Proc Natl Acad Sci USA* 1997;**94**(7):3284–9.

15. Taams LS, van Rensen AJ, Poelen MC, van Els CA, Besseling AC, Wagenaar JP, et al. Anergic T cells actively suppress T cell responses via the antigen-presenting cell. *Eur J Immunol* 1998;**28**(9):2902–12.

16. James JA, Gross T, Scofield RH, Harley JB. Immunoglobulin epitope spreading and autoimmune disease after peptide immunization: Sm B/B′-derived PPPGMRPP and PPPGIRGP induce spliceosome autoimmunity. *J Exp Med* 1995;**181**(2):453–61.

17. Topfer F, Gordon T, McCluskey J. Intra- and intermolecular spreading of autoimmunity involving the nuclear self-antigens La (SS-B) and Ro (SS-A). *Proc Natl Acad Sci USA* 1995;**92**(3):875–9.

18. Kaliyaperumal A, Mohan C, Wu W, Datta SK. Nucleosomal peptide epitopes for nephritis-inducing T helper cells of murine lupus. *J Exp Med* 1996;**183**(6):2459–69.

19. Singh RR, Hahn BH. Reciprocal T–B determinant spreading develops spontaneously in murine lupus: implications for pathogenesis. *Immunol Rev* 1998;**164**:201–8.

20. Kaliyaperumal A, Michaels MA, Datta SK. Antigen-specific therapy of murine lupus nephritis using nucleosomal peptides: tolerance spreading impairs pathogenic function of autoimmune T and B cells. *J Immunol* 1999;**162**(10):5775–83.

21. Vincent A, Willcox N, Hill M, Curnow J, MacLennan C, Beeson D. Determinant spreading and immune responses to acetylcholine receptors in myasthenia gravis. *Immunol Rev* 1998;**164**:157–68.

22. Zhu J, Pelidou SH, Deretzi G, Levi M, Mix E, van der Meide P, et al. P0 glycoprotein peptides 56–71 and 180–199 dose-dependently induce acute and chronic experimental autoimmune neuritis in Lewis rats associated with epitope spreading. *J Neuroimmunol* 2001;**114**(1–2):99–106.

23. Deeg CA, Thurau SR, Gerhards H, Ehrenhofer M, Wildner G, Kaspers B. Uveitis in horses induced by interphotoreceptor retinoid-binding protein is similar to the spontaneous disease. *Eur J Immunol* 2002;**32**(9):2598–606.

24. Alderuccio F, Toh BH, Tan SS, Gleeson PA, van Driel IR. An autoimmune disease with multiple molecular targets abrogated by the transgenic expression of a single autoantigen in the thymus. *J Exp Med* 1993;**178**(2):419–26.

25. Lou YH, McElveen MF, Garza KM, Tung KS. Rapid induction of autoantibodies by endogenous ovarian antigens and activated T cells: implication in autoimmune disease pathogenesis and B cell tolerance. *J Immunol* 1996;**156**(9):3535–40.

26. Dai YD, Carayanniotis G, Sercarz E. Antigen processing by autoreactive B cells promotes determinant spreading. *Cell Mol Immunol* 2005;**2**(3):169–75.

27. Tuohy VK, Yu M, Weinstock-Guttman B, Kinkel RP. Diversity and plasticity of self recognition during the development of multiple sclerosis. *J Clin Invest* 1997;**99**(7):1682–90.

28. Tuohy VK, Yu M, Yin L, Kawczak JA, Kinkel PR. Regression and spreading of self-recognition during the development of autoimmune demyelinating disease. *J Autoimmun* 1999;**13**(1):11–20.
29. Tuohy VK, Yu M, Yin L, Kawczak JA, Kinkel RP. Spontaneous regression of primary autoreactivity during chronic progression of experimental autoimmune encephalomyelitis and multiple sclerosis. *J Exp Med* 1999;**189**(7):1033–42.
30. Bonifacio E, Scirpoli M, Kredel K, Fuchtenbusch M, Ziegler AG. Early autoantibody responses in prediabetes are IgG1 dominated and suggest antigen-specific regulation. *J Immunol* 1999;**163**(1):525–32.
31. Bonifacio E, Lampasona V, Bernasconi L, Ziegler AG. Maturation of the humoral autoimmune response to epitopes of GAD in preclinical childhood type 1 diabetes. *Diabetes* 2000;**49**(2):202–8.
32. Sohnlein P, Muller M, Syren K, Hartmann U, Bohm BO, Meinck HM, et al. Epitope spreading and a varying but not disease-specific GAD65 antibody response in type I diabetes. The Childhood Diabetes in Finland Study Group. *Diabetologia* 2000;**43**(2):210–17.
33. Brooks-Worrell B, Gersuk VH, Greenbaum C, Palmer JP. Intermolecular antigen spreading occurs during the preclinical period of human type 1 diabetes. *J Immunol* 2001;**166**(8):5265–70.
34. Alam A, Lambert N, Lule J, Coppin H, Mazieres B, de Preval C, et al. Persistence of dominant T cell clones in synovial tissues during rheumatoid arthritis. *J Immunol* 1996;**156**(9):3480–5.
35. Roth EB, Stenberg P, Book C, Sjoberg K. Antibodies against transglutaminases, peptidylarginine deiminase and citrulline in rheumatoid arthritis – new pathways to epitope spreading. *Clin Exp Rheumatol* 2006;**24**(1):12–18.
36. van de Stadt LA, de Koning MH, van de Stadt RJ, Wolbink G, Dijkmans BA, Hamann D, et al. Development of the anti-citrullinated protein antibody repertoire prior to the onset of rheumatoid arthritis. *Arthritis Rheum* 2011;**63**(11):3226–33.
37. van der Woude D, Rantapaa-Dahlqvist S, Ioan-Facsinay A, Onnekink C, Schwarte CM, Verpoort KN, et al. Epitope spreading of the anti-citrullinated protein antibody response occurs before disease onset and is associated with the disease course of early arthritis. *Ann Rheum Dis* 2010;**69**(8):1554–61.
38. Fisher DE, Reeves WH, Wisniewolski R, Lahita RG, Chiorazzi N. Temporal shifts from Sm to ribonucleoprotein reactivity in systemic lupus erythematosus. *Arthritis Rheum* 1985;**28**(12):1348–55.
39. Neu E, Hemmerich PH, Peter HH, Krawinkel U, von Mikecz AH. Characteristic epitope recognition pattern of autoantibodies against eukaryotic ribosomal protein L7 in systemic autoimmune diseases. *Arthritis Rheum* 1997;**40**(4):661–71.
40. Arbuckle MR, Reichlin M, Harley JB, James JA. Shared early autoantibody recognition events in the development of anti-Sm B/B′ in human lupus. *Scand J Immunol* 1999;**50**(5):447–55.
41. Ueki A, Isozaki Y, Tomokuni A, Hatayama T, Ueki H, Kusaka M, et al. Intramolecular epitope spreading among anti-caspase-8 autoantibodies in patients with silicosis, systemic sclerosis and systemic lupus erythematosus, as well as in healthy individuals. *Clin Exp Immunol* 2002;**129**(3):556–61.
42. Wucherpfennig KW, Strominger JL. Molecular mimicry in T cell-mediated autoimmunity: viral peptides activate human T cell clones specific for myelin basic protein. *Cell* 1995;**80**(5):695–705.
43. Swanborg RH. Experimental autoimmune encephalomyelitis in the rat: lessons in T-cell immunology and autoreactivity. *Immunol Rev* 2001;**184**:129–35.
44. Kuchroo VK, Anderson AC, Waldner H, Munder M, Bettelli E, Nicholson LB. T cell response in experimental autoimmune encephalomyelitis (EAE): role of self and

cross-reactive antigens in shaping, tuning, and regulating the autopathogenic T cell repertoire. *Annu Rev Immunol* 2002;**20**:101–23.

45. Lehmann PV, Sercarz EE, Forsthuber T, Dayan CM, Gammon G. Determinant spreading and the dynamics of the autoimmune T-cell repertoire. *Immunol Today* 1993;**14**(5):203–8.

46. Vanderlugt CL, Neville KL, Nikcevich KM, Eagar TN, Bluestone JA, Miller SD. Pathologic role and temporal appearance of newly emerging autoepitopes in relapsing experimental autoimmune encephalomyelitis. *J Immunol* 2000;**164**(2):670–8.

47. Miller SD, Vanderlugt CL, Lenschow DJ, Pope JG, Karandikar NJ, Dal Canto MC, et al. Blockade of CD28/B7-1 interaction prevents epitope spreading and clinical relapses of murine EAE. *Immunity* 1995;**3**(6):739–45.

48. Howard LM, Miga AJ, Vanderlugt CL, Dal Canto MC, Laman JD, Noelle RJ, et al. Mechanisms of immunotherapeutic intervention by anti-CD40L (CD154) antibody in an animal model of multiple sclerosis. *J Clin Invest* 1999;**103**(2):281–90.

49. Getts DR, Chastain EM, Terry RL, Miller SD. Virus infection, antiviral immunity, and autoimmunity. *Immunol Rev* 2013;**255**(1):197–209.

50. Tuohy VK, Yu M, Yin L, Mathisen PM, Johnson JM, Kawczak JA. Modulation of the IL-10/IL-12 cytokine circuit by interferon-beta inhibits the development of epitope spreading and disease progression in murine autoimmune encephalomyelitis. *J Neuroimmunol* 2000;**111**(1–2):55–63.

51. Stevens DB, Gold DP, Sercarz EE, Moudgil KD. The Wistar Kyoto (RT1(l)) rat is resistant to myelin basic protein-induced experimental autoimmune encephalomyelitis: comparison with the susceptible Lewis (RT1(l)) strain with regard to the MBP-directed CD4+ T cell repertoire and its regulation. *J Neuroimmunol* 2002;**126**(1–2):25–36.

52. Klehmet J, Shive C, Guardia-Wolff R, Petersen I, Spack EG, Boehm BO, et al. T cell epitope spreading to myelin oligodendrocyte glycoprotein in HLA-DR4 transgenic mice during experimental autoimmune encephalomyelitis. *Clin Immunol* 2004;**111**(1):53–60.

53. Robinson WH, Fontoura P, Lee BJ, de Vegvar HE, Tom J, Pedotti R, et al. Protein microarrays guide tolerizing DNA vaccine treatment of autoimmune encephalomyelitis. *Nat Biotechnol* 2003;**21**(9):1033–9.

54. Getts DR, Martin AJ, McCarthy DP, Terry RL, Hunter ZN, Yap WT, et al. Microparticles bearing encephalitogenic peptides induce T-cell tolerance and ameliorate experimental autoimmune encephalomyelitis. *Nat Biotechnol* 2012;**30**(12):1217–24.

55. Smith CE, Miller SD. Multi-peptide coupled-cell tolerance ameliorates ongoing relapsing EAE associated with multiple pathogenic autoreactivities. *J Autoimmun* 2006;**27**(4):218–31.

56. Badawi AH, Siahaan TJ. Suppression of MOG- and PLP-induced experimental autoimmune encephalomyelitis using a novel multivalent bifunctional peptide inhibitor. *J Neuroimmunol* 2013;**263**(1–2):20–7.

57. Cavone L, Aldinucci A, Ballerini C, Biagioli T, Moroni F, Chiarugi A. PARP-1 inhibition prevents CNS migration of dendritic cells during EAE, suppressing the encephalitogenic response and relapse severity. *Mult Scler* 2011;**17**(7):794–807.

58. Chen Y, Langrish CL, McKenzie B, Joyce-Shaikh B, Stumhofer JS, McClanahan T, et al. Anti-IL-23 therapy inhibits multiple inflammatory pathways and ameliorates autoimmune encephalomyelitis. *J Clin Invest* 2006;**116**(5):1317–26.

59. Ho PP, Fontoura P, Platten M, Sobel RA, DeVoss JJ, Lee LY, et al. A suppressive oligodeoxynucleotide enhances the efficacy of myelin cocktail/IL-4-tolerizing DNA vaccination and treats autoimmune disease. *J Immunol* 2005;**175**(9):6226–34.

60. Genain CP, Hauser SL. Experimental allergic encephalomyelitis in the New World monkey *Callithrix jacchus*. *Immunol Rev* 2001;**183**:159–72.

61. Boon L, Brok HP, Bauer J, Ortiz-Buijsse A, Schellekens MM, Ramdien-Murli S, et al. Prevention of experimental autoimmune encephalomyelitis in the common marmoset

(*Callithrix jacchus*) using a chimeric antagonist monoclonal antibody against human CD40 is associated with altered B cell responses. *J Immunol* 2001;**167**(5):2942–9.

62. Laman JD, t Hart BA, Brok H, Meurs M, Schellekens MM, Kasran A, et al. Protection of marmoset monkeys against EAE by treatment with a murine antibody blocking CD40 (mu5D12). *Eur J Immunol* 2002;**32**(8):2218–28.

63. Zechel MA, Elliott JF, Atkinson MA, Singh B. Characterization of novel T-cell epitopes on 65 kDa and 67 kDa glutamic acid decarboxylase relevant in autoimmune responses in NOD mice. *J Autoimmun* 1998;**11**(1):83–95.

64. Holoshitz J, Matitiau A, Cohen IR. Arthritis induced in rats by cloned T lymphocytes responsive to mycobacteria but not to collagen type II. *J Clin Invest* 1984;**73**(1):211–15.

65. van Eden W, Thole JE, van der Zee R, Noordzij A, van Embden JD, Hensen EJ, et al. Cloning of the mycobacterial epitope recognized by T lymphocytes in adjuvant arthritis. *Nature* 1988;**331**(6152):171–3.

66. Gaston JS, Life PF, Bailey LC, Bacon PA. In vitro responses to a 65-kilodalton myco-bacterial protein by synovial T cells from inflammatory arthritis patients. *J Immunol* 1989;**143**(8):2494–500.

67. Quayle AJ, Wilson KB, Li SG, Kjeldsen-Kragh J, Oftung F, Shinnick T, et al. Peptide recognition, T cell receptor usage and HLA restriction elements of human heat-shock protein (hsp) 60 and mycobacterial 65-kDa hsp-reactive T cell clones from rheumatoid synovial fluid. *Eur J Immunol* 1992;**22**(5):1315–22.

68. Moudgil KD. Diversification of response to hsp65 during the course of autoimmune arthritis is regulatory rather than pathogenic. *Immunol Rev* 1998;**164**:175–84.

69. Durai M, Gupta RS, Moudgil KD. The T cells specific for the carboxyl-terminal deter-minants of self (rat) heat-shock protein 65 escape tolerance induction and are involved in regulation of autoimmune arthritis. *J Immunol* 2004;**172**(5):2795–802.

70. Durai M, Kim HR, Moudgil KD. The regulatory C-terminal determinants within mycobacterial heat shock protein 65 are cryptic and cross-reactive with the dominant self homologs: implications for the pathogenesis of autoimmune arthritis. *J Immunol* 2004;**173**(1):181–8.

71. Benoist C, Mathis D. Autoimmunity. The pathogen connection. *Nature* 1998;**394** (6690):227–8.

72. Zandman-Goddard G, Shoenfeld Y. Novel approaches to therapy for SLE. *Clin Rev Allergy Immunol* 2003;**25**(1):105–12.

73. Via CS, Handwerger BS. B-cell and T-cell function in systemic lupus erythematosus. *Curr Opin Rheumatol* 1993;**5**(5):570–4.

74. Tsokos GC. Systemic lupus erythematosus. A disease with a complex pathogenesis. *Lancet* 2001;**358**(Suppl.):S65.

75. Deshmukh US, Lewis JE, Gaskin F, Kannapell CC, Waters ST, Lou YH, et al. Immune responses to Ro60 and its peptides in mice. I. The nature of the immunogen and endog-enous autoantigen determine the specificities of the induced autoantibodies. *J Exp Med* 1999;**189**(3):531–40.

76. Scofield RH, Pierce PG, James JA, Kaufman KM, Kurien BT. Immunization with peptides from 60 kDa Ro in diverse mouse strains. *Scand J Immunol* 2002;**56** (5):477–83.

77. Eilat E, Dayan M, Zinger H, Mozes E. The mechanism by which a peptide based on complementarity-determining region-1 of a pathogenic anti-DNA auto-Ab ameliorates experimental systemic lupus erythematosus. *Proc Natl Acad Sci USA* 2001;**98**(3):1148–53.

78. Matsumoto Y, Park IK, Kohyama K. B-cell epitope spreading is a critical step for the switch from C-protein-induced myocarditis to dilated cardiomyopathy. *Am J Pathol* 2007;**170**(1):43–51.

79. Sercarz EE, Lehmann PV, Ametani A, Benichou G, Miller A, Moudgil K. Dominance and crypticity of T cell antigenic determinants. *Annu Rev Immunol* 1993;**11**:729–66.

80. Cibotti R, Kanellopoulos JM, Cabaniols JP, Halle-Panenko O, Kosmatopoulos K, Sercarz E, et al. Tolerance to a self-protein involves its immunodominant but does not involve its subdominant determinants. *Proc Natl Acad Sci USA* 1992;**89**(1):416–20.

81. Moudgil KD, Sercarz EE. Dominant determinants in hen eggwhite lysozyme correspond to the cryptic determinants within its self-homologue, mouse lysozyme: implications in shaping of the T cell repertoire and autoimmunity. *J Exp Med* 1993;**178** (6):2131–8.

82. Mamula MJ. The inability to process a self-peptide allows autoreactive T cells to escape tolerance. *J Exp Med* 1993;**177**(2):567–71.

83. Anderton SM, Viner NJ, Matharu P, Lowrey PA, Wraith DC. Influence of a dominant cryptic epitope on autoimmune T cell tolerance. *Nat Immunol* 2002;**3**(2):175–81.

84. Lanzavecchia A. How can cryptic epitopes trigger autoimmunity? *J Exp Med* 1995;**181** (6):1945–8.

85. Di Rosa F, Barnaba V. Persisting viruses and chronic inflammation: understanding their relation to autoimmunity. *Immunol Rev* 1998;**164**:17–27.

86. Bottazzo GF, Pujol-Borrell R, Hanafusa T, Feldmann M. Role of aberrant HLA-DR expression and antigen presentation in induction of endocrine autoimmunity. *Lancet* 1983;**2**(8359):1115–19.

87. Sarvetnick N, Shizuru J, Liggitt D, Martin L, McIntyre B, Gregory A, et al. Loss of pancreatic islet tolerance induced by beta-cell expression of interferon-gamma. *Nature* 1990;**346**(6287):844–7.

88. Oldstone MB. Molecular mimicry as a mechanism for the cause and a probe uncovering etiologic agent(s) of autoimmune disease. *Curr Top Microbiol Immunol* 1989;**145**:127–35.

89. Zhao ZS, Granucci F, Yeh L, Schaffer PA, Cantor H. Molecular mimicry by herpes simplex virus-type 1: autoimmune disease after viral infection. *Science* 1998;**279**(5355):1344–7.

90. Soloski MJ, Metcalf ES. The involvement of class Ib molecules in the host response to infection with Salmonella and its relevance to autoimmunity. *Microbes Infect* 2001;**3** (14–15):1249–59.

91. Rose NR. Viral damage or 'molecular mimicry'-placing the blame in myocarditis. *Nat Med* 2000;**6**(6):631–2.

92. Fairweather D, Rose NR. Type 1 diabetes: virus infection or autoimmune disease? *Nat Immunol* 2002;**3**(4):338–40.

93. Rose NR, Hill SL. Autoimmune myocarditis. *Int J Cardiol* 1996;**54**(2):171–5.

94. Hill SL, Rose NR. The transition from viral to autoimmune myocarditis. *Autoimmunity* 2001;**34**(3):169–76.

95. Casciola-Rosen LA, Anhalt G, Rosen A. Autoantigens targeted in systemic lupus erythematosus are clustered in two populations of surface structures on apoptotic keratinocytes. *J Exp Med* 1994;**179**(4):1317–30.

96. Casciola-Rosen L, Rosen A. Ultraviolet light-induced keratinocyte apoptosis: a potential mechanism for the induction of skin lesions and autoantibody production in LE. *Lupus* 1997;**6**(2):175–80.

97. Griffiths HR. Is the generation of neo-antigenic determinants by free radicals central to the development of autoimmune rheumatoid disease? *Autoimmun Rev* 2008;**7**(7):544–9.

98. Kidd BA, Ho PP, Sharpe O, Zhao X, Tomooka BH, Kanter JL, et al. Epitope spreading to citrullinated antigens in mouse models of autoimmune arthritis and demyelination. *Arthritis Res Ther* 2008;**10**(5):R119.

99. Kurien BT, Scofield RH. Autoimmunity and oxidatively modified autoantigens. *Autoimmun Rev* 2008;**7**(7):567–73.

100. Scofield RH, Kurien BT, Ganick S, McClain MT, Pye Q, James JA, et al. Modification of lupus-associated 60-kDa Ro protein with the lipid oxidation product 4-hydroxy-2-nonenal increases antigenicity and facilitates epitope spreading. *Free Radic Biol Med* 2005;**38**(6):719–28.

101. Harrington CJ, Paez A, Hunkapiller T, Mannikko V, Brabb T, Ahearn M, et al. Differential tolerance is induced in T cells recognizing distinct epitopes of myelin basic protein. *Immunity* 1998;**8**(5):571–80.
102. Mamula MJ, Janeway Jr. CA. Do B cells drive the diversification of immune responses? *Immunol Today* 1993;**14**(4):151–2, discussion 153–4.
103. Lyons JA, Ramsbottom MJ, Mikesell RJ, Cross AH. B cells limit epitope spreading and reduce severity of EAE induced with PLP peptide in BALB/c mice. *J Autoimmun* 2008;**31**(2):149–55.
104. Salinas GF, Braza F, Brouard S, Tak PP, Baeten D. The role of B lymphocytes in the progression from autoimmunity to autoimmune disease. *Clin Immunol* 2013;**146** (1):34–45.
105. Simitsek PD, Campbell DG, Lanzavecchia A, Fairweather N, Watts C. Modulation of antigen processing by bound antibodies can boost or suppress class II major histocompatibility complex presentation of different T cell determinants. *J Exp Med* 1995;**181** (6):1957–63.
106. Ji Q, Castelli L, Goverman JM. MHC class I-restricted myelin epitopes are cross-presented by Tip-DCs that promote determinant spreading to CD8(+) T cells. *Nat Immunol* 2013;**14**(3):254–61.
107. McMahon EJ, Bailey SL, Castenada CV, Waldner H, Miller SD. Epitope spreading initiates in the CNS in two mouse models of multiple sclerosis. *Nat Med* 2005;**11** (3):335–9.
108. van Zwam M, Huizinga R, Heijmans N, van Meurs M, Wierenga-Wolf AF, Melief MJ, et al. Surgical excision of CNS-draining lymph nodes reduces relapse severity in chronic-relapsing experimental autoimmune encephalomyelitis. *J Pathol* 2009;**217**(4):543–51.
109. Voskuhl RR. Myelin protein expression in lymphoid tissues: implications for peripheral tolerance. *Immunol Rev* 1998;**164**:81–92.
110. Kumar V. Determinant spreading during experimental autoimmune encephalomyelitis: is it potentiating, protecting or participating in the disease? *Immunol Rev* 1998;**164**:73–80.
111. Takacs K, Altmann DM. The case against epitope spread in experimental allergic encephalomyelitis. *Immunol Rev* 1998;**164**:101–10.
112. Jones RE, Bourdette D, Moes N, Vandenbark A, Zamora A, Offner H. Epitope spreading is not required for relapses in experimental autoimmune encephalomyelitis. *J Immunol* 2003;**170**(4):1690–8.
113. Steinman L. Despite epitope spreading in the pathogenesis of autoimmune disease, highly restricted approaches to immune therapy may still succeed [with a hedge on this bet]. *J Autoimmun* 2000;**14**(4):278–82.

CHAPTER 5

CD5-Expressing B-1 Cells and Infection

Yves Renaudineau[*,†,1], **Christophe Viale**[†], **Pierre Youinou**[*]
[*]Immunologie et Pathologie, LabEx IGO, SFR ScInBioS, Université de Brest et Université Européenne de Bretagne, Brest, France
[†]Laboratory of Immunology and Immunotherapy, CHRU, Brest, France
[1]Corresponding Author: yves.renaudineau@univ-brest.fr

1 INTRODUCTION

The 67-kDa T cell marker CD5 was originally identified on malignant human B cells[1] and subsequently shown to act as a co-receptor on a subpopulation of normal B lymphocytes in humans[2] and mice.[3] These have been classified into B-2 cells, representing the conventional cells, and B-1 cells, predominating in coelomic cavities.[4] The latter population comprises B-1a cells, which express CD5 (Figure 1), and B-1b subpopulations, which do not express CD5 but share all the other attributes of B-1 cells,[5] such as the presence of messenger RNA for CD5, the expression of the myelomonocytic marker Mac-1, and the reduced density of the high-molecular-weight isoform of the common leukocyte antigen (Ag) CD45-RA.

Accumulating evidence suggests that B-1 lymphocytes are key in the defence against infectious agents. For example, they produce much of the immunoglobulin (Ig), almost all natural antibodies (Abs) reactive with lipopolysaccharide,[6] and up to 80% of the innate Ab in serum,[7] although they constituting only a minor fraction of the B compartment. Furthermore, they contribute significantly to the IgA-producing plasma cells in the lamina propria of the gut.[8] Indeed, in germ-free conditions, few peritoneal B-1 cells are detected in mice, while a number of them exist in specific pathogen-free conditions, indicating that bacterial infections are necessary for their generation.[9]

The finding that numerous autoimmune conditions are associated with elevated levels of circulating B-1 cells and the demonstration that such lymphocytes accumulate in chronic lymphocytic leukemia (CLL) and other B cell malignancies because of their resistance to apoptosis have sparked a great

Infection and Autoimmunity
http://dx.doi.org/10.1016/B978-0-444-63269-2.00004-0

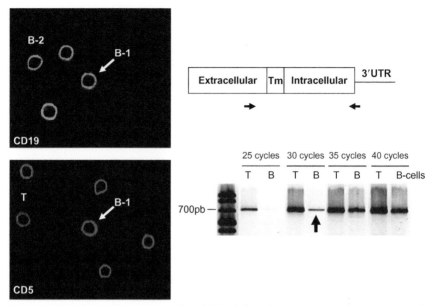

Figure 1 Double-staining of peripheral blood lymphocytes using the CD19 B cell marker and the CD5 T cell marker (left) permits identification of B cells that express CD5 (i.e., B-1 cells [arrows]), as opposed to conventional B-2 cells. Polymerase chain reaction of the transcripts for CD5 followed by electrophoresis and blots (right) show the message in T cells and, to a lesser degree, in B cells.

deal of interest in the possibility of a role of B-1 cells in the pathophysiology of a number of diseases, including infectious conditions. However, the function of these cells in different disease states remains unclear.

2 CHARACTERIZATION OF CD5+ B CELLS

2.1 Origins of the Cells

On one hand, there is evidence in support of a different lineage. Early experiments showed that irradiated mice could be reconstituted with CD5$^+$ B cells if the graft contained bone marrow stem cells together with peritoneal cells.[10] Additional support came from studies of severe combined immunodeficiency mice. These animals fail to develop either T or B cells because of a genetic deficiency in the enzyme required for rearrangements of Ag receptor genes. Immunological reconstitution with CD5$^+$ B cells can be achieved by injecting fetal liver but not adult bone marrow.[11] The B-1 cell progenitor has been characterized recently, as well as the key role played by the foetal microRNA Lin28b in driving B-1 cell development.[12,13]

On the other hand, the selection model, which argues against the notion that CD5$^+$ B cells are a separate lineage, supports the general view that such cells are just an activated subpopulation. One clue is that human CD5$^-$ B cells can be induced in vitro to become CD5$^+$ by activation with phorbol myristate acetate (PMA),[14] and several cytokines modulate the expression of this molecule.[15] Similar data from mouse models are now available, showing that anti–IgM and interleukin (IL)-6 treatment increased CD5 expression on splenic B cells.

To account for these opposing viewpoints we proposed a reconciliation of the divergent theses[16] by postulating two different classes of CD5$^+$ B cells (Figure 2): those in which CD5 expression is constitutive ("classic" CD5$^+$ B cells), particularly in the fetal liver and in cord blood (CB); and conventional B-2 cells induced to express CD5 upon appropriate activation ("induced" CD5$^+$ B cells), which usually are located in the germinal centre of any secondary lymphoid organ.

In humans, B-1 cells overlap imperfectly with CD5$^+$ B cells in part because CD5 can be detected in activated and regulatory B cells. According to Griffin et al.,[17] the B-1 cell subset is referred to as the CD20$^+$ CD27$^+$ CD43$^+$ B cell subset. However, controversy exists because this subset is suspected to overlap with CD3$^+$ T cells, plasmablasts, and T–B cell doublets.[17–20]

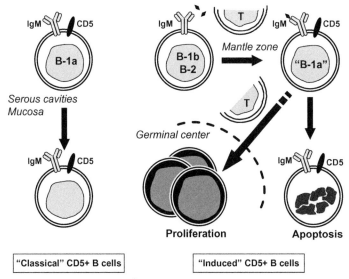

Figure 2 Innate or "classical" CD5$^+$ B cells in cord blood are distinct from acquired or "induced" CD5$^+$ B cells in the germinal centre of a secondary lymphoid organ. B-1a refers to CD5-positive and B-1b to CD5-negative B-1 cells as opposed to conventional B-2 cells.

2.2 Functions of CD5[+] B Cells

This question of the function of CD5[+] B cells has been approached using immortalized CB clones. There seems to be a propensity for B-1 lymphocytes to produce low-affinity, polyreactive Ab binding to both self and exogenous Ags, including several bacteria.[21] Some positive clones were reactive with the I/i carbohydrate red blood cell Ags,[22] which are accessible to B lymphocytes in the CB. This observation suggests that the CD5[+] clones have been driven by such autoAg and therefore are selected in vivo; it also agrees with the previous finding that, at least in the *Hemophilus influenza* model, innate (B-1 cells) and acquired (B-2 cells) humoral immunities are mediated by distinct arms of the system.[23] In line with the assertion that B-1 cells are Ag selected, B-1 cells are characterized by the utilization of specific V_{H11} and V_{H12} germ-line genes[22] and the expression of cross-reactive idiotypes.[21] As a consequence, it is not surprising to observe that anti-phosphorylcholine-specific B cells represent 5–8% of the peritoneal CD5[+] B cell repertoire in normal mice.[24] Natural derived CD5[+] B cell natural anti-phosphorylcholine Abs are protective against infections[25] and have been implicated in the clearance of apoptotic cells.[26,27]

2.3 Control of the CD5[+] B Cell Population

In monozygotic twins[28] and family members of patients with rheumatoid arthritis (RA),[29] the size of B cell subsets seems to be controlled by the major histocompatibility complex, as established in mice.[30] The distribution of B cells into B-1a, B-1b, and B-2 would thus be genetically regulated, whereas IL-10 rescues B-1a cells from apoptosis and encourages B-1b cell proliferation.[31] Interestingly, an Ig-independent regulating feedback mechanism of the B-1 cell compartments has been described in mice.[32,33]

3 CD5[+] B CELLS AND DISEASE

3.1 Connective Tissue Diseases

Several groups have reported that the CD5[+] B cell subset may be expanded in patients with RA. Using double-fluorochrome ultraviolet light microscopy, the CD5[+] B cell subset was originally found to comprise an average of 20% of the B cells in 16 patients with RA compared to a maximum of 3% in 8 normal controls, although the average absolute numbers of circulating B cells were comparable in these two groups of subjects.[29] Although CD5 molecules are present at a low density on B lymphocytes, this is increased[14]

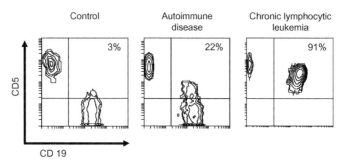

Figure 3 The level of CD5$^+$ B cells is increased in some non-organ-specific diseases as well as infectious states. These cells accumulate in chronic lymphocytic leukemia.

following treatment of B lymphocyte–enriched cell suspensions with PMA. These results were subsequently confirmed by flow cytometry analysis (Figure 3). Thus it was possible to detect coexpression of CD5 on a larger population of B cells from patients with RA and controls than earlier studies, but the mean proportions of B cells that express CD5 were still greater in patients than in controls. These data conflict with some reports showing no significant differences in percentages of circulating CD5$^+$ B cells in patients with RA compared with normal individuals. In fact, they fall into two categories: two-thirds have CD5$^+$ B cell levels within the normal range, and one third has elevated levels. Clearly, the elevation of CD5$^+$ B cells per se is insufficient to give rise to RA. The corollary is that a high level of this B cell subpopulation is not a prerequisite for developing the disease.

The number of circulating CD5$^+$ B cells does, however, correlate with the titer of rheumatoid factor (RF). While there are reports of elevated frequencies of these cells in patients with RA with extremely high titers of RF, other studies claim that increased levels of CD5$^+$ B cells were associated with RF and antinuclear Ab in such patients. The level of CD5$^+$ B cells also was elevated in patients with primary Sjögren syndrome,[34] particularly in those patients with associated monoclonal Ig.

Surprisingly, in most cases of systemic lupus erythematosus (SLE), there are not elevated numbers of CD5$^+$ B cells. Decreased expression has, however, been described,[35] suggesting that CD5 control of the B cell receptor (BCR) may be affected in these patients (see 4.3.1).

3.2 Lymphoid Malignancies

CLL comprises a heterogeneous group of disorders, in which three main conditions have emerged: CLL, pro-lymphocytic leukemia, and hairy cell leukemia. The malignant cells from approximately 95% of the patients with CLL co-express CD5 and other B cell surface markers.[36] Thus, in most cases of CLL there is a proliferation of a B cell clone characterized by low amounts of surface Ig and increased expression of the CD5 Ag. It has been claimed that the B cells of CLL with a particularly indolent character are more frequently CD5$^+$ than those B cells in patients with more aggressive CLL,[37] but no correlation between the expression of CD5 and surface Ig class or type, clinical stage, disease activity, or age at diagnosis was definitively established by other investigators.

It is well documented that surface Ig receptors on CLL B cells exhibit specificity for a variety of self Ag. This concept has been extended[38] by studies of IgM Ab secreted by leukemia B cells after stimulation with PMA, which results in the production of low-affinity polyreactive autoAbs.

3.3 Infectious States

3.3.1 Viruses

Elevated levels of circulating CD5$^+$ B cells also have been reported in a great number of infectious diseases, especially those of viral origin (Table 1). Surprisingly, this has been described in infectious mononucleosis[40] but never confirmed, because the Epstein-Barr virus reduces the expression of CD5. On the other hand, CD5$^+$ B cells have repeatedly been enhanced in chronic hepatitis C virus (HCV) infection compared with patients with

Table 1 CD5 B Cells and Human Infections

Infection	CD5$^+$ B cell	References
Virus		
Cytomegalovirus	Reduction	39
Epstein-Barr	Reduction	40
Hepatitis C	Increase	41
Hepatitis B	Increase	42
Human imunodeficiency	Increase	43
Parasites		
Schistosoma sp.	Increase	44
Bacteria		
Mycobacterium tuberculosis	Increase (CD1d$^+$ CD5$^+$ Breg)	45
Vaccination		
Pneumococeal polysaccharide	Increase after vaccination	46

resolved infection.[47] In fact, chronic infection with HCV is associated with the disturbance of B lymphocyte activation and function, leading to serological abnormalities, such as autoAb production, mixed cryoglobulinemia, and B cell lymphomas.[48] A recent study demonstrated that CD5 is essential for HCV infection and cellular entry.[49] CD81, which is upregulated in CD5$^+$ B cells, also is suspected to contribute to HCV entry.[50]

3.3.2 Parasites

Furthermore, several parasites, particularly worms, have been associated with an expansion of CD5$^+$ B cells, including *Toxoplasma gondii*,[51] *Trypanosoma evansi*,[52] and *Schistosiamis mansoni*.[53] In the latest parasitemia, whether B-1a cells are responsible for Ab against egg Ag polylactosamine sugars, as previously described for a mouse model, has not yet been determined.

3.3.3 Fungus

CD5 can bind to β-glucan present on both saprophytic and pathogenic fungal cells, including *Saccharomyces pombe*, *Saccharomyces cerevisiae*, *Aspergillus fumigatus*, *Candida albicans*, and *Criptococcus neoformans*.[54] Similar to CD5,[55] CD6 has evolved to recognize bacterial lipopolysaccharide.[56] Following binding to the three extracellular domains of CD5, zymosan induces mitogen–activated protein kinase activation and IL-8 production.

4 CD5 MOLECULE

4.1 CD5 Gene and Transcripts

The CD5 protein is encoded by a single gene in both T and B cells, mapping to chromosome 11q12.2 located between CD6 and vps37c and consisting of at least 11 exons.[57] These 11 exons, as well as most of their transcription regulatory elements, are conserved in size and number in mice.

A novel exon 1 that is exclusively transcribed in B cells has been discovered.[58] Intriguingly, the existence of this new exon is due to a defective human endogenous retrovirus.[59] The data also provide attractive evidence for a reciprocal expression of this alternative exon 1, designated exon 1B, with the conventional exon 1, referred to as exon 1A. Exon 1B-type transcripts are translated into a truncated variant of the CD5 molecule devoid of leader peptide. As a consequence, whereas exon 1A promotes the expression of membrane CD5 protein in T cells and a subset of B cells (Figure 4), exon 1B acts to reduce CD5 protein expression in B cells and, therefore, possibly reduce the

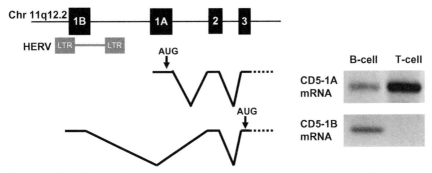

Figure 4 The *CD5* gene is made up of 11 exons. Exon 1 associates the classical exon 1, termed 1A, and the alternative exon 1, designated 1B. The former is expressed in B and T cells, and the latter is present exclusively in B cells. When exon 1A splices to exon 2, the initiation site AUG is located within exon 1, and the resulting CD5 molecule is full length, whereas when exon 1B splices out exon 1A and binds to AUG-free exon 2, the first initiation site AUG is located within exon 3, and the resulting CD5 molecule is truncated because the 5′ segment of exon 3 is not transcribed into messenger RNA (mRNA).

signalling functions of CD5, such as the production of Abs against infectious agents and autoAbs.[60] This balance between the two exons 1 might be important in the regulation of membrane expression of CD5, although both proteins are able to induce IL-10 expression when transfected in B cell lines.[35,61]

4.2 CD5 Regulation

Several lines of evidence indicate that the expression of CD5 is tightly regulated. Thus, membrane density of CD5 is ~30-fold higher in T cells than in B cells, and the expression of CD5 is developmentally regulated because the membrane density of CD5 is higher on mature T cells than on thymocytes. CD5-expressing B cells represent the majority of B lineage cells during foetal and neonatal life, but the number of CD5$^+$ B cells declines in relative number with age.[62] Further evidence supporting tight CD5 regulation comes from experiments showing that ex vivo B cells downregulate their membrane CD5 expression when cultured in the presence of IL-4,[15] but they upregulate CD5 following activation with PMA[14,63] or when their membrane IgM is cross-linked in the presence of IL-6.[64] Consistent with this view are findings that, despite their loss of membrane expression of CD5-, B-1b cells retain CD5 messenger RNA, albeit at lower levels than B-1a cells.[5] Finally, feedback regulation of murine B-1a cells also has been advocated.[32] In apparent contrast to these findings, a recent report suggested that all B cells constitutively express CD5 but the level of expression varies considerably, from B-1a cells at one end of the spectrum to B-2 cells at the other.[65] All in all, these observations imply that multiple mechanisms regulating CD5 expression exist.

CD5 internalization, which is enhanced in T cells but inhibited in B cells, upon Ag receptor cross-linking is another mechanism known to be involved in CD5 regulation,[66] even though the spontaneous turnover of this molecule is rather low. At the post-translational level, shedding of the molecule has been described and suggested to be exaggerated in non-organ-specific autoimmune and infectious diseases.[67] Cell-free CD5 could even bind to cells endowed with the related receptors, leading to an over-estimation of CD5$^+$ B cells.

4.3 Functions

4.3.1 Control of BCR Signalling

CD5 is physically[68] and functionally[69] associated with the BCR. Increased numbers of CD5$^+$ B cells might thus reflect defective regulation of B cell function through CD5 itself (Figure 5). There is now a growing body of evidence that CD5 is essential in modulating signals downstream of the

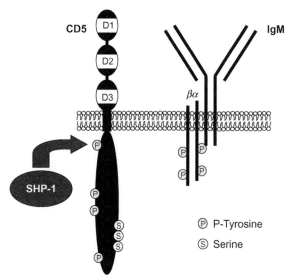

Figure 5 The B cell receptor (BCR) comprises membrane immunoglobulin (Ig) M, with Igα/Igβ as transducing molecules. CD5 is made up of three extra-cytoplasmic domains (D1–D3) and is associated with the BCR and brings about the *src*-homology 2 domain-containing phosphatase (SHP-1) to dampen the transducing cascade. The tyrosine residues are phorphorylated (P) by phosphorylases but not serine residues.

BCR. In this respect, we showed that ligation of CD5 or IgM on tonsillar B cells but not blood T cells resulted in apoptosis.[70] This observation has since been confirmed in a group of patients with CLL[71] and shown to take the BCR pathway.[72] In addition, anti-CD5 sustains the proliferation of tonsillar B cells pre-activated with anti-IgM Ab and IL-2.[73] This is in contrast to CB CD5$^+$ B cells, which do not apoptose in response to anti-CD5, but rather might reflect the fact these CB B cells are continuously exposed to autoAg in vivo. It is important to note that the *src*-homology 2 domain-containing protein tyrosine phosphatase (SHP-1) is constitutively linked with the Igα/Igβ chains of the BCR through the immunoregulatory tyrosine-based inhibitory motif of CD5.[72] The tyrosine residues, but not the serine residues, are phosphorylated. It has thus been suggested that such interaction with CD5 "sequesters" SHP-1 and limits its role with important molecules in positive signalling through the BCR.[74]

4.3.2 Control of Tolerance

The role of CD5 in the maintenance of clonal anergy has been addressed by the elegant experiments by Hippen et al. using hen egg lysosyme (HEL)–Ig transgenic (Tg) mice.[75] In this model, mice Tg for HEL-Ig and the membrane-bound form of the self Ag HEL produce apoptosis in anti-HEL B cells, whereas those Tg for HEL-Ig and the soluble form of HEL initiate anergy through SHP-1. Breeding of the latter Tg mice onto a CD5-/- background results in loss of tolerance. These data indicate that the presence of CD5 increases the threshold required for activation of self-reactive B cells in such a way that it determines their ultimate fate. Consistent with this role for CD5 is a more recent model in which CD5$^-$ spleen cells from mice made Tg for anti-ribonucleoprotein, a common autoAb in SLE and other connective tissue diseases, were injected into irradiated naïve mice. They migrated to the peritoneal cavity, where most CD5$^+$ B cells are found, and began to express CD5, which prevented their production of anti-ribonucleoprotein autoAb.[76] In addition to CD5 being important in this negative regulation of auto-reactive B cells, other molecules have been shown to play a role. For example, CD19 amplifies BCR signalling by favoring the activity of phosphorylases, such that a modest 10–20% increase in CD19 expression may be sufficient to shift the balance between tolerance and immunity to autoimmunity.[77] In contrast, CD22 dampens the signals by recruiting SHP-1, so that a CD22 deficiency encourages the development of autoimmunity.[78] Furthermore, defective signalling through the BCR has already been demonstrated for B cells from patients with SLE.[79]

4.3.3 Regulatory B Cell Functions

Regulatory B cells were initially characterized in an experimental auto-immune encephalomyelitis mouse model that mimics multiple sclerosis in humans (reviewed by Jamin et al.[80]). The phenotype of regulatory B cells was further explored, revealing that the CD1d^{high} CD5^{high} B cell subset affected T cell proliferation and differentiation, mainly through its abilities to produce IL-10.[81] These abilities were recently confirmed in humans.[82]

5 CONCLUSION

The bar mitzvah of B-1 cells is being celebrated.[83] We are indeed close to understanding the way they operate in autoimmunity and infection. Paradoxically, in light of recent findings of the modulation of B cell signalling by CD5, this and other molecules play a crucial role in preventing autoimmunity. Aberrations of transduction through CD5 are thought to exist and could lead to autoimmune disorders. Hence, the current views on the potential functions of CD5$^+$ B cells in autoimmunity are quite different from the rather naïve interpretation that the increased levels of CD5 B cells in patients with non-organ-specific autoimmune diseases represented a direct source of autoAbs, leading to pathogenesis.

ACKNOWLEDGMENTS

Studies mentioned in this review were supported by the "Ligue contre le cancer" and the "Cancéropôle Grand Ouest". The secretarial assistance of Simone Forest and Geneviève Michel is appreciated.

REFERENCES

1. Boumsell L, Bernard A, Lepage V, Degos L, Lemerle J, Dausset J. Some chronic lymphocytic leukemia cells bearing surface immunoglobulins share determinants with T cells. *Eur J Immunol* 1978;**8**:900–4.
2. Caligaris-Cappio F, Gobbi M, Bofill M, Janossy G. Infrequent normal B lymphocytes express features of B-chronic lymphocytic leukemia. *J Exp Med* 1982;**155**:623–8.
3. Ledbetter JA, Evans RL, Lipinski M, Cunningham-Rundles C, Good RA, Herzenberg LA. Evolutionary conservation of surface molecules that distinguish T lymphocyte helper/inducer and cytotoxic/suppressor subpopulations in mouse and man. *J Exp Med* 1981;**153**:310–23.
4. Kantor A. A new nomenclature for B cells. *Immunol Today* 1991;**12**:388.
5. Kasaian MT, Ikematsu H, Casali P. Identification and analysis of a novel human surface CD5- B lymphocyte subset producing natural antibodies. *J Immunol* 1992;**148**:2690–702.

6. Su SD, Ward MM, Apicella MA, Ward RE. The primary B cell response to the O/core region of bacterial lipopolysaccharide is restricted to the Ly-1 lineage. *J Immunol* 1991;**146**:327–31.

7. Kaveri SV, Silverman GJ, Bayry J. Natural IgM in immune equilibrium and harnessing their therapeutic potential. *J Immunol* 2012;**188**:939–45.

8. Murakami M, Honjo T. Involvement of B-1 cells in mucosal immunity and autoimmunity. *Immunol Today* 1995;**16**:534–9.

9. Murakami M, Nakajima K, Yamazaki K, Muraguchi T, Serikawa T, Honjo T. Effects of breeding environments on generation and activation of autoreactive B-1 cells in anti-red blood cell autoantibody transgenic mice. *J Exp Med* 1997;**185**:791–4.

10. Hayakawa K, Hardy RR, Herzenberg LA. Progenitors for Ly-1 B cells are distinct from progenitors for other B cells. *J Exp Med* 1985;**161**:1554–68.

11. Godin IE, Garcia-Porrero JA, Coutinho A, Dieterlen-Lievre F, Marcos MA. Para-aortic splanchnopleura from early mouse embryos contains B1a cell progenitors. *Nature* 1993;**364**:67–70.

12. Yoshimoto M, Montecino-Rodriguez E, Ferkowicz MJ, Porayette P, Shelley WC, Conway SJ, et al. Embryonic day 9 yolk sac and intra-embryonic hemogenic endothelium independently generate a B-1 and marginal zone progenitor lacking B-2 potential. *Proc Natl Acad Sci U S A* 2011;**108**:1468–73.

13. Yuan J, Nguyen CK, Liu X, Kanellopoulou C, Muljo SA. Lin28b reprograms adult bone marrow hematopoietic progenitors to mediate fetal-like lymphopoiesis. *Science* 2012;**335**:1195–200.

14. Youinou P, Mackenzie L, Jouquan J, Le Goff P, Lydyard PM. CD5 positive B cells in patients with rheumatoid arthritis: phorbol ester mediated enhancement of detection. *Ann Rheum Dis* 1987;**46**:17–22.

15. Defrance T, Vanbervliet B, Durand I, Banchereau J. Human interleukin 4 down-regulates the surface expression of CD5 on normal and leukemic B cells. *Eur J Immunol* 1989;**19**:293–9.

16. Youinou P, Jamin C, Lydyard PM. CD5 expression in human B-cell populations. *Immunol Today* 1999;**20**:312–16.

17. Griffin DO, Holodick NE, Rothstein TL. Human B1 cells are CD3-: A reply to "A human equivalent of mouse B-1 cells?" and "The nature of circulating CD27 +CD43 + B cells". *J Exp Med* 2011;**208**:2566–9.

18. Henry C, Ramadan A, Montcuquet N, Pallandre JR, Mercier-Letondal P, Deschamps M, et al. CD3+CD20 + cells may be an artifact of flow cytometry: comment on the article by Wilk et al. *Arthritis Rheum* 2010;**62**:2561–3, Author reply 3–5.

19. Descatoire M, Weill JC, Reynaud CA, Weller S. A human equivalent of mouse B-1 cells? *J Exp Med* 2011;**208**:2563–4.

20. Perez-Andres M, Grosserichter-Wagener C, Teodosio C, van Dongen JJ, Orfao A, van Zelm MC. The nature of circulating CD27+CD43 + B cells. *J Exp Med* 2011;**208**:2565–6.

21. Lydyard PM, MacKenzie LE, Youinou PY, Deane M, Jefferis R, Mageed RA. Specificity and idiotope expression of IgM produced by CD5 + and CD5 − cord blood B-cell clones. *Ann N Y Acad Sci* 1992;**651**:527–39.

22. Deane M, Mackenzie LE, Stevenson FK, Youinou PY, Lydyard PM, Mageed RA. The genetic basis of human VH4 gene family-associated cross-reactive idiotype expression in CD5 + and CD5- cord blood B-lymphocyte clones. *Scand J Immunol* 1993;**38**:348–58.

23. Baumgarth N, Herman OC, Jager GC, Brown L, Herzenberg LA. Innate and acquired humoral immunities to influenza virus are mediated by distinct arms of the immune system. *Proc Natl Acad Sci U S A* 1999;**96**:2250–5.

24. Wang H, Clarke SH. Positive selection focuses the VH12 B-cell repertoire towards a single B1 specificity with survival function. *Immunol Rev* 2004;**197**:51–9.

25. Briles DE, Forman C, Hudak S, Claflin JL. The effects of idiotype on the ability of IgG1 anti-phosphorylcholine antibodies to protect mice from fatal infection with Streptococcus pneumoniae. *Eur J Immunol* 1984;**14**:1027–30.
26. Tsiantoulas D, Gruber S, Binder CJ. B-1 cell immunoglobulin directed against oxidation-specific epitopes. *Front Immunol* 2012;**3**:415.
27. Wang C, Turunen SP, Kummu O, Veneskoski M, Lehtimaki J, Nissinen AE, et al. Natural antibodies of newborns recognize oxidative stress-related malondialdehyde acetaldehyde adducts on apoptotic cells and atherosclerotic plaques. *Int Immunol* 2013;**25**:575–87.
28. Kipps TJ, Vaughan JH. Genetic influence on the levels of circulating CD5 B lymphocytes. *J Immunol* 1987;**139**:1060–4.
29. Youinou P, Mackenzie L, Katsikis P, Merdrignac G, Isenberg DA, Tuaillon N, et al. The relationship between CD5-expressing B lymphocytes and serologic abnormalities in rheumatoid arthritis patients and their relatives. *Arthritis Rheum* 1990;**33**:339–48.
30. Pers JO, Jamin C, Lydyard PM, Charreire J, Youinou P. The H2 haplotype regulates the distribution of B cells into B-1a, B-1b and B-2 subsets. *Immunogenetics* 2002;**54**:208–11.
31. Pers JO, Jamin C, Youinou P, Charreire J. Role of IL-10 in the distribution of B cell subsets in the mouse B-1 cell population. *Eur Cytokine Netw* 2003;**14**:178–85.
32. Lalor PA, Herzenberg LA, Adams S, Stall AM. Feedback regulation of murine Ly-1 B cell development. *Eur J Immunol* 1989;**19**:507–13.
33. Lino MM, Paulo CS, Vale AC, Vaz MF, Ferreira LS. Antifungal activity of dental resins containing amphotericin B-conjugated nanoparticles. *Dent Mater* 2013;**29**:e252–62.
34. Youinou P, Mackenzie L, le Masson G, Papadopoulos NM, Jouquan J, Pennec YL, et al. CD5-expressing B lymphocytes in the blood and salivary glands of patients with primary Sjogren's syndrome. *J Autoimmun* 1988;**1**:185–94.
35. Garaud S, Morva A, Lemoine S, Hillion S, Bordron A, Pers JO, et al. CD5 promotes IL-10 production in chronic lymphocytic leukemia B cells through STAT3 and NFAT2 activation. *J Immunol* 2011;**186**:4835–44.
36. Martin PJ, Hansen JA, Siadak AW, Nowinski RC. Monoclonal antibodies recognizing normal human T lymphocytes and malignant human B lymphocytes: a comparative study. *J Immunol* 1981;**127**:1920–3.
37. Caligaris-Cappio F, Gobbi M, Bergui L, Campana D, Lauria F, Fierro MT, et al. B-chronic lymphocytic leukaemia patients with stable benign disease show a distinctive membrane phenotype. *Br J Haematol* 1984;**56**:655–60.
38. Broker BM, Klajman A, Youinou P, Jouquan J, Worman CP, Murphy J, et al. Chronic lymphocytic leukemic (CLL) cells secrete multispecific autoantibodies. *J Autoimmun* 1988;**1**:469–81.
39. Chidrawar S, Khan N, Wei W, McLarnon A, Smith N, Nayak L, et al. Cytomegalovirus-seropositivity has a profound influence on the magnitude of major lymphoid subsets within healthy individuals. *Clin Exp Immunol* 2009;**155**:423–32.
40. Hassan J, Feighery C, Bresnihan B, Whelan A. Increased CD5+ B cells in infectious mononucleosis. *Br J Haematol* 1990;**74**:375–6.
41. Mizuochi T, Ito M, Takai K, Yamaguchi K. Differential susceptibility of peripheral blood CD5+ and CD5- B cells to apoptosis in chronic hepatitis C patients. *Biochem Biophys Res Commun* 2009;**389**:512–15.
42. Sun H, Lv J, Tu Z, Hu X, Yan H, Pan Y, et al. Antiviral treatment improves disrupted peripheral B lymphocyte homeostasis in chronic hepatitis B virus-infected patients. *Exp Biol Med (Maywood)* 2013;**238**:1275–83.
43. Franceschi C, Franceschini MG, Boschini A, Trenti T, Nuzzo C, Castellani G, et al. Phenotypic characteristics and tendency to apoptosis of peripheral blood mononuclear cells from HIV+ long term non progressors. *Cell Death Differ* 1997;**4**:815–23.

44. Seydel LS, Petelski A, van Dam GJ, van der Kleij D, Kruize-Hoeksma YC, Luty AJ, et al. Association of in utero sensitization to Schistosoma haematobium with enhanced cord blood IgE and increased frequencies of CD5- B cells in African newborns. *Am J Trop Med Hyg* 2012;**86**:613–19.

45. Zhang M, Zheng X, Zhang J, Zhu Y, Zhu X, Liu H, et al. CD19(+)CD1d(+)CD5(+) B cell frequencies are increased in patients with tuberculosis and suppress Th17 responses. *Cell Immunol* 2012;**274**:89–97.

46. Leggat DJ, Khaskhely NM, Iyer AS, Mosakowski J, Thompson RS, Weinandy JD, et al. Pneumococcal polysaccharide vaccination induces polysaccharide-specific B cells in adult peripheral blood expressing CD19(+)CD20(+)CD3(-)CD70(-)CD27(+)IgM(+) CD43(+)CD5(+/-). *Vaccine* 2013;**31**:4632–40.

47. Curry MP, Golden-Mason L, Nolan N, Parfrey NA, Hegarty JE, O'Farrelly C. Expansion of peripheral blood CD5 + B cells is associated with mild disease in chronic hepatitis C virus infection. *J Hepatol* 2000;**32**:121–5.

48. Curry MP, Golden-Mason L, Doherty DG, Deignan T, Norris S, Duffy M, et al. Expansion of innate CD5pos B cells expressing high levels of CD81 in hepatitis C virus infected liver. *J Hepatol* 2003;**38**:642–50.

49. Sarhan MA, Pham TN, Chen AY, Michalak TI. Hepatitis C virus infection of human T lymphocytes is mediated by CD5. *J Virol* 2012;**86**:3723–35.

50. Dutra WO, Martins-Filho OA, Cancado JR, Pinto-Dias JC, Brener Z, Freeman Junior GL, et al. Activated T and B lymphocytes in peripheral blood of patients with Chagas' disease. *Int Immunol* 1994;**6**:499–506.

51. Chen M, Aosai F, Norose K, Mun HS, Yano A. The role of anti-HSP70 autoantibody-forming V(H)1-J(H)1 B-1 cells in Toxoplasma gondii-infected mice. *Int Immunol* 2003;**15**:39–47.

52. Onah DN, Hopkins J, Luckins AG. Increase in CD5 + B cells and depression of immune responses in sheep infected with Trypanosoma evansi. *Vet Immunol Immunopathol* 1998;**63**:209–22.

53. El-Cheikh MC, Bonomo AC, Rossi MI, Pinho Mde F, Borojevic R. Experimental murine schistosomiasis mansoni: modulation of the B-1 lymphocyte distribution and phenotype expression. *Immunobiology* 1998;**199**:51–62.

54. Vera J, Fenutria R, Canadas O, Figueras M, Mota R, Sarrias MR, et al. The CD5 ectodomain interacts with conserved fungal cell wall components and protects from zymosan-induced septic shock-like syndrome. *Proc Natl Acad Sci U S A* 2009;**106**:1506–11.

55. Alonso-Ramirez R, Loisel S, Buors C, Pers JO, Montero E, Youinou P, et al. Rationale for Targeting CD6 as a Treatment for Autoimmune Diseases. *Arthritis* 2010;**2010**:130646.

56. Sarrias MR, Farnos M, Mota R, Sanchez-Barbero F, Ibanez A, Gimferrer I, et al. CD6 binds to pathogen-associated molecular patterns and protects from LPS-induced septic shock. *Proc Natl Acad Sci USA* 2007;**104**:11724–9.

57. Padilla O, Calvo J, Vila JM, Arman M, Gimferrer I, Places L, et al. Genomic organization of the human CD5 gene. *Immunogenetics* 2000;**51**:993–1001.

58. Renaudineau Y, Hillion S, Saraux A, Mageed RA, Youinou P. An alternative exon 1 of the CD5 gene regulates CD5 expression in human B lymphocytes. *Blood* 2005;**106**:2781–9.

59. Renaudineau Y, Vallet S, Le Dantec C, Hillion S, Saraux A, Youinou P. Characterization of the human CD5 endogenous retrovirus-E in B lymphocytes. *Genes Immun* 2005;**6**:663–71.

60. Garaud S, Le Dantec C, Berthou C, Lydyard PM, Youinou P, Renaudineau Y. Selection of the alternative exon 1 from the cd5 gene down-regulates membrane level of the protein in B lymphocytes. *J Immunol* 2008;**181**:2010–18.

61. Garaud S, Le Dantec C, de Mendoza AR, Mageed RA, Youinou P, Renaudineau Y. IL-10 production by B cells expressing CD5 with the alternative exon 1B. *Ann N Y Acad Sci* 2009;**1173**:280–5.

62. Bergler W, Adam S, Gross HJ, Hormann K, Schwartz-Albiez R. Age-dependent altered proportions in subpopulations of tonsillar lymphocytes. *Clin Exp Immunol* 1999;**116**:9–18.

63. Miller RA, Gralow J. The induction of Leu-1 antigen expression in human malignant and normal B cells by phorbol myristic acetate (PMA). *J Immunol* 1984;**133**:3408–14.

64. Cong YZ, Rabin E, Wortis HH. Treatment of murine CD5- B cells with anti-Ig, but not LPS, induces surface CD5: two B-cell activation pathways. *Int Immunol* 1991;**3**:467–76.

65. Kaplan D, Smith D, Meyerson H, Pecora N, Lewandowska K. CD5 expression by B lymphocytes and its regulation upon Epstein-Barr virus transformation. *Proc Natl Acad Sci U S A* 2001;**98**:13850–3.

66. Lu X, Axtell RC, Collawn JF, Gibson A, Justement LB, Raman C. AP2 adaptor complex-dependent internalization of CD5: differential regulation in T and B cells. *J Immunol* 2002;**168**:5612–20.

67. Jamin C, Magadur G, Lamour A, Mackenzie L, Lydyard P, Katsikis P, et al. Cell-free CD5 in patients with rheumatic diseases. *Immunol Lett* 1992;**31**:79–83.

68. Lankester AC, van Schijndel GM, Cordell JL, van Noesel CJ, van Lier RA. CD5 is associated with the human B cell antigen receptor complex. *Eur J Immunol* 1994;**24**:812–16.

69. Jamin C, Lydyard PM, Le Corre R, Youinou PY. CD5+B cells: differential capping and modulation of IgM and CD5. *Scand J Immunol* 1996;**43**:73–80.

70. Pers JO, Jamin C, Le Corre R, Lydyard PM, Youinou P. Ligation of CD5 on resting B cells, but not on resting T cells, results in apoptosis. *Eur J Immunol* 1998;**28**:4170–6.

71. Pers JO, Berthou C, Porakishvili N, Burdjanadze M, Le Calvez G, Abgrall JF, et al. CD5-induced apoptosis of B cells in some patients with chronic lymphocytic leukemia. *Leukemia* 2002;**16**:44–52.

72. Sen G, Bikah G, Venkataraman C, Bondada S. Negative regulation of antigen receptor-mediated signaling by constitutive association of CD5 with the SHP-1 protein tyrosine phosphatase in B-1 B cells. *Eur J Immunol* 1999;**29**:3319–28.

73. Jamin C, Le Corre R, Lydyard PM, Youinou P. Anti-CD5 extends the proliferative response of human CD5+ B cells activated with anti-IgM and interleukin-2. *Eur J Immunol* 1996;**26**:57–62.

74. Bikah G, Carey J, Ciallella JR, Tarakhovsky A, Bondada S. CD5-mediated negative regulation of antigen receptor-induced growth signals in B-1 B cells. *Science* 1996;**274**:1906–9.

75. Hippen KL, Tze LE, Behrens TW. CD5 maintains tolerance in anergic B cells. *J Exp Med* 2000;**191**:883–90.

76. Qian Y, Santiago C, Borrero M, Tedder TF, Clarke SH. Lupus-specific antiribonucleoprotein B cell tolerance in nonautoimmune mice is maintained by differentiation to B-1 and governed by B cell receptor signaling thresholds. *J Immunol* 2001;**166**:2412–19.

77. Sato S, Hasegawa M, Fujimoto M, Tedder TF, Takehara K. Quantitative genetic variation in CD19 expression correlates with autoimmunity. *J Immunol* 2000;**165**:6635–43.

78. Smith KG, Tarlinton DM, Doody GM, Hibbs ML, Fearon DT. Inhibition of the B cell by CD22: a requirement for Lyn. *J Exp Med* 1998;**187**:807–11.

79. Liossis SN, Kovacs B, Dennis G, Kammer GM, Tsokos GC. B cells from patients with systemic lupus erythematosus display abnormal antigen receptor-mediated early signal transduction events. *J Clin Invest* 1996;**98**:2549–57.

80. Jamin C, Morva A, Lemoine S, Daridon C, de Mendoza AR, Youinou P. Regulatory B lymphocytes in humans: a potential role in autoimmunity. *Arthritis Rheum* 2008;**58**:1900–6.

81. Fillatreau S, Sweenie CH, McGeachy MJ, Gray D, Anderton SM. B cells regulate auto-immunity by provision of IL-10. *Nat Immunol* 2002;**3**:944–50.
82. Lemoine S, Morva A, Youinou P, Jamin C. Human T cells induce their own regulation through activation of B cells. *J Autoimmun* 2011;**36**:228–38.
83. Tarakhovsky A. Bar Mitzvah for B-1 cells: how will they grow up? *J Exp Med* 1997;**185**:981–4.

CHAPTER 6

T Cells and Autoimmunity

Vaishali R. Moulton[1], Kamalpreet Nagpal, George C. Tsokos
Division of Rheumatology, Department of Medicine, Beth Israel Deaconess Medical Center, Harvard Medical School, Boston, Massachusetts, USA
[1]Corresponding Author: vmoulton@bidmc.harvard.edu

1 INTRODUCTION

T lymphocytes are important in the pathogenesis of systemic autoimmune diseases such as systemic lupus erythematosus (SLE). A combination of genetic predisposition, environmental factors such as infections and hormones such as estrogen leads to a breakdown of immune tolerance, resulting in autoantibody production and unchecked expansion of self-reactive T cells, ultimately leading to tissue destruction. Altered T cell signalling events couple with defective gene expression and aberrant cytokine production, thus leading to the abnormal phenotype of T cells in SLE. T cells from patients with SLE are unique in that they bear some features of naïve T cells, such as their low interleukin (IL)-2 production, and yet certain characteristics are reminiscent of an activated/memory cell phenotype such as the rewired T cell receptor (TCR) signalling subunits and aberrant cytokine production.[2] The following sections describe the role and regulation of T cells in the pathophysiology of the prototype autoimmune disease SLE.

2 ROLE OF HORMONES

Hormones are a crucial component in the pathogenesis of autoimmune disease, as evidenced by the predominant affliction of women: 90% of patients with SLE are women, and the disease is mainly seen among women of reproductive age.[3] The role of female hormones in autoimmune disease, specifically in SLE, has been studied both in clinical trials and in mouse models. While the precise cellular and molecular mechanisms of the hormonal contribution to disease are not clear, estrogen is implicated in disease pathophysiology. Most cells including immune cells and T cells express estrogen receptors (ERs) α and β. Estrogen binds to ERs and form dimers that subsequently recognize and

Infection and Autoimmunity
http://dx.doi.org/10.1016/B978-0-444-63269-2.00005-2

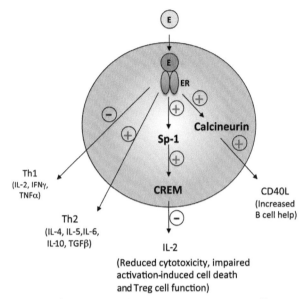

Figure 1 Select roles of estrogen and estrogen receptors in T cells in SLE.

bind to estrogen response elements within target genes and regulate gene transcription (Figure 1). ERs are emerging as important contributors to autoimmune disease pathogenesis.[4] In lupus–prone mice models, ER-α deficiency attenuated disease and prolonged survival.[5,6] Estrogen was shown to increase CD40L expression in T cells from patients with SLE compared to healthy individuals.[7] Estrogen treatment of T cells from healthy individuals increased expression of the transcriptional repressor cAMP response element modulator (CREM) and suppressed IL-2 production.[8]

Estrogen is associated with regulation of cytokines, promoting a T helper (Th) 2 cytokine profile and suppressing Th1 cytokines. Mice treated with estrogen were susceptible to infection by *Listeria monocytogenes*, which correlated with their splenocytes, which produced reduced amounts of IL-2 necessary for cytotoxicity.[9] Estrogen was recently found to increase IL-17 production in splenocytes from wild-type mice treated with.[10] Estrogen suppresses the expression of FasL affecting T cell apoptosis, suggesting that it may permit the persistence of autoreactive T cells.[11] Estrogen administration to peripheral blood mononuclear cell (PBMC)–induced expression of calcineurin messenger RNA (mRNA) expression and encoded enzyme PP2B phosphatase activity in an ER-dependent manner.[12]

3 ROLE OF INFECTIONS

Environmental influences are an important contributor to SLE pathogenesis, and infectious agents are a crucial component. Pathogenic mechanisms involving infections and autoimmunity include molecular mimicry, lymphocyte bystander activation, superantigens, polyclonal activation, and epitope spreading.[13] Viral infections such as the Epstein–Barr virus have long been associated with the triggering of autoimmunity, specifically SLE. Evidence for this connection includes the molecular similarity of the Epstein–Barr nuclear antigen (EBNA) 1 to the common lupus autoantigen Ro and of EBNA-1 and EBNA-2 with an SmD epitope. This cross-reactivity of antibodies is important in the initiation of lupus autoimmunity. Following autoantibody production, self-antigens are processed and epitope spreading begins. Patients with SLE show accelerated seroconversion to the Epstein–Barr virus and have higher viral titers compared to healthy individuals; this results from defective CD8 cytotoxic responses that are unable to control viral load. Aberrant T cell responses are observed in patients with SLE with increased interferon-γ-producing CD4-positive cells and dysfunctional CD8 T cells.[14] Superantigens are proteins produced by bacteria (such as staphylococci and streptococci) or viruses and are capable of binding to the TCR and also with high avidity to major histocompatibility complex class II molecules independent of antigen specificity. Therefore, they can activate large numbers of CD4 T cells, including self-reactive T cells, to aberrantly produce inflammatory cytokines and eventual B cell activation. Inflammatory cytokines can mediate the bystander activation and proliferation of T cells to propagate the autoimmune process and pathology.

4 T CELL SIGNALLING: T CELL RECEPTOR (TCR)–CD3 COMPLEX

TCR engagement feeds into an intricate signalling network culminating in gene expression, cytokine production and effector function. TCR signal transduction commences upon the recognition of the cognate peptide–MHC molecule on the surface of antigen-presenting cells (APCs).[15,16] The TCR consists of the highly variable α and β chains as part of a complex with the CD3 δ, ε, γ and ζ chains to form the TCR-CD3 complex.[17] While the δ, ε, and γ chains each bear a single immunoreceptor tyrosine activation motif (ITAM), each of the ζ chains has three ITAMs; thus the ζζ homodimer has a total of six motifs, making it a critical signal transducer of T cells.[18] In naïve T cells, antigen recognition is followed by a clustering of the TCR, the co-receptor molecule (CD4 or CD8) as well as CD45 into lipid-rich micro-domains called lipid rafts.[2] The TCR lacks any intrinsic enzymatic activity and instead relies on the Src family of kinases, particularly Lck, to initiate signalling by phosphorylating the six ITAMs on CD3ζ chains.[19–21] This renders the CD3 zeta-chain capable of binding zeta-associated protein (ZAP70) kinase, which is also phosphorylated by Lck. This causes a conformational change and an increase in the enzymatic activity of ZAP70, leading to phosphorylation of its target molecules, including the adaptor molecules linker for activation in T cells (LAT) and SLP-76.[22] The phosphorylated LAT molecules, in turn, recruit and activate a number of downstream signalling molecules, forming the LAT signalosome and transmitting the signal downstream into distinct pathways. Ras–mitogen-activated protein kinase (MAPK) is activated through the guanine nucleotide exchange factor. In addition the enzyme phospholipase Cγ is activated.[23,24] The activation of these pathways ultimately causes an increase in intracellular calcium and the activation of various transcription factors such as nuclear factor (NF)-κB, NF of activated T cells (NFAT) and activator protein (AP) 1. The activation of these transcription factors is followed by their nuclear translocation and induction of target gene transcription, T cell growth, and differentiation. Signalling initiated from the TCR also leads to actin mobilization, cytoskeletal rearrangements as well as activation of integrins by inside-out signalling.[25,26] T cells from patients with SLE present with abnormal attributes and characteristics that contribute to disease progression and pathology, with distinct aberrations in early and late signalling (Figure 2).

4.1 Defects in Early T-Cell Signalling

T cells isolated from patients with SLE display amplified activation in response to antigen recognition. These cells show increased tyrosine phosphorylation of signalling proteins as well as an enhanced calcium influx.[27] In contrast to cells from healthy individuals, lipid rafts in SLE T cells are pre-clustered and ready for activation.[28] In addition, they have an abnormal representation of some of the key molecules involved in signalling. Defective expression and activity of the tyrosine phosphatase CD45 leads to a decreased expression of the kinase Lck in lipid rafts in SLE T cells. In addition, there is increased expression of Fc receptor (FcR) γ, spleen tyrosine kinase (Syk), and phospholipase Cγ.[29] The importance of lipid raft clustering is demonstrated by a study where cholera toxin, an agent that forces the clustering of lipid rafts, exacerbated the disease in a mouse model of lupus.[30]

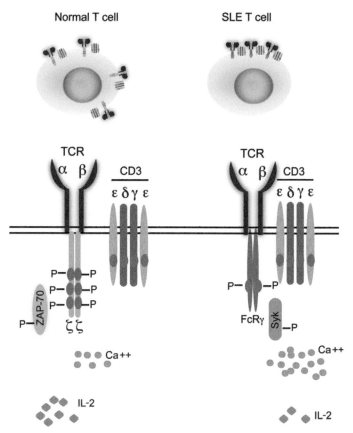

Figure 2 T cell receptor in normal and SLE T cells.

The increased calcium response is due at least in part to the reorganization/rewiring of the TCR complex in SLE T cells. In these cells, the expression of the CD3ζ chain is decreased compared to healthy individuals.[31] This decrease is accompanied by an increase in the levels of FcRγ, a homologous protein that structurally and functionally replaces the CD3ζ molecule in the TCR–CD3 complex.[32] FcRγ has only one ITAM (compared to three in CD3ζ) and couples to Syk instead of ZAP70. This leads to defective signalling through the TCR, culminating in increased calcium influx. The decreased expression of CD3ζ is attributed to a number of different defects: abnormal transcription, decreased mRNA stability, alternate splicing and protein degradation. The key role that this rewiring plays in SLE T cells is shown by the inhibition of Syk, wherein the defective calcium influx in SLE T cells is corrected.[33] In another study, restoring the levels of CD3ζ in SLE T cells restored the IL-2 production, thus emphasizing the importance of the CD3ζ chain in T cell signalling.[34]

4.2 Defects in Downstream Signalling Events

SLE T cells have defects in the MAPK signalling pathways, especially extracellular signal–regulated kinase (ERK) signalling pathway. Defective Ras signalling, decreased levels of ras guanyl nucleotide releasing protein 1 (RasGRP1) and abnormal protein kinase Cδ activation are some of the factors contributing to this defect.[35–37] SLE T cells also exhibit increased levels of the protein phosphatase (PP) 2A, which contributes to defective ERK signalling.[38] Abnormalities in the ERK cascade ultimately contribute to DNA hypomethylation via its effect on the enzyme DNA methyltransferase (DNMT) 1. DNA hypomethylation is one of the hallmarks of T cells from patients with SLE and a key feature contributing to the development of disease.[39]

Dysfunction of mitochondria is another anomaly seen in SLE T cells, with hyperpolarization and excessive production of reactive oxygen species, leading to oxidative stress. Mammalian target of rapamycin (mTOR) is a kinase that acts as a sensor of the mitochondrial membrane potential. SLE T cells exhibit higher levels of mTOR.[40] In addition to its effect on mitochondrial polarization, high levels and activation of mTOR lead to lower levels of CD3ζ through lysosomal degradation.[41]

4.3 Increased Cell Death in SLE T Cells

Mitochondrial hyperpolarization also leads to increased death of T cells by necrosis, as opposed to spontaneous apoptosis in the absence of oxidizing agents.[42,43] Mitochondrial hyperpolarization as well as increased reactive oxygen species modify the expression of cytokines such as IL-10 and tumor necrosis factor (TNF)-α, thus leading to increased death of SLE T cells by necrosis.[44] Increased cell death of SLE T cells by apoptosis as well as necrosis exacerbates the inflammation by providing extracellular nuclear material.

4.4 Defects in Gene Expression

The expression and function of various transcription factors is altered in T cells isolated from patients with SLE, affecting gene expression of many different signalling intermediates as well as effector molecules that are key to the optimal functioning of the T cell.

CD3ζ/FcR1γ

Aberrant expression and activity of Elf-1, a transcription factor belonging to the Ets family of transcription factors, is responsible for skewing the CD3ζ-to-FcR1γ ratio in SLE T cells.[45] Elf-1 reciprocally regulates CD3ζ and FcR1γ, leading to reduced levels of the former and higher expression of the latter.[46]

CREB/CREM

cAMP-controlled transcription factors CREB (cAMP response element binding protein) and CREM are two antagonistic transcription factors that are defectively regulated in SLE T cells.[47] Phosphorylated (p) CREB acts as a transcriptional activator, whereas pCREM is a repressor of transcription. The ratio of these two proteins at a specific site within the *IL-2* promoter determines the expression levels of IL-2. In the case of SLE T cells, the highly expressed PP2A causes dephosphorylation of CREB, whereas increased activity of the calcium-activated calmodulin kinase (CAMK) IV leads to increased pCREM levels and increased binding to the target gene.[48] The result is a reduction in the levels of the cytokine IL-2 produced by SLE T cells upon activation.[49]

4.5 Epigenetic Changes in SLE

Epigenetics comprise stable and heritable changes that modify gene expression without changing the underlying genomic sequence.[50] Such changes broadly include CpG DNA methylation and histone modifications.

DNA methylation

One of the most efficient methods of gene silencing is DNA methylation by the DNMT enzymes to the 5′ carbon position of cytosine in CpG dinucleotides.[51] Abnormalities in the DNA methylation system can lead to an increase or decrease in the expression of that particular gene. A generally hypomethylated state of T cells has been reported in SLE.[52] It has been shown that defective protein kinase Cδ activity, as well as enhanced PP2Ac levels, lead to abnormal ERK/MAPK pathway activation and ultimately reduced DNMT1 expression and activity[53,3838]. Some examples of methylation-sensitive genes that are hypomethylated in lupus T cells include *CD40L*, *CD11a*, cytokines *IL-4*, *IL-6*, *IL-10*, and the serine threonine phosphatase *PP2A*.[54–56]

Histone modifications

Histones are the building blocks of chromatin and are amenable to various post-translational modifications that can affect the functional abilities of chromatin. Some of the modifications include acetylation, methylation, phosphorylation, sumoylation, and ADP-ribosylation.[57] The silencing of the *IL-2* locus by the recruitment of histone deacetylase 1 by the transcriptional repressor CREMα is an example of a histone modification that plays a role in SLE.[58] Acetylation of histone residues is associated with transcriptional activation and their removal by repressing transcription.

4.6 Alternative Splicing

A common theme in the aberrant gene expression observed in T cells from patients with SLE is the abnormal processing of mRNA, resulting in abnormal expression and/or activity of proteins encoded by these variants. For example, abnormal alternative splicing of the CD3 zeta 3′ untranslated region results in the deletion of a large 500-bp fragment that contains elements essential for the stability of the transcript.[59] Increased expression of this aberrant isoform contributes to the reduced expression of the CD3ζ chain and therefore to the rewired TCR.[60] By mass spectrometry discovery approaches, the serine arginine-rich splicing factor (SRSF) 1 or splicing factor 2/alternative splicing factor was found to bind and regulate alternative splicing of the *CD3ζ* 3′ untranslated region. Interestingly, reduced expression of SRSF1 correlated with CD3ζ expression in T cells from patients with SLE.[61] *CD44*, an important adhesion and differentiation molecule in T cells, has a very complex gene structure and bears numerous spliced isoforms, of which specifically the variable (v) 3 and v6 variants were found to be increased in SLE T cells and conferred increased migration capacity.[62] The *CREM* gene bears multiple promoters and produces distinct products with opposing functions in gene transcription. CREMα is a repressor, whereas CREM tau2α is an activator. Inducible cAMP early repressor isoforms are also isoforms of the *CREM* gene and are repressors. Increased expression and activity of CREMα contributes to the defect in *IL-2* transcription and low IL-2 production in SLE T cells.[63]

5 COSTIMULATORY PATHWAYS

APCs capture, process, and present antigen-specific sequences to T cells through the interaction of the cognate peptide–MHC complex on the surface of APCs and the TCR on the T cell. This interaction is, however, insufficient to propagate downstream signals and requires help from other costimulatory pathways to continue and sustain the signal (Figure 3). In addition to propagating the signal, costimulatory signals also are required to keep the signalling in check and attenuate it when necessary so that

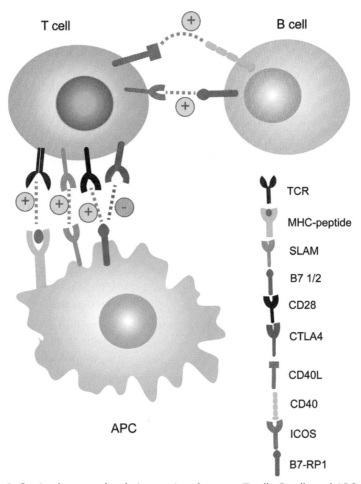

Figure 3 Costimulatory molecule interactions between T cells, B cells and APCs.

immune tolerance is not breached. Some of the well-characterized costimu-latory molecules and their role in the pathophysiology of SLE are presented in the following sections.

5.1 CD28–CD80/86

During the early stages of T cell activation, CD28, which is expressed on T cells, couples to the CD80 (B7-1)/CD86 (B7-2) molecules on APCs.[64] CD80/86 are constitutively expressed on dendritic cells but are inducible in B cells as well as other APCs such as monocytes. Activation of the CD28-B7 interaction provides a potent signal (in addition to the

TCR–MHC interaction) for the production of various cytokines such as IL-2 and IL-6.[65] The interaction between CD28 and CD80/86 has received much attention with respect to SLE. A number of studies have demonstrated amelioration of the disease upon blockade of this interaction in murine models of lupus.[66]

Cytotoxic T-lymphocyte antigen 4 (CTLA4) is a receptor present on the surface of T cells and transmits an inhibitory signal to T cells. It is similar in structure to CD28 and can bind to both CD80 as well as CD86. However, CTLA4 binds to CD80/86 with much higher affinity, thus outcompeting CD28 and attenuating the signal. Abatacept (a CTLA4–immunoglobulin fusion molecule) has been used in clinical studies to block the CD28: CD80/86 stimulation and led to the amelioration of autoimmune-driven inflammation.[67]

5.2 Inducible Costimulator–B7RP1

Another costimulatory pathway related to CD28-CD80/86 is the inducible co-stimulator (ICOS) B7–related protein 1 (B7RP1) pathway.[68] ICOS is structurally functional to CD28 and is expressed on activated T cells. It binds to B7RP1, which is expressed on B cells as well as dendritic cells and monocytes. ICOS activation induces class switching and antibody production by B cells. It has been reported that ICOS is highly expressed on the CD4 + T cells of patients with autoimmune diseases such as rheumatoid arthritis and SLE.[69]

5.3 CD40L-CD40

Activated T cells express CD40L on their surface, which binds to CD40 on the surface of B cells, APCs, and non-immune cells such as epithelial, endothelial, and renal tubular cells.[70] The ligation of CD40 and CD40L can deliver strong signals, which can drive B cell differentiation, maturation, and isotype switching.[71] A number of autoimmune diseases exhibit an increased surface expression of CD40L on their T cells, and this is correlated with increased autoantibody production.[72,73] Moreover, in lupus-prone mice, blockade of CD40L has been shown to prevent the development of SLE.[74]

5.4 Signalling Lymphocytic Activation Molecules

The signalling lymphocytic activation molecule (SLAM) family comprises nine members that are type I transmembrane receptors belonging to the immunoglobulin superfamily.[75] These receptor molecules provide potent co-stimulatory signals and are recognized as important immunomodulatory molecules with roles in T cell function and B cell activation as well as lineage commitment during hematopoiesis, cell survival and cell adhesion.[76,77] SLAM molecules have a tyrosine-rich motif through which they can interact with SH2 domain–containing proteins such as the SLAM-associated protein.[76] Genome-wide association studies of the families of patients with SLE have identified a susceptibility locus on chromosome 1 that harbors the SLAM genes.[78,79] Among the SLAM family members, SLAMF3 and SLAMF6 are expressed at higher levels in SLE T cells compared to T cells from healthy individuals.[80]

5.5 CD44 And Cell Adhesion/Migration

CD44 is a glycoprotein expressed on the T cell surface and is involved in cell adhesion, migration, and signalling. It binds to its ligand, hyaluronic acid, in tissues and helps T cells to migrate into peripheral tissues. In cells it functions in association with its signalling partners ezrin, radixin, moiesin (ERM) and requires pERM for its adhesive capacity.[81] SLE T cells have an elevated surface expression of certain isoforms of CD44 and are found in aggregated lipid rafts along with ERM.[82] High levels of CD44 as well as pERM have been reported in kidney infiltrates of patients with lupus, suggesting that signalling through CD44 enables the migration of T cells into kidneys.[62] ERM signalling molecules are phosphorylated by rho-associated protein kinase. Inhibiting rho-associated protein kinase or blocking the activation of CD44 pathways inhibits the migration of T cells.

6 CYTOKINES

Cytokines are small proteins secreted by cells in both the innate and adaptive immune systems and can regulate diverse functions in the immune response. Dysregulation of cytokines and their consequent signalling networks are an important component of the pathogenesis of autoimmune disease. In SLE, a number of cytokines are aberrantly expressed and, through their effects on immune cells, facilitate abnormal cellular and humoral responses; they also directly mediate tissue pathology and damage.[83] CD4 Th cell differentiation is driven by specific cytokines: IL-12 drives a Th1 differentiation important for cell-mediated immunity against intracellular pathogens, IL-4 is required for a Th2 differentiation necessary for a humoral response against extracellular pathogens and a combination of IL-6, transforming growth factor (TGF)-β, IL-23 and IL-21 drive Th17 differentiation, which is important for certain types of bacterial and fungal infections.[84] TGF-β in the absence of inflammation drives regulatory T cell (Treg) generation, and IL-6 with IL-21 lead to T follicular helper cell differentiation (Figure 4). The differentiation into these specific cell types is controlled by lineage-specific transcription factors. T-bet and GATA-3 are important for Th1 and Th2 differentiation, respectively. Retinoid-related orphan receptor (ROR) γt and RORα are activating factors for *IL-17* transcription. FoxP3 is the transcription factor important for Tregs, whereas Bcl-6 is important for T follicular helper cell differentiation.

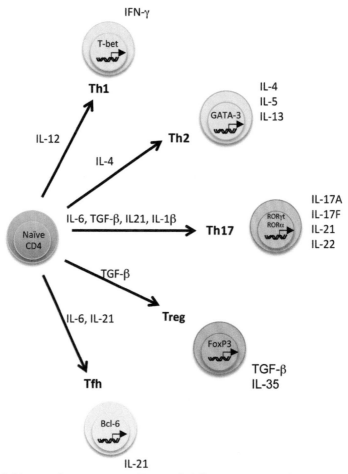

Figure 4 Diagram depicting naïve CD4 T cell differentiation into Th1, Th2, Th17, Treg and Tfhsubsets. Cytokines and transcription factors involved in lineage-specific differentiation are indicated.

6.1 IL-2

T cells from patients with SLE produce aberrantly low amounts of the vital cytokine IL-2. IL-2 is important in autoimmune disease because it is not only necessary for the proliferation and function of Tregs but also vital for activation-induced cell death, which is important for the deletion of autoreactive T cells. In addition, IL-2 is important for cell-mediated immunity, which is crucial because patients with autoimmune disease are susceptible to infections caused by either immunosuppressive therapy or dysregulated immune responses. Tregs qualified by the CD4+ CD25+ or CD4+CD25+FoxP3+ phenotype are impaired in proliferation in human autoimmune disease accounting for their reduced numbers and function.[85] Studies of IL-2 and IL-2 receptor knockout mice have shown that these mice develop severe spontaneous autoimmune disease and succumb to lymphoproliferative disease.[86] A deficiency of Tregs in these mice is thought to account for the unchecked proliferation of lymphocytes, leading to lymphadenopathy.[87]

Whereas IL-2 production is reduced and is protective for autoimmunity, it also has been ascribed a pro-inflammatory role in selective target tissues, rendering its role in disease complicated.[88] IL-2 knockout and FoxP3-deficient scurfy mice both develop multi-organ inflammation, but the IL-2 knockout mice do not develop skin and lung inflammation. It was shown that IL-2 controls the migration and localization of both Th1 and Th2 CD4 T cells in an organ-specific manner. IL-2-deficient mice demonstrated a lack of trafficking receptors and Th2 cytokines (IL-4, IL-5, IL-13) important for skin and lung inflammation, revealing a target organ-specific pro-inflammatory role for IL-2.

IL-2 gene expression is controlled mainly at the transcriptional and post-transcriptional levels. Transcription factors NFAT, AP1, and NF-κB, among others, are key factors that bind to cognate sites within the *IL-2* promoter (Figure 5). Upon T cell activation, TCR signalling induces intracellular signalling cascades that ultimately lead to the translocation of NFAT and NF-κB into the nucleus and initiate transcription of *IL-2*. In SLE T cells, reduced amounts and activity of NF-κB and AP1 are thought to contribute to lower *IL-2* expression. Whereas NFAT is increased in SLE T cells, hence activating CD40L expression, NFAT in conjunction with AP1 is necessary for *IL-2* transcriptional activation.[89] Therefore, the lack of AP1 is important in the *IL-2* defect. A role for SRSF1, an RNA binding protein, was recently identified in *IL-2* production by indirectly activating IL-2 transcription. SRSF1 expression was reduced in patients with SLE, more so in patients

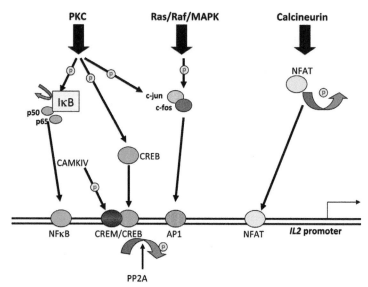

Figure 5 Signalling pathways and transcription factors involved in IL-2 production in T cells.

with active disease. Interestingly, forced expression of SRSF1 into SLE T cells rescued IL-2 production.[90] In addition to these factors, a balance between the transcription factors CREM and CREB is important in IL-2 regulation. Both factors compete for binding to a cAMP response element site at the –180 position within the *IL-2* promoter. In SLE T cells, disruption of this balance is thought to contribute to the reduced IL-2 expression. Protein kinase A phosphorylates and PP2A dephosphorylates CREB. Reduced activity of protein kinase A and increased expression of PP2A leads to reduced availability of pCREB. Increased expression of CREM is attributed to the increase in transcription mediated by the SP1 transcription factor and binding to the *CREM* promoter. CREM is phosphorylated by the calcium-regulated kinase CAMKIV. CAMKIV is increased in SLE T cells, and therefore increased pCREM leads to *IL-2* repression. Serum from patients with SLE induced the increased binding of CREM to the *IL-2* promoter through activation of CAMKIV,[91] and T cells from MRL/lpr lupus-prone mice also showed increased levels of CAMKIV. CAMKIV inhibitor treatment was able to prevent and correct autoimmunity and disease pathology in lupus-prone mice.[92]

6.2 IL-17

IL-17 (IL-17A, IL-17F) is a pro-inflammatory cytokine that is essential for host defence against bacteria and fungi. Its importance in autoimmune disease pathogenesis was recently uncovered in both human patients and animal models. IL-17 is produced by a subset of activated CD4 T cells under inflammatory conditions. Increased levels of IL-17 in the serum and increased numbers of IL-17-producing cells were demonstrated in patients with SLE. Increased IL-17 was found in target organs such as skin, lungs kidneys, indicating the role of IL-17 in local tissue damage. Patients with lupus nephritis had increased numbers of IL-17-producing double-negative T cells in the kidneys.[93] Increased expression also was noted in muscle tissue from patients with autoimmune myositis.[85] IL-17 recently has emerged as an important driver of pathogenic inflammation and is considered a key underlying element in the pathogenesis of autoimmune diseases such as SLE, multiple sclerosis and others.

IL-17 gene transcription is controlled by the RORγt and RORα transcription factors. RORγt drives differentiation of Th17 cells and is exclusively expressed by them. IL-17 is thought to be the key cytokine mediating inflammation, as demonstrated in numerous autoimmune diseases including SLE and multiple sclerosis . In addition to its role in inflammation, it also affects other cell types such as B cells. When treated with IL-17, PBMCs from patients with lupus nephritis produced increased amounts of double stranded DNA autoantibodies and IL-6, suggesting the role of IL-17 in B cell regulation. When stimulated under pro-inflammatory conditions, CD4 T cells, including cytokines IL-6, IL-23, IL-21, and TGF-β, differentiate into the Th17 phenotype and produce IL-17. IL-21 is necessary to initiate IL-17 production, whereas IL-23 is required to maintain IL-17. An IL-23 receptor deficiency lowered IL-17 production in lupus-prone mice; more important, these mice were protected from the development of disease.[94] IL-6, IL-21, and IL-23 bind to their respective receptors and, through the JAK–signal activator and transducer (STAT) signalling pathway, activate the same transcription factor, STAT3, which can directly bind to the *IL-17* and *IL-21* genes. T cells from patients with SLE were found to have increased STAT3 activity. This also was associated with their enhanced capacity for chemokine-mediated migration.[83]

6.3 IL-6

IL-6 is a pleiotropic cytokine secreted by a large variety of cells and mediates its effects through activation and differentiation of immune cells including

T and B lymphocytes.[95] IL-6 exerts its effects on target cells via the IL-6 receptor, which has two components: the 80-kDa IL-6R α chain, which is the IL-6 binding chain, and the IL-6R β chain (glycoprotein 130), which is the signal transducing chain. The pathogenic role of IL-6 has been demonstrated in both human SLE and murine lupus disease. IL-6-deficient MRL/lpr mice show delayed disease development and reduced renal pathology, including immunoglobulin G and C3 complement deposition.[96] In pristane-induced lupus, IL-6-deficient mice showed less-severe kidney disease and reduced levels of autoantibodies.[97] In other mice models such as BWF mice, administration of IL-6 increases, but blocking IL-6 reduces, the production of anti-DNA autoantibodies. In addition, an acceleration of renal pathology, increased expression of MHC class II on mesangial cells and increased expression of glomerular ICAM-1 was observed in female BWF mice administered the human IL-6 cytokine. As in mice, elevated levels of IL-6 have been observed in patients with SLE and have been shown to correlate variably with disease severity or anti–double strand DNA autoantibodies. Increased numbers of IL-6-producing cells in the PBMCs of patients with SLE correlates with disease severity; autoreactive T cell clones from patients produce large amounts of IL-6, which in turn mediates effects on B cells. IL-6 is known to promote B cell activation and autoantibody production in SLE, as evidenced by exogenous administration of IL-6 as well as by neutralizing antibodies.[98]

6.4 TNF-α

TNF-α is secreted by activated macrophages and other immune cells including monocytes and T cells. TNF-α mediates its effects through two distinct receptors—TNFR1 (p55) and TNFR2 (p75)—and can induce either pro-inflammatory or anti-inflammatory pathways, depending on receptor engagement. Through the TNF receptor 1, apoptosis and anti-inflammatory pathways are triggered via the Fas-associated death domain and caspase cascade.[95] Alternatively, recruitment of TNF receptor-associated factor 2 is pro-inflammatory via activation of NF-κB and JNK and MAPK pathways. These pathways also are activated when TNF-α engages TNF receptor 2. The effects of these opposing functions of TNF-α—as a pro-inflammatory or an immunoregulatory cytokine—have been demonstrated in autoimmune disease as well. Many studies have shown the pathogenic role of TNF-α in mice. MRL/lpr mice were found to have increased TNF-α levels in serum and in kidneys, which correlated with disease,[99,100] and TNF blockade treatment proved advantageous in this mouse strain. Anti-TNF treatment also led to reduced development of autoantibodies, proteinuria and immuno-globulin G deposition in the kidneys of lupus-prone mice.[101,102] On the other hand, TNF-α-deficient SLE mice showed exacerbated disease, and recombinant TNF-α administration in BWF mice was beneficial. These contradictory roles of TNF-α in disease reflect the dual function of this cytokine in pro- and anti-inflammatory processes. Similar to the studies in mice, data from human studies are complicated. While some studies found elevated levels of TNF-α in serum and disease correlation in patients with SLE, others did not.[103,104] In addition to the circulating TNF-α, tissue-specific cytokine expression may contribute locally to tissue pathology in SLE. Increased expression of the TNF-α gene and protein was demonstrated in kidney biopsies from 52% of patients with lupus nephritis.[105] Reduced expression of TNF adaptor proteins—TNF receptor-associated factor 2, TNF receptor 1–associated DEATH domain, Fas-associated death domain and receptor interacting protein 1—in PBMCs from patients with SLE may contribute to the anti-apoptotic effects and increased survival of autoreactive cells,[106] whereas increased expression of these adaptor proteins was found in kidneys from patients with lupus nephritis,[107] which may account for the local inflammatory effect of TNF-α. Thus the systemic and local effects of TNF-α may be uncoupled via the distinct actions on TNF receptors and adaptor molecules such that it has a systemic immune modulatory function and a local pro-inflammatory effect.

REFERENCES

1. Tsokos GC. Systemic lupus erythematosus. *N Engl J Med* 2011;**365**(22):2110–21.
2. Moulton VR, Tsokos GC. Abnormalities of T cell signaling in systemic lupus erythematosus. *Arthritis Res Ther* 2011;**13**(2):207.
3. Lahita RG. Gender and age in lupus. In: Lahita RG, editor. *Systemic Lupus Erythematosus.* 5th ed. Elsevier: Philadelphia, PA, USA, 2011. p. 405–23.
4. Cunningham M, Gilkeson G. Estrogen receptors in immunity and autoimmunity. *Clin Rev Allergy Immunol* 2011;**40**(1):66–73.
5. Bynote KK, Hackenberg JM, Korach KS, Lubahn DB, Lane PH, Gould KA. Estrogen receptor-alpha deficiency attenuates autoimmune disease in (NZB x NZW)F1 mice. *Genes Immun* 2008;**9**(2):137–52.
6. Svenson JL, EuDaly J, Ruiz P, Korach KS, Gilkeson GS. Impact of estrogen receptor deficiency on disease expression in the NZM2410 lupus prone mouse. *Clinical Immun* 2008;**128**(2):259–68.
7. Rider V, Jones S, Evans M, Bassiri H, Afsar Z, Abdou NI. Estrogen increases CD40 ligand expression in T cells from women with systemic lupus erythematosus. *J Rheumatol* 2001;**28**(12):2644–9.

8. Moulton VR, Holcomb DR, Zajdel MC, Tsokos GC. Estrogen upregulates cyclic AMP response element modulator alpha expression and downregulates interleukin-2 production by human T lymphocytes. *Mol Med* 2012;**18**:370–8 [Research Support, N.I.H., Extramural Research Support, Non-U.S. Gov't].

9. Pung OJ, Tucker AN, Vore SJ, Luster MI. Influence of estrogen on host resistance: increased susceptibility of mice to Listeria monocytogenes correlates with depressed production of interleukin 2. *Infect Immun* 1985;**50**(1):91–6.

10. Khan D, Dai R, Karpuzoglu E, Ahmed SA. Estrogen increases, whereas IL-27 and IFN-gamma decrease, splenocyte IL-17 production in WT mice. *Eur J Immunol* 2010;**40**(9):2549–56.

11. Kim WU, Min SY, Hwang SH, Yoo SA, Kim KJ, Cho CS. Effect of estrogen on T cell apoptosis in patients with systemic lupus erythematosus. *Clin Exp Immunol* 2010;**161**(3):453–8.

12. Rider V, Jones SR, Evans M, Abdou NI. Molecular mechanisms involved in the estrogen-dependent regulation of calcineurin in systemic lupus erythematosus T cells. *Clinical Immun* 2000;**95**(2):124–34.

13. Vista ES, Farris AD, James JA. Role for infections in systemic lupus erythematosus pathogenesis. In: Lahita RG, editor. *Systemic Lupus Erythematosus*. 5th ed. Elsevier: Philadelphia, PA, USA, 2011. p. 425–35.

14. Gross AJ, Hochberg D, Rand WM, Thorley-Lawson DA. EBV and systemic lupus erythematosus: a new perspective. *J Immunol* 2005;**174**(11):6599–607 [Comparative Study Research Support, N.I.H., Extramural Research Support, Non-U.S. Gov't Research Support, U.S. Gov't, P.H.S.].

15. Smith-Garvin JE, Koretzky GA, Jordan MS. T cell activation. *Ann Rev Immunol* 2009;**27**:591–619 [Review].

16. Brownlie RJ, Zamoyska R. T cell receptor signalling networks: branched, diversified and bounded. *Nat Rev Immunol* 2013;**13**(4):257–69 [Research Support, Non-U.S. Gov't Review].

17. Call ME, Pyrdol J, Wiedmann M, Wucherpfennig KW. The organizing principle in the formation of the T cell receptor-CD3 complex. *Cell* 2002;**111**(7):967–79 [Research Support, U.S. Gov't, P.H.S.].

18. Abram CL, Lowell CA. The expanding role for ITAM-based signaling pathways in immune cells. *Sci STKE* 2007;**2007**(377):re2 [Review].

19. Palacios EH, Weiss A. Function of the Src-family kinases, Lck and Fyn, in T-cell development and activation. *Oncogene* 2004;**23**(48):7990–8000.

20. Salmond RJ, Filby A, Qureshi I, Caserta S, Zamoyska R. T-cell receptor proximal signaling via the Src-family kinases, Lck and Fyn, influences T-cell activation, differentiation, and tolerance. *Immunol Rev* 2009;**228**(1):9–22 [Research Support, Non-U.S. Gov't Review].

21. Parsons SJ, Parsons JT. Src family kinases, key regulators of signal transduction. *Oncogene* 2004;**23**(48):7906–9 [Review].

22. Deindl S, Kadlecek TA, Brdicka T, Cao X, Weiss A, Kuriyan J. Structural basis for the inhibition of tyrosine kinase activity of ZAP-70. *Cell* 2007;**129**(4):735–46.

23. Finco TS, Kadlecek T, Zhang W, Samelson LE, Weiss A. LAT is required for TCR-mediated activation of PLCgamma1 and the Ras pathway. *Immunity* 1998;**9**(5):617–26 [Research Support, U.S. Gov't, P.H.S.].

24. Zhang W, Sommers CL, Burshtyn DN, Stebbins CC, DeJarnette JB, Trible RP, et al. Essential role of LAT in T cell development. *Immunity* 1999;**10**(3):323–32 [Research Support, Non-U.S. Gov't].

25. Dustin ML, Cooper JA. The immunological synapse and the actin cytoskeleton: molecular hardware for T cell signaling. *Nat Immunol* 2000;**1**(1):23–9 [Research Support, U.S. Gov't, P.H.S. Review].

26. Burbach BJ, Medeiros RB, Mueller KL, Shimizu Y. T-cell receptor signaling to integrins. *Immunol Rev* 2007;**218**:65–81 [Research Support, N.I.H., Extramural Research Support, Non-U.S. Gov't Review].

27. Crispin JC, Kyttaris VC, Juang YT, Tsokos GC. How signaling and gene transcription aberrations dictate the systemic lupus erythematosus T cell phenotype. *Trends Immunol* 2008;**29**(3):110–5 [Research Support, N.I.H., Extramural Review].

28. Jury EC, Kabouridis PS, Flores-Borja F, Mageed RA, Isenberg DA. Altered lipid raft-associated signaling and ganglioside expression in T lymphocytes from patients with systemic lupus erythematosus. *J Clinical Invest* 2004;**113**(8):1176–87.

29. Krishnan S, Nambiar MP, Warke VG, Fisher CU, Mitchell J, Delaney N, et al. Alterations in lipid raft composition and dynamics contribute to abnormal T cell responses in systemic lupus erythematosus. *J Immunol* 2004;**172**(12):7821–31.

30. Deng GM, Tsokos GC. Cholera toxin B accelerates disease progression in lupus-prone mice by promoting lipid raft aggregation. *J Immunol* 2008;**181**(6):4019–26 [Research Support, N.I.H., Extramural].

31. Liossis SN, Ding XZ, Dennis GJ, Tsokos GC. Altered pattern of TCR/CD3-mediated protein-tyrosyl phosphorylation in T cells from patients with systemic lupus erythematosus. Deficient expression of the T cell receptor zeta chain. *J Clinical Invest* 1998;**101**(7):1448–57.

32. Enyedy EJ, Nambiar MP, Liossis SN, Dennis G, Kammer GM, Tsokos GC. Fc epsilon receptor type I gamma chain replaces the deficient T cell receptor zeta chain in T cells of patients with systemic lupus erythematosus. *Arthritis Rheumatism* 2001;**44**(5):1114–21.

33. Krishnan S, Juang YT, Chowdhury B, Magilavy A, Fisher CU, Nguyen H, et al. Differential expression and molecular associations of Syk in systemic lupus erythematosus T cells. *J Immunol* 2008;**181**(11):8145–52.

34. Nambiar MP, Fisher CU, Warke VG, Krishnan S, Mitchell JP, Delaney N, et al. Reconstitution of deficient T cell receptor zeta chain restores T cell signaling and augments T cell receptor/CD3-induced interleukin-2 production in patients with systemic lupus erythematosus. *Arthritis Rheumatism* 2003;**48**(7):1948–55.

35. Yasuda S, Stevens RL, Terada T, Takeda M, Hashimoto T, Fukae J, et al. Defective expression of Ras guanyl nucleotide-releasing protein 1 in a subset of patients with systemic lupus erythematosus. *J Immunol* 2007;**179**(7):4890–900 [Research Support, N.I. H., Extramural Research Support, Non-U.S. Gov't].

36. Gorelik G, Fang JY, Wu A, Sawalha AH, Richardson B. Impaired T cell protein kinase C delta activation decreases ERK pathway signaling in idiopathic and hydralazine-induced lupus. *J Immunol* 2007;**179**(8):5553–63 [Research Support, N.I.H., Extramural Research Support, U.S. Gov't, Non-P.H.S.].

37. Oelke K, Lu Q, Richardson D, Wu A, Deng C, Hanash S, et al. Overexpression of CD70 and overstimulation of IgG synthesis by lupus T cells and T cells treated with DNA methylation inhibitors. *Arthritis Rheumatism* 2004;**50**(6):1850–60 [Research Support, Non-U.S. Gov't Research Support, U.S. Gov't, Non-P.H.S. Research Support, U.S. Gov't, P.H.S.].

38. Sunahori K, Nagpal K, Hedrich CM, Mizui M, Fitzgerald LM, Tsokos GC. The catalytic subunit of protein phosphatase 2A (PP2Ac) promotes DNA hypomethylation by suppressing the phosphorylated mitogen-activated protein kinase/extracellular signal-regulated kinase (ERK) kinase (MEK)/phosphorylated ERK/DNMT1 protein pathway in T-cells from controls and systemic lupus erythematosus patients. *J Biol Chem* 2013;**288**(30):21936–44.

39. Richardson B. DNA methylation and autoimmune disease. *Clinical Immun* 2003;**109**(1):72–9 [In Vitro Research Support, U.S. Gov't, P.H.S. Review].

40. Fernandez D, Perl A. mTOR signaling: a central pathway to pathogenesis in systemic lupus erythematosus? *Discov Med* 2010;**9**(46):173–8.

41. Fernandez D, Perl A. Metabolic control of T cell activation and death in SLE. *Autoimmunity Rev* 2009;**8**(3):184–9.

42. Emlen W, Niebur J, Kadera R. Accelerated in vitro apoptosis of lymphocytes from patients with systemic lupus erythematosus. *J Immunol* 1994;**152**(7):3685–92 [Research Support, Non-U.S. Gov't].

43. Gergely Jr. P, Grossman C, Niland B, Puskas F, Neupane H, Allam F, et al. Mitochondrial hyperpolarization and ATP depletion in patients with systemic lupus erythematosus. *Arthritis Rheumatism* 2002;**46**(1):175–90 [Research Support, Non-U.S. Gov't Research Support, U.S. Gov't, P.H.S.].

44. Gergely Jr. P, Niland B, Gonchoroff N, Pullmann Jr. R, Phillips PE, Perl A. Persistent mitochondrial hyperpolarization, increased reactive oxygen intermediate production, and cytoplasmic alkalinization characterize altered IL-10 signaling in patients with systemic lupus erythematosus. *J Immunol* 2002;**169**(2):1092–101 [Research Support, Non-U.S. Gov't Research Support, U.S. Gov't, P.H.S.].

45. Juang YT, Tenbrock K, Nambiar MP, Gourley MF, Tsokos GC. Defective production of functional 98-kDa form of Elf-1 is responsible for the decreased expression of TCR zeta-chain in patients with systemic lupus erythematosus. *J Immunol* 2002;**169**(10):6048–55.

46. Juang YT, Sumibcay L, Tolnay M, Wang Y, Kyttaris VC, Tsokos GC. Elf-1 binds to GGAA elements on the FcRgamma promoter and represses its expression. *J Immunol* 2007;**179**(7):4884–9.

47. Kyttaris VC, Wang Y, Juang YT, Weinstein A, Tsokos GC. CAMP response element modulator a expression in patients with systemic lupus erythematosus. *Lupus* 2006;**15**(12):840–4.

48. Katsiari CG, Kyttaris VC, Juang YT, Tsokos GC. Protein phosphatase 2A is a negative regulator of IL-2 production in patients with systemic lupus erythematosus. *J Clinical Invest* 2005;**115**(11):3193–204.

49. Tenbrock K, Juang YT, Tolnay M, Tsokos GC. The cyclic adenosine 5'-monophosphate response element modulator suppresses IL-2 production in stimulated T cells by a chromatin-dependent mechanism. *J Immunol* 2003;**170**(6):2971–6.

50. Ballestar E. An introduction to epigenetics. *Adv Exp Med Biol* 2011;**711**:1–11 [Research Support, Non-U.S. Gov't Review].

51. Hedrich CM, Tsokos GC. Epigenetic mechanisms in systemic lupus erythematosus and other autoimmune diseases. *Trends Mol Med* 2011;**17**(12):714–24 [Research Support, N.I.H., Extramural Review].

52. Renaudineau Y, Youinou P. Epigenetics and autoimmunity, with special emphasis on methylation. *Keio J Med* 2011;**60**(1):10–16 [Review].

53. Stevens MM, Scribano PV, Gorelick MH. Screening for poor short-term outcome in acute pediatric asthma. *Ann Allergy Asthma Immunol* 2007;**98**(5):432–9 [Research Support, U.S. Gov't, P.H.S.].

54. Lu Q, Kaplan M, Ray D, Zacharek S, Gutsch D, Richardson B. Demethylation of ITGAL (CD11a) regulatory sequences in systemic lupus erythematosus. *Arthritis Rheumatism* 2002;**46**(5):1282–91 [Research Support, Non-U.S. Gov't Research Support, U.S. Gov't, Non-P.H.S. Research Support, U.S. Gov't, P.H.S.].

55. Sunahori K, Juang YT, Tsokos GC. Methylation status of CpG islands flanking a cAMP response element motif on the protein phosphatase 2Ac alpha promoter determines CREB binding and activity. *J Immunol* 2009;**182**(3):1500–8.

56. Sunahori K, Juang YT, Kyttaris VC, Tsokos GC. Promoter hypomethylation results in increased expression of protein phosphatase 2A in T cells from patients with systemic lupus erythematosus. *J Immunol* 2011;**186**(7):4508–17 [Comparative Study Research Support, N.I.H., Extramural Research Support, Non-U.S. Gov't].

57. Dieker J, Muller S. Epigenetic histone code and autoimmunity. *Clinical Rev Allergy Immunol* 2010;**39**(1):78–84 [Research Support, Non-U.S. Gov't Review].

58. Tenbrock K, Juang YT, Leukert N, Roth J, Tsokos GC. The transcriptional repressor cAMP response element modulator alpha interacts with histone deacetylase 1 to repress promoter activity. *J Immunol* 2006;**177**(9):6159–64 [Research Support, N.I.H., Extramural Research Support, Non-U.S. Gov't].

59. Moulton VR, Kyttaris VC, Juang YT, Chowdhury B, Tsokos GC. The RNA-stabilizing protein HuR regulates the expression of zeta chain of the human T cell receptor-associated CD3 complex. *J Biol Chem* 2008;**283**(29):20037–44.

60. Chowdhury B, Tsokos CG, Krishnan S, Robertson J, Fisher CU, Warke RG, et al. Decreased stability and translation of T cell receptor zeta mRNA with an alternatively spliced 3'-untranslated region contribute to zeta chain down-regulation in patients with systemic lupus erythematosus. *J Biol Chem* 2005;**280**(19):18959–66.

61. Moulton VR, Tsokos GC. Alternative splicing factor/splicing factor 2 regulates the expression of the zeta subunit of the human T cell receptor-associated CD3 complex. *J Biol Chem* 2010;**285**(17):12490–6.

62. Crispin JC, Keenan BT, Finnell MD, Bermas BL, Schur P, Massarotti E, et al. Expression of CD44 variant isoforms CD44v3 and CD44v6 is increased on T cells from patients with systemic lupus erythematosus and is correlated with disease activity. *Arthritis Rheumatism* 2010;**62**(5):1431–7.

63. Tenbrock K, Juang YT, Gourley MF, Nambiar MP, Tsokos GC. Antisense cyclic adenosine 5'-monophosphate response element modulator up-regulates IL-2 in T cells from patients with systemic lupus erythematosus. *J Immunol* 2002;**169**(8):4147–52.

64. Riha P, Rudd CE. CD28 co-signaling in the adaptive immune response. *Self Nonself* 2010;**1**(3):231–40.

65. Bour-Jordan H, Esensten JH, Martinez-Llordella M, Penaranda C, Stumpf M, Bluestone JA. Intrinsic and extrinsic control of peripheral T-cell tolerance by costimulatory molecules of the CD28/ B7 family. *Immunol Rev* 2011;**241**(1):180–205 [Research Support, N.I.H., Extramural Research Support, Non-U.S. Gov't Review].

66. Finck BK, Linsley PS, Wofsy D. Treatment of murine lupus with CTLA4Ig. *Science* 1994;**265**(5176):1225–7 [Research Support, U.S. Gov't, Non-P.H.S.].

67. Davidson A, Diamond B, Wofsy D, Daikh D. Block and tackle: CTLA4Ig takes on lupus. *Lupus* 2005;**14**(3):197–203 [Review].

68. Aicher A, Hayden-Ledbetter M, Brady WA, Pezzutto A, Richter G, Magaletti D, et al. Characterization of human inducible costimulator ligand expression and function. *J Immunol* 2000;**164**(9):4689–96 [Research Support, Non-U.S. Gov't Research Support, U.S. Gov't, P.H.S.].

69. Ruth JH, Rottman JB, Kingsbury GA, Coyle AJ, Haines 3rd. GK, Pope RM, et al. ICOS and B7 costimulatory molecule expression identifies activated cellular subsets in rheumatoid arthritis. *Cytometry A* 2007;**71**(5):317–26.

70. Karmann K, Hughes CC, Schechner J, Fanslow WC, Pober JS. CD40 on human endothelial cells: inducibility by cytokines and functional regulation of adhesion molecule expression. *Proc Natl Acad Sci USA* 1995;**92**(10):4342–6 [Research Support, Non-U. S. Gov't Research Support, U.S. Gov't, P.H.S.].

71. Van Gool SW, Vandenberghe P, de Boer M, Ceuppens JL. CD80, CD86 and CD40 provide accessory signals in a multiple-step T-cell activation model. *Immunol Rev* 1996;**153**:47–83 [Research Support, Non-U.S. Gov't Review].

72. Liu MF, Chao SC, Wang CR, Lei HY. Expression of CD40 and CD40 ligand among cell populations within rheumatoid synovial compartment. *Autoimmunity* 2001;**34** (2):107–13 [Research Support, Non-U.S. Gov't].

73. Katsiari CG, Liossis SN, Dimopoulos AM, Charalambopoulo DV, Mavrikakis M, Sfikakis PP. CD40L overexpression on T cells and monocytes from patients with systemic lupus erythematosus is resistant to calcineurin inhibition. *Lupus* 2002;**11** (6):370–8.

74. Early GS, Zhao W, Burns CM. Anti-CD40 ligand antibody treatment prevents the development of lupus-like nephritis in a subset of New Zealand black x New Zealand white mice. Response correlates with the absence of an anti-antibody response. *J Immunol* 1996;**157**(7):3159–64 [Research Support, Non-U.S. Gov't].

75. Crispin JC, Hedrich CM, Tsokos GC. Gene-function studies in systemic lupus erythematosus. *Nat Rev Rheumatol* 2013;**9**(8):476–84 [Research Support, N.I.H., Extramural Research Support, Non-U.S. Gov't].

76. Cannons JL, Tangye SG, Schwartzberg PL. SLAM family receptors and SAP adaptors in immunity. *Ann Rev Immunol* 2011;**29**:665–705 [Review].

77. Detre C, Keszei M, Romero X, Tsokos GC, Terhorst C. SLAM family receptors and the SLAM-associated protein (SAP) modulate T cell functions. *Seminars Immunopathol* 2010;**32**(2):157–71 [Research Support, N.I.H., Extramural Research Support, Non-U.S. Gov't Review].

78. Tsao BP. An update on genetic studies of systemic lupus erythematosus. *Current Rheumatol Rep* 2002;**4**(4) [Research Support, Non-U.S. Gov't Research Support, U.S. Gov't, P.H.S. Review].

79. Shai R, Quismorio Jr. FP, Li L, Kwon OJ, Morrison J, Wallace DJ, et al. Genome-wide screen for systemic lupus erythematosus susceptibility genes in multiplex families. *Hum Mol Genet* 1999;**8**(4):639–44 [Research Support, U.S. Gov't, P.H.S.].

80. Chatterjee M, Rauen T, Kis-Toth K, Kyttaris VC, Hedrich CM, Terhorst C, et al. Increased expression of SLAM receptors SLAMF3 and SLAMF6 in systemic lupus erythematosus T lymphocytes promotes Th17 differentiation. *J Immunol* 2012;**188**(3):1206–12 [Research Support, N.I.H., Extramural Research Support, Non-U.S. Gov't].

81. Li Y, Harada T, Juang YT, Kyttaris VC, Wang Y, Zidanic M, et al. Phosphorylated ERM is responsible for increased T cell polarization, adhesion, and migration in patients with systemic lupus erythematosus. *J Immunol* 2007;**178**(3):1938–47.

82. Estess P, DeGrendele HC, Pascual V, Siegelman MH. Functional activation of lymphocyte CD44 in peripheral blood is a marker of autoimmune disease activity. *J Clinical Invest* 1998;**102**(6):1173–82 [Research Support, Non-U.S. Gov't Research Support, U.S. Gov't, P.H.S.].

83. Apostolidis SA, Lieberman LA, Kis-Toth K, Crispin JC, Tsokos GC. The dysregulation of cytokine networks in systemic lupus erythematosus. *J Interferon Cytokine Res* 2011;**31**(10):769–79 [Research Support, N.I.H., Extramural Review].

84. Korn T, Bettelli E, Oukka M, Kuchroo VK. IL-17 and Th17 cells. *Ann Rev Immunol* 2009;**27**:485–517 [Research Support, Non-U.S. Gov't Review].

85. Wahren-Herlenius M, Dorner T. Immunopathogenic mechanisms of systemic autoimmune disease. *Lancet* 2013;**382**(9894):819–31 [Research Support, Non-U.S. Gov't Review].

86. Ma A, Koka R, Burkett P. Diverse functions of IL-2, IL-15, and IL-7 in lymphoid homeostasis. *Ann Rev Immunol* 2006;**24**:657–79 [Research Support, N.I.H., Extramural Review].

87. Setoguchi R, Hori S, Takahashi T, Sakaguchi S. Homeostatic maintenance of natural Foxp3(+) CD25(+) CD4(+) regulatory T cells by interleukin (IL)-2 and induction of autoimmune disease by IL-2 neutralization. *J Exp Med* 2005;**201**(5):723–35 [Research Support, Non-U.S. Gov't].

88. Ju ST, Sharma R, Gaskin F, Fu SM, Ju ST, Sharma R, et al. IL-2 controls trafficking receptor gene expression and Th2 response for skin and lung inflammation. *Clinical Immunol* 2012;**145**(1):82–8 [Research Support, N.I.H., Extramural Research Support, Non-U.S. Gov't Review].

89. Kyttaris VC, Wang Y, Juang YT, Weinstein A, Tsokos GC. Increased levels of NF-ATc2 differentially regulate CD154 and IL-2 Genes in T cells from patients with systemic lupus erythematosus. *J Immunol* 2007;**178**(3):1960–6.

90. Moulton VR, Grammatikos AP, Fitzgerald LM, Tsokos GC. Splicing factor SF2/ASF rescues IL-2 production in T cells from systemic lupus erythematosus patients by activating IL-2 transcription. *Proc Natl Acad Sci U S A* 2013;**110**(5):1845–50.

91. Juang YT, Wang Y, Solomou EE, Li Y, Mawrin C, Tenbrock K, et al. Systemic lupus erythematosus serum IgG increases CREM binding to the IL-2 promoter and suppresses IL-2 production through CaMKIV. *J Clinical Invest* 2005;**115**(4):996–1005.

92. Ichinose K, Juang YT, Crispin JC, Kis-Toth K, Tsokos GC. Suppression of autoimmunity and organ pathology in lupus-prone mice upon inhibition of calcium/calmodulin-dependent protein kinase type IV. *Arthritis Rheumatism* 2011;**63**(2):523–9 [Research Support, N.I.H., Extramural].

93. Crispin JC, Oukka M, Bayliss G, Cohen RA, Van Beek CA, Stillman IE, et al. Expanded double negative T cells in patients with systemic lupus erythematosus produce IL-17 and infiltrate the kidneys. *J Immunol* 2008;**181**(12):8761–6.

94. Kyttaris VC, Zhang Z, Kuchroo VK, Oukka M, Tsokos GC. Cutting edge: IL-23 receptor deficiency prevents the development of lupus nephritis in C57BL/6-lpr/lpr mice. *J Immunol* 2010;**184**(9):4605–9.

95. Jacob N, Stohl W. Cytokine disturbances in systemic lupus erythematosus. *Arthritis Res Therapy* 2011;**13**(4):228 [Research Support, N.I.H., Extramural Review].

96. Cash H, Relle M, Menke J, Brochhausen C, Jones SA, Topley N, et al. Interleukin 6 (IL-6) deficiency delays lupus nephritis in MRL-Faslpr mice: the IL-6 pathway as a new therapeutic target in treatment of autoimmune kidney disease in systemic lupus erythematosus. *J Rheumatol* 2010;**37**(1):60–70 [Research Support, Non-U.S. Gov't].

97. Richards HB, Satoh M, Shaw M, Libert C, Poli V, Reeves WH. Interleukin 6 dependence of anti-DNA antibody production: evidence for two pathways of autoantibody formation in pristane-induced lupus. *J Exp Med* 1998;**188**(5):985–90 [Research Support, Non-U.S. Gov't Research Support, U.S. Gov't, P.H.S.].

98. Linker-Israeli M, Deans RJ, Wallace DJ, Prehn J, Ozeri-Chen T, Klinenberg JR. Elevated levels of endogenous IL-6 in systemic lupus erythematosus. A putative role in pathogenesis. *J Immunol* 1991;**147**(1):117–23.

99. Boswell JM, Yui MA, Burt DW, Kelley VE. Increased tumor necrosis factor and IL-1 beta gene expression in the kidneys of mice with lupus nephritis. *J Immunol* 1988;**141** (9):3050–4 [Research Support, Non-U.S. Gov't Research Support, U.S. Gov't, P.H.S.].

100. Yokoyama H, Kreft B, Kelley VR. Biphasic increase in circulating and renal TNF-alpha in MRL-lpr mice with differing regulatory mechanisms. *Kidney Int* 1995;**47** (1):122–30 [Comparative Study Research Support, Non-U.S. Gov't Research Support, U.S. Gov't, P.H.S.].

101. Edwards CK, Zhou T, Zhang J, Baker TJ, De M, Long RE, et al. Inhibition of superantigen-induced proinflammatory cytokine production and inflammatory arthritis in MRL-lpr/lpr mice by a transcriptional inhibitor of TNF-alpha. *J Immunol* 1996;**157**(4):1758–72 [Research Support, Non-U.S. Gov't Research Support, U.S. Gov't, P.H.S.].

102. Segal R, Dayan M, Zinger H, Mozes E. Suppression of experimental systemic lupus erythematosus (SLE) in mice via TNF inhibition by an anti-TNFalpha monoclonal antibody and by pentoxiphylline. *Lupus* 2001;**10**(1):23–31.

103. Gabay C, Cakir N, Moral F, Roux-Lombard P, Meyer O, Dayer JM, et al. Circulating levels of tumor necrosis factor soluble receptors in systemic lupus erythematosus are significantly higher than in other rheumatic diseases and correlate with disease activity. *J Rheumatol* 1997;**2**:303–8 [Comparative Study Research Support, Non-U.S. Gov't].

104. Gomez D, Correa PA, Gomez LM, Cadena J, Molina JF, Anaya JM. Th1/Th2 cytokines in patients with systemic lupus erythematosus: is tumor necrosis factor alpha protective? *Seminars Arthritis Rheumatism* 2004;**33**(6):404–13 [Research Support, Non-U.S. Gov't].

105. Herrera-Esparza R, Barbosa-Cisneros O, Villalobos-Hurtado R, Avalos-Diaz E. Renal expression of IL-6 and TNFalpha genes in lupus nephritis. *Lupus* 1998;**7**(3):154–8 [Research Support, Non-U.S. Gov't].

106. Zhu L, Yang X, Chen W, Li X, Ji Y, Mao H, et al. Decreased expressions of the TNF-alpha signaling adapters in peripheral blood mononuclear cells (PBMCs) are correlated with disease activity in patients with systemic lupus erythematosus. *Clin Rheumatol* 2007;**26**(9):1481–9 [Research Support, Non-U.S. Gov't].

107. Zhu L, Yang X, Ji Y, Chen W, Guan W, Zhou SF, et al. Up-regulated renal expression of TNF-alpha signalling adapter proteins in lupus glomerulonephritis. *Lupus* 2009;**18** (2):116–27 [Research Support, Non-U.S. Gov't].

CHAPTER 7

Lymphocytes and Infection in Autoimmune Diseases

Graziela Carvalheiras[*,1], Mariana Brandão[*], Vital Domingues[†],
Esmeralda Neves[*], Júlia Vasconcelos[*], Isabel Almeida[‡],
Carlos Vasconcelos[*]
[*]Internal Medicine Assistant in Medicine Service and Clinical Immunology Unit—Centro Hospitalar do Porto and Unit for Multidisciplinary Research in Biomedicine (UMIB/ICBAS)—Porto University, Portugal
[†]Internal Medicine Resident in Medicine Service—Centro Hospitalar do Porto, Portugal
[‡]Internal Medicine Senior Graduated Assistant in Medicine Service and Clinical Immunology Unit—Centro Hospitalar do Porto and Unit for Multidisciplinary Research in Biomedicine (UMIB/ICBAS)—Porto University, Portugal
[1]Corresponding Author: gcarvalheiras@gmail.com

1 INTRODUCTION

The paradigm of autoimmune diseases (AIDs) is complex and still poorly understood. The best scenery to characterize the immunopathology underlining autoimmunity is an intricate network of humoral and cellular interactions, where the boundaries between immune deregulation, hypersensitivity and immunodeficiency are unclear.

Lymphopenia is a frequent finding in AID and is one of the causes for the increased risk of infection. In many cases it is difficult to identify the best target and treatment to control lymphopenia because of its diverse etiology, where a reciprocal relationship of cause and effect may be observed.

Intensive research has been performed in recent years, but there are still few consensual recommendations to deal with lymphopenia and its related infections in AID, which reveals the complexity of this issue.

This chapter consists of a review of the current knowledge about lymphocytes and infection in AID and is particularly directed to the role and function of lymphocytes subsets and their relation to infection in pathologic autoimmunity. The main causes of lymphopenia and its management in preventing infection in AID is also described.

2 LYMPHOCYTES AND ITS SUBSETS IN AIDs

2.1 T-Cells in AIDs

T lymphocytes are key players in AID, with both regulatory and effector functions. The model proposed by Mossman and Coffman in 1986, which

Infection and Autoimmunity
http://dx.doi.org/10.1016/B978-0-444-63269-2.00015-5
109

classifies long-term effector $CD4^+$ T lymphocytes into Th1 and Th2 cells, with different polarized functional properties based on the ability for interferon-gamma (IFN-γ), interleukin (IL)-2, and tumor necrosis factor (TNF)-β or IL-4, IL-5, IL-10, and IL-13 production, proved to be incomplete.[1]

Further research showed that $CD4^+$ T-cells include a larger group of distinct cell populations. New effector lymphocytes subsets have been described, with different phenotypes, transcription factors, pattern of cytokines and functions, including Th9, Th17, Th22, and T follicular helper cells.

Advances were also observed concerning T lymphocytes with regulatory function, mostly resulting from studies in humans and animal models with AID.

The ability to control other cells' function, either through cytokine production or by cell contact-dependent mechanisms, is the main feature of regulatory T-cells (Tregs), a group that includes IL-10-secreting $CD4^+$ T regulatory-1 (Tr1) cells, TGF-β-secreting $CD4^+$ (Th3) cells, $CD8^+CD28/Foxp3^+$ cells, γ/δ TCR^+ cells, and $CD4^+/CD25^{high}/Foxp3^+$ cells, the last widely accepted as naturally occurring regulatory T-cells (nTregs).

The concept of immune deregulation is linked to autoimmunity and to the implicit imbalance between effector and Tregs. All of them have already been proved to participate in autoimmune reactions and their role and interactions are among the most studied subjects in the past years, particularly as they concern Th17 and nTregs in multisystem AID such as systemic lupus erythematosus (SLE).

$CD8^+$ lymphocytes are recognized as less important players in autoimmune pathology but have been strongly implicated in specific diseases such as multiple sclerosis, as effector cells that can directly damage central nervous system target cells, and in polymyosistis, where directed cytotoxic action of $CD8^+$ T-cells against muscle fibres is observed and considered the main mechanism for necrosis.

The dichotomy between different T lymphocytes subsets in autoimmunity is not complete.[2]

A new concept of cell plasticity that changes the image of these cells has emerged and has given even more complexity to the mechanisms of control and maintenance of immune homeostasis. The phenotype of effector T-cells is more flexible; they can have overlap phenotypes and functions and can interconvert from one subset to another, depending on multiple factors, including tissue microenvironment and cytokine network.[3]

2.2 B-Cells in AIDs

B lymphocytes are also important effector cells involved in abnormal autoimmune immunological responses.

They are particularly implicated in autoantibody production, with or without direct pathological effects, but they are also effective antigen-presenting cells and stimulate T lymphocytes though cytokine production and co-stimulatory molecules.

Some intrinsic defects related with B-cell development and maturation are connected with autoimmunity, including impaired negative selection, production of autoreactive immunoglobulins due to somatic hypermutation, overexpression or deficiency of molecules belonging to B-cell receptor signalling pathways, and increased survival of autoreactive B-cells controlled by the B-cell activation factor (BAFF), among others. Some of these defects may be the target for new therapeutic strategies.[4,5]

It has been recently recognized that, like T lymphocytes, the existence of regulatory B-cells with suppressor activity for cellular immune responses and inflammation are mostly mediated by IL-10 in a different setting.

2.3 Natural Killer Cells

Natural killer (NK) cells are implicated in the pathogenesis of AID, with both regulatory and inducer activity, even in the same disease.

They may be decreased in number, have deregulated production of cytokines or impaired cytotoxic function. Patients with active SLE display phenotypic and functional features associated with NK activation that has the capacity to produce large amounts of IFN-γ.

NK cells express many receptors that can be either inhibitors or activators. Aberrant expression of NK cell activation receptor ligands in inflamed tissues, which promote pro-inflammatory cytokine production by CD56[bright] NK cells, may be observed in some cases, and genetic studies have provided evidence that specific combinations of killer immunoglobulin-like receptors with some human leukocyte antigen genotypes may also favor activation of NK cells.[6,7]

NK cells can also prevent and limit adaptive autoimmune responses by killing autologous lymphoid cells.

2.4 NK T Cells

NK T-cells are a subset of T lymphocytes with important regulatory functions that control peripheral tolerance. They are capable of secreting large quantities of cytokines in a short period of time and can regulate B lymphocyte activity and function.

Changes in the number of invariant NK T-cells (iNKT) are associated with many autoimmune disorders in humans, such as SLE, psoriasis, rheumatoid arthritis, and myasthenia gravis. Reductions in the number and activity of iNKT cells have been observed in patients with SLE, suggesting its suppressive role.[8]

Therapeutic applications of NK T-cells have already been reported in type 1 diabetes, experimental autoimmune encephalomyelitis, SLE, scleroderma, rheumatoid arthritis, and Sjögren's syndrome.[9]

2.5 Lymphocytes Subsets and Infection in AIDs

Lymphocytes are central effector cells regarding the host defense against infection and other threats.

The relationship between altered immune function and infections have multiple effects, in which microbes can act not only as inductors or triggers but also as protectors, depending on the interactions between them and the host immune system.

Patients with AID are more susceptible to infection, due in part to the underlying immune deregulation and the chronicity of these disorders. Although the defective immune functions are not universal, humoral and cellular defects usually coexist.

Cellular immune defects are not restricted to lymphocytes, but T-cell lymphopenia is the most common quantitative disorder observed, particularly in patients with lupus. It is considered a major contributor for the increased risk of infection and also correlates with disease flares and immunosuppressive therapy, particularly $CD4^+$ T lymphopenia.

T-cell function can also be affected. $CD8^+$ T-cell deficiency is a general feature of chronic AID and may be an important factor linked to infection susceptibility.[10] It can also be observed in patients' healthy relatives, suggesting an underlying genetically determined defect.

Cytotoxic $CD8^+$ T-cells are considered of major importance for the control of Epstein–Barr virus infection, a major agent that can induce autoimmunity.[11]

B-cell functions are preserved in the majority of cases. Hypergammaglobulinemia is common in patients with Sjögren's syndrome, rheumatoid arthritis, and SLE. Antibody production and immunization responses are usually maintained, although in some cases a decreased primary humoral immune response and an altered recall of antigens may be observed.

During the course of the diseases, autoreactive activated B-cells can contribute, in an indirect way, to increasing patients' infection susceptibility, though the production of autoantibodies that can neutralize key components of the immune system that are essential in mounting antimicrobial responses.

One example is the development of neutralizing antibodies against cytokines or it receptors, affecting cellular functions and the clearance of pathogens.[12] NK cell number and function may be also affected in patients with AID, reducing the defence against intracellular bacteria and viruses, such as papilloma virus in patients with lupus.

3 CAUSES OF LYMPHOPENIA IN AIDs

The causes of lymphopenia in AIDs vary and can be the result of iatrogenic factors, congenital immunodeficiency disorders, infections, and the AID itself, among others. The reduction in the total number of circulating lymphocytes can be transient and a deficiency of a selective lymphocyte subpopulation may also occur (e.g. T-cells, B-cells, NK cells).

3.1 Autoimmune Diseases

Hematological involvement is common in AID, especially in SLE, where usually it is the third most frequent clinical manifestation, but it can be the most common.[13] It occurs more frequently with increasing age, seems to be more common in men[14] and its frequency varies among ethnic populations.[15]

The most typical feature of the hematological involvement in SLE is leukopenia and may occur primarily as a result of lymphopenia; it can, however, also result from neutropenia, or a combination of the two. T-cell lymphopenia, particularly $CD4^+$ T-cells, is frequently found in patients with SLE.[16–19] Studies demonstrate that lymphotoxic antibodies,[20–22] elevated serum concentrations of IFN-α,[23] and reduced surface expression of complement regulatory proteins CD55 and CD59[24,25] may be implicated in the pathogenesis of lymphopenia in SLE. However, it is difficult to determine whether lymphopenia is the cause or the consequence because peripheral blood cell counts can also reflect organ involvement of the underlying disease, systemic disease activity or immunosuppressive therapy.

Lymphopenia is associated with several clinical and immunologic manifestations, leading to diagnostic and prognostic implications of patients with SLE. In fact, the main clinical usefulness of lymphopenia in SLE is its inclusion as one of the hematologic criteria for SLE classification according to the American College of Rheumatology.[26] In addition, the degree of lymphopenia itself correlates and is one of the clinical parameters used to assess disease activity, such as those found in the Systemic Lupus Activity Measure, British Isles Lupus Assessment Group, and European Consensus Activity Measurement.[18,27–30] Lymphopenia was also found to predict flares,[29] to correlate with damage accrual[31] and to be predictive of decreased survival in SLE.[32] Several studies show lymphopenia to be associated with particular manifestations of SLE, such as arthritis, neuropsychiatric involvement, vasculitis, renal disease, and levels of anti-double-stranded DNA and anti-Ro antibodies.[31,33–36]

Lymphopenia also raises the propensity of patients to infectious diseases, in which we include several microorganisms, not necessarily opportunistic.[31,37,38] Related or not with lymphopenia, infections are a major cause of morbidity and mortality in patients with SLE.[39,40] The risk of infection is dependent on several immunological abnormalities associated with lymphopenia, including a decreased number of T-cells, $CD4^+$ T-cells, B-cells, and dendritic cells.[31,41–44] T-helper cell activity against viral antigens, toxoids, and alloantigens is impaired in patients with SLE, particularly in flares, and in patients long exposed to glucocorticoids.[45]

Lymphopenia is also commonly found in other AIDs such as Sjögren's syndrome, where it is more frequent in patients who are anti-SSA positive and comprises the patients group at risk for development of non-Hodgkin malignant lymphoma,[46–48] rheumatoid arthritis, diabetes mellitus, Crohn's disease, and primary vasculitis.[49,50]

In conclusion, lymphopenia is commonly manifested and may have serious clinical implications in patients with autoimmunity.

3.2 Primary Immunodeficiency Diseases

Primary immunodeficiencies (PIDs) are a heterogeneous group of diseases caused by defects in the development and maturation of immune cells. Defects can occur in the adaptative immune system with involvement of B- and/or T-cells and in the innate immune system.[51] PIDs are associated with increased susceptibility to infections, and the type of infection is determined by the immune cells affected.

Autoimmunity has long been known to be a part of the presenting symptoms and clinical course of many PIDs. Autoimmune manifestations are the second most common clinical manifestation apart from infections.[52] A significant proportion of patients presenting with an autoimmune condition have an underlying PID.[53] The association of PIDs and autoimmune conditions may imply diagnostic and therapeutic challenges for physicians.

The spectrum of severe combined immunodeficiencies (SCIDs) is very large. The most severe forms include a group of disorders that affected T, B, or NK lymphocyte development and may cause severely decreased numbers of these cells in lymphoid organs and in the peripheral blood. Autoimmune complications have been noted in Omenn syndrome, a subtype of SCID. Patients have susceptibility to infections from birth due to severely low peripheral T- and B-cells, as well as lymphadenopathy, splenomegaly, erythroderma, and autoimmune hepatic dysfunction.[51,54,55]

Idiopathic $CD4^+$ lymphopenia (ICL) is not usually included in the group of PIDs, although it shares some features with SCID and autoimmunity. It is diagnosed in patients who manifest opportunistic infections and in whom evaluation demonstrates $CD4^+$ T lymphopenia ($CD4^+$ T-cells counts <300 cells/mm^3) without human immunodeficiency virus (HIV) infection or other known lymphotropic virus, and in the absence of any other defined immunodeficiency or therapy capable of lowering $CD4^+$ T-cell levels.[56] Low counts of other lymphocytes subsets are observed, and several studies suggest that factors related to $CD4^+$ T lymphocyte function play a role in the disease.[57] In addition to opportunistic infections, AID are commonly associated in these patients.[58,59]

Common variable immunodeficiency has heterogeneous clinical manifestations; patients suffer only a few or no infections until severe recurrent sinopulmonary and gastrointestinal infections and even structural lung damage occur. Clinical manifestations of AIDs are common, such as autoimmune cytopenias (thrombocytopenia and hemolytic anemia), rheumatoid arthritis, and inflammatory bowel disease. Some patients with common variable immunodeficiency have defective antibody production and underlying T-cell defects.[51,60–64] Wiskott Aldrich syndrome is a PID that affects many aspects of immune cell function (NK, B- and T-cells, mast cells, platelets, and neutrophil functions) and is associated with a remarkably high prevalence of autoimmune manifestations (70%) such as vasculitis, autoimmune hemolytic anemia, and glomerulonephritis.[51,62,63,65,66] Multiple mechanisms may contribute to autoimmune complications. Patients have reduced responses to polysaccharide vaccines and increased susceptibility to bacterial, viral, and fungal infections.

3.3 Infections

Infection has long been implicated in the pathogenesis of SLE. The relation between deregulated immune function and infections in SLE is complex because infectious agents can interact with the immune system in different ways, such as triggering autoimmunity via structural or functional molecular mimicry, codification of proteins that induce cross-reactive immune responses to self-antigens or modulate antigen processing, and activation or even apoptosis of B- and T-cells, macrophages, or dendritic cells.[67] Infections may mimic exacerbations of SLE, making diagnosis and appropriate treatment more difficult.[68]

There are four typical infections (bacterial, viral, fungal, and parasitic) that may lower lymphocytes counts.

Tuberculosis is a common infection seen in SLE.[69] Hematologic abnormalities are common and considered poor prognostic signs in these patients.[70] The hematologic abnormalities include leukopenia and lymphopenia.[71] CD4[+] T lymphopenia was found in 9.6% of hospitalized HIV-negative patients with tuberculosis and in 4.2% of patients with ambulatory tuberculosis.[72] Lymphopenia is frequently found in brucellosis and can be significantly correlated with the severity of clinical manifestations of the disease.[73,74] Disturbances in immune homeostasis are found in patients with typhoid fever and manifested by T lymphopenia, which has a prognostic value.[75,76]

Within viral infections, hematopoietic abnormalities, including anemia, cytopenias, and changes of the stem cell plasticity in the bone marrow microenvironment, commonly occur in HIV-infected patients.[77] The association with SLE can occur despite the loss of immunocompetence caused by HIV infection; these two diseases influence each other through immunologic mechanisms and determining abnormal manifestations.[78]

Cytomegalovirus infection can also depress CD4[+] T-cells and cause a great increase in CD8[+] T-cell counts.[79] A major characteristic of acute measles is lymphopenia, resulting from depletion, which can occur at any stage of lymphocyte development.[80] Lymphopenia is a risk factor for a poor outcome.[81] Concerning SLE, physicians should be aware that, in rare cases, measles might present with a butterfly-like rash.[82]

Within fungal infections, histoplasmosis usually occurs in immunocompromised patients from endemic regions. Hematologic abnormalities such as T-cell deficiency that resolve with treatment and association with AIDs were reported.[46,83] Lymphopenia also has frequently been described in patients with malaria.[84]

3.4 Immunosuppressive Therapy and Other Drugs

Chronic immunosuppressive therapy has beneficial effects on disease progression. Severe AID requires aggressive regimens. However, at some stage, the weapons to control disease and inflammation may lead to infectious complications due to an impaired response against infectious agents.

Several studies have investigated the risk of lymphopenia caused by immunosuppressive therapy, throughout the course of AID, although it is difficult to distinguish the main cause because lymphopenia can be caused by the disease itself.

3.4.1 Glucocorticoids

Glucocorticoids are considered powerful immunosuppressants at pharmacologic doses. Yet, at physiologic concentrations, they are immunomodulators. They play a crucial role in regulating the immune response. Besides skin atrophy, easy bruising, and delayed wound healing, steroids use leads to neutrophilia, decreased migration of neutrophils to sites of inflammation, inhibition of chemotaxis, decreased phagocytosis, and intracellular killing.[85] Chronic use also leads to lymphopenia, decreased IgG serum concentrations, and suppression of normal delayed hypersensitivity reactions. Defective phagocytic function and diminished cell-mediated immunity are the main reasons for infections in steroid-treated patients.[86] Ferreira et al. published a series of SLE cases and described a relation between CD4$^+$ T-cell counts and use of steroids, among other variables. The authors documented normal CD4$^+$ T-cell counts in only 31% of steroid-treated patients and in 18% of non-steroid-treated patients, similar to those with CD4$^+$ T-cell counts less than 200/mm^3 (37% in steroid-treated and 19% in non-steroid-treated patients).[18] We add that SLE disease itself, and not only the use of steroids, may increase the risk for infection.

It is known that the risk of infection in glucocorticoid-treated patients increases with dose and duration of treatment and tends to remain low in patients exposed to lower doses of glucocorticoids, even if the cumulative doses are high.[87]

3.4.2 Methotrexate

Methotrexate is immunosuppressive in high doses, but low doses can inhibit immunoglobulin synthesis and neutrophil chemotaxis and may cause bone marrow suppression. Low doses are associated with opportunistic infections as early as a few weeks to several years after starting therapy.[88] Szalay et al. documented a decrease in Th17 prevalence in patients treated with methotrexate in addition to glucocorticoids, which contributes to infectious risk.[89]

3.4.3 Anti-Calcineurinic Agents

Cyclosporine A and tacrolimus inhibit the activity of calcineurin-causing inhibition of T-cell proliferation and function (T-helper, T-suppressor, and T-cytotoxic cells), production of IL-2 and infections related to defective cell–mediated immunity.[88]

3.4.4 Azathioprine

Azathioprine causes lymphopenia and suppresses immunoglobulin synthesis in a dose-dependent way, while neutrophil function seems to remain intact. The risk of infection is lower than with cyclophosphamide or methotrexate.[88] Gomez-Martin et al. found that patients with SLE with azathioprine-associated lymphopenia had a decreased number of CD4$^+$/D69$^+$ T-cells and CD4$^+$/IL17$^+$ T-cells compared to patients with disease activity-associated lymphopenia; it also affected Treg proliferation and suppressive capacity.[90]

3.4.5 Leflunomide

Leflunomide has an antiproliferative and inflammatory effect, inhibiting the synthesis of pyrimidine. The drug is usually used in psoriatic or reactive rheumatoid arthritis and causes mainly agranulocytosis. Oh et al. found that leflunomide, such as sulphasalazine, inhibits the antiproliferative function of Tregs on cocultured effector T-cells and reduced Treg expression of Foxp3 mRNA, but no further studies were done to demonstrate an increased risk of infection.[91]

3.4.6 Mycophenolate Mofetil

Mycophenolate mofetil, widely used in AIDs as off-label treatment, causes mainly leucopenia and neutropenia, inhibits the proliferation of T- and B-cells and expression of adhesion molecules, induces T-activated cells apoptosis and decreases immunoglobulin synthesis. Most published studies are related to immunosuppression in transplantation and few report infection risk in AIDs; instead, most report respiratory tract infections, cytomegalovirus and herpes zoster infections.[92]

3.4.7 Cyclophosphamide

Cyclophosphamide causes mainly lymphopenia and neutropenia, which results from decreased production of neutrophils as well as its increased destruction documented serious infections in 46% of treated patients with SLE, the risk of serious infection being dose-dependent.[88] Cyclophosphamide is a well-documented cause of lymphopenia. Morton et al. identified lymphopenia as a risk factor for major infection, in particular respiratory tract infections, in patients followed after treatment with methylprednisolone and cyclophosphamide for granulomatosis with polyangiitis and SLE.[93]

Vilá et al. testified that lymphopenia was more likely in patients with SLE who received glucocorticoids, azathioprine, mycophenolate mofetil, and methotrexate. Although this study was done to understand the SLE-induced lymphopenia, the authors discussed its role and found higher disease activity and damage accrual related to lymphopenia.[31] Lymphopenia with resulting impairment in cellular immunity is a stronger predictor for herpes zoster infection than leucopenia, as stated by Chu–Sung Hu et al. The use of cytotoxic drugs may worsen the immune suppression that is already inherent in patients with SLE, which in turn may increase the risk of infection.[94]

Finally, Scholmerich et al. analyzed the immune status and risk for infection in patients receiving chronic immunosuppressive therapy and found a decrease in total lymphocyte count in patients receiving steroids (doses >10 mg prednisolone per day) or immunosuppressive therapy combinations with cytotoxic drugs and steroids at various doses, especially among those treated with cyclophosphamide and steroids. However, no significant effect was seen in $TCD4^+/TCD8^+$ ratio in those treated with cytotoxic drugs and/or steroids. Significantly lower levels of IL-2, but not IFN-γ, was another finding seen in treated patients who subsequently developed infections compared to those without infections. Lower incidence of infections was seen in patients receiving methotrexate with or without steroids, azathioprine with or without steroids, or steroids alone, compared to those receiving cyclophosphamide with or without steroids. Cyclophosphamide-treated patients were those who most often experienced infectious complications. $CD4^+$ T-cell count was found to be the only independent predictive variable for subsequent hospitalization for infections, in values around the same magnitude typically seen in patients with advanced HIV infection. Then, Scholmerich et al. suggest that lower T-helper cell counts can serve as a useful indicator to assess risk for infections, regardless of their pathogenesis.[95]

3.4.8 Biologic Therapy

Biologic therapy is becoming an alternative to the traditional disease-modifying anti-rheumatic drugs (DMARDs). Anti-TNF drugs, such as infliximab, etarnecept, adalimumab, golimumab, and certolizumab, cause cytopenia, not only by the mechanism itself but especially as a result of secondary viral or bacterial infections. Then, various infections have to be routinely excluded.

Tocilizumab, a recombinant monoclonal IgG1 anti-human IL-6 receptor antibody used in rheumatoid arthritis after failure with anti-TNF usually has a higher risk to infections, mostly of the upper respiratory tract and gastrointestinal tract. Blocking IL-6, the inflammatory cascade is inhibited, as well as T- and B-helper cell and B-cell differentiation, causing leucopenia and neutropenia.[96,97]

Belimumab, a human monoclonal immunoglobulin (IgG1) that binds to and inhibits the soluble form of the BlyS protein, has been shown to be safe, although it may be associated with leucopenia and severe infections. Some authors have shown that adverse effects were not higher and were independent of the dose.[98]

Abatacept competes with endogenous CD28[+] T-cell and CTLA4 for binding to TCD80/86 complex, inhibiting the biological co-stimulation of T-cells by these molecules. The main adverse effect of this drug is infection through leucopenia, T-cell proliferation reduction, and cytokine inhibition (TNF, IFN-α, and IL-2).[99,100]

Alemtuzumab, a monoclonal antibody against CD52[+] surface glycoprotein has been found to be associated with profound and long-lasting lymphopenia; however, it does not excessively increase mortality, nor does it have an unusual spectrum of infections, at least during a medium-term follow-up.[101]

Rituximab, a chimeric human monoclonal antibody against CD20[+] protein found on naïve, mature, and memory B-cells, is associated with a decrease of gamma–globulin concentrations, depending on the cumulative dose; however, it does not seem to lead to higher risk of infection.[102] Some authors suggest that progressive multifocal leukoencephalopathy (PML) may be secondary to rituximab and induces lymphopenia, but PML has been described in systemic diseases independent of the use of any treatment.[103] Many patients with PML and SLE have records of modest levels of immunosuppression, suggesting that SLE itself may be a predisposing factor.[42,104]

3.4.9 Immunoglobulins

Immunoglobulins act through a complex mechanism involving immunomodulation, specifically neutralizing pathogenic autoantibodies, the expression and function of Fc-γ receptors, complement activation, and release of inflammatory cytokines. They also inhibit B- and T-cell function and differentiation.[105] They have a protective role for infections and, so far, no described risk of lymphopenia.

3.4.10 Hydroxychloroquine and Sulphasalazine

Hydroxychloroquine is commonly used in AIDs. Its mechanism is wide, including inhibition of T- and B-cell proliferation, migration of neutrophils and production of several pro-inflammatory cytokines. It may cause agranulocytosis and leucopenia, complications that also were observed with sulphasalazine. Hydroxychloroquine and sulphasalazine are not associated with an increased risk for infection.[87] Ferreira et al. did not find any correlation between hydroxychloroquine intake and CD4 T-cell levels.[18]

3.4.11 Gold Salts

Gold salts were used in juvenile and rheumatoid arthritis through an unknown mechanism. They have seriously hematologic effects, namely agranulocytosis, pancytopenia, and eosinophilia. No study was found focussing on the risk of infection and hematologic effects caused by gold salts.

3.4.12 Vitamin D

Experimental and epidemiological observations accrued over the past few decades implicate vitamin D deficiency as a risk factor for AID. Vitamin D induces a preferential increase of naïve $CD4^+$ T-cells, an increase of Tregs, a decrease of effector Th1 and Th17 cells, and a decrease of memory B-cells and anti-DNA antibodies.[106] A significant correlation between higher SLE activity and lower serum 25-hydroxyvitamin D levels was shown.[107] Recent studies demonstrated that vitamin D deficiency is related to the incidence and severity of infection.[108,109]

4 MANAGEMENT OF LYMPHOPENIA IN PREVENTING INFECTION IN AIDs

As stated earlier, the causes of lymphopenia in AIDs are multiple and can result from the AID itself, congenital immunodeficiency disorders, infections, immunosuppressive therapy, or other drugs. Given that there is no specific treatment for lymphopenia, primary attention should be paid to the diagnosis and treatment of the underlying condition, and causative drugs should be withdrawn or their dose reduced whenever possible. In addition to the latter, there are no guidelines to determine which subgroups of patients may benefit from prophylaxis treatment against infective pathogens, the antimicrobials that should be used or the best timing to start it, in opposition to HIV management.[17,110,111]

Lymphopenia by itself is not indicated for therapeutic intervention.

The risk of infection related to immunosuppressive drugs increases with dose and duration of treatment and tends to remain low in patients exposed to low doses, even if the cumulative doses are high.[87,112] Therefore, we should try to optimize treatment using the lowest effective dosage, according to the disease activity and to the patient's general condition.

In 1998 Le Moing and Leport recommended starting cotrimoxazole as primary prophylaxis against *Pneumocystis jirovecii* pneumonia (PCP), in all patients with SLE with marked lymphopenia.[113]

Immune deregulation related to chronic immunosuppressive therapy may involve impaired cytokine release and lymphopenia that involves all subsets. Glück et al. showed in a multiple logistic regression analysis that in patients with an AID treated with different immunosuppressive drugs, T-helper lymphopenia less than $250/mm^3$ was the best predictor of infections, with a positive predictive value of 0.53 and a negative predictive value of 0.97. Corticosteroids more than 10 mg/day were also predictive of infections. The authors conclude that $CD4^+$ T-cell counts associated with infection in AIDs are in the same range as in patients with HIV and conclude that antibiotic prophylaxis may be warranted in select patients receiving chronic immunosuppressive treatment.[95]

Other authors showed that lymphopenia $\leq 1.0 \times 10^9/L$ at lupus diagnosis is strongly predictive of the occurrence of infection.[37]

Nevertheless, the appropriate prescription of PCP primary prophylaxis for immunocompromised patients without HIV infection has not been established, and whether all patients in a recognized risk category for PCP should receive prophylaxis remains controversial.[114,115]

The overall incidence of PCP in AID is low, related to 1–2%, with rates of up to 6% in Wegener's granulomatosis.[116] Patients with Wegener's granulomatosis and polyarteritis nodosa may be at greater risk for PCP because high-dose immunosuppressive treatment is more commonly used in this AID.[117–119] Although PCP in AID is uncommon, the mortality rate is high, ranging from 39% to 59%, compared to 10–15% in patients with HIV with PCP.[120]

Administration of prophylaxis to all autoimmune patients would unnecessarily expose patients to drug side effects and potentially encourage drug resistance.

Mansharamani et al. suggest that $CD4^+$ T-cells less than 300 cells/mm^3 and corticosteroids more than 16–20 mg/day (alone or in combination) for more than 1 month may potentially guide the initiation of prophylaxis in immunocompromised persons without HIV infection, including those with AIDs, although the specific $CD4^+$ T-cell cutoff that confers protection requires further study.[115]

Sowden and Carmichael proposed evaluating $CD4^+$ T-cell counts after 1 month of immunosuppression only in patients who fulfill all the following criteria: corticosteroid dosage more than 15 mg prednisolone or equivalent per day, corticosteroid treatment proposed for more than 3 months, total lymphocyte counts less than 600 cells/mm^3. A CD4$^+$ T-cell count less than 200 cells/mm^3 might then warrant the use of prophylactic cotrimoxazole.[121]

Demoruelle et al. more recently suggested prophylaxis in autoimmune patients that meet more than two of the following risk factors: corticosteroids equal or more than 20 mg for more than 4 weeks, current use of equal or more than two DMARDs, which include biologic agents, absolute lymphocyte count less than 350 cell/mm^3 and underlying parenchymal lung disease.[122]

Patients with lupus receiving cyclophosphamide are at risk of PCP, with substantial morbidity and mortality. Gupta et al. demonstrate that routine use of cotrimoxazole in this population does not seem to be warranted, except in those with elevated risk, such as those with severe leucopenia, lymphopenia, high-dose corticosteroids, hypocomplementemia, active renal disease, and higher mean SLEDAI score.[123]

Consensus guidelines addressing prophylactic antibiotics in these patients are needed, and no primary prevention is suggested for other opportunistic infections.

As in the case of patients with HIV receiving highly active antiretroviral therapy and who discontinue prophylaxis to PCP when CD4$^+$ T-cells are more than 200 cells/mm^3 in two evaluations, we could take this strategy to other autoimmune patients. However, studies defining the adequate sustained level of CD4$^+$ T-cell counts before discontinuation of PCP prophylaxis are lacking.[115]

In autoimmune patients with underlying ICL, the management is well defined, based on HIV management experience. In most cases monitoring CD4$^+$ T-cell counts every 3–6 months might be enough. In rare cases, patients may normalize CD4$^+$ T-cell counts, enabling them to discontinue any prophylaxis initially given.[57,59] In selected patients with ICL, therapeutic options used to increase CD4$^+$ T-cells and/or improve immune deregulation may be used, including IL-2 and IFN-γ. Many successful cases have been reported.[59,124–126] IL-7 also has been investigated as a potential therapy aimed to improve CD4$^+$ T-cells and CD8$^+$ T-cells.[59,127]

Recently published reports describe the potential role of vitamin D in prevention and adjunct treatment of infection.[108,109] Vitamin D modulates the immune system responses and inflammatory cascade. Terrier et al. proved that in patients with SLE, vitamin D induced a preferential increase of naïve CD4$^+$ T-cells and Treg cells and a decrease of effector Th1 and Th17 cells.[107] Based on this finding, its supplementation may prevent the risk of infection associated to lymphopenia. Data from double-blind, randomized, controlled trials are still lacking.

It is also of general consensus that all patients should receive annual influenza vaccination, pneumococcal vaccination every 5 years and regular Papanicoloau tests. Live vaccines should not be used in patients taking immunosuppressive drugs until a few months after their cessation. It is also recommended that when non-live vaccines are given, an assessment of immune response should be evaluated and a booster considered when antibody titers are low. Before using immunosuppressive therapy, including high dosage of corticosteroids, patients should be screened for *Mycobacterium tuberculosis* and for some viral infections, including HIV, HCV, and HBV, and adequate prophylaxis should be given when indicated.[69,112,128–130] Serology for *Strongyloides stercolaris* is also indicated in endemic areas.[128]

Table 1 summarizes the management approach intended to reduce risk infection associated with lymphopenia in AIDs.

Table 1 Management Approach to Reduce Risk of Infection Associated with Lymphopenia in AID

General approach

1. Optimize treatment in AID using corticosteroids and immunosuppressants at the lowest effective dosage
2. Screen for *Mycobacterium tuberculosis* infection (active or latent), HIV1/2, HCV, and HBV, particularly before using immunosuppressants, and treat accordingly
3. Influenza vaccine annually
4. Pneumococcal vaccine every 5 years until 65 years old; if 65 years old or older, give only one dose
5. Immunosuppressants should be withdrawn 3 months before vaccination and reintroduced 2–4 weeks after vaccination
6. Avoid live attenuated vaccines, particularly with immunosuppressant or prednisolone at a dose of more than 20 mg
7. Regular Papanicolaou tests

Related to lymphopenia

1. PCP prophylaxis
    1.1. $CD4^+$ T-cells <300 cells/mm^3 and corticosteroids >16–20 mg/day (alone or in combination) for more than 1 month
    1.2. Patients meet more than two of the following risk factors: corticosteroids ≥ 20 mg for more than 4 weeks, current use of two or more disease-modifying anti-rheumatic drugs (DMARDs) including biologic agents, absolute lymphocyte count <350 cells/mm^3 and underlying parenchymal lung disease
2. Idiopathic $CD4^+$ T lymphopenia (ICL)
    2.1. PCP prophylaxis based on HIV management experience
    2.2. IL-2, IL-7, and IFN-γ in selected patients with ICL
3. Vitamin D supplementation

REFERENCES

1. Mosmann TR, Cherwinski H, Bond MW, Giedlin MA, Coffman RL. Two types of murine helper T cell clone. I. Definition according to profiles of lymphokine activities and secreted proteins. *J Immunol* 1986;**136**(7):2348–57.
2. Zheng SG. Regulatory T, cells vs Th17: differentiation of Th17 versus Treg, are the mutually exclusive? *Am J Clin Exp Immunol* 2013;**2**(1):94–106.
3. Muranski P, Restifo NP. Essentials of Th17 cell commitment and plasticity. *Blood* 2013;**121**(13):2402–14.
4. Grimaldi CM, Hicks R, Diamond B. B cell selection and susceptibility to autoimmunity. *J Immunol* 2005;**174**(4):1775–81.
5. Vincent FB, Saulep-Easton D, Figgett WA, Fairfax KA, Mackay F. The BAFF/APRIL system: emerging functions beyond B cell biology and autoimmunity. *Cytokine Growth Factor Rev* 2013;**24**(3):203–15.
6. Henriques A, Teixeira L, Ines L, Carvalheiro T, Goncalves A, Martinho A, et al. NK cells dysfunction in systemic lupus erythematosus: relation to disease activity. *Clin Rheumatol* 2013;**32**(6):805–13.
7. Green MR, Kennell AS, Larche MJ, Seifert MH, Isenberg DA, Salaman MR. Natural killer T cells in families of patients with systemic lupus erythematosus: their possible role in regulation of IGG production. *Arthritis Rheum* 2007;**56**(1):303–10.
8. Chuang YP, Wang CH, Wang NC, Chang DM, Sytwu HK. Modulatory function of invariant natural killer T cells in systemic lupus erythematosus. *Clin Dev Immunol* 2012;**2012**:478429.
9. Parekh VV, Wu L, Olivares-Villagomez D, Wilson KT, Van Kaer L. Activated invariant NKT cells control central nervous system autoimmunity in a mechanism that involves myeloid-derived suppressor cells. *J Immunol* 2013;**190**(5):1948–60.
10. Draborg AH, Duus K, Houen G. Epstein–Barr virus in systemic autoimmune diseases. *Clin Dev Immunol* 2013;**2013**:535738.
11. Pender MP. CD8+ T-cell deficiency, Epstein–Barr virus infection, vitamin D deficiency, and steps to autoimmunity: a unifying hypothesis. *Autoimmune Dis* 2012;**2012**:189096.
12. Puel A, Casanova JL. Autoantibodies against cytokines: back to human genetics. *Blood* 2013;**121**(8):1246–7.
13. Al Arfaj AS, Khalil N. Clinical and immunological manifestations in 624 SLE patients in Saudi Arabia. *Lupus* 2009;**18**(5):465–73.
14. Cooper GS, Parks CG, Treadwell EL, St Clair EW, Gilkeson GS, Cohen PL, et al. Differences by race, sex and age in the clinical and immunologic features of recently diagnosed systemic lupus erythematosus patients in the southeastern United States. *Lupus* 2002;**11**(3):161–7.
15. Pons-Estel BA, Catoggio LJ, Cardiel MH, Soriano ER, Gentiletti S, Villa AR, et al. The GLADEL multinational Latin American prospective inception cohort of 1,214 patients with systemic lupus erythematosus: ethnic and disease heterogeneity among "Hispanics". *Medicine* 2004;**83**(1):1–17.
16. Arce-Salinas CA, Rodriguez-Garcia F, Gomez-Vargas JI. Long-term efficacy of anti-CD20 antibodies in refractory lupus nephritis. *Rheumatol Int* 2012;**32**(5):1245–9.
17. Hepburn AL, Narat S, Mason JC. The management of peripheral blood cytopenias in systemic lupus erythematosus. *Rheumatology* 2010;**49**(12):2243–54.
18. Ferreira S, Vasconcelos J, Marinho A, Farinha F, Almeida I, Correia J, et al. CD4 lymphocytopenia in systemic lupus erythematosus. *Acta Reumatol Port* 2009;**34**(2A):200–6.
19. Martinez-Banos D, Crispin JC, Lazo-Langner A, Sanchez-Guerrero J. Moderate and severe neutropenia in patients with systemic lupus erythematosus. *Rheumatology* 2006;**45**(8):994–8.
20. Mittal KK, Rossen RD, Sharp JT, Lidsky MD, Butler WT. Lymphocyte cytotoxic antibodies in systemic lupus erythematosus. *Nature* 1970;**225**(5239):1255–6.

21. Butler WT, Sharp JT, Rossen RD, Lidsky MD, Mittal KK, Gard DA. Relationship of the clinical course of systemic lupus erythematosus to the presence of circulating lymphocytotoxic antibodies. *Arthritis Rheum* 1972;**15**(3):251–8.

22. Winfield JB, Winchester RJ, Kunkel HG. Association of cold-reactive antilymphocyte antibodies with lymphopenia in systemic lupus erythematosus. *Arthritis Rheum* 1975;**18**(6):587–94.

23. Bengtsson AA, Sturfelt G, Truedsson L, Blomberg J, Alm G, Vallin H, et al. Activation of type I interferon system in systemic lupus erythematosus correlates with disease activity but not with antiretroviral antibodies. *Lupus* 2000;**9**(9):664–71.

24. Garcia-Valladares I, Atisha-Fregoso Y, Richaud-Patin Y, Jakez-Ocampo J, Soto-Vega E, Elias-Lopez D, et al. Diminished expression of complement regulatory proteins (CD55 and CD59) in lymphocytes from systemic lupus erythematosus patients with lymphopenia. *Lupus* 2006;**15**(9):600–5.

25. Ruiz-Arguelles A, Llorente L. The role of complement regulatory proteins (CD55 and CD59) in the pathogenesis of autoimmune hemocytopenias. *Autoimmun Rev* 2007;**6**(3):155–61.

26. Tan EM, Cohen AS, Fries JF, Masi AT, McShane DJ, Rothfield NF, et al. The 1982 revised criteria for the classification of systemic lupus erythematosus. *Arthritis Rheum* 1982;**25**(11):1271–7.

27. Worrall JG, Snaith ML, Batchelor JR, Isenberg DA. SLE: a rheumatological view. Analysis of the clinical features, serology and immunogenetics of 100 SLE patients during long-term follow-up. *Q J Med* 1990;**74**(275):319–30.

28. Nossent JC, Swaak AJ. Prevalence and significance of haematological abnormalities in patients with systemic lupus erythematosus. *Q J Med* 1991;**80**(291):605–12.

29. Mirzayan MJ, Schmidt RE, Witte T. Prognostic parameters for flare in systemic lupus erythematosus. *Rheumatology* 2000;**39**(12):1316–19.

30. Lam GK, Petri M. Assessment of systemic lupus erythematosus. *Clin Exp Rheumatol* 2005;**23**(5 Suppl. 39):S120–32.

31. Vila LM, Alarcon GS, McGwin Jr. G, Bastian HM, Fessler BJ, Reveille JD, et al. Systemic lupus erythematosus in a multiethnic US cohort, XXXVII: association of lymphopenia with clinical manifestations, serologic abnormalities, disease activity, and damage accrual. *Arthritis Rheum* 2006;**55**(5):799–806.

32. Halberg P, Alsbjorn B, Balslev JT, Lorenzen I, Gerstoft J, Ullman S, et al. Systemic lupus erythematosus. Follow-up study of 148 patients. II: predictive factors of importance for course and outcome. *Clin Rheumatol* 1987;**6**(1):22–6.

33. Rivero SJ, Diaz-Jouanen E, Alarcon-Segovia D. Lymphopenia in systemic lupus erythematosus. Clinical, diagnostic, and prognostic significance. *Arthritis Rheum* 1978;**21**(3):295–305.

34. Drenkard C, Villa AR, Reyes E, Abello M, Alarcon-Segovia D. Vasculitis in systemic lupus erythematosus. *Lupus* 1997;**6**(3):235–42.

35. Silva LM, Garcia AB, Donadi EA. Increased lymphocyte death by neglect-apoptosis is associated with lymphopenia and autoantibodies in lupus patients presenting with neuropsychiatric manifestations. *J Neurol* 2002;**249**(8):1048–54.

36. Yu HH, Wang LC, Lee JH, Lee CC, Yang YH, Chiang BL. Lymphopenia is associated with neuropsychiatric manifestations and disease activity in paediatric systemic lupus erythematosus patients. *Rheumatology* 2007;**46**(9):1492–4.

37. Ng WL, Chu CM, Wu AK, Cheng VC, Yuen KY. Lymphopenia at presentation is associated with increased risk of infections in patients with systemic lupus erythematosus. *QJM* 2006;**99**(1):37–47.

38. Merayo-Chalico J, Gomez-Martin D, Pineirua-Menendez A, Santana-De Anda K, Alcocer-Varela J. Lymphopenia as risk factor for development of severe infections in patients with systemic lupus erythematosus: a case-control study. *QJM* 2013;**106**(5):451–7.

39. Cervera R, Khamashta MA, Font J, Sebastiani GD, Gil A, Lavilla P, et al. Morbidity and mortality in systemic lupus erythematosus during a 10-year period: a comparison of early and late manifestations in a cohort of 1,000 patients. *Medicine* 2003;**82**(5):299–308.

40. Edwards CJ, Lian TY, Badsha H, Teh CL, Arden N, Chng HH. Hospitalization of individuals with systemic lupus erythematosus: characteristics and predictors of outcome. *Lupus* 2003;**12**(9):672–6.

41. Wouters CH, Diegenant C, Ceuppens JL, Degreef H, Stevens EA. The circulating lymphocyte profiles in patients with discoid lupus erythematosus and systemic lupus erythematosus suggest a pathogenetic relationship. *Br J Dermatol* 2004;**150**(4):693–700.

42. Brandao M, Damasio J, Marinho A, da Silva AM, Vasconcelos J, Neves E, et al. Systemic lupus erythematosus, progressive multifocal leukoencephalopathy, and T-CD4$^+$ lymphopenia. *Clin Rev Allergy Immunol* 2012;**43**(3):302–7.

43. Odendahl M, Jacobi A, Hansen A, Feist E, Hiepe F, Burmester GR, et al. Disturbed peripheral B lymphocyte homeostasis in systemic lupus erythematosus. *J Immunol* 2000;**165**(10):5970–9.

44. Robak E, Smolewski P, Wozniacka A, Sysa-Jedrzejowska A, Robak T. Clinical significance of circulating dendritic cells in patients with systemic lupus erythematosus. *Mediators Inflamm* 2004;**13**(3):171–80.

45. Bermas BL, Petri M, Goldman D, Mittleman B, Miller MW, Stocks NI, et al. T helper cell dysfunction in systemic lupus erythematosus (SLE): relation to disease activity. *J Clin Immunol* 1994;**14**(3):169–77.

46. Rodrigo HF, Stavile RN, Deleo S. Disseminated histoplasmosis, lymphopenia and Sjogren's syndrome. *Medicina* 2012;**72**(5):435–8.

47. Mandl T, Bredberg A, Jacobsson LT, Manthorpe R, Henriksson G. CD4$^+$ T-lymphocytopenia—a frequent finding in anti-SSA antibody seropositive patients with primary Sjogren's syndrome. *J Rheumatol* 2004;**31**(4):726–8.

48. Henriksson G, Manthorpe R, Bredberg A. Antibodies to CD4 in primary Sjogren's syndrome. *Rheumatology* 2000;**39**(2):142–7.

49. Schulze-Koops H. Lymphopenia and autoimmune diseases. *Arthritis Res Ther* 2004;**6**(4):178–80.

50. Kirtava Z, Blomberg J, Bredberg A, Henriksson G, Jacobsson L, Manthorpe R. CD4$^+$ T-lymphocytopenia without HIV infection: increased prevalence among patients with primary Sjogren's syndrome. *Clin Exp Rheumatol* 1995;**13**(5):609–16.

51. Goyal R, Bulua AC, Nikolov NP, Schwartzberg PL, Siegel RM. Rheumatologic and autoimmune manifestations of primary immunodeficiency disorders. *Curr Opin Rheumatol* 2009;**21**(1):78–84.

52. Coutinho A, Carneiro-Sampaio M. Primary immunodeficiencies unravel critical aspects of the pathophysiology of autoimmunity and of the genetics of autoimmune disease. *J Clin Immunol* 2008;**28**(Suppl. 1):S4–S10.

53. Barsalou J, Saint-Cyr C, Drouin E, Le Deist F, Haddad E. High prevalence of primary immune deficiencies in children with autoimmune disorders. *Clin Exp Rheumatol* 2011;**29**(1):125–30.

54. Milner JD, Fasth A, Etzioni A. Autoimmunity in severe combined immunodeficiency (SCID): lessons from patients and experimental models. *J Clin Immunol* 2008;**28**(Suppl. 1):S29–33.

55. Elhasid R, Bergman R, Etzioni A. Autoimmunity in severe combined immunodeficiency (SCID). *Blood* 2002;**100**(7):2677–8, author reply 8–9.

56. Haider S, Nafziger D, Gutierrez JA, Brar I, Mateo N, Fogle J. Progressive multifocal leukoencephalopathy and idiopathic CD4$^+$ lymphocytopenia: a case report and review of reported cases. *Clin Infect Dis* 2000;**31**(4):E20–2.

57. Ahmad DS, Esmadi M, Steinmann WC. Idiopathic CD4 lymphocytopenia: spectrum of opportunistic infections, malignancies, and autoimmune diseases. *Avicenna J Med* 2013;**3**(2):37–47.

58. Walker UA, Warnatz K. Idiopathic CD4 lymphocytopenia. *Curr Opin Rheumatol* 2006;**18**(4):389–95.
59. Zonios DI, Falloon J, Bennett JE, Shaw PA, Chaitt D, Baseler MW, et al. Idiopathic CD4⁺ lymphocytopenia: natural history and prognostic factors. *Blood* 2008;**112** (2):287–94.
60. Castigli E, Wilson SA, Garibyan L, Rachid R, Bonilla F, Schneider L, et al. TACI is mutant in common variable immunodeficiency and IgA deficiency. *Nat Genet* 2005;**37**(8):829–34.
61. Salzer U, Chapel HM, Webster AD, Pan-Hammarstrom Q, Schmitt-Graeff A, Schlesier M, et al. Mutations in TNFRSF13B encoding TACI are associated with common variable immunodeficiency in humans. *Nat Genet* 2005;**37**(8):820–8.
62. Cunningham-Rundles C, Bodian C. Common variable immunodeficiency: clinical and immunological features of 248 patients. *Clin Immunol* 1999;**92**(1):34–48.
63. Uluhan A, Sager D, Jasin HE. Juvenile rheumatoid arthritis and common variable hypogammaglobulinemia. *J Rheumatol* 1998;**25**(6):1205–10.
64. Webster AD. Clinical and immunological spectrum of common variable immunodeficiency (CVID). *Iran J Allergy Asthma Immunol* 2004;**3**(3):103–13.
65. Sullivan KE, Mullen CA, Blaese RM, Winkelstein JA. A multiinstitutional survey of the Wiskott–Aldrich syndrome. *J Pediatr* 1994;**125**(6 Pt. 1):876–85.
66. Dupuis-Girod S, Medioni J, Haddad E, Quartier P, Cavazzana-Calvo M, Le Deist F, et al. Autoimmunity in Wiskott–Aldrich syndrome: risk factors, clinical features, and outcome in a single-center cohort of 55 patients. *Pediatrics* 2003;**111**(5 Pt. 1):e622–7.
67. Francis L, Perl A. Infection in systemic lupus erythematosus: friend or foe? *Int J Clin Rheumatol* 2010;**5**(1):59–74.
68. Zandman-Goddard G, Shoenfeld Y. Infections and SLE. *Autoimmunity* 2005;**38** (7):473–85.
69. Danza A, Ruiz-Irastorza G. Infection risk in systemic lupus erythematosus patients: susceptibility factors and preventive strategies. *Lupus* 2013;**22**(12):1286–94.
70. Hasibi M, Rasoulinejad M, Hosseini SM, Davari P, Sahebian A, Khashayar P. Epidemiological, clinical, laboratory findings, and outcomes of disseminated tuberculosis in Tehran, Iran. *South Med J* 2008;**101**(9):910–13.
71. Singh KJ, Ahluwalia G, Sharma SK, Saxena R, Chaudhary VP, Anant M. Significance of haematological manifestations in patients with tuberculosis. *J Assoc Physicians India* 2001;**49**(788):90–4.
72. Djomand G, Diaby L, N'Gbichi JM, Coulibaly D, Kadio A, Yapi A, et al. Idiopathic CD4⁺ T-lymphocyte depletion in a west African population. *Aids* 1994;**8**(6):843–7.
73. Crosby E, Llosa L, Miro Quesada M, Carrillo C, Gotuzzo E. Hematologic changes in brucellosis. *J Infect Dis* 1984;**150**(3):419–24.
74. al-Eissa Y, al-Nasser M. Haematological manifestations of childhood brucellosis. *Infection* 1993;**21**(1):23–6.
75. Iushchuk ND, Akhmedov DR, Frolov VM, Peresadin NA, Khomutianskaia NI. The immune status of patients with typhoid fever. *Zh Mikrobiol Epidemiol Immunobiol* 1994 Jul-Aug;(4):92–6.
76. Abdool Gaffar MS, Seedat YK, Coovadia YM, Khan Q. The white cell count in typhoid fever. *Trop Geogr Med* 1992;**44**(1–2):23–7.
77. Koka PS, Reddy ST. Cytopenias in HIV infection: mechanisms and alleviation of hematopoietic inhibition. *Curr HIV Res* 2004;**2**(3):275–82.
78. Carugati M, Franzetti M, Torre A, Giorgi R, Genderini A, Strambio de Castilla F, et al. Systemic lupus erythematosus and HIV infection: a whimsical relationship. Reports of two cases and review of the literature. *Clin Rheumatol* 2013;**32**(9):1399–405.
79. Laurence J. T-cell subsets in health, infectious disease, and idiopathic CD4⁺ T lymphocytopenia. *Ann Intern Med* 1993;**119**(1):55–62.

80. Schneider-Schaulies S, Schneider-Schaulies J. Measles virus-induced immunosuppression. *Curr Top Microbiol Immunol* 2009;**330**:243–69.

81. Takizawa Y, Inokuma S, Tanaka Y, Saito K, Atsumi T, Hirakata M, et al. Clinical characteristics of cytomegalovirus infection in rheumatic diseases: multicentre survey in a large patient population. *Rheumatology* 2008;**47**(9):1373–8.

82. Tsuruta D, Kobayashi H, Kurokawa I, Ishii M, Takekawa KE. Letter: adult measles with a butterfly rash-like appearance. *Dermatol Online J* 2010;**16**(3):16.

83. Odio CM, Navarrete M, Carrillo JM, Mora L, Carranza A. Disseminated histoplasmosis in infants. *Pediatr Infect Dis J* 1999;**18**(12):1065–8.

84. van Wolfswinkel ME, Vliegenthart-Jongbloed K, de Mendonca Melo M, Wever PC, McCall MB, Koelewijn R, et al. Predictive value of lymphocytopenia and the neutrophil-lymphocyte count ratio for severe imported malaria. *Malar J* 2013;**12**:101.

85. Saag KG. Short-term and long-term safety of glucocorticoids in rheumatoid arthritis. *Bull NYU Hosp Jt Dis* 2012;**70**(Suppl. 1):21–5.

86. Tait AS, Butts CL, Sternberg EM. The role of glucocorticoids and progestins in inflammatory, autoimmune, and infectious disease. *J Leukoc Biol* 2008;**84**(4):924–31.

87. Sfriso P, Ghirardello A, Botsios C, Tonon M, Zen M, Bassi N, et al. Infections and autoimmunity: the multifaceted relationship. *J Leukoc Biol* 2010;**87**(3):385–95.

88. Greenberg SB. Infections in the immunocompromised rheumatologic patient. *Crit care Clin* 2002;**18**(4):931–56.

89. Szalay B, Vasarhelyi B, Cseh A, Tulassay T, Deak M, Kovacs L, et al. The impact of conventional DMARD and biological therapies on CD4$^+$ cell subsets in rheumatoid arthritis: a follow-up study. *Clin Rheumatol* 2014;**33**(2):175–85.

90. Gomez-Martin D, Diaz-Zamudio M, Vanoye G, Crispin JC, Alcocer-Varela J. Quantitative and functional profiles of CD4$^+$ lymphocyte subsets in systemic lupus erythematosus patients with lymphopenia. *Clin Exp Immunol* 2011;**164**(1):17–25.

91. Oh JS, Kim YG, Lee SG, So MW, Choi SW, Lee CK, et al. The effect of various disease-modifying anti-rheumatic drugs on the suppressive function of CD4(+)CD25(+) regulatory T cells. *Rheumatol Int* 2013;**33**(2):381–8.

92. Chakravarty EF, Michaud K, Katz R, Wolfe F. Increased incidence of herpes zoster among patients with systemic lupus erythematosus. *Lupus* 2013;**22**(3):238–44.

93. Morton M, Edmonds S, Doherty AM, Dhaygude A, Helbert M, Venning M. Factors associated with major infections in patients with granulomatosis with polyangiitis and systemic lupus erythematosus treated for deep organ involvement. *Rheumatol Int* 2012;**32**(11):3373–82.

94. Hu SC, Lin CL, Lu YW, Chen GS, Yu HS, Wu CS, et al. Lymphopaenia, anti-Ro/anti-RNP autoantibodies, renal involvement and cyclophosphamide use correlate with increased risk of herpes zoster in patients with systemic lupus erythematosus. *Acta Derm Venereol* 2013;**93**(3):314–18.

95. Gluck T, Kiefmann B, Grohmann M, Falk W, Straub RH, Scholmerich J. Immune status and risk for infection in patients receiving chronic immunosuppressive therapy. *J Rheumatol* 2005;**32**(8):1473–80.

96. Rosman Z, Shoenfeld Y, Zandman-Goddard G. Biologic therapy for autoimmune diseases: an update. *BMC Med* 2013;**11**:88.

97. Hashizume M, Mihara M. The roles of interleukin-6 in the pathogenesis of rheumatoid arthritis. *Arthritis* 2011;**2011**:765624.

98. Navarra SV, Guzman RM, Gallacher AE, Hall S, Levy RA, Jimenez RE, et al. Efficacy and safety of belimumab in patients with active systemic lupus erythematosus: a randomised, placebo-controlled, phase 3 trial. *Lancet* 2011;**377**(9767):721–31.

99. Kremer JM, Dougados M, Emery P, Durez P, Sibilia J, Shergy W, et al. Treatment of rheumatoid arthritis with the selective costimulation modulator abatacept: twelve-

month results of a phase iib, double-blind, randomized, placebo-controlled trial. *Arthritis Rheum* 2005;**52**(8):2263–71.

100. Kremer JM, Russell AS, Emery P, Abud-Mendoza C, Szechinski J, Westhovens R, et al. Long-term safety, efficacy and inhibition of radiographic progression with abatacept treatment in patients with rheumatoid arthritis and an inadequate response to methotrexate: 3-year results from the AIM trial. *Ann Rheum Dis* 2011;**70**(10):1826–30.

101. Isaacs JD, Greer S, Sharma S, Symmons D, Smith M, Johnston J, et al. Morbidity and mortality in rheumatoid arthritis patients with prolonged and profound therapy-induced lymphopenia. *Arthritis Rheum* 2001;**44**(9):1998–2008.

102. Isvy A, Meunier M, Gobeaux-Chenevier C, Maury E, Wipff J, Job-Deslandre C, et al. Safety of rituximab in rheumatoid arthritis: a long-term prospective single-center study of gammaglobulin concentrations and infections. *Joint Bone Spine* 2012;**79**(4):365–9.

103. Tavazzi E, Ferrante P, Khalili K. Progressive multifocal leukoencephalopathy: an unexpected complication of modern therapeutic monoclonal antibody therapies. *Clin Microbiol Infect* 2011;**17**(12):1776–80.

104. Molloy ES, Calabrese LH. Progressive multifocal leukoencephalopathy associated with immunosuppressive therapy in rheumatic diseases: evolving role of biologic therapies. *Arthritis Rheum* 2012;**64**(9):3043–51.

105. Gelfand EW. Intravenous immune globulin in autoimmune and inflammatory diseases. *N Engl J Med* 2013;**368**(8):777.

106. Schwalfenberg GK. A review of the critical role of vitamin D in the functioning of the immune system and the clinical implications of vitamin D deficiency. *Mol Nutr Food Res* 2011;**55**(1):96–108.

107. Terrier B, Derian N, Schoindre Y, Chaara W, Geri G, Zahr N, et al. Restoration of regulatory and effector T cell balance and B cell homeostasis in systemic lupus erythematosus patients through vitamin D supplementation. *Arthritis Res Ther* 2012;**14**(5):R221.

108. Gunville CF, Mourani PM, Ginde AA. The role of vitamin D in prevention and treatment of infection. *Inflamm Allergy Drug Targets* 2013;**12**(4):239–45.

109. Bartley J. Vitamin D: emerging roles in infection and immunity. *Expert Rev Anti Infect Ther* 2010;**8**(12):1359–69.

110. Newman K, Owlia MB, El-Hemaidi I, Akhtari M. Management of immune cytopenias in patients with systemic lupus erythematosus – old and new. *Autoimmun Rev* 2013;**12** (7):784–91.

111. Keeling DM, Isenberg DA. Haematological manifestations of systemic lupus erythematosus. *Blood Rev* 1993;**7**(4):199–207.

112. Doria A, Canova M, Tonon M, Zen M, Rampudda E, Bassi N, et al. Infections as triggers and complications of systemic lupus erythematosus. *Autoimmun Rev* 2008;**8** (1):24–8.

113. Le Moing V, Leport C. Infections and lupus. *Rev Prat* 1998;**48**(6):637–42.

114. Yale SH, Limper AH. *Pneumocystis carinii* pneumonia in patients without acquired immunodeficiency syndrome: associated illness and prior corticosteroid therapy. *Mayo Clin Proc* 1996;**71**(1):5–13.

115. Mansharamani NG, Balachandran D, Vernovsky I, Garland R, Koziel H. Peripheral blood CD4$^+$ T-lymphocyte counts during *Pneumocystis carinii* pneumonia in immuno-compromised patients without HIV infection. *Chest* 2000;**118**(3):712–20.

116. Sepkowitz KA. Opportunistic infections in patients with and patients without acquired immunodeficiency syndrome. *Clin Infect Dis* 2002;**34**(8):1098–107.

117. Godeau B, Coutant-Perronne V, Le Thi Huong D, Guillevin L, Magadur G, De Bandt M, et al. *Pneumocystis carinii* pneumonia in the course of connective tissue disease: report of 34 cases. *J Rheumatol* 1994;**21**(2):246–51.

118. Ognibene FP, Shelhamer JH, Hoffman GS, Kerr GS, Reda D, Fauci AS, et al. *Pneumocystis carinii* pneumonia: a major complication of immunosuppressive therapy in

patients with Wegener's granulomatosis. *Am J Respir Crit Care Med* 1995;**151**(3 Pt. 1):795–9.

119. Ward MM, Donald F. *Pneumocystis carinii* pneumonia in patients with connective tissue diseases: the role of hospital experience in diagnosis and mortality. *Arthritis Rheum* 1999;**42**(4):780–9.

120. Mansharamani NG, Garland R, Delaney D, Koziel H. Management and outcome patterns for adult *Pneumocystis carinii* pneumonia, 1985 to 1995: comparison of HIV-associated cases to other immunocompromised states. *Chest* 2000;**118**(3):704–11.

121. Sowden E, Carmichael AJ. Autoimmune inflammatory disorders, systemic corticosteroids and pneumocystis pneumonia: a strategy for prevention. *BMC Infect Dis* 2004;**4**:42.

122. Demoruelle MK, Kahr A, Verilhac K, Deane K, Fischer A, West S. Recent-onset systemic lupus erythematosus complicated by acute respiratory failure. *Arthritis Care Res* 2013;**65**(2):314–23.

123. Gupta D, Zachariah A, Roppelt H, Patel AM, Gruber BL. Prophylactic antibiotic usage for *Pneumocystis jirovecii* pneumonia in patients with systemic lupus erythematosus on cyclophosphamide: a survey of US rheumatologists and the review of literature. *J Clin Rheumatol* 2008;**14**(5):267–72.

124. Trojan T, Collins R, Khan DA. Safety and efficacy of treatment using interleukin-2 in a patient with idiopathic CD4(+) lymphopenia and *Mycobacterium avium*-intracellulare. *Clin Exp Immunol* 2009;**156**(3):440–5.

125. Cunningham-Rundles C, Murray HW, Smith JP. Treatment of idiopathic CD4 T lymphocytopenia with IL-2. *Clin Exp Immunol* 1999;**116**(2):322–5.

126. Sternfeld T, Nigg A, Belohradsky BH, Bogner JR. Treatment of relapsing *Mycobacterium avium* infection with interferon-gamma and interleukin-2 in an HIV-negative patient with low CD4 syndrome. *Int J Infect Dis* 2010;**14**(Suppl. 3):e198–201.

127. Ponchel F, Cuthbert RJ, Goeb V. IL-7 and lymphopenia. *Clin Chim Acta* 2011;**412** (1–2):7–16.

128. Doria A, Arienti S, Rampudda M, Canova M, Tonon M, Sarzi-Puttini P. Preventive strategies in systemic lupus erythematosus. *Autoimmun Rev* 2008;**7**(3):192–7.

129. Solovic I, Sester M, Gomez-Reino JJ, Rieder HL, Ehlers S, Milburn HJ, et al. The risk of tuberculosis related to tumour necrosis factor antagonist therapies: a TBNET consensus statement. *Eur Respir J* 2010;**36**(5):1185–206.

130. Thalayasingam N, Isaacs JD. Anti-TNF therapy. *Best Pract Res Clin Rheumatol* 2011;**25** (4):549–67.

CHAPTER 8

Endothelial Cell Autoreactivity and Infection

Christophe Jamin[*,†], Laurent Simonin[†], Christophe Viale[†], Pierre Youinou[*], Yves Renaudineau[*,†,1]

[*]EA2216 Immunologie et Pathologie, LabEx IGO, SFR ScInBioS, Université de Brest et Université Européenne de Bretagne, Brest, France
[†]Laboratory of Immunology and Immunotherapy, CHRU Brest, Brest, France
[1]Corresponding Author: yves.renaudineau@univ-brest.fr

1 INTRODUCTION

Because of their permanent contact with circulating immune effectors, endothelial cells (ECs) have long been suspected of being a target for antibody (Ab)-mediated assault. In spite of incredibly wide variations in the results,[1] it is not surprising that antiendothelial cell antibodies (AECAs) have been reported in a variety of clinical settings that are accompanied by vascular changes.[2] These include not only most non–organ-specific autoimmune diseases but also numerous infectious states.

AECAs were first detected by indirect immunofluorescence (IIF) analysis[3,4] and subsequently characterized using purified IgG and F(ab')$_2$ fragments.[5] The disorders associated with AECAs are impressively diverse,[6] and sera apparently negative for this autoAb on a given cell type may become positive if appropriate substrate cells are used instead.[7] Thus, AECAs certainly represent a heterogeneous family of autoAbs. As a corollary, the antigens (Ags) recognized by AECAs may be inferred to be multiple, although we have hitherto been unable to identify any of these EC Ags.[8] Furthermore, the presence of such autoAbs does not imply causation because it may follow rather than precede EC damage. There is nonetheless compelling evidence that AECAs are pathogenic. At this time, the most persuasive argument for this interpretation is that from the development of an idiotypic experimental model of systemic vasculitis.[9] A number of recent findings have indeed kindled a new debate on their pathogenicity.

Concomitantly, the interest for further analysis of infection-induced AECAs has been revived by the finding that infectious agents, such as *Mycobacterium leprae*, cytomegalovirus (CMV), and dengue virus[10–12] colonize

Infection and Autoimmunity
http://dx.doi.org/10.1016/B978-0-444-63269-2.00006-4

133

ECs and contribute to the pathophysiology of vasculitis. Evidence also has been presented that some AECAs recognize the membrane, whereas others react with components of their cytosol.[13] The former may be involved in pathogenesis, but the latter would merely constitute a disease marker. Such findings support the view that AECAs are also functionally heterogeneous, depending on their specificity.

2 PITFALLS IN AECA DETECTION

The methods of detecting AECAs can be classified into those requiring fixation of the cells and those using suspensions of ECs. The group requiring fixation includes IIF of tissue sections, cytotoxicity of ECs labeled with Cr^{51} or I^{111}, radioimmunoassay and cell enzyme-linked immunosorbent assay (ELISA). There are, in fact, some major pitfalls in the ELISA method developed by Hashemi et al.[14] We reported that heterophile Ab against fetal calf serum (FCS) may be mistaken for AECA.[15] Such interference can be eliminated simply by absorption of dilution buffer containing FCS. Given that antinuclear Ab and rheumatoid factor may interfere with AECA, these may also be detected by an ELISA using Abs from EC lysate.[16] In addition, considering that false-negative AECAs may result from the lack of expression of specific Ags, analysis of infectious or other AECAs[17] dictates the use of several EC types, including microvascular ECs. However, because fixation with glutaraldehyde permeabilizes the cells, autoAbs to non–EC-specific cytosolic components can been detected in these assays, as reported in malaria.[13]

ECs may rather be used as a suspension. Fluorescence-activated cell sorting (FACS) analysis, immunoprecipitation (IP), and Western blotting (WB) have thus been developed.[18] Human umbilical vein endothelial cells (HUVECs) remain the most widely used substrate cells. Hybrid cell lines, such as EA.hy926, are occasionally used.[19] However, it must be stressed that HUVECs have a limited use on a routine basis because there are so few of them (approximately 10^6 cells are eluted from a cord) that the procedure becomes extremely tedious. In addition, the phenotype of the cells is not stable, and ECs die at the third or fourth passage. EA.hy926 cells have the advantage (one of limited value) of consisting of an unlimited number of cells, of which the phenotype remains the same until 50 passages or more. It may be necessary to absorb the sera with the mother epithelial cells A-549 before use. However, although "AECA" has long been used as a designation for these autoAbs, this does not necessarily mean that they recognize only ECs. Numerous other human, bovine, and murine cell lines are available.

With regard to the practical development of AECA binding, the most accurate method is the cell ELISA.[18] It is quantitative because ECs are used only once they are confluent. It is therefore possible to test a large number of sera at the same time. IIF, a semiquantitative test, is not recommended, given that it does not permit adequate follow-up of the AECA levels. Cytotoxicity tests and radioimmunoassay are not used anymore.

FACS is a technique where the cells do not adhere to a matrix but are suspended in a buffer.[18,19] It has been claimed to be the most suitable method to measure membrane-specific AECAs,[20] and we showed that such autoAbs detected that way predominate in leprosy.[13] Yet standardization has not been achieved, and creating a suspension of adherent cells may underestimate the expression of certain Ags.[21] The results of ongoing programs could standardize the test and perhaps bring about more insights into the understanding of these autoAbs. At present they have to be compared with those obtained by ELISA. ECs display different Ag distributions on their surface, depending on whether they are in contact with the solid support (subendothelial matrix or plastic) or flooding in the supernatant. AutoAbs against the extracellular matrix can masquerade as AECAs[22] and have pathological significance in vascular damage. IP and WB are too complicated to be applied on a routine basis. An additional problem is that cytoplasmic proteins, along with surface glycoproteins, can be precipitated. Because of the uncertainly of such results, we have evaluated the same sera using in-house cell ELISA, FACS analysis, and WB completed by densitometric quantitation and have identified AECA using these three different methods.[18] We came to the conclusion that, ideally, the three methods should be used.

It is equally important to agree on the way to express results.[23] Given the variations in the number of cells in a well, they should not be expressed as optical densities but as a binding index, using the formula: $100 \times (S - A) (B - A)$, where S is the result of the disease, A is the negative value and B is the positive value.

3 DETECTION OF AECAs

3.1 Viral Infections

Despite obvious differences in their pathophysiology, similar AECAs have been reported in a vast array of diseases (Table 1). For example, IgG and IgM AECAs have long been described[24] in Kawasaki syndrome (KS) and are claimed to be involved in the development of its acute phases.[31] Such a statement has been subsequently challenged,[32] so still very little is known

Table 1 Prevalence of Antiendothelial Cell Antibodies in Infectious Disease

Infectious Diseases	Antiendothelial Cell Antibodies Not Positive/Not Tested (% Positive)	References
Viral infections		
Kawasaki disease	13/16 (81)	[24]
Puumala virus	3/17 (18)	[25]
Behçet disease	13/72 (18)	[26]
Cytomegalovirus	10/23 (43)	[27]
Hepatitis C virus	28/69 (41)	[28]
Bacterial infections		
Infective endocarditis	7/15 (47)	[29]
Leprosy	35/68 (51)	[13]
Streptococcus A	56/140 (40%)	[30]
Parasitic infections		
Malaria	30/34 (88)	[13]
Toxocara infection	3/5 (60)	Unpublished
Amebiasis	4/5 (80)	Unpublished
Echinococcus	4/6 (67)	Unpublished
Schistosomiasis	5/5 (100)	Unpublished

about the etiology of the syndrome. AECAs have been detected in 18% of the cases of Behçet disease, which is also of unknown origin but possibly triggered by a virus , and were found to be associated with thrombotic events and therefore suspected to be pathogenic.[26]

There is increasing evidence that AECAs are associated with various viral infections. AutoAbs have thus been reported in nephropathia epidemica, one of the milder forms of hemorrhagic fever caused by the Puumala virus in 3 of 17 patients, as well as in 4 of 9 sera and 2 of 19 sera from patients with influenza A and influenza B, respectively.[25] Interestingly, AECAs are a common finding in hepatitis C virus (HCV) infection, but not in non–HCV chronic liver diseases.[28] It might be a risk factor for vascular rejection in CMV–infected recipients of cardiac,[27] renal, or liver[33] allograft. In this respect, the dengue virus is another particular case because ECs are cellular reservoirs to this virus and AECAs are generated in the majority of the patients.[34]

3.2 Other Infections

AECAs also have been found in less than half of the sera from infective endocarditis[29] and more than half of those from leprosy.[13] In the latter disease, more patients with lepromatous and the borderline lepromatous forms were positive compared with patients with the tuberculoid and the borderline tuberculoid forms, and the truly specific autoAbs to the membrane of ECs were preferentially associated with multibacillary than with paucibacillary leprosy. Other bacteria, including *Chlamydia pneumoniae* and *Helicobacter pylori*, activate ECs, although, for unknown reasons, they do not promote the synthesis of AECAs.[35] Finally, the cell ELISA for these autoAbs was recorded positive in 30 of 34 patients with malaria compared with 17 of 50 local controls.[13] This baseline production in healthy African individuals is relatively high, as would be expected in an area where parasitic infection is endemic. Consistent with this view is the high level of AECAs in toxocara infection (60%), amebiasis (80%), echinococcus (67%), and schistosomiasis (100%).

4 PATHOGENIC EFFECTS OF AECAs

The pathogenicity of AECAs remains uncertain. The likelihood of such an effect was first suggested by the observation that autoAb levels fluctuate with disease activity in patients with systemic lupus erythematosus (SLE), Wegener granulomatosis (WG), and KS. The AECA test can even identify subsets of systemic sclerosis (SSc),[36] vasculitides,[37] or inflammatory myopathies[38] with differing prognoses. Interestingly, the production of AECAs is complicated by renal failure in SLE,[39] vasculitis in rheumatoid arthritis (RA)[40] and lung fibrosis in dermatomyositis.[41] Some AECAs cause complement-mediated killing of ECs in SLE,[5] KS[31] and hemolytic-uremic syndrome[42] or induce Ab-dependent cellular cytotoxicity in WG.[43] Thrombomodulin, an EC-specific glycoprotein, is released by damage to these cells in WG and other systemic vasculitides.[44]

Plasma from patients with thrombotic thrombocytopenic purpura and sporadic hemolytic-uremic syndrome induces apoptosis in restricted lineages of human microvascular EC, although the agents responsible for initiating EC injury and the exact role played by AECAs are elusive.[45] Also supporting an apoptotic process in these thrombotic microangiopathies are the EC detachment from affected vessels, their appearance in the periphery[46] and the clear absence of inflammatory changes. The finding that EC apoptosis is one of the earliest events in a chicken model of SSc[47] may be highly relevant to this problem. Similar endothelial changes also are found in the initial phase of human generalized and local scleroderma.

In addition, speculation about the mechanism of vascular conditions associated with AECAs has focused on increased expression of adhesion molecules, such as E-selectin, intercellular adhesion molecule 1, and vascular cell adhesion molecule 1, by ECs.[48] This enhancement, together with the production of chemotactic cytokines (e.g. interleukin [IL]-1β, IL-6, IL-8, and monocyte chemotatic protein 1), would facilitate adhesion of leukocytes to the inflamed vessel walls, followed by their extravascular migration and granuloma formation. A different group of AECAs has been shown to induce tissue factor in ECs.[49]

Another appealing possibility is that EC apoptosis is initiated by AECAs. In this study, incubation of ECs with AECAs derived from patients with vasculitis or mouse monoclonal AECAs resulted in the expression of phosphatidylserine (PS) on the surface of the cells, as established through the binding of cationic annexin V.[50] Hypoploid cell enumeration, DNA fragmentation study, optical immunofluorescence, and confocal and electron microscopy analysis confirmed apoptosis of ECs (Figure 1). In some but not all sera, a subgroup of AECAs may thus be pathogenic that way. Such a complication has been described in leprosy[13] and dengue virus infection.[51] We therefore addressed the issue of whether activation is a prerequisite for AECA-mediated apoptosis of ECs,[52] showed that the ability of some AECAs to activate the cells was irrelevant to the nature of the underlying disorder and established that activation does not play a role in the advent of apoptosis.

We have since extended these studies and found that AECAs binding to HUVECs makes anionic phospholipids (PLs) accessible to the

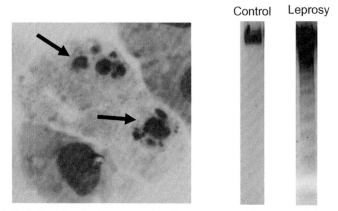

Figure 1 Endothelial cells (EC) stained with May-Grünwald–Giemsa (left) exhibit the typical morphological aspect of apoptosis (arrows). Agarose gel electrophoresis (right) shows ECs incubated with control IgG or with apoptosis-inducing autoantibodies. These generate fragmentation of DNA.

anti-glycoprotein I (β_2GPI) Ab.[53] A mechanism by which some anti-PL (aPL) Abs bind to ECs has thus been proposed. Should PS become available, following the binding of AECAs, circulating β_2GPI would attach to ECs, thereby allowing the β_2GPI/PL complex to be recognized by autoimmune aPLs. It is not yet known whether the anti-β_2GPI Ab from patients with primary aPL syndrome recognizes new epitopes formed after binding of the molecule to anionic structures displayed by native β_2GPI when available at increased density, as one would expect for a low-affinity Ab.[54] In line with the first interpretation is the report by Pittoni et al. that a monoclonal Ab from a patient with SLE reacts with a cryptic epitope on β_2GPI following binding to apoptotic cells.[55]

Thus, not only AECAs encourage the binding of pre-existing aPLs to apoptotic ECs but the exposure to PS might result in de novo production of aPLs. It may be argued that, if AECAs were essential to the production of aPLs, they should be present in all patients with aPLs. However, a proportion of sera contain aPLs but not AECAs. One possibility is that by the time a patient is investigated for autoAbs, AECAs may have already disappeared, so that the serum, while being aPL positive, has become AECA negative. As suggested by Shoenfeld,[56] aPLs may be infectiously induced. Inasmuch as there are plenty of infectious diseases associated with AECAs, it is tempting to speculate a role for these infection-related autoAbs in the production of aPLs.

5 MECHANISMS OF AECA PRODUCTION IN INFECTIOUS DISEASE

5.1 Direct Involvement of ECs

Four mechanisms of AECA production in infectious disease deserve to be considered. The first refers to molecular mimicry, as described in dengue virus infection where Abs cross-react with ECs and their binding is inhibited by pre-treatment of the cells with nonstructural protein 1 from the virus.[34] Human heat-shock protein (HSP)70, which is a chaperone molecule, is recognized by some autoAbs from some lepromatous sera.[13] This target Ag of AECA reproduces the C-terminal half of the *M. leprae* HSP70.[57] Accordingly, it may initiate cross-reactive autoAbs, either singularly or through interaction with any chaperoned autoAg. Alternatively, AECAs may represent one of many serological hallmarks of polyclonal B cell activation. This second mechanism, well established in SLE, has been demonstrated in the production of malarial AECAs.[13,58] The third option is related to the capacity of circulating EC microparticles to induce AECAs, but this option was recently ruled out.[59] The fourth possibility is the induction of cell proliferation and morphological changes through colonization of ECs. One example is *M. leprae*, most notably in cells lining epineurial and perineurial blood vessels.[10] Dengue virus–EC interaction also has been studied in depth using differential display reverse transcription and real-time polymerase chain reaction and Affymetrix oligonucleotide microarrays.[60] Striking changes in gene expression were seen after infection of HUVECs with the virus.

5.2 Indirect Involvement of ECs

Several indirect mechanisms have been suspected to initiate the production of AECAs. These include activation of ECs by IL-1α released by epithelial cells infected with the respiratory syncytial virus[61] and upregulation of CD40 expression on ECs infected with CMV.[62]

6 THE TARGET AG OF AECAs

6.1 Cell Membrane Specificity

Early studies have excluded anti–ABO and anti–human leukocyte Ag Abs from the AECAs.[63] Specificity for the membrane that cannot be absorbed with cytosolic lysates predominates over that for cytosolic components in leprosy.[13] WB analysis, expression bank evaluation, and two-dimensional electrophoresis have revealed that calreticulin, vimentin, tubulin, and HSP70 are recognized by AECAs from patients with leprosy, but numerous proteins remain unidentified (Table 2). In SLE, which is the prototype vasculitis-associated disease, 19 bands ranging from 15 to 200 kDa were identified by van der Zee et al.[64] using WB, and Abs against 38-, 41-, and 150-kDa proteins were shown to be tightly associated with lupus nephritis. Li et al.,[65] however, reported that patients with SLE with nephritis, vasculitis, and hypocomplement raise IgG-AECA against a 66-kDa membrane Ag, whereas a 55-kDa Ag would be the specific target for AECAs in patients with thrombocytopenia and another 18-kDa component the target in patients with pleuritis. Other groups have demonstrated that ribosomal P protein is an EC target for autoAbs. It may be involved in the pathogenesis of lupus nephritis.[66] Although the AECA epitopes vary from one patient to another, a subgroup can be immunoprecipitated only by SLE sera, suggesting that the way AECAs react might be specific for each disease.[67]

Table 2 Membrane Components Recognized by Antiendothelial Cell Antibodies

Disease	Components
Leprosy	Calreticulin, vimentin, tubulin, heat-shock protein (HSP)-70
Streptococcus A	Vimentin, HSP-70, streptopain
Systemic lupus erythematosus	Ribosomal P protein
Systemic vasculitides	Triose phosphate isomerase
Systemic sclerosis	Heparan sulphate
Granulomatosis with polyangiitis	70-kDa protein (HSP-70) ATP synthase

It also has been established that AECAs from patients with renal diseases and kidney transplantation with systemic vasculitis recognize 30–35-kDa Ag. In contrast, a 28-kDa Ag has been claimed to be specific for vasculitis and to share 93% amino-acid sequence with triose phosphate isomerase.[68] Interestingly, Wheeler et al.[69] demonstrated the association of these anti-triose phosphate isomerase Abs with IgM anti-vimentin Abs in transplant-associated coronary artery disease in humans. This observation might be a clue to the concept that a fraction of AECAs enter the cells.

In RA, 12 proteins, ranging from 16 to 48 kDa, have been identified by WB and IP. In patients with RA vasculitis, IgG-AECAs were as directed towards a 44-kDa EC membrane Ag.[40] This is reminiscent of the intriguing finding that a 44-kDa protein was targeted by AECAs from patients with Behçet disease when human dermal microvascular ECs were used.[70] Del Papa et al.[67] found that any one of five proteins in WG reacts with AECAs (180, 155, 125, 38, and 25 kDa). Ab binding to an as yet unknown 43-kDa component in the cytosol and the nucleus of human microvascular renal ECs have been identified in hemolytic-uremic syndrome and thrombotic thrombocytopenic purpura.[71] In heparin-induced thrombocytopenia, some circulating Abs react with platelet factor 4 complexed with heparin, and others react with heparan sulphate incorporated into the membrane of ECs. Thus, it is not unreasonable to assume that AECAs may play an active role in the development of thrombosis.[72] Similar reactions have been reported to occur[73] in connective tissue diseases associated with vasculitis. Finally, an 18-kDa EC membrane Ag was shown to be important for auto-Abs from patients with SSc. It should be stressed that the related AECAs are associated with the CREST (Calcinosis, Raynaud phenomenon, Esophageal dysmotility, Sclerodactyly, and Telangiectasia) variant of this disorder. Finally, the possibility exists that murine monoclonal AECAs produced by idiotypic manipulation with human Ab recognizes HSP70.[74]

6.2 HSP Autoantibodies

HSPs belong to danger signal protein known as alarmin, which can be recognized by the immune system. In physiologic conditions, HSPs have an intracellular localization, and in inflammatory processes they are exposed on the plasma membrane. HSPs derive from mitochondria and share both sequence and three-dimensional homology with bacterial HSPs. Thus explaining that autoAbs against endogenous endothelial HSP70 result from cross-reactivity with *M. leprae* during leprosy.[13] In a similar way, classical vaccination against *Mycobacterium tuberculosis* also leads to an increase of anti-HSP60 autoAb. In addition, cross-reactivity between streptococcal A protein Abs and streptococcal anti-HSP70 Abs were recently described with anti-vimentin Abs and AECAs in rheumatic heart disease. The pathogenicity of anti-HSPs have been explored, revealing at least two pathways. First, anti-HSP60 Ab can bind to an HSP60/GRP75 complex present on ECs and in turn trigger a proapoptotic pathway via CCR5 activation.[75] Second, the HSP60/ATP synthase complex is recognized by anti-HSP60, and the Ab-induced pathogenicity comes from a perturbation of the capacity of the cells to maintain a neutral pH to stay alive.[76] Anti-HSP60 Abs are more frequently observed in carotid or coronary diseases, whereas anti-HSP70 Abs are found in aortic and perivascular diseases.[77]

6.3 Other Ags Possibly Recognized by AECAs

It seems that most AECA-positive malarian sera react with the cytosol but not with the membrane of ECs.[13] This is substantiated (Figure 2) by our finding that sera negative in FACS analysis become positive once ECs have been permeabilized with saponin. Clearly, the target Ag of these pseudo-AECAs are specific neither for malaria nor for ECs.

The majority of AECAs that bind to Ags seem to be EC membrane proteins. Yet the demonstration that extensive washes of radiolabeled preparations with highly molar buffers result in the reduction of AECAs from SLE sera indicates that some of these Abs are able to recognize non-constitutive proteins. This is further supported by the description of monoclonal and polyclonal anti-DNA Ab binding in vitro to ECs through DNA or DNA/histone complexes attached to the cell membrane.[78]

To conclude, there is compelling evidence identifying more and more specific proteins and epitopes recognized by apoptosis-inducing AECAs. Still, clarification of the function of target Ag is required to achieve a better understanding of the effects of AECAs on associated infectious diseases.

Leprosy

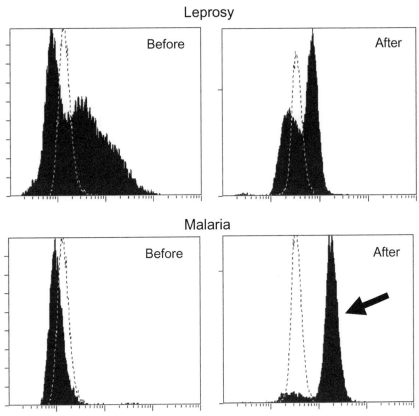

Figure 2 Detection of antiendothelial cell (EC) antibodies (Abs) from lepromatous (top) and malarial (bottom) sera using flow cytometry analysis. The serum from the patient with leprosy is positive before permeabilization of the cells because Abs bind to the membrane, whereas the serum from the patient with malaria needs ECs to be incubated with saponin to encounter cytosolic antigens (arrow).

ACKNOWLEDGMENT

The secretarial assistance of Simone Forest and Geneviève Michel is appreciated.

REFERENCES

1. Youinou P, Meroni PL, Khamashta MA, Shoenfeld Y. A need for standardization of the anti-endothelial-cell antibody test. *Immunol Today* 1995;**16**:363–4.
2. Youinou P. Antiendothelial cell autoantibodies and disease. *Intern Med Clin Lab* 1995;**3**:7–10.
3. Lindqvist KJ, Osterland CK. Human antibodies to vascular endothelium. *Clin Exp Immunol* 1971;**9**:753–60.

4. Tan EM, Pearson CM. Rheumatic disease sera reactive with capillaries in the mouse kidney. *Arthritis Rheum* 1972;**15**:23–8.
5. Cines DB, Lyss AP, Reeber M, Bina M, DeHoratius RJ. Presence of complement-fixing anti-endothelial cell antibodies in systemic lupus erythematosus. *J Clin Invest* 1984;**73**:611–25.
6. Meroni PL, Youinou P. Endothelial cell antibodies. In: Peter JB, Shoenfeld Y, editors. *Autoantibodies*. Amsterdam: Elsevier; 1996. p. 245–52.
7. Praprotnik S, Blank M, Meroni PL, Rozman B, Eldor A, Shoenfeld Y. Classification of anti-endothelial cell antibodies into antibodies against microvascular and macrovascular endothelial cells: the pathogenic and diagnostic implications. *Arthritis Rheum* 2001;**44**:1484–94.
8. Castillo S, Revelen R, Bordron A, Renaudineau Y, Dueymes M, Youinou P. Anti-endothelial cell reactivity, the unresolved enigma. *Int J Immunopathol Pharmacol* 2001;**14**:109–18.
9. Damianovich M, Gilburd B, George J, Del Papa N, Afek A, Goldberg I, et al. Pathogenic role of anti-endothelial cell antibodies in vasculitis. An idiotypic experimental model. *J Immunol* 1996;**156**:4946–51.
10. Fite GL. The vascular lesions of leprosy. *Int J Lepr* 1941;**9**:193–202.
11. Ho DD, Rota TR, Andrews CA, Hirsch MS. Replication of human cytomegalovirus in endothelial cells. *J Infect Dis* 1984;**150**:956–7.
12. Funahara Y, Ogawa K, Fujita N, Okuno Y. Three possible triggers to induce thrombocytopenia in dengue virus infection. *Southeast Asian J Trop Med Public Health* 1987;**18**:351–5.
13. Dugue C, Perraut R, Youinou P, Renaudineau Y. Effects of anti-endothelial cell antibodies in leprosy and malaria. *Infect Immun* 2004;**72**:301–9.
14. Hashemi S, Smith CD, Izaguirre CA. Anti-endothelial cell antibodies: detection and characterization using a cellular enzyme-linked immunosorbent assay. *J Lab Clin Med* 1987;**109**:434–40.
15. Revelen R, Bordron A, Dueymes M, Youinou P, Arvieux J. False positivity in a cyto-ELISA for anti-endothelial cell antibodies caused by heterophile antibodies to bovine serum proteins. *Clin Chem* 2000;**46**:273–8.
16. Drouet C, Nissou MF, Ponard D, Arvieux J, Dumestre-Perard C, Gaudin P, et al. Detection of antiendothelial cell antibodies by an enzyme-linked immunosorbent assay using antigens from cell lysate: minimal interference with antinuclear antibodies and rheumatoid factors. *Clin Diagn Lab Immunol* 2003;**10**:934–9.
17. Renaudineau Y, Revelen R, Levy Y, Salojin K, Gilburg B, Shoenfeld Y, et al. Anti-endothelial cell antibodies in systemic sclerosis. *Clin Diagn Lab Immunol* 1999;**6**:156–60.
18. Revelen R, D'Arbonneau F, Guillevin L, Bordron A, Youinou P, Dueymes M. Comparison of cell-ELISA, flow cytometry and Western blotting for the detection of antiendothelial cell antibodies. *Clin Exp Rheumatol* 2002;**20**:19–26.
19. Edgell CJ, McDonald CC, Graham JB. Permanent cell line expressing human factor VIII-related antigen established by hybridization. *Proc Natl Acad Sci USA* 1983;**80**:3734–7.
20. Westphal JR, Boerbooms AM, Schalwijk CJ, Kwast H, De Weijert M, Jacobs C, et al. Anti-endothelial cell antibodies in sera of patients with autoimmune diseases: comparison between ELISA and FACS analysis. *Clin Exp Immunol* 1994;**96**:444–9.
21. Forsyth KD, Talbot V. Assessment of endothelial immunophenotype—limitation of flow cytometric analysis. *J Immunol Methods* 1991;**144**:93–9.
22. Direskeneli H, D'Cruz D, Khamashta MA, Hughes GR. Autoantibodies against endothelial cells, extracellular matrix, and human collagen type IV in patients with systemic vasculitis. *Clin Immunol Immunopathol* 1994;**70**:206–10.
23. Rosenbaum J, Pottinger BE, Woo P, Black CM, Loizou S, Byron MA, et al. Measurement and characterisation of circulating anti-endothelial cell IgG in connective tissue diseases. *Clin Exp Immunol* 1988;**72**:450–6.

24. Leung DY, Collins T, Lapierre LA, Geha RS, Pober JS. Immunoglobulin M antibodies present in the acute phase of Kawasaki syndrome lyse cultured vascular endothelial cells stimulated by gamma interferon. *J Clin Invest* 1986;**77**:1428–35.

25. Wangel AG, Temonen M, Brummer-Korvenkontio M, Vaheri A. Anti-endothelial cell antibodies in nephropathia epidemica and other viral diseases. *Clin Exp Immunol* 1992;**90**:13–17.

26. Aydintug AO, Tokgoz G, D'Cruz DP, Gurler A, Cervera R, Duzgun N, et al. Antibodies to endothelial cells in patients with Behcet's disease. *Clin Immunol Immunopathol* 1993;**67**:157–62.

27. Costa C, Touscoz GA, Bergallo M, Terlizzi ME, Astegiano S, Sidoti F, et al. Non-organ-specific and anti-endothelial antibodies in relation to CMV infection and acute rejection in renal transplant recipients. *Clin Transplant* 2010;**24**:488–92.

28. Cacoub P, Ghillani P, Revelen R, Thibault V, Calvez V, Charlotte F, et al. Anti-endothelial cell auto-antibodies in hepatitis C virus mixed cryoglobulinemia. *J Hepatol* 1999;**31**:598–603.

29. Portig I, Beck V, Pankuweit S, Maisch B. Antiendothelial antibodies in sera of patients with infective endocarditis. *Basic Res Cardiol* 2001;**96**:75–81.

30. Scalzi V, Hadi HA, Alessandri C, Croia C, Conti V, Agati L, et al. Anti-endothelial cell antibodies in rheumatic heart disease. *Clin Exp Immunol* 2010;**161**:570–5.

31. Leung DY, Geha RS, Newburger JW, Burns JC, Fiers W, Lapierre LA, et al. Two monokines, interleukin 1 and tumor necrosis factor, render cultured vascular endothelial cells susceptible to lysis by antibodies circulating during Kawasaki syndrome. *J Exp Med* 1986;**164**:1958–72.

32. Nash MC, Shah V, Reader JA, Dillon MJ. Anti-neutrophil cytoplasmic antibodies and anti-endothelial cell antibodies are not increased in Kawasaki disease. *Br J Rheumatol* 1995;**34**:882–7.

33. Varani S, Muratori L, De Ruvo N, Vivarelli M, Lazzarotto T, Gabrielli L, et al. Auto-antibody appearance in cytomegalovirus-infected liver transplant recipients: correlation with antigenemia. *J Med Virol* 2002;**66**:56–62.

34. Lin CF, Lei HY, Shiau AL, Liu CC, Liu HS, Yeh TM, et al. Antibodies from dengue patient sera cross-react with endothelial cells and induce damage. *J Med Virol* 2003;**69**:82–90.

35. Schumacher A, Seljeflot I, Lerkerod AB, Sommervoll L, Otterstad JE, Arnesen H. Does infection with *Chlamydia pneumoniae* and/or *Helicobacter pylori* increase the expression of endothelial cell adhesion molecules in humans? *Clin Microbiol Infect* 2002;**8**:654–61.

36. Salojin KV, Le Tonqueze M, Saraux A, Nassonov EL, Dueymes M, Piette JC, et al. Anti-endothelial cell antibodies: useful markers of systemic sclerosis. *Am J Med* 1997;**102**:178–85.

37. Salojin KV, Le Tonqueze M, Nassovov EL, Blouch MT, Baranov AA, Saraux A, et al. Anti-endothelial cell antibodies in patients with various forms of vasculitis. *Clin Exp Rheumatol* 1996;**14**:163–9.

38. Salojin KV, Bordron A, Nassonov EL, Shtutman VZ, Guseva NG, Baranov AA, et al. Anti-endothelial cell antibody, thrombomodulin, and von Willebrand factor in idiopathic inflammatory myopathies. *Clin Diagn Lab Immunol* 1997;**4**:519–21.

39. D'Cruz DP, Houssiau FA, Ramirez G, Baguley E, McCutcheon J, Vianna J, et al. Antibodies to endothelial cells in systemic lupus erythematosus: a potential marker for nephritis and vasculitis. *Clin Exp Immunol* 1991;**85**:254–61.

40. Heurkens AH, Hiemstra PS, Lafeber GJ, Daha MR, Breedveld FC. Anti-endothelial cell antibodies in patients with rheumatoid arthritis complicated by vasculitis. *Clin Exp Immunol* 1989;**78**:7–12.

41. Cervera R, Ramirez G, Fernandez-Sola J, D'Cruz D, Casademont J, Grau JM, et al. Antibodies to endothelial cells in dermatomyositis: association with interstitial lung disease. *BMJ* 1991;**302**:880–1.

42. Leung DY, Moake JL, Havens PL, Kim M, Pober JS. Lytic anti-endothelial cell antibodies in haemolytic-uraemic syndrome. *Lancet* 1988;**2**:183–6.
43. del Papa N, Meroni PL, Barcellini W, Sinico A, Radice A, Tincani A, et al. Antibodies to endothelial cells in primary vasculitides mediate in vitro endothelial cytotoxicity in the presence of normal peripheral blood mononuclear cells. *Clin Immunol Immunopathol* 1992;**63**:267–74.
44. Boehme MW, Schmitt WH, Youinou P, Stremmel WR, Gross WL. Clinical relevance of elevated serum thrombomodulin and soluble E-selectin in patients with Wegener's granulomatosis and other systemic vasculitides. *Am J Med* 1996;**101**:387–94.
45. Raife TJ, Atkinson B, Aster RH, McFarland JG, Gottschall JL. Minimal evidence of platelet and endothelial cell reactive antibodies in thrombotic thrombocytopenic purpura. *Am J Hematol* 1999;**62**:82–7.
46. George F, Poncelet P, Laurent JC, Massot O, Arnoux D, Lequeux N, et al. Cytofluorometric detection of human endothelial cells in whole blood using S-Endo 1 monoclonal antibody. *J Immunol Methods* 1991;**139**:65–75.
47. Sgonc R, Gruschwitz MS, Dietrich H, Recheis H, Gershwin ME, Wick G. Endothelial cell apoptosis is a primary pathogenetic event underlying skin lesions in avian and human scleroderma. *J Clin Invest* 1996;**98**:785–92.
48. Del Papa N, Guidali L, Sironi M, Shoenfeld Y, Mantovani A, Tincani A, et al. Anti-endothelial cell IgG antibodies from patients with Wegener's granulomatosis bind to human endothelial cells in vitro and induce adhesion molecule expression and cytokine secretion. *Arthritis Rheum* 1996;**39**:758–66.
49. Kornberg A, Renaudineau Y, Blank M, Youinou P, Shoenfeld Y. Anti-beta 2-glycoprotein I antibodies and anti-endothelial cell antibodies induce tissue factor in endothelial cells. *Isr Med Assoc J* 2000;**2**(Suppl.):27–31.
50. Bordron A, Dueymes M, Levy Y, Jamin C, Leroy JP, Piette JC, et al. The binding of some human antiendothelial cell antibodies induces endothelial cell apoptosis. *J Clin Invest* 1998;**101**:2029–35.
51. Avirutnan P, Malasit P, Seliger B, Bhakdi S, Husmann M. Dengue virus infection of human endothelial cells leads to chemokine production, complement activation, and apoptosis. *J Immunol* 1998;**161**:6338–46.
52. Bordron A, Revelen R, D'Arbonneau F, Dueymes M, Renaudineau Y, Jamin C, et al. Functional heterogeneity of anti-endothelial cell antibodies. *Clin Exp Immunol* 2001;**124**:492–501.
53. Bordron A, Dueymes M, Levy Y, Jamin C, Ziporen L, Piette JC, et al. Anti-endothelial cell antibody binding makes negatively charged phospholipids accessible to antiphospholipid antibodies. *Arthritis Rheum* 1998;**41**:1738–47.
54. Ronda N, Haury M, Nobrega A, Kaveri SV, Coutinho A, Kazatchkine MD. Analysis of natural and disease-associated autoantibody repertoires: anti-endothelial cell IgG autoantibody activity in the serum of healthy individuals and patients with systemic lupus erythematosus. *Int Immunol* 1994;**6**:1651–60.
55. Pittoni V, Ravirajan CT, Donohoe S, Machin SJ, Mackie IJ, Lydyard PM, et al. Human monoclonal antiphospholipid antibodies bind to membrane phospholipids and a cryptic epitope of beta2-glycoprotein I on apoptotic cells. *Arthritis Rheum* 1998;**41**(Suppl. 12): S166 [Abstract].
56. Shoenfeld Y. Etiology and pathogenetic mechanisms of the anti-phospholipid syndrome unraveled. *Trends Immunol* 2003;**24**:2–4.
57. Janson AA, Klatser PR, van der Zee R, Cornelisse YE, de Vries RR, Thole JE, et al. A systematic molecular analysis of the T cell-stimulating antigens from *Mycobacterium leprae* with T cell clones of leprosy patients. Identification of a novel *M. leprae* HSP 70 fragment by *M. leprae*-specific T cells. *J Immunol* 1991;**147**:3530–7.

58. Adebajo AO, Charles P, Maini RN, Hazleman BL. Autoantibodies in malaria, tuberculosis and hepatitis B in a west African population. *Clin Exp Immunol* 1993;**92**:73–6.
59. Duval A, Helley D, Capron L, Youinou P, Renaudineau Y, Dubucquoi S, et al. Endothelial dysfunction in systemic lupus patients with low disease activity: evaluation by quantification and characterization of circulating endothelial microparticles, role of anti-endothelial cell antibodies. *Rheumatology (Oxford)* 2010;**49**:1049–55.
60. Warke RV, Xhaja K, Martin KJ, Fournier MF, Shaw SK, Brizuela N, et al. Dengue virus induces novel changes in gene expression of human umbilical vein endothelial cells. *J Virol* 2003;**77**:11822–32.
61. Chang CH, Huang Y, Anderson R. Activation of vascular endothelial cells by IL-1alpha released by epithelial cells infected with respiratory syncytial virus. *Cell Immunol* 2003;**221**:37–41.
62. Maisch T, Kropff B, Sinzger C, Mach M. Upregulation of CD40 expression on endothelial cells infected with human cytomegalovirus. *J Virol* 2002;**76**:12803–12.
63. Ferraro G, Meroni PL, Tincani A, Sinico A, Barcellini W, Radice A, et al. Anti-endothelial cell antibodies in patients with Wegener's granulomatosis and micropolyarteritis. *Clin Exp Immunol* 1990;**79**:47–53.
64. van der Zee JM, Heurkens AH, van der Voort EA, Daha MR, Breedveld FC. Characterization of anti-endothelial antibodies in patients with rheumatoid arthritis complicated by vasculitis. *Clin Exp Rheumatol* 1991;**9**:589–94.
65. Li JS, Liu MF, Lei HY. Characterization of anti-endothelial cell antibodies in the patients with systemic lupus erythematosus: a potential marker for disease activity. *Clin Immunol Immunopathol* 1996;**79**:211–6.
66. Reichlin M, Wolfson-Reichlin M. Evidence for the participation of anti-ribosomal P antibodies in lupus nephritis. *Arthritis Rheum* 1999;**42**:2728–9.
67. Del Papa N, Conforti G, Gambini D, La Rosa L, Tincani A, D'Cruz D, et al. Characterization of the endothelial surface proteins recognized by anti-endothelial antibodies in primary and secondary autoimmune vasculitis. *Clin Immunol Immunopathol* 1994;**70**:211–6.
68. Moriya S, Khouri NA, Cameron JS, Frampton G. Preliminary report of a vasculitis associated 28 kD endothelial cell autoantigen which shares a 93% identity with triose phosphate isomerase. *Lupus* 1995;**4**:99 [Abstract].
69. Wheeler CH, Collins A, Dunn MJ, Crisp SJ, Yacoub MH, Rose ML. Characterization of endothelial antigens associated with transplant-associated coronary artery disease. *J Heart Lung Transplant* 1995;**14**:S188–97.
70. Lee KH, Bang D, Choi ES, Chun WH, Lee ES, Lee S. Presence of circulating antibodies to a disease-specific antigen on cultured human dermal microvascular endothelial cells in patients with Behcet's disease. *Arch Dermatol Res* 1999;**291**:374–81.
71. Koenig DW, Barley-Maloney L, Daniel TO. A western blot assay detects autoantibodies to cryptic endothelial antigens in thrombotic microangiopathies. *J Clin Immunol* 1993;**13**:204–11.
72. Visentin GP, Ford SE, Scott JP, Aster RH. Antibodies from patients with heparin-induced thrombocytopenia/thrombosis are specific for platelet factor 4 complexed with heparin or bound to endothelial cells. *J Clin Invest* 1994;**93**:81–8.
73. Renaudineau Y, Revelen R, Bordron A, Mottier D, Youinou P, Le Corre R. Two populations of endothelial cell antibodies cross-react with heparin. *Lupus* 1998;**7**:86–94.
74. Levy Y, Gilburd B, George J, Del Papa N, Mallone R, Damianovich M, et al. Characterization of murine monoclonal anti-endothelial cell antibodies (AECA) produced by idiotypic manipulation with human AECA. *Int Immunol* 1998;**10**:861–8.
75. Alard JE, Dueymes M, Mageed RA, Saraux A, Youinou P, Jamin C. Mitochondrial heat shock protein (HSP) 70 synergizes with HSP60 in transducing endothelial cell apoptosis induced by anti-HSP60 autoantibody. *FASEB J* 2009;**23**:2772–9.

76. Alard JE, Hillion S, Guillevin L, Saraux A, Pers JO, Youinou P, et al. Autoantibodies to endothelial cell surface ATP synthase, the endogenous receptor for hsp60, might play a pathogenic role in vasculatides. *PLoS One* 2011;**6**:e14654.
77. Mehta TA, Greenman J, Ettelaie C, Venkatasubramaniam A, Chetter IC, McCollum PT. Heat shock proteins in vascular disease—a review. *Eur J Vasc Endovasc Surg* 2005;**29**:395–402.
78. Chan TM, Frampton G, Staines NA, Hobby P, Perry GJ, Cameron JS. Different mechanisms by which anti-DNA MoAbs bind to human endothelial cells and glomerular mesangial cells. *Clin Exp Immunol* 1992;**88**:68–74.

CHAPTER 9

Microbiota and Autoimmunity

Dimitrios P. Bogdanos[*,†], **Daniel S. Smyk**[*], **Lazaros I. Sakkas**[†],
Yehuda Shoenfeld[‡,1]

[*]Division of Transplantation Immunology and Mucosal Biology, King's College London School of Medicine at King's College Hospital, Denmark Hill Campus, London, UK
[†]Department of Rheumatology, School of Health Sciences, University of Thessaly, Larissa, Greece
[‡]Zabludowicz Center for Autoimmune Diseases, Sheba Medical Center, Tel Hashomer affiliated with Sackler Faculty of Medicine, Tel Aviv University, Ramat Aviv, Tel Aviv, Israel
[1]Corresponding Author: shoenfel@post.tau.ac.il

1 INFECTIONS, THE MICROBIOME AND AUTOIMMUNITY

Infections have long been considered triggers of autoimmunity, but the study of microbial-induced autoimmunity has been limited to an approach of a single infections causing a single autoimmune disease because it has been difficult to trace and study the vast number of infectious agents etiologically linked with an autoimmune disease. While the human genome comprises approximately 20,500 genes, that of the microbiome accounts for several millions.[1] The dynamic interplay of microbiota with human genes governs homeostasis and affects most of the body processes in healthy as well as in disease states, including autoimmunity. The study of foreign and host protein interactions has led to the understanding that a single infection can alter the expression of approximately 500 genes.[2] This number is likely multiplied by thousands during the lifetime of an individual, who is exposed to hundreds of infectious agents. While 10 years ago fewer than 300 bacterial genomes were completed and published, today this has increased to a striking number in excess of 2,000, and approximately 20,000 more are in the process of completion. This information has considerably changed the way we can design studies investigating the role of the microbiome in the induction of autoimmunity. Thus, we are now in a much better position to study the influence of microbial/self interactions leading to immunological breakdown and the induction of autoimmunity—and indeed that of overt autoimmune disease. For example, we are aware now that he microbiomes of patients with autoimmune gastrointestinal diseases such as Crohn's disease (CD) or ulcerative colitis (UC) significantly differs from

149

patients with insulin–dependent diabetes mellitus (IDDM), as well as those not affected with an autoimmune disease.[3,4] Elegant data have demonstrated the dynamic intravariability of the human microbiome over time (even within days) at different body sites such as skin, gut (feces) and mouth.[5] Intrinsic and extrinsic factors participate in the temporal variation of the human microbiome within a body site. The outcome of efficient or insufficient adaptive immune responses largely affects the microbiota and is one of the major intrinsic factors, whereas changes in diet or alterations in medications and exposure to various xenobiotics are some of the extrinsic factors participating in the variability of an individual's microbiome. If we wish to delineate the complex mechanisms that are responsible for the development of autoimmune diseases, we must understand the influence of these factors on an individual's microbiota. Another challenging issue it that there is a significant subject–to–subject variability in microbiome studies conducted so far, suggesting that microbiomes are dynamic 'fingerprints' that are unique for an individual but can evolve over time, depending on the environment.[5,6] Data stemming from the investigation of biological fluids indicate that a large number of proteins remain the same among individuals, narrowing down to few hundred that are changing. Among those, the microbial ones reflect alterations of the human microbiome and can be directly or indirectly linked to the pathogenesis of an autoimmune disease if the individual is evaluated before the onset of the disease.[7] Because most autoimmune diseases are preceded by long preclinical stages, alterations of the microbiome that potentially play role in the induction of autoimmunity need to be documented at various time points. What has been missed by the approach to studying autoimmunity-related microbiomes is that a better understanding of the induction of autoimmune diseases requires better knowledge of the fine specificity of immune responses against specific microbial antigens. An infectious burden in autoimmunity has been documented in the form of infection-specific antibody and cellular responses against numerous antigens originating from bacteria, viruses, parasites, and fungi.[8–10] Geo-epidemiological, microbiological, and immunological data indicate the existence of infectious burdens varying from one autoimmune disease to another. Autoantibody burdens in infected individuals also have been noted, but these individuals have not been followed up for long, and it is not clear how many of those autoantibodies have been induced by pathogenetically linked pathogens or are mere consequences of the progression of the autoimmune processes in susceptible individuals.[11] Thus, if we want to study, for example, the mechanism of molecular mimicry between viruses and autoantigens, we need to take into account that such investigation requires an in-depth knowledge of the epitope specificity of B- (CD4 and CD8) and T-cell responses that accumulate over time in an infected individual. This topic has not been tackled by the scientific community as much as necessary. To this end, we introduce the concept of the infectome/autoinfectome.[12,13] We define the disease-linked infections as the "infectome" and the totality of the autoimmune disease-causing infections as its autoinfectome.[12,13] Thus, while the gut microbiome identifies all microorganisms in the intestine, the autoinfectome is the part of the microbiome that causes immune-mediated inflammatory bowel diseases (IBDs) such as CD and UC. Figure 1 illustrates the possible time points from which we can trace infectious agents during the processes that lead to the loss of immunological tolerance. Most studies investigating the role of the microbiome in the perpetuation of autoimmunity focus on the role of the gut microbiome because the gut microbiota is the largest reservoir of microbes in the human body. Hence, this chapter mainly discusses the role of the gut microbiome in the induction of autoimmune diseases. However, the microbiomes populating human skin, the oral cavity, airways, and the genitourinary tract are also sources of microbial-induced autoimmune diseases, and their role is discussed in the case of rheumatoid arthritis. A list of the major terms frequently quoted in this chapter is provided in Table 1. Figure 2 illustrates common links between the gut, lung, skin, and oral microbiomes with diseases, including autoimmune disorders.

2 GUT MICROBIOME AND IBD

The risk for developing IBD has long been considered mainly genetic; family history was a well-known factor for developing the disease, and recent genome-wide association studies (GWASs) identified several loci conferring susceptibility to or protection from the disease.[3] A partial overlap between loci for CD and UC, as well as a significant degree of loci that are common among IBD and other autoimmune diseases, have been noted. The same studies, however, made clear that susceptibility alleles per se are insufficient to fully explain the immunopathogenesis of IBD. GWASs have brought up novel pathways pathogenetically linked with IBD, and one of those previously unnoticed demonstrated that IBD genetic risk loci substantially overlap with risk loci conferring susceptibility to mycobacterial infection. Whether this risk partly explains the apparent link between CD and *Mycobacterium avium* subsp. *paratuberculosis*–induced Johne's disease, a CD-like

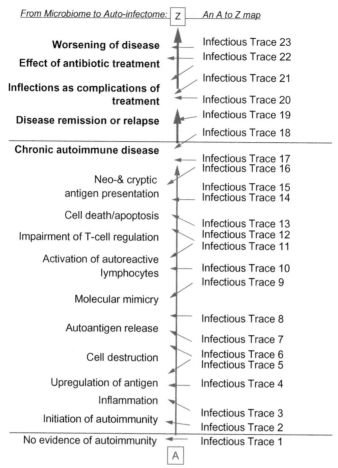

Figure 1 From microbiome to autoinfectome: an A to Z map. The study of the infectome requires the in-depth analysis of infectious traces at various time points long before onset, at onset and during the course of the autoimmune disease. A key element of this study is the screening of individuals at high risk or the first-degree relatives of affected individuals. Traces of the infectious agent and the study of its fine specificity in terms of antigen-specific immune responses may shed light on the exact mechanisms that play role in the induction of the disease. Microbiome-/genome-wide associations studies can reveal the genes and their protein products that are temporarily or consistently involved in the induction of autoimmunity. Narrowing down to few dozen those that are consistently identified as frequent triggers of autoimmunity can help us to better design studies focusing on specific agents rather than 'fishing exhibitions' or 'out of the box' approaches.

Table 1 Terminology Regularly Used in Studies Investigating the Role of Microbial–Host Mechanisms Inducing Autoimmunity.

Term	Definition	Description
Genome	The genetic material of an organism	The human genome is made up of 23 chromosome pairs, with a total of about 3 billion DNA base pairs and an estimated 20,000–25,000 human protein-coding genes.
Genomics	The study of all the genes of a cell or a tissue	Genome studies are conducted at the DNA (genotype), messenger RNA (transcriptome) or protein (proteome) levels.
Proteome	The entire set of proteins expressed by a genome, cell, tissue or organism	The proteomes are dynamic and describe the proteins expressed from a cell at a given time.
Interactome	The set of protein-to-protein interactions that occurs in a cell	Unlike the genome, the interactome is in a continuous dynamic state. The pathogen–host interactome has been used as a term to study the complex interactions between host and microbial organisms.
Microbiome	The sum of the microbes existing within the host	The human microbiome is the totality of the microbes that persist in the human body.
Virome	All viruses and bacteriophages infecting an organism	The human virome encompasses all viruses and bacteriophages and considerably contributes to the human microbe.
Microbiota	The microorganisms that typically inhabit a bodily organ or a specific region, also known as microbial flora	Gut microbiota describes the microbe population living in the gastrointestinal system. Microbiota differ among different sites (e.g., the blood, oral cavity, mucosal surfaces, endometrium).
Symbiosis	The natural microbial flora is in balance	The relationship or association between the host and the microbial flora is harmful to neither.
Dysbiosis	The state that results when the natural microbial flora of the gut are thrown out of balance	Dysbiosis is most prominent in the digestive tract and is particularly evident when antibiotics are taken.
Exposome	All environmental factors, both exogenous and endogenous, to which one is exposed during a lifetime	It can be used as a tool to study infectious and noninfectious agents causing autoimmunity.
Autoinfectome	A term used to describe the part of the exposome referring to the collection of an individual's exposures to infectious agents which can cause autoimmunity	The microbiome fails to identify those few infectious agents that cause autoimmunity. The infectome describes the totality of those pathogens (among thousands) that directly or indirectly induce autoimmune disease. The infectome pays attention to the immune responses at a specific antigen level that participate in the loss of immunological tolerance.

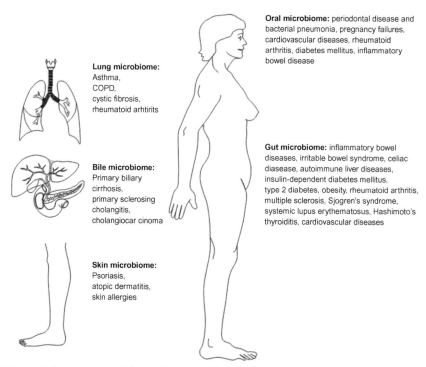

Figure 2 An overview of the major connections between our body's microbiomes and diseases, particularly autoimmune disorders. COPD, chronic obstructive pulmonary disease.

disease noted in ruminants, remains to be seen.[14,15] The paradoxical link between susceptibility to mycobacterial infection and the development of IBD may stem from an impaired autophagy of invasive mycobacteria or other commensal bacteria that allows them to become pathogenic. The nucleotide oligomerization domain 2 (*NOD2*) is one of the strongest CD susceptibility genes.[16] This gene induces autophagy in dendritic cells and is necessary for the proper function of *ATG16L*, the autophagy-related 16-like 1 gene, which is another strong susceptibility gene for both CD and UC.[17,18] *NOD2* is a potent stimulator of immune responses upon recognition of the cell wall peptidoglycan muramyl dipeptide of Gram-positive and Gram-negative bacteria, and *NOD2* mutations in patients with IBD are closely linked with increased numbers of mucosa-adherent bacteria, including *Escherichia coli*.[19] Several of the 160 loci conferring susceptibility to CD are directly or indirectly linked with the close interplay of microbiota and the establishment of dysbiosis. Most of them are linked to an impairment of immunity (innate and adaptive) to commensal bacteria and other pathogens, increased production of T-helper 17 cells and decreased integrity of the mucosal barrier (reviewed by Kostic et al.[3]). These processes are closely linked to a taxonomic and metabolic dysbiosis that is a characteristic feature of IBD bearing pathogenic potential. It needs to be noted that diet and nutrients shape the gut microbiome and are likely regulators of host–pathogen interactions.[20] For example, consumption of saturated fats and subsequent increase of taurocholic acid lead to an increase of organic sulfur in the bile and an imbalance of sulfite-reducing *Bilophila wadsworthia*, the expansion of which is closely linked with increased rates of colitis in interleukin (IL)-10–deficient mice.[21] The role of the Western diet in autoimmune diseases is the focus of ongoing studies, and a better understanding of the changes seen in the gut microbiome as a result of this diet have started to emerge.[20] It has become apparent that high-fat diets shape the composition of the microbiome, even in nonobese individuals. All together, host genetic associations in IBD described to date are closely linked with microbiome interactions with gut homeostasis. In addition to GWASs, microbiome-wide association studies may shed light to the pathogenesis of IBD.

2.1 Gut Microbiome and ExtraIntestinal Autoimmune Diseases

It has become apparent that alterations of the gut microbiome are closely linked to the pathogenesis of autoimmune diseases, unrelated to the intestine, that affect the liver, pancreas or even the central nervous system. Such studies have indicated that the development of extraintestinal autoimmune diseases is closely related to alterations of the gut microbiome, which seems to play a vital role mainly in the balance of T-helper 17/T regulatory cells, as well as the induction of functional T regulatory cells by specific human bacteria,[22–24] such as IDDM and multiple sclerosis.

2.2 Gut Microbiome and Autoimmune Liver Diseases

Immunoglobulin G3 antibodies against the β-galactosidase of *Lactobacillus delbrueckii* cross-react with the primary biliary cirrhosis–specific mitochondrial autoantigen;[25] lactobacillus vaccination can also induce the disease in susceptible individuals.[26] Also, *Novosphingobium aromaticivorans* is found in the feces of more than 25% of affected individuals, and antibodies against this pathogen are specifically present in the great majority of patients with primary biliary cirrhosis and their first-degree relatives. This pathogen can also induce the disease in experimental animals, further reinforcing the concept that gut microbiome–related infectious agents are probably involved in the pathogenesis of this disease, along with *E. coli* and other pathogens.[27] The close association of primary sclerosing cholangitis (PSC) with UC, which coexist in most patients with PSC, has led investigators to consider the possibility that intestinal microbiota and inflammation are associated with the development of this cholestatic autoimmune disease. In support of this view, there is a strong positive association between intestinal inflammation and PSC induction.[28] Also, PSC-related atypical perinuclear antineutrophil cytoplasmic antibodies react with β-tubulin and cross-react with the bacterial cytoskeletal FtsZ protein.[29]

2.3 Gut Microbiome and IDDM

Many of the same shifts in function of the gut microbiota have been noted, especially in type 2 diabetes.[30] The interaction of the gut microbiome with the innate immune system is well documented and significantly alters susceptibility to IDDM,.[31] Recent data suggest that androgens influence gut microbiota and exert a protective effect on the development of diabetes in germ-free nonobese diabetic mice colonized with specific microbiota.[32] The reverse is also true: colonization by commensal microbes leads to an increase of serum testosterone concentrations and protects nonobese diabetic male mice from the development of IDDM; transfer of specific gut microbiota from males to females not only alters the microbiota of the recipient but also results in an androgen receptor activity–dependent increase in testosterone concentrations, reduced pancreatic β-cell inflammation, IDDM autoantibody production and subsequent protection from IDDM.[33]

2.4 Gut Microbiome and Multiple Sclerosis

The conventional understanding of infection-induced multiple sclerosis (MS) perceives this disease as closely linked with the Epstein-Barr virus and human herpesvirus 6. These viruses have been linked with MS at various levels, based on serological, immunological and experimental data, suggesting that experimental autoimmune encephalomyelitis (EAE), the animal model of MS, can be induced in virus-infected animals. Recent data have elegantly demonstrated that EAE cannot be developed in the absence of intestinal commensal bacteria.[34] Thus, commensal microbiota are critical for the development of EAE in epitope-specific myelin oligodendrocyte glycoprotein T-cell receptor transgenic mice.[34] Germ-free B6 mice develop only mild EAE compared with that induced by the commensal microbiota, the former form of the disease characterized by increased Foxp3$^+$ T regulatory cells and decreased interferon-γ and IL-17 responses.[35] Several studies assessed the role of probiotic treatment in the induction of and/or prevention of EAE.[36] For example, a mixture of lactobacilli suppresses the progression and reverses the histological and clinical signs of EAE.[37] Dietary nutrients also play a role in the development of EAE, possibly through the regulation of gut microbiome interactions with the host.

The role of the gut microbiome in other autoimmune demyelinating disorders, such as Devic's disease (neuromyelitis optica), is poorly defined, and a direct link between microbiome and this disease remains to be identified. Nevertheless, indirect links have been made based on the fact that patients with autoantibodies against the central nervous system water channel aquaporin 4 (AQP4) protein, the hallmark autoantibody marker of neuromyelitis optica, have much higher levels of antigliadin antibodies as well as anti–*Saccharomyces cerevisiae* antibodies compared with healthy controls. Also, HLA-DRB1*0301 AQP4-specific CD4 T cells recognizing specific peptides seem to cross-reactively recognize a microbial mimic originating from *Clostridium perfringens* adenosine triphosphate–binding cassette transporter permease, which shows 90% homology with the AQP4 epitope.[38] These data support the notion that molecular mimicry could be involved in the pathogenesis of neuromyelitis optica and further support the role of the gut microbiome in the pathogenesis of the disease.

3 MICROBIOME AND RHEUMATOID ARTHRITIS

Rheumatoid arthritis (RA) has been considered a disease caused by environmental factors. Among the possible environmental triggers necessary for the development of RA, the microbiomes of the gut, the oral cavity and the lung have been considered potential inflicting factors.[39] The gut is the largest reservoir from which the immune system encounters antigens, and it is logical to consider that infectious triggers of inflammatory arthritis stem from the gut microbiome. Early studies convincingly showed that certain mucosal microbes are necessary for the induction of RA in rat models of adjuvant-induced and streptococcal cell wall–induced arthritis.[39] Germ-free environments protect against the development of arthritis. Colonization of IL-1 receptor antagonist knockout and the K/BxN mouse models of arthritis with *Lactobacillus* and segmented filamentous bacteria makes them susceptible to inflammatory arthritis in a T-helper 17–dependent manner.[40] The microbiome of arthritis-susceptible *0401 transgenic mice has been compared with the microbiome of arthritis-resistant *0402 transgenic mice. The *0401 mice seem to be dominated by *Clostridium* bacteria, whereas *Porphyromonadaceae* and *Bifidobacteria* families predominate in the arthritis-resistant *0402 mice.[41] Such studies are extremely informative and need to be carried out in other experimental models of autoimmune diseases.

A pathogenic role for the microbiota of the oral cavity, in particular that of the gingival tissue, has long been considered in the development of RA. Several decades ago, a link was established between RA and infection-induced periodontal disease mainly caused by *Porphyromonas gingivalis*, *Treponema denticola*, and *Tannerella forsythia*. More recent studies provide support to this link, demonstrating an increased incidence and severity of periodontal disease in patients with RA. However, whether this association is epiphenomenal remains unclear. *P. gingivalis* encodes for peptidyl arginine deiminase, an enzyme that converts arginine residues into citrulline, and it has been postulated that this bacterium supplies the immune system with the antigenic material necessary for the induction of anticitrullinated protein antibodies present in patients with RA.[42] In fact, efficient treatment (hygiene instruction and supragingival scaling) of periodontal disease decreases the levels of both anti–*P. gingivalis* antibodies and anticyclic citrullinated peptide antibodies.[43]

RA serves as an ideal model to study the role of the lung microbiome in the induction of an autoimmune disease, but more work needs to be done in this matter. The lung seems to be an early site of immune-mediated injury characterised by the presence of periodontal tissue–derived proinflammatory microbiota, which can be responsible for the citrullination of proteins and the induction of RA-related autoimmunity. The ZAP-70 single-point mutation mouse model, SKG, which is genetically prone to developing autoimmune arthritis, failed to develop the disease under a microbially clean condition. In these mice, a single intraperitoneal injection of zymosan, a crude fungal β-glucan, or purified β-glucans such as curdlan and laminarin can trigger severe chronic arthritis in SKG, suggesting that fungal organisms residing in the lungs can play a role in the induction of arthritis, especially since SKG mice harbor a larger respiratory fungal load.

Table 2 provides an overview of the techniques that can be used to study the microbiome and microbiome-induced autoimmunity in the form of an infectious and autoimmune burden.

Table 2 An Overview of Techniques Used for the Multiparametric Analysis of Infectious and Autoimmune Burden.[44–46]

Immunological assays	• Multiparametric ELISA, line blots/dots • Multiparametric IFA chips • Triplex lateral flow immunoassay • Magnetic and nonmagnetic bead multiplex immunoassays • Lateral flow immunochromatography • Assays optical immunosensor systems • Electrochemical-based ELISA

Molecular detection

Multiplex real-time PCR	• Real-time PCR and highly specific melting point analyses, e.g., LightCycler Septi*Fast* (can study up to 25 pathogens)
Molecular hybridization	• Commercially available platforms are already in use for the simultaneous detection of multiple viral types and subtypes from nasopharyngeal swabs and simultaneous detection of viral, bacterial and protozoan parasites causing gastrointestinal diseases
Nucleotide sequencing	• Nucleotide (pyro)sequencing • Next-generation sequencing: highly massive pyrosequencing technology, sequencing by synthesis, sequencing by oligonucleotide ligation and detection (SOLiD) system
Mass spectrometry	• Microbial identification by MALDI-TOF after culture
Integrated fluidic systems	• Microbial identification by PCR-ESI after PCR

ELISA, enzyme-linked immunosorbant assay; ESI, electrospray ionization; IFA, immunofluorescence assay; MALDI-TOF, matrix-assisted laser desorption/ionization time of flight; PCR, polymerase chain reaction.

REFERENCES

1. Aagaard K, Petrosino J, Keitel W, Watson M, Katancik J, Garcia N, et al. The Human Microbiome Project strategy for comprehensive sampling of the human microbiome and why it matters. *FASEB J* 2012;**27**(3):1012–22.
2. Xu Y, Xie J, Li Y, Yue J, Chen J, Chunyu L, et al. Using a cDNA microarray to study cellular gene expression altered by Mycobacterium tuberculosis. *Chin Med J (Engl)* 2003;**116**(7):1070–3.
3. Kostic AD, Xavier RJ, Gevers D. The Microbiome in Inflammatory Bowel Diseases: Current Status and the Future Ahead. *Gastroenterology* 2014;**146**(6):1489–99.
4. Giongo A, Gano KA, Crabb DB, Mukherjee N, Novelo LL, Casella G, et al. Toward defining the autoimmune microbiome for type 1 diabetes. *ISME J* 2010;**5**(1):82–91.

5. Booijink CC, El-Aidy S, Rajilic-Stojanovic M, Heilig HG, Troost FJ, Smidt H, et al. High temporal and inter-individual variation detected in the human ileal microbiota. *Environ Microbiol* 2010;**12**(12):3213–27.

6. Caporaso JG, Lauber CL, Costello EK, Berg-Lyons D, Gonzalez A, Stombaugh J, et al. Moving pictures of the human microbiome. *Genome Biol* 2011;**12**(5):R50.

7. Schutzer SE, Angel TE, Liu T, Schepmoes AA, Clauss TR, Adkins JN, et al. Distinct cerebrospinal fluid proteomes differentiate post-treatment lyme disease from chronic fatigue syndrome. *PLoS One* 2011;**6**(2):e17287.

8. Kivity S, Agmon-Levin N, Blank M, Shoenfeld Y. Infections and autoimmunity–friends or foes? *Trends Immunol* 2009;**30**(8):409–14.

9. Shapira Y, Agmon-Levin N, Renaudineau Y, Porat-Katz BS, Barzilai O, Ram M, et al. Serum markers of infections in patients with primary biliary cirrhosis: evidence of infection burden. *Exp Mol Pathol* 2012;**93**(3):386–90.

10. Shapira Y, Agmon-Levin N, Shoenfeld Y. Defining and analyzing geoepidemiology and human autoimmunity. *J Autoimmun* 2010;**34**(3):J168–77.

11. Berlin T, Zandman-Goddard G, Blank M, Matthias T, Pfeiffer S, Weis I, et al. Auto-antibodies in nonautoimmune individuals during infections. *Ann NY Acad Sci* 2007;**1108**:584–93.

12. Bogdanos DP, Smyk DS, Invernizzi P, Rigopoulou EI, Blank M, Pouria S, et al. Infectome: a platform to trace infectious triggers of autoimmunity. *Autoimmun Rev* 2012;**12** (7):726–40.

13. Bogdanos DP, Smyk DS, Invernizzi P, Rigopoulou EI, Blank M, Sakkas L, et al. Tracing environmental markers of autoimmunity: introducing the infectome. *Immunol Res* 2013;**56**(2–3):220–40.

14. Polymeros D, Bogdanos DP, Day R, Arioli D, Vergani D, Forbes A. Does cross-reactivity between mycobacterium avium paratuberculosis and human intestinal antigens characterize Crohn's disease? *Gastroenterology* 2006;**131**(1):85–96.

15. Liaskos C, Spyrou V, Roggenbuck D, Athanasiou LV, Orfanidou T, Mavropoulos A, et al. Crohn's disease-specific pancreatic autoantibodies are specifically present in ruminants with paratuberculosis: implications for the pathogenesis of the human disease. *Autoimmunity* 2013;**46**(6):388–94.

16. Ogura Y, Bonen DK, Inohara N, Nicolae DL, Chen FF, Ramos R, et al. A frameshift mutation in NOD2 associated with susceptibility to Crohn's disease. *Nature* 2001;**411** (6837):603–6.

17. Cooney R, Baker J, Brain O, Danis B, Pichulik T, Allan P, et al. NOD2 stimulation induces autophagy in dendritic cells influencing bacterial handling and antigen presentation. *Nat Med* 2010;**16**(1):90–7.

18. Jostins L, Ripke S, Weersma RK, Duerr RH, McGovern DP, Hui KY, et al. Host-microbe interactions have shaped the genetic architecture of inflammatory bowel disease. *Nature* 2012;**491**(7422):119–24.

19. Frank DN, Robertson CE, Hamm CM, Kpadeh Z, Zhang T, Chen H, et al. Disease phenotype and genotype are associated with shifts in intestinal-associated microbiota in inflammatory bowel diseases. *Inflamm Bowel Dis* 2011;**17**(1):179–84.

20. Manzel A, Muller DN, Hafler DA, Erdman SE, Linker RA, Kleinewietfeld M. Role of "Western diet" in inflammatory autoimmune diseases. *Curr Allergy Asthma Rep* 2014;**14** (1):404.

21. Devkota S, Wang Y, Musch MW, Leone V, Fehlner-Peach H, Nadimpalli A, et al. Dietary-fat-induced taurocholic acid promotes pathobiont expansion and colitis in Il10-/- mice. *Nature* 2012;**487**(7405):104–8.

22. Atarashi K, Tanoue T, Shima T, Imaoka A, Kuwahara T, Momose Y, et al. Induction of colonic regulatory T cells by indigenous Clostridium species. *Science* 2011;**331** (6015):337–41.

23. Atarashi K, Tanoue T, Oshima K, Suda W, Nagano Y, Nishikawa H, et al. Treg induction by a rationally selected mixture of Clostridia strains from the human microbiota. *Nature* 2011;**500**(7461):232–6.

24. Esplugues E, Huber S, Gagliani N, Hauser AE, Town T, Wan YY, et al. Control of TH17 cells occurs in the small intestine. *Nature* 2011;**475**(7357):514–18.

25. Bogdanos DP, Baum H, Okamoto M, Montalto P, Sharma UC, Rigopoulou EI, et al. Primary biliary cirrhosis is characterized by IgG3 antibodies cross-reactive with the major mitochondrial autoepitope and its Lactobacillus mimic. *Hepatology* 2005;**42**(2):458–65.

26. Bogdanos D, Pusl T, Rust C, Vergani D, Beuers U. Primary biliary cirrhosis following Lactobacillus vaccination for recurrent vaginitis. *J Hepatol* 2008;**49**(3):466–73.

27. Bogdanos DP, Baum H, Vergani D, Burroughs AK. The role of E. coli infection in the pathogenesis of primary biliary cirrhosis. *Dis Markers* 2011;**29**(6):301–11.

28. Joo M, Abreu-e-Lima P, Farraye F, Smith T, Swaroop P, Gardner L, et al. Pathologic features of ulcerative colitis in patients with primary sclerosing cholangitis: a case-control study. *Am J Surg Pathol* 2009;**33**(6):854–62.

29. Terjung B, Sohne J, Lechtenberg B, Gottwein J, Muennich M, Herzog V, et al. p-ANCAs in autoimmune liver disorders recognise human beta-tubulin isotype 5 and cross-react with microbial protein FtsZ. *Gut* 2010;**59**(6):808–16.

30. Larsen N, Vogensen FK, van den Berg FW, Nielsen DS, Andreasen AS, Pedersen BK, et al. Gut microbiota in human adults with type 2 diabetes differs from non-diabetic adults. *PLoS One* 2010;**5**(2):e9085.

31. Wen L, Ley RE, Volchkov PY, Stranges PB, Avanesyan L, Stonebraker AC, et al. Innate immunity and intestinal microbiota in the development of Type 1 diabetes. *Nature* 2008;**455**(7216):1109–13.

32. Yurkovetskiy L, Burrows M, Khan AA, Graham L, Volchkov P, Becker L, et al. Gender bias in autoimmunity is influenced by microbiota. *Immunity* 2013;**39**(2):400–12.

33. Markle JG, Frank DN, Mortin-Toth S, Robertson CE, Feazel LM, Rolle-Kampczyk U, et al. Sex differences in the gut microbiome drive hormone-dependent regulation of autoimmunity. *Science* 2013;**339**(6123):1084–8.

34. Berer K, Mues M, Koutrolos M, Rasbi ZA, Boziki M, Johner C, et al. Commensal microbiota and myelin autoantigen cooperate to trigger autoimmune demyelination. *Nature* 2011;**479**(7374):538–41.

35. Lee YK, Menezes JS, Umesaki Y, Mazmanian SK. Proinflammatory T-cell responses to gut microbiota promote experimental autoimmune encephalomyelitis. *Proc Natl Acad Sci USA* 2011;**108**(Suppl 1):4615–22.

36. Wang Y, Kasper LH. The role of microbiome in central nervous system disorders. *Brain Behav Immun* 2014;**38**:1–12.

37. Lavasani S, Dzhambazov B, Nouri M, Fak F, Buske S, Molin G, et al. A novel probiotic mixture exerts a therapeutic effect on experimental autoimmune encephalomyelitis mediated by IL-10 producing regulatory T cells. *PLoS One* 2010;**5**(2):e9009.

38. Varrin-Doyer M, Spencer CM, Schulze-Topphoff U, Nelson PA, Stroud RM, Cree BA, et al. Aquaporin 4-specific T cells in neuromyelitis optica exhibit a Th17 bias and recognize Clostridium ABC transporter. *Ann Neurol* 2012;**72**(1):53–64.

39. Brusca SB, Abramson SB, Scher JU. Microbiome and mucosal inflammation as extra-articular triggers for rheumatoid arthritis and autoimmunity. *Curr Opin Rheumatol* 2014;**26**(1):101–7.

40. Wu HJ, Ivanov II, Darce J, Hattori K, Shima T, Umesaki Y, et al. Gut-residing segmented filamentous bacteria drive autoimmune arthritis via T helper 17 cells. *Immunity* 2010;**32**(6):815–27.

41. Gomez A, Luckey D, Yeoman CJ, Marietta EV, Berg Miller ME, Murray JA, et al. Loss of sex and age driven differences in the gut microbiome characterize arthritis-susceptible 0401 mice but not arthritis-resistant 0402 mice. *PLoS One* 2012;**7**(4):e36095.

42. Wegner N, Wait R, Sroka A, Eick S, Nguyen KA, Lundberg K, et al. Peptidylarginine deiminase from Porphyromonas gingivalis citrullinates human fibrinogen and alpha-enolase: implications for autoimmunity in rheumatoid arthritis. *Arthritis Rheum* 2010;**62**(9):2662–72.
43. Okada M, Kobayashi T, Ito S, Yokoyama T, Abe A, Murasawa A, et al. Periodontal treatment decreases levels of antibodies to Porphyromonas gingivalis and citrulline in patients with rheumatoid arthritis and periodontitis. *J Periodontol* 2013;**84**(12):e74–84.
44. Gordon J, Michel G. Discerning trends in multiplex immunoassay technology with potential for resource-limited settings. *Clin Chem* 2012;**58**(4):690–8.
45. Bissonnette L, Bergeron MG. Next revolution in the molecular theranostics of infectious diseases: microfabricated systems for personalized medicine. *Expert Rev Mol Diagn* 2006;**6**(3):433–50.
46. Bissonnette L, Bergeron MG. Multiparametric technologies for the diagnosis of syndromic infections. *Clin Microbiol Newsl* 2012;**34**(20):159–68.

CHAPTER 10

Infection, Autoimmunity, and Vitamin D

Amy D. Proal[*,1], **Paul J. Albert**[†], **Trevor G. Marshall**[*]
[*]Autoimmunity Research Foundation, Thousand Oaks, California, USA
[†]Weill Cornell Medical College, New York, USA
[1]Corresponding Author: amy.proal@gmail.com

1 INTRODUCTION

For decades, researchers have noted the presence of culturable pathogens in patients with a wide range of chronic inflammatory diseases. These pathogens include Epstein–Barr virus (EBV), cytomegalovirus, hepatitis C virus, *Chlamydia pneumoniae*, *Mycobacteriaceae*, and *Borrelia* spp. Yet the prevalence of any one pathogen in a particular cohort varies widely depending on the methodology of the study, and no single pathogen has been reliably detected in all patients with a particular inflammatory diagnosis.

However, genome-based microbial detection methods that have emerged during the past decade revealed vast communities of bacteria, viruses, and fungi now known to persist in nearly every body site, called the human microbiome. This discovery has uncovered thousands of new microbial species capable of contributing to autoimmune and inflammatory disease processes. In lieu of a single pathogen causing a single disease, many of these microbes instead seem to generate dysfunction by continually interacting with other species in a shared intra-phagocytic environment. Yet to persist inside host immune cells, the microbiome must necessarily degrade the host's innate immune defences. In doing so, the pathogens also dysregulate other aspects of human metabolism by directly altering the expression of human genes. This chapter describes how the cumulative effect of these changes to the human metabolome and interactome may lead to the catastrophic failure of human metabolism so often observed in chronic idiopathic disease.

Infection and Autoimmunity
http://dx.doi.org/10.1016/B978-0-444-63269-2.00007-6

2 THE FIELD OF METAGENOMICS IS BORN

After completion of the Human Genome Project in 2003, researchers began to use many of the DNA-based technologies that had been developed to decode the human genome to explore the microbial genomes now being found in the human body. The results were unprecedented. Thousands of microbes that had never been identified by culture-based laboratory techniques were readily detected in human tissue and blood.

Two large-scale, multi-center collaborations spearheaded use of the genome-based technologies to better identify and characterize these previously undiscovered microbes. One was the Human Microbiome Project (HMP) (2008–2012), a US-based initiative funded by the US National Institutes of Health.[1] The Project, which sampled the microbial populations of 242 healthy adults across 15–18 body sites, eventually generated more than 3.5 terabases of metagenomic sequences.[2] The second initiative was the European-based project MetaHIT (2008–2012), which focused primarily on better characterizing the microbiome of the gut.[3] In concert with a number of private research teams also focused on microbiome research, these projects succeeded in identifying so many novel microbes in *Homo sapiens* that today at least 90% of cells in the human body are estimated to be bacterial, viral, fungal, or otherwise non-human in origin.

As the HMP and related projects moved forward, research shifted from the study of a dozen or so well-characterized human pathogens to the exploration of myriad microbial species that have now been identified across nearly all body sites. Metagenomic communities of microbes were shown to persist not just on the body's mucosal surfaces but also in tissue and blood. Polybacterial and chronic infections have been detected in atherosclerotic plaque.[4] Microbial RNA has been detected even in healthy human blood.[5] The lungs are now understood to harbor a microbiome as well, the composition of which differs in patients with chronic lung conditions.[6] Even the biofilm removed from prosthetic hip joints during revision arthroplasties has been shown to harbor dozens of distinct bacterial phylotypes.[7]

As of October 2013, the Genomes Online database lists 2337 completed and published bacterial genomes, with another 24,303 in progress.[8] Even so, each new metagenomic analysis continues to allow researchers to identify previously unknown microbes. For example, an analysis by Nasidze et al. of the human oral cavity identified 101 bacterial genera in the mouth as well as 64 genera previously unknown to science.[9]

Similarly, our knowledge of the chronic viruses that persist in *H. sapiens* (the virome) also has evolved rapidly. We have known for some time that several well-characterized viruses such as polyomaviruses infect and remain with most humans throughout life. Yet entirely new persistent viral populations have now been discovered. After analyzing the fecal virome of monozygotic twins and their mothers, Reyes et al. found that 81% of the reads generated from this virome did not match those of any known viruses.[10] In 2011, Pride et al. reported that previously uncharacterized bacteriophages dominate the oral cavity, and several phages serve as reservoirs for pathogenic gene function.[11]

3 THE HUMAN SUPERORGANISM

The approximately 20,500 genes expressed by the human genome are vastly outnumbered by the millions of genes expressed by our microbial inhabitants. The human gut microbiome alone expresses at least 9 million unique genes.[12] It follows that we cannot study disease by studying the human genome in isolation. The millions of proteins and metabolites expressed by the microbiome continually interact with the human genome, altering the manner in which human genes are subsequently expressed. For example, one analysis demonstrated that the expression of at least 463 human genes is changed during a single infection with *Mycobacterium tuberculosis*.[13]

This new understanding redefines what it means to be human – human beings are now most accurately described as superorganisms. The metabolism of the human superorganism represents a combination of microbial and human attributes. For example, the human angiotensin-converting enzyme (*ACE*) has been associated with myocardial infarction, Alzheimer's disease, diabetes mellitus, and sarcoidosis.[14] Yet the expression of *ACE* also has been shown to be downregulated by *Lactobacillus* and *Bifdobacteria*, microbes commonly found in dairy products.[15] The ability of these and other microbes to directly alter human gene expression significantly affects the pathogenesis of inflammatory conditions, albeit in ways not yet fully understood.

Proteins and metabolites generated by the microbiome permeate the body. Of the small molecules found in healthy human blood, 36% are created by the human gut microbiome.[16] The myriad interactions between these foreign and host proteins in the body, referred to as the interactome, affect an array of human metabolic processes. For example, the presence or absence of particular microbial metabolites in the blood of any individual cause the medication acetaminophen to be metabolized differently from person to person.[17]

These transgenomic interactions are complicated by the fact that the structures of many microbial proteins are identical or very similar to those expressed by the human genome. For example, some bacteria metabolize folate and glucose with a metabolism similar to that of their human hosts. Because of this overlap, the human superorganism may have great difficulty distinguishing proteins and metabolites created by the microbes from those recognized as "self".

This "molecularly mimicry" is extremely common. Tens of thousands of protein–protein interactions have been documented between the genomes of *Yersinia, Salmonella, Escherichia coli*, and the human genome.[18] Kusalik et al. identified 19,605 pentamers from the hepatitis C virus polyprotein with a high level of similarity to the human proteome.[19] This high level of similarity persisted even when the team used longer peptide motifs as probes for identity scanning.

4 THE MICROBIOME IN HEALTH AND DISEASE

An increasing body of research demonstrates that microbiome composition often changes over time in patients with a range of chronic inflammatory diseases. This disturbance in the body's microbial populations, or dysbiosis, is associated with a growing number of chronic conditions including types 1[20] and 2[21] diabetes, Crohn's disease, ulcerative colitis[22] and psoriasis.[23] For example, Amar et al. recently demonstrated that 16S recombinant DNA blood serum concentrations were significantly elevated in 3280 subjects without obesity or diabetes at baseline but who later developed diabetes.[24]

The composition of the microbiome has even been shown to shift in patients with cancer. Kostic et al. analyzed whole genome sequences from patients with colorectal carcinomas.[25] The Bacteroidetes and Firmicutes phyla were depleted in tumors, whereas *Fusobacterium* sequences were enriched in carcinomas. Patients with chronic lyme disease and chronic fatigue syndrome exhibited greatly altered cerebrospinal proteomes, which also differ from those of healthy individuals.[26] Considering that almost all of the atypical proteins in the human body are microbial in origin, these proteomic differences directly reflect shifts in microbiome composition.

These alterations of the microbiome in health and disease involve entire microbial ecosystems. Thus, chronic disease processes driven by infection are likely due to changes in complex microbial communities rather than the acquisition of a single pathogen. It follows that Koch's postulates, which dictate that a single infectious disease must be caused by a single pathogen, are no longer tenable in the current era of the metagenome.

Unfortunately, studies of microbiome composition in health and disease are complicated by a host of environmental variables that can also cause significant shifts in the body's microbial populations. These include geographic location, food consumption, water intake, and the use of medications and supplements. These additional environmental factors contribute to significant variability in the microbiome across months, weeks, and even days – so much so that even the microbiomes of monozygotic twins are no more similar than those of fraternal twins.[27]

It follows that while the identification of the species present in patients with a given inflammatory condition can provide valuable clues about disease, we cannot focus simply on population-based studies. Instead, we must examine what the microbial genomes actually *do* to persist and to influence the body's metabolic processes.

5 VITAMIN D NUCLEAR RECEPTOR DYSREGULATION

Those pathogens most successful at causing disease tend to persist inside the cells of the immune system. *M. tuberculosis* and the EBV are two examples. The ability of these intracellular pathogens to persist in nucleated cells allows them to directly interfere with transcription, translation, and DNA repair processes. If the accumulation of errors resulting from this interference exceeds the capacity of cellular repair mechanisms, the interactome can become significantly dysregulated. For example, *Helicobacter pylori* infection generates significant genetic instability in gastric epithelial cells by disrupting their DNA repair mechanisms.[28]

Some intracellular pathogens (e.g. *M. tuberculosis* and EBV) survive by dysregulating gene expression by the vitamin D nuclear receptor (VDR). Just a decade ago, the VDR was studied almost solely in the context of calcium metabolism. Today, however, this receptor has been shown to express at least 1000 genes, with many more putative gene candidates in the pipeline.[29] VDR promoters are ubiquitous throughout the human genome, and genes already associated with VDR regulation are directly connected to autoimmune and inflammatory processes.[29] The receptor also expresses genes related to cancer, including metastasis suppressor protein 1 (*MTSS1*), which plays a key role in promoting apoptosis and repressing the cell cycle in cancerous cells.[29]

In addition to its key role in transcription regulation, the VDR also lies at the heart of the human innate immune response. It expresses TLR2, which allows the immune system to recognize bacterial polysaccharides. In addition, it regulates expression of the cathelicidin and β-antimicrobial peptides (AMPs), which play vital roles in targeting intracellular pathogens.

Thus, any microbe capable of dysregulating VDR activity would significantly disable the innate immune response, facilitating its persistence. Indeed, several of the pathogens most often linked to inflammatory disease have in fact evolved to survive in exactly this fashion. Persistent *M. tuberculosis* has evolved to slow VDR activity. When lymphoblastoid cell lines are infected with EBV, activity of the VDR is downregulated as much as 15 times.[30] *Mycobacterium leprae*,[31] cytomegalovirus,[32] and *Borrelia burgdorferi*[33] also inhibit VDR activity to varying degrees. The fungus *Aspergillus fumigatus*, common in cystic fibrosis, secretes a gliotoxin that significantly downregulates VDR expression.[34] In addition, bacterial species in biofilm often secrete the sulphonolipid capnine,[35] which we have demonstrated can inhibit VDR activation.[36] Indeed, disabling the innate immune response via the VDR pathway is such a logical pathogen survival mechanism that many more species capable of persisting in the same or similar fashion will likely be identified in the coming years.

6 FLOW-ON EFFECTS OF VDR DYSREGULATION

VDR dysregulation generates a number of imbalances that further compromise homeostasis and immunity. The activated VDR is responsible for expressing *CYP24A1*, an enzyme primarily responsible for deactivating the active vitamin D metabolite 1,25-dihydroxyvitamin D (1,25-D).[37] In addition, inflammation associated with persistent intracellular microbes causes excess production of the enzyme *CYP27B1*. This results in increased conversion of 25-hydroxyvitamin D (25-D) into 1,25-D. Both processes cause 1,25-D concentrations to increase. Indeed, elevated concentrations of 1,25-D leaking into the bloodstream have been demonstrated in several inflammatory conditions, including tuberculosis and rheumatoid arthritis.[38] Our analysis found that 85 of 100 patients with autoimmune and inflammatory conditions had elevated concentrations of 1,25-D, ranging from 110 pmol/L to a high of 350 pmol/L.[39]

Our data indicate that, as its concentration rises, 1,25-D may also dysregulate gene expression via nuclear receptors other than the VDR.[40] These include the androgen receptor, the glucocorticoid receptor, and the α- and β-thyroid receptors.[41] Each of these nuclear receptors also controls multiple families of AMPs (20, 17, and 15 families, respectively, of the 22 analyzed by Brahmachary et al.[42]). Thus, as 1,25-D accumulates within infected cells, it may disable the activity of these AMPs as well, leaving the host increasingly immunocompromised.

7 SUCCESSIVE INFECTION

As acquired pathogens slow activity of the VDR and related receptors, an individual's microbiome gradually shifts towards a state that promotes overt disease. During this process of "successive infection", the host microbiome gradually shifts away from a homeostatic state. Opportunistic pathogens are progressively incorporated into the microbiome, where they alter the expression of the human genome. As a result, the interactome becomes increasingly dysregulated. Infected human cells fail to correctly express human metabolites in the presence of the proteins, enzymes, and metabolites generated by the accumulating pathogenic genomes.

In addition, any pathogen that decreases nuclear receptor AMP expression slows the innate immune response so that the host more easily acquires even more microbes, some of which may well symbiotically suppress AMP. This creates a snowball effect, in which it becomes progressively easier for the host to acquire pathogens as the strength of the immune response wanes.

As an increasing number of pathogens become incorporated into the microbiome, a patient may eventually begin to present with clinically evident symptoms characteristic of an inflammatory diagnosis. Each individual's unique symptoms vary depending on the location, species, and virulence of the pathogens they have accumulated into their microbiome. Symptoms vary between individuals because of the semi-infinite number of ways in which the microbial proteins and metabolites can interfere with those of the host.

While successive infection leads to the acquisition of more pathogens over time, the diversity of microbes in a particular niche may not necessarily increase. Microbes are highly competitive, meaning that certain pathogens often successfully outcompete larger populations of other less aggressive species. Higher levels of dysfunction may result if keystone species are lost. Indeed, some studies show that microbiome diversity is diminished in patients who are already ill. For example, lower microbial diversity has been reported in the guts of infants with atopic eczema.[43] In other cases, successive infection may lead to greater species diversity. In women who suffer from bacterial vaginosis, for example, the vaginal microbiome composition often shifts to become more taxon-rich than that of healthy subjects.[44]

8 COMORBIDITY

Patients with one inflammatory diagnosis are at higher risk for developing a second. For example, the Prospective Epidemiological Study of Myocardial Infarction (PRIME) study found that baseline depressive symptoms were associated with an increased risk of coronary heart disease in the short term and stroke over the long term in otherwise healthy, European, middle-aged men.[45] The overlap between the symptoms and disease presentation associated with comorbid conditions directly reflects the variability inherent to the process of successive infection. No two people exposed to pathogens over time ever acquire the exact same mix of species in their microbiome. Therefore, no two individuals will ever develop an identical disease presentation, and the symptoms of patients with similar diagnoses can be expected to overlap and fluctuate with time. Figure 1 shows the extent to which patients with one inflammatory disease often suffer from other comorbid conditions.

This suggests that various inflammatory diagnoses are best studied together. Current pragma often dictates that one inflammatory condition is directly causal of a second, although the mechanisms behind these assumptions remain unclear. For example, obesity is generally believed to cause diabetes. Yet, increasing evidence shows that the gut microbiome is significantly altered in patients with both conditions.[46] It may be more likely, then, that both obesity and diabetes gradually occur together because of successive infection or a common underlying pathogenesis.

In the same vein, patients suffering from physical inflammatory conditions are at greater risk for developing neurological dysfunction and vice versa. This suggests that neurological and autoimmune diagnoses, which are currently separated into different medical specialties, may indeed arise from similar underlying infectious processes. Indeed, dysbiosis of the microbiome has been documented in patients with a range of neurological conditions including multiple sclerosis,[47] autism and obsessive-compulsive disorder.[48]

9 FAMILIAL AGGREGATION

Familial aggregation must be reexamined in light of comorbid disposition. A host of studies show that the relatives of patients with inflammatory disease are more likely to be ill themselves. For example, a 2006 study by Anaya et al. of families who have a member with primary Sjögren's syndrome showed that 38% had at least one first-degree relative with an autoimmune disease versus 22% of control families.[49]

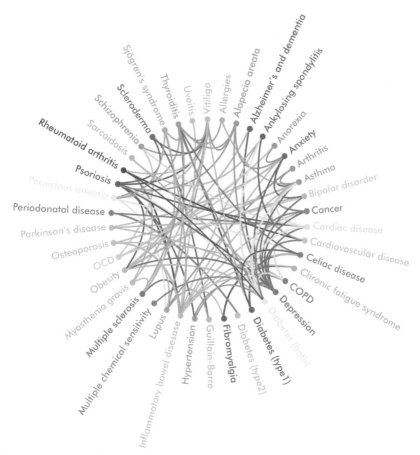

Figure 1 Comorbidities among common inflammatory diseases. Each "spoke" of this wheel represents a published study appearing in MEDLINE, which shows a significant statistical relationship between one disease and another.

While this clustering of inflammatory diseases in families could be explained by the sharing of common genes, any such genes confer no known survival advantage and should subsequently have been weeded from the population. Instead, familial aggregation likely results from the sharing of common microbes. For example, infected mothers, fathers, and siblings are all major sources for *H. pylori* acquisition among young children; the infected mother serves as the main source for childhood acquisition of microbes.[50] Certain pathogens have been shown to cross the placental barrier and even persist in the amniotic fluid, sperm and egg.[51] These microbes can thus be passed easily from generation to generation.

Pathogens passed down the maternal line seem to have a particularly strong effect on the microbiome of subsequent generations. The founding microbial populations of an infant delivered by vaginal birth closely mirror those of its mother's vagina. In addition, after Cesarean delivery, differences in infants' founding microbial populations can persist for months.[52] Breast milk is now understood to deliver a microbiome that varies among women and depends on a host of factors. Cabrera-Rubio et al. found that the composition of the breast milk microbiome significantly changed over the course of at least the first 6 months of lactation.[53] The weight of the mother further affects the composition of her breast milk microbiome. Milk from obese mothers tended to contain a different and less diverse bacterial community than that obtained from healthy subjects. In addition, those mothers who underwent elective Cesarean delivery displayed different bacterial communities in their milk samples then those subjects who gave birth by vaginal delivery.

10 IMMUNOSUPPRESSIVE THERAPIES MAY PALLIATE SYMPTOMS BUT INCREASE DISEASE OVER THE LONG TERM

The standard of care for most autoimmune and inflammatory conditions is immunosuppression. Commonly used immunosuppressive treatments include corticosteroids, methotrexate, and tumor necrosis factor-α antagonists. While these therapeutic options often provide short-term symptom palliation, they have poor long-term associations with stability and relapse. Indeed, no definitive studies have identified corticosteroids capable of enhancing long-term prognosis or reducing mortality rates. For example, Gottlieb et al. reported that in sarcoidosis, steroid use leads to relapse and contributes to prolongation of disease by delaying resolution.[54] To date there have been nearly 150 clinical trials testing prospective agents designed to block inflammation in patients with sepsis, and all have failed.[55]

Most immunosuppressive medications were developed to slow what is historically believed to be an overactive immune response. However, as the inflammation and autoantibodies associated with these conditions are becoming increasingly tied to infection, the efficacy of these drugs must be reexamined. By slowing the immune response, immunosuppressive medications cause a decrease in inflammation and cytokine release. While this decrease in inflammation may allow a patient to *feel* better in the short term, the immune system may well become compromised to a point where it can no longer correctly maintain microbiome homeostasis. This exacerbates the underlying disease state and leaves patients more vulnerable to the acquisition of new pathogens.

11 VITAMIN D SUPPLEMENTS ARE IMMUNOSUPPRESSIVE: 25-D PALLIATES SYMPTOMS BUT DOES NOT CURE INFLAMMATORY DISEASE

One of the most common supplements used to palliate inflammatory symptoms is cholecalciferol, a precursor for the secosteroid 25-D. While vitamin D has long been viewed solely as a nutrient, vitamin D metabolites are actually potent secosteroids. In 2008 we described some of the complexity inherent in the actions of these metabolites.[37] While the metabolism of a vitamin is characterized by a first-order mass-action model, metabolism of the vitamin D secosteroids is instead governed by layers of feedback and feed-forward transcriptional pathways that are tightly regulated in *H. sapiens*. This calls into question whether the word *vitamin* accurately communicates any of the primary activities of this supplement.

While proper functioning of the VDR is vital to a plethora of activities necessary for optimal human health, an increasing number of studies show that artificial supplementation of vitamin D metabolites does not result in optimal VDR activity. Under conditions of health, the VDR is activated by 1,25-D. Yet, as previously described, if 1,25-D concentrations increase in patients as they become ill, the elevated metabolite can interfere with the ability of key nuclear receptors to correctly express the AMPs under their control.[40]

Elevated concentrations of 25-D in the blood cause additional immunosuppression by a number of mechanisms. Dickie et al. found that 25-D slows the activity of several toll-like receptors including TLR2, TLR4, and TLR9.[56] A study of multiple sclerosis demonstrated that the supplement effectively slowed the immune activity of peripheral blood mononuclear cells.[57] Indeed, Arnson et al. argued that vitamin D has multiple immunosuppressant properties and that, on the whole, vitamin D confers an immunosuppressive effect.[58]

Over the past decade we performed several *in silico* experiments that suggest that blood-borne 25-D is able to directly bind into the VDR binding pocket to slow receptor activity.[37] Much like the microbial ligands that slow innate immunity by interfering with VDR activity, this antagonism would result in a significant decrease in the expression of AMP and TLR2. This immunosuppressive effect progressively increases as higher doses of vitamin D are administered, resulting in the J- or U-shaped curves evident in so many of the clinical trials.[59,60] The resulting decrease in innate immune activity enhances pathogen survival, and homeostasis of the microbiome is more easily disrupted.

We have subsequently argued, with increasing urgency, that any subjective or objective improvements associated with vitamin D supplementation in the short term result from its ability to decrease the immunopathology associated with an effective innate immune response to elements of a patient's microbiome.[61] Blood-borne 25-D likely provides symptomatic relief by acting in a manner similar to the immunosuppressive medications described earlier, the use of which has been associated with high rates of relapse and instability over time.

Thus, while we are accustomed to the hypothesis that high levels of vitamin D supplementation are necessary to curb the current epidemic of chronic disease, the opposite may instead be true. Vitamin D is added to an increasing variety of food products and is more frequently used in the clinic, but the incidence of nearly every chronic condition has, in fact, increased. To minimize potential harm, we believe that blood-borne 25-D must be kept *below* the consensus immunosuppressive level of approximately 50–60 nmol/L to optimize innate immune function and overall health.

12 HARM FROM VITAMIN D IS INCREASINGLY SUPPORTED BY HIGH-QUALITY STUDIES

Description of vitamin D as the "sunshine vitamin" has led many to assume that the secosteroid is not likely to cause any serious harm (despite the fact that solar exposure can cause skin cancer). Yet vitamin D supplementation is increasingly being associated with a host of negative health outcomes including brain lesions,[62] kidney stones,[63] increased bone fractures[64] and increased incidence of allergy and atopy.[65]

Despite these reports, many researchers still believe that vitamin D is a panacea. The majority of studies referenced to support these assumptions, however, rely largely on surrogate outcomes and speculation. Most also fail to provide a basis in human molecular biology for the apparent benefits observed in their analyses. Some researchers assume that ancient man obtained high concentrations of vitamin D from the sun on the plains of

Africa and conclude that modern humans should do the same. However, anthropologists have no definitive data on the sun exposure of early *H. sapiens*. Other studies discuss instances in which people who live at sunnier latitudes display a lower incidence of some inflammatory diseases. Nonetheless, myriad other variables confound their analyses, and even a quick search of the literature reveals numerous, but less frequently cited, counterexamples. Others have argued for increased vitamin D supplementation on the basis that sunscreens block the production of vitamin D in the skin, but even the hypothesis that vitamin D is primarily produced by irradiation of the skin is now being questioned[66] and, in any case, sunscreen does not seem to block vitamin D production.[67]

In 2009, the US and Canadian governments commissioned the Tufts Evidence-based Practice Center to compile a report on vitamin D for the Institute of Medicine (IOM).[68] In an effort to address the discrepancies observed in the vitamin D literature, this report assessed all studies relating to health outcomes and vitamin D and/or calcium intake. After an evidence-based analysis, the Tufts researchers were able to support a positive association only between vitamin D intake and bone health. In the case of all other chronic or inflammatory conditions analyzed, they found no evidence to support an association between vitamin D intake and improved health. The IOM committee therefore decided not to increase the Daily Recommended Intake of vitamin D and further noted that intake of the secosteroid is associated with adverse health outcomes.

Given that the IOM report was released, the results of randomized controlled trials evaluating the use of vitamin D in a variety of inflammatory conditions continue to demonstrate little benefit, and even harm, from vitamin D supplementation. Well-designed studies recently determined that supplemental vitamin D does not significantly improve cardiovascular disease risk factors,[69] isolated systolic hypertension,[70] tuberculosis[71] and upper respiratory infections.[72] Several studies have called into question the one positive association between vitamin D intake and bone health that the IOM committee was able to support in 2010. In 2013, McAlindon et al. published the results of a randomized placebo-controlled trial showing that vitamin D3 supplementation for a period of 2 years did not reduce knee pain or loss of cartilage volume in patients with symptomatic knee osteoarthritis.[73] Another such study found increased risk of fracture among elderly women taking vitamin D.[64] A second systematic review found that vitamin D supplementation failed to improve bone health in women with breast cancer.[74]

13 THE CONCEPT OF VITAMIN D DEFICIENCY IS FLAWED: LOW BLOOD CONCENTRATIONS OF 25-D LIKELY RESULT FROM THE INFLAMMATORY DISEASE PROCESS

Despite the data discussed above, vitamin D supplementation is routinely justified based on a plethora of studies that report low concentrations of 25-D in the blood of patients with a wide variety of inflammatory conditions. Thus far, the consensus on these findings has been to assume that the low concentrations of 25-D are driving or contributing to the pathogenesis of these diseases.

However, the low concentrations of 25-D often detected in patients with inflammatory conditions may be a *result* of the inflammatory disease process rather than the cause of the inflammation. Indeed, our data suggest that under conditions of microbiome and interactome dysregulation, the body uses multiple mechanisms to naturally downregulate intracellular production of 25-D.[37]

Expression of the enzyme *CYP24A1* normally controls excess concentrations of 1,25-D. However, if VDR activity is slowed by the intra-phagocytic microbiome, the enzyme cannot be expressed as robustly. In addition, when 1,25-D increases, it downregulates the amount of previtamin D converted into 25-D. One of these mechanisms is antagonism of the PXR nuclear receptor and expression of the enzyme *CYP27A1*. The result is that blood concentrations of 25-D, the metabolite most commonly measured in the clinic, decrease.

The concept of vitamin D "deficiency" has been further complicated by the arbitrary ranges used to define insufficiency and deficiency. Vitamin D supplementation has become so prevalent that individuals who choose not to ingest extra amounts of the secosteroid may be deemed deficient simply because they eat unfortified foods.[75] Indeed, it is difficult to find unsupplemented populations to study. Nevertheless, studies of healthy individuals in populations that do not heavily supplement their food supplies with vitamin D have demonstrated that subjects' 25-D concentrations are naturally found to be in the range we today have labeled as "deficient".

Saudi Arabia does not yet add vitamin D to their food supply. It is not surprising, then, that one study found that 100% of Saudi medical students receiving standard amounts sunlight and eating a normal diet were vitamin D insufficient or deficient according to conventional standards.[75] Similarly, a study of healthy Bangladeshi women not supplementing with vitamin D found that approximately 80% had 25-D concentrations less than 16 ng/mL.[76] A separate study of premenopausal Bangladeshi women came to a similar conclusion.[77] A study of young healthy adults from the west of India, also not consuming supplemental vitamin D, found the average serum concentration of 25-D to be 17.4 ng/mL.[78] In 1992, before vitamin D supplementation became more common in China, a study found that healthy full-term Chinese infants had serum concentrations of 25-D ranging from an average of 5 to 14 ng/mL, a level that would be regarded as "highly deficient" by current dogma.[79]

It is tempting to argue that the individuals in these studies do not receive adequate exposure to sunlight. (Whether people require a certain amount of sunlight also remains a matter of debate.) Yet in each instance the authors clearly ascertain that their subjects are healthy and quite functional. Instead of assuming that these healthy subjects should be given extra vitamin D, as the current standard of care indicates, it may be prudent to consider whether the ranges we have created for vitamin D deficiency and insufficiency have a basis in human molecular science.

14 DISCUSSION

In just a decade, the discovery of the human microbiome has uncovered the presence of thousands of microbes capable of contributing to chronic infectious processes. Indeed, dysbiosis of the microbiome has been tied to an increasing number of inflammatory disease states. In lieu of a single pathogen causing a single chronic infectious disease, the microbiome as a whole gradually shifts away from a state of homeostasis as people become ill. Those pathogens capable of persisting inside nucleated cells are able to extensively dysregulate human metabolism by directly interfering with gene expression. A number of key pathogens associated with autoimmune disease persist by inhibiting the VDR and subsequently the innate immune response. This allows them to more easily accumulate into the microbiome over time.

Anti-inflammatory treatments that slow the immune response may provide short-term symptomatic improvement, but they do so at the expense of long-term microbiome stability. This leads to relapse and increases the likelihood of comorbid conditions over time. The secosteroid we call vitamin D is immunosuppressive. In patients with chronic inflammatory disease, low concentrations of 25-D in the bloodstream are likely a result of the disease process, rather than its cause. To allow the immune system to keep control of the microbiome, concentrations of blood-borne 25-D should be kept below the immunosuppressive threshold of 50–60 nmol/L.

REFERENCES

1. Turnbaugh PJ, Ley RE, Hamady M, Fraser-Liggett CM, Knight R, Gordon JI. The human microbiome project. *Nature* 2007;**449**(7164):804–10.
2. Methé BA, Nelson KE, Pop M, Creasy HH, Giglio MG, Huttenhower C, et al. A framework for human microbiome research. *Nature* 2012;**486**(7402):215–21.
3. Ehrlich SD. *MetaHIT: The European Union Project on metagenomics of the human intestinal tract.* New York: Springer; 2011, p. 307–16.
4. Kozarov E. Bacterial invasion of vascular cell types: vascular infectology and atherogenesis. *Future Cardiol* 2012;**8**(1):123–38.
5. McLaughlin RW, Vali H, Lau PCK, Palfree RGE, De Ciccio A, Sirois M, et al. Are there naturally occurring pleomorphic bacteria in the blood of healthy humans? *J Clin Microbiol* 2002;**40**(12):4771–5.
6. Erb-Downward JR, Thompson DL, Han MK, Freeman CM, McCloskey L, Schmidt LA, et al. Analysis of the lung microbiome in the "healthy" smoker and in COPD. *PLoS ONE* 2011;**6**(2):e16384–e.
7. Dempsey KE, Riggio MP, Lennon A, Hannah VE, Ramage G, Allan D, et al. Identification of bacteria on the surface of clinically infected and non-infected prosthetic hip joints removed during revision arthroplasties by 16S rRNA gene sequencing and by microbiological culture. *Arthritis Res Ther* 2007;**9**(3):R46.
8. Pagani I, Liolios K, Jansson J, Chen IM, Smirnova T, Nosrat B, et al. The Genomes OnLine Database (GOLD) v. 4: status of genomic and metagenomic projects and their associated metadata. *Nucleic Acids Res* 2012;**40**(Database issue):D571–9.
9. Nasidze I, Li J, Quinque D, Tang K, Stoneking M. Global diversity in the human salivary microbiome. *Genome Res* 2009;**19**(4):636–43.
10. Reyes A, Haynes M, Hanson N, Angly FE, Heath AC, Rohwer F, et al. Viruses in the faecal microbiota of monozygotic twins and their mothers. *Nature* 2010;**466**(7304):334–8.
11. Pride DT, Salzman J, Haynes M, Rohwer F, Davis-Long C, White 3rd RA, et al. Evidence of a robust resident bacteriophage population revealed through analysis of the human salivary virome. *ISME J* 2012;**6**(5):915–26.
12. Yang X, Xie L, Li Y, Wei C. More than 9,000,000 unique genes in human gut bacterial community: estimating gene numbers inside a human body. *PLoS One* 2009;**4**(6):e6074.
13. Xu Y, Xie J, Li Y, Yue J, Chen J, Chunyu L, et al. Using a cDNA microarray to study cellular gene expression altered by *Mycobacterium tuberculosis*. *Chin Med J* 2003;**116**(7):1070–3.
14. Goh KI, Cusick ME, Valle D, Childs B, Vidal M, Barabasi AL. The human disease network. *Proc Natl Acad Sci USA* 2007;**104**(21):8685–90.
15. Ramchandran L, Shah NP. Proteolytic profiles and angiotensin-I converting enzyme and alpha-glucosidase inhibitory activities of selected lactic acid bacteria. *J Food Sci* 2008;**73**(2):M75–81.
16. Hood L. Tackling the microbiome. *Science* 2012;**336**(6086):1209.
17. Clayton TA, Baker D, Lindon JC, Everett JR, Nicholson JK. Pharmacometabonomic identification of a significant host-microbiome metabolic interaction affecting human drug metabolism. *Proc Natl Acad Sci USA* 2009;**106**(34):14728–33.
18. Krishnadev O, Srinivasan N. Prediction of protein–protein interactions between human host and a pathogen and its application to three pathogenic bacteria. *Int J Biol Macromol* 2011;**48**(4):613–9.
19. Kusalik A, Bickis M, Lewis C, Li Y, Lucchese G, Marincola FM, et al. Widespread and ample peptide overlapping between HCV and *Homo sapiens* proteomes. *Peptides* 2007;**28**(6):1260–7.
20. Giongo A, Gano KA, Crabb DB, Mukherjee N, Novelo LL, Casella G, et al. Toward defining the autoimmune microbiome for type 1 diabetes. *ISME J* 2010;**5**(1):82–91.

21. Larsen N, Vogensen FK, van den Berg FW, Nielsen DS, Andreasen AS, Pedersen BK, et al. Gut microbiota in human adults with type 2 diabetes differs from non-diabetic adults. *PLoS One* 2010;**5**(2):e9085.
22. Morgan XC, Tickle TL, Sokol H, Gevers D, Devaney KL, Ward DV, et al. Dysfunction of the intestinal microbiome in inflammatory bowel disease and treatment. *Genome Biol* 2012;**13**(9):R79.
23. Gao Z, Tseng CH, Strober BE, Pei Z, Blaser MJ. Substantial alterations of the cutaneous bacterial biota in psoriatic lesions. *PLoS One* 2008;**3**(7):e2719.
24. Amar J, Serino M, Lange C, Chabo C, Iacovoni J, Mondot S, et al. Involvement of tissue bacteria in the onset of diabetes in humans: evidence for a concept. *Diabetologia* 2011;**54**(12):3055–61.
25. Kostic AD, Gevers D, Pedamallu CS, Michaud M, Duke F, Earl AM, et al. Genomic analysis identifies association of Fusobacterium with colorectal carcinoma. *Genome Res* 2012;**22**(2):292–8.
26. Schutzer SE, Angel TE, Liu T, Schepmoes AA, Clauss TR, Adkins JN, et al. Distinct cerebrospinal fluid proteomes differentiate post-treatment lyme disease from chronic fatigue syndrome. *PLoS One* 2011;**6**(2):e17287.
27. Stahringer SS, Clemente JC, Corley RP, Hewitt J, Knights D, Walters WA, et al. Nurture trumps nature in a longitudinal survey of salivary bacterial communities in twins from early adolescence to early adulthood. *Genome Res* 2012;**22**(11):2146–52.
28. Machado AM, Figueiredo C, Touati E, Maximo V, Sousa S, Michel V, et al. *Helicobacter pylori* infection induces genetic instability of nuclear and mitochondrial DNA in gastric cells. *Clin Cancer Res* 2009;**15**(9):2995–3002.
29. Wang TT, Tavera-Mendoza LE, Laperriere D, Libby E, MacLeod NB, Nagai Y, et al. Large-scale *in silico* and microarray-based identification of direct 1,25-dihydroxyvitamin D3 target genes. *Mol Endocrinol* 2005;**19**(11):2685–95.
30. Yenamandra SP, Lundin A, Arulampalam V, Yurchenko M, Pettersson S, Klein G, et al. Expression profile of nuclear receptors upon Epstein–Barr virus induced B cell transformation. *Exp Oncol* 2009;**31**(2):92–6.
31. Liu PT, Wheelwright M, Teles R, Komisopoulou E, Edfeldt K, Ferguson B, et al. MicroRNA-21 targets the vitamin D-dependent antimicrobial pathway in leprosy. *Nat Med* 2012;**18**(2):267–73.
32. Chan G, Bivins-Smith ER, Smith MS, Smith PM, Yurochko AD. Transcriptome analysis reveals human cytomegalovirus reprograms monocyte differentiation toward an M1 macrophage. *J Immunol* 2008;**181**(1):698–711.
33. Salazar JC, Duhnam-Ems S, La Vake C, Cruz AR, Moore MW, Caimano MJ, et al. Activation of human monocytes by live *Borrelia burgdorferi* generates TLR2-dependent and -independent responses which include induction of IFN-beta. *PLoS Pathog* 2009;**5**(5):e1000444.
34. Coughlan CA, Chotirmall SH, Renwick J, Hassan T, Low TB, Bergsson G, et al. The effect of *Aspergillus fumigatus* infection on vitamin D receptor expression in cystic fibrosis. *Am J Respir Crit Care Med* 2012;**186**(10):999–1007.
35. White RH. Biosynthesis of the sulfonolipid 2-amino-3-hydroxy-15-methylhexadecane-1-sulfonic acid in the gliding bacterium *Cytophaga johnsonae*. *J Bacteriol* 1984;**159**(1):42–6.
36. Marshall TG. Bacterial capnine blocks transcription of human antimicrobial peptides, In: Third international conference on metagenomics, San Diego, CA, July 11–13; 2007.
37. Marshall TG. Vitamin D, discovery outpaces FDA decision making. *BioEssays* 2008;**30**(2):173–82.
38. Bell NH. Renal and nonrenal 25-hydroxyvitamin D-1alpha-hydroxylases and their clinical significance. *J Bone Miner Res* 1998;**13**(3):350–3.
39. Blaney GP, Albert PJ, Proal AD. Vitamin D metabolites as clinical markers in autoimmune and chronic disease. *Ann NY Acad Sci* 2009;**1173**:384–90.

40. Proal AD, Albert PJ, Marshall TG. Dysregulation of the vitamin D nuclear receptor may contribute to the higher prevalence of some autoimmune diseases in women. *Ann NY Acad Sci* 2009;**1173**:252–9.
41. Marshall TG, Lee RE, Marshall FE. Common angiotensin receptor blockers may directly modulate the immune system via VDR, PPAR and CCR2b. *Theor Biol Med Model* 2006;**3**:1.
42. Brahmachary M, Schonbach C, Yang L, Huang E, Tan SL, Chowdhary R, et al. Computational promoter analysis of mouse, rat and human antimicrobial peptide-coding genes. *BMC Bioinformatics* 2006;**7**(Suppl. 5):S8.
43. Abrahamsson TR, Jakobsson HE, Andersson AF, Björkstén B, Engstrand L, Jenmalm MC. Low diversity of the gut microbiota in infants with atopic eczema. *J Allergy Clin Immunol* 2012;**129**(2):434–40, 40.e1–2.
44. Oakley BB, Fiedler TL, Marrazzo JM, Fredricks DN. Diversity of human vaginal bacterial communities and associations with clinically defined bacterial vaginosis. *Appl Environ Microbiol* 2008;**74**(15):4898–909.
45. Majed B, Arveiler D, Bingham A, Ferrieres J, Ruidavets J-B, Montaye M, et al. Depressive symptoms, a time-dependent risk factor for coronary heart disease and stroke in middle-aged men: the PRIME study. *Stroke* 2012;**43**(7):1761–7.
46. Kinross JM, Darzi AW, Nicholson JK. Gut microbiome–host interactions in health and disease. *Genome Med* 2011;**3**(3):14.
47. Berer K, Mues M, Koutrolos M, Rasbi ZA, Boziki M, Johner C, et al. Commensal microbiota and myelin autoantigen cooperate to trigger autoimmune demyelination. *Nature* 2011;**479**(7374):538–41.
48. Gonzalez A, Stombaugh J, Lozupone C, Turnbaugh PJ, Gordon JI, Knight R. The mind-body-microbial continuum. *Dialogues Clin Neurosci* 2011;**13**(1):55–62.
49. Anaya JM, Tobon GJ, Vega P, Castiblanco J. Autoimmune disease aggregation in families with primary Sjogren's syndrome. *J Rheumatol* 2006;**33**(11):2227–34.
50. Weyermann M, Rothenbacher D, Brenner H. Acquisition of *Helicobacter pylori* infection in early childhood: independent contributions of infected mothers, fathers, and siblings. *Am J Gastroenterol* 2009;**104**(1):182–9.
51. DiGiulio DB, Romero R, Amogan HP, Kusanovic JP, Bik EM, Gotsch F, et al. Microbial prevalence, diversity and abundance in amniotic fluid during preterm labor: a molecular and culture-based investigation. *PLoS One* 2008;**3**(8):e3056.
52. Grönlund MM, Lehtonen OP, Eerola E, Kero P. Fecal microflora in healthy infants born by different methods of delivery: permanent changes in intestinal flora after cesarean delivery. *J Pediatr Gastroenterol Nutr* 1999;**28**(1):19–25.
53. Cabrera-Rubio R, Collado MC, Laitinen K, Salminen S, Isolauri E, Mira A. The human milk microbiome changes over lactation and is shaped by maternal weight and mode of delivery. *Am J Clin Nutr* 2012;**96**(3):544–51.
54. Gottlieb JE, Israel HL, Steiner RM, Triolo J, Patrick H. Outcome in sarcoidosis. The relationship of relapse to corticosteroid therapy. *Chest* 1997;**111**(3):623–31.
55. Seok J, Warren HS, Cuenca AG, Mindrinos MN, Baker HV, Xu W, et al. Genomic responses in mouse models poorly mimic human inflammatory diseases. *Proc Natl Acad Sci USA* 2013;**110**(9):3507–12.
56. Dickie LJ, Church LD, Coulthard LR, Mathews RJ, Emery P, McDermott MF. Vitamin D3 down-regulates intracellular Toll-like receptor 9 expression and Toll-like receptor 9-induced IL-6 production in human monocytes. *Rheumatology (Oxford)* 2010;**49**(8):1466–71.
57. Kimball S, Vieth R, Dosch HM, Bar-Or A, Cheung R, Gagne D, et al. Cholecalciferol plus calcium suppresses abnormal PBMC reactivity in patients with multiple sclerosis. *J Clin Endocrinol Metab* 2011;**96**(9):2826–34.

58. Arnson Y, Amital H, Shoenfeld Y. Vitamin D and autoimmunity: new aetiological and therapeutic considerations. *Ann Rheum Dis* 2007;**66**(9):1137–42.
59. Durup D, Jørgensen HL, Christensen J, Schwarz P, Heegaard AM, Lind B. A reverse J-shaped association of all-cause mortality with serum 25-hydroxyvitamin D in general practice, the CopD study. *J Clin Endocrinol Metab* 2012;**97**(8):2644–52.
60. Ahn J, Peters U, Albanes D, Purdue MP, Abnet CC, Chatterjee N, et al. Serum vitamin D concentration and prostate cancer risk: a nested case-control study. *J Natl Cancer Inst* 2008;**100**(11):796–804.
61. Albert PJ, Proal AD, Marshall TG. Vitamin D: the alternative hypothesis. *Autoimmun Rev* 2009;**8**(8):639–44.
62. Payne ME, Anderson JJ, Steffens DC. Calcium and vitamin D intakes may be positively associated with brain lesions in depressed and nondepressed elders. *Nutr Res* 2008;**28**(5):285–92.
63. Bjelakovic G, Gluud LL, Nikolova D, Whitfield K, Wetterslev J, Simonetti RG, et al. Vitamin D supplementation for prevention of mortality in adults. *Cochrane Database Syst Rev* 2011;(7):CD007470.
64. Sanders KM, Stuart AL, Williamson EJ, Simpson JA, Kotowicz MA, Young D, et al. Annual high-dose oral vitamin D and falls and fractures in older women: a randomized controlled trial. *JAMA* 2010;**303**(18):1815–22.
65. Hypponen E, Sovio U, Wjst M, Patel S, Pekkanen J, Hartikainen AL, et al. Infant vitamin d supplementation and allergic conditions in adulthood: northern Finland birth cohort 1966. *Ann NY Acad Sci* 2004;**1037**:84–95.
66. Becklund BR, Severson KS, Vang SV, DeLuca HF. UV radiation suppresses experimental autoimmune encephalomyelitis independent of vitamin D production. *Proc Natl Acad Sci USA* 2010;**107**(14):6418–23.
67. Diehl JW, Chiu MW. Effects of ambient sunlight and photoprotection on vitamin D status. *Dermatol Ther* 2010;**23**(1):48–60.
68. Chung M, Balk EM, Brendel M, Ip S, Lau J, Lee J, et al. Vitamin D and calcium: a systematic review of health outcomes. *Evid Rep Technol Assess (Full Rep)* 2009;(183):1–420.
69. Wood AD, Secombes KR, Thies F, Aucott L, Black AJ, Mavroeidi A, et al. Vitamin D3 supplementation has no effect on conventional cardiovascular risk factors: a parallel-group, double-blind, placebo-controlled RCT. *J Clin Endocrinol Metab* 2012;**97**(10):3557–68.
70. Witham MD, Price RJ, Struthers AD, Donnan PT, Messow CM, Ford I, et al. Cholecalciferol treatment to reduce blood pressure in older patients with isolated systolic hypertension: the VitDISH randomized controlled trial. *JAMA Intern Med* 2013;**173**(18):1672–9.
71. Wejse C, Gomes VF, Rabna P, Gustafson P, Aaby P, Lisse IM, et al. Vitamin D as supplementary treatment for tuberculosis: a double-blind, randomized, placebo-controlled trial. *Am J Respir Crit Care Med* 2009;**179**(9):843–50.
72. Murdoch DR, Slow S, Chambers ST, Jennings LC, Stewart AW, Priest PC, et al. Effect of vitamin D3 supplementation on upper respiratory tract infections in healthy adults: the VIDARIS randomized controlled trial. *JAMA* 2012;**308**(13):1333–9.
73. McAlindon T, LaValley M, Schneider E, Nuite M, Lee JY, Price LL, et al. Effect of vitamin D supplementation on progression of knee pain and cartilage volume loss in patients with symptomatic osteoarthritis: a randomized controlled trial. *JAMA* 2013;**309**(2):155–62.
74. Datta M, Schwartz GG. Calcium and vitamin D supplementation and loss of bone mineral density in women undergoing breast cancer therapy. *Crit Rev Oncol Hematol* 2013;**88**(3):613–24.
75. Al-Elq AH. The status of Vitamin D in medical students in the preclerkship years of a Saudi medical school. *J Fam Commun Med* 2012;**19**(2):100–4.

76. Islam MZ, Akhtaruzzaman M, Lamberg-Allardt C. Hypovitaminosis D is common in both veiled and nonveiled Bangladeshi women. *Asia Pac J Clin Nutr* 2006;**15**(1):81–7.
77. Islam MZ, Shamim AA, Kemi V, Nevanlinna A, Akhtaruzzaman M, Laaksonen M, et al. Vitamin D deficiency and low bone status in adult female garment factory workers in Bangladesh. *Br J Nutr* 2008;**99**(6):1322–9.
78. Shivane VK, Sarathi V, Bandgar T, Menon P, Shah NS. High prevalence of hypovitaminosis D in young healthy adults from the western part of India. *Postgrad Med J* 2011;**87**(1030):514–18.
79. Specker BL, Ho ML, Oestreich A, Yin TA, Shui QM, Chen XC, et al. Prospective study of vitamin D supplementation and rickets in China. *J Pediatr* 1992;**120**(5):733–9.

CHAPTER 11

Seasonality and Autoimmunity

Luciana Parente Costa Seguro[1], Sandra Gofinet Pasoto

Rheumatology Division, Hospital das Clínicas da Universidade de São Paulo, São Paulo, Brazil
[1]Corresponding Author: lucianapc@gmail.com

1 INTRODUCTION

Several diseases with a well-known autoimmune pathogenesis have a seasonal pattern of clinical manifestations, disease onset, and/or month of birth of affected individuals, such as multiple sclerosis, type 1 diabetes mellitus, and narcolepsy. The seasonal features of these diseases may reflect the role of environmental factors, including infectious agents and environmental pollutants, triggering abnormal autoimmune regulation in genetically predisposed subjects. Indeed, different seasons have peculiar characteristics that may influence exposure to these environmental agents. In addition, vitamin D (of which production in the skin is dependent on exposure to sunlight) and melatonin (the secretion of which by the pineal gland experiences seasonal variations) have been implicated in the risk of developing autoimmune diseases because both hormones have effects on immune system regulation.[1] In this chapter, we revise the possible mechanisms involved in the seasonality of autoimmune diseases as well as the seasonal characteristics of human immune function.

2 SEASONALITY AND IMMUNE SYSTEM

The effect of environmental factors on the immune system has been described in animals, in healthy subjects, and in patients with autoimmune diseases. Some parameters of the immune system in healthy individuals present seasonal variations. The numbers of immune cells and the concentrations of cytokines change during the year according to the seasons. The number of leukocytes; neutrophils; monocytes; lymphocytes; CD4+, CD8+, and CD25+ T cells; CD20+ B cells; the CD4+-to-CD8+ ratio and serum concentrations of interleukin (IL)-6 have seasonal variations.[2] Higher concentrations of pro-inflammatory cytokines such as interferon (IFN)-α and IFN-γ were detected during the winter compared to summer.[3]

Infection and Autoimmunity
http://dx.doi.org/10.1016/B978-0-444-63269-2.00009-X

Similarly, elevated IFN-γ and decreased concentrations of IL-10 (which have anti-inflammatory effects) were reported in a study performed during an Antarctic winter.[4] In healthy adults and healthy children or children with rheumatic fever, lymphocyte response fluctuates during different seasons of the year, with the maximum in summer.[5]

Also, the functional seasonality of the immune system has been demonstrated, exemplified by differences in seroconversion response to vaccines at different seasons. In a double-blind, placebo-controlled study in the former Soviet Union, febrile reactions and an increase in antibody titers after influenza vaccination were higher among volunteers inoculated in January compared to other months.[6]

3 SEASONALITY, INFECTIONS, AND AUTOIMMUNITY

Observations, especially from epidemiological studies, support the hypothesis that some seasonal patterns in autoimmune diseases can be explained by seasonal infections. Multiple sclerosis and central nervous system demyelination have been associated with Epstein-Barr virus (EBV) infections.[7,8] Type 1 diabetes and subclinical β-cell autoimmunity (appearance of autoantibodies) have been associated with enterovirus infections.[9] Narcolepsy has been associated with *Streptococcus pyogenes* and influenza A H1N1 infection and H1N1 vaccination.[10] Also, a possible infectious etiology has been suggested for juvenile arthritis (JA), temporal arteritis, polymyalgia rheumatic, and celiac disease autoimmunity.[11–13]

In addition to the suspected examples cited above, some infections are known to trigger an autoimmune process and cause reactive seasonal diseases. Acute rheumatic fever, acute post-streptococcal glomerulonephritis, Sydenham's chorea, and pediatric autoimmune neuropsychiatric disorders associated with streptococcal infections (PANDAS) are expressions of immune-mediated response to streptococcal infections.

4 VITAMIN D, SUN EXPOSURE, AND AUTOIMMUNITY

Epidemiological studies show that the prevalence of certain autoimmune diseases such as multiple sclerosis, type 1 diabetes, rheumatoid arthritis (RA), and inflammatory bowel disease varies with latitude; higher rates occur where sun exposure is reduced. These findings lead to the theory that sunlight exposure, and therefore vitamin D, may play a role in the pathogenesis of these diseases.[14,15]

Vitamin D is synthesized from cholesterol in the skin (80–90%) under solar ultraviolet radiation and then metabolized to 25-hydroxyvitamin D in the liver and to its active form, 1,25-dihydroxyvitamin D, in the kidneys.[16] Consequently, vitamin D concentrations are lower in winter and peak in summer; this circannual rhythm is associated with changes in the human peripheral T-cell compartment in healthy adult males[17] and with the clinical status of some autoimmune diseases.

In healthy adult males, elevated serum vitamin D concentrations in summer are associated with a higher number of peripheral CD4+ and CD8+ T cells, an increase in naive T cells and a decrease in memory T cells. The percentage of T regulatory cells is reduced in summer but increases the expression of forkhead box protein 3 (Foxp3). Skin, gut, and lymphoid tissue homing potential is increased during summer, exemplified by increased concentrations of chemokine receptor (CCR) 4, CCR6, cutaneous lymphocyte antigen, CCR9, and CCR7. Also, in summer, CD4+ and CD8+ T cells reveal a reduced capacity to produce pro-inflammatory cytokines.[17]

Vitamin D modulates T-cell, B-cell, and antigen-presenting cell function and immunoglobulin production, switches the immune profile from T helper (Th) 1/Th17 to Th2/T regulatory cells and thus affects innate and adaptive immune responses, which result in prevention of and protection from autoimmune diseases in humans and in animal models.[18–23] Activation of vitamin D receptor, present in immune cells, affects messenger RNA expression, T-cell, and B-cell proliferation and antibody production.[24] In addition, 1α-hydroxylase was detected in B cells, indicating a possible role for B cells in autocrine and paracrine production and response to vitamin D.[25]

Moreover, the effects on the immune system of deprivation of sunlight and vitamin D at higher latitudes further impairs the control of certain viruses, such as EBV, that also are implicated in the development of autoimmune diseases.[26] Polymorphisms in the vitamin D receptor gene have been associated with increased risk of several autoimmune diseases including multiple sclerosis, type 1 diabetes, autoimmune thyroid disease, systemic lupus erythematosus (SLE), and RA.[27–31]

5 MELATONIN, SEASONALITY, AND THE IMMUNE SYSTEM

Melatonin may regulate the seasonal variability of the immune system because its secretion by the pineal gland presents circadian and seasonal rhythms; this hormone has confirmed effects on cellular and humoral immune responses in addition to participating in various body functions. Also, it can be secreted by lymphoid organs such as the bone marrow, thymus, and lymphocytes.[32,33]

Melatonin secretion is closely correlated with the seasons of the year, with an earlier peak in summer than in winter; the regulatory function of melatonin on the immune system also presents a seasonal pattern.[33,34] Melatonin has an immunomodulatory effect on the regulation of cellular and humoral immunity.[35,36] Melatonin enhances the production of natural killer cells, monocytes, and leukocytes. Furthermore, melatonin alters the balance of Th1 and Th2 cells, mainly concerning Th1 responses, and increases the production of IL-2, IL-6, IL-12, and IFN-γ.[33] Of note, melatonin stimulates production of granulocytes and macrophages, which are important components of the innate immune system.[37] The seasonal pattern of immune function regulation by melatonin may in part account for the annual cyclic pattern of incidence and symptom expression of some infectious and autoimmune diseases, as well as affective disorders.

6 SEASONALITY IN AUTOIMMUNE DISEASES: INFECTIOUS AGENTS, VITAMIN D, AND MELATONIN

6.1 Multiple Sclerosis

The etiology of multiple sclerosis, an autoimmune disease of the central nervous system, is still unknown, but some risk factors have been implicated in its pathogenesis, including an association of genetic susceptibility and environmental agents. Season of birth, EBV infection, vitamin D deficiency, and smoking are strongly involved in the development of multiple sclerosis.[38–42] In this regard, seasonality is directly involved with exposure to environmental agents, and seasonal factors may act even before birth, affecting the structure and function of embryonic/fetal tissues. The births of patients with multiple sclerosis follow a seasonal distribution, being more frequent during the spring and winter and less frequent during the autumn; it is hypothesized that this could reflect low maternal vitamin D during pregnancy.[38,39] Past infection with EBV is associated with increased risk of central nervous system demyelination. The risk of developing multiple sclerosis following EBV infections is increased at least fourfold after 10 years and persists for more than 30 years.[40,41]

Moreover, concentrations of vitamin D are lower in patients with multiple sclerosis than in controls and, among patients with multiple sclerosis, lower concentrations of vitamin D are associated with progressive forms of the disease, increased disability, and clinical activity and risk of relapse. Multiple sclerosis relapses are inversely associated with ultraviolet radiation and serum vitamin D concentrations, positively associated with upper respiratory tract infections and occur mostly during the winter.[42,43] Interestingly, polymorphisms of vitamin D receptor in the promoter region of the human leukocyte antigen (HLA) DRB1*1501 are associated with response to vitamin D and with multiple sclerosis susceptibility in Caucasians.[27,43]

6.2 Type 1 Diabetes Mellitus

Enterovirus has been implicated as a possible environmental trigger for type 1 diabetes. These viruses were detected in diabetic patients more frequently than in control individuals, and they may induce diabetes in animal models. Likewise, in enterovirus infection, seasonality was observed in both the onset of clinical diabetes and subclinical β-cell autoimmunity (detection of autoantibodies). Furthermore, prospective studies suggest the occurrence of enterovirus infection before clinical diabetes.[9,44]

The prevalence of cord islet autoantibodies in newborns consistently varied with the seasons over 4 years: the highest prevalence occurred in July, August, and September, and the lowest prevalence occurred between January and April in a Swedish study. Children with type 1 diabetes with significant β-cell-specific autoimmunity (high autoantibody titers or positivity for several β-cell-specific autoantibodies) showed a different pattern of month of birth compared with type 1 diabetic children with low β-cell autoimmunity and the general population.[44] Also, in patients newly diagnosed with type 1 diabetes, β-cell cytotoxic cytokines levels tend to be higher during summer, especially IL-1β and tumor necrosis factor-α.[45]

Regarding vitamin D, lower concentrations are seen in patients than in controls and are associated with decompensated diabetes, ketoacidosis, incipient nephropathy, and tubulointerstitial damage.[46–48]

6.3 Narcolepsy

Another intriguing example is narcolepsy. The loss of hypothalamic hypocretin/orexin (HCRT)-producing neurons causes narcolepsy with cataplexy. There is evidence for an autoimmune pathogenesis for this disease. Narcolepsy with HCRT deficiency is known to be associated with HLA and T-cell receptor (TCR) polymorphisms, suggesting the occurrence of an autoimmune process directed to a peptide of the HCRT cells via specific HLA-peptide-TCR interactions.[49]

Notable seasonality of disease onset in children and associations with *S. pyogenes*, influenza A H1N1-infection, and H1N1-vaccination was observed. Upper airway infections may be common precipitants of a whole host of central nervous system autoimmune complications, including narcolepsy.[10] Also, a higher frequency of vitamin D deficiency is found in narcolepsy with cataplexy.[50]

6.4 Autoimmune Thyroid Disorders

Environmental and genetic factors are thought to be involved in the pathogenesis of autoimmune thyroid diseases, which include Graves' disease and Hashimoto's thyroiditis.[51] Vitamin D deficiency is higher in patients with autoimmune thyroid diseases compared to controls and correlates to the presence of antithyroid antibodies and abnormal thyroid function tests.[51] Also, polymorphisms of vitamin D receptor are implicated in the risk for autoimmune thyroid disorders.[29]

6.5 Systemic Lupus Erythematosus

In SLE, there are seasonal variations in disease activity that likely reflect environmental factors, including ultraviolet light and infections. There is an increased incidence of photosensitive skin rashes and joint pain in the spring and summer and the winter.[52,53] Also, a significantly higher prevalence of class V lupus nephritis was observed in the winter and spring compared with the summer and autumn. A similar seasonal distribution was seen for class III lupus nephritis. These findings were not confirmed in other series. Evaluation of the seasonality of lupus nephritis may contribute to understanding its pathogenesis, which may be multifactorial, because the different classes of nephritis represent different types of glomerular injury. Further studies are needed to clarify this potentially important observation.[54,55]

The risk of SLE is influenced by the season of birth, as described in a study from the United Kingdom. The distributions of births differed from that of the general population, with a peak in April. The risk of SLE was inversely correlated with maternal predicted second-trimester ultraviolet B exposure and predicted third-trimester vitamin D status.[56]

Vitamin D deficiency is prevalent in patients and is associated with activity parameters such as activity scores, anti–double-stranded DNA antibody titers and complement levels.[18,57–61] Interestingly, vitamin D deficiency is associated with antinuclear antibody (ANA) positivity in healthy controls.[62]

Vitamin D deficiency is associated with higher concentrations of IFN-α and higher B-cell activation in patients with SLE. in vitro exposure to vitamin D inhibits proliferation and induces apoptosis of activated B cells in patients with SLE and decreases plasma cell generation and differentiation. In a murine lupus model, mice supplemented with vitamin D for 22 weeks did not develop dermatologic lesions such as alopecia, necrosis of the ear and scab formation and had less proteinuria than non-supplemented mice.[63]

6.6 Rheumatoid Arthritis

There are seasonal differences in RA symptoms and disease activity assessed both subjectively and objectively with activity, health quality, and pain assessment scores; serum markers of inflammation (C-reactive protein and erythrocyte sedimentation rate) and rheumatoid factor levels, which were higher in spring and lower during autumn.[64]

RA onset is commoner in the winter.[65,66] Also, the risk of RA is influenced by the season of birth and is inversely correlated with maternal predicted second-trimester ultraviolet B exposure and predicted third-trimester vitamin D status.[56]

Vitamin D deficiency correlates with increase of autoimmune aggression in RA and exacerbation of clinical symptoms.[67] Lower serum vitamin D concentrations were observed in patients with RA from North versus South Europe with a circannual rhythm in winter and summer.[68] In addition, vitamin D values show a negative correlation with the clinical status of RA as assessed by the Health Assessment Questionnaire quality of life score and the Disease Activity Score in 28 Joints; the lowest values were in patients with high disease activity. In addition, a meta-analysis of 215,757 participants suggested that low vitamin D intake is associated with an elevated risk of RA development and reinforced that lower vitamin D concentrations are associated with RA activity.[69] Interestingly, the onset of symptoms of early arthritis during winter or spring have been associated with greater radiographic evidence of disease progression at 12 months, possibly related to seasonal lower vitamin D serum concentrations. Seasonal factors at disease onset may relate to short-term radiographic severity but do not seem to affect long-term radiographic joint damage in RA.[70,71]

Some studies suggest pathogenic pathways for vitamin D in inflammation-induced bone destruction in RA. Vitamin D modulates the mammalian target of rapamycin pathway, which is critical for osteoclast differentiation and survival.[72] Also, vitamin D binding protein (VDBP) expression is decreased in synovial membranes from patients with RA. Of note, VDBP modulates bone resorption by osteoclasts and is involved in vitamin D actions of inhibiting cell proliferation, producing immunoglobulin and releasing cytokines.[73] Furthermore, vitamin D receptor polymorphisms have been associated with RA and, in some cases, this association is strongest in shared epitope-positive patients with RA.[74]

Also, the seasonal effects of melatonin on the production of pro-inflammatory cytokines in human monocytes and T cells may act as a trigger for RA. In fact, melatonin activates the production of pro-inflammatory cytokines by acting on specific nuclear receptors present in monocytes and T cells. In addition, patients with RA have greater nocturnal melatonin concentrations in serum and synovial fluid than healthy controls.[75,76]

6.7 Spondyloarthritis and Uveitis

Spondyloarthritis symptoms may present seasonal differences. In patients with ankylosing spondylitis, the Bath Ankylosing Spondylitis Disease Activity Index score is higher in winter than in summer. Also, there is a link between health status and perceived quality of life and season and weather conditions. Higher lumbar spine flexibility (Schober index) was associated with higher climatic temperature and lower wind speed. Physical quality of life and social interaction improved in summer.[77,78] Patients with psoriatic arthritis graded their disease as being worse in winter compared with summer, but the change in season did not affect disease activity outcomes.[79] An increase in the incidence of anterior uveitis cases in the warm and transitional seasons compared with the cold season was observed in southwestern Finland.[80]

6.8 Juvenile Arthritis

Seasonal variations were observed in systemic JA. Changes in the incidence of childhood arthritis over time also were detected, suggesting that environmental factors influence disease frequency, whereas familial aggregations indicate the relevance of genetic susceptibility. A possible infectious etiology has been suggested from observational studies. In a Canadian province, a significant correlation was found between the incidence of JA and the number of *Mycoplasma pneumoniae* infections.[11]

Vitamin D insufficiency is common in patients with JA, but there is no evidence of association with disease activity. A truncated isoform of VDBP is present at significantly reduced concentrations in the synovial fluid of patients with oligoarticular JA who are at risk of disease extension relative to other subgroups.[82,83]

6.9 Rheumatic Fever and PANDAS

Some infections are known to trigger an autoimmune process and cause reactive seasonal diseases. Acute rheumatic fever, acute post-streptococcal glomerulonephritis, Sydenham's chorea, and PANDAS are clinical presentations of immune-mediated response to streptococcal infections. Rheumatic fever has a seasonal pattern; it is more common during the cold months, and hospital admissions also vary with the season. Also, seasonal fluctuations were noted in the distribution of serogroups among healthy children. PANDAS have seasonal occurrence (September through April) which is comparable to the seasonality of streptococcal tonsillopharyngitis.[84–87] There is an association between vitamin D binding protein polymorphism and rheumatic fever.[88]

6.10 Polymyalgia Rheumatica and Temporal Arteritis

Epidemiological studies suggested a regular cyclical pattern of incidence of polymyalgia rheumatica (PMR), whereas others do not confirm this finding. Some studies showed a higher incidence in winter, whereas others showed a higher incidence in summer. No seasonal rhythm was detected in patients with temporal arteritis (TA), although 58% of the biopsy-proven cases of TA, compared with 39.3% of the biopsy-negative cases, were diagnosed during the autumn or winter. Biopsy-proven cases seem to be more severe than biopsy-negative cases at the time of diagnosis. Seasonal difference at diagnosis may suggest a different etiological origin.[89]

A Danish study suggests that an infectious factor influences the incidence of TA and PMR. Close concurrence of epidemics of *M. pneumoniae*, parvovirus B19, and *Chlamydia pneumoniae* with peak incidences of TA and PMR suggest that they may be triggered by certain virus and/or bacterial agents.[12,90]

6.11 Myositis

Seasonal birth patterns were identified in subgroups of patients with myositis, suggesting an etiologic role of early environmental exposures. Some subgroups of patients with juvenile myositis had seasonal birth distributions. Patients with juvenile dermatomyositis with the p155 autoantibody had a birth distribution that differed significantly from that of patients with p155 antibody-negative juvenile dermatomyositis. Patients with juvenile myositis with the HLA risk factor allele DRB1*0301 and patients with myositis with the linked allele DQA1*0501 had a birth distribution significantly different from those without the alleles. Birth distributions seem to have greater seasonality in juvenile than in adult myositis subgroups, suggesting greater influence of perinatal exposures in childhood-onset illness.[91]

6.12 Cutaneous Diseases

In bullous pemphigoid, the onset of disease and the extension of skin involvement are associated with sunlight and air temperature. Autoantibody response also is correlated to both environmental factors.[92] Pityriasis rosea has long been suspected to be triggered by an infectious agent because of its seasonal variation and association with respiratory tract infections. Alternative etiological hypotheses are autoimmunity, atopy, and genetic predisposition.[93]

6.13 Allergy

Patients with respiratory allergy have a seasonal variation in immunoglobulin E responses to autoallergens, which may be boosted by seasonal exposure to pollen allergens.[94]

6.14 Others

Season of birth also is associated with increased risk for later celiac disease and ulcerative colitis, suggesting that environmental factors (e.g. gluten introduction, ultraviolet B exposure, vitamin D status) and perinatal infections can be plausible candidates for the primary trigger.[95] Frequent rotavirus infections may increase the risk of celiac disease autoimmunity during childhood in genetically predisposed individuals.[13]

7 CONCLUSION

The influences of seasonality on autoimmunity may reflect the effects of (protective or triggering) environmental factors, including infectious agents, on genetically predisposed subjects. In addition, vitamin D (the production of which is dependent on exposure to sunlight) and melatonin (the secretion of which varies by season) have been implicated in the risk of developing autoimmune diseases, because the both hormones have effects on immune system regulation. Seasonal characteristics may include worsening of symptoms and an increase in disease activity that should be considered in the management of patients with these autoimmune diseases.

REFERENCES

1. Shapira Y, Agmon-Levin N, Shoenfeld Y. Geoepidemiology of autoimmune rheumatic diseases. *Nat Rev Rheumatol* 2010;**6**:468–76.
2. Maes M, Stevens W, Scharpé S, Bosmans E, De Meyer F, D'Hondt P, et al. Seasonal variation in peripheral blood leukocyte subsets and in serum interleukin-6, and soluble interleukin-2 and -6 receptor concentrations in normal volunteers. *Experientia* 1994;**50**:821–9.
3. Katila H, Cantell K, Appelberg B, Rimón R. Is there a seasonal variation in the interferon-producing capacity of healthy subjects? *J Interferon Res* 1993;**13**:233–4.
4. Shearer WT, Lee BN, Cron SG, Rosenblatt HM, Smith EO, Lugg DJ, et al. Suppression of human anti-inflammatory plasma cytokines IL-10 and IL-1RA with elevation of proinflammatory cytokine IFN-gamma during the isolation of the Antarctic winter. *J Allergy Clin Immunol* 2002;**109**:854–7.
5. Sofronov BN, Nazarov PG, Purin VI. Some characteristics of human lymphocyte responsibility to stimulation in vitro. *Allerg Immunol (Leipz)* 1976;**22**:383–6.
6. Shadrin AS, Marinich IG, Taros LY. Experimental and epidemiological estimation of seasonal and climato-geographical features of non-specific resistance of the organism to influenza. *J Hyg Epidemiol Microbiol Immunol* 1977;**21**:155–61.
7. Thacker EL, Mirzaei F, Ascherio A. Infectious mononucleosis and risk for multiple sclerosis: a meta-analysis. *Ann Neurol* 2006;**59**:499–503.
8. Lucas RM, Hughes AM, Lay ML, Ponsonby AL, Dwyer DE, Taylor BV, et al. Epstein-Barr virus and multiple sclerosis. *J Neurol Neurosurg Psychiatry* 2011;**82**:1142–8.
9. Tauriainen S, Salminen K, Hyöty H. Can enteroviruses cause type 1 diabetes? *Ann N Y Acad Sci* 2003;**1005**:13–22.
10. Kornum BR, Faraco J, Mignot E. Narcolepsy with hypocretin/orexin deficiency, infections and autoimmunity of the brain. *Curr Opin Neurobiol* 2011;**21**:897–903.
11. Oen K, Fast M, Postl B. Epidemiology of juvenile rheumatoid arthritis in Manitoba, Canada, 1975-92: cycles in incidence. *J Rheumatol* 1995;**22**:745–50.
12. Elling H, Olsson AT, Elling P. Human Parvovirus and giant cell arteritis: a selective arteritic impact? *Clin Exp Rheumatol* 2000;**18**:S12–4.
13. Stene LC, Honeyman MC, Hoffenberg EJ, Haas JE, Sokol RJ, Emery L, et al. Rotavirus infection frequency and risk of celiac disease autoimmunity in early childhood: a longitudinal study. *Am J Gastroenterol* 2006;**101**:2333–40.
14. Antico A, Tampoia M, Tozzoli R, Bizzaro N. Can supplementation with vitamin D reduce the risk or modify the course of autoimmune diseases? A systematic review of the literature. *Autoimmun Rev* 2012;**12**:127–36.
15. Schwalfenberg GK. Solar radiation and vitamin D: mitigating environmental factors in autoimmune disease. *J Environ Public Health* 2012;**2012**:619381.
16. Holick MF. Vitamin D, deficiency. *N Engl J Med* 2007;**357**:266–81.
17. Khoo AL, Koenen HJ, Chai LY, Sweep FC, Netea MG, van der Ven AJ, et al. Seasonal variation in vitamin D levels is paralleled by changes in the peripheral blood human T cell compartment. *PLoS One* 2012;**7**:e29250.
18. Casella CB, Seguro LP, Takayama L, Medeiros D, Bonfa E, Pereira RM. Juvenile onset systemic lupus erythematosus: a possible role for vitamin D in disease status and bone health. *Lupus* 2012;**21**:1335–42.
19. Guillot X, Semerano L, Saidenberg-Kermanac'h N, Falgarone G, Boissier MC. Vitamin D and inflammation. *Joint Bone Spine* 2010;**77**:552–7.
20. Cutolo M, Pizzorni C, Sulli A. Vitamin D endocrine system involvement in autoimmune rheumatic diseases. *Autoimmun Rev* 2011;**11**:84–7.
21. Ginanjar E. Sumariyono, Setiati S, Setiyohadi B. Vitamin D and autoimmune disease. *Acta Med Indones* 2007;**39**:133–41.

22. Cutolo M, Otsa K, Uprus M, Paolino S, Seriolo B. Vitamin D in rheumatoid arthritis. *Autoimmun Rev* 2007;**7**:59–64.

23. Ponsonby AL, Lucas RM, van der Mei IA. UVR, vitamin D and three autoimmune diseases – multiple sclerosis, type 1 diabetes, rheumatoid arthritis. *Photochem Photobiol* 2005;**81**:1267–75.

24. Adorini L. Immunomodulatory effects of vitamin D receptor ligands in autoimmune diseases. *Int Immunopharmacol* 2002;**2**:1017–28.

25. Chen S, Sims GP, Chen XX, Gu YY, Chen S, Lipsky PE. Modulatory effects of 1,25-dihydroxyvitamin D3 on human B cell differentiation. *J Immunol* 2007;**179**:1634–47.

26. Pender MP. CD8+ T-cell deficiency, Epstein-Barr virus infection, vitamin D deficiency, and steps to autoimmunity: a unifying hypothesis. *Autoimmune Dis* 2012;**2012**:189096.

27. Handunnetthi L, Ramagopalan SV, Ebers GC. Multiple sclerosis, vitamin D, and HLA-DRB1*15. *Neurology* 2010;**74**:1905–10.

28. Frederiksen B, Liu E, Romanos J, Steck AK, Yin X, Kroehl M, et al. Investigation of the vitamin D receptor gene (VDR) and its interaction with protein tyrosine phosphatase, non-receptor type 2 gene (PTPN2) on risk of islet autoimmunity and type 1 diabetes: the Diabetes Autoimmunity Study in the Young (DAISY). *J Steroid Biochem Mol Biol* 2013;**133**:51–7.

29. Feng M, Li H, Chen SF, Li WF, Zhang FB. Polymorphisms in the vitamin D receptor gene and risk of autoimmune thyroid diseases: a meta-analysis. *Endocrine* 2013;**43**:318–26.

30. Monticielo OA, Teixeira Tde M, Chies JA, Brenol JC, Xavier RM. Vitamin D and polymorphisms of VDR gene in patients with systemic lupus erythematosus. *Clin Rheumatol* 2012;**31**:1411–21.

31. Karray EF, Ben Dhifallah I, Ben Abdelghani K, Ben Ghorbel I, Khanfir M, Houman H, et al. Associations of vitamin D receptor gene polymorphisms FokI and BsmI with susceptibility to rheumatoid arthritis and Behçet's disease in Tunisians. *Joint Bone Spine* 2012;**79**:144–8.

32. Nelson RJ, Drazen DL. Melatonin mediates seasonal changes in immune function. *Ann NY Acad Sci* 2000;**917**:404–15.

33. Srinivasan V, Spence DW, Trakht I, Pandi-Perumal SR, Cardinali DP, Maestroni GJ. Immunomodulation by melatonin: its significance for seasonally occurring diseases. *Neuroimmnunomodulation* 2008;**15**:93–101.

34. Honma K, Honma S, Kohsaka M, Fukuda N. Seasonal variation in the human circadian rhythm: dissociation between sleep and temperature rhythm. *Am J Physiol* 1992;**262**: R885–91.

35. Champney TH, Prado J, Youngblood T, Appel K, McMurray DN. Immune responsiveness of splenocytes after chronic daily melatonin administration in male Syrian hamsters. *Immunol Lett* 1997;**58**:95–100.

36. Akbulut KG, Gonul B, Akbulut H. The effects of melatonin on humoral immune responses of young and aged rats. *Immunol Invest* 2001;**30**:17–20.

37. Maestroni GJ, Conti A. Melatonin and the immune-hematopoietic system therapeutic and adverse pharmacological correlates. *Neuroimmunomodulation* 1996;**3**:325–32.

38. Willer CJ, Dyment DA, Sadovnick AD, Rothwell PM, Murray TJ, Ebers GC. Timing of birth and risk of multiple sclerosis: population based study. *Br Med J* 2005;**330**:120.

39. Saastamoinen KP, Auvinen MK, Tienari PJ. Month of birth is associated with multiple sclerosis but not with HLA-DR15 in Finland. *Mult Scler* 2012;**18**:563–8.

40. Nielsen TR, Rostgaard K, Nielsen NM, Koch-Henriksen N, Haahr S, Sørensen PS, et al. Multiple sclerosis after infectious mononucleosis. *Arch Neurol* 2007;**64**:72–5.

41. Ramagopalan SV, Valdar W, Dyment DA, DeLuca GC, Yee IM, G Giovannoni, et al. Association of infectious mononucleosis with multiple sclerosis. A population-based study. *Neuroepidemiology* 2009;**32**:257–62.
42. Tremlett H, van der Mei IA, Pittas F, Blizzard L, Paley G, Mesaros D, et al. Monthly ambient sunlight, infections and relapse rates in multiple sclerosis. *Neuroepidemiology* 2008;**31**:271–9.
43. Milo R, Kahana E. Multiple sclerosis: geoepidemiology, genetics and the environment. *Autoimmun Rev* 2010;**9**:A387–94.
44. Lewy H, Hampe CS, Kordonouri O, Haberland H, Landin-Olsson M, Torn C, et al. Seasonality of month of birth differs between type 1 diabetes patients with pronounced beta-cell autoimmunity and individuals with lesser or no beta-cell autoimmunity. *Pediatr Diabetes* 2008;**9**:46–52.
45. Svensson J, Eising S, Hougaard DM, Mortensen HB, Skogstrand K, Simonsen LB, et al. Danish Childhood Diabetes Registry. Few differences in cytokines between patients newly diagnosed with type 1 diabetes and their healthy siblings. *Hum Immunol* 2012;**73**:1116–26.
46. Singh DK, Winocour P, Summerhayes B, Viljoen A, Sivakumar G, Farrington K. Are low erythropoietin and 1,25-dihydroxyvitamin D levels indicative of tubulo-interstitial dysfunction in diabetes without persistent microalbuminuria? *Diabetes Res Clin Pract* 2009;**85**:258–64.
47. Verrotti A, Basciani F, Carle F, Morgese G, Chiarelli F. Calcium metabolism in adolescents and young adults with type 1 diabetes mellitus without and with persistent microalbuminuria. *J Endocrinol Invest* 1999;**22**:198–202.
48. Huynh T, Greer RM, Nyunt O, Bowling F, Cowley D, Leong GM, et al. The association between ketoacidosis and 25(OH)-vitamin D levels at presentation in children with type 1 diabetes mellitus. *Pediatr Diabetes* 2009;**10**:38–43.
49. Mahlios J, De la Herrán-Arita AK, Mignot E. The autoimmune basis of narcolepsy. *Curr Opin Neurobiol* 2013;**23**:767–73.
50. Carlander B, Puech-Cathala AM, Jaussent I, Scholz S, Bayard S, Cochen V, et al. Low vitamin D in narcolepsy with cataplexy. *PLoS One* 2011;**6**:e20433.
51. Kivity S, Agmon-Levin N, Zisappl M, Shapira Y, Nagy EV, Dankó K, et al. Vitamin D and autoimmune thyroid diseases. *Cell Mol Immunol* 2011;**8**:243–7.
52. Duarte-García A, Fang H, To CH, Magder LS, Petri M. Seasonal variation in the activity of systemic lupus erythematosus. *J Rheumatol* 2012;**39**:1392–8.
53. Chiche L, Jourde N, Ulmann C, Mancini J, Darque A, Bardin N, et al. Seasonal variations of systemic lupus erythematosus flares in southern France. *Eur J Intern Med* 2012;**23**:250–4.
54. Krause I, Shraga I, Molad Y, Guedj D, Weinberger A. Seasons of the year and activity of SLE and Behcet's disease. *Scand J Rheumatol* 1997;**26**:435–9.
55. Schlesinger N, Schlesinger M, Seshan SV. Seasonal variation of lupus nephritis: high prevalence of class V lupus nephritis during the winter and spring. *J Rheumatol* 2005;**32**:1053–7.
56. Disanto G, Chaplin G, Morahan JM, Giovannoni G, Hypponen E, Ebers GC, et al. Month of birth, vitamin D and risk of immune mediated disease: a case control study. *BMC Med* 2012;**10**:69.
57. Cutolo M, Otsa K, Paolino S, Yprus M, Veldi T, Seriolo B. Vitamin D involvement in rheumatoid arthritis and systemic lupus erythaematosus. *Ann Rheum Dis* 2009;**68**:446–7.
58. Huisman AM, White KP, Algra A, Harth M, Vieth R, Jacobs JW, et al. Vitamin D levels in women with systemic lupus erythematosus and fibromyalgia. *J Rheumatol* 2001;**28**:2535–9.

59. Cutillas-Marco E, Morales-Suárez-Varela M, Marquina-Vila A, Grant W. Serum 25-hydroxyvitamin D levels in patients with cutaneous lupus erythematosus in a Mediterranean region. *Lupus* 2010;**19**:810–4.

60. Kamen DL, Cooper GS, Bouali H, Shaftman SR, Hollis BW, Gilkeson GS. Vitamin D deficiency in systemic lupus erythematosus. *Autoimmun Rev* 2006;**5**:114–17.

61. Bonakdar ZS, Jahanshahifar L, Jahanshahifar F, Gholamrezaei A. Vitamin D deficiency and its association with disease activity in new cases of systemic lupus erythematosus. *Lupus* 2011;**20**:1155–60.

62. Ritterhouse LL, Crowe SR, Niewold TB, Kamen DL, Macwana SR, Roberts VC, et al. Vitamin D deficiency is associated with an increased autoimmune response in healthy individuals and in patients with systemic lupus erythematosus. *Ann Rheum Dis* 2011;**70**:1569–74.

63. Lemire JM, Ince A, Takashima M. 1,25-Dihydroxyvitamin D3 attenuates the expression of experimental murine lupus of MRL/l mice. *Autoimmunity* 1992;**12**:143–8.

64. Iikuni N, Nakajima A, Inoue E, et al. What's in season for rheumatoid arthritis patients? Seasonal fluctuations in disease activity. *Rheumatology (Oxford)* 2007;**46**:846–8.

65. Jacoby RK, Jayson MI, Cosh JA. Onset, early stages, and prognosis of rheumatoid arthritis: a clinical study of 100 patients with 11-year follow-up. *Br Med J* 1973;**2**:96–100.

66. Fleming A, Crown JM, Corbett M. Early rheumatoid disease. I Onset Ann Rheum Dis 1976;**35**:357–60.

67. Varenna M, Manara M, Cantatore FP, Del Puente A, Di Munno O, Malavolta N, et al. Determinants and effects of vitamin D supplementation on serum 25-hydroxy-vitamin D levels in patients with rheumatoid arthritis. *Clin Exp Rheumatol* 2012;**30**:714–19.

68. Cutolo M, Otsa K, Laas K, Yprus M, Lehtme R, Secchi ME, et al. Circannual vitamin d serum levels and disease activity in rheumatoid arthritis: Northern versus Southern Europe. *Clin Exp Rheumatol* 2006;**24**:702–4.

69. Song GG, Bae SC, Lee YH. Association between vitamin D intake and the risk of rheumatoid arthritis: a meta-analysis. *Clin Rheumatol* 2012;**31**:1733–9.

70. Mouterde G, Lukas C, Logeart I, Flipo RM, Rincheval N, Daurès JP, et al. Predictors of radiographic progression in the ESPOIR cohort: the season of first symptoms may influence the short-term outcome in early arthritis. *Ann Rheum Dis* 2011;**70**:1251–6.

71. de Rooy DP, Andersson ML, Knevel R, Huizinga TW, Svensson B, van der Helm-van Mil AH. Does the season at symptom onset influence the long-term severity of radiographic joint destruction in rheumatoid arthritis? *Ann Rheum Dis* 2012;**71**:2055–6.

72. Kim TH, Choi SJ, Lee YH, Song GG, Ji JD. Combined therapeutic application of mTOR inhibitor and vitamin D(3) for inflammatory bone destruction of rheumatoid arthritis. *Med Hypotheses* 2012;**79**:757–60.

73. Yan X, Zhao Y, Pan J, Fang K, Wang Y, Li Z, et al. Vitamin D-binding protein (group-specific component) has decreased expression in rheumatoid arthritis. *Clin Exp Rheumatol* 2012;**30**:525–33.

74. Hitchon CA, Sun Y, Robinson DB, Peschken CA, Bernstein CN, Siminovitch KA, et al. Vitamin D receptor polymorphism rs2228570 (Fok1) is associated with rheumatoid arthritis in North American natives. *J Rheumatol* 2012;**39**:1792–7.

75. Maestroni GJ, Sulli A, Pizzorni C, Villaggio B, Cutolo M. Melatonin in rheumatoid arthritis: a disease-promoting and modulating hormone? *Clin Exp Rheumatol* 2002;**20**:872–3.

76. Maestroni GJ, Cardinali DP, Esquifino AI, Pandi-Perumal SR. Does melatonin play a disease-promoting role in rheumatoid arthritis? *J Neuroimmunol* 2005;**158**:106–11.

77. Yazmalar L, Ediz L, Alpayci M, Hiz O, Toprak M, Tekeoglu I. Seasonal disease activity and serum vitamin D levels in rheumatoid arthritis, ankylosing spondylitis and osteoarthritis. *Afr Health Sci* 2013;**13**:47–55.

78. Challier B, Urlacher F, Vançon G, Lemelle I, Pourel J, Guillemin F. Is quality of life affected by season and weather conditions in ankylosing spondylitis? *Clin Exp Rheumatol* 2001;**19**:277–81.
79. Touma Z, Thavaneswaran A, Chandran V, Gladman DD. Does the change in season affect disease activity in patients with psoriatic arthritis? *Ann Rheum Dis* 2012;**71**:1370–3.
80. Päivönsalo-Hietanen T, Tuominen J, Saari KM. Seasonal variation of endogenous uveitis in south-western Finland. *Acta Ophthalmol Scand* 1998;**76**:599–602.
81. Andersson Gäre B. Juvenile arthritis – who gets it, where and when? A review of current data on incidence and prevalence. *Clin Exp Rheumatol* 1999;**17**:367–74.
82. Pelajo CF, Lopez-Benitez JM, Kent DM, Price LL, Miller LC, Dawson-Hughes B. 25-hydroxyvitamin D levels and juvenile idiopathic arthritis: is there an association with disease activity? *Rheumatol Int* 2012;**32**:3923–9.
83. Gibson DS, Newell K, Evans AN, Finnegan S, Manning G, Scaife C, et al. Vitamin D binding protein isoforms as candidate predictors of disease extension in childhood arthritis. *J Proteomics* 2012;**75**:5479–92.
84. Halfon ST. Epidemiologic aspects of rheumatic fever and rheumatic heart disease in Israel. *Isr J Med Sci* 1979;**15**:999–1002.
85. Miyake CY, Gauvreau K, Tani LY, Sundel RP, Newburger JW. Characteristics of children discharged from hospitals in the United States in 2000 with the diagnosis of acute rheumatic fever. *Pediatrics* 2007;**120**:503–8.
86. Tewodros W, Muhe L, Daniel E, Schalén C, Kronvall G. A one-year study of streptococcal infections and their complications among Ethiopian children. *Epidemiol Infect* 1992;**109**:211–25.
87. Murphy ML, Pichichero ME. Prospective identification and treatment of children with pediatric autoinmune neuropsychiatric disorder associated with group A streptococcal infection (PANDAS). *Arch Pediatr Adolesc Med* 2002;**156**:356–61.
88. Bahr GM, Eales LJ, Nye KE, Majeed HA, Yousof AM, Behbehani K, et al. An association between Gc (vitamin D-binding protein) alleles and susceptibility to rheumatic fever. *Immunology* 1989;**67**:126–8.
89. Petursdottir V, Johansson H, Nordborg E, Nordborg C. The epidemiology of biopsy-positive giant cell arteritis: special reference to cyclic fluctuations. *Rheumatology (Oxford)* 1999;**38**:1208–12.
90. Duhaut P, Bosshard S, Ducroix JP. Is giant cell arteritis an infectious disease? Biological and epidemiological evidence. *Presse Med* 2004;**33**:1403–8.
91. Vegosen LJ, Weinberg CR, O'Hanlon TP, Targoff IN, Miller FW, Rider LG. Seasonal birth patterns in myositis subgroups suggest an etiologic role of early environmental exposures. *Arthritis Rheum* 2007;**56**:2719–28.
92. Kyriakis KS, Panteleos DN, Tosca AD. Sunlight and air temperature affect autoantibody activity and skin involvement of bullous pemphigoid. *Int J Dermatol* 1996;**35**:498–501.
93. Chuh A, Chan H, Zawar V. Pityriasis rosea—evidence for and against an infectious aetiology. *Epidemiol Infect* 2004;**132**:381–90.
94. Seiberler S, Natter S, Hufnagl P, Binder BR, Valenta R. Characterization of IgE-reactive autoantigens in atopic dermatitis. 2. A pilot study on IgE versus IgG subclass response and seasonal variation of IgE autoreactivity. *Int Arch Allergy Immunol* 1999;**120**:117–25.
95. Tanpowpong P, Obuch JC, Jiang H, McCarty CE, Katz AJ, Leffler DA, et al. Multicenter study on season of birth and celiac disease: evidence for a new theoretical model of pathogenesis. *J Pediatr* 2013;**162**:501–4.

CHAPTER 12

The Protective Role of Helminths in Autoimmunity

Tomer Bashi[*], Tom Konikoff[*], Miri Blank[*], Yehuda Shoenfeld[*,1]
[*]Zabludowicz Center For Autoimmune Diseases; Sheba Medical Center; Tel-Aviv University; Ramat Gan, Israel
[1]Corresponding Author: Yehuda.shoenfeld@sheba.health.gov.il

1 INTRODUCTION

For the past several decades, Western industrialized countries are facing a high rate of autoinflammatory disorders, which are being expressed by higher prevalence of autoimmune diseases and allergies.[1,2] The lifestyle in industrialized countries had led to a decrease of infectious burden; however, a reverse correlation has been seen with the prevalence of autoimmune diseases.[3] Limited exposure to microorganisms such as helminths and microbes during childhood eventually leads to an off-balanced immune system. This theory, known as the Hygiene Theory or the Hygiene Hypothesis, was first proposed by Strachan, who observed an inverse correlation between hay fever and the number of older siblings while following more than 17,000 British children born in 1958.[4–6]

In addition to the eradication of worms in the Western world, eradication of helminths increased atopic skin sensitization in Venezuela,[7] in Gabon,[8] and in Vietnam.[9] For example, the prevalence of malaria is in reverse correlation to autoimmune diseases; several sources of epidemiological and immunogenetic evidence link the disappearance of malaria because of societies' eradication programs with the increase of multiple sclerosis (MS) in Sardinia, due to the high genetic susceptibility of human leukocyte antigen DR3 within the island.[10–13]

Moreover, the contribution of helminths to the development of autoimmune diseases also was demonstrated in the Karelian region. Finland's Karelian maintains have one of the highest prevalences of autoimmune and allergic diseases, whereas the prevalence in the Russian Karelian region is far lower. The fact that the Russian section is rife with infections and the Finnish part is dramatically cleaner has a large impact on the difference in prevalence.[14,15]

Infection and Autoimmunity
http://dx.doi.org/10.1016/B978-0-444-63269-2.00012-X

Helminths aim is to survive in the host; therefore they try to induce a tolerance scenario. Yet it is important to keep in mind that immunomodulation is affected by several key elements such as the burden of the infection and the host's immune system. In most cases helminths induce tolerance, but in some scenarios they may cause an inflammatory response. The spectrum of affliction in chronic helminthic tissue infection contains low pathology with high parasite burden and chronic disease with low parasite burden. For example, in areas where schistosomiasis and filarial diseases are endemic, some individuals develop chronic debilitating pathologies and others show a tolerant phenotype. The tolerant phenotype is characterized by the production of anti-inflammatory cytokines such as transforming growth factor (TGF)-β and interleukin (IL)-10 and increased number of FoxP3^{+} T regulatory cells (Tregs). These cytokines lead to suppressed parasite-specific T-cell proliferation in peripheral blood mononuclear cells, reduced levels of T helper (Th) 2 cytokines, and ablated Th1 cytokines. Thus, the parasite survives productively in the host with minimal collateral damage.[16,17]

2 THE PROTECTIVE ROLE OF HELMINTHS IN AUTOIMMUNE DISEASES

2.1 Helminths and Inflammatory Bowel Disease

Ulcerative colitis (UC) and Crohn's disease (CD) are two medical conditions collectively called inflammatory bowel disease (IBD). They involve an excess Th1 immune response towards the intestinal cells.[18,19] UC and CD are classified as separate diseases because each exhibits several distinguishing clinical and pathological features. UC has higher incidence of rectal involvement and the lesions are continuous, whereas CD contains skipped regions of lesions, terminal ileal ulceration, fistulization and/or anal fissuring and longitudinal ulcerations.

In the late 1990s, Elliott et al.[20] raised the IBD 'hygiene hypothesis' based on the increasing prevalence of IBDs in the United States and the fact it is in contrast to the prevalence of helminths in the USA. They proposed that exposure to helminths might protect against IBDs.

In sub-Saharan Africa, low incidence and prevalence of IBD was observed and cannot be explained by genetic factors because in black populations in the USA and the UK, the incidence of IBDs is approaching that of white populations.[21] Researchers attribute this fact to the ability of helminths to influence the composition of the microbiome, downmodulate the secretion of proinflammatory cytokines, upregulate Tregs and switch the immune response from Th1 to Th2, thus reducing inflammation in IBDs.[22–29]

Helminths, their ova and their antigens have been used in many studies that tried to treat IBDs in murine models and in human cases. Colonization of *Heligmosomoides polygyrus* in IL-10 knockout mice with piroxicam–induced colitis suppressed the production of IL-17 by lamina propria mononuclear cells and improved colitis.[30–32] Schistosome ova exposure attenuated 2,4,6-trinitrobenzene sulfonic acid colitis and protected mice from lethal inflammation. Interferon (IFN)-γ levels were reduced, whereas IL-4 and IL-10 messenger RNA levels were enhanced because of production by αCD3-stimulated spleen and mesenteric lymph node.[33–36]

Murine studies have led to human therapy trials with helminth ova:

(1) A study conducted in the early 2000s suggested that *Trichuris suis* (pig whipworm) seemed to be safe and possibly effective in the treatment of IBD. *T. suis* met safety requirements. The pig is a natural host for *T. suis;* it can colonize people but only for a short length of time.[37] A single dose of *T. suis* ova (TSO; up to 7500 ova) was well tolerated and did not result in short- or long-term treatment-related side effects.[38]

(2) Summers et al.[39] studied four patients with active CD and three with UC. In an initial treatment and observation period, a single dose of 2500 live TSO was given orally, and patients were followed every 2 weeks for 12 weeks. To assess safety and efficacy with subsequent doses, two patients with CD and two with UC were given 2500 ova at 3-week intervals as maintenance. Patients with UC experienced a reduction of the Clinical Colitis Activity Index to 57% of baseline. According to the IBD Quality of Life Index, 6 of 7 patients (86%) achieved remission. The benefit was temporary in some patients with a single dose, but it could be prolonged with maintenance therapy every 3 weeks.

(3) Another study using TSO also conducted by Summers et al.,[40] involved 29 patients with active CD. All patients ingested 2500 live TSO every 3 weeks for 24 weeks, and disease activity was monitored using the Crohn's Disease Activity Index (CDAI). The results were impressive: At week 24, 23 patients (79.3%) responded (decrease in CDAI by >100 points or a CDAI <150) and 21 of 29 patients (72.4%) remitted (CDAI <150).

(4) In a randomized, double blind, placebo-controlled trial including 54 patients with active colitis, defined by Disease Activity Index (DAI)

of ≥ 4, patients received 2500 TSO or placebo orally at 2-week intervals for 12 weeks. The primary efficacy variable was improvement of the DAI to ≥ 4. After 12 weeks of therapy, improvement according to the intent-to-treat principle occurred in 13 of 30 patients (43.3%) receiving ova treatment compared with 4 of 24 patients (16.7%) given placebo ($P = .04$). Improvement also occurred with the Simple Index, which was significant by week 6.[41,42]

It is important to mention one case report regarding iatrogenic infection by *T. suis* in a 16-year-old adolescent with CD who was treated with TSO. He received 5 oral doses of 2500 TSO off protocol. When admitted to the hospital, pathologic evaluation showed several round helminthic forms directly beneath attenuated ileocecal mucosal epithelium—the helminths from the TSO had evolved in his intestine.[43]

As for antigens, treatment with *Trichinella spiralis* frozen skeletal muscle larvae before inducing colitis with dinitrobenzene sulfonic acid significantly reduced the severity of colitis; downregulated myeloperoxidase activity, IL-1β production, and inducible nitric oxide synthase expression; and an upregulated IL-13 and TGF-β production in the colon in a mouse model.[44]

Furthermore, the use of antagonists of Toll-like receptor (TLR) signaling and agonists of their negative regulators from helminths or helminth products should be considered for the treatment of IBD because TLR signaling may contribute to destructive host responses and chronic inflammation, whereas helminths may play an important role in the downregulation of gene activation in controlling overwhelming inflammation and proinflammatory cytokine production.[45]

2.2 Helminths and Multiple Sclerosis

MS is an inflammatory, demyelinating, neurodegenerative disorder of the central nervous system (CNS) of unknown etiology. The most common clinical signs and symptoms, occurring in isolation or in combination, include sensory disturbance of the limbs ($\sim$30%), partial or complete visual loss ($\sim$15%), acute and subacute motor dysfunction of the limbs ($\sim$13%), diplopia (7%) and gait dysfunction (5%). The impact of MS on an individual is variable, but one constant feature is the uncertainty of this disease.[46,47]

The incidence of MS has significantly increased during the second half of the 20th century. Caucasian individuals from Northern Europe are more prone to have the disease, while it is rare among Asians and Africans, with a low prevalence in tropical regions, indicating the importance of environmental factors such as helminths. The incidence increases as distance north of the equator lengthens.[48,49] It was mentioned earlier that the eradication of malaria in Sardinia was preceded by the increase in the prevalence of MS on the island because of the high genetic susceptibility of human leukocyte antigen DR3 there.[10,11]

The most frequently studied animal model of MS is experimental autoimmune encephalitis (EAE), which mimics several of the key clinical and pathological features of the human disease, such as paralysis and demyelination.[50] Percutaneously infection of *Schistosoma mansoni* cercariae in mice significantly reduced the incidence and delayed the onset of EAE in a mouse model. Production of IFN-γ, nitric oxide, and tumor necrosis factor (TNF)-α by splenocytes was significantly reduced.[51]

Taenia crassiceps cysticerci (a 40 metacestodes infection load) also was able to reduce the severity of EAE. Only 50% of *T. crassiceps*-infected mice displayed EAE symptoms, which were significantly ($P < 0.05$) less severe than in uninfected mice. This effect was associated with both decreased myelin oligodendrocyte glycoprotein–specific splenocyte proliferation and IL-17 production and limited leukocyte infiltration into the spinal cord. Infection with *T. crassiceps* induced an anti-inflammatory cytokine microenvironment, including decreased TNF-α production and high myelin oligodendrocyte glycoprotein–specific production of IL-4 and IL-10.[52]

To prove the beneficial effect of helminths on patients with MS, Correale and Farez performed several studies. In a prospective double-cohort study, 12 patients (8 female and 4 male patients) with a clinical diagnosis of MS were assessed. The 12 patients with MS were infected with several helminth species (*Hymenolepis nanan*, *Trichiuris trichura*, *Ascaris lumbricoides*, *Strongyloides stercoralis* and *Enterobius vermicularis*); each patient was infected with one species. A control group containing healthy subjects was also infected with helminths, and another 12 uninfected patients with MS in remission matched for age, sex, and disease duration served as control subjects. It was shown that parasite-infected patients with MS had significantly fewer exacerbations, minimal variation in disability scores, as well as fewer magnetic resonance imaging (MRI) changes when compared with uninfected patients with MS.[53,54]

Moreover, responses to myelin basic protein peptide–specific T-cell clones were tested for cytokine secretion in peripheral blood and showed a significant increase ($P < 0.0001$) in the anti-inflammatory cytokines

IL-10 and TGF-β and a decrease in cells secreting proinflammatory cytokines IL-12 and IFN-γ in infected patients with MS compared with noninfected patients. Myelin basic protein–specific T-cells cloned from infected subjects were characterized by the absence of IL-2 and IL-4 production but high IL-10 and/or TGF-β secretion. In addition, the cloning frequency of CD4+ CD25+ FoxP3+ Tregs from those patients was increased ($P < 0.0001$) in infected patients compared with uninfected subjects with MS.[53,54]

Investigation of B-cell-mediated control mechanisms occurring during parasite infections in patients with MS demonstrated that helminthic infections (*H. nanan, T. trichura, A. lumbricoides, S. stercoralis* and *E. vermicularis*) cause a B-cell population producing high levels of IL-10, thus inhibiting harmful autoinflammatory immune responses. Moreover, B cells isolated from patients with MS infected with helminths also produced greater amounts of brain-derived neurotrophic factor and nerve growth factor, which is a type of protein that is important for the growth, maintenance, and survival of nerve cells, compared with healthy subjects and uninfected individuals with MS, raising the possibility that these cells may exert certain neuroprotective functions on the CNS. Hence, in addition to their immune-modulatory effect, helminths possess other beneficial aspects, such as promoting the growth of nerve cells.[55]

A latter study by this group using the same patients with MS with helminthic infection compared with noninfected patients showed that surface expression of TLR2 on both B cells and dendritic cells (DCs) was significantly higher in infected patients with MS. Stimulation of myelin-specific T-cell lines with a TLR2 agonist induced inhibition of T-cell proliferation; suppressed IFN-γ, IL-12, and IL-17 secretion; as well as increased IL-10 production, suggesting the functional responses observed correlate with TLR2 expression patterns.[56]

Helminths' ova were introduced to mice with EAE and were found to reduce disease severity. Mice treated with *S. mansoni* ova 2 weeks before EAE induction underwent disease assessment, and the severity of EAE was reduced when measured by decreased clinical scores and CNS cellular infiltrates.[57]

TSO is a preliminary therapy in MS (phase 1 helminth-induced immunomodulatory therapy), a Th1/Th17-associated autoimmune disease. Slight downregulation of the Th1-associated cytokine pattern occurred and was especially relevant in IL-2 ($P < 0.05$ after 2 months of therapy), with a temporary increase of Th2-associated cytokines such as IL-4.[58,59] In addition, the mean number of new gadolinium-enhanced MRI lesions decreased from 6.6 at baseline to 2.0 at the end of TSO administration, and 2 months after TSO was discontinued the mean number of new gadolinium-enhanced MRI lesions increased to 5.8, and no significant adverse effects were observed. Furthermore, mild eosinophilia and changes in the amounts of CD4+ and CD8+ T cells and natural killer CD56 bright cells were observed. The findings observed in this group of patients suggest that TSO therapy has a moderate immunomodulatory impact in MS.[58,59] Nevertheless, it is important to take into account the potential for unrelated gastrointestinal events.

Excretory-secretory muscle larvae (ES L1) products of the parasite *T. spiralis* successfully ameliorate EAE in Dark Agouti rats. Prophylactic application of ES L1 caused significant ($P < 0.05$) amelioration of EAE by a shift to the Th2-type response in the periphery and the CNS, as well as activation of regulatory mechanisms. Unconventional CD4+CD25-Foxp3 + regulatory cells were identified in increased proportion ($P < 0.001$) both in the periphery and the CNS of rats treated with ES L1 before the induction of EAE, and a possible role for these cells in amelioration of the disease was suggested.[60]

Treatment with soluble egg product homogenate from the nematodes *T. suis*, *S. mansoni* and *T. spiralis* was demonstrated to suppress TNF-α and IL-12 secretion by TLR-activated human DCs and induced significant suppression of symptoms in a murine EAE model.[61] Parasite antigens such as omega-1, a glycoprotein derived from *S. mansoni* eggs, helminth cystatins from *Acanthocheilonema viteae*, *Brugia malayi*, *Nippostrongylus braisliensis* and *Onchocerca volvulus* were able to induce TLR2 expression on both B cells and DCs.[56]

It is important to remember the requirement for early treatment to gain therapeutic effect. This is mostly because the symptomatic phase of EAE is characterized by extensive tissue damage, much of which may be irreversible. Also, the treatment must be continuous.[62]

2.3 Helminths and Lupus

Systemic lupus erythematosus (SLE) is a multiorgan chronic autoimmune disease. Most patients have skin lesions (the most common is a butterfly rash) and over 90 % of patients suffer from joint involvement such as inflammatory arthritis. SLE may, however, affect the kidneys, lungs, nervous system and other organs as well. It is a multifactorial disease that depends on genetic and environmental factors (including exposure to ultraviolet light and infections).[63,64]

Similarity between parasitic infections and autoimmune disorders was found.[65] Autoantibodies such as antinuclear antibodies, double-stranded DNA, and anti-Smith antibodies, which are present in SLE, have been identified in the serum of patients infected with *Schistosoma*.[66] Furthermore, anti-ribosomal P protein antibodies present in chronic Chagas heart disease, caused by *Trypanosoma cruzi*, were shown to cross-react with anti-Smith antibodies, which are present in early SLE.[67]

Genetic polymorphisms conferring susceptibility to SLE, more specifically the inhibitory receptor FcγRIIb, has been identified in African and Asian populations living in areas considered to be endemic to malaria (*Plasmodium falciparum*). This lupus-associated FcγRIIb polymorphism enhances phagocytosis of the parasite-infected erythrocytes. This suggests that a polymorphism predisposing to SLE may be gained through reduced susceptibility to malaria.[68] Moreover, one study using a experimental lupus model of NZB/NZWXF1 mice showed that female mice infected with *Toxoplasma gondii* developed milder renal involvement and had a longer life span than noninfected mice. Lower amounts of IL-10 and IFN-γ were found in spleen cells of the infected mice.[69]

2.4 Helminths and Type 1 Diabetes

Type 1 diabetes (T1D) is considered a Th1-mediated autoimmune disease and is influenced by both genetic and environmental factors. These factors lead to the development of autoantibodies directed at various islet cell components including glutamic acid decarboxylase antibodies (GAD65), islet cell antibodies (ICA512/IA-2) and insulin antibodies, which eventually leads to the destruction of pancreatic insulin-secreting β-cells. The subsequent lack of insulin leads to increased blood and urine glucose. Classical symptoms are polyuria, polydipsia, polyphagia and weight loss.[70]

The incidence of T1D has dramatically increased in the developed world over the past several decades. A linkage between the high prevalence of T1D and improved sanitation was proposed and was discussed previously in the hygiene theory.[1] During the past two decades the potential use of helminths and helminth-derived products in the prevention of T1D has gained attention.

Following the discovery of the role of Tregs in maintaining self-tolerance,[71,72] the correlation between Th1 cells (IL-2 and IFN-γ) and the pathogenesis of T1D was established. The role of Th2 cells (IL-4 and IL-10) and Tregs (IL-10 and TGF-β) in protection against T1D was demonstrated as well.[73]

The elevated number of Tregs in helminthic infection attenuates inflammatory response and subsequent tissue damage. Based on the hypothesis that the pathomechanism of T1D is related to the impaired immunoregulatory activity of diabetogenic T cells, leading to the development of autoimmunity, early work in the field showed helminthic infections can prevent T1D. This is based on the assumption that the Th2 immune bias would ultimately attenuate the Th1-mediated response that triggers diseases such as T1D.[74]

Infection by the gastrointestinal helminths *T. spiralis* and *Heligmosomoides polygyrus* among 4- to 6-week-old nonobese diabetic (NOD) mice, which is a model of T1D, elicited a Th2 response, demonstrated by increased IL-4 and immunoglobulin (Ig) E levels. This is in contrast to the Th1 response that accompanies the development of diabetes in NOD mice and suggests that the Th2 response induced by *T. spiralis* and *H. polygyrus* infection might protect the mice from the effects of Th1-mediated β-cell destruction. NOD mice infected with *H. polygyrus* remained free of diabetes over the entire experimental time course (36 to 37 weeks).[75]

Litomosoides sigmodontis filarial worms prevent the onset of diabetes in infected NOD mice. Six-week-old female NOD mice were infected with either 40 L3-stage larvae, adult female worms or adult male worms, and glucose concentrations were monitored over time. The onset of diabetes (glucose concentration >230 mg/dL) was prevented in all mice tested until the end of the experiment, when they were 25 weeks old. Protection against diabetes was associated with a Th2 shift, as IL-4 and IL-5 released from α-CD3/α-CD28-stimulated splenocytes was greater in mice infected with *L. sigmodontis* than in uninfected mice.[76] A subsequent study tested whether infection with *L. sigmodontis* prevents diabetes onset in IL-4-deficient NOD mice and whether depletion or absence of Tregs, IL-10, or TGF-β alters helminth-mediated protection.[77] The study demonstrated that *L. sigmodontis*–mediated protection against diabetes in NOD mice is not dependent on the induction of a type 2 immune shift but does require TGF-β. Helminthic infection prevented the development of diabetes in NOD mice, even in the absence of IL-4 ($P < 0.01$).

S. mansoni eggs have been shown to prevent T1D when administered to 4- to 6-week-old NOD mice. None of the injected mice developed diabetes, whereas the control mice developed diabetes with a 70% incidence by 27 weeks of age ($p < 0.005$).[78] Insulin autoantibodies spontaneously develop in NOD mice and prediabetic humans. Infected mice had insulin autoantibodies that were predominantly of the IgM isotype. Infection with *S. mansoni* prevented the class switch of anti-insulin antibody, which is normally seen in most NOD mice as they approach overt diabetes.[79] The live eggs of *S. mansoni* actively secrete the glycoprotein omega-1, which has been shown to be capable of conditioning human monocyte-derived DCs in vitro to induce a Th2 response,[80] thus regulating (shifting) the host immune response and aiding in the parasite's survival as well as migration.[79] The glycoprotein omega-1 alone has been shown to directly elicit human DCs to induce Th2 development from naïve CD4+ T cells and, furthermore, inhibit the release of IL-12, therefore reducing the differentiation of Th1 cells.[80] Omega-1 also has been shown to induce IL-4 production as well as to prime Foxp3+ Tregs in NOD mice CD4+ cells.[81]

Antigen-nonspecific IgE was purified from the roundworm *Dirofilaria immitis*, which induces IgE in mice and rats. Recombinant *D. immitis* antigen treatment of 6-week-old NOD female mice completely prevented insulitis and diabetes. It was also associated with a switching of the response from a Th1 to a Th2 profile,[82] as was shown in the previously presented studies.

2.5 Helminths and Rheumatoid Arthritis

Rheumatoid arthritis (RA) is a chronic inflammatory arthritis with an autoimmune mechanism. It is the most common inflammatory arthritis, affecting about 1 % of the population.[83] Like other autoimmune diseases, it comprises genetic as well as environmental factors, of which smoking is the most prominent.[84] The disease is typically polyarticular and manifests as stiffness, pain and swelling. Extra-articular involvement includes anemia, subcutaneous nodules (rheumatoid nodules), neuropathy, Sjögren's syndrome, vasculitis, renal disease and other extra-articular features. An immunological hallmark of the disease is the development of anticitrullinated protein antibodies.[85] Moreover, there is a predominance of Th1 cells, mostly CD4+, and a deficiency of Th2 and Tregs. The T cells, and consequently the anticitrullinated protein antibodies, target the deaminated areas within rheumatoid joints.[86,87]

The first study associating helminthic infection and joint disease, dating back to 1975, was a surprising observation that rats infected with the nematode *Syphacia obvelata* developed milder complete Freund's adjuvant–induced arthritis.[88] Since then, studies have used various helminth models for investigating joint inflammation.

The most commonly used model of arthritis is the type II collagen (Col II) model, which provokes multijoint inflammation. One such study demonstrated that infection with *S. mansoni* reduces the severity of Col

II–induced arthritis in male DBA/1 mice. *S. mansoni* infection suppresses systemic and local proinflammatory mediators, thus leading to significantly less synovial hyperplasia, inflammatory cell recruitment and bone/cartilage destruction. Levels of IgG2a, which is involved in the pathology of Col II–induced arthritis, were decreased and polyclonal-stimulated splenic T cells expressed lower amounts of IFN-γ, IL-17A and TNF-α. Higher amounts of IL-4 and IL-10 also were measured in comparison with naïve mice immunized with Col II.[89]

C57BL/6 mice prophylactically infected with the rat intestinal tapeworm *Hymenolepis diminuta* (10 cysticercoids in 100 μm of phosphate-buffered saline) showed significantly ($P < 0.05$) attenuated complete Freund's adjuvant–induced arthritis. Treatment with helminthic infection was as effective as treatment with dexamethasone or indomethacin ($P < 0.05$), the mainstay of treatment for arthritis. The infected mice showed reduced knee swelling, and, in addition, activated splenic T cells showed the expression of higher levels of IL-4 and IL-10.[90]

RA is associated with a Th1 response and a general increase in proinflammatory cytokines such as IL-6, IFN-γ and TNF-α. Moreover, *H. polygyrus* excretory-secretory antigen induces the de novo expression of Foxp3 Tregs[91,92] and induces the activity of alternatively activated macrophages.[93]

Early studies showed that the rodent filarial nematode *A. viteae* secretes ES-62, an immunomodulatory glycoprotein surrounded by a phosphorylcholine moiety attached to the protein by glycans.[94] ES-62 induced a shift from a Th1 to a Th2 response and attenuated an RA-like disease in collagen-induced arthritis (CIA). It elevated the production of the anti-inflammatory cytokine IL-10 and reduced levels of IFN-γ and IL-12, which are proinflammatory cytokines.[95–97] Cultures of human patients with RA synovial fluid showed reduced levels ($P < 0.05$) of TNF-α and IFN-γ secretion in the presence of ES-62, whereas peripheral blood smears from the patients exhibited mononuclear cells with low IFN-γ secretion after treatment with ES-62.[98,99] Use of recombinant ES-62, the whole ES-62 molecule and a synthetic phosphorylcholine–ovalbumin conjugate showed that the clinical score of CIA was affected only PC-OVA or ES-62 but not recombinant ES-62. This fact led to the idea that the common denominator inducing tolerance is phosphorylcholine.[100] Furthermore, Al-Riyami et al.[101] designed a small-molecule analogue—a sulfone-containing phosphorylcholine analogue (11a)—and provided proof of concept in a murine CIA model. 11a Was as effective as ES-62 in protecting DBA/1 mice from developing CIA and mirrored its mechanism of action as an anti-inflammatory antigen.

2.6 Helminths and Graves' Disease

Graves' disease is considered an autoimmune syndrome in which hyperthy-roidism is present in almost all patients. This thyroid disease is characterized by the presence of thyroid-stimulating hormone receptor (TSHR) anti-bodies,[102] leading to follicular dysplasia, lymphocytic infiltration and, in most cases, diffuse enlargement of the gland. TSHR antibodies are detect-able in almost all patients with Graves' disease.[103] A murine model of Graves' disease has been described by the immunization of mice with thyrotropin receptor complementary DNA.[104] From reviewing the literature, we found only one study that examined the association between helminthic infection and Graves' disease. Graves' disease was once thought to be a Th2-type immune response, but recent studies have described an Th1-type as well as a Th2-type response.[105,106]

Based on the ability of helminthic infection to polarize the immune response towards a Th2 type, a soluble homogenate of *S. mansoni* worm product and α-galactosylceramide (α-GalCer) has been used prophylacti-cally in a murine model. α-GalCer is one of many glycoconjugates expressed by *S. mansoni* worms and live eggs.[107] α-GalCer stimulates natural killer T cells to rapidly produce both Th1 and Th2 cytokines, but at a later time point and with repeated doses, α-GalCer promotes the development of a Th2 immune response, thus protecting against various autoimmune diseases. The results showed that both *S. mansoni* products and α-GalCer protected from Grave's disease, mainly by suppressing a Th1-type anti-TSHR immune response at the time of antigen priming. This occurred by increas-ing the levels of the anti-inflammatory cytokine IL-10.[108]

3 CONCLUSION

In Western countries a strong correlation exists between improved sanita-tion and hygiene and the significant increase in the prevalence of autoim-mune and autoinflammatory diseases. Moreover, a reverse correlation was reported between the high prevalence of helminths and autoimmune dis-eases in certain geographic areas. Different helminths were proven to secrete different molecules that enhance tolerance in the human immune system to survive. Therefore, many researchers harness helminth secretory mole-cules to develop novel therapeutic compounds to treat autoimmune diseases.

REFERENCES

1. Moroni L, Bianchi I, Lleo A. Geoepidemiology, gender and autoimmune disease. *Autoimmun Rev* 2012;**11**:A386–92.
2. Okada H, Kuhn C, Feillet H, Bach JF. The 'hygiene hypothesis' for autoimmune and allergic diseases: an update. *Clin Exp Immunol* 2010;**160**:1–9.
3. van Panhuis WG, Grefenstette J, Jung SY, Chok NS, Cross A, Eng H, et al. Contagious diseases in the united states from 1888 to the present. *N Engl J Med* 2013;**369**:2152–8.
4. von Mutius E. Allergies, infections and the hygiene hypothesis—the epidemiological evidence. *Immunobiology* 2007;**212**:433–9.
5. Strachan DP. Hay fever, hygiene, and household size. *BMJ* 1989;**299**:1259–60.
6. Carpenter L, Beral V, Strachan D, Ebi-Kryston KL, Inskip H. Respiratory symptoms as predictors of 27 year mortality in a representative sample of British adults. *BMJ* 1989;**299**:357–61.
7. Lynch NR, Hagel I, Perez M, Di Prisco MC, Lopez R, Alvarez N. Effect of anthelmintic treatment on the allergic reactivity of children in a tropical slum. *J Allergy Clin Immunol* 1993;**92**:404–11.
8. van den Biggelaar AH, Rodrigues LC, van Ree R, van der Zee JS, Hoeksma-Kruize YC, Souverijn JH, et al. Long-term treatment of intestinal helminths increases mite skin-test reactivity in Gabonese schoolchildren. *J Infect Dis* 2004;**189**:892–900.
9. Flohr C, Tuyen LN, Lewis S, Quinnell R, Minh TT, Liem HT, et al. Poor sanitation and helminth infection protect against skin sensitization in Vietnamese children: a cross-sectional study. *J Allergy Clin Immunol* 2006;**118**:1305–11.
10. Bitti PP, Murgia BS, Ticca A, Ferrai R, Musu L, Piras ML, et al. Association between the ancestral haplotype hla a30b18dr3 and multiple sclerosis in central Sardinia. *Genet Epidemiol* 2001;**20**:271–83.
11. Sotgiu S, Angius A, Embry A, Rosati G, Musumeci S. Hygiene hypothesis: innate immunity, malaria and multiple sclerosis. *Med Hypotheses* 2008;**70**:819–25.
12. Francis L, Perl A. Infection in systemic lupus erythematosus: friend or foe? *Int J Clin Rheumtol* 2010;**5**:59–74.
13. Butcher GA, Clark IA. Sle and malaria: another look at an old idea. *Parasitol Today* 1990;**6**:259–61.
14. Kondrashova A, Seiskari T, Ilonen J, Knip M, Hyoty H. The 'hygiene hypothesis' and the sharp gradient in the incidence of autoimmune and allergic diseases between Russian karelia and Finland. *APMIS* 2013;**121**:478–93.
15. Seiskari T, Kondrashova A, Viskari H, Kaila M, Haapala AM, Aittoniemi J, et al. Allergic sensitization and microbial load—a comparison between Finland and Russian karelia. *Clin Exp Immunol* 2007;**148**:47–52.
16. McSorley HJ, Maizels RM. Helminth infections and host immune regulation. *Clin Microbiol Rev* 2012;**25**:585–608.
17. Ben-Ami Shor D, Harel M, Eliakim R, Shoenfeld Y. The hygiene theory harnessing helminths and their ova to treat autoimmunity. *Clin Rev Allergy Immunol* 2013;**45**:211–16.
18. Assadsangabi A, Lobo AJ. Diagnosing and managing inflammatory bowel disease. *Practitioner* 2013;**257**:13–82.
19. Mayer L. Evolving paradigms in the pathogenesis of ibd. *J Gastroenterol* 2010;**45**:9–16.
20. Elliott DE, Urban JJ, Argo CK, Weinstock JV. Does the failure to acquire helminthic parasites predispose to Crohn's disease? *FASEB J* 2000;**14**:1848–55.
21. Fiasse R, Latinne D. Intestinal helminths: a clue explaining the low incidence of inflammatory bowel diseases in subsaharan Africa? Potential benefits and hazards of helminth therapy. *Acta Gastroenterol Belg* 2006;**69**:418–22.

22. Walk ST, Blum AM, Ewing SA, Weinstock JV, Young VB. Alteration of the murine gut microbiota during infection with the parasitic helminth heligmosomoides polygyrus. *Inflamm Bowel Dis* 2010;**16**:1841–9.
23. Weinstock JV. Autoimmunity: the worm returns. *Nature* 2012;**491**:183–5.
24. Hang L, Setiawan T, Blum AM, Urban J, Stoyanoff K, Arihiro S, et al. Heligmosomoides polygyrus infection can inhibit colitis through direct interaction with innate immunity. *J Immunol* 2010;**185**:3184–9.
25. Elliott DE, Setiawan T, Metwali A, Blum A, Urban Jr. JF, Weinstock JV. Heligmosomoides polygyrus inhibits established colitis in il-10-deficient mice. *Eur J Immunol* 2004;**34**:2690–8.
26. Wang LJ, Cao Y, Shi HN. Helminth infections and intestinal inflammation. *World J Gastroenterol* 2008;**14**:5125–32.
27. Cassinotti A, Sarzi-Puttini P, Fichera M, Shoenfeld Y, de Franchis R, Ardizzone S. Immunity, autoimmunity and inflammatory bowel disease. *Autoimmun Rev* 2014;**13**:1–2.
28. Weinstock JV, Summers RW, Elliott DE. Role of helminths in regulating mucosal inflammation. *Springer Semin Immunopathol* 2005;**27**:249–71.
29. Scholmerich J. Trichuris suis ova in inflammatory bowel disease. *Dig Dis* 2013;**31**:391–5.
30. Elliott DE, Metwali A, Leung J, Setiawan T, Blum AM, Ince MN, et al. Colonization with heligmosomoides polygyrus suppresses mucosal il-17 production. *J Immunol* 2008;**181**:2414–9.
31. Fitzpatrick LR. Inhibition of il-17 as a pharmacological approach for ibd. *Int Rev Immunol* 2013;**32**:544–55.
32. Mohammadi M, Zahedi MJ, Nikpoor AR, Baneshi MR, Hayatbakhsh MM. Interleukin-17 serum levels and tlr4 polymorphisms in ulcerative colitis. *Iran J Immunol* 2013;**10**:83–92.
33. Elliott DE, Li J, Blum A, Metwali A, Qadir K, Urban Jr. JF, et al. Exposure to schistosome eggs protects mice from TNBS-induced colitis. *Am J Physiol Gastrointest Liver Physiol* 2003;**284**:G385–91.
34. Moreels TG, Nieuwendijk RJ, De Man JG, De Winter BY, Herman AG, Van Marck EA, et al. Concurrent infection with schistosoma mansoni attenuates inflammation induced changes in colonic morphology, cytokine levels, and smooth muscle contractility of trinitrobenzene sulphonic acid induced colitis in rats. *Gut* 2004;**53**:99–107.
35. Ruyssers NE, De Winter BY, De Man JG, Loukas A, Pearson MS, Weinstock JV, et al. Therapeutic potential of helminth soluble proteins in TNBS-induced colitis in mice. *Inflamm Bowel Dis* 2009;**15**:491–500.
36. Ruyssers NE, De Winter BY, De Man JG, Ruyssers ND, Van Gils AJ, Loukas A, et al. Schistosoma mansoni proteins attenuate gastrointestinal motility disturbances during experimental colitis in mice. *World J Gastroenterol* 2010;**16**:703–12.
37. Beer RJ. The relationship between trichuris trichiura (linnaeus 1758) of man and trichuris suis (schrank 1788) of the pig. *Res Vet Sci* 1976;**20**:47–54.
38. Sandborn WJ, Elliott DE, Weinstock J, Summers RW, Landry-Wheeler A, Silver N, et al. Randomised clinical trial: the safety and tolerability of trichuris suis ova in patients with Crohn's disease. *Aliment Pharmacol Ther* 2013;**38**:255–63.
39. Summers RW, Elliott DE, Qadir K, Urban Jr. JF, Thompson R, Weinstock JV. Trichuris suis seems to be safe and possibly effective in the treatment of inflammatory bowel disease. *Am J Gastroenterol* 2003;**98**:2034–41.
40. Summers RW, Elliott DE, Urban Jr. JF, Thompson R, Weinstock JV. Trichuris suis therapy in Crohn's disease. *Gut* 2005;**54**:87–90.
41. Summers RW, Elliott DE, Urban Jr. JF, Thompson RA, Weinstock JV. Trichuris suis therapy for active ulcerative colitis: a randomized controlled trial. *Gastroenterology* 2005;**128**:825–32.

42. Summers RW, Elliott DE, Weinstock JV. Is there a role for helminths in the therapy of inflammatory bowel disease? *Nat Clin Pract Gastroenterol Hepatol* 2005;**2**:62–3.

43. Kradin RL, Badizadegan K, Auluck P, Korzenik J, Lauwers GY. Iatrogenic trichuris suis infection in a patient with Crohn disease. *Arch Pathol Lab Med* 2006;**130**:718–20.

44. Motomura Y, Wang H, Deng Y, El-Sharkawy RT, Verdu EF, Khan WI. Helminth antigen-based strategy to ameliorate inflammation in an experimental model of colitis. *Clin Exp Immunol* 2009;**155**:88–95.

45. Sun S, Wang X, Wu X, Zhao Y, Wang F, Liu X, et al. Toll-like receptor activation by helminths or helminth products to alleviate inflammatory bowel disease. *Parasit Vectors* 2011;**4**:186.

46. *Multiple sclerosis: national clinical guideline for diagnosis and management in primary and secondary care.* NICE Clinical Guidelines, No. 8. London: National Collaborating Centre for Chronic Conditions (UK); 2004.

47. Stuve O, Oksenberg J. Multiple sclerosis overview. In: Pagon RA, Adam MP, Bird TD, Dolan CR, Fong CT, Stephens K, editors. *Genereviews;* 1993, *GeneReviews®* [Internet]. Seattle (WA): University of Washington, Seattle; 1993–2014. Available from: http://www.ncbi.nlm.nih.gov/books/NBK1316/.

48. Correale J, Farez MF. The impact of environmental infections (parasites) on ms activity. *Mult Scler* 2011;**17**:1162–9.

49. Rosati G. The prevalence of multiple sclerosis in the world: an update. *Neurol Sci* 2001;**22**:117–39.

50. Rangachari M, Kuchroo VK. Using eae to better understand principles of immune function and autoimmune pathology. *J Autoimmun* 2013;**45**:31–9.

51. La Flamme AC, Ruddenklau K, Backstrom BT. Schistosomiasis decreases central nervous system inflammation and alters the progression of experimental autoimmune encephalomyelitis. *Infect Immun* 2003;**71**:4996–5004.

52. Reyes JL, Espinoza-Jimenez AF, Gonzalez MI, Verdin L, Terrazas LI. Taenia crassiceps infection abrogates experimental autoimmune encephalomyelitis. *Cell Immunol* 2011;**267**:77–87.

53. Correale J, Farez M. Association between parasite infection and immune responses in multiple sclerosis. *Ann Neurol* 2007;**61**:97–108.

54. Correale J, Farez MF. The impact of parasite infections on the course of multiple sclerosis. *J Neuroimmunol* 2011;**233**:6–11.

55. Correale J, Farez M, Razzitte G. Helminth infections associated with multiple sclerosis induce regulatory b cells. *Ann Neurol* 2008;**64**:187–99.

56. Correale J, Farez MF. Does helminth activation of toll-like receptors modulate immune response in multiple sclerosis patients? *Front Cell Infect Microbiol* 2012;**2**:112.

57. Sewell D, Qing Z, Reinke E, Elliot D, Weinstock J, Sandor M, et al. Immunomodulation of experimental autoimmune encephalomyelitis by helminth ova immunization. *Int Immunol* 2003;**15**:59–69.

58. Benzel F, Erdur H, Kohler S, Frentsch M, Thiel A, Harms L, et al. Immune monitoring of trichuris suis egg therapy in multiple sclerosis patients. *J Helminthol* 2012;**86**:339–47.

59. Fleming JO, Isaak A, Lee JE, Luzzio CC, Carrithers MD, Cook TD, et al. Probiotic helminth administration in relapsing-remitting multiple sclerosis: a phase 1 study. *Mult Scler* 2011;**17**:743–54.

60. Sofronic-Milosavljevic LJ, Radovic I, Ilic N, Majstorovic I, Cvetkovic J, Gruden-Movsesijan A. Application of dendritic cells stimulated with trichinella spiralis excretory-secretory antigens alleviates experimental autoimmune encephalomyelitis. *Med Microbiol Immunol* 2013;**202**:239–49.

61. Kuijk LM, Klaver EJ, Kooij G, van der Pol SM, Heijnen P, Bruijns SC, et al. Soluble helminth products suppress clinical signs in murine experimental autoimmune

encephalomyelitis and differentially modulate human dendritic cell activation. *Mol Immunol* 2012;**51**:210–18.
62. Fleming JO. Helminth therapy and multiple sclerosis. *Int J Parasitol* 2013;**43**:259–74.
63. Shoenfeld Y, Zandman-Goddard G, Stojanovich L, Cutolo M, Amital H, Levy Y, et al. The mosaic of autoimmunity: hormonal and environmental factors involved in autoimmune diseases—2008. *Isr Med Assoc J* 2008;**10**:8–12.
64. Sherer Y, Gorstein A, Fritzler MJ, Shoenfeld Y. Autoantibody explosion in systemic lupus erythematosus: more than 100 different antibodies found in sle patients. *Semin Arthritis Rheum* 2004;**34**:501–37.
65. Zandman-Goddard G, Shoenfeld Y. Parasitic infection and autoimmunity. *Lupus* 2009;**18**:1144–8.
66. Rahima D, Tarrab-Hazdai R, Blank M, Arnon R, Shoenfeld Y. Anti-nuclear antibodies associated with schistosomiasis and anti-schistosomal antibodies associated with sle. *Autoimmunity* 1994;**17**:127–41.
67. Levitus G, Hontebeyrie-Joskowicz M, Van Regenmortel MH, Levin MJ. Humoral autoimmune response to ribosomal p proteins in chronic chagas heart disease. *Clin Exp Immunol* 1991;**85**:413–7.
68. Clatworthy MR, Willcocks L, Urban B, Langhorne J, Williams TN, Peshu N, et al. Systemic lupus erythematosus-associated defects in the inhibitory receptor fcγriib reduce susceptibility to malaria. *Proc Natl Acad Sci USA* 2007;**104**:7169–74.
69. Chen M, Aosai F, Norose K, Mun HS, Ishikura H, Hirose S, et al. Toxoplasma gondii infection inhibits the development of lupus-like syndrome in autoimmune (New Zealand black x New Zealand white) f1 mice. *Int Immunol* 2004;**16**:937–46.
70. Donath MY, Hess C, Palmer E. What is the role of autoimmunity in type 1 diabetes? A clinical perspective. *Diabetologia* 2014;**57**:653–5.
71. Hori I, Kishida Y. Quantitative changes in nuclear pores and chromatoid bodies induced by neuropeptides during cell differentiation in the planarian dugesia japonica. *J Submicrosc Cytol Pathol* 2003;**35**:439–44.
72. Wing K, Sakaguchi S. Regulatory t cells exert checks and balances on self tolerance and autoimmunity. *Nat Immunol* 2010;**11**:7–13.
73. Kikodze N, Pantsulaia I, Rekhviashvili K, Iobadze M, Jakhutashvili N, Pantsulaia N, et al. Cytokines and t regulatory cells in the pathogenesis of type 1 diabetes. *Georgian Med News* 2013;**222**:29–35.
74. Taylor MD, van der Werf N, Maizels RM. T cells in helminth infection: the regulators and the regulated. *Trends Immunol* 2012;**33**:181–9.
75. Saunders KA, Raine T, Cooke A, Lawrence CE. Inhibition of autoimmune type 1 diabetes by gastrointestinal helminth infection. *Infect Immun* 2007;**75**:397–407.
76. Hubner MP, Stocker JT, Mitre E. Inhibition of type 1 diabetes in filaria-infected non-obese diabetic mice is associated with a t helper type 2 shift and induction of foxp3+ regulatory t cells. *Immunology* 2009;**127**:512–22.
77. Hubner MP, Shi Y, Torrero MN, Mueller E, Larson D, Soloviova K, et al. Helminth protection against autoimmune diabetes in nonobese diabetic mice is independent of a type 2 immune shift and requires tgf-beta. *J Immunol* 2012;**188**:559–68.
78. Zaccone P, Fehervari Z, Jones FM, Sidobre S, Kronenberg M, Dunne DW, et al. Schistosoma mansoni antigens modulate the activity of the innate immune response and prevent onset of type 1 diabetes. *Eur J Immunol* 2003;**33**:1439–49.
79. Cooke A, Tonks P, Jones FM, O'Shea H, Hutchings P, Fulford AJ, et al. Infection with schistosoma mansoni prevents insulin dependent diabetes mellitus in non-obese diabetic mice. *Parasite Immunol* 1999;**21**:169–76.
80. Everts B, Perona-Wright G, Smits HH, Hokke CH, van der Ham AJ, Fitzsimmons CM, et al. Omega-1, a glycoprotein secreted by schistosoma mansoni eggs, drives th2 responses. *J Exp Med* 2009;**206**:1673–80.

81. Zaccone P, Burton OT, Gibbs SE, Miller N, Jones FM, Schramm G, et al. The s. Mansoni glycoprotein omega-1 induces foxp3 expression in nod mouse cd4(+) t cells. *Eur J Immunol* 2011;**41**:2709–18.
82. Imai S, Tezuka H, Fujita K. A factor of inducing ige from a filarial parasite prevents insulin-dependent diabetes mellitus in nonobese diabetic mice. *Biochem Biophys Res Commun* 2001;**286**:1051–8.
83. Rothschild BM, Turner KR, DeLuca MA. Symmetrical erosive peripheral polyarthritis in the late archaic period of Alabama. *Science* 1988;**241**:1498–501.
84. Lundstrom E, Kallberg H, Alfredsson L, Klareskog L, Padyukov L. Gene-environment interaction between the drb1 shared epitope and smoking in the risk of anti-citrullinated protein antibody-positive rheumatoid arthritis: all alleles are important. *Arthritis Rheum* 2009;**60**:1597–603.
85. Wegner N, Lundberg K, Kinloch A, Fisher B, Malmstrom V, Feldmann M, et al. Autoimmunity to specific citrullinated proteins gives the first clues to the etiology of rheumatoid arthritis. *Immunol Rev* 2010;**233**:34–54.
86. De Rycke L, Nicholas AP, Cantaert T, Kruithof E, Echols JD, Vandekerckhove B, et al. Synovial intracellular citrullinated proteins colocalizing with peptidyl arginine deiminase as pathophysiologically relevant antigenic determinants of rheumatoid arthritis-specific humoral autoimmunity. *Arthritis Rheum* 2005;**52**:2323–30.
87. Takizawa Y, Suzuki A, Sawada T, Ohsaka M, Inoue T, Yamada R, et al. Citrullinated fibrinogen detected as a soluble citrullinated autoantigen in rheumatoid arthritis synovial fluids. *Ann Rheum Dis* 2006;**65**:1013–20.
88. Pearson DJ, Taylor G. The influence of the nematode syphacia oblevata on adjuvant arthritis in the rat. *Immunology* 1975;**29**:391–6.
89. Osada Y, Shimizu S, Kumagai T, Yamada S, Kanazawa T. Schistosoma mansoni infection reduces severity of collagen-induced arthritis via down-regulation of proinflammatory mediators. *Int J Parasitol* 2009;**39**:457–64.
90. Shi M, Wang A, Prescott D, Waterhouse CC, Zhang S, McDougall JJ, et al. Infection with an intestinal helminth parasite reduces Freund's complete adjuvant-induced monoarthritis in mice. *Arthritis Rheum* 2011;**63**:434–44.
91. Grainger JR, Smith KA, Hewitson JP, McSorley HJ, Harcus Y, Filbey KJ, et al. Helminth secretions induce de novo t cell foxp3 expression and regulatory function through the tgf-beta pathway. *J Exp Med* 2010;**207**:2331–41.
92. Carranza F, Falcon CR, Nunez N, Knubel C, Correa SG, Bianco I, et al. Helminth antigens enable cpg-activated dendritic cells to inhibit the symptoms of collagen-induced arthritis through foxp3+ regulatory t cells. *PLoS One* 2012;**7**:e40356.
93. Espinoza-Jimenez A, Rivera-Montoya I, Cardenas-Arreola R, Moran L, Terrazas LI. Taenia crassiceps infection attenuates multiple low-dose streptozotocin-induced diabetes. *J Biomed Biotechnol* 2010;**2010**:850541.
94. Harnett W, Harnett MM, Leung BP, Gracie JA, McInnes IB. The anti-inflammatory potential of the filarial nematode secreted product, es-62. *Curr Top Med Chem* 2004;**4**:553–9.
95. Marshall FA, Grierson AM, Garside P, Harnett W, Harnett MM. Es-62, an immunomodulator secreted by filarial nematodes, suppresses clonal expansion and modifies effector function of heterologous antigen-specific t cells in vivo. *J Immunol* 2005;**175**:5817–26.
96. Stepek G, Auchie M, Tate R, Watson K, Russell DG, Devaney E, et al. Expression of the filarial nematode phosphorylcholine-containing glycoprotein, es62, is stage specific. *Parasitology* 2002;**125**:155–64.
97. Harnett W, Harnett MM. Filarial nematode secreted product es-62 is an anti-inflammatory agent: therapeutic potential of small molecule derivatives and es-62 peptide mimetics. *Clin Exp Pharmacol Physiol* 2006;**33**:511–18.

98. McInnes IB, Leung BP, Harnett M, Gracie JA, Liew FY, Harnett W. A novel therapeutic approach targeting articular inflammation using the filarial nematode-derived phosphorylcholine-containing glycoprotein es-62. *J Immunol* 2003;**171**:2127–33.

99. McInnes IB, Schett G. Cytokines in the pathogenesis of rheumatoid arthritis. *Nat Rev Immunol* 2007;**7**:429–42.

100. Harnett MM, Kean DE, Boitelle A, McGuiness S, Thalhamer T, Steiger CN, et al. The phosphorycholine moiety of the filarial nematode immunomodulator es-62 is responsible for its anti-inflammatory action in arthritis. *Ann Rheum Dis* 2008;**67**:518–23.

101. Al-Riyami L, Pineda MA, Rzepecka J, Huggan JK, Khalaf AI, Suckling CJ, et al. Designing anti-inflammatory drugs from parasitic worms: a synthetic small molecule analogue of the acanthocheilonema viteae product es-62 prevents development of collagen-induced arthritis. *J Med Chem* 2013;**56**:9982–10002.

102. Latif R, Morshed SA, Zaidi M, Davies TF. The thyroid-stimulating hormone receptor: impact of thyroid-stimulating hormone and thyroid-stimulating hormone receptor antibodies on multimerization, cleavage, and signaling. *Endocrinol Metab Clin North Am* 2009;**38**:319–41, viii.

103. Lytton SD, Kahaly GJ. Bioassays for tsh-receptor autoantibodies: an update. *Autoimmun Rev* 2010;**10**:116–22.

104. Costagliola S, Many MC, Denef JF, Pohlenz J, Refetoff S, Vassart G. Genetic immunization of outbred mice with thyrotropin receptor cdna provides a model of Graves' disease. *J Clin Invest* 2000;**105**:803–11.

105. Dogan RN, Vasu C, Holterman MJ, Prabhakar BS. Absence of il-4, and not suppression of the th2 response, prevents development of experimental autoimmune Graves' disease. *J Immunol* 2003;**170**:2195–204.

106. Nagayama Y, Mizuguchi H, Hayakawa T, Niwa M, McLachlan SM, Rapoport B. Prevention of autoantibody-mediated graves'-like hyperthyroidism in mice with il-4, a th2 cytokine. *J Immunol* 2003;**170**:3522–7.

107. Makaaru CK, Damian RT, Smith DF, Cummings RD. The human blood fluke schistosoma mansoni synthesizes a novel type of glycosphingolipid. *J Biol Chem* 1992;**267**:2251–7.

108. Nagayama Y, Watanabe K, Niwa M, McLachlan SM, Rapoport B. Schistosoma mansoni and alpha-galactosylceramide: prophylactic effect of th1 immune suppression in a mouse model of Graves' hyperthyroidism. *J Immunol* 2004;**173**:2167–73.

CHAPTER 13

Vaccination and Autoimmunity

Carlo Perricone[*,1], Fabrizio Conti[*], Nancy Agmon-Levin[†,‡],
Guido Valesini[*], Yehuda Shoenfeld[†,‡,§]

[*]Reumatologia, Dipartimento di Medicina Interna e Specialità Mediche, Sapienza Università di Roma,
Roma, Italy
[†]The Zabludowicz Center for Autoimmune Diseases, Sheba Medical Center, Tel-Hashomer, Israel
[‡]Sackler Faculty of Medicine, Tel-Aviv University, Tel-Aviv, Israel
[§]Incumbent of the Laura Schwarz-Kipp Chair for Research of Autoimmune Diseases, Tel-Aviv University,
Tel-Aviv, Israel
[1]Corresponding Author: carlo.perricone@gmail.com

1 INTRODUCTION

Vaccines have significantly improved the prevention of infectious diseases, especially in specific groups of patients such as the elderly and immunocompromised patients. Currently, millions of children and adults are immunized regularly, and it is evident that the benefits of preventing suffering and death from infectious diseases outweigh the adverse effects of immunization. Vaccines have changed the occurrence of concurrent infectious diseases in patients with autoimmune diseases (AIDs).[1] The history of vaccines goes back to 1798, when Edwards Jenner inoculated 12 people with cowpox material and prevented the deadly disease smallpox. During the third decade of the twentieth century, vaccination against measles, mumps, diphtheria, rubella, polio, and others was introduced, reducing the morbidity from these diseases by close to 100% by the end of the century.[2] Thus, the benefits of immunization are irrefutable; however, during the past 15 years or so, several reports of adverse autoimmune reactions to various vaccines have raised concerns. The connection between vaccination and autoimmune reaction was mostly temporal and causality could not be confirmed. Indeed, it is imperative to emphasize that so far no causal connection has been demonstrated between any one vaccine and an autoimmune syndrome, even though strong evidence exists to suggest such a connection in regard to reactive arthritis following rubella vaccine[3,4] and Guillain-Barré syndrome (GBS) following swine flu vaccine.[5]

Furthermore, it has been suggested that some vaccines might trigger autoimmune diseases, and thus the safety as well as the efficacy of vaccines in rheumatic patients is still a matter of concern. A potential new syndrome, namely, autoimmune/inflammatory syndrome induced by adjuvants (ASIA syndrome),

Infection and Autoimmunity
http://dx.doi.org/10.1016/B978-0-444-63269-2.00014-3

217

has been recently described comprising four medical conditions: siliconosis, the Gulf War syndrome, the macrophagic myofasciitis syndrome and the post-vaccination phenomena, and is characterized by hyperactive immune responses accompanied by a similar complex of signs and symptoms. Most relevant is that these conditions share a linkage: adjuvants, such those contained in some vaccines.[6] This commonality may induce autoimmune or inflammatory diseases in humans, as was demonstrated in different animal models. The evidence that those vaccines containing adjuvants are only associated with occurrence of autoimmune response is not only intriguing but also provocative and may help unravel novel pathogenic mechanisms, preventive measures and therapeutic targets.

To clarify the issue of safety and immunogenicity of vaccines in patients with rheumatic diseases, the European League Against Rheumatism (EULAR) recently published recommendations supporting the use of inactivated vaccines in most patients while their disease is stable.[7] Notably, in rare cases, especially in untreated or unstable disease, flare-ups can occur after immunization.[8]

All together it seems that individualized considerations have to be made before administrating a vaccine, including the risk of infection, infection morbidity and mortality, the immunogenicity of the vaccine (induction of a protective antibody level) and its plausible toxicity. In the case of patients with autoimmune-rheumatic diseases, the EULAR committee issued further recommendations, namely[7]:

1. vaccination status should be assessed during the initial investigation of patients with AD;
2. vaccination in patients with AD should ideally be administered during stable disease;
3. live attenuated vaccines should be avoided whenever possible in immunosuppressed patients with AD;
4. in patients with AD, vaccines can be administered during the use of disease modifying anti-rheumatic drugs and TNF-α blocking agents but should ideally be administered before starting B-cell-depleting biological therapy;
5. influenza vaccination should be strongly considered for patients with AD;
6. 23-valent polysaccharide pneumococcal vaccination should be strongly considered for patients with AD;
7. patients with AD should receive tetanus toxoid vaccination in accordance with recommendations for the general population;

8. in the case of major and/or contaminated wounds in patients who received rituximab within the past 24 weeks, passive immunization with tetanus immunoglobulin should be administered;

9. Herpes zoster vaccination may be considered in patients with AD;

10. Human papillomavirus (HPV) vaccination should be considered in selected patients with AD;

11. in hyposplenic/asplenic patients with AD, influenza, pneumococcal, Hemophilus influenzae B and meningococcal C vaccinations are recommended;

12. Hepatitis A and/or B vaccination is only recommended in patients with AD who are at risk for hepatitis;

13. patients with AD who plan to travel are recommended to receive their vaccinations according to general rules, except for live attenuated vaccines, which should be avoided whenever possible in immunosuppressed patients with AD; and

14. BCG vaccination is not recommended in patients with AD.

Thus, it has been suggested that upon the initial evaluation of a patient with an autoimmune disease, vaccination status should be assessed. This should consider missed vaccinations that are recommended for the general population as well as enquire about adverse events and flares following previous immunizations. However, in this group of patients the role of each vaccine should be addressed individually. For instance, the inactivated influenza vaccination should be strongly considered for patients with AD because it reduces morbidity and mortality from influenza-associated diseases and was found to be efficacious in patients with rheumatoid arthritis (RA), systemic lupus erythematosus (SLE), ANCA-associated vasculitis and systemic sclerosis, even while they are being treated with disease-modifying anti-rheumatic drugs and biological therapies. The 23-valent polysaccharide pneumococcal vaccination should also be strongly considered for rheumatic patients because pulmonary infections represent a significant source of morbidity and mortality among this group. Similar considerations are accepted regarding tetanus toxoid. On the other hand, vaccination against herpes zoster virus, although highly recommended for patients with autoimmune diseases, is considered only for patients with very mild or no immune suppression because it is a live vaccine. Another controversial vaccine is the new one against HPV. This is an efficacious vaccine that is recommended for young patients. However, several concerns were raised regarding the risk of autoimmune phenomena and thromboembolic events following HPV immunization. Another issue of concern is the hepatitis B vaccine, which is currently recommended only for patients at risk of acquiring this viral disease.

The faction raises the concern that immunizations may be hazardous because vaccines, like infectious agents, activate both the innate and adaptive immune systems. Furthermore, inoculation often leads to acute and transient adverse events, such as fever, rash, flu-like symptoms, lymphadenopathy and local swelling, as well as other less common adverse events such as allergic reactions and the induction of infectious disease. Hypothetically, live attenuated vaccines may induce infections among immunosuppressed patients. Last, but not least, some vaccines seem to be less efficacious in patients with AD, and immunizing patients with AD during stable disease has been recommended because mostly stable patients were enrolled in the studies.[7] The medical community has accepted the link between vaccines and autoimmunity for certain vaccines but remains suspicious of others. Thus the individual decision regarding each patient and each vaccine has become very complex in recent years.

To assess this, we should keep in mind the criteria suggested by the WHO to address the safety of vaccines by taking into consideration the consistency of reports (different areas, different times), the specificity of association (the adverse event does not occur commonly and spontaneously in association with other external stimuli) and the temporal issue (vaccination should precede the adverse event), as well as the biological plausibility and the strength of association. Nonetheless, as stated by the WHO committee, it is not necessary that all these criteria be present together. Furthermore, some associations are difficult to ascertain, such as time relationship, because of the long latency, which may be required for the development of an AD. On the other hand, autoantibodies following vaccination may appear after only 6 months.[9] Reported association between vaccines and autoimmune diseases mainly come from case reports. These include patients developing SLE after vaccination against tetanus serum, streptococcal toxin, diphtheria toxin, typhoid-paratyphoid, hepatitis B virus (HBV), hepatitis A virus, multi-vaccine and anthrax. Following a polio virus vaccine programme in 1988 in Israel, 4 of 73 patients with SLE who were vaccinated experienced an exacerbation of the disease in the 3 months following vaccination compared to none of 37 control patients with SLE who were not vaccinated.[10] Similarly, several cases of RA have been described following HBV vaccination, whereas the influenza and pneumococcal vaccines were shown to exacerbate flare-ups of RA.[11–13]

2 VACCINATION AND ARTHRITIS

The occurrence of arthritis has been described following administration of several vaccines (Table 1). The arthritis resembles the features of reactive arthritis with poly- or monoarticular involvement; the onset of a well-defined RA has been described as well.[12,13]

2.1 Rheumatoid Arthritis

It has been estimated that patients affected by RA have almost a double risk of developing an infection, mainly respiratory ones, compared with age- and sex-matched subjects.[13]

2.1.1 Rheumatoid Arthritis, Influenza, and Pneumococcal Vaccination

Several studies, only two of which used a randomized design, investigated the safety and immunogenicity of influenza immunization in patients with RA (Table 2). All together, in these studies more than 500 patients with RA

Table 1 Vaccines Associated with Post-Vaccination Reactive Arthritis and Rheumatoid Arthritis

Disease	Vaccine	No. of Cases	Additional Symptoms
Reactive arthritis	HBV	1	Erythema nodosum
	HBV	1	Migratory arthritis, urticaria, oedema of the glottis
	HBV	1	Hypercalcaemia, lytic bone lesions
	HBV	4	Myalgia
	HBV	3	Vasculitis
	HBV	1	Adult-onset Still's disease
	HBV	>10	Reactive arthritis alone
	Rubella	>100	
	Mumps and measles	1	
	Influenza	1	
	DPT	2	
	Typhoid	2	
Rheumatoid arthritis	HBV	15	
	HBV	1	
	HBV	6	
	HBV	5	
	Tetanus	13	

HBV, hepatitis B virus; DPT, diphtheria–pertussis–tetanus.

Table 2 Safety and Immunogenicity of Influenza Immunization in Patients with Rheumatoid Arthritis

Authors	Type of Study	Subjects	Follow-up (wks)	Safety	Immuno-genicity
Herron et al.[13]	Controlled	17 RA; 32 NHS	16	6 Flare-ups	Quite similar
Chalmers et al.[14]	Randomized, controlled	63 RA cases; 63 RA controls; 64 NHS	4	No differences	Similar
Del Porto et al.[15]	Controlled	10 RA cases; 10 RA controls; 10 NHS	24	No differences	Quite similar
Fomin et al.[16]	Controlled	82 RA (27 on anti-TNF); 30 NHS	6	No major flare-ups	Slightly reduced
Kaine et al.[17]	Randomized, ADA vs. placebo	99 RA cases; 109 RA controls	4	No differences	Quite similar
Kubota et al.[18]	Controlled	27 RA on anti-TNF; 36 RA controls; 52 NHS	4-6	–	Similar
Gelinck et al.[19]	Controlled	4 RA on anti-CD20; 19 RA on anti-TNF, 20 NHS	4	–	Reduced with anti-CD20
Oren et al.[20]	Controlled	14 RA on anti-CD20; 29 RA DMARDs; 21 NHS	4	No differences	Reduced with anti-CD20
Elkayam et al.[21]	Controlled	20 RA on anti-TNF; 23 RA on DMARDs; 17 NHS	4	No differences	Similar
Salemi et al.[22]	Controlled (3 seasons)	28 RA on anti-TNF; 20 RA controls; 20 NHS	4-24	No differences	Quite similar
van Assen et al.[23]	Controlled	23 RA on anti-CD20; 20 RA on MTX; 29 NHS	4	No differences	Reduced with anti-CD20

ADA, adalimumab; DMARD, disease-modifying anti-rheumatic drug; MTX, methotrexate; NHS, normal healthy sera; RA, rheumatoid arthritis; TNF, tumor necrosis factor.

were immunized and only 14 flare-ups were reported; based on data emerging from randomized controlled trials it seems that there is no difference in the incidence of flares between immunized and non-immunized patients. However, it should be noted that the length of follow-up was very short in the majority of these studies (4 weeks), whereas flare-ups may be diagnosed later. The antibody response to the vaccine was similar in patients and controls regardless of immunosuppressive therapy or glucocorticoid dose.[24] Interestingly, medications seem not to affect the immune response.[15] Conversely, in patients treated with the anti-CD20 drug rituximab, a decreased response to different vaccines occurred. For instance, the humoral response to the influenza vaccine was significantly lower in the rituximab group compared to the non-rituximab group (21% vs. 67%, respectively; $p = 0.006$), although a substantial proportion of the patients treated with rituximab responded to immunization despite B-cell depletion.[25] Notably, several cases of RA have been described after immunization, mostly following HBV vaccination,[12,13] although a causal relationship has not been established yet.

2.1.2 Rheumatoid Arthritis and Pneumococcal Vaccination

Few studies evaluated safety and immunogenicity of pneumococcal immunization in patients with RA. The 23-valent pneumococcal vaccine was proved to be immunogenic in the patients evaluated, although those treated with TNF-α blockers showed a lower increase in antibodies. In another study, antibody titer after vaccination among patients treated with TNF blockers and healthy controls showed similar responses to vaccination; conversely, the immune response was reduced in patients treated with methotrexate.[18,22]

2.1.3 Arthritis and Hepatitis B Vaccine

Over the past 2 decades more than 30 cases of arthritis following vaccination with the HBV recombinant vaccine have been reported. Of these, some were cases of isolated inflammation of the joints, whereas others turned out to be harbingers of frank RA. In 1990 two cases of arthritis were reported shortly following immunization with HBV vaccines.[23,26] One of the patients developed poly-arthritis and erythema nodosum and the other reactive arthritis only. The symptoms receded in both patients, and there was no evidence of a systemic autoimmune illness later on. During the next decade more reports of people developing arthritis after HBV vaccination were published.[27–32] Some of the described patients were found to have high titers of rheumatoid factor (RF) in their sera without fulfilling other American College of Rheumatology criteria for RA.[28] Others were carriers of genetic markers predisposing to autoimmune disease.[13] In 1998, 11 patients who developed arthritis after receiving HBV recombinant vaccine were reported.[13] Ten of these patients fulfilled the American College of Rheumatology criteria for RA, nine of whom required disease-modifying drugs. Five of the subjects were carriers of the HLA DR4 haplotype. Nine of the 11 patients genotyped for HLA-DR and DQ expressed the RA shared motif in their HLA class II genes. The findings from this report suggested that the HBV recombinant vaccine might trigger RA in genetically prone individuals. An additional case report supports this hypothesis to a certain extent.[30] This is the case of a 44-year-old man who had had myasthenia gravis 20 years earlier and developed arthritis shortly after administration of the HBV vaccine. Overall, the occurrence of arthritis, and especially RA, after anti-HBV immunization is rare.[21] Moreover, studies that examined the response of patients with known RA to HBV vaccination showed that the administration of the vaccine was not associated with an appreciable deterioration of any laboratory or clinical parameters of the disease[33] and that 68% of patients produced antibodies. Older age and higher scores of daytime pain were associated with a lower rate of antibody production after vaccination. Thus it seems that HBV vaccines may be safe for most patients with stable, treated RA. For others the plausible association may have different explanations,[34] and it may represent the chance occurrence of two common phenomena: immunization precipitates a specific form of arthritis that is distinct from RA and that is usually self-limited (arthritis after immunization), or immunization is one of the factors that can trigger the manifestation of RA, as can infection, in susceptible subjects.

2.1.4 Arthritis and Rubella Vaccine

Joint manifestations have been documented often in connection with rubella vaccine, as well as with the wild virus itself.[35,36] In 1991, the Institute of Medicine released a report examining adverse effects of the diphtheria-pertussis-tetanus vaccine and the rubella vaccine (strain 27/3). The report concluded that the evidence suggests a causal relation between the rubella vaccine and acute arthritis in adult women.[37,38] In a large study[39] that included 2658 immunized and 2359 non-immunized children, there was an increased risk of arthralgia or arthritis 6 weeks after immunization with the measles-mumps-rubella vaccine.

3 VACCINATION AND SLE

Vaccines have been proved to be of great benefit in patients with SLE because infections are still among the major causes of morbidity in these patients.[40,41] The occurrence of SLE after immunization has been rarely reported in the medical literature, and the articles are mainly case reports related to old vaccines. In 1948, Ayvazian and Badger[42] raised several concerns after observing the onset of fatal SLE in three nurses after multiple vaccinations, and this report induced a worldwide fear of vaccinating patients with SLE.

3.1 SLE and Influenza Vaccination

Since 1978, several studies examined the risk-to-benefit ratio of influenza vaccination in patients with SLE (Table 3). Only one study used a randomized, controlled, double-blinded design[43] and showed that the vaccination was well tolerated with a low incidence of serious flare-ups. Moreover, no significant change in complement and autoantibody concentrations occurred after vaccination. Overall, seroconversion was similar or quite similar in comparison to normal subjects and decreased only in one study.[48–49] Abu-Shakra et al.[50] showed that disease activity was decreased within each group (cases and controls) compared with the pre-vaccination assessment, and influenza vaccine did not exacerbate renal conditions. Their data also suggested that the response of patients with SLE to vaccination might be lower than that expected in the general population, in particular among older patients (age ≥ 50 years) and in those treated with azathioprine or prednisone ≥ 10 mg/day.

3.2 SLE and Pneumococcal Vaccination

Pneumococcal vaccination was first assessed in patients with SLE during the 1970s, showing no clinical or serologic difference between patients treated with placebo or vaccine. Moreover, patients showed a significant increase, although lower than that in healthy subjects, in specific antipneumococcal antibody concentrations. More recent studies demonstrated that oral cyclophosphamide, azathioprine, or a combination of the two drugs given in low doses had no effect on immunization with pneumococcal vaccine.[53] Sporadic occurrence of disease flare-ups was reported by Elkayam et al..[21] Thus, as stated in the EULAR recommendations, it seems that, for patients with SLE with stable disease, this vaccine is relatively safe, although further studies are needed.

Table 3 Safety and Immunogenicity of Influenza Vaccine in Patients with Systemic Lupus Erythematosus (SLE)

Authors	Type of Study	Subjects	Follow-up (weeks)	Safety	Immunogenicity
Williams et al.[43]	Randomized, placebo-controlled, double-blind	19 SLE cases; 21 SLE controls; 36 NHS	20	1 Disease flare-up in each group	Reduced
Brodman et al.[44]	Controlled	46 patients; 58 NHS	8	No major flare-ups	Similar
Louie et al.[45]	Controlled	11 patients; 8 NHS	12	1 Diffuse proliferative GN	Similar
Ristow et al.[46]	Controlled	29 patients; 29 NHS	8	1 Focal GN	Quite similar
Herron et al.[13]	Controlled	20 patients; 32 NHS	16	1 Major flare-up	Similar
Turner-Stokes and Isenberg[47]	Retrospective, controlled *in vitro*	28 patients; 35 NHS	–	–	Reduced
Abu-Shakra et al.[48–50]	Controlled	24 SLE cases; 24 SLE controls	12	Decrease of mean SLEDAI in cases and controls	Reduced
Mercado et al.[51]	Controlled	18 patients; 18 NHS	8	Decrease of mean Mex-SLEDAI	Reduced
Holvast et al.[52]	Controlled	56 patients; 18 NHS	4	No increased SLEDAI	Reduced
Del Porto et al.[15]	Controlled	14 SLE cases; 14 SLE controls; 10 NHS	24	2 Flare-ups in cases, 1 flare-up in controls; no increased	Quite similar
Mercado et al.[51]	Controlled	18 SLE; 18 NHS	8	Decrease of Mex-SLEDAI	Reduced
Holvast et al.[52]	Controlled	56 SLE; 18 NHS	4	No increased SLEDAI	Reduced

Del Porto et al.[15]	Controlled	14 SLE cases; 14 SLE controls; 10 NHS	24	No increased SLEDAI	Quite similar
Holvast et al.[52a]	Controlled	52 SLE (II booster); 28 NHS	8	No increased SLEDAI	II Booster useless
Holvast et al.[52b]	Randomized, controlled	54 SLE; 26 SLE controls; 54 NHS	4	No increased SLEDAI	Reduced
Więsik-Szewczyk et al.[52c]	Controlled	62 SLE; 47 NHS	12	1 Severe flare, 6 mild flares; no increased SLEDAI	Reduced
Mathian et al.[52d]	Prospective	111 SLE	7	No increased SELENA-SLEDAI	Reduced by immunosuppressed lymphopenia
Saad et al.[52e]	Controlled	1668 Patients with AIIRD 572 SLE; 234 NHS	3	–	Reduced

GN = glomerulonephritis, NHS = normal human sera, SELENA, SLE = disease activity index.

3.3 SLE and Hepatitis B Vaccine

The HBV vaccine has been relatively frequently associated with manifestations of SLE in both sexes and all age groups.[54–59] It is interesting to note familial "clustering" of cases of lupus after vaccination.[55] The issue of the safety of HBV immunization in patients with SLE has been addressed so far only in retrospective studies. The safety of such immunization has yet to be definitively determined, and prospective studies are needed. It seems that most patients mount an adequate immune response to vaccination, even though it may be quantitatively and qualitatively less than in healthy controls.[59] All together, it has been recommended that only individuals at risk of exposure to hepatitis B should be immunized.

4 VACCINATION AND NEUROLOGICAL AUTOIMMUNE MANIFESTATIONS

Several neurologic demyelinating diseases have been reported following vaccination, the main being GBS. This is an acute polyradiculoneuropathy that usually manifests as a rapidly evolving symmetric and ascending motor paralysis with loss of tendon reflexes. It has been shown that the neurological symptoms of GBS are preceded by an acute infection in two-thirds of cases. GBS is an autoimmune disease, and autoantibodies to gangliosides, as well as T-cells reactivity, which cross-react to nerve components, can be detected in patients with GBS. Several vaccines have been related to the appearance of GBS, including influenza, tetanus toxoid, BCG, rabies, smallpox, mumps, rubella, oral poliovirus vaccine, hepatitis B vaccines, either plasma-derived or recombinant vaccine, and diphtheria vaccine. In 1976, the "swine flu" or New Jersey 76 vaccine caused a marked increase in GBS occurrence during the 6–8 weeks after vaccination. The reported relative risk of GBS associated with vaccination, adjusted for age, sex, and vaccine season, was 1.7.[5] Over a total of 3,623,046 person-years of observation, De Wals et al.[60] more recently identified 83 GBS cases during the 6 months of follow-up. Of these, 25 had been vaccinated against 2009 influenza A (H1N1), with an adjusted relative risk of 1.80 (95% CI, 1.12–2.87). The number of GBS cases attributable to vaccination was approximately 2 per 1 million doses, concluding that the risk was small and significant but is outweighed by the benefits of immunization.[60]

Moreover, Baxter et al.[61] did not observe recurrence of GBS that could be considered associated with vaccination. The main limitation of this study was the relatively small size, due to the rarity if the disease. Another demyelinating disease associated with vaccines is acute disseminated encephalomyelitis (ADEM).[62] This is an inflammatory disease of the central nervous system frequently occurring after vaccination. Rabies, diphtheria-tetanus-polio, smallpox, measles, mumps, rubella, Japanese B encephalitis, pertussis, influenza, hepatitis B and the Hog vaccines have been suggested as being involved. Huynh et al.[63] focused on the precipitating factor, suggesting the presence of mutations in the SCN1A gene; the re-infection theory (a vaccination with an attenuated virus strain may cause problems only if administered in patients suffering from a previous infection) may be responsible but yet not sufficient for the development of the syndrome. The worldwide use of the novel influenza type A virus in 2009, trivalent vaccines against H1N1 (pandemic) 09 and seasonal influenza gave rise to the description of a number of cases of ADEM, suggesting the existence of a component of the vaccine that is more likely to trigger this condition.[64] Similar concerns were raised by the use of the anti-HPV vaccine, specifically Gardasil, which is different from Cervarix in that it contains yeast.[65] Nonetheless, Schäffer et al.[66] reported another case of ADEM following HPV vaccination, but the vaccine used was not specified. The same Gardasil vaccine was associated with the onset of five cases of inflammatory demyelination that occurred within the "clinically isolated syndrome/multiple sclerosis" diagnostic spectrum occurring within 21 days of vaccination. The multifocal and atypical nature of these reports suggested that the vaccine might influence the nature and the severity of central nervous system inflammation.[67] Vaccines can also trigger other rare neurological conditions such as transverse myelitis. A recent article reported 37 cases of transverse myelitis that were associated with different vaccines including anti-HBV, measles-mumps-rubella and diphtheria-pertussis-tetanus. The authors found a temporal association between several days and 3 months, although a longer time frame of up to several years also was suggested.[68] Ablin et al.[69] addressed the issue of infections and vaccination with the development of another disorder characterized mainly by asthenia and muscle pain: fibromyalgia. The authors pointed the finger towards rubella and Lyme vaccines, although current data are insufficient to establish a causal relationship.[69]

The association between HBV and demyelination has been recently demonstrated in a nested case-control study conducted in the United Kingdom. The study had 163 patients and 1604 controls, showing an odds ratio within 3 years of developing multiple sclerosis of 3.1 (95% CI, 1.5-6.3).[70] Another paper by Mikaeloff et al.[71] showed that HBV (Engerix B) administered 3 years earlier was associated with an increased risk of CNS demyelinating event and a slightly higher risk of having a confirmed diagnosis of multiple sclerosis in a population of 349 children.

4.1 Vaccination and Neurolepsy

Narcolepsy is another interesting disease that has been associated with vaccines, in particular with the AS03 adjuvant H1N1 2009 vaccination (Pandemrix).[72–74] Interestingly, the pathogenesis of narcolepsy has been suggested to involve autoimmune mechanisms[75]; indeed, several antibodies have been found in these patients. More recently, the anti-Tribbles antibodies were demonstrated in a higher percentage of patients with narcolepsy, and experimental models suggest potential pathogenic role.[76,77] Furthermore, it was recently shown that the H1N1 virus infection itself did not contribute to the sudden increase in the incidence of childhood narcolepsy observed in Finland in 2010, and a direct role has been attributed to the AS03-adjuvant Pandemrix vaccination.[78]

5 VACCINATION AND OTHER AUTOIMMUNE CONDITIONS

HPV vaccination has been associated with several autoimmune disorders including SLE.[79,80] Gatto and coll.[81] recently described six cases of SLE and SLE-like disease following HPV immunization. Several common features were observed, such as personal or familial susceptibility to autoimmunity, as well as an adverse response to a prior dose of the same vaccine. Not only potentially life-threatening but also disabling conditions have been related with HPV vaccination, including premature ovarian failure (POF). A recent case of a young girl who developed POF after she was immunized with three quadrivalent HPV recombinant vaccinations was described. The authors stressed the need for detailed information concerning ovarian histology and ongoing fecundity after HPV vaccination.[82] Furthermore, the cases of three women – including two sisters – who developed secondary amenorrhea following HPV vaccine were recently described.[83] Interestingly, anti-ovarian and anti-thyroperoxidase antibodies were detected following the vaccine in two of three cases. Moreover, given that POF developed in siblings, a genetic susceptibility predisposing to post-vaccination POF has been hypothesized.[83] HPV vaccine has been related with the *de novo* onset of postural tachycardia orthostatic syndrome (POTS), an autonomic disorder of uncertain origin in which the detection of ganglionic acetylcholine receptor antibodies suggested the hypothesis of an autoimmune origin in some cases.[84] The case of 20-year-old woman developing POTS 2 weeks following HPV immunization—in the absence of both further risk factors and events preceding the illness—was reported by Blitshteyn,[85] who suggested for the first time a plausible temporal relationship between POTS and the HPV vaccine. Taken together, this evidence led researchers to hypothesize that the HPV vaccine may trigger an autoimmune response.

The HBV vaccine has been used routinely for almost 20 years. Although most of the adverse reactions are local and transient, major side effects may include protean autoimmune phenomena. Erythema nodosum, lichen planus, vasculitis, glomerulonephritis, Evan's syndrome, thrombocytopenic purpura, RA and reactive arthritis have been described as post-vaccination singularities.[86,87] McMahon et al.[88] suggested that adverse events caused by the plasma-derived HBV vaccine could be due both to the preservative material thimerosal (a mercurial compound that was found to be neurotoxic but that is not included anymore in the HBV vaccines since 1999) and to alum-hydroxide when used as an adjuvant.[88] Other components of the vaccine, such as yeast, also have been indicted. Yeast can, for instance, reduce the number and function of T regulatory cells, a mechanism that is involved in the generation of autoimmunity. The largest cohort of cases diagnosed with immune-mediated diseases following immunization HBV vaccine has been described by Zafrir et al.[89] Another autoimmune disease that can be triggered by vaccinations, specifically HBV, is pemphigus. This is caused by autoantibodies against epithelial intercellular components, and there are reports associating the disease with influenza and tetanus with diphtheria vaccination. Nonetheless, the first case of pemphigus following HBV vaccination (EngerixB) was reported by Berkun et al.[90] The patients developed pemphigus only three months after the vaccination, suggesting a possible temporal association and that the vaccine *per se* or its adjuvant may cause a non-specific activation of the immune system and unmask already existent but dormant pemphigus.[90] The association between HBV vaccine and the onset of undifferentiated connective tissue disease (UCTD) also has been described recently.[91] It has been hypothesized that some components of the HBV vaccine, such as yeast and alum, may contribute to the unbalance of the T regulatory cell-to-Th17 cell ratio toward a Th17 response, which is found to have a role in the pathogenesis of UCTD.[92] Nonetheless, HBV vaccine can trigger other even rarer autoimmune conditions such as dermatomyositis[93] and systemic polyarteritis nodosa.[94]

6 POSSIBLE MECHANISMS OF VACCINE-RELATED AUTOIMMUNITY

Many common infections can induce a transient increase in autoantibody production. A similar increase in autoantibody production has been observed after various vaccinations. Such autoantibodies usually resolve within a period of two months[95] but can persist in rare cases. Several studies indicate that stimulation of autoantibody production has become one of the criteria of establishing the safety of vaccines. It is to be remembered, however, that although autoantibodies are a characteristic of autoimmune disease, it often is unclear whether they are an epiphenomena or represent the causal agents of the illness. The human immune system is highly complex; it displays both specificity and memory and is designed to provide protection against almost all infections. The drawback of such a complex and broadly responding immune system is that in responding to infection, the immune system of a few individuals will lose self-tolerance and cause autoimmunity.[96] An infection (or vaccine, for that matter) can induce autoimmunity via two mechanisms: antigen specific or antigen non-specific. An autoimmune condition will arise, however, only if the individual is genetically predisposed to that condition. A common explanation of how an infectious agent can cause autoimmunity via an antigen-specific mechanism is the molecular mimicry theory. Antigenic determinants of infections can thus be recognized by the host immune system as being similar to antigenic determinants of the host itself.[96] The situation is more complex for molecular mimicry that involves T lymphocytes. These cells recognize their antigen as short peptides bound to MHC molecules. To serve as a molecular mimic, an infectious agents' antigen must copy the shape of a self-antigenic epitope bound to the appropriate MHC molecule. Experimental findings have shown that a single T-cell receptor can recognize a broad range of sequences,[97,98] including peptides with totally different sequences. It has been calculated that each individual T cell should be able to recognize more than one million distinct peptide epitopes.[99] Another mechanism whereby microorganisms (or vaccines) may cause autoimmunity involves bystander activation. This is an antigen–non-specific mechanism. In this instance the infectious agent causes the release of previously sequestered self-antigens or stimulates the innate immune response, resulting in activation of self-antigen-expressing antigen-presenting cells. Evidence for this mechanism has come from several studies of transgenic mice.[99,100] Autoimmune disease is most likely to be induced in the infected organ. For example, mice that harbor high numbers of islet antigen-specific T cells developed diabetes only when infected with an islet-cell tropic virus.[101] The effect of this virus has been reproduced by an islet cell-damaging drug but not by non-specific T-cell activation.[102] These findings imply that viruses can precipitate disease by damaging tissue and causing the release and presentation of previously sequestered self-antigens. So far we can conclude that there is a high probability for infectious agents' antigen to cross-react with self-antigens and that autoimmune disorders can be triggered by the innate immune response to microorganisms. The fact that autoimmune disease does not occur more frequently is probably due to a "fail-safe" mechanism that the immune system has evolved to prevent extensive tissue damage in response to infection. The immune system is controlled by homeostatic mechanisms.[103] Lymphocytes have to compete with each other for antigen and growth factors. Furthermore, T-cell reaction to an antigen is limited by activation-induced cell death.[104] These mechanisms are designed to keep the lymphocyte population at an optimal predetermined level, thus limiting the expansion of self-reactive lymphocytes.[104] In a lymphopenic setting, self-reactive lymphocytes undergo homeostatic proliferation and are released from peripheral tolerance, thus causing autoimmune disease.[105–111] The immune system is equipped with a wide variety of lymphocytes bearing receptors with varying affinity to antigen.[107] The immune response to a given antigen selects only a strictly limited set of these lymphocytes. The selection depends on several mechanisms: (a) the role of antigen-processing and MHC-peptide complex formation, (b) selective binding of antigenic epitopes to specific MHC molecules, and (c) selective depletion of specific lymphocytes by overstimulation (clonal exhaustion or deletion).[110] Also, the fact that the threshold for activation of T cells is close to the threshold for activation-induced cell death results in a highly focused reaction of the immune system to any antigen.[109,111] These mechanisms limit the immune response to antigen and prevent activation of cells bearing high-affinity receptors. As high-affinity receptors are more likely to be cross-reactive, it is probable that this mechanism evolved to prevent collateral tissue damage, which occurs during the immune response to infection, and to limit the likelihood of self-reactive lymphocyte activation during infection.[96] An additional control mechanism is imposed on the immune system by regulatory T cells. The best-characterized subset of T cells is the CD4+CD25+ cell,[112,113] which arise in the thymus, where they are positively selected by recognition of self-antigen.[114] Unlike the majority of the T-cell population, which leaves the thymus as naive lymphocytes, the CD25+ cells emigrate from the thymus but do not proliferate in response to antigen. They are capable of suppressing the response to self-antigens. These cells were first described by Sakaguchi et al.,[115] who noted that thymectomy of young mice prevented their generation and resulted in widespread autoimmune disease in adult animals. Additional examples of the role and importance of these cells exist.[116] The physiological role of T regulatory type I cells is probably to moderate the immune response to infection and thereby limit the collateral damage that results from the immune response to an infectious agent.[117] These combined homeostatic and regulatory mechanisms have evolved to ensure that the immune response is focused and controlled, and they prevent the individual from developing autoimmune disease during the course of infection.[96] These mechanisms also apply to the host response to vaccination. It is probable that a killed vaccine would be less likely to activate the innate response to infection and to cause tissue disruption than a live-attenuated one, thereby reducing the risk of autoimmune disease. Nevertheless, the degree of activation achieved by an attenuated organism is much less than that induced by the wild strain. Every new vaccine should therefore be assessed on a case-by-case basis, giving extreme consideration to the potential benefit in terms of public health provision.

7 ANIMAL MODELS

Animal studies have confirmed that vaccines may induce an autoimmune response in experimental models of disease. For instance, autoantibodies (including SLE-associated autoantibodies such as anti-laminin and anti-fibronectin) were produced in immunized dogs.[118] Human vaccines against pertussis and Hemophilus influenzae B increased the incidence of diabetes in non-obese diabetic mice and biobreeding rats,[119] and wild and farm-raised Atlantic salmon vaccinated with oil-based vaccines developed autoantibodies (such as anti-single-stranded DNA, anti-double-stranded DNA, anti-SSA and anti-SSB antibodies) and autoimmune diseases with involvement of the kidney and liver.[120] In another experimental model, the recombinant hepatitis B vaccine was capable of initiating alopecia areata in predisposed mice.[121]

Furthermore, glucan, a polysaccharide from the yeast *Saccharomyces cerevisiae*, was able to increase disease activity and caused early death in New Zealand brown/New Zealand white F1 mice.[122] In a study from 1973, *S. cerevisiae* injected into rabbits was able to provoke the onset of acute hematogenous pyelonephritis.[123] Alum was found in tissues, indicating the presence of the adjuvant in the nervous tissue of experimental animals.[124] An isoprenoid adjuvant, pristane, has been shown to promote lupus-like syndromes and pathologic nephritis in both autoimmune-prone and non-susceptible mouse strains after a single intra-peritoneal administration.[123–125] Furthermore, squalene, a triterpene, and Freunds' adjuvants (complete and incomplete) could also provoke lupus-like syndromes in non-autoimmune prone BALB/c mice.[126,127]

8 CONCLUSION

Thus, if it seems that immunization can be associated with the development of an autoimmune response, the real strength of such *association* and the mechanisms by which autoimmunity takes place are still a matter of discussion. Nonetheless, vaccines still represent an important prophylactic intervention, and the risk-to-benefit ratio clearly leans towards the advantages of infectious disease prevention. It does not seem that, besides the above-mentioned recommendations, vaccination routines should be changed in the healthy population or in patients with known autoimmune disorders.[128–131] We should consider post-vaccination autoimmunity as a rare phenomenon in many patients. The ethical problem is limited to the possibility of provoking the development of an AD in an otherwise healthy subject. The practical problem is the risk of triggering a flare-up of disease in a patient with a rheumatologic condition, with the knowledge that that vaccine could be less efficacious than in the general population. Even if some cause-and-effect mechanism were proven, most of the data against the use of vaccines come from the case reports, and there is the feeling that well-conducted epidemiological studies are missing. The future will see the design of less immunogenic/more efficacious vaccines, personalized according to the individual's susceptibility (a field covered by vaccinomics, e.g. vaccine-genomics), and exploration of the role of adjuvants in the determination of autoimmune processes.

REFERENCES

1. Conti F, Rezai S, Valesini G. Vaccination and autoimmune rheumatic diseases. *Autoimmun Rev* 2008;**8**(2):124–8.
2. Nass M. Safety of the smallpox vaccine among military recipients. *JAMA* 2003;**290**:2123–4.
3. Nossal GJV. Vaccination and autoimmunity. *J Autoimmun* 2000;**14**:15–22.
4. Shoenfeld Y, Aron-Maor A, Sherer Y. Vaccination as an additional player in the mosaic of autoimmunity. *Clin Exp Rheumatol* 2000;**18**(2):181–4.

5. Lasky T, Terracciano GJ, Magder L, Koski CL, Ballesteros M, Nash D, et al. The Guillain-Barré syndrome and the 1992-1993 and 1993-1994 influenza vaccines. *N Engl J Med* 1998;**339**:1797–802.

6. van Assen S, Agmon-Levin N, Elkayam O, Cervera R, Doran MF, Dougados M, et al. EULAR recommendations for vaccination in adult patients with autoimmune inflammatory rheumatic diseases. *Ann Rheum Dis* 2011;**70**(3):414–22.

7. van Assen S, Elkayam O, Agmon-Levin N, Cervera R, Doran MF, Dougados M, et al. Vaccination in adult patients with auto-immune inflammatory rheumatic diseases: a systematic literature review for the European league against rheumatism evidence-based recommendations for vaccination in adult patients with auto-immune inflammatory rheumatic diseases. *Autoimmun Rev* 2011;**10**(6):341–52.

8. Toplak N, Kveder T, Trampus-Bakija A, Subelj V, Cucnik S, Avcin T. Autoimmune response following annual influenza vaccination in 92 apparently healthy adults. *Autoimmun Rev* 2008;**8**(2):134–8. http://dx.doi.org/10.1016/j.autrev.2008.07.008.

9. Molina V, Shoenfeld Y. Infection, vaccines and other environmental triggers of autoimmunity. *Autoimmunity* 2005;**38**(3):235–45.

10. Doran MF, Crowson CS, Pond GR, O'Fallon WM, Gabriel SE. Frequency of infection in patients with rheumatoid arthritis compared with controls: a population-based study. *Arthritis Rheum* 2002;**46**:2287–93.

11. Vautier G, Carty JE. Acute sero-positive rheumatoid arthritis occurring after hepatitis B vaccination. *Br J Rheumatol* 1994;**33**:991–8.

12. Pope JE, Stevens A, Howson W, Bell DA. The development of rheumatoid arthritis after recombinant hepatitis B vaccination. *J Rheumatol* 1998;**25**:1687–93.

13. Herron A, Dettleff G, Hixon B, Brandwin L, Ortbals D, Hornick R, et al. Influenza vaccination in patients with rheumatic diseases. *JAMA* 1979;**242**:53–6.

14. Chalmers A, Scheifele D, Patterson C, Williams D, Weber J, Shuckett R. etal. Immunization of patients with rheumatoid arthritis against influenza: a study of vaccine safety and immunogenicity. *J Rheumatol* 1994;**21**:1203–6.

15. Del Porto F, Laganá B, Biselli R, Donatelli I, Campitelli L, Nisini R, et al. Influenza vaccine administration in patients with systemic lupus erythematosus and rheumatoid arthritis: safety and immunogenicity. *Vaccine* 2006;**24**:3217–23.

16. Fomin I, Caspi D, Levy V, Varsano N, Shalev Y, Paran D, et al. Vaccination against influenza in rheumatoid arthritis: the effect of disease modifying drugs, including TNF a blockers. *Ann Rheum Dis* 2006;**65**:191–4.

17. Kaine JL, Kivitz AJ, Birbara C, Luo AY. Immune responses following administration of influenza and pneumococcal vaccines to patients with rheumatoid arthritis receiving adalimumab. *J Rheumatol* 2007;**34**:272–9.

18. Kubota T, Nii T, Nanki T, Kohsaka H, Harigai M, Komano Y, et al. Anti-tumor necrosis factor therapy does not diminish the immune response to influenza vaccine in Japanese patients with rheumatoid arthritis. *Mod Rheumatol* 2007;**17**:531–3.

19. Gelinck LB, Teng YK, Rimmelzwaan GF, van den Bemt BJ, Kroon FP, van Laar JM. Poor serological responses upon influenza vaccination in patients with rheumatoid arthritis treated with rituximab. *Ann Rheum Dis* 2007;**66**:1402–3.

20. Oren S, Mandelboim M, Braun-Moscovici Y, Paran D, Ablin J, Litinsky I, et al. Vaccination against influenza in rheumatoid arthritis patients: the effect of rituximab on the humoral response. *Ann Rheum Dis* 2008;**67**:937–41.

21. Elkayam O, Yaron M, Caspi D. Safety and efficacy of vaccination against hepatitis B in patients with rheumatoid arthritis. *Ann Rheum Dis* 2002;**61**:623–5.

22. Salemi S, Picchianti-Diamanti A, Germano V, et al. Influenza vaccine administration in rheumatoid arthritis patients under treatment with TNF alpha blockers: safety and immunogenicity. *Clin Immunol* 2010;**134**:113–20.

23. van Assen S, Holvast A, Benne CA, et al. Humoral responses after influenza vaccination are severely reduced in patients with rheumatoid arthritis treated with rituximab. *Arthritis Rheum* 2010;**62**:75–81.

24. Cimmino MA, Seriolo B, Accardo S. Influenza vaccination in rheumatoid arthritis. *J Rheumatol* 1995;**22**:1802–3.

25. Kapetanovic MC, Saxne T, Sjöholm A, Truedsson L, Jönsson G, Geborek P. Influenza of methotrexate, TNF blockers and prednisolone on antibody responses to pneumococcal polysaccharide vaccine in patients with rheumatoid arthritis. *Rheumatology* 2006;**45**:106–11.

26. Biasi D, De Sandre G, Bambara LM, Carletto A, Caramaschi P, Zanoni G, et al. A new case of reactive arthritis after hepatitis B vaccination. *Clin Exp Rheumatol* 1993;**11**:215.

27. Biasi D, Carletto A, Caramaschi P, Frigo A, Pacor ML, Bezzi D, et al. Rheumatological manifestations following hepatitis B vaccination. A report of two clinical cases. *Recenti Prog Med* 1994;**85**:438–40.

28. Gross K, Combe C, Kruger K, Schattenkirschner M. Arthritis after hepatitis B vaccination. Report of three cases. *Scand J Rheumatol* 1995;**24**:50–2.

29. Cathebras P, Cartry O, Lafage-Proust MH, Lauwers A, Acquart S, Thomas T, et al. Arthritis, hypercalcemia and lytic bone lesions after hepatitis B vaccination. *J Rheumatol* 1996;**23**:558–60.

30. Maillefert JF, Sibilia J, Toussirot E, Vignon E, Eschard JP, Lorcerie B, et al. Rheumatic disorders developed after hepatitis B vaccination. *Rheumatology (Oxford)* 1999;**38**: 978–83.

31. Grasland A, Le Maitre F, Pouchot J, Hazera P, Bazin C, Vinceneux P. Adult-onset Still's disease after hepatitis A and B vaccination. *Rev Med Interne* 1998;**91**:134–6.

32. Sibilia J, Maillefert JF. Vaccination and rheumatoid arthritis. *An Rheum Dis* 2002;**61**:575–6.

33. Symmons DPM, Chakravarty K. Can immunization trigger rheumatoid arthritis. *Ann Rheum Dis* 1993;**52**:843–4.

34. Weibel RE, Bemor DE. Chronic arthropathy and musculoskeletal symptoms associated with rubella vaccine. A review of 124 claims submitted to the National Vaccine Injury Compensation Program. *Arthritis Rheum* 1996;**39**:1529–34.

35. Ray P, Black S, Shinefield H, Dillon A, Schwalbe J, Holmes S, et al. Risk of chronic arthropathy among women after rubella vaccination. Vaccine safety datalink team. *JAMA* 1997;**278**:551–6.

36. Howson CP, Fineberg HV. Adverse events following pertussis and rubella vaccines. Summary of a report of the Institute of Medicine. *JAMA* 1992;**267**:392–6.

37. Howson CP, Katz M, Johnston Jr. RB, Fineberg HV. Chronic arthritis after rubella vaccination. *Clin Infect Dis* 1992;**15**:307–12.

38. Benjamin CM, Chew CG, Silman AJ. Joint and limb symptoms in children after immunization with measles, mumps and rubella vaccine. *BMJ* 1992;**304**:1075–7.

39. Urowitz MB, Gladman DD, Abu-Shakra M, Farewell VT. Mortality studies in systemic lupus erythematosus. Results from a single center. III. Improved survival over 24 years. *J Rheumatol* 1997;**24**:1061–5.

40. Petri M. Infection in systemic lupus erythematosus. *Rheum Dis Clin North Am* 1996;**24**:423–56.

41. Conti F, Rezai S, Valesini G. Vaccination and rheumatic diseases: is there still a dilemma? *Curr Rheumatol Rev* 2007;**3**:79–91.

42. Ayvazian LF, Badger TL. Disseminated lupus erythematosus occurring among student nurses. *N Engl J Med* 1948;**239**:565–70.

43. Williams GW, Steinberg AD, Reinertsen JR, Klassen LW, Decker JL, Dolin R. Influenza immunization systemic lupus erythematosus. *Ann Intern Med* 1978;**88**:729–35.

44. Brodman R, Gilfillan R, Glass D, Schur PH. Influenza vaccine response in SLE. *Ann Intern Med* 1978;**88**:735–40.

45. Louie JS, Nies KM, Shoji KT, Fraback RC, Abrass C, Border W, et al. Clinical and antibody responses after influenza immunization in systemic lupus erythematosus. *Ann Intern Med* 1978;**88**:790–2.

46. Ristow SC, Douglas RG, Condemi JJ. Influenza vaccination of patients with systemic lupus erythematosus. *Ann Intern Med* 1978;**88**:786–9.

47. Turner-Stokes L, Isenberg DA. Leading article: immunisation of patients with rheumatoid arthritis and systemic lupus erythematosus. *Ann Rheum Dis* 1988;**47**:529–31.

48. Abu-Shakra M, Zalmanson S, Neumann L, Flusser D, Sukenik S, Buskila D. Influenza virus vaccination of patients with SLE: effects on the disease activity. *J Rheumatol* 2000;**27**:1681–5.

49. Abu-Shakra M, Press J, Varsano N, Levy V, Mendelson E, Sukenik S, et al. Specific antibody response after influenza immunization in systemic lupus erythematosus. *J Rheumatol* 2002;**29**:2555–7.

50. Abu-Shakra M, Press J, Sukenik S, Buskila D. Influenza virus vaccination of patient with SLE: effects on generation of autoantibodies. *Clin Rheumatol* 2002;**21**:369–72.

51. Mercado U, Acosta H, Avendano L. Influenza vaccination of patients with systemic lupus erythematosus. *Rev Invest Clin* 2004;**56**(1):16–20.

52. Holvast A, Huckriede AL, Wilschut J, Horst G, De Vries JJ, Benne CA, et al. Safety and efficacy of influenza vaccination in systemic lupus erythematosus patients with quiescent disease. *Ann Rheum Dis* 2006;**65**:913–18.

52a. Holvast A, van Assen S, de Haan A, Huckriede A, Benne CA, Westra J, et al. Effect of a second, booster, influenza vaccination on antibody responses in quiescent systemic lupus erythematosus: an open, prospective, controlled study. *Rheumatology (Oxford)* 2009;**48**(10):1294–9.

52b. Holvast A, van Assen S, de Haan A, Huckriede A, Benne CA, Westra J, et al. Studies of cell-mediated immune responses to influenza vaccination in systemic lupus erythematosus. *Arthritis Rheum* 2009;**60**(8):2438–47.

52c. Wiesik-Szewczyk E, Romanowska M, Mielnik P, Chwalińska-Sadowska H, Brydak LB, Olesińska M, et al. Anti-influenza vaccination in systemic lupus erythematosus patients: an analysis of specific humoral response and vaccination safety. *Clin Rheumatol* 2010;**29**(6):605–13.

52d. Mathian A, Devilliers H, Krivine A, Costedoat-Chalumeau N, Haroche J, Huong DB, et al. Factors influencing the efficacy of two injections of a pandemic 2009 influenza A (H1N1) nonadjuvanted vaccine in systemic lupus erythematosus. *Arthritis Rheum* 2011;**63**(11):3502–11.

52e. Saad CG, Borba EF, Aikawa NE, et al. Immunogenicity and safety of the 2009 non-adjuvanted influenza A/H1N1 vaccine in a large cohort of autoimmune rheumatic diseases. *Ann Rheum Dis* 2011;**70**:1068–73.

53. Tudela P, Marti S, Bonal J. Systemic lupus erythematosus and vaccination against hepatitis B. *Nephron* 1992;**62**:236.

54. Finielz P, Lam-Kam-Sang LF, Guiserix J. Systemic lupus erythematosus and thrombocytopenic purpura in two members of the same family following hepatitis B vaccine. *Nephrol Dial Transplant* 1998;**13**:2420–1.

55. Guiserix J. Systemic lupus erythematosus following hepatitis B vaccine. *Nephron* 1996;**74**:441.

56. Mamoux V, Dumont C. Lupus erythemateux dissemine et vaccination contrel'hepatite B. *Arch Pediatr* 1994;**1**:307–8.

57. Grezard P, Chaff M, Philippot V, Perrot H, Faisnat M. Cutaneous lupus erythematosus and buccal aphthosis after hepatitis B vaccination in a 6 year old child. *Ann Dermatol Venereol* 1996;**123**:657–9.

58. Ioannou Y, Isenberg DA. Immunization of patients with systemic lupus erythematosus: the current state of play. *Lupus* 1999;**8**:497–501.
59. Kuruma KA, Borba EF, Lopes MH, de Carvalho JF, Bonfá E. Safety and efficacy of hepatitis B vaccine in systemic lupus erythematosus. *Lupus* 2007;**16**(5):350–4.
60. De Wals P, Deceuninck G, Toth E, Boulianne N, Brunet D, Boucher RM, et al. Risk of Guillain-Barré syndrome following H1N1 influenza vaccination in Quebec. *JAMA* 2012;**308**:175–81.
61. Baxter R, Lewis N, Bakshi N, Vellozzi C, Klein NP, CISA Network. Recurrent Guillain-Barre syndrome following vaccination. *Clin Infect Dis* 2012;**54**:800–4.
62. Ozawa H, Noma S, Yoshida Y, Sekine H, Hashimoto T. Acute disseminated encephalomyelitis associated with poliomyelitis vaccine. *Pediatr Neurol* 2000;**23**(2):177–9.
63. Huynh W, Cordato DJ, Kehdi E, Masters LT, Dedousis C. Post-vaccination encephalomyelitis: literature review and illustrative case. *J Clin Neurosci* 2008;**15**:1315–22.
64. Maeda K, Idehara R. Acute disseminated encephalomyelitis following 2009 H1N1 influenza vaccination. *Intern Med* 2012;**51**:1931–3.
65. Mendoza Plasencia Z, González López M, FernándezSanfiel ML, Muñiz Montes JR. Acute disseminated encephalomyelitis with tumefactive lesions after vaccination against human papillomavirus. *Neurologia* 2010;**25**:58–9.
66. Schäffer V, Wimmer S, Rotaru I, Topakian R, Haring HP, Aichner FT. HPV vaccine: a cornerstone of female health a possible cause of ADEM? *J Neurol* 2008;**255**:1818–20.
67. Sutton I, Lahoria R, Tan I, Clouston P, Barnett M. CNS demyelination and quadrivalent HPV vaccination. *Mult Scler* 2009;**15**:116–9.
68. Agmon-Levin N, Kivity S, Szyper-Kravitz M, Shoenfeld Y. Transverse myelitis and vaccines: a multi-analysis. *Lupus* 2009;**18**:1198–204.
69. Ablin JN, Shoenfeld Y, Buskila D. Fibromyalgia, infection and vaccination: two more parts in the etiological puzzle. *J Autoimmun* 2006;**27**:145–52.
70. Hernán MA, Jick SS, Olek MJ, Jick H. Recombinant hepatitis B vaccine and the risk of multiple sclerosis: a prospective study. *Neurology* 2004;**63**:838–42.
71. Mikaeloff Y, Caridade G, Suissa S, Tardieu M. Hepatitis B vaccine and the risk of CNS inflammatory demyelination in childhood. *Neurology* 2009;**72**:873–80. http://dx.doi.org/10.1212/01.wnl.0000335762.42177.07.
72. Persson I, Granath F, Askling J, Ludvigsson JF, Olsson T, Feltelius N. Risks of neurological and immune-related diseases, including narcolepsy, after vaccination with Pandemrix: a population- and registry-based cohort study with over 2 years of follow-up. *J Intern Med* 2014;**275**:172–90.
73. Nohynek H, Jokinen J, Partinen M, Vaarala O, Kirjavainen T, Sundman J, et al. AS03 adjuvanted AH1N1 vaccine associated with an abrupt increase in the incidence of childhood narcolepsy in Finland. *PLoS One* 2012;**7**(3):e33536.
74. Szakács A, Darin N, Hallböök T. Increased childhood incidence of narcolepsy in western Sweden after H1N1 influenza vaccination. *Neurology* 2013;**80**(14):1315–21.
75. Overeem S, Black 3rd. JL, Lammers GJ. Narcolepsy: immunological aspects. *Sleep Med Rev* 2008;**12**(2):95–107.
76. Katzav A, Arango MT, Kivity S, Tanaka S, Givaty G, Agmon-Levin N, et al. Passive transfer of narcolepsy: anti-TRIB2 autoantibody positive patient IgG causes hypothalamic orexin neuron loss and sleep attacks in mice. *J Autoimmun* 2013; **45**:24–30.
77. Cvetkovic-Lopes V, Bayer L, Dorsaz S, Maret S, Pradervand S, Dauvilliers Y, et al. Elevated tribbles homolog 2-specific antibody levels in narcolepsy patients. *J Clin Invest* 2010;**120**(3):713–19. http://dx.doi.org/10.1172/JCI41366.
78. Melén K, Partinen M, Tynell J, Sillanpää M, Himanen SL, Saarenpää-Heikkilä O, et al. No serological evidence of influenza A H1N1pdm09 virus infection as a contributing factor in childhood narcolepsy after Pandemrix vaccination campaign in Finland. *PLoS One* 2013;**8**(8):e68402. http://dx.doi.org/10.1371/journal.pone.0068402. eCollection 2013.

79. Slade BA, Leidel L, Vellozzi C, Woo EJ, Hua W, Sutherland A, et al. Postlicensure safety surveillance for quadrivalent human papillomavirus recombinant vaccine. *JAMA* 2009;**302**(7):750–7. http://dx.doi.org/10.1001/jama.2009.1201.
80. Soldevilla HF, Briones SF, Navarra SV. SLE Systemic lupus erythematosus following HPV immunization or infection? *Lupus* 2012;**21**:158–61.
81. Gatto M, Agmon-Levin N, Soriano A, Manna R, Maoz-Segal R, Kivity S, et al. Human papillomavirus vaccine and systemic lupus erythematosus. *Clin Rheumatol* 2013;**32**: 1301–7.
82. Little DT, Ward HR. Premature ovarian failure 3 years after menarche in a 16-year-old girl following human papillomavirus vaccination. *BMJ Case Rep* 2012;**2012**. http://dx. doi.org/10.1136/bcr-2012-006879, pii: bcr2012006879.
83. Colafrancesco S, Perricone C, Tomljenovic L, Shoenfeld Y. Human papilloma virus vaccine and primary ovarian failure: another facet of the autoimmune/inflammatory syndrome induced by adjuvants. *Am J Reprod Immunol* 2013;**70**:309–16.
84. Thieben MJ, Sandroni P, Sletten DM, Benrud-Larson LM, Fealey RD, Vernino S, et al. Postural orthostatic tachycardia syndrome: the Mayo clinic experience. *Mayo Clin Proc* 2007;**82**:308–13.
85. Blitshteyn S. Postural tachycardia syndrome after vaccination with Gardasil. *Eur J Neurol* 2010;**17**:e52.
86. Geier DA, Geier MR. A case-control study of serious autoimmune adverse events following hepatitis B immunization. *Autoimmunity* 2005;**38**(4):295–301.
87. Israeli E, Agmon-Levin N, Blank M, Shoenfeld Y. Adjuvants and autoimmunity. *Lupus* 2009;**18**(13):1217–25.
88. McMahon AW, Iskander JK, Haber P, Braun MM, Ball R. Inactivated influenza vaccine (IIV) in children <2 years of age: examination of selected adverse events reported to the Vaccine Adverse Event Reporting System (VAERS) after thimerosal-free or thimerosal-containing vaccine. *Vaccine* 2008;**26**(3):427–9.
89. Zafrir Y, Agmon-Levin N, Paz Z, Shilton T, Shoenfeld Y. Autoimmunity following hepatitis B vaccine as part of the spectrum of 'autoimmune (auto-inflammatory) syndrome induced by adjuvants' (ASIA): analysis of 93 cases. *Lupus* 2012;**21**:146–52.
90. Berkun Y, Mimouni D, Shoenfeld Y. Pemphigus following hepatitis B vaccination—coincidence or causality? *Autoimmunity* 2005;**38**:117–19.
91. Bruzzese V, Zullo A, Hassan C. Connective tissue disease following epatitis B vaccination. *J Clin Rheumatol* 2013;**19**:280–1.
92. Perricone C, Shoenfeld Y. Hepatitis B vaccination and undifferentiated connective tissue disease: another brick in the wall of the autoimmune/inflammatory syndrome induced by adjuvants (Asia). *J Clin Rheumatol* 2013;**19**:231–3.
93. Salvetti M, Pisani A, Bastianello S, Millefiorini E, Buttinelli C, Pozzilli C. Clinical and MRI assessment of disease activity in patients with multiple sclerosis after influenza vacciniation. *J Neurol* 1995;**242**:143–6.
94. Williams GW, Steinberg AD, Reinertsen JL, Klassen LW, Decker JL, Dolin R. Influenza immunization in systemic lupus erythematosus. A double blind trial. *Ann Intern Med* 1978;**88**:729–34.
95. Borchers AT, Keen CL, Shoenfeld Y, Silva J, Gershwin ME. Vaccines, viruses and voodoo. *J Investig Allergol Clin Immunol* 2002;**12**:155–68.
96. Wraith DC, Goldman M, Lambert PH. Vaccination and autoimmune disease: what is the evidence? *Lancet* 2003;**362**:1659–66.
97. Hemmer B, Jacobsen M, Somner M. Degeneracy in T-cell antigen recognition: implications for the pathogenesis of autoimmune diseases. *J Neuroimmunol* 2000;**107**:148–53.
98. Mason D. A very high level of crossreactivity is an essential feature of the T-cell receptor. *Immunol Today* 1998;**19**:395–404.

99. Kissler S, Anderton SM, Wraith DC. Antigen-presenting cell activation: a link between infection and autoimmunity. *J Autoimmun* 2001;**16**:303–8.

100. Kissler S, Anderton SM, Wraith DC. Cross-reactivity and T-cell receptor antagonism of myelin basic protein reactive T cells is modulated by the activation state of the antigen-presenting cell. *J Autoimmun* 2002;**19**:183–93.

101. Horwitz MS, Bradley LM, Harbertson J. Diabetes induced by coxsackie virus: initiation by bystander damage and not molecular mimicry. *Nat Med* 1998;**4**:781–5.

102. Horwitz MS, Ilic A, Fine C, Rodriguez E, Sarvetnick N. Presented antigen from damaged pancreatic beta cells activates autoreactive T-cells in virus mediated autoimmune diabetes. *J Clin Invest* 2002;**109**:79–87.

103. Theophilopoulos AN, Durraner W, Kono DW. T cell homeostasis of systemic autoimmunity. *J Clin Invest* 2001;**108**:335–40.

104. Walker LS, Abbas AK. The enemy within: keeping self-reactive T cells at bay in the periphery. *Nat Rev Immunol* 2002;**2**:11–19.

105. Bucy RP, Xu XY, Li J, Huang G. Cyclosporin A-induced autoimmune disease in mice. *J Immunol* 1993;**151**:1039–50.

106. Sakauchi N, Miyai K, Sakaguchi S. Ionizing radiation and autoimmunity: induction of autoimmune disease in mice by high dose fractionated total lymphoid irradiation and its prevention by inoculating normal T cells. *J Immunol* 1994;**152**:2586–95.

107. Morse SS, Sakaguchi N, Sakaguchi S. Virus and autoimmunity: induction of autoimmune disease in mice by mouse T lymphotropic virus (MTLV) destroying CD4+ T cells. *J Immunol* 1999;**162**:5309–16.

108. Kono DH, Balomenos D, Pearson DL. The prototypic Th2 autoimmunity induced by mercury is dependent on WN-gamma and not Thl/Th2 imbalance. *J Immunol* 1998;**161**:234–40.

109. Anderton SM, Radu CG, Lowrey PA, Ward ES, Wrait DC. Negative selection during the peripheral immune response to antigen. *J Exp Med* 2001;**193**:1–11.

110. Sercarz EE, Lehmann PV, Ametani A. Dominance and crypticity of T cell antigenic determinants. *Annu Rev Immunol* 1993;**11**:729–66.

111. Anderton SM, Wraith DC. Selection and fine-tuning of the autoimmuune T cell repertoire. *Nat Rev Immunol* 2002;**2**:487–98.

112. Maloy KJ, Powrie F. Regulatory T cells in the control of immune pathology. *Nat Imunol* 2001;**2**:816–22.

113. SEM Certified Professionals. CD4+ CD25+ suppressor T cells. *J Exp Med* 2001;**193**:41–5.

114. Itoh M, Takahashi T, Sakaguchi N. Thymus and autoimmunity: production of CD25 +CD4+ naturally anergic and suppressive T cells as a key function of the thymus in maintaining immunologic self tolerance. *J Immunol* 1999;**162**:5317–26.

115. Sakaguchi S, Sakaguchi N, Assano M, Itoh M, Toda M. Immunologic self tolerance maintained by activated T cells expressing IL-2 receptor alpha-chains (CD25): breakdown of a single mechanism of self-tolerance causes various autoimmune diseases. *J Immunol* 1995;**155**:1151–64.

116. Olivares-Villagomez D, Wang Y, Lafaille JJ. Regulatory CD4+ cells expressing endogenous T cell receptor chains protect myelin basic protein-specific transgenic mice from spontaneous autoimmune encephalomyelitis. *J Exp Med* 1998;**188**:1883–94.

117. Trinchieri G. Regulatory role of T cells producing both interferon gamma and interleukin 10 in persistent infection. *J Exp Med* 2001;**194**:53–7.

118. Tishler M, Shoenfeld Y. Vaccination may be associated with autoimmune diseases. *Isr Med Assoc J* 2004;**6**:430–2.

119. Agmon-Levin N, Paz Z, Israeli E, Shoenfeld Y. Vaccines and autoimmunity. *Nat Rev Rheumatol* 2009;**5**:648–52.

120. Koppang EO, Bjerkås I, Haugarvoll E, Chan EK, Szabo NJ, Ono N, et al. Vaccination-induced systemic autoimmunity in farmed Atlantic salmon. *J Immunol* 2008;**181**(7):4807–14.

121. Sundberg JP, Silva KA, Zhang W, Sundberg BA, Edwards K, King LE, et al. Recombinant human hepatitis B vaccine initiating alopecia areata: testing the hypothesis using the C3H/HeJ mouse model. *Vet Dermatol* 2009;**20**(2):99–104.

122. Harima HA, Mendes NF, Mamizuka EM, Mariano M. Effect of glucan on murine lupus evolution and on host resistance to Klebsiella pneumoniae. *J Clin Lab Anal* 1997;**11**:175–8.

123. Johnston WH, Latta H. Acute hematogenous pyelonephritis induced in the rabbit with *Saccharomyces cerevisiae*. An electron microscopic study. *Lab Invest* 1973;**29**:495–505.

124. Satoh M, Reeves WH. Induction of lupus-associated autoantibodies in BALB/c mice by intraperitoneal injection of pristane. *J Exp Med* 1994;**180**:2341–6.

125. Satoh M, Kumar A, Kanwar YS, Reeves WH. Anti-nuclear antibody production and immune-complex glomerulonephritis in BALB/c mice treated with pristane. *Proc Natl Acad Sci USA* 1995;**92**:10934–8.

126. Satoh M, Richards HB, Shaheen VM, Yoshida H, Shaw M, Naim JO, et al. Widespread susceptibility among inbred mouse strains to the induction of lupus autoantibodies by pristane. *Clin Exp Immunol* 2000;**121**:399–405.

127. Kuroda Y, Nacionales DC, Akaogi J, Reeves WH, Satoh M. Autoimmunity induced by adjuvant hydrocarbon oil components of vaccine. *Biomed Pharmacother* 2004;**58**:325–37.

128. Cruz-Tapias P, Agmon-Levin N, Israeli E, Anaya JM, Shoenfeld Y. Autoimmune (auto-inflammatory) syndrome induced by adjuvants (ASIA)—animal models as a proof of concept. *Curr Med Chem* 2013;**20**:4030–6.

129. Colafrancesco S, Agmon-Levin N, Perricone C, Shoenfeld Y. Unraveling the soul of autoimmune diseases: pathogenesis, diagnosis and treatment adding dowels to the puzzle. *Immunol Res* 2013;**56**(2–3):200–5.

130. Perricone C, Agmon-Levin N, Valesini G, Shoenfeld Y. Vaccination in patients with chronic or autoimmune rheumatic diseases: the ego, the id and the superego. *Joint Bone Spine* 2012;**79**(1):1–3.

131. Atzeni F, Bendtzen K, Bobbio-Pallavicini F, Conti F, Cutolo M, Montecucco C, et al. Infections and treatment of patients with rheumatic diseases. *Clin Exp Rheumatol* 2008;**26**(1 Suppl. 48):S67–73.

CHAPTER 14

BCG Vaccination

Moshe Tishler[1]
Department of Medicine B, Asaf Harofe Medical Center, Zrifin, Israel
Tel Aviv University, Sackler School of Medicine, Tel Aviv, Israel
[1]Corresponding Author: tishlerm@netvision.net.il

1 INTRODUCTION

Although vaccination is a very effective tool to prevent infectious diseases, it has a powerful stimulation on the immune system, which has created some fears concerning its role in creating autoimmune phenomena.

This issue has been discussed extensively in the literature for the past decade, both in case reports and in reviews. The relationship between vaccination and autoimmunity is bidirectional. On the one hand, vaccination can prevent autoimmune diseases that might be triggered by infectious agents. On the other hand, many case reports and clinical studies, most of them observational, have described both post-vaccination autoimmune phenomena and full-blown diseases. Establishing a causal relationship between vaccination and autoimmune disease induction is difficult to prove in humans because the need to perform large complex and expensive epidemiological studies will limit their availability.[1]

Moreover, the criteria for such causality are not well defined, because safety cannot be measured directly and such a link can be suspected only indirectly by a temporal relationship of these two events.[2]

Bacillus Calmette–Guérin (BCG) vaccine was derived from an attenuated strain of *Mycobacterium bovis*, and was first administered to humans in 1921. This vaccine, which is almost one century old, remains today the only available vaccine against tuberculosis (TB). It is routinely administered to infants in many countries worldwide with high TB prevalence and to health care employees in endemic areas. This vaccine is also used intravesically as an adjuvant treatment for intermediate- and high-risk superficial bladder cancer with impressive efficacy.

In this chapter the relationship between BCG vaccination, BCG immunotherapy, and autoimmunity is discussed.

Infection and Autoimmunity
http://dx.doi.org/10.1016/B978-0-444-63269-2.00017-9

2 MYCOBACTERIA AND AUTOIMMUNITY

Mycobacteria have long been found to be immunogenic, and many auto-antibodies can be detected with high frequency in patients infected by mycobacteria.[3]

These included ds-DNA, Sm, RNP, Ro, IgM-ACA, and β^2 glycoprotein-1, many of which were above the normal serum concentrations. A similarity between human and mycobacterial antigens has been proven both in humoral and cellular mechanisms.

Monoclonal anti-DNA antibodies derived from both patients and mice with systemic lupus erythematosus (SLE) were found to bind to three glycoproteins extracted from mycobacterial cell walls.[4] The inhibition of such a binding could be inhibited by the prior incubation of antibodies with glycolipid antigens and with anti-SS DNA, thus indicating a sharing of common antigens between human tissue and mycobacteria. Studies performed in the early 1980s in a model of rat with adjuvant arthritis have found a T-cell clone specific for *Mycobacterium tuberculosis*, which was arthritogenic.[5] There is ample evidence which suggests that TB reactive T-cells can potentially recognize self-antigens. This evidence came from both animal models and affected individuals with arthritis. In a model of adjuvant arthritis in rat cross antigenicity between *M. tuberculosis* and human cartilage, proteoglycans have been demonstrated.[6] Furthermore, T-cells responding to the 65-kDa antigen of *M. tuberculosis* have been shown to be present in the synovial fluid of patients with early chronic arthritis.[7]

The immunogenic effect of mycobacteria has not been limited to the strain of the bacteria or to the adjuvant arthritis model. In a pre-diabetic non–obese diabetic (NOD) mice model, a single injected dose of *M. bovis* resulted in the prevention of type 1 diabetes but the appearance of a systemic autoimmune disease similar to SLE manifested by hemolytic anemia, sialadenitis, and glomerulonephritis.[8] Furthermore, a proof-of-concept randomized controlled study done in adults with type 1 diabetes who received BCG vaccine has shown transient elevation of c-peptide, which suggests that BCG stimulates host innate immunity.[9]

Sarcoidosis is another granulomatous disorder of unknown etiology in which autoimmunity probably plays a role. A recent hypothesis suggests that in genetically different individuals the same mycobacterial heat shock proteins may induce different immune responses. This hypothesis is supported by the fact that in epidemiological worldwide studies the distribution of TB is approximately opposite to that of sarcoidosis.[10]

This molecular mimicry between mycobacteria and self-antigens that causes autoimmune responses can be used as a conceptual basis for a potential use of a number of *M. tuberculosis*-specific T-cell epitopes as potential vaccines for therapeutic purposes.[11]

3 BCG IN CLINICAL PRACTICE

BCG is used both as a vaccine for the prevention of TB, and as intravesical instillation for treatment of superficial bladder cancer.

BCG vaccination is routinely used in children worldwide, especially in countries with endemic TB. Reported side effects of vaccination are extremely uncommon. In a study that followed 5.5 million vaccinated children in six European countries, the incidence of systemic side effects was 2.8 cases per million.[12] These systemic side effects were mainly disseminated to organs (bones, joints, liver, meninges) via lymphatic or blood circulation. Miliary spread was exceedingly rare and was seen only in immunocompromised children.

Another complication reported in immunocompetent children is osteoarticular infection with *M. bovis*. The prevalence of such infection varies across Europe and is high in Scandinavian countries (6.4/100,000) while very low in France (0.39/1,000,000).[13]

The explanation of this variation can be explained by many factors, such as age of vaccination, vaccine preparation, and different manufactures. Osteoarticular complications usually occur 20 months after vaccination (range 3–60 months), and the lower limbs are selectively affected with a typical solitary lesion in the metaphyses of long bones.

Given that *M. bovis* strains are usually resistant to a single-drug regimen, combination therapy with rifampin, isoniazide, and ethambutol is given for the first 2 months, followed by rifampin and isoniazide for another 10 months.[14]

A small number of other complications, such as aseptic polyarthritis, sarcoidosis, dermatomyositis, and anterior uveitis,[15–18] have been reported as case reports associated with BCG vaccination.

4 INTRAVESICAL BCG INSTILLATION

Intravesical instillation of BCG has been used successfully since 1976. This method of treatment is given for superficial bladder carcinoma and does not destroy tumor cells directly, but rather increases local immune response against the tumor. Recently updated guidelines of the European Association of Urology recommended that patients with non-muscle-invasive urothelial bladder carcinoma with intermediate- and high-risk tumor should be treated with BCG instillation for 1–3 years accordingly.[19] In most patients, treatment has no serious side effects, and the most common adverse effects such as malaise, low-grade fever, cystitis, and hematuria are self-limited. More serious side effects that have been reported include rash, renal and prostatic abscesses, epididymitis, pneumonitis, hepatitis, and osteoarticular side effects.[20]

Also, various musculoskeletal side effects have been reported, with a prevalence ranging from 0.5% to 1%.[13,21]

Most reviews have shown that patients' complaints were due to arthralgia, but arthritis has not been common. Arthritis secondary to intravesical BCG instillation has been mainly documented as case reports. Two reviews published in 2006 reported 43 and 59 patients, respectively,[11,20] who were compared to patients with a classic pattern of reactive arthritis.

A recent article reviewed 73 papers present in the world literature with a total of 112 patients, but it focused only on 61 papers with a total of 89 patients suitable for evaluation.[21] Most of the reported cases (80%) were males with a mean age of 62.1 ± 10.8 years, and the onset of arthritis from the last instillation was 14 days on average. The clinical manifestation of arthritis was symmetrical polyarticular in about 55%, oligoarticular in about 33%, and monoarticular in 8% of patients.

Although polyarthritis was symmetric in half of the reported cases in those with oligoarthritis, it was symmetric in only 33% of reported cases. The most frequently affected joints were those of the lower limbs, mainly the knees, ankles, and feet. When arthritis presented as monoarticular disease, the only involved joints were knees and ankles, whereas in the polyarticular presentation, the small joints of hands and feet were more frequently affected. Neither the duration of the arthritis nor the levels of inflammatory markers were significantly related to the number, size, or site of the involved joints.

Spinal pain was present in 8% of reported cases and bilateral sacroiliitis in 9% of patients. The mean duration of symptoms in affected patients was about 2 months, and more than 90% of patients recovered completely within 6 months. The prevalence of human leukocyte antigen (HLA) B27 is reported in about 50% of affected patients and was more prevalent in those with polyarticular involvement. The erythrocyte sedimentation rate (ESR) was reported to be elevated in more than 90% of cases, synovial cultures were negative in all patients and radiographic evaluation usually revealed no specific abnormalities.

Treatment regimen, according to reported cases, included mainly NSAIDs; a minority of patients with severe polyarthritis were treated with corticosteroids as well. Overall, arthritis has a favorable course, and pharmacologic treatment is effective in nearly all cases.[26]

5 BCG AND ARTHRITIS: MECHANISM OF ACTION

The exact mechanism of BCG-induced arthritis is not clear and well defined. Studies of animals have shown that the antineoplastic effect of BCG requires an intact host immune system.[22] Clinical and laboratory evidence suggests that the antitumor activity of the vaccine seems to be confined to the site of administration. BCG does not act by the direct killing of the neoplastic cells, but rather by stimulating local inflammatory response and local cytokine production. It has been shown that, following sequential instillation of BCG into the bladder, large quantities of various cytokines can be detected in the urine, including IL-1β, IL-2, IL-6, IL-8, IL-10, TNF-α, IFN-γ, and soluble ICAM-1.[23]

Although response has been reported to be heterogeneous between patients at baseline, the concentration of the various cytokines are increased with repeated BCG instillation. The most likely mechanism involved in BCG arthritis is that of molecular mimicry, as suggested by the shared homology between mycobacterial heat shock protein 65 and cartilage proteoglycans.[6] Moreover, serial biopsies obtained during treatment revealed induction of strong HLA-DR expression by urothelial cells that persisted for several months after completion of therapy.[24]

It is presumed that penetration of the bacteria or bacterial antigens through the wall of the inflamed bladder tissue into the circulation can generate a systemic immune response with the joints as a target. An attack on the joints can take place in genetically susceptible individuals such as those with specific HLA antigens.

Such genetic susceptibility has been found in subjects positive to HLA B27 antigen who were treated with BCG instillation.[22]

Indeed, more than 50% of patients with arthritis after BCG therapy were carrying the HLA B27 antigen, particularly those with more severe polyarthritis.

The effect of generating an effect on a host organism from within has been given the name "Trojan horse"[25] and is not unique to BCG vaccination, but rather to a large number of autoimmune phenomena occurring after vaccination.

6 CONCLUSION

BCG immunization has proved to be a powerful tool both in preventing TB in endemic areas and as a treatment for superficial bladder carcinoma when given intravesically. Side effects of such immunization using both methods have been infrequently recorded and are usually mild and self-limited.

Nevertheless, immunization, especially by intravesical instillation, can act as "a double-edged sword"[27] and trigger autoimmune phenomena and even a full-blown autoimmune disease. This link between mycobacteria and autoimmunity is probably a consequence of molecular mimicry, although genetic and environmental factors might play an important role as well.

REFERENCES

1. Wraith DC, Goldman M, Lambert PH. Vaccination and autoimmune diseases: what is the evidence. *Lancet* 2003;**362**:1659–66.
2. WHO Global advisory committee on vaccine safety. Causality assessment of adverse events following immunization. *Wkly Epidemiol Rec* 2001;**76**:85–9.
3. Elkayam O, Caspi D, Lidgi M, Segal R. Autoantibody profiles in patients with active pulmonary tuberculosis. *Int J Tuberc Lung Dis* 2007;**11**:306–10.
4. Shoenfeld Y, Volmar Y, Coates ARM, Rauch J, Shaul D, Pinhas J. Monoclonal anti-tuberculosis antibodies react with DNA, and monoclonal anti-DNA and autoantibodies react with *M. Tuberculosis*. *Clin Exp Immunol* 1986;**66**:255–61.
5. Holoshitz J, Matitiahu A, Cohen IR. Arthritis induced in rats by cloned T lymphocyte responsive to mycobacteria but not to collagen type II. *J Clin Invest* 1984;**73**:211–15.
6. Van Eden W, Holoshitz J, Nevo Z, Frenkel A, Klujman A, Cohen IR. Arthritis induced by a T-lymphocyte clone that responds to M. tuberculosis and to cartilage proteglycans. *Proc Natl Acad Sci USA* 1985;**82**:5113–20.
7. Pes PC, Schaar CG, Breedveld FC, Van Eden W, Van Embaden JD, de Cohen IR, et al. Synovial fluid T-cell reactivity against 65 kD heat shock protein of mycobacteria in early chronic arthritis. *Lancet* 1988;**2**(8609):478–80.
8. Baxter AG, Horsfall AC, Healy D, Ozegbe P, Day S, Williams DG, et al. Mycobacteria precipitate an SLE-like syndrome in diabetes-prone NOD mice. *Immmunology* 1994;**83**:227–31.
9. Faustman DL, Wang L, Okubo Y, Burger D, Ban L, Man G, et al. Proof-of-concept randomized, controlled clinical trial of Bacillus-Calmette-Guerin for the treatment of long-term type 1 diabetes. *PLoS One* 2012;**7**(8):e41756.
10. Dubaniewicz A. *Mycobacterium tuberculosis* heat shock proteins and autoimmunity in sarcoidosis. *Autoimmun Rev* 2010;**9**:419–24.
11. Mustafa AS, Al-Attiyah R, Hanif SN, Shaban FA. Efficient testing of large pools of M. tuberculosis RD1 peptides and identification of major antigens and immunodominant peptides recognized by human Th1 cells. *Clin Vaccine Immunol* 2008;**15**:916–24.
12. Lotte A, Wasz-Hockert O, Poisson N, Engbaek H, Landmann H, Quast U, et al. Second IUATLD study on complications induced by intradermal BCG-vaccination. *Bull Int Union Tuberc Lung Dis* 1988;**63**:47–59.
13. Clavel G, Grados F, Lefauveau P, Fardellone P. Osteoarticular side effects of BCG therapy. *Joint Bone Spine* 2006;**73**:24–8.

14. Kroger L, Korppi M, Brander E, Kroger H, Wasz-Hockert O, Backman A, et al. Osteitis caused by BCG vaccination a retrospective analysis of 222 cases. *J Infect Dis* 1995;**172**:574–6.
15. Koduli VR, Clague BB. Arthritis after BCG vaccine in a healthy woman. *J Intern Med* 1998;**244**:183–4.
16. Osborne G, Mallon E, Mayon S. Juvenile sarcoidosis after BCG vaccination. *J Am Acad Dermatol* 2003;**48**:99–102.
17. Kass E, Straume S, Munthe E. Dermatomyositis after BCG vaccination. *Lancet* 1978;**1**:772.
18. Spratt A, Key T, Vivian AJ. Chronic anterior uveitis following BCG vaccination: molecular mimicry in action? *J Pediatr Ophtalmol Strabismus* 2008;**45**:252–3.
19. Babjuk M, Burger M, Zigeuner R, Shariat SF, van Rhijn BW, Comperat E, et al. EAU guidelines of non-muscle invasive urothelial carcinoma of bladder: update 2013. *EUR Urol* 2013;**64**:639–53.
20. Sylvester RJ, van der Meijden AP, Lamom DL, Intraversical BCG reduces the risk of progression in patients with superficial bladder cancer: a meta-analysis of the published results of randomized clinical trials. *J Urol* 2002;**168**:1964–70.
21. Lamm D, Stogdill V, Stogdill B, Crispen R. Complications of immunotherapy in 1278 patients with bladder cancer. *J Urol* 1986;**135**:272–4.
22. Tinazzi E, Ficarra V, Simeoni S, Artibani W, Lunardi C. Reactive arthritis following BCG immune therapy for urinary bladder carcinoma: a systematic review. *Rheumatol Int* 2006;**26**:481–8.
23. Jackson AN, Alexandroff AB, Kelly RW, Shibinska A, Esuvaranathan K, et al. Changes in urinary cytokines and soluble intracellular adhesion molecule-1 (ICAM-1) in bladder cancer patients after BCG immunotherapy. *Clin Exp Immunol* 1995;**991**:369–75.
24. Prescott S, James K, Busuttil A, Hargreave TB, Chrisholm GD, Smyth JF. HLA-DR expression by high grade superficial bladder cancer treated with BCG. *Br J Urol* 1989;**63**:264–9.
25. Aron-Maor A, Shoenfeld Y. BCG immunization and the "Trojan Horse" phenomenon of vaccination. *Clin Rheumatol* 2003;**22**:6–7.
26. Bernini L, Manzini CU, Giuggioli D, Sebastian M, Ferri C. Reactive arthritis induced by intravesical BCG therapy for bladder cancer: our clinical experience and systematic review of the literature. *Autoimmun Rev* 2013;**12**:1150–9.
27. Shoenfeld Y, Aron-Maor A, Tania A, Eherenfeld M. BCG and autoimmunity: another two edged sword. *J Autoimmun* 2001;**16**:235–40.

CHAPTER 15

Opportunistic Infections and Autoimmune Diseases

Raquel Faria[*,1], **Cláudia Pereira**[†], **Rute Alves**[†], **Teresa Mendonça**[‡],
Fátima Farinha[‡], **Carlos Vasconcelos**[§]

[*]Internal Medicine Assistant in Medicine Service and Clinic Immunology Unit, Centro Hospitalar do Porto and Unit for Multidisciplinary Research in Biomedicine (UMIB/ICBAS), Porto University, PORTUGAL
[†]Internal Medicine Resident in Medicine Service, Centro Hospitalar do Porto, PORTUGAL
[‡]Internal Medicine Senior Assistant in Medicine Service and Clinic Immunology Unit, Centro Hospitalar do Porto and Unit for Multidisciplinary Research in Biomedicine (UMIB/ICBAS), Porto University, PORTUGAL
[§]Internal Medicine Senior Graduate Assistant and Head of Clinic Immunology Unit, Centro Hospitalar do Porto and Unit for Multidisciplinary Research in Biomedicine (UMIB/ICBAS), Porto University, PORTUGAL
[1]Corresponding Author: raqfaria@gmail.com

1 INTRODUCTION

Infections are common causes of morbidity and mortality in autoimmune diseases, and opportunistic infections are the tip of this problem, emerging as one main causes of morbidity in these patients.

Opportunistic infections may be defined as infection caused by non-pathogenic microorganisms (bacterial, viral, fungal, or protozoan) which become pathogenic when the immune system is systemically or locally impaired by an unrelated disease such as cancer, diabetes, HIV infection, and other immunodeficiencies or immunosuppression therapy.[1,2] Even so, grey areas can be identified with respect to some microorganisms such as *Mycobacteria*, which can cause diseases that are considered definitely opportunistic (e.g. disseminated tuberculosis (TB)) and at the same time can cause other diseases that are not considered opportunistic (e.g. pulmonary and pleural TB). This highlights the need for the addition of a "defective" host to the definition of opportunistic infection.

Several hypotheses explaining the pathogenesis of autoimmune diseases have been described, among them the deregulation of the immune system, the breakdown of the idiotype–anti-idiotype network of antibodies[3] and primary immunodeficiencies based on real-life clinical models: monogenetic immunodeficiencies that lead to secondary autoimmune diseases.[4]

Infection and Autoimmunity
http://dx.doi.org/10.1016/B978-0-444-63269-2.00018-0

Opportunistic infections have been linked to therapy more than diseases itself ever since immunosuppressors were first used to treat autoimmune diseases, but special interest arose with new biologic therapies, which linked specific microorganism infection pathways and cytokines, and the drastic increase in the incidence of very rare diseases.

We revised the mechanism by which autoimmune diseases and exposure to specific therapy increase susceptibility to opportunistic infection and the particularities of some opportunistic infections in autoimmune diseases.

2 METHODS

The PRISMA statement[5] was used as the review protocol (www.plosmedicine.org) based on a search of PubMed and Cochrane databases from inception through October 2013, applying the terms *opportunistic infections, autoimmune diseases, systemic lupus erythematosus (SLE), rheumatoid arthritis (RA), ankylosing spondylitis, vasculitis, myositis, Sjögren syndrome, Toxoplasmosis, Pneumocystis carinii jirovecii, cytomegalovirus (CMV), cryptococcus, histoplasma, John Cunningham (JC) virus, TB, non-tuberculous mycobacteria,* and combinations of these. We reviewed evidence from meta-analyses, randomized controlled trials, and retrospective studies; however, because of the paucity of data regarding some associations, case–control studies, case series, and case reports also were reviewed. We excluded articles written in languages other than English, Spanish, Italian, French, and Portuguese and those that referred to HIV-seropositive patients, cancer patients, post-transplant patients, and patients receiving chemotherapy.

In addition, the references cited in these articles were examined to identify additional reports. We also added some not previously reported cases from our cohort when appropriate.

3 AUTOIMMUNE DISEASE AND SUSCEPTIBILITY TO OPPORTUNISTIC INFECTION

Specific autoimmune diseases cause different susceptibility to opportunistic infections because of their physiopathology, common morbidities, or a different kind of immunosuppression than commonly used (Table 1).[6–18]

Infections and autoimmune diseases have multi-faceted and multi-directional relationships.[19] Some infections, namely viral ones, have pathogenic similarities and share several clinical and laboratory findings with autoimmune diseases.[20–23] As an example, the clinical presentation of some virus-associated vasculitides may be indistinguishable from idiopathic ANCA vasculitis; the

Table 1 Mechanisms of Immunological Dysfunction in Rheumatic Diseases

Disease	Associated Mechanism(s) of Immunological Dysfunction
Rheumatoid arthritis	• Defects in cellular immunity ○ Hyperproduction of IL-17 cells and IL-23 with perpetuation of local inflammation, induction of angiogenesis, osteoclastogenesis and, ultimately, destruction of cartilage and bone ○ Altered regulatory T cells: these cells express TNF-receptor II, which make them susceptible to the deleterious effect of TNF-α • Defects in humoral immunity ○ Hyperproduction of inflammatory cytokines TNF-α and IL-6, contributing to the perpetuation of inflammation and auto-activation of B cells ○ Antibodies against the formation of the self- and immune complex in response to debris of dead cells in RA synovium ○ Formation of tertiary lymphoid structures in synovium by hyperstimulation of B cells by synovium secreted factors such as B-cell activating factor (BAFF) ○ Altered regulatory B cells: these cells overproduce IL-10, probably down-regulating immune response by tolerizing T cells • Chronic hyperinflammatory state ○ Excess production of pro-inflammatory cytokines such as TNF-α
Systemic lupus erythematosus	• Dysfunction of phagocytic activity of monocytes ○ Decreased production of TNF-α; deficit in the generation of superoxide • Dysfunction of B lymphocytes ○ Hypogammaglobulinemia ○ Antibodies against neutrophil cytoplasmic components ○ Antibodies against Fc-γ receptor • Defects in cellular immunity, quantitative and functional alterations of T lymphocytes and its subtypes ○ Lymphopenia ○ Decreased T CD4+ counts ○ Reduced cytokine production (namely IL-2 and IFN-γ) ○ Decreased and altered regulatory T cell population • Functional asplenia

(Continued)

Table 1 Mechanisms of Immunological Dysfunction in Rheumatic Diseases—cont'd

Disease	Associated Mechanism(s) of Immunological Dysfunction

	○ Impaired reticuloendothelial system, with defect in the removal of circulating immune complexes and organisms' elimination
	• Complement low levels and dysfunction
	  ○ Depletion of C1q and C1r/C1s and other complement components: C3, C5–C9
	  ○ Deficit of mannose-binding lectin
	  ○ Opsonization dysfunction (formation of anti-C1q antibodies)
	  ○ alteration of receptor Fc-γ RIIa
	• Decreased production of immunoglobulin

Sjögren's syndrome	• T CD4+ lymphocytopenia • Low levels of complement, especially C4 (either genetically determined or secondary to consumption)

Table 2 Induction and Perpetuation of Autoimmune Diseases by Infections

Antigen-Specific Mechanisms	Non-Specific Mechanisms
1. Molecular mimicry	1. Bystander activation
2. Expression of modified, cryptic, or new antigen determinants 3. Superantigens	

experienced gained from studying hepatitis C virus-associated cryoglobulinemic vasculitis suggests that treating the accompanying viral infections can lead to remission of vasculitis.[20,21]

Infections can not only induce or precipitate autoimmune diseases (Table 2),[6,7] but may also protect from autoimmunity or even abolish an ongoing autoimmune process depending on the interaction between the microorganism and host.[6,7,23] Therefore, we should also look at microorganisms as potential agents able to modulate the immune system.[6,7,24–27]

Molecular mimicry represents a shared immunologic epitope between a microbe and the host.[28] Pathogens bear elements that are similar enough in amino acid sequence or structure to self-antigen. Immune response can eventually turn towards the self-peptide as a result of cross-reactivity, leading to the activation of naïve, auto-reactive T cells specific to the corresponding self-molecule. Molecular mimicry can be responsible for initiating an autoimmune phenomenon in various diseases including rheumatic fever, SLE[24] and systemic sclerosis,[25] but many other factors are necessary to develop autoimmunity.[6]

Bystander activation of auto-reactive immune T cells by virus–activated antigen-presenting cells can initiate autoimmune diseases.[6,7]

There are some case reports of a inaugural diagnosis of autoimmune disease being preceded by a viral infection, namely, CMV esophagitis and SLE[29] and CMV myocarditis and SLE.[23] Challenging and possible model cases are also those in which one episode of an autoimmune disease happens at the same time as an infection and remission of the disease occurs after resolving the infection: *Helicobacter pylori* infection and immune thrombocytopenia,[30] CMV infection and ANCA positive vasculitis,[21,31] or ganglionic TB and uni-episodic SLE (not reported case from our cohort).

3.1 Rheumatoid Arthritis

RA is the most common systemic autoimmune disease, occurring in about 1% of population. Unresolved systemic inflammation and immune deregulation (Table 1) is mainly seen in joints, but involvement of several other organs usually occurs (e.g. the lungs in accelerated atherosclerosis).

In patients with RA, diminished survival is associated with comorbidities of the disease itself,[32,33] cardiovascular accelerated disease or infection. Common and opportunistic infections in RA occur mainly associated with immunosuppression or when intrinsic effects of RA on certain organ systems develop, specifically the musculoskeletal systems[34–38] and lungs (related or not to RA).

Propensity scores have been proposed to evaluate the risk of some opportunistic infection in RA,[39] mainly for *Pneumocystis* pneumonia (PCP),[40] herpes zoster (HZ),[41] and TB.[39] They all share as risk factors age older than 65 years, structural lung disease and previous exposure to specific immunosuppressive therapies (dose and duration of steroid use and methotrexate [MTX]).

Different classes of immunosuppressive drugs have been used to treat autoimmune diseases. They act in different pathways of the immune system, resulting in different susceptibilities to particular infective agents (Table 3).[12,36,42]

The steroid-related risk of infection is dependent on dose and duration (increases 1.6-fold when 20–40 mg/day are used for 4–6 weeks) and is due to its ubiquitous depression of the immune system.[42,43] Classical disease-modifying anti-rheumatic drugs (DMARDs) also increase susceptibility to infection, but the actual relative risk is confounded by the association with steroids.[42]

Biologic DMARDs are generally safer than classical immunosuppressors, but specific concerns should be kept in mind. Anti-TNF drugs favor opportunistic infection by intracellular pathogens and reactivation of chronic latent infections such as TB, histoplasmosis, *Listeria,* and hepatitis

Table 3 Immunological Dysfunction Mechanisms and Their Relationship with Pharmacologic Agents and Infectious Pathogens in Autoimmune Diseases

Immunological Abnormality	Pharmacologic Agent	Bacteria	Fungus	Virus	Protozoal
Cellular immunity dysfunction	Corticosteroids Methotrexate Azathioprine Cyclosporine A	*Mycobacterium* spp. *Listeria* spp. *Nocardia* spp. *Salmonella* spp.	*Pneumocystis jirovecii* *Cryptococcus neoformans*	Cytomegalovirus Epstein–Barr virus Varizella zoster virus	*Toxoplasma gondii* *Strongyloides stercoralis*
Humoral immunity dysfunction	Corticosteroids (high dose) Azathioprine Cyclophosphamide and other alkylating agents	*Streptococcus pneumoniae* *Hemophilus influenzae* *Neisseria* spp.			
Quantitative or functional neutropenia and/or qualitative defect of phagocytic function	Corticosteroids Azathioprine Methotrexate Cyclophosphamide and other alkylating agents	*Staphylococcus aureus* *Streptococcus* spp. *Nocardia* spp. *Escherichia coli* *Pseudomonas aeruginosa* *Klebsiella pneumoniae* Other Enterobactericeae	*Candida* spp. *Aspergillus* spp.		
Tumor necrosis factor blockage	Infliximab Adalimumab Etanercept Golimumab	*Mycobacterium* spp. *Listeria* spp.	*Histoplasma* spp.		

B virus. They usually occur in the first 12 months of therapy.[42] Opportunistic infections are very rare with rituximab and tocilizumab and were not reported with abatacept, anakinra, or the more recent tofacitinib. The risk that might be caused by biological treatment is probably related to association therapy with cyclophosphamide, MTX, or other DMARDs.[42]

3.2 Systemic Lupus Erythematosus

SLE is a multisystemic, heterogeneous, chronic inflammatory disease of unknown etiology. Among patients with SLE the leading causes of death are infections,[44–50] cardiovascular diseases, and renal failure.[51,52] Different organs may have different mechanisms of injury mediated by autoantibodies, immunocomplex production, and probably direct cytotoxicity.[51,53] The etiopathogenic pathways of SLE have been extensively studied in the last two decades, and several mechanisms seem to be involved (Table 1); viral and bacterial infections can work as a trigger for the development and/or exacerbation of SLE.[54]

Most infections are caused by common pathogens, frequently bacteria,[50,55] and increasing evidence shows opportunistic infections contribute to mortality in patients with SLE.[14,56] In addition to being an important cause of morbidity and mortality, infections are a cause for hospitalization: up to 30% of patients with infections are hospitalized.[14]

Factors associated with the occurrence of infection in patients with SLE are previous infection – almost 50% of patients have recurrent episodes of infection – and defects in clearance of immunocomplexes by the spleen, resulting in functional asplenia, which is present in 5% of patients with SLE and seems to correlate with disease activity,[57] renal lupus investment,[14] immunosuppressive therapy,[54] and invasive medical procedures.[58] Genetic alterations that predispose to SLE are described in Table 1.

It is important to highlight that the presence of infection in patients with SLE poses a real challenge to the physicians because the distinction between infection and flare-up of disease can be difficult to distinguish or can coexist.[14]

In our cohort of 672 patients with lupus, 17 cases (2.5%) of opportunistic infections were identified: extrapulmonary TB (7 cases); invasive fungal infections (2 pulmonary aspergillosis, 2 cryptococcal meningitis, 1 invasive *Microsporum canis*, 1 *Pneumocystis jiroveci* pneumonia); viral infections (2 JC virus, 2 CMV); and 1 bacterial infection (disseminated salmonellosis).

3.3 Sjögren's Syndrome

Primary Sjögren's syndrome (pSS) is a chronic autoimmune disorder primarily characterized by mononuclear cell infiltration of exocrine glands and leading to parenchymal damage and secretory impairment. The spectrum of this disease extends from an autoimmune exocrinopathy to more widespread and systemic involvement with chronic B-cell lymphocyte hyperstimulation.[59] Hematologic abnormalities such as cytopenias, monoclonal gammopathies, lymphoproliferative disorders (mainly non-Hodgkin's lymphoma),[6,59] and type II cryoglobulinemia are commonly present. The development of cryoglobulinemia seems to be a consequence of B-cell hyperstimulation and rheumatoid factor production. Although its pathway is not fully understood, one hypothesis was introduced by showing "occult" hepatitis C and hepatitis B virus infection as possible triggers (with antibodies and viral load below the threshold of detection).[6]

T CD4+ lymphocytopenia also is found in 5% of patents with pSS, is associated with anti-Ro/SSA antibody positivity and can predispose to opportunistic infections, but there are only anecdotal case reports of opportunistic infections in patients with pSS.[60]

4 OPPORTUNISTIC INFECTIONS

Recognition and treatment of opportunistic infections may be delayed because the clinical manifestations of infections often are indistinguishable from the underlying autoimmune disease.[61,62] We review here the most relevant opportunistic infections in autoimmune diseases.

4.1 Mycobacteria

Mycobacterium spp. are organized in two groups: slow-growing species (including *M. tuberculosis* complex, *M. avium* complex, *M. escrofulaceum*, *M. xenopi*, *M. hekershornense*, *M. gordonae,* and *M. kansasii*) and rapidly growing ones (*M. chelonae*, *M. mucogenicum*, *M. marinum*, *M. fortuitum*, *M. parafortuitum*). They are ubiquitous and aerobic, and some are pathogenic to humans. Although the most known mycobacteria is *M. tuberculosis*, most of them colonize an asymptomatic host and cause infection in susceptible patients with local or systemic dysfunction of immune mechanisms caused by factors such as HIV infection, immunosuppressive therapies, organ transplant, autoimmune diseases, malnutrition, and alcohol use.[63]

The most well-known mechanism by which *Mycobacteria* provokes disease is the formation of granuloma deficits.[64,65] This is highly dependent on TNF and the costimulation between T cells and the monocyte–macrophage system.[65]

4.1.1 Mycobacterium tuberculosis

Patients with RA are at increased risk for TB all over the world, especially in countries with medium to high prevalence of TB. There are factors favoring TB in RA: administration of immunosuppressive drugs (steroids and nonbiologic and biologic DMARDs), a latent or active history of TB, and endemic area of origin.[66]

In the United States, the incidence of TB in patients with RA is 6.2 in 100,000 patients; after the introduction of anti-TNF therapy, this incidence rose to 52.5 in 100,000.[63] In Japan, the incidence among the general population is 25.8 in 100,000 people and is increased 3.21-fold in patients with RA.[63]

TB incidence among the general Spanish population was 21 in 100,000 people per year. In the Spanish registry, there is a fourfold increased risk of TB in patients with RA,[67] even before exposure to anti-TNF. Among these patients, the incidence was 143 in 100,000 patients per year for those treated with MTX, 2703 in 100,000 patients per year in those treated with azathioprine, and 4878 in 100,000 patients per year in those treated with anti-TNF-α therapy.[68] With these biologics, *Mycobacteria* represents the most commonly reported opportunistic infection,[69] increasing the risk of active TB up to five times.[65]

According to the FDA database, the rates of TB in patients treated with infliximab and etanercept were 54 and 28 per 100,000, respectively,[70,71] pointing to a decreased risk with the anti-TNF receptor.

In our cohort, we audited the TB incidence in steroid-treated patients attending the clinic in a 3-month period. Four TB cases (3 pulmonary and 1 pleural TB) were identified in 186 patients exposed to steroids independent of additional immunosuppressive therapies, representing an overall incidence of 183 in 100,000 steroid-treated patients per year (with a medium daily dose of steroid of 8.8 mg/day). The mean daily dose of steroids was the same as that in the overall group, but they showed nearly twice the length of treatment and underlying disease duration. The incidence observed was much higher than the general population incidence in our geographic area (45.4 in 100,000).

This highlights the role of the geographic prevalence of the disease and endemic areas.[72]

Although these data are from RA studies, similar incidence and risk were established for ankylosing spondylitis[73,74] and bowel inflammatory disease exposed to anti-TNF.[75] These findings have important implications for the monitoring of these patients and indicate that even atypical signs and symptoms of TB should be investigated carefully.[76]

The risk of developing TB can be minimized by screening for exposure risks and latent TB before the start of therapy.[76] Recommendations are different between countries because of diverse incidence rates for TB, as well as the vaccination status, among the various populations; both of these factors influence the interpretation of screening test results.[76] In Spain,[77] after the induction of official recommendations for the screening and management of latent TB, the rates for active TB in patients treated with biologics decreased by 78% in total, and among patients with RA, it dropped by 83%.

The incidence of all kinds of mycobacteriosis is also increased in patients with SLE; this is attributable to multiple immune abnormalities, as well as to immunosuppressive therapy.[78–80] A Spanish study[81] found a sixfold higher incidence of TB compared to the general population.

Predisposing factors for TB in patients with SLE include highly active SLE, particularly active lupus nephritis, chronic corticosteroid treatment,[82] and the use of immunosuppressive drugs.[78,80,82–84]

Extrapulmonary TB is more frequent in autoimmune diseases. In RA, shortly after the start of anti-TNF therapy,[66] 65% of TB cases manifest as extrapulmonary TB and 25% as disseminated disease.[66,73,76,85–87] This probably represents a reactivation of a latent infection, whereas when it appears later it usually is a new infection that progresses directly to active disease.[65]

In patients with SLE, serious local and disseminated infection are more likely, and extrapulmonary involvement is more frequent,[88,89] including meningitis,[90] abdominal TB and cutaneous,[91–93] joint[94] and spine involvement.[95,96]

Curiously, it seems that mycobacteriosis in SLE is mainly caused by *M. tuberculosis* early in the course of disease, but in later years non-tuberculous *Mycobacteria* infection predominates, more frequently involving skin and soft tissue.[51,82]

4.1.2 Non-Tuberculous Mycobacteria

M. avium complex and *Mycobacterium kansasii* account for most episodes of non-tuberculous systemic disease, particularly since the arrival of the AIDS epidemic; the lungs and lymph nodes are the most common sites of infection.

In contrast, in autoimmune diseases, most of the rapid or slow-growth non-tuberculous *Mycobacteria* infections are cutaneous or subcutaneous (*M. mucogenicum*,[91] *M. chelonae*,[92,97] *M. marinum*,[98] *M. escrofulaceum*[93]), but infections at other sites such as breast implant (*M. fortuitum*[99]), spondylodisciitis (*M. hekershornense*[95]), and lung (*M. xenopi*[100]) also were described.

4.2 Cytomegalovirus

CMV infection has evolved from an endemic disease worldwide[101] (prevalence between 40% and 100%)[102] to be considered one of the most common serious viral opportunistic pathogens. Its reactivation is common, unpredictable and potentially severe[101] and it causes significant morbidity and mortality in immunocompromised patients.[103]

Different studies have suggested that lymphopenia,[104] SLE,[105,106] dermatomyositis,[105] hypogammaglobulinemia,[107] reactivation with elevated viral loads,[108] and intensive immunosuppressive therapies[109] are poor prognostic factors and/or contribute to patients being highly susceptible to CMV infection and disease. Besides classical systemic autoimmune diseases, some reports also highlight the challenging diagnosis and management of CMV gut infection in bowel inflammatory diseases.[101,110]

Depletion of TNF by treatment with TNF-α blockade may facilitate the risk of reactivation of viral infection,[111,112] but in a 2010 literature review of 125 cases of CMV infection following TNF-α blocking therapy in rheumatic diseases (124 were taking infliximab), most were using more than one immunosuppressive drug[112] in addition to anti-TNF. In autoimmune diseases, the most common organ affected by CMV is the lung,[101,113–116] sometimes with bizarre pulmonary cavitation;[113,117–119] fewer patients have gastrointestinal involvement,[107,110,120,121] pancreatitis,[122,123] retinitis,[124] and severe life-threatening manifestations.[125–127]

Some authors suggest that patients complicated by CMV antigenemia are susceptible to combined opportunistic infections such as PCP.[109]

4.3 John Cunningham Virus

The JC virus is ubiquitous in the general population, and asymptomatic infection is thought to occur during childhood.[128,129] A healthy immune system maintains the latent virus in several organs and restrains it from causing disease. There is some doubt whether the central nervous system (CNS) is an actual site of latency.[128]

JC virus reactivation causes progressive multifocal leukoencephalopathy (PML), which is a rare progressive demyelinating disease of the CNS. It is usually fatal (20–50% of patients die within 3 months) or causes incapacitating neurological impairments.[128,130] Although there is no clear threshold of CD4+ lymphocytes below which JC virus reactivates, some authors consider measuring CD4+ lymphocyte levels before initiating rituximab.[13]

Most reported cases occurred in HIV infection, but it also has been reported in patients with lymphoproliferative malignancies and transplant recipients taking immunosuppressive therapy.[131,132] In the past decade, PML has been described in patients after taking natalizumab and rituximab, although some patients with SLE, RA, and vasculitis[131] had not been previously exposed to biologics.[13] Despite being a rare disease, PML should be suspected in immunosuppressed patients with gradual uncommon neurological manifestations.[13]

Patients with RA have twice the incidence of PML as the general population (0.4 in 100,000), rising to 10 times (4 in 100,000) among those treated with rituximab. To date, no cases have been reported after treatment with TNF-α antagonists.[129,133]

PML prevalence is the highest in SLE (4 in 100,000),[132] and it can be found in patients taking only mild immunosuppressive therapy (≤ 15 mg/day prednisone or antimalarial agents) as well as those taking MTX, mycofenolate mofetil,[134] calcineurin inhibitors, cyclophosphamide, azathioprine, chlorambucil, anti-TNF therapy, or other monoclonal antibodies. However, there are reported cases among patients not undergoing any immunosuppressive therapy.[53,128,132,135–138] Furthermore, PML may mimic neuropsychiatric lupus involvement, which makes this interaction even more complex.[13]

Of interest, natalizumab, a biological agent approved for multiple sclerosis[139,140] and Crohn's disease, shows the most pronounced risk association: the PML prevalence after 2 years of treatment in multiple sclerosis is 100 in 100,000.[140]

4.4 Varicella Zoster Virus

Varicella zoster virus is a human herpesvirus that causes chickenpox during primary infection, stays latent in sensory ganglia, and may reactivate as HZ.[141] HZ is a common condition (affecting 10–30% of people throughout their lifetime)[112,142–144] that causes substantial pain and morbidity:[41] 18% of cases result in postherpetic neuralgia and 10–15% involve ocular tissues, with the potential for permanent vision loss.[141,145]

It is more clearly associated with ageing,[41] but people with decreased cell-mediated immunity, such as those with HIV or malignancies or taking immunosuppressors, are also at a higher risk for HZ and its severe disseminated forms.[41,146,147] In addition to a direct association with specific rheumatic disorders, namely SLE and its clinical activity,[141] therapies that decrease cell-mediated immunity increase the risk of HZ:[41] prednisolone has the highest estimated risk,[41,148] and association with DMARDs (cyclophosphamide,[149,150] azathioprine, and leflunomide[41]) increases that risk.

In the 5000 patients within the German RABBIT registry,[151] 86 HZ episodes were found, with crude incidence rates of 11.1, 8.9, and 5.6 per 1000 patient-years for monoclonal antibodies, etanercept and conventional DMARDs, respectively. In an international rituximab clinical trial of RA (2578 patients with 5013 patient-years of follow-up), HZ infections occurred in 49 patients (2%), a rate of 0.98 events per 100 patient-years.[152] Thus, HZ is nowadays one of the most common opportunistic infection related to immunosuppression.

4.5 Pneumocystis jirovecii

P. jirovecii (formerly *P. carinii*) is a yeast-like fungus asymptomatically present in the lungs of up to 65% of adults,[153,154] but it leads to clinical disease and tissue damage only in the setting of cell-mediated immune dysfunction, predominantly CD4 T lymphocyte counts of $<200/\text{mm}^{3}$.[153] PCP is an uncommon but serious life-threatening complication in immunocompromised hosts, such as those receiving intensive immunosuppressant therapies.[155,156]

The overall incidence of PCP infection in autoimmune diseases is approximately 1–2%.[157] Interestingly, the frequency of PCP differed substantially among patients with different autoimmune diseases:[153,158] Wegener's granulomatosis (WG) and polyarteritis nodosa seemed to have the greatest susceptibility to PCP[158]—up to 6% of patients with WG had PCP.[157] In a meta-analysis of PCP infection in 11,905 autoimmune patients, 12% of patients with WG, 6% with dermatomyositis, 5% with SLE, and 1% with RA developed PCP.[159] Although it is controversial, it seems that prophylaxis is only recommended in vasculitis.[21,31,160–162]

Several risk factors for PCP have been described in individuals with autoimmune diseases: age older than 65 years;[40,163] lymphopenia[158,164] and decreased CD4 counts;[153] underlying lung disease;[165,166] corticosteroid use (both increased dose and duration have been associated with an elevated risk); and use of more than one immunosuppressive agent.[158,164,167] In Japan, several studies showed that PCP is probably due to new infection rather than reactivation of a previous one.[168] One of the causes of reinfection could be airborne contact with outpatients in the clinic waiting room.[169,170]

It is important to know that PCP in patients without HIV, particularly those with autoimmune diseases, often presents with a more severe and fulminant course,[153,171] with higher morbidity and mortality rates (30–60% in autoimmune diseases[158,159] vs. 10–15% in HIV[171]). Furthermore, the quantitative fungal burden of *P. jirovecii* in the lungs of individuals with PCP infection was found to be significantly lower in patients without HIV, supporting that the increased severity of the disease may be the result of an immune-mediated inflammatory process and not a pathogen-driven mechanism of tissue damage.[168,172] The serological tests β-D-glucan has been shown to be useful in early diagnosis and prognostic assessment.[173]

4.6 *Cryptococcus* Species

Cryptococcus spp. are yeast-like encapsulated organisms, widespread in soils. The most common species is *C. neoformans*, which is found in the feces of wild birds (mostly pigeons) that is inhaled when dust is stirred up. It causes infection after pulmonary colonization and spreads through the blood to other organs.[174]

Cell-mediated immunity seems to be responsible for host defence against *Cryptococcus*,[175] so most cases of cryptococcosis are associated with AIDS, but it is increasingly found in organ transplant recipients and patients with other conditions associated with immunosuppression therapy, cancer, diabetes, and SLE.[176]

Cryptococcus is a rare opportunistic infection in autoimmune diseases, and organ involvement seems to be different across connective tissue diseases. In inflammatory arthritis, the lungs[177,178] are the main organs involved, and it occurs more often after anti-TNF agents;[177] one case occurred after tofacitinib.[178] In SLE, the CNS[160,175,179–183] is mainly infected with or without immunosuppression and can be completely asymptomatic or present with unspecific features that may be mistaken for manifestations of SLE activity.[184] The main risk factor identified was the cumulative dose of prednisolone in the previous year.[175] Kidney infection, disseminated cryptococcosis,[185] and tenosynovitis cryptococcosis[186] have been anecdotally reported.

4.7 Toxoplasma gondii

T. gondii is a ubiquitous intracellular protozoan, and infection is mainly acquired by ingesting food or water contaminated with oocysts shed by cats or by eating undercooked or raw meat carrying cysts in the tissue.[187] Toxoplasmosis is among the most prevalent chronic parasitic infections in humans and is emerging as an important opportunistic pathogen in immunocompromised patients.[188] The role of toxoplasmosis in autoimmune diseases has not received as much focus as that of other microbial pathogens, although cellular immunity is essential for protection against its infection.[189,190] TNF is an important mediator of resistance to this parasite,[191] but there are only a few reported cases presenting mainly as chorioretinitis in patients treated with anti-TNF-α therapies.[187,192–194]

4.8 Histoplasmosis

Histoplasma capsulatum is a dimorphic fungus that causes infection almost exclusively in endemic areas. Its infection is usually insidious and subclinical, and the fungus can remain quiescent in granulomas.[195] It affects mainly immunocompromised hosts[196] and has a poor outcome (95% mortality).[197]

The three major clinical presentations are, by order of frequency, pulmonary, primary cutaneous, and progressive disseminated histoplasmosis; the latter is responsible for about 10% of cases.[198]

Histoplasmosis is rare in patients with SLE.[196] Disseminated presentations mostly affect lungs, liver, and bone marrow; diagnosis may be challenging because it may mimic an SLE flare.[199] The risk of developing histoplasmosis is associated with not only immunosuppressive therapy[196,200] but also inherent defects in humoral and cellular immunity; these may put patients with SLE per se at higher risk,[199] even without immunosuppressive agents.[201,202] Interestingly, when compared to controls taking similar amounts of steroids (patients with RA or nephrotic syndrome), patients with SLE are still at a higher risk.[203]

Anti-TNF therapies in RA[195] seem to increase patient susceptibility (especially infliximab),[204–206] although the majority of patients were taking a second immunomodulating drug when histoplasmosis developed.[195,207–212]

5 CONCLUSIONS

Autoimmune diseases have several mechanisms by which they make patients more susceptible to common and opportunistic infections. These might be related either to genetic or acquired immune defects because of the disease itself or immunosuppressive therapy.

Some opportunistic infections are more common and related to specific deficits such as *M. tuberculosis* and anti-TNF biologic therapies. HZ is nowadays one of the most common opportunistic infections related to immunosuppression. PCP and *Cryptococcus* infection also have been reported, and their clinical manifestations are different from the more common AIDS-related situations, which should increase doctors' awareness. Other rarer infections such as PML are more common in autoimmune diseases and probably more related to exposure to natalizumab and rituximab.

Furthermore, it is important to highlight that the presence of infection in autoimmune patients poses a real challenge to physicians because the distinction between infection and a flare-up of disease can be difficult to distinguish or can coexist.

REFERENCES

1. Mosby Inc. *Mosby's medical dictionary*. 8th ed. St. Louis, MO: Mosby; 2009, xiv, A1–A43, 1998.
2. Longe JL, Blanchfield DS. *Gale Research Company. Gale encyclopedia of medicine*. 2nd ed. Detroit, MI: Gale Group; 2002.
3. Lindenmann J. Homobodies: do they exist? *Ann Immunol (Paris)* 1979;**130**(2):311–18.
4. Cheng MH, Anderson MS. Monogenic autoimmunity. *Annu Rev Immunol* 2012;**30**:393–427.
5. Moher D, Liberati A, Tetzlaff J, Altman DG, Group P. Preferred reporting items for systematic reviews and meta-analyses: the PRISMA statement. *PLoS Med* 2009;**6**(7): e1000097.
6. Sfriso P, Ghirardello A, Botsios C, Tonon M, Zen M, Bassi N, et al. Infections and autoimmunity: the multifaceted relationship. *J Leukoc Biol* 2010;**87**(3):385–95.
7. Fujinami RS, von Herrath MG, Christen U, Whitton JL. Molecular mimicry, bystander activation, or viral persistence: infections and autoimmune disease. *Clin Microbiol Rev* 2006;**19**(1):80–94.
8. Al-Hadithy H, Isenberg DA, Addison IE, Goldstone AH, Snaith ML. Neutrophil function in systemic lupus erythematosus and other collagen diseases. *Ann Rheum Dis* 1982;**41**(1):33–8.
9. Iliopoulos AG, Tsokos GC. Immunopathogenesis and spectrum of infections in systemic lupus erythematosus. *Semin Arthritis Rheum* 1996;**25**(5):318–36.
10. Ng WL, Chu CM, Wu AK, Cheng VC, Yuen KY. Lymphopenia at presentation is associated with increased risk of infections in patients with systemic lupus erythematosus. *QJM* 2006;**99**(1):37–47.
11. Ehrenfeld M, Urowitz MB, Platts ME. Selective C4 deficiency, systemic lupus erythematosus, and Whipple's disease. *Ann Rheum Dis* 1984;**43**(1):91–4.

12. Greenberg SB. Infections in the immunocompromised rheumatologic patient. *Crit Care Clin* 2002;**18**(4):931–56.

13. Brandao M, Damasio J, Marinho A, da Silva AM, Vasconcelos J, Neves E, et al. Systemic lupus erythematosus, progressive multifocal leukoencephalopathy, and T-CD4+ lymphopenia. *Clin Rev Allergy Immunol* 2012;**43**(3):302–7.

14. Enberg GM, Kahn ChM, Goity FC, Villalon SM, Zamorano RJ, Figueroa EF. Infections in patients with systemic lupus erythematosus. *Rev Med Chil* 2009;**137** (10):1367–74.

15. Garred P, Voss A, Madsen HO, Junker P. Association of mannose-binding lectin gene variation with disease severity and infections in a population-based cohort of systemic lupus erythematosus patients. *Genes Immun* 2001;**2**(8):442–50.

16. Salmon JE, Pricop L. Human receptors for immunoglobulin G: key elements in the pathogenesis of rheumatic disease. *Arthritis Rheum* 2001;**44**(4):739–50.

17. Salmon JE, Millard SS, Brogle NL, Kimberly RP. Fc gamma receptor IIIb enhances Fc gamma receptor IIa function in an oxidant-dependent and allele-sensitive manner. *J Clin Invest* 1995;**95**(6):2877–85.

18. Burmester GR, Pratt AG, Scherer HU, van Laar JM. Rheumatoid arthritis: pathogenesis and clinical features. In: Biljsma JWJ, editor. *EULAR textbook on rheumatic diseases.* 1st ed. United Kingdom: BMJ Group; 2012. p. 206–31.

19. Doria A, Sarzi-Puttini P, Shoenfeld Y. Infections, rheumatism and autoimmunity: the conflicting relationship between humans and their environment. *Autoimmun Rev* 2008;**8**(1):1–4.

20. Gross WL. New concepts in treatment protocols for severe systemic vasculitis. *Curr Opin Rheumatol* 1999;**11**(1):41–6.

21. Meyer MF, Hellmich B, Kotterba S, Schatz H. Cytomegalovirus infection in systemic necrotizing vasculitis: causative agent or opportunistic infection? *Rheumatol Int* 2000;**20** (1):35–8.

22. Cunha BA, Gouzhva O, Nausheen S. Severe cytomegalovirus (CMV) community-acquired pneumonia (CAP) precipitating a systemic lupus erythematosus (SLE) flare. *Heart Lung* 2009;**38**(3):249–52.

23. Hachfi W, Laurichesse JJ, Chauveheid MP, Houhou N, Bonnet D, Longuet P, et al. Acute cytomegalovirus infection revealing systemic lupus erythematosus. *Rev Med Interne* 2011;**32**(1):e6–8.

24. Doria A, Canova M, Tonon M, Zen M, Rampudda E, Bassi N, et al. Infections as triggers and complications of systemic lupus erythematosus. *Autoimmun Rev* 2008;**8** (1):24–8.

25. Randone SB, Guiducci S, Cerinic MM. Systemic sclerosis and infections. *Autoimmun Rev* 2008;**8**(1):36–40.

26. Kallenberg CG, Tadema H. Vasculitis and infections: contribution to the issue of auto-immunity reviews devoted to "autoimmunity and infection" *Autoimmun Rev* 2008;**8** (1):29–32.

27. Patole PS, Pawar RD, Lichtnekert J, Lech M, Kulkarni OP, Ramanjaneyulu A, et al. Coactivation of Toll-like receptor-3 and -7 in immune complex glomerulonephritis. *J Autoimmun* 2007;**29**(1):52–9.

28. Fujinami RS, Oldstone MB, Wroblewska Z, Frankel ME, Koprowski H. Molecular mimicry in virus infection: crossreaction of measles virus phosphoprotein or of herpes simplex virus protein with human intermediate filaments. *Proc Natl Acad Sci USA* 1983;**80**(8):2346–50.

29. Kellermayer R, Kim ST, Perez M, Tatevian N, Dishop M, Abrams S, et al. Cytomegalovirus esophagitis preceding the diagnosis of systemic lupus erythematosus. *Endoscopy* 2007;**39**(Suppl. 1):E218.

30. Teawtrakul N, Sawadpanich K, Sirijerachai C, Chansung K, Wanitpongpun C. Clinical characteristics and treatment outcomes in patients with *Helicobacter pylori*-positive chronic immune thrombocytopenic purpura. *Platelets* 2013; http://dx.doi.org/10.3109/09537104.2013.841883.

31. Palsson R, Choi HK, Niles JL. Opportunistic infections are preceded by a rapid fall in antineutrophil cytoplasmic antibody (ANCA) titer in patients with ANCA associated vasculitis. *J Rheumatol* 2002;**29**(3):505–10.

32. Vaughan JH. Infection and rheumatic diseases: a review (2). *Bull Rheum Dis* 1990;**39**(2):1–8.

33. Doran MF, Crowson CS, Pond GR, O'Fallon WM, Gabriel SE. Frequency of infection in patients with rheumatoid arthritis compared with controls: a population-based study. *Arthritis Rheum* 2002;**46**(9):2287–93.

34. Riise T, Jacobsen BK, Gran JT, Haga HJ, Arnesen E. Total mortality is increased in rheumatoid arthritis. A 17-year prospective study. *Clin Rheumatol* 2001;**20**(2):123–7.

35. Venables PJ. Infection and rheumatoid arthritis. *Curr Opin Rheumatol* 1989;**1**(1):15–20.

36. Segal BH, Sneller MC. Infectious complications of immunosuppressive therapy in patients with rheumatic diseases. *Rheum Dis Clin North Am* 1997;**23**(2):219–37.

37. Rowe IF, Deans AC, Keat AC. Pyogenic infection and rheumatoid arthritis. *Postgrad Med J* 1987;**63**(735):19–22.

38. Symmons DP, Jones MA, Scott DL, Prior P. Longterm mortality outcome in patients with rheumatoid arthritis: early presenters continue to do well. *J Rheumatol* 1998;**25**(6):1072–7.

39. Winthrop KL. Serious infections with antirheumatic therapy: are biologicals worse? *Ann Rheum Dis* 2006;**65**(Suppl. 3):iii54–7.

40. Mori S, Cho I, Ichiyasu H, Sugimoto M. Asymptomatic carriage of *Pneumocystis jiroveci* in elderly patients with rheumatoid arthritis in Japan: a possible association between colonization and development of *Pneumocystis jiroveci* pneumonia during low-dose MTX therapy. *Mod Rheumatol* 2008;**18**(3):240–6.

41. Wolfe F, Michaud K, Chakravarty EF. Rates and predictors of herpes zoster in patients with rheumatoid arthritis and non-inflammatory musculoskeletal disorders. *Rheumatology (Oxford)* 2006;**45**(11):1370–5.

42. Van Delden C. Infectious risks of immunomodulating therapies in rheumatology. *Rev Med Suisse* 2006;**2**(57):738–40, 43–5.

43. Fabre S, Gibert C, Lechiche C, Dereure J, Jorgensen C, Sany J. Visceral leishmaniasis infection in a rheumatoid arthritis patient treated with infliximab. *Clin Exp Rheumatol* 2005;**23**(6):891–2.

44. Bellomio V, Spindler A, Lucero E, Berman A, Santana M, Moreno C, et al. Systemic lupus erythematosus: mortality and survival in Argentina. A multicenter study. *Lupus* 2000;**9**(5):377–81.

45. Hoffman GS, Kerr GS, Leavitt RY, Hallahan CW, Lebovics RS, Travis WD, et al. Wegener granulomatosis: an analysis of 158 patients. *Ann Intern Med* 1992;**116**(6):488–98.

46. Jonsson H, Nived O, Sturfelt G. Outcome in systemic lupus erythematosus: a prospective study of patients from a defined population. *Medicine (Baltimore)* 1989;**68**(3):141–50.

47. Mok CC, Lee KW, Ho CT, Lau CS, Wong RW. A prospective study of survival and prognostic indicators of systemic lupus erythematosus in a southern Chinese population. *Rheumatology (Oxford)* 2000;**39**(4):399–406.

48. Ward MM, Pyun E, Studenski S. Causes of death in systemic lupus erythematosus. Long-term followup of an inception cohort. *Arthritis Rheum* 1995;**38**(10):1492–9.

49. Yeap SS, Chow SK, Manivasagar M, Veerapen K, Wang F. Mortality patterns in Malaysian systemic lupus erythematosus patients. *Med J Malaysia* 2001;**56**(3):308–12.

50. Zonana-Nacach A, Camargo-Coronel A, Yanez P, Sanchez L, Jimenez-Balderas FJ, Fraga A. Infections in outpatients with systemic lupus erythematosus: a prospective study. *Lupus* 2001;**10**(7):505–10.
51. Prabu V, Agrawal S. Systemic lupus erythematosus and tuberculosis: a review of complex interactions of complicated diseases. *J Postgrad Med* 2010;**56**(3):244–50.
52. Avihingsanon Y, Hirankarn N. Major lupus organ involvement: severe lupus nephritis. *Lupus* 2010;**19**(12):1391–8.
53. Ferreira S, Vasconcelos J, Marinho A, Farinha F, Almeida I, Correia J, et al. CD4 lymphocytopenia in systemic lupus erythematosus. *Acta Reumatol Port* 2009;**34**(2A):200–6.
54. Strasser C, Wolf EM, Kornprat P, Hermann J, Munch A, Langner C. Opportunistic cytomegalovirus infection causing colonic perforation in a patient with systemic lupus erythematosus. *Lupus* 2012;**21**(4):449–51.
55. Fessler BJ. Infectious diseases in systemic lupus erythematosus: risk factors, management and prophylaxis. *Best Pract Res Clin Rheumatol* 2002;**16**(2):281–91.
56. Paton NI. Infections in systemic lupus erythematosus patients. *Ann Acad Med Singapore* 1997;**26**(5):694–700.
57. Villaseñor-Ovies CAA-SaP. Infections and systemic lupus erythematosus. In: Almoallim H, editor. *Systemic lupus erythematosus.* InTech; 2012. p. 554.
58. Gardner GC, Weisman MH. Pyarthrosis in patients with rheumatoid arthritis: a report of 13 cases and a review of the literature from the past 40 years. *Am J Med* 1990;**88** (5):503–11.
59. Malladi AS, Sack KE, Shiboski SC, Shiboski CH, Baer AN, Banushree R, et al. Primary Sjogren's syndrome as a systemic disease: a study of participants enrolled in an international Sjogren's syndrome registry. *Arthritis Care Res (Hoboken)* 2012;**64** (6):911–18.
60. Rodrigo HF, Stavile RN, Deleo S. Disseminated histoplasmosis, lymphopenia and Sjogren's syndrome. *Medicina (B Aires)* 2012;**72**(5):435–8.
61. Moore PM, Cupps TR. Neurological complications of vasculitis. *Ann Neurol* 1983;**14** (2):155–67.
62. Mraz-Gernhard SM, Bush TM, Riebman JB. Clinical images: Libman-Sacks endocarditis. *Arthritis Rheum* 2001;**44**(9):2111.
63. Yamada T, Nakajima A, Inoue E, Tanaka E, Hara M, Tomatsu T, et al. Increased risk of tuberculosis in patients with rheumatoid arthritis in Japan. *Ann Rheum Dis* 2006;**65** (12):1661–3.
64. Martinez S, Sellam V, Marco S, Sanfiorenzo C, Macone F, Marquette CH. Tuberculosis and pneumocystis: an unusual co-infection. *Rev Mal Respir* 2011;**28**(1):92–6.
65. Blanco Perez JJ, Aranda Torres A, Pego Reigosa JM, Nunez Delgado M, Temes Montes E, Guerra Vales JL. Pulmonary tuberculosis associated to adalimumab: a study of 3 cases. *Arch Bronconeumol* 2010;**46**(4):203–5.
66. Keane J, Gershon S, Wise RP, Mirabile-Levens E, Kasznica J, Schwieterman WD, et al. Tuberculosis associated with infliximab, a tumor necrosis factor alpha-neutralizing agent. *N Engl J Med* 2001;**345**(15):1098–104.
67. Furst DE. The risk of infections with biologic therapies for rheumatoid arthritis. *Semin Arthritis Rheum* 2010;**39**(5):327–46.
68. Vadillo Font C, Hernandez-Garcia C, Pato E, Morado IC, Salido M, Judez E, et al. Incidence and characteristics of tuberculosis in patients with autoimmune rheumatic diseases. *Rev Clin Esp* 2003;**203**(4):178–82.
69. Winthrop KL, Baxter R, Liu L, McFarland B, Austin D, Varley C, et al. The reliability of diagnostic coding and laboratory data to identify tuberculosis and nontuberculous mycobacterial disease among rheumatoid arthritis patients using anti-tumor necrosis factor therapy. *Pharmacoepidemiol Drug Saf* 2011;**20**(3):229–35.

70. Wallis RS, Broder MS, Wong JY, Hanson ME, Beenhouwer DO. Granulomatous infectious diseases associated with tumor necrosis factor antagonists. *Clin Infect Dis* 2004;**38**(9):1261–5.

71. Liote H. Respiratory complications of new treatments for rheumatoid arthritis. *Rev Mal Respir* 2004;**21**(6 Pt 1):1107–15.

72. Falagas ME, Voidonikola PT, Angelousi AG. Tuberculosis in patients with systemic rheumatic or pulmonary diseases treated with glucocorticosteroids and the preventive role of isoniazid: a review of the available evidence. *Int J Antimicrob Agents* 2007;**30** (6):477–86.

73. van der Klooster JM, Bosman RJ, Oudemans-van Straaten HM, van der Spoel JI, Wester JP, Zandstra DF. Disseminated tuberculosis, pulmonary aspergillosis and cutaneous herpes simplex infection in a patient with infliximab and methotrexate. *Intensive Care Med* 2003;**29**(12):2327–9.

74. Baeten D, Kruithof E, Van den Bosch F, Van den Bossche N, Herssens A, Mielants H, et al. Systematic safety follow up in a cohort of 107 patients with spondyloarthropathy treated with infliximab: a new perspective on the role of host defence in the pathogenesis of the disease? *Ann Rheum Dis* 2003;**62**(9):829–34.

75. Van Assche G, Lewis JD, Lichtenstein GR, Loftus EV, Ouyang Q, Panes J, et al. The London position statement of the World Congress of Gastroenterology on Biological Therapy for IBD with the European Crohn's and Colitis Organisation: safety. *Am J Gastroenterol* 2011;**106**(9):1594–602, quiz 3, 603.

76. Strangfeld A, Listing J. Infection and musculoskeletal conditions: bacterial and opportunistic infections during anti-TNF therapy. *Best Pract Res Clin Rheumatol* 2006;**20** (6):1181–95.

77. Carmona L, Gomez-Reino JJ, Rodriguez-Valverde V, Montero D, Pascual-Gomez E, Mola EM, et al. Effectiveness of recommendations to prevent reactivation of latent tuberculosis infection in patients treated with tumor necrosis factor antagonists. *Arthritis Rheum* 2005;**52**(6):1766–72.

78. Tam LS, Li EK, Wong SM, Szeto CC. Risk factors and clinical features for tuberculosis among patients with systemic lupus erythematosus in Hong Kong. *Scand J Rheumatol* 2002;**31**(5):296–300.

79. Balakrishnan C, Mangat G, Mittal G, Joshi VR. Tuberculosis in patients with systemic lupus erythematosus. *J Assoc Physicians India* 1998;**46**(8):682–3.

80. Feng PH, Tan TH. Tuberculosis in patients with systemic lupus erythematosus. *Ann Rheum Dis* 1982;**41**(1):11–14.

81. Erdozain JG, Ruiz-Irastorza G, Egurbide MV, Martinez-Berriotxoa A, Aguirre C. High risk of tuberculosis in systemic lupus erythematosus? *Lupus* 2006;**15**(4):232–5.

82. Mok MY, Wong SS, Chan TM, Fong DY, Wong WS, Lau CS. Non-tuberculous mycobacterial infection in patients with systemic lupus erythematosus. *Rheumatology (Oxford)* 2007;**46**(2):280–4.

83. Jick SS, Lieberman ES, Rahman MU, Choi HK. Glucocorticoid use, other associated factors, and the risk of tuberculosis. *Arthritis Rheum* 2006;**55**(1):19–26.

84. Mok MY, Lo Y, Chan TM, Wong WS, Lau CS. Tuberculosis in systemic lupus erythematosus in an endemic area and the role of isoniazid prophylaxis during corticosteroid therapy. *J Rheumatol* 2005;**32**(4):609–15.

85. Melboucy-Belkhir S, Flexor G, Stirnemann J, Morin AS, Boukari L, Polliand C, et al. Prolonged paradoxical response to anti-tuberculous treatment after infliximab. *Int J Infect Dis* 2010;**14**(Suppl. 3):e333–4.

86. Dimakou K, Papaioannides D, Latsi P, Katsimboula S, Korantzopoulos P, Orphanidou D. Disseminated tuberculosis complicating anti-TNF-alpha treatment. *Int J Clin Pract* 2004;**58**(11):1052–5.

87. Contini S, Raimondi G, Graziano P, Saltini C, Bocchino M. Difficult diagnosis of infliximab-related miliary tuberculosis. *Monaldi Arch Chest Dis* 2004;**61** (2):128–30.

88. Hou CL, Tsai YC, Chen LC, Huang JL. Tuberculosis infection in patients with systemic lupus erythematosus: pulmonary and extra-pulmonary infection compared. *Clin Rheumatol* 2008;**27**(5):557–63.

89. Zhang L, Wang DX, Ma L. A clinical study of tuberculosis infection in systemic lupus erythematosus. *Zhonghua Nei Ke Za Zhi* 2008;**47**(10):808–10.

90. Yang CD, Wang XD, Ye S, Gu YY, Bao CD, Wang Y, et al. Clinical features, prognostic and risk factors of central nervous system infections in patients with systemic lupus erythematosus. *Clin Rheumatol* 2007;**26**(6):895–901.

91. Shehan JM, Sarma DP. Mycobacterium mucogenicum: report of a skin infection associated with etanercept. *Dermatol Online J* 2008;**14**(1):5.

92. Diaz F, Urkijo JC, Mendoza F, de la Viuda JM, Blanco M, Unzurrunzaga A, et al. Mycobacterium chelonae infection associated with adalimumab therapy. *Scand J Rheumatol* 2008;**37**(2):159–60.

93. Lai J, Abbey BV, Jakubovic HR. Epithelioid histiocytic infiltrate caused by *Mycobacterium scrofulaceum* infection: a potential mimic of various neoplastic entities. *Am J Dermatopathol* 2013;**35**(2):266–9.

94. Brown A, Grubbs P, Mongey AB. Infection of total hip prosthesis by *Mycobacterium tuberculosis* and *Mycobacterium chelonae* in a patient with rheumatoid arthritis. *Clin Rheumatol* 2008;**27**(4):543–5.

95. Elyousfi AA, Leiter JR, Goytan MJ, Robinson DB. Mycobacterium heckeshornense lumbar spondylodiskitis in a patient with rheumatoid arthritis receiving etanercept treatment. *J Rheumatol* 2009;**36**(9):2130–1.

96. Hodkinson B, Musenge E, Tikly M. Osteoarticular tuberculosis in patients with systemic lupus erythematosus. *QJM* 2009;**102**(5):321–8.

97. Lamb SR, Stables GI, Merchant W. Disseminated cutaneous infection with *Mycobacterium chelonae* in a patient with steroid-dependent rheumatoid arthritis. *Clin Exp Dermatol* 2004;**29**(3):254–7.

98. Dare JA, Jahan S, Hiatt K, Torralba KD. Reintroduction of etanercept during treatment of cutaneous *Mycobacterium marinum* infection in a patient with ankylosing spondylitis. *Arthritis Rheum* 2009;**61**(5):583–6.

99. Lizaso D, Garcia M, Aguirre A, Esposto A. Breast implant infection by *Mycobacterium fortuitum* in a patient with systemic lupus erythematosus. *Rev Chilena Infectol* 2011;**28** (5):474–8.

100. Maimon N, Brunton J, Chan A, Marras TK. Fatal pulmonary *Mycobacterium xenopi* in a patient with rheumatoid arthritis receiving etanercept. *Thorax* 2007;**62** (8):739–40.

101. Tnani N, Massoumi A, Lortholary O, Soussan P, Prinseau J, Baglin A, et al. Management of cytomegalovirus infections in patients treated with immunosuppressive drugs for chronic inflammatory diseases. *Rev Med Interne* 2008;**29**(4):305–10.

102. Krech U. Complement-fixing antibodies against cytomegalovirus in different parts of the world. *Bull World Health Organ* 1973;**49**(1):103–6.

103. Mori T, Mori S, Kanda Y, Yakushiji K, Mineishi S, Takaue Y, et al. Clinical significance of cytomegalovirus (CMV) antigenemia in the prediction and diagnosis of CMV gastrointestinal disease after allogeneic hematopoietic stem cell transplantation. *Bone Marrow Transplant* 2004;**33**(4):431–4.

104. Takizawa Y, Inokuma S, Tanaka Y, Saito K, Atsumi T, Hirakata M, et al. Clinical characteristics of cytomegalovirus infection in rheumatic diseases: multicentre survey in a large patient population. *Rheumatology (Oxford)* 2008;**47**(9):1373–8.

105. Fujimoto D, Matsushima A, Nagao M, Takakura S, Ichiyama S. Risk factors associated with elevated blood cytomegalovirus pp 65 antigen levels in patients with autoimmune diseases. *Mod Rheumatol* 2013;**23**(2):345–50.
106. Barber C, Gold WL, Fortin PR. Infections in the lupus patient: perspectives on prevention. *Curr Opin Rheumatol* 2011;**23**(4):358–65.
107. Ozaki T, Yamashita H, Kaneko S, Yorifuji H, Takahashi H, Ueda Y, et al. Cytomegalovirus disease of the upper gastrointestinal tract in patients with rheumatic diseases: a case series and literature review. *Clin Rheumatol* 2013;**32**(11):1683–90.
108. Hanaoka R, Kurasawa K, Maezawa R, Kumano K, Arai S, Fukuda T. Reactivation of cytomegalovirus predicts poor prognosis in patients on intensive immunosuppressive treatment for collagen-vascular diseases. *Mod Rheumatol* 2012;**22**(3):438–45.
109. Yoda Y, Hanaoka R, Ide H, Isozaki T, Matsunawa M, Yajima N, et al. Clinical evaluation of patients with inflammatory connective tissue diseases complicated by cytomegalovirus antigenemia. *Mod Rheumatol* 2006;**16**(3):137–42.
110. Vallet H, Houitte R, Azria A, Mariette X. Cytomegalovirus colitis and hypo-IgG after rituximab therapy for rheumatoid arthritis. *J Rheumatol* 2011;**38**(5):965–6.
111. Guidotti LG, Chisari FV. Noncytolytic control of viral infections by the innate and adaptive immune response. *Annu Rev Immunol* 2001;**19**:65–91.
112. Kim SY, Solomon DH. Tumor necrosis factor blockade and the risk of viral infection. *Nat Rev Rheumatol* 2010;**6**(3):165–74.
113. Ayyappan AP, Thomas R, Kurian S, Christopher DJ, Cherian R. Multiple cavitating masses in an immunocompromised host with rheumatoid arthritis-related interstitial lung disease: an unusual expression of cytomegalovirus pneumonitis. *Br J Radiol* 2006;**79**(947):e174–6.
114. Clerc D, Brousse C, Mariette X, Bennet P, Bisson M. Cytomegalovirus pneumonia in a patient with rheumatoid arthritis treated with low dose methotrexate and prednisone. *Ann Rheum Dis* 1991;**50**(1):67.
115. Tokunaga Y, Takenaka K, Asayama R, Shibuya T. Cytomegalovirus-induced interstitial pneumonitis in a patient with systemic lupus erythematosus. *Intern Med* 1996;**35**(6):517–20.
116. Sanchez-Roman J, Varela-Aguilar JM, Fraile I, Andreu-Alvarez J, Fernandez Alonso J. Cytomegalic inclusion disease in a patient with systemic lupus. *Rev Clin Esp* 1991;**188**(1):34–6.
117. Azuma N, Hashimoto N, Yasumitsu A, Fukuoka K, Yokoyama K, Sawada H, et al. CMV infection presenting as a cavitary lung lesion in a patient with systemic lupus erythematosus receiving immunosuppressive therapy. *Intern Med* 2009;**48**(24):2145–9.
118. Najjar M, Siddiqui AK, Rossoff L, Cohen RI. Cavitary lung masses in SLE patients: an unusual manifestation of CMV infection. *Eur Respir J* 2004;**24**(1):182–4.
119. Katagiri A, Ando T, Kon T, Yamada M, Iida N, Takasaki Y. Cavitary lung lesion in a patient with systemic lupus erythematosus: an unusual manifestation of cytomegalovirus pneumonitis. *Mod Rheumatol* 2008;**18**(3):285–9.
120. Vilaichone RK, Mahachai V, Eiam-Ong S, Kullavanuaya P, Wisedopas N, Bhattarakosol P. Necrotizing ileitis caused by cytomegalovirus in patient with systemic lupus erythematosus: case report. *J Med Assoc Thai* 2001;**84**(Suppl. 1):S469–73.
121. Sackier JM, Kelly SB, Clarke D, Rees AJ, Wood CB. Small bowel haemorrhage due to cytomegalovirus vasculitis. *Gut* 1991;**32**(11):1419–20.
122. Perdan-Pirkmajer K, Koren-Kranjc M, Tomsic M. A successfully treated pancreatitis caused by a CMV infection in a lupus patient. *Lupus* 2011;**20**(10):1104–5.
123. Ikura Y, Matsuo T, Ogami M, Yamazaki S, Okamura M, Yoshikawa J, et al. Cytomegalovirus associated pancreatitis in a patient with systemic lupus erythematosus. *J Rheumatol* 2000;**27**(11):2715–7.

124. Kelkar A, Kelkar J, Kelkar S, Bhirud S, Biswas J. Cytomegalovirus retinitis in a sero-negative patient with systemic lupus erythematosus on immunosuppressive therapy. *J Ophthalmic Inflamm Infect* 2011;**1**(3):129–32.

125. Yoon KH, Fong KY, Tambyah PA. Fatal cytomegalovirus infection in two patients with systemic lupus erythematosus undergoing intensive immunosuppressive therapy: role for cytomegalovirus vigilance and prophylaxis? *J Clin Rheumatol* 2002;**8**(4):217–22.

126. Iwasaki T, Satodate R, Masuda T, Kurata T, Hondo R. An immunofluorescent study of generalized infection of human cytomegalovirus in a patient with systemic lupus erythematosus. *Acta Pathol Jpn* 1984;**34**(4):869–74.

127. Ku SC, Yu CJ, Chang YL, Yang PC. Disseminated cytomegalovirus disease in a patient with systemic lupus erythematosus not undergoing immunosuppressive therapy. *J Formos Med Assoc* 1999;**98**(12):855–8.

128. Calabrese LH, Molloy ES, Huang D, Ransohoff RM. Progressive multifocal leukoen-cephalopathy in rheumatic diseases: evolving clinical and pathologic patterns of disease. *Arthritis Rheum* 2007;**56**(7):2116–28.

129. Boren EJ, Cheema GS, Naguwa SM, Ansari AA, Gershwin ME. The emergence of progressive multifocal leukoencephalopathy (PML) in rheumatic diseases. *J Autoimmun* 2008;**30**(1–2):90–8.

130. Major EO. Progressive multifocal leukoencephalopathy in patients on immunomodu-latory therapies. *Annu Rev Med* 2010;**61**:35–47.

131. Palazzo E, Yahia SA. Progressive multifocal leukoencephalopathy in autoimmune diseases. *Joint Bone Spine* 2012;**79**(4):351–5.

132. Molloy ES, Calabrese LH. Progressive multifocal leukoencephalopathy: a national esti-mate of frequency in systemic lupus erythematosus and other rheumatic diseases. *Arthri-tis Rheum* 2009;**60**(12):3761–5.

133. Koralnik IJ, Schellingerhout D, Frosch MP. Case records of the Massachusetts General Hospital. Weekly clinicopathological exercises. Case 14-2004. A 66-year-old man with progressive neurologic deficits. *N Engl J Med* 2004;**350**(18):1882–93.

134. Lefevre G, Queyrel V, Maurage CA, Laurent C, Launay D, Lacour A, et al. Effective immune restoration after immunosuppressant discontinuation in a lupus patient presenting progressive multifocal leukoencephalopathy. *J Neurol Sci* 2009;**287**(1–2):246–9.

135. Molloy ES. PML and rheumatology: the contribution of disease and drugs. *Cleve Clin J Med* 2011;**78**(Suppl. 2):S28–32.

136. Graff-Radford J, Robinson MT, Warsame RM, Matteson EL, Eggers SD, Keegan BM. Progressive multifocal leukoencephalopathy in a patient treated with etanercept. *Neurologist* 2012;**18**(2):85–7.

137. Epker JL, van Biezen P, van Daele PL, van Gelder T, Vossen A, van Saase JL. Progres-sive multifocal leukoencephalopathy, a review and an extended report of five patients with different immune compromised states. *Eur J Intern Med* 2009;**20**(3):261–7.

138. Tavazzi E, Ferrante P, Khalili K. Progressive multifocal leukoencephalopathy: an unex-pected complication of modern therapeutic monoclonal antibody therapies. *Clin Microbiol Infect* 2011;**17**(12):1776–80.

139. Berger JR. Progressive multifocal leukoencephalopathy and newer biological agents. *Drug Saf* 2010;**33**(11):969–83.

140. Calabrese LH, Molloy ES. Progressive multifocal leucoencephalopathy in the rheu-matic diseases: assessing the risks of biological immunosuppressive therapies. *Ann Rheum Dis* 2008;**67**(Suppl. 3):iii64–5.

141. Park HB, Kim KC, Park JH, Kang TY, Lee HS, Kim TH, et al. Association of reduced CD4 T cell responses specific to varicella zoster virus with high incidence of herpes zoster in patients with systemic lupus erythematosus. *J Rheumatol* 2004;**31**(11):2151–5.

142. Thomas SL, Hall AJ. What does epidemiology tell us about risk factors for herpes zoster? *Lancet Infect Dis* 2004;**4**(1):26–33.

143. Brisson M, Edmunds WJ, Law B, Gay NJ, Walld R, Brownell M, et al. Epidemiology of varicella zoster virus infection in Canada and the United Kingdom. *Epidemiol Infect* 2001;**127**(2):305–14.

144. Schmader KE. Epidemiology and impact on quality of life of postherpetic neuralgia and painful diabetic neuropathy. *Clin J Pain* 2002;**18**(6):350–4.

145. Insinga RP, Itzler RF, Pellissier JM, Saddier P, Nikas AA. The incidence of herpes zoster in a United States administrative database. *J Gen Intern Med* 2005;**20** (8):748–53.

146. Yawn BP, Saddier P, Wollan PC, St Sauver JL, Kurland MJ, Sy LS. A population-based study of the incidence and complication rates of herpes zoster before zoster vaccine introduction. *Mayo Clin Proc* 2007;**82**(11):1341–9.

147. Harpaz R, Ortega-Sanchez IR, Seward JF, Advisory Committee on Immunization Practices Centers for Disease C, Prevention. Prevention of herpes zoster: recommendations of the Advisory Committee on Immunization Practices (ACIP). *MMWR Recomm Rep* 2008;**57**(RR-5):1–30, quiz CE2-4.

148. Winthrop KL, Furst DE. Rheumatoid arthritis and herpes zoster: risk and prevention in those treated with anti-tumour necrosis factor therapy. *Ann Rheum Dis* 2010;**69** (10):1735–7.

149. Kang TY, Lee HS, Kim TH, Jun JB, Yoo DH. Clinical and genetic risk factors of herpes zoster in patients with systemic lupus erythematosus. *Rheumatol Int* 2005;**25**(2):97–102.

150. Takada K, Illei GG, Boumpas DT. Cyclophosphamide for the treatment of systemic lupus erythematosus. *Lupus* 2001;**10**(3):154–61.

151. Strangfeld A, Listing J, Herzer P, Liebhaber A, Rockwitz K, Richter C, et al. Risk of herpes zoster in patients with rheumatoid arthritis treated with anti-TNF-alpha agents. *JAMA* 2009;**301**(7):737–44.

152. van Vollenhoven RF, Emery P, Bingham 3rd CO, Keystone EC, Fleischmann R, Furst DE, et al. Longterm safety of patients receiving rituximab in rheumatoid arthritis clinical trials. *J Rheumatol* 2010;**37**(3):558–67.

153. Demoruelle MK, Kahr A, Verilhac K, Deane K, Fischer A, West S. Recent-onset systemic lupus erythematosus complicated by acute respiratory failure. *Arthritis Care Res (Hoboken)* 2013;**65**(2):314–23.

154. Ponce CA, Gallo M, Bustamante R, Vargas SL. Pneumocystis colonization is highly prevalent in the autopsied lungs of the general population. *Clin Infect Dis* 2010;**50** (3):347–53.

155. Thomas Jr. CF, Limper AH. Pneumocystis pneumonia. *N Engl J Med* 2004;**350** (24):2487–98.

156. Catherinot E, Lanternier F, Bougnoux ME, Lecuit M, Couderc LJ, Lortholary O. *Pneumocystis jirovecii* pneumonia. *Infect Dis Clin North Am* 2010;**24**(1):107–38.

157. Sepkowitz KA. Opportunistic infections in patients with and patients without Acquired Immunodeficiency Syndrome. *Clin Infect Dis* 2002;**34**(8):1098–107.

158. Ward MM, Donald F. Pneumocystis carinii pneumonia in patients with connective tissue diseases: the role of hospital experience in diagnosis and mortality. *Arthritis Rheum* 1999;**42**(4):780–9.

159. Falagas ME, Manta KG, Betsi GI, Pappas G. Infection-related morbidity and mortality in patients with connective tissue diseases: a systematic review. *Clin Rheumatol* 2007;**26** (5):663–70.

160. Iwazu K, Iwazu Y, Takeda S, Akimoto T, Yumura W, Takahashi H, et al. Successful treatment of serial opportunistic infections including disseminated nocardiosis and

cryptococcal meningitis in a patient with ANCA-associated vasculitis. *Intern Med* 2012;**51**(21):3051–6.

161. Lapraik C, Watts R, Bacon P, Carruthers D, Chakravarty K, D'Cruz D, et al. BSR and BHPR guidelines for the management of adults with ANCA associated vasculitis. *Rheumatology (Oxford)* 2007;**46**(10):1615–16.

162. Charles P, Guillevin L. S3. Rituximab for ANCA-associated vasculitides: the French experience. *Presse Med* 2013;**42**(4 Pt 2):534–6.

163. Tanaka M, Sakai R, Koike R, Komano Y, Nanki T, Sakai F, et al. *Pneumocystis jirovecii* pneumonia associated with etanercept treatment in patients with rheumatoid arthritis: a retrospective review of 15 cases and analysis of risk factors. *Mod Rheumatol* 2012;**22** (6):849–58.

164. Soejima M, Sugiura T, Kawaguchi Y, Kawamoto M, Katsumata Y, Takagi K, et al. Association of the diplotype configuration at the N-acetyltransferase 2 gene with adverse events with co-trimoxazole in Japanese patients with systemic lupus erythematosus. *Arthritis Res Ther* 2007;**9**(2):R23.

165. Camus P, Bonniaud P, Fanton A, Camus C, Baudaun N, Foucher P. Drug-induced and iatrogenic infiltrative lung disease. *Clin Chest Med* 2004;**25**(3):479–519, vi.

166. Kameda H, Tokuda H, Sakai F, Johkoh T, Mori S, Yoshida Y, et al. Clinical and radiological features of acute-onset diffuse interstitial lung diseases in patients with rheumatoid arthritis receiving treatment with biological agents: importance of *Pneumocystis pneumonia* in Japan revealed by a multicenter study. *Intern Med* 2011;**50**(4):305–13.

167. Roblot F, Godet C, Le Moal G, Garo B, Faouzi Souala M, Dary M, et al. Analysis of underlying diseases and prognosis factors associated with *Pneumocystis carinii* pneumonia in immunocompromised HIV-negative patients. *Eur J Clin Microbiol Infect Dis* 2002;**21** (7):523–31.

168. Tokuda H, Sakai F, Yamada H, Johkoh T, Imamura A, Dohi M, et al. Clinical and radiological features of *Pneumocystis pneumonia* in patients with rheumatoid arthritis, in comparison with methotrexate pneumonitis and *Pneumocystis pneumonia* in acquired immunodeficiency syndrome: a multicenter study. *Intern Med* 2008;**47**(10):915–23.

169. Wissmann G, Morilla R, Martin-Garrido I, Friaza V, Respaldiza N, Povedano J, et al. *Pneumocystis jirovecii* colonization in patients treated with infliximab. *Eur J Clin Invest* 2011;**41**(3):343–8.

170. Prekates A, Kyprianou T, Paniara O, Roussos C. *Pneumocystis carinii* pneumonia in a HIV-seronegative patient with untreated rheumatoid arthritis and CD4+ T-lymphocytopenia. *Eur Respir J* 1997;**10**(5):1184–6.

171. Mansharamani NG, Garland R, Delaney D, Koziel H. Management and outcome patterns for adult *Pneumocystis carinii pneumonia*, 1985 to 1995: comparison of HIV-associated cases to other immunocompromised states. *Chest* 2000;**118**(3):704–11.

172. Festic E, Gajic O, Limper AH, Aksamit TR. Acute respiratory failure due to pneumocystis pneumonia in patients without human immunodeficiency virus infection: outcome and associated features. *Chest* 2005;**128**(2):573–9.

173. Yoshida M, Ishibashi K, Hida S, Yoshikawa N, Nakabayashi I, Akashi M, et al. Rapid decrease of anti-beta-glucan antibody as an indicator for early diagnosis of carinii pneumonitis and deep mycotic infections following immunosuppressive therapy in antineutrophil cytoplasmic antibody-associated vasculitis. *Clin Rheumatol* 2009;**28**(5):565–71.

174. Fessel WJ. Cryptococcal meningitis after unusual exposures to birds. *N Engl J Med* 1993;**328**(18):1354–5.

175. Kim JM, Kim KJ, Yoon HS, Kwok SK, Ju JH, Park KS, et al. Meningitis in Korean patients with systemic lupus erythematosus: analysis of demographics, clinical features

and outcomes; experience from affiliated hospitals of the Catholic University of Korea. *Lupus* 2011;**20**(5):531–6.

176. Kiertiburanakul S, Wirojtananugoon S, Pracharktam R, Sungkanuparph S. Cryptococcosis in human immunodeficiency virus-negative patients. *Int J Infect Dis* 2006;**10** (1):72–8.

177. Shrestha RK, Stoller JK, Honari G, Procop GW, Gordon SM. Pneumonia due to *Cryptococcus neoformans* in a patient receiving infliximab: possible zoonotic transmission from a pet cockatiel. *Respir Care* 2004;**49**(6):606–8.

178. Kremer J, Li ZG, Hall S, Fleischmann R, Genovese M, Martin-Mola E, et al. Tofacitinib in combination with nonbiologic disease-modifying antirheumatic drugs in patients with active rheumatoid arthritis: a randomized trial. *Ann Intern Med* 2013;**159**(4):253–61.

179. Mora DJ, da Cunha Colombo ER, Ferreira-Paim K, Andrade-Silva LE, Nascentes GA, Silva-Vergara ML. Clinical, epidemiological and outcome features of patients with cryptococcosis in Uberaba, Minas Gerais, Brazil. *Mycopathologia* 2012;**173**(5–6):321–7.

180. Tristano AG. Cryptococcal meningitis and systemic lupus erythematosus: a case report and review. *Rev Chilena Infectol* 2010;**27**(2):155–9.

181. Matsumura M, Kawamura R, Inoue R, Yamada K, Kawano M, Yamagishi M. Concurrent presentation of cryptococcal meningoencephalitis and systemic lupus erythematosus. *Mod Rheumatol* 2011;**21**(3):305–8.

182. Huang JL, Chou ML, Hung IJ, Hsieh KH. Multiple cryptococcal brain abscesses in systemic lupus erythematosus. *Br J Rheumatol* 1996;**35**(12):1334–5.

183. Hung JJ, Ou LS, Lee WI, Huang JL. Central nervous system infections in patients with systemic lupus erythematosus. *J Rheumatol* 2005;**32**(1):40–3.

184. Fong KY, Thumboo J. Neuropsychiatric lupus: clinical challenges, brain-reactive autoantibodies and treatment strategies. *Lupus* 2010;**19**(12):1399–403.

185. David VG, Korula A, Choudhrie L, Michael JS, Jacob S, Jacob CK, et al. Cryptococcal granulomatous interstitial nephritis and dissemination in a patient with untreated lupus nephritis. *Nephrol Dial Transplant* 2009;**24**(10):3243–5.

186. Horcajada JP, Pena JL, Martinez-Taboada VM, Pina T, Belaustegui I, Cano ME, et al. Invasive Cryptococcosis and adalimumab treatment. *Emerg Infect Dis* 2007;**13**(6):953–5.

187. Azevedo VF, Pietrovski CF, de Almeida Jr. Santos M. Acute toxoplasmosis infection in a patient with ankylosing spondylitis treated with adalimumab: a case report. *Reumatismo* 2010;**62**(4):283–5.

188. Fischer S, Agmon-Levin N, Shapira Y, Porat Katz BS, Graell E, Cervera R, et al. Toxoplasma gondii: bystander or cofactor in rheumatoid arthritis. *Immunol Res* 2013;**56**(2–3):287–92.

189. Suzuki Y, Sher A, Yap G, Park D, Neyer LE, Liesenfeld O, et al. IL-10 is required for prevention of necrosis in the small intestine and mortality in both genetically resistant BALB/c and susceptible C57BL/6 mice following peroral infection with *Toxoplasma gondii*. *J Immunol* 2000;**164**(10):5375–82.

190. Denkers EY, Gazzinelli RT, Hieny S, Caspar P, Sher A. Bone marrow macrophages process exogenous *Toxoplasma gondii* polypeptides for recognition by parasite-specific cytolytic T lymphocytes. *J Immunol* 1993;**150**(2):517–26.

191. Johnson LL. A protective role for endogenous tumor necrosis factor in Toxoplasma gondii infection. *Infect Immun* 1992;**60**(5):1979–83.

192. Korner H, McMorran B, Schluter D, Fromm P. The role of TNF in parasitic diseases: still more questions than answers. *Int J Parasitol* 2010;**40**(8):879–88.

193. Lassoued S, Zabraniecki L, Marin F, Billey T. Toxoplasmic chorioretinitis and antitumor necrosis factor treatment in rheumatoid arthritis. *Semin Arthritis Rheum* 2007;**36** (4):262–3.

194. Caporali R, Caprioli M, Bobbio-Pallavicini F, Montecucco C. DMARDS and infections in rheumatoid arthritis. *Autoimmun Rev* 2008;**8**(2):139–43.
195. Bourre-Tessier J, Fortin C, Belisle A, Desmarais E, Choquette D, Senecal JL. Disseminated *Histoplasma capsulatum* infection presenting with panniculitis and focal myositis in rheumatoid arthritis treated with etanercept. *Scand J Rheumatol* 2009;**38**(4):311–16.
196. Franca CM, Cavalcante EG, Ribeiro AS, Oliveira GT, Litvinov N, Silva CA. Disseminated histoplasmosis in a juvenile lupus erythematosus patient. *Acta Reumatol Port* 2012;**37**(3):276–9.
197. Ceccato F, Gongora V, Zunino A, Roverano S, Paira S. Unusual manifestation of histoplasmosis in connective tissue diseases. *Clin Rheumatol* 2007;**26**(10):1717–19.
198. Joshi SA, Kagal AS, Bharadwaj RS, Kulkarni SS, Jadhav MV. Disseminated histoplasmosis. *Indian J Med Microbiol* 2006;**24**(4):297–8.
199. Lim SY, Kijsiricharenchai K, Winn R. Progressive disseminated histoplasmosis in systemic lupus erythematosus-an unusual presentation of acute tenosynovitis and a literature review. *Clin Rheumatol* 2013;**32**(1):135–9.
200. Cairoli E, Tafuri J, Olivari D. Laryngeal histoplasmosis in systemic lupus erythematosus: first reported case. *Lupus* 2010;**19**(11):1354–5.
201. Sullivan AA, Benson SM, Ewart AH, Hogan PG, Whitby RM, Boyle RS. Cerebral histoplasmosis in an Australian patient with systemic lupus erythematosus. *Med J Aust* 1998;**169**(4):201–2.
202. Goodwin Jr. RA, Shapiro JL, Thurman GH, Thurman SS, Des Prez RM. Disseminated histoplasmosis: clinical and pathologic correlations. *Medicine (Baltimore)* 1980;**59**(1):1–33.
203. Staples PJ, Gerding DN, Decker JL, Gordon Jr. RS. Incidence of infection in systemic lupus erythematosus. *Arthritis Rheum* 1974;**17**(1):1–10.
204. Burmester GR, Mease P, Dijkmans BA, Gordon K, Lovell D, Panaccione R, et al. Adalimumab safety and mortality rates from global clinical trials of six immune-mediated inflammatory diseases. *Ann Rheum Dis* 2009;**68**(12):1863–9.
205. Frank KM, Hogarth DK, Miller JL, Mandal S, Mease PJ, Samulski RJ, et al. Investigation of the cause of death in a gene-therapy trial. *N Engl J Med* 2009;**361**(2):161–9.
206. Asrani NS. Disseminated histoplasmosis associated with the treatment of rheumatoid arthritis with anticytokine therapy. *Ann Intern Med* 2008;**149**(8):594–5.
207. Arunkumar P, Crook T, Ballard J. Disseminated histoplasmosis presenting as pancytopenia in a methotrexate-treated patient. *Am J Hematol* 2004;**77**(1):86–7.
208. LeMense GP, Sahn SA. Opportunistic infection during treatment with low dose methotrexate. *Am J Respir Crit Care Med* 1994;**150**(1):258–60.
209. Sawalha AH, Lutz BD, Chaudhary NA, Kern W, Harley JB, Greenfield RA. Panniculitis: a presenting manifestation of disseminated histoplasmosis in a patient with rheumatoid arthritis. *J Clin Rheumatol* 2003;**9**(4):259–62.
210. Galandiuk S, Davis BR. Infliximab-induced disseminated histoplasmosis in a patient with Crohn's disease. *Nat Clin Pract Gastroenterol Hepatol* 2008;**5**(5):283–7.
211. Colombel JF, Loftus Jr. EV, Tremaine WJ, Egan LJ, Harmsen WS, Schleck CD, et al. The safety profile of infliximab in patients with Crohn's disease: the Mayo clinic experience in 500 patients. *Gastroenterology* 2004;**126**(1):19–31.
212. Wood KL, Hage CA, Knox KS, Kleiman MB, Sannuti A, Day RB, et al. Histoplasmosis after treatment with anti-tumor necrosis factor-alpha therapy. *Am J Respir Crit Care Med* 2003;**167**(9):1279–82.

CHAPTER 16

Can Antibiotics Cure Autoimmune Diseases?

Cristina Rosário[1]
Internal Medicine Department, Hospital Pedro Hispano, Matosinhos, Portugal
[1]Corresponding Author: tina.rosario@gmail.com

1 INTRODUCTION

Autoimmune diseases are characterized by dysregulation of the immune system, resulting in a loss of tolerance to self-antigen. A combination of genetic, immunologic, hormonal, and environmental factors is required, comprising what is known as "the mosaic of autoimmunity".[1] Infections play a preponderant role on the development of autoimmunity; in fact, almost every autoimmune disease investigated is linked to one or more specific infectious agents. Several mechanisms have been proposed as possible links between the development of autoimmunity and exposure to infectious agents, namely polyclonal lymphocyte activation, molecular antigen mimicry, epitope spreading, bystander activation and activation by a superantigen. Discussion of these mechanisms has been previously detailed in the literature[1,2] and is beyond the scope of this chapter. One of the best-recognized examples of the relationship between infection and autoimmunity is acute rheumatic fever (RF), which presents several weeks after infection with group A *Streptococcus*. In this specific example the treatment of streptococcal infections of the pharynx with antibiotics is well known to prevent an episode of acute RF.[3] It is possible to prevent the development of the autoimmune disease by treating the infection that precedes it. Actually, several studies report prevalence of serology of infectious agents in many autoimmune diseases, but few report attempts to eradicate the infectious agent.

2 RHEUMATIC FEVER AND GROUP A *STREPTOCOCCUS*

RF is a systemic inflammatory condition occurring in response to a group A streptococcal infection. It commonly occurs after group A streptococcal

Infection and Autoimmunity
http://dx.doi.org/10.1016/B978-0-444-63269-2.00008-8

pharyngitis. Involvement of the heart, joints, nervous system, skin and immune systems is usual, although all of these are not universally seen in all patients. After the initial attack of acute RF, repeated group A strepto-coccal infections can lead to rheumatic recurrences.[3] The pathogenesis of RF is complex, and both environmental and genetic factors contribute to its etiology. Molecular mimicry between streptococcal and human proteins is considered the triggering factor leading to autoimmunity in RF and rheu-matic heart disease.[4] A meta-analysis showed that the treatment of group A streptococcal infections of the pharynx with antibiotics prevented epi-sodes of acute RF (primary prevention). The overall protective effect was 70%, with a confidence interval of 95% and a relative risk of 0.32. This has dramatically reduced the incidence of RF in the developed world. Sec-ondary prevention with long-term antibiotic prophylaxis has reduced the recurrence rate of RF and its most serious component, rheumatic heart dis-ease.[3] Nowadays, all guidelines recommend oral or intramuscular penicillin as the preferred therapy for streptococcal pharyngitis. In individuals allergic to penicillin, the choices are azithromycin, clindamycin, a cephalosporin, and clarithromycin.[3,5]

3 HELICOBACTER PYLORI

Of the various infectious agents triggering autoimmunity, *Helicobacter pylori* is one of the most widely studied, although its precise role in many autoimmune diseases is still controversial.[6] *H. pylori* is a curved gram-negative bacillus; it most commonly colonizes the gastric mucosa in early childhood and can per-sist throughout life if no antibiotic therapy is given.[6] Since its initial discovery as a human pathogen in 1983, *H. pylori* has been implicated in numerous diseases.[7] There are contradictory data about the role of *H. pylori* effects on the human immune response. On one side there is evidence indicating an overall downregulation of the host immune response in *H. pylori*-infected individuals. On the other, the persistent presence of *H. pylori* in gastric mucosa results in chronic immune system activation with cytokine signalling, infiltra-tion of gastric mucosa by neutrophils, macrophages and lymphocytes and production of antibodies and effector T-cells.[6] There are several proposed mechanisms by which *H. pylori* may cause loss of self-tolerance and therefore autoimmunity, including molecular mimicry, polyclonal activation, epitope spread, bystander activation and superantigen phenomena.[6]

3.1 *H. pylori* and Immune Thrombocytopenic Purpura

Immune thrombocytopenic purpura (ITP) is an autoimmune disease result-ing from antibodies against platelet glycoproteins. The worldwide preva-lence of *H. pylori* in patients with ITP is estimated to be 62.3%, similar to the prevalence among the healthy population (matched by age and geo-graphic area).[6] The association with ITP is supported by the fact that erad-ication of *H. pylori* improves thrombocytopenia in some patients with ITP, but the pathogenic role of *H. pylori* is largely unknown. Several mechanisms have been proposed to explain the association between *H. pylori* and ITP. The most prevailing hypothesis suggests molecular mimicry between one of the *H. pylori* antigens (cytotoxin-associated gene A [CagA] protein) and platelet glycoproteins producing cross-reacting autoantibodies.[8] Clini-cal studies demonstrate a platelet count response in approximately 50% of patients with ITP following *H. pylori* eradication. This response rate corre-lates with the prevalence of *H. pylori* in the population being treated, with higher response rates reported from Japan and much lower rates in the United States. This observed variability in treatment effect by country may be explained by the fact that CagA-positive strains of *H. pylori* are more prevalent in Japan than in North America.[6,8] Interesting, in a review by Stasi et al.,[9] the most consistently reported characteristic associated with better chances of response was a shorter duration of ITP.[6,8] It could be that erad-ication therapy led to the improvement of thrombocytopenia by mecha-nisms independent of *H. pylori*, including the immune-modulating effects of the treatment itself or the removal of other commensal bacteria. To clarify this, Arnold et al.,[8] performed a systematic review using *H. pylori*-negative patients as controls and concluded that the effect of *H. pylori* treatment is indeed due to eradication of the bacteria and not to the treatment itself.[8] In this review, they also found that the rate of complete response (platelet count $>150 \times 10^9$/L) was low in both *H. pylori*-positive and -negative patients following eradication therapy (35.1% vs. 11.1%, respectively), sug-gesting that while treatment may improve platelet counts, it may not reverse the autoimmune process.[8] Additional prospective studies are needed to clar-ify the regional differences observed, and extended follow-up is needed to address the durability of the platelet count response. Nevertheless, based on the current evidence for a relationship between *H. pylori* and chronic ITP, the European Helicobacter Study Group consensus 2007 recommended the eradication of *H. pylori* infection in affected patients.[10]

3.2 *H. pylori* and Rheumatoid Arthritis

Rheumatoid arthritis (RA) is an autoimmune inflammatory disorder primarily characterized by a symmetric destructive polyarthritis affecting small, medium and large joints. A number of genetic and environmental factors, including bacterial pathogens, may play a role in disease pathogenesis.[11] In-vitro studies suggest a role for *H. pylori* in the development of autoimmunity, but the clinical correlation between *H. pylori* infection and RA is less convincing.[7] Variable rates of *H. pylori* antibodies and *H. pylori* infection are reported in patients with RA. Data regarding the association of *H. pylori* infection with the onset or severity of RA remains unclear. Some studies suggested some clinical improvement in RA symptoms after eradication of *H. pylori*, but many others have been unable to corroborate these findings.[7]

3.3 *H. pylori* and Vasculitis

Henoch-Schonlein purpura (HSP) is a systemic vasculitis of small vessels, resulting in skin, joint, gastrointestinal, and renal involvement. The pathogenesis of HSP remains poorly understood, but it is postulated that an unknown antigenic stimulus causes elevation of circulating immunoglobulin A and that complement activation leads to necrotizing vasculitis. A wide variety of conditions such as infections, vaccinations, drugs, and other environmental exposures may be responsible for the onset.[12] Increased prevalence of serum antibody to *H. pylori* has been found in patients with HSP compared to adult controls; however, the rate of active infection documented by urease test or histology was lower.[13] In 1995 Reinauer et al.[14] described the first case of HSP associated with gastric *H. pylori*. The symptoms of HSP disappeared after *H. pylori* eradication, then recurred 10 months later due to reinfection with the bacteria. After the second eradication treatment, the clinical manifestations faded again. Since then, several single case reports have been published showing resolution of HSP symptoms coinciding with the eradication of *H. pylori* infection.[6,12]

Behçet's disease (BD) is a systemic vasculitic disorder consisting of recurrent aphthous stomatitis, genital ulcerations and relapsing uveitis. Although the etiology of BD is still unknown, various environmental, and genetic factors have been implicated in its pathogenesis. *H. pylori* infection is endemic in most countries in which BD is also highly prevalent.[15] Variable rates of *H. pylori* positivity were reported: from 85% (higher than controls) to 73% (lower than controls).[6] In a study with a cohort of 91 patients with BD, the prevalence of *H. pylori* seropositivity was similar to that of controls; however, the prevalence of CagA positivity was significantly higher in patients with BD. The pathogenic role of *H. pylori* in BD is still unknown. Two different studies showed that the eradication of *H. pylori* significantly decreased the clinical manifestations of BD, such as oral and genital ulcerations, arthritis/arthralgia and cutaneous manifestations. It is suggested that patients with BD should be screened for possible *H. pylori* infection in endemic areas, and prompt treatment should be instituted.[15]

3.4 *H. pylori* and Primary Raynaud's Phenomenon

Raynaud's phenomenon is an intermittent vasospasm of the arterioles of the distal limbs which occurs mostly following exposure to cold or emotional stimuli.[16] There have been contradictory results about the seroprevalence of *H. pylori* infection in patients with Raynaud's phenomenon.[17] The association between *H. pylori* infection and Raynaud's phenomenon has been attributed to an increased level of cytokines and acute phase reactants, resulting in vasospasm and platelet aggregation.[15] In two different clinical studies with patients with primary Raynaud's phenomenon, eradication of *H. pylori* infection was associated with complete disappearance of the episodes of Raynaud's phenomenon in 17–18% of treated patients and a reduction in symptoms in an additional 68–72%. It is remarkable that symptoms of Raynaud's phenomenon did not improve in those patients in whom eradication of *H. pylori* failed. Another study showed that the eradication of *H. pylori* improved the frequency and duration of Raynaud's attacks compared to the group in whom *H. pylori* was not eradicated.[16]

3.5 *H. pylori* and Chronic Urticaria

Chronic urticaria (CU) is a mucocutaneous disease characterized by erythematous, edematous, and pruritic lesions of the dermis and/or hypodermis lasting more than 6 weeks.[15] It results from the degranulation of mast cells and basophils and the release of inflammatory mediators, mainly histamine.[18] The pathogenesis of CU has not yet been fully elucidated, and a triggering factor can be indentified in only a minority of cases. A possible association between *H. pylori* infection and CU has been proposed.[15] Several pathophysiologic mechanisms have been suggested to explain this association.[15] One of those is that the presence of the *H. pylori* in the gastric mucosa stimulates the activated eosinophils to release cytotoxic proteins, which are involved in the pathophysiology of urticaria and interfere with the production of pro-inflammatory cytokines and with the expression of epitopes of adhesion to the endothelial cells, triggering a systemic immune response.[18] Conflicting reports regarding the effect of *H. pylori* eradication on CU symptoms have been published. There are studies suggesting that *H. pylori* eradication in patients with CU leads to an improvement in the symptoms of CU, including a case report of total remission of the symptoms of CU when the proper antibiotic treatment was instituted for both the first episode as well as the reinfection.[18] Otherwise, other publications showed no improvement of CU symptoms with *H. pylori* treatment. In 2010, Shakouri et al.[19] evaluated 19 studies and noticed that 10 of them showed a beneficial effect of bacterial eradication on the resolution of the symptoms of CU. This result did not allow definitive conclusions because of the observational nature of the studies, the small number of patients, and the short-term follow-up. Anyway, to cure at least some patients from quality of life-reducing CU, it seems worthwhile to eradicate *H. pylori* in all patients with CU and *H. pylori* infection.[15,20]

3.6 *H. pylori* and Alopecia Areata

Alopecia areata is a common condition causing nonscarring hair loss and is hypothesized to be an autoimmune, organ-specific, T-cell-mediated reaction directed against the human hair follicle. One study found no significant difference in the seroprevalence of *H. pylori* infection between patients with alopecia areata and healthy controls. In contrast, another one found that the seroprevalence of *H. pylori* infection was higher among patients with alopecia areata compared to age-matched controls.[15] There is only a single case report of a patient that went into remission from Alopecia areata after *H. pylori* eradication.[21]

3.7 *H. pylori* and Psoriasis

Psoriasis is an inflammatory skin disease that affects 1–3% of Caucasians.[15] Recent genetic and immunological advances have greatly increased understanding of the pathogenesis of psoriasis as a chronic, immune-mediated inflammatory disorder. Despite being controversial, it has been suggested that *H. pylori* may be one of the organisms capable of triggering psoriasis.[22] Seroprevalence studies of *H. pylori* infection in psoriatic patients are controversial. In an uncontrolled study of 33 patients with psoriasis but without any history of chronic gastrointestinal tract complaints, the seroprevalence of *H. pylori* infection was 27%. In another recent study of 50 psoriatic patients, the prevalence of *H. pylori* seropositivity was significantly higher than in the control group. Also, there does not seem to be a relation with the more virulent CagA strain and psoriasis. There are contradicting reports of the benefits of *H. pylori* eradication in patients with chronic psoriasis.[15,23] A recent study of 300 psoriasis patients showed correlations between *H. pylori* infection and the severity of psoriasis.[22] Most patients with positive *H. pylori* tests belonged to the moderate and severe psoriasis groups, and the eradication of *H. pylori* enhanced the effectiveness of psoriasis treatment.

3.8 *H. pylori* and Autoimmune Gastritis

Autoimmune gastritis is characterized by the presence of autoantibodies against gastric parietal cells and/or the intrinsic factor. Clinically, patients may have pernicious anemia, hypergastrinemia, and low pepsinogen concentrations. In the past it was believed that autoimmune gastritis was independent from *H. pylori* infection. It is now widely accepted that long-term infection by *H. pylori* is probably involved in autoimmune gastritis and body atrophy because the inflammation caused by *H. pylori* extends to all gastric mucosa, and the active infection process is gradually replaced by an immune process. Different studies report that about two-thirds of patients with autoimmune gastritis have evidence of *H. pylori* infection. Importantly, it should be noticed that, with the progress of the disease and consequently the development of body atrophy, the *H. pylori* disappears from gastric mucosa.[16] Evidence supports the conclusion that activated CD4+ T helper 1 cells, which infiltrate the gastric mucosa in response to *H. pylori* infection, cross-recognize epitopes of the K+/H+ ATPase proton pump and various *H. pylori* proteins.[24] It has been shown that eradication therapy of *H. pylori* seems to reverse some adverse effects on gastric function and regression in body atrophy.[16]

3.9 *H. pylori* and Anti-phospholipid Syndrome

The classic anti-phospholipid syndrome (APS) is characterized by the presence of anti-phospholipid antibodies (aPL), which bind target phospholipid molecules, mainly through β2-glycoprotein I, and are associated with recurrent fetal loss and thromboembolic phenomena. Many infections may be accompanied by increases in aPL, and, in some, these increases may be accompanied by clinical manifestations of the APS. Two reports point to the effectiveness of antibiotics treatment in APS. In the first, a patient with APS associated with *H. pylori*, all disease manifestations disappeared upon eradication of the bacteria. In the other—an experimental model of APS—the manifestations were abrogated by parallel treatment with ciprofloxacin.[25]

In conclusion, eradication of *H. pylori* infection in patients with ITP has been shown to be effective in improving platelet counts in 50% of cases, and there is consensus in the recommendation to eradicate *H. pylori* in chronic ITP. There is conflicting and controversial data regarding the association of *H. pylori* infection with other autoimmune diseases. Single or few case reports have documented associations between *H. pylori* infection and several autoimmune diseases, but these are only descriptive in nature.

4 GRANULOMATOSIS WITH POLYANGIITIS AND *STAPHYLOCOCCUS AUREUS*

Granulomatosis with polyangiitis (GPA), formerly known as Wegener's granulomatosis, is a small-vessel vasculitis characterized by granulomatous and necrotizing inflammation affecting the upper and lower respiratory tracts and, often, the kidneys.[26] Chronic nasal carriage of *Staphylococcus aureus* occurs in around 63% of patients with GPA, in contrast to around 25% of healthy controls.[27] Furthermore, chronic nasal carriage concurs with a strongly increased risk (relative risk of 7.2) for disease relapse and is associated with persistent positivity for proteinase 3 (PR3)—anti-neutrophil cytoplasmic antibody (ANCA). Similar results were reported from several other studies.[28] Various mechanistic explanations for this relationship are supported by experimental and clinical data, but the exact mechanism in which *S. aureus* modulates disease expression in GPA is not known. One hypothesis relates to persistent low-grade inflammation in the nasal cavity with the release of pro-inflammatory cytokines that prime neutrophils and monocytes for ANCA-induced full neutrophil activation. Also, superantigens from *S. aureus* may stimulate autoreactive lymphocytes to a PR3-directed immune response. Recent studies even suggest that *S. aureus*-derived peptides may induce PR3-ANCA via idiotypic–anti-idiotypic interactions. This notorious relationship between nasal colonization with *S. aureus* and relapsing GPA underscores a possible role for antibiotic treatment in this disease. Different studies support that prophylactic treatment with co-trimoxazole (960 mg b.i.) is effective in reducing the rate of GPA relapse. This effect was particularly apparent in patients with locoregional GPA occurring in the upper airways. Indeed, it was observed that disease progression stopped in 10 patients with GPA with locoregional disease treated with co-trimoxazole; however, among 24 patients with generalized GPA in remission, relapses occurred in more than 50%. In addition, this treatment was not curative in many cases, as demonstrated by recurrent disease activity after stopping it.[28] In another study of 31 patients with limited GPA treated with co-trimoxazole, only 18 patients reached complete remission and 9 partial remission at a median treatment time of 3 months, but 11 patients relapsed, particularly patients without carriage of *S. aureus* or disease outside the ear, nose, and throat region.[28] A double-blind, placebo-controlled study was performed to test the hypothesis that maintenance prophylactic treatment with co-trimoxazole could prevent the occurrence of relapses in patients with GPA. It showed that the treatment led to a 60% decrease in the incidence of relapses (relative risk, 0.40) and a strong decrease in the incidence of (mostly respiratory) infections.[27] Unfortunately, no data were available on *S. aureus* carriage in this study. There is a need for prospective randomized controlled studies in which intervention in *S. aureus* carriage is related to recurrent disease activity.[28]

5 CROHN'S DISEASE AND ENTERIC INFECTIONS

Crohn's disease (CD) is an inflammatory bowel disease characterized by an altered composition of the intestinal commensal bacteria (dysbiosis). Dysbiosis is considered to have an important role in CD pathogenesis, inducing an abnormal immune response in genetically susceptible individuals.[29] A number of intestinal pathogens including *Mycobacterium avium* subspecies *paratuberculosis* (MAP), adherent-invasive *Escherichia coli*, and *Campylobacter* species are associated at high prevalence with CD. The involvement of bacteria in CD inflammation has provided the rationale for including antibiotics in the therapeutic regimen. However, randomized controlled trials have failed to demonstrate an efficacy of these drugs in patients with active uncomplicated CD, even if a subgroup of patients with colonic location seems to benefit from antibiotics. Metronidazole and ciprofloxacin are recommended in perianal disease, and the use of nitroimidazole compounds have been shown to be efficacious in decreasing CD recurrence rates in operated patients. However, to treat this chronic relapsing disease the use of antibiotics must be for long-term periods which leads to the appearance of more systemic side effects, limiting their use. Rifaximin, characterized by an excellent safety profile, has provided promising results in inducing remission of CD, but larger studies are needed.[29,30] A recent randomized, double-blind, placebo-controlled trial in 8 Dutch hospitals enrolling 76 patients with CD with active perianal fistulizing disease showed that combination therapy of adalimumab and ciprofloxacin is more effective than adalimumab monotherapy to achieve fistula closure in CD. However, after discontinuing antibiotic therapy, the beneficial effect of initial co-administration is not maintained.[31]

Of the intestinal pathogens known to be associated with CD, MAP has been subject of several studies.[32] MAP is more prevalent among patients with CD compared with controls, although the pathogenic role of this bacterium in CD remains uncertain.[33] The resemblance of CD to tuberculous enteritis and Johne's disease of ruminants, caused by MAP, and the isolation of atypical mycobacteria from blood and tissue of patients with CD, lead to the evaluation of the efficacy of anti-mycobacterial drugs in these patients. However, the results of the randomized controlled trials performed with antibiotics active against atypical Mycobacteria for obtaining and maintaining CD remission are conflicting. A meta-analysis that considered several trials using different associations of anti-mycobacterial drugs showed that these drugs seem to be ineffective for inducing remission without a course of steroid therapy.[29] However, because of the heterogeneity of the trials, which used a wide range of antibiotic combinations administered for variable periods to a small number of patients, no definitive conclusion could be drawn. Those studies also were criticized because they used earlier tuberculosis drugs, such as ethambutol and isoniazid, which are not effective against MAP infection, and fewer than three antibiotics (a number considered critical for preventing development of drug resistance). Clarithromycin and azithromycin, macrolide compounds that are considered to be the most effective drugs for treatment of MAP, were used in four subsequent studies with encouraging results.[34] In a large study,[35] 213 Australian patients were randomized to receive a combination of clarithromycin plus rifabutin and clofazimine (active against MAP) or placebo for up to 2 years, in addition to a 16-week course of corticosteroids. It showed a significant benefit only at 16 weeks, when the antibiotic combination was added to steroids, confirming the data founded by the meta-analysis and suggesting that the short-term advantage could be related to a generic antibacterial effect. The authors concluded that this study does not support a significant role for MAP in CD pathogenesis; however, several objections to this conclusion have been raised.[29] Namely, the trial suffered profoundly from the problem of treating a very slow-growing mycobacterium with drug dosages that were not only suboptimal, but one of the drugs was only partially bioavailable because of faulty capsule design.[36,37] At the moment the mycobacterial hypothesis cannot be completely ruled out, and it continues to be reasonable that an infectious agent could start the inflammatory process and adequate antibiotic therapy can add benefit to therapy of CD.[29]

6 REACTIVE ARTHRITIS AND GASTROINTESTINAL/ GENITOURINARY INFECTION

Reactive arthritis (ReA) has traditionally been described as a nonseptic arthritis occurring following an extra-articular bacterial infection. This concept became clinically associated with antecedent infections of either the gastrointestinal or genitourinary tract.[38] The onset of joint symptoms is typically 1–4 weeks post-enteric. The joint disease may be monoarticular but is more commonly polyarticular, and the clinical spectrum varies from slight transient arthralgias to long-standing debilitating arthritis.[39] ReA has been reported to occur in up to 62% of people following an enteric infection caused by any one of a variety of microbes. The enteric bacterial species most often associated with ReA are *Salmonella enteritidis*, *Shigella* spp., *Campylobacter* spp., and *Yersinia* spp.[39] During active infection, enteric bacteria invade the intestinal mucosa, enter the systemic circulation, and are transported to the joint. Once there, the bacterial antigens invoke a local and persistent immune response leading to the inflammation associated with ReA. There are two possible mechanisms to explain this localized inflammatory response. One is that the immune system may be directly activated by recurrent infection or delivery of a bacterial antigen to the joint; the other is that the immune response to the initial infection may result in production of antibody epitopes with cross-reactivity with bacterial and human antigens.[39] Antibiotics did not seem to decrease the risk of ReA for patients treated with fluoroquinolones for *S. enteritidis*, and ReA may be slightly increased in those treated with antibiotics. Postulated reasons for this include antibiotic-induced alteration of the microbe and prolonged carriage of the microorganism, or it may simply be a marker of more severe disease. However, in another study of patients who developed ReA after infection with *Salmonella hadar*, antibiotic therapy seemed to be protective.[39] A recent systematic review and meta-analysis of randomized controlled trials of antibiotics for treatment of ReA concluded that these trials have produced heterogeneous results that may be related to differences in study design. As such, in this moment the efficacy of the treatment of enteric infection with antibiotics to prevent ReA is still uncertain.[40]

7 GUILLAIN-BARRÉ SYNDROME AND *CAMPYLOBACTER* INFECTION

Guillain-Barré syndrome (GBS) is an immune-mediated demyelinating polyneuropathy of the peripheral nervous system characterized by global weakness affecting both proximal and distal limbs, areflexia and sensory abnormalities.[41] Among numerous microbial infections, only *Campylobacter jejuni* (which is a leading cause of gastroenteritis worldwide) is firmly established as a causative agent of GBS. Up to 40% of patients with GBS worldwide suffer from *C. jejuni* infection 1–3 weeks before the illness. However, only 1 in 1000 patients who are exposed to *Campylobacter* infection develops GBS. The isolation rate of *C. jejuni* from stool culture of patients with GBS ranges from 8% to 50%, and seropositivity ranges from 24% to 76%. GBS results from autoimmune-driven nerve damage. This seems to occur by a cross-reactive immune response due to molecular mimicry between sialylated lipooligosaccharide structures on the cell envelope of these bacteria and ganglioside epitopes on the human nerves.[41] Despite the recognition of the association between GBS and *C. jejuni*, there are no studies about the efficacy of antibiotic use in enteric infections and prevention of GBS.

8 IMMUNE THROMBOCYTOPENIC PURPURA AND DAPSONE

Dapsone is an antibacterial sulfonamide with an anti-inflammatory property, but the mechanism of this anti-inflammatory effect is not fully understood.[42] Several studies highlighted the therapeutic activity of dapsone as salvage therapy in primary ITP, with a 40–60% overall response rate and a 15–50% complete response (platelet count $\geq 100 \times 10^9$/L) rate. The platelet increase was generally treatment dependent, even if the persistence of response after dapsone was discontinued occurred in some patients. Interestingly, the response to dapsone was unaffected by characteristics such as sex, age, platelet count or duration of ITP.[43,44] These studies suggest that dapsone may be a safe and effective second-line agent for patients with steroid-dependent or refractory ITP.[43] Furthermore, a more recent study evaluated the effect of dapsone in 20 consecutive adult patients with primary ITP previously treated at least with steroids and rituximab.[42] It documented a 55% response rate (platelet count $\geq 30 \times 10^9$/L) and a complete response (platelet count $\geq 100 \times 10^9$/L) rate of 20%. All responders were able to interrupt any other specific anti-ITP treatment. The median duration of dapsone therapy in responders and the median response duration were 31 and 42 months, respectively. Therapy was well tolerated overall, and none of the patients interrupted the treatment because of toxicity. None of the responders lost response during treatment. These results highlight the therapeutic activity and good safety profile of dapsone in patients with ITP who previously failed rituximab treatment.[42] A better understanding of ITP pathophysiology and of the dapsone mechanism of action will allow a better and rational integration of this agent into the treatment algorithm of primary ITP in the future.

9 DISCUSSION

When we talk about curing autoimmune diseases with antibiotics, we expect complete resolution of the clinical manifestations and analytical parameters of disease after antibiotic treatment. Indeed, there are few examples of documented cure of an autoimmune disease with antibiotics. Few patients with ITP can be cured with the eradication of *H. pylori*, and there are some isolated case reports of cure with antibiotics in other autoimmune diseases (Table 1). A little different is the case of RF, which cannot be cured but, even better, can be prevented with antibiotic treatment of the streptococcal pharyngitis.

In other cases antibiotic treatment can improve, both clinically and analytically, some autoimmune diseases without curing them. This supports the idea that, in those cases, antibiotics may not reverse the autoimmune process. In fact, in some of those cases, the improvement is treatment dependent, and autoimmune diseases recur after the stopping treatment with the antibiotics. Some anti-inflammatory action intrinsic to antibiotics may be responsible for disease improvement, as with the effect of dapsone in ITP or co-trimoxazole in *S. aureus*-negative patients with GPA. Even so, antibiotics are recommended in the treatment of different autoimmune conditions (Table 1), and in the majority of them are intended to eradicate a specific infectious agent.

Many different aspects have to be considered when speaking of curing an autoimmune process with antibiotics. For instance, the duration of the autoimmune disease when the antibiotic therapy is instituted can be relevant. In fact, in ITP, it has been shown that *H. pylori* eradication induced better response rates if ITP had a shorter duration. Similarly, co-trimoxazole prophylaxis is more effective in reducing relapses in patients with GPA with localized disease compared to patients with a more generalized disease. So, do we treat patients too late? After they already have too much damage to their immune system? An interesting theory being discussed is that an

Table 1 Evidence of the Use of Antibiotics in Autoimmune Diseases

Autoimmune Disease	Infectious Agent/ Infection/Antibiotic	Prevalence of the Infection in Patients with the Autoimmune Disease	Benefits of Antibiotic Treatment
Rheumatic fever (RF)	*Streptococcus* group A	RF always occurs after group A streptococcal infection	Treatment of streptococcal pharyngitis prevents RF (70% overall protection). Long-term antibiotic prophylaxis reduces the recurrence rate of RF in patients that already had a first acute attack.[3]
Immune thrombocytopenic purpura (ITP)	*H. pylori*	62.3% (Similar to the healthy population)	Platelet count responds in approximately 50% of patients with ITP following *H. pylori* eradication; very low rates of complete response (cure). The eradication of *H. pylori* infection is recommended in affected patients.[10]
Rheumatoid arthritis	*H. pylori*	Variable rates described (from lower to higher than controls)	Contradictory results[7]
Henoch–Schonlein purpura (HSP)	*H. pylori*	Increased rate of antibodies to *H. pylori*, but lower rate of active infection, in patients with HSP[13]	Several case reports of clinical disappearance of symptoms with *H. pylori* eradication.[6,12]
Behçet's disease	*H. pylori*	Variable rates described (from lower to higher than controls)[6]	Different studies suggest clinical improvement of BD manifestations with *H. pylori* eradication.[15]
Raynaud's disease	*H. pylori*	Variable rates described (from lower to higher than controls)[17]	Different studies showed cure in approximately 18% of patients and improvement of symptoms in 68–72% with *H. pylori* eradication.[16]

Disease	Bacteria		Comments
Chronic urticaria (CU)	H. pylori	Not reported	Contradictory results It has been suggested that in patients with quality of life-reducing CU, it seems worthwhile to eradicate H. pylori.[15,18,20]
Alopecia areata	H. pylori	Variable rates described (similar or higher than controls)[15]	One single case report of alopecia areata cure with H. pylori eradication.[21]
Psoriasis	H. pylori	Variable rates described (from lower to higher than controls)[15]	Contradictory results.[15]
Autoimmune gastritis	H. pylori	66% (Similar to the healthy population)[16]	Reversal of some adverse effects on gastric function and regression of body atrophy with H. pylori eradication.[16]
Anti-phospholipid syndrome (APS)	H. pylori	Not reported	One single case report of cure of APS with H. pylori eradication.[25]
Granulomatosis with polyangiitis (GPA)	Staphylococcus aureus	65% of patients (versus 25% of healthy controls)[27]	Different studies demonstrated a reduction of relapse rate of GPA with co-trimoxazole treatment, mainly in patients with localized disease.[27,28] Some reports of recurrence of the disease activity after stopping antibiotic treatment.[28]
Crohn's disease (CD)	Enteric bacteria		The use of metronidazol and ciprofloxacin is recommended in perianal disease. Nitroimidazole compounds have been shown to be efficacious in

(Continued)

Table 1 Evidence of the Use of Antibiotics in Autoimmune Diseases—cont'd

Autoimmune Disease	Infectious Agent/ Infection/Antibiotic	Prevalence of the Infection in Patients with the Autoimmune Disease	Benefits of Antibiotic Treatment
			decreasing CD recurrence rates in operated patients.[29,30] Contradictory results about the use of antibiotics in other forms of CD, as well as the use of antibiotics against *Mycobacterium avium* subspecies *paratuberculosis*.[29,36,37]
Reactive arthritis	Gastrointestinal or genitourinary infections	Reactive arthritis is usually preceded by a gastrointestinal or genitourinary infection[38]	Contradictory results[40]
Guillain-Barré syndrome	*Campylobacter jejuni*	8–50% isolation rate of *C. jejuni* from stool culture 24–76% seropositivity of *C. jejuni*.[41]	Not reported
ITP	Dapsone		Dapsone has anti-inflammatory properties. It is effective as a second-line agent for steroid-dependent or refractory ITP, even in those who failed rituximab treatment.[42,43] Most patients relapse after stopping the treatment.[43]

infection-induced immune response continues after the pathogen has been eradicated.[45] Maybe there is a time in which this process is still reversible. This could explain why some patients get cured and in others the autoimmune disease recurs.

Another important point is the possible role of intrinsic characteristics of the bacteria, of which the best example is the CagA-positive strains of *H. pylori*. In countries where CagA-positive strains of *H. pylori* are more prevalent, a higher response rate to antibiotic eradication in ITP has been noticed.[8] Being so, it is possible that specific intrinsic characteristics of the bacteria may be determinants in the development of an autoimmune disease, and consequently in the response to an antibiotic treatment.

Finally, an aspect that is also crucial for the understanding of the possibility of curing autoimmune diseases with antibiotics is that *not all autoimmune conditions are the same*, that is, they derive from different mechanisms. For instance, in RF there is a direct cause and effect in which the infection leads to the autoimmune disease; however, it seems that APS is derived through "two hit mechanisms", that is, the infections might have occurred long before the autoimmune manifestation emerges.[1] Moreover, it is known that triggering autoimmunity is sometimes a cumulative process, as in atherosclerosis. The immune system is affected by repeated infections from childhood, and in immune-sensitive individuals, a breakthrough point might occur when the infection burden crosses a crucial level.[1] Being so, it would be crucial to identify which mechanism is responsible for a specific autoimmune disease so it would be possible to determine which ones can be prevented/cured with antibiotics.

Despite the large body of evidence to support the contention that infections cause autoimmunity, as described above, in some cases infections can actually protect individuals from autoimmune diseases.[1] For instance, recent data suggest a protective effect of *H. pylori* against several autoimmune diseases, namely, inflammatory bowel disease, multiple sclerosis, and systemic lupus erythematosus.[6] As such, the idea of treating every bacterial infection with antibiotics to prevent the development of autoimmune diseases does not seem reasonable.

The possible role of antibiotics in curing autoimmune diseases is a very complex subject and at present their use is recommended in very few cases. Systematic studies examining different aspects of the relationship between autoimmune diseases and treatment with antibiotics are needed to further our understanding of this topic.

REFERENCES

1. Kivity S, Agmon-Levin N, Blank M, Shoenfeld Y. Infections and autoimmunity—friends or foes? *Trends Immunol* 2009;**30**(8):409–14, PubMed PMID: 19643667.
2. Getts MT, Miller SD. 99th Dahlem conference on infection, inflammation and chronic inflammatory disorders: triggering of autoimmune diseases by infections. *Clin Exp Immunol* 2010;**160**(1):15–21, PubMed PMID: 20415846. Pubmed Central PMCID: 2841830.
3. Chang C. Cutting edge issues in rheumatic fever. *Clin Rev Allergy Immunol* 2012 Apr;**42**(2):213–37, PubMed PMID: 21597903.
4. Guilherme L, Ramasawmy R, Kalil J. Rheumatic fever and rheumatic heart disease: genetics and pathogenesis. *Scand J Immunol* 2007;**66**(2–3):199–207, PubMed PMID: 17635797.
5. Wessels MR. Clinical practice. Streptococcal pharyngitis. *New Eng J Med* 2011 Feb 17;**364**(7):648–55, PubMed PMID: 21323542.
6. Hasni SA. Role of Helicobacter pylori infection in autoimmune diseases. *Curr Opin Rheumatol* 2012;**24**(4):429–34, PubMed PMID: 22617822. Pubmed Central PMCID: 3643302.
7. Hasni S, Ippolito A, Illei GG. Helicobacter pylori and autoimmune diseases. *Oral Dis* 2011 Oct;**17**(7):621–7, PubMed PMID: 21902767. Pubmed Central PMCID: 3653166.
8. Arnold DM, Bernotas A, Nazi I, Stasi R, Kuwana M, Liu Y, et al. Platelet count response to H pylori treatment in patients with immune thrombocytopenic purpura with and without H pylori infection: a systematic review. *Haematologica* 2009;**94**(6):850–6, PubMed PMID: 19483158. Pubmed Central PMCID: 2688577.
9. Stasi R, Sarpatwari A, Segal JB, Osborn J, Evangelista ML, Cooper N, et al. Effects of eradication of Helicobacter pylori infection in patients with immune thrombocytopenic purpura: a systematic review. *Blood* 2009;**113**(6):1231–40, PubMed PMID: 18945961.
10. Malfertheiner P, Megraud F, O'Morain C, Bazzoli F, El-Omar E, Graham D, et al. Current concepts in the management of Helicobacter pylori infection: the Maastricht III Consensus Report. *Gut* 2007;**56**(6):772–81, PubMed PMID: 17170018. Pubmed Central PMCID: 1954853.
11. Pordeus V, Szyper-Kravitz M, Levy RA, Vaz NM, Shoenfeld Y. Infections and autoimmunity: a panorama. *Clin Rev Allergy Immunol* 2008;**34**(3):283–99, PubMed PMID: 18231878.
12. Ulas T, Tursun I, Dal MS, Eren MA, Buyukhatipoglu H. Rapid improvement of Henoch-Schonlein purpura associated with the treatment of Helicobacter pylori infection. *J Res Med Sci* 2012;**17**(11):1086–8, PubMed PMID: 23833587. Pubmed Central PMCID: 3702094.
13. Novak J, Szekanecz Z, Sebesi J, Takats A, Demeter P, Bene L, et al. Elevated levels of anti-Helicobacter pylori antibodies in Henoch-Schonlein purpura. *Autoimmunity* 2003;**36**(5):307–11, PubMed PMID: 14567560.
14. Reinauer S, Megahed M, Goerz G, Ruzicka T, Borchard F, Susanto F, et al. Schonlein-Henoch purpura associated with gastric Helicobacter pylori infection. *J Am Acad Dermatol* 1995;**33**(5 Pt 2):876–9, PubMed PMID: 7593800.
15. Hernando-Harder AC, Booken N, Goerdt S, Singer MV, Harder H. Helicobacter pylori infection and dermatologic diseases. *Europ J Dermatol* 2009;**19**(5):431–44, PubMed PMID: 19527988.
16. Faria C, Zakout R, Araujo M. Helicobacter pylori and autoimmune diseases. *Biomed Pharmacother Biomed Pharmacotherapie* 2013;**67**(4):347–9, PubMed PMID: 23583190.
17. Herve F, Cailleux N, Benhamou Y, Ducrotte P, Lemeland JF, Denis P, et al. Prevalence des infections a Helicobacter pylori au cours de la maladie de Raynaud [Helicobacter pylori prevalence in Raynaud's disease]. *Rev Med Interne* 2006;**27**(10):736–41, PubMed PMID: 16978744.
18. Bruscky DM, da Rocha LA, Costa AJ. Recurrence of chronic urticaria caused by reinfection by Helicobacter pylori. *Rev Paul Pediatr* 2013;**31**(2):272–5, PubMed PMID: 23828067.

19. Shakouri A, Compalati E, Lang DM, Khan DA. Effectiveness of Helicobacter pylori eradication in chronic urticaria: evidence-based analysis using the Grading of Recommendations Assessment, Development, and Evaluation system. *Curr Opin Allergy Clin Immunol* 2010;**10**(4):362–9, PubMed PMID: 20610979.

20. Akashi R, Ishiguro N, Shimizu S, Kawashima M. Clinical study of the relationship between Helicobacter pylori and chronic urticaria and prurigo chronica multiformis: effectiveness of eradication therapy for Helicobacter pylori. *J Dermatol* 2011;**38** (8):761–6, PubMed PMID: 21352335.

21. Campuzano-Maya G. Cure of alopecia areata after eradication of Helicobacter pylori: a new association? *World J Gastroenterol* 2011;**17**(26):3165–70, PubMed PMID: 21912461. Pubmed Central PMCID: 3158418.

22. Onsun N, Arda Ulusal H, Su O, Beycan I, Biyik Ozkaya D, Senocak M. Impact of Helicobacter pylori infection on severity of psoriasis and response to treatment. *Eur J Dermatol* 2012;**22**(1):117–20, PubMed PMID: 22063790.

23. Martin Hubner A, Tenbaum SP. Complete remission of palmoplantar psoriasis through Helicobacter pylori eradication: a case report. *Clin Exp Dermatol* 2008;**33**(3):339–40, PubMed PMID: 18201263.

24. Bergman MP, Vandenbroucke-Grauls CM, Appelmelk BJ, D'Elios MM, Amedei A, Azzurri A, et al. The story so far: Helicobacter pylori and gastric autoimmunity. *Int Rev Immunol* 2005;**24**(1–2):63–91, PubMed PMID: 15763990.

25. Shoenfeld Y, Blank M, Cervera R, Font J, Raschi E, Meroni PL. Infectious origin of the antiphospholipid syndrome. *Ann Rheum Dis* 2006;**65**(1):2–6, PubMed PMID: 16344491. Pubmed Central PMCID: 1797971.

26. Jennette JC, Falk RJ, Bacon PA, Basu N, Cid MC, Ferrario F, et al. 2012 revised International Chapel Hill Consensus Conference Nomenclature of Vasculitides. *Arthritis Rheum* 2013;**65**(1):1–11, PubMed PMID: 23045170.

27. Kallenberg CG, Tadema H. Vasculitis and infections: contribution to the issue of autoimmunity reviews devoted to "autoimmunity and infection" *Autoimmun Rev* 2008;**8** (1):29–32, PubMed PMID: 18703171.

28. Kallenberg CG. What is the evidence for prophylactic antibiotic treatment in patients with systemic vasculitides? *Curr Opin Rheumatol* 2011;**23**(3):311–6, PubMed PMID: 21346576.

29. Scribano ML, Prantera C. Use of antibiotics in the treatment of Crohn's disease. *World J Gastroenterol* 2013;**19**(5):648–53, PubMed PMID: 23429474. Pubmed Central PMCID: 3574590.

30. Kale-Pradhan PB, Zhao JJ, Palmer JR, Wilhelm SM. The role of antimicrobials in Crohn's disease. *Expert Rev Gastroenterol Hepatol* 2013;**7**(3):281–8, PubMed PMID: 23445237.

31. Dewint P, Hansen BE, Verhey E, Oldenburg B, Hommes DW, Pierik M, et al. Adalimumab combined with ciprofloxacin is superior to adalimumab monotherapy in perianal fistula closure in Crohn's disease: a randomised, double-blind, placebo controlled trial (ADAFI). *Gut* 2013, PubMed PMID: 23525574.

32. Feller M, Huwiler K, Stephan R, Altpeter E, Shang A, Furrer H, et al. Mycobacterium avium subspecies paratuberculosis and Crohn's disease: a systematic review and meta-analysis. *Lancet Inf Dis* 2007 Sep;**7**(9):607–13, PubMed PMID: 17714674.

33. Abubakar I, Myhill D, Aliyu SH, Hunter PR. Detection of Mycobacterium avium subspecies paratuberculosis from patients with Crohn's disease using nucleic acid-based techniques: a systematic review and meta-analysis. *Inflamm Bowel Dis* 2008;**14** (3):401–10, PubMed PMID: 17886288.

34. Peyrin-Biroulet L, Neut C, Colombel JF. Antimycobacterial therapy in Crohn's disease: game over? *Gastroenterology* 2007;**132**(7):2594–8, PubMed PMID: 17570230.

35. Selby W, Pavli P, Crotty B, Florin T, Radford-Smith G, Gibson P, et al. Two-year combination antibiotic therapy with clarithromycin, rifabutin, and clofazimine for Crohn's disease. *Gastroenterology* 2007;**132**(7):2313–19, PubMed PMID: 17570206.

36. Gitlin L, Biesecker J. Australian Crohn's antibiotic study opens new horizons. *Gastroenterology* 2007;**133**(5):1743–4, author reply 5–6. PubMed PMID: 17983826.
37. Lipton JE, Barash DP. Flawed Australian CD study does not end MAP controversy. *Gastroenterology* 2007;**133**(5):1742, author reply 5–6. PubMed PMID: 17983825.
38. Morris D, Inman RD. Reactive arthritis: developments and challenges in diagnosis and treatment. *Curr Rheumatol Rep* 2012;**14**(5):390–4, PubMed PMID: 22821199.
39. Connor BA, Riddle MS. Post-infectious sequelae of travelers' diarrhea. *J Travel Med* 2013;**20**(5):303–12, PubMed PMID: 23992573.
40. Barber CE, Kim J, Inman RD, Esdaile JM, James MT. Antibiotics for treatment of reactive arthritis: a systematic review and metaanalysis. *J Rheumatol* 2013 Jun;**40**(6):916–28, PubMed PMID: 23588936.
41. Nyati KK, Nyati R. Role of Campylobacter jejuni infection in the pathogenesis of Guillain-Barre syndrome: an update. *BioMed Res Int* 2013;**2013**:852195, PubMed PMID: 24000328. Pubmed Central PMCID: 3755430.
42. Zaja F, Marin L, Chiozzotto M, Puglisi S, Volpetti S, Fanin R. Dapsone salvage therapy for adult patients with immune thrombocytopenia relapsed or refractory to steroid and rituximab. *Am J Hematol* 2012;**87**(3):321–3, PubMed PMID: 22190262.
43. Vancine-Califani SM, De Paula EV, Ozelo MC, Orsi FL, Fabri DR, Annichino-Bizzacchi JM. Efficacy and safety of dapsone as a second-line treatment in non-splenectomized adults with immune thrombocytopenic purpura. *Platelets* 2008;**19**(7):489–95, PubMed PMID: 18979360.
44. Damodar S, Viswabandya A, George B, Mathews V, Chandy M, Srivastava A. Dapsone for chronic idiopathic thrombocytopenic purpura in children and adults—a report on 90 patients. *Eur J Haematol* 2005;**75**(4):328–31, PubMed PMID: 16146539.
45. Radic M, Kaliterna DM, Radic J. Helicobacter pylori infection and systemic sclerosis—is there a link? *Joint Bone Spine* 2011;**78**(4):337–40, PubMed PMID: 21145276.

PART 2

Viruses and Autoimmunity

CHAPTER 17

Anti-Viral Therapy, Epstein–Barr Virus, Autoimmunity, and Chaos (The Butterfly Effect)

David H. Dreyfus[1]
Associate Clinical Professor, Department of Pediatrics, Yale SOM, New Haven, Connecticut, USA
[1]Corresponding Author: dhdreyfusmd@gmail.com

1 INTRODUCTION: NON-LINEAR EQUATIONS, CHAOS, AND THE "BUTTERFLY EFFECT"

More than a century ago, the mathematician H. Poincare (1854–1912) proved that seemingly simple and apparently deterministic astronomical systems, such as the combined orbits of the sun, earth, and moon, could not be characterized using simple mathematical equations.[1–3] Later, other mathematicians studying complicated phenomena such as the weather also found the seemingly simple interactions of more than three or more forces, such as solar heating, humidity, atmospheric pressure, and the tides could not be solved for similar reasons. Given that each variable affects all the other variables in these systems, small differences in starting conditions may lead to large or non-linear consequences, and a simple account of these systems behavior cannot be absolutely determined.[4]

This new mathematics is commonly associated with the so-called butterfly effect in which a very small change such as the wind generated by butterfly wings may in theory unpredictably alter the course of global weather on a very large scale.[1–3] These sorts of problems have led to a new mathematics of non-linear equations also termed chaos theory (Figures 1 and 2). Autoimmune diseases, like the solar system and the weather, seem to result from interactions between many different cofactors, including host parameters such as diet, genetic inheritance, as well as acquired differences in vaccination and microbiome, including endogenous viral replication (Figure 3). As in other chaotic systems, all of these factors may interact with each other, and the combined effects determine disease onset and outcome. The

Infection and Autoimmunity
http://dx.doi.org/10.1016/B978-0-444-63269-2.00019-2

Periodic oscillation

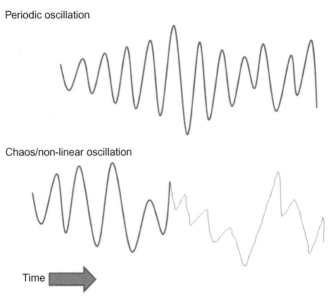

Chaos/non-linear oscillation

Time

Figure 1 In non-chaotic systems (top), a regular continuous curve mapping input into the system and output from the system is evident (blue line). In chaotic systems (bottom), discontinuous output is evident (red line) after the point of transition from a non-chaotic system (blue line). Chaotic systems are not random, but they lack a continuous or smooth transition from point to point; thus small changes in input can result in large changes in output.

Non-linear or chaotic systems

- Small changes in input conditions can lead to large and unpredictable changes in output the "butterfly effect"
- Not random but follow different and more complicated patterns than a linear or simple oscillating system
- Simple addition or subtraction of variable inputs are inadequate to explain outcomes

Figure 2 Properties of chaotic systems.

resulting chaos is not random but obeys a different set of laws and patterns that can be useful, yielding unexpected order.[5,6]

A critical and often neglected factor is that the Epstein–Barr virus (EBV) genome, like other herpes viruses, encodes approximately 100 regulated genes, some of which interact with expression of host genes such as

Complex interactions between
autoimmunity, infection, hygiene, and the genome

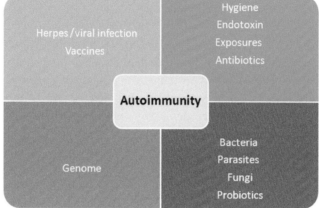

Figure 3 Autoimmunity can be modeled as a chaotic system because multiple factors, including viral infections and vaccines, host factors, environmental exposures and toxins, and other components of the microbiome, such as gut bacteria, interact with each other and affect disease onset and progression.

cytokines and other aspects of the host immune system.[7] These viral genes are exciting targets for new therapies but also increase the complexity of autoimmune diseases. The remainder of this review summarizes evidence that the butterfly effect is relevant to autoimmune disease because infectious agents such as EBV evolve over time and interact with the host and environment in multiple pathways that are not independent of each other and thus can only be modeled using non-linear concepts derived from chaos theory.

For example, the EBV genome contains phenocopies of host transcription factors and cytokines, as well as variable repeat elements similar to the V (D)J and somatic immunoglobulin and T-cell receptor recombination sequences, which apparently play essential roles in viral replication and produce a population of divergent viruses in the infected host from a single or small number of infecting viral genomes.[8,9] Chaotic interactions between an evolving viral population in a host and differing host genes and environmental factors described previous for other viruses, such as human immunodeficiency virus (HIV) and HTLV (human T-cell lymphoma virus), can help to model EBV-related autoimmune diseases and also suggest targets for anti-viral therapy and vaccines.[10–14]

2 EBV AND MS: A PARADIGM FOR ANTI-VIRAL THERAPY AND VACCINES, CHAOS THEORY, AND THE "BUTTERFLY EFFECT"

2.1 Current Models of EBV Pathogenesis in MS

EBV has been extensively studied as a cofactor in the neurological condition multiple sclerosis (MS).[15-20] While host genes, such as the major histocompatibility complex (MHC) and proteins regulating dietary sodium, and epidemiologic factors, such as vitamin D and dietary sodium, have been identified using genomic and epidemiologic analyses, evidence from studies of twins suggests that these factors can only account for less than half of the risk of autoimmune diseases.[20,21] Recent reviews summarized the many significant therapeutic options that can alter the risk of disease and progression of disease, and one may be left with the impression that there are an excess of observations combined with a shortage of a unifying theory.[22,23]

An informative and comprehensive recent review summarizes many of the variables, including EBV, that affect MS and suggests a novel unifying hypothesis that a particular melanoma–associated protein expressed in epithelial cells is a key or even causal variable because of its effects on oxidative stress.[24,25] In this model, oxidative stress triggers inflammatory changes in the brain epithelium that, in turn, trigger other observed pathology such as auto-antibodies. Rather than seeking to characterize evidence that EBV is a also causative factor in MS, this review proposes that rather than a single "cause" of MS there are a number of interacting cofactors, all of which are necessary but not sufficient to trigger the disease. As in the three-body problem found in astronomy and the weather, it is evident that many or all of these cofactors, including EBV, interact with non–linear dynamics because they are all constantly influencing each other.

2.2 Evidence for Chaotic Interactions Between EBV and Multiple Factors in MS

Dietary factors such as vitamin D and sodium have been proposed as a central factor in MS, and cigarette smoking and stress also affect the host and promote disease.[20,21,26,27] Certainly, adding vitamin D and other nutritional factors, limiting sodium intake, ceasing smoking, and reducing stress should be a part of any autoimmune therapy and are undoubtedly the most cost-effective therapy available. However, other variables associated with MS, such as EBV replication, cytokines, and the HLA locus, as well as multiple other immune factors of the host that contribute to anti-viral immunity may also interact directly or indirectly with melanocyte-associated proteins through effects on replication of EBV and expression of human endogenous retrovirus (HERV).[28–30]

More than any single factor, it must be recognized that in chaotic systems, once a certain threshold is crossed (Figures 1 and 2), the onset and progression of the disease may obey chaotic rules of progression different than those existing before the onset of illness. Thus, for example, while vitamin D or other dietary measures implemented in the population would normally be of benefit in preventing disease, it would be perhaps less effective after the onset of disease. Conversely, immunologic therapy such as interferons, while essential in preventing progression of established disease, may have little or no role in the prevention of disease. In chaotic systems, unlike in the Newtonian universe, the clock does not run the same backwards as forwards.[3]

3 EBV AND SLE, RA, MG: DIFFERENT TARGET ORGANS AND DIFFERENT DISEASES, SAME VIRUS?

3.1 Tissue-Specific Effects of EBV

EBV is a cofactor in common autoimmune disease in addition to MS, most extensively studied in systemic lupus erythematosus (SLE), rheumatoid arthritis (RA), and myasthenia gravis (MG). How can the same virus serve as a cofactor in multiple diseases? Is the difference in the host, in the virus or in the complex interactions between both? One possibility suggested by models such a molecular mimicry between viral and host gene products may explain the differing pathology in the case of SLE and RA, because different viral antigens mimic different host tissues.[17,18,31–34] Different tissues may have different expression of HERV.[28–30] Replication of the virus in target organs such as the T cells or the thymus in MG or SLE may also alter host pathology.[35,36] As with MS, consideration of cofactors such as heredity, environment, diet, and infectious pathogens may affect the outcome of the disease because all of these cofactors can influence the incidence, target organ, and progression of the disease through complex and chaotic interactions. Based on other viral systems, another important implication of the ability of EBV to alter itself is that the virus may be a "moving target", changing itself in response to therapy.[10,13,14,37] The host immune system also changes with time.[11]

3.2 Tissue-Specific Mutations in the EBV Viral Capsid Protein

Considering that most in vitro EBV research has been conducted in the laboratory using the B-958 strain, which is adapted for growth in vitro in non-human cell lines and highly tropic for B lymphocytes, it may come as a surprise to find that EBV isolated from the human lymphoblastoid Akata cell line infects a wide range of human cell types.[38] Mutation of a single viral gene product in the viral capsid—termed VCA (the viral capsid antigen)—is sufficient to completely alter the tissues bound and infected by EBV.[38] In humans, differences in viral tropism also are evident in different host populations; some types of cancer, such as T-cell lymphoma and nasopharyngeal carcinoma affecting T-lymphocytes and oropharyngeal epithelial cells, are common in Japanese and Chinese populations, respectively, but are rare in other host populations. Interestingly, in one study no evidence of polymorphisms in the EBNA (Epstein–Barr virus nuclear activator) gene were identified as effecting MS prognosis.[39] However, with advances in DNA sequencing it may be possible in the future to analyse entire viral genome populations in individuals at risk for a specific autoimmune syndrome and determine their risk not only through host factors but also through viral profiles.[40]

3.3 Additional Mutations in EBV Transcription Factors may Alter Tissue-Specific Viral Replication

I identified a polymorphism in the viral BZLF-1 or ZEBRA protein, which is a viral-encoded critical switch between viral latency and lytic growth (Figure 4). This polymorphism alters a serine at amino acid 205 in the Akata strain to an alanine in the B-958 strain. As noted earlier, B-958 adapts to tissue and has an altered range of target tissues.[41] The region of ZEBRA altered by this mutation is in a residue (serine) that is a target of host enzyme phosphorylation and regulation during viral replication; it is also in a region of the virus termed ZANK (ZEBRA ANKyrin-like) that binds to host transcription factors NF-κB and tumor suppressor p53. ZANK also is adjacent to another region of ZEBRA that binds viral and host AP-1 transcription sites. Because viral replication proceeds in different host tissues and environments, selection for different viral genes and proteins, such as VCA and ZEBRA, is also ongoing, altering, and affecting both host cell tropisms and viral growth parameters as in other viral host systems.

A polymorphism in the EBV BZLF-1 protein ZEBRA between viral strains B-958 and Akata is in a critical structural element termed ZANK (ZEBRA ANKyrin-like region)

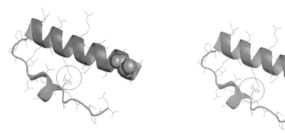

Figure 4 Viruses such as the EBV are not a uniform population; they contain complex genomes that interact with the host. The viral transcription factor encoded by the EBV BZLF-1 open reading frame, termed ZEBRA, is a multifunctional protein binding to host and viral DNA sites also recognized by the host AP-1 transcription factors. ZEBRA also binds to the host NF-κB transcription factors through a carboxyl ankyrin-like region termed ZANK. I propose that polymorphisms in ZANK and ZEBRA may alter viral replication and interactions with host transcription factors. A strain polymorphism in ZANK altering a serine to an alanine in ZANK is shown: ZANK with B-958 residue alanine 205 (orange) is indicated on the left; ZANK with Akata residue serine 205 (serine, green; hydroxyl, pink) is shown on the right. The position of contact between the ZANK system and loop residues is circled.

3.4 EBV Interacts with Both RAG-Mediated V(D)J Recombination, accelerating Viral Evolution in Response to Therapy

As shown in Figure 5, EBV contains in its genome host recombination signals that seem to be targets of host and viral DDE recombinases. DDE recombinases are a widely dispersed family of enzymes including transposases, retroviral integrases, and the recombination activating genes (RAGs) that may serve to increase viral and host variation in infected cells. The virus carries in its genome a linear phenocopy of the host immunoglobulin locus, including sequences that are targeted by adenosine deaminase, required for somatic mutation of immunoglobulin.[8,42] EBV internal and terminal sequences, termed LTR (long terminal repeats), are apparently targets of a recombinase resembling the vertebrate RAG protein (recombination activating gene-1).[8,43] These sequence seem to recombine through a process similar to vertebrate immunoglobulin and T–cell receptor gene recombination to generate a variable population of latent and lytic viral progeny genomes. EBV also encodes its own V(D)J-like recombinase, similar to the host RAG-1 recombinase.[44]

DDE recombination signals

- Tc1:   **CAGTG**CTGGCC<u>AAAAG</u>ATATCCAC<u>TTTTG</u>
- Tc3:   **CAGTG**TGGG<u>AAAG</u>TTCTATAGGACCCCCC

- EBV: **CACAG**GCAACCCTGA<u>CAAAG</u>GCCCCCCAGG<u>AAAGA</u>
- HSUb: **CACA**CCCCCCGGGGGTCGCGCGCGGCGCCCTTT<u>AAAG</u>
- HSUC:* **CAC**GCCGCCCGGACCGCCGCCCGCCT<u>TTTTTG</u>

- R12:   **CACAGTG**CTACAGACTGGA<u>ACAAAAACC</u>
- R23:   **CACAGTG**GTAGTACTCCACTGTCTGGCTGT<u>ACAAAAAC</u>

- TSib: **CACAGTG**GGCAATTGGCCGAATT<u>TTTTTTG</u>GAA<u>AAAAAG</u>CAA

Figure 5 Herpes virus genomes contain repeating units resembling the V(D)J recombination signals required for recombination of vertebrate immunoglobulin and T-cell receptors by recombinases in the DDE recombinase family. Herpes viruses also encode a copy of a DDE recombinase similar to the vertebrate recombination activating gene (RAG)-1 DDE recombinase that cuts and recombines V(D)J recombination sites in vertebrate immunoglobulin and T-cell receptor genes. Viral DDE recombinases are coregulated with RAG gene expression and viral replication, and herpes viruses may use a process similar to V(D)J recombination to generate viral diversity during genome replication. Here, heptamer sequences are bold, nonamer-like sequences are underlined. *Sequences of the Epstein–Barr virus and herpes simplex virus.

It is likely that mutation and recombination in ongoing EBV infection over time—rather than duplicate copies of the input virus—result in a population of progeny viruses differing rapidly in tissue tropism and other properties specific to the viral host.[45–47] These variant viral progeny, in turn, are at the same time selected for differences in host tissues and host genetic factors. Thus, it is not surprising that over time differences in viral dynamics, as well as host factors, interact chaotically to result in different diseases. These recombination processes that generate viral and host variation are not random and could be blocked by pharmacologic intervention. For example, the retroviral integrase inhibitors that block HIV integration are also effective inhibitors of herpes-encoded proteins required for viral replication, including the herpes-encoded homologs of RAG-1.[17,44]

4 EBV INTERACTIONS WITH ATOPIC AND VIRAL-ENCODED CYTOKINES IN AUTOIMMUNE PATHOGENESIS

Another factor that suggests chaotic dynamics of the virus–host relationship during chronic EBV infection is the ability of the host to alter its cytokines and inflammatory pathways. All herpes viruses replicate more effectively in a Th2 rather than a Th1 cytokine environment.[7] Remarkably, EBV and other herpes viruses also actively manipulate the host cytokine profile, for example, through viral-encoded cytokines.[7] Conversely, Th1 cytokines such as interferons play a significant role in MS therapy, although predicting who will respond to interferon and related Th1 cytokines is challenging.[22,48] If Th2 cytokines play a significant role in some patients with identified triggers to allergy, immunotherapy and/or allergen avoidance could alter both the progression of disease and the response to Th1 cytokine therapy such as interferon and other Th1 cytokines.[16,33,49–52] Conversely, alterations in host allergen exposures and Th2 gene expression could interact chaotically with diet and other environmental factors.

5 EBV REPLICATION, COMMON VARIABLE IMMUNODEFICIENCY, AND AUTOIMMUNITY: WHICH COMES FIRST?

Immunodeficient hosts are at increased risk of both EBV-related autoimmune diseases and malignancy. For example, common variable immunodeficiency (CVID) seems to have two phenotypes: one associated with autoimmune disease and a second associated with increased infection but not autoimmunity.[52–57] These observations could suggest that some forms of hereditary immunodeficiency such as CVID predispose to increased viral replication by EBV and related herpes viruses and thus to autoimmune syndromes.[52] Conversely, increased replication of EBV could cause CVID by killing or inactivating lymphocytes important in the immune response.[9,36] As our understanding of the various forms of hereditary immunodeficiency increase through whole exome sequencing and other technology, it may be possible to identify subtle genetic defects in syndromes such as CVID that can be targeted through gene therapy of the host, simultaneously curing both the CVID and the associated autoimmune syndromes. Oscillation between normal and abnormal immune function in CVID and other immunodeficiency is therefore apparently another component of autoimmune chaos, because host immune function is, in turn, dependent on infection, host nutrition, cytokines, and other factors that vary with time.[12,50,58]

6 DOES THE BUTTERFLY EFFECT MATTER?

6.1 Chaos: Implications for Animal Models of Autoimmune Disease

Chaos theory can provide a means of understanding the limitations of current animal models of autoimmune disease. In most animal models, a single variable, such as the absence of a mutation, the presence of an environmental factor or use of drug therapy, in genetic autoimmunity is studied. One can imagine scenarios in which widely different or opposing results of these variables could occur through unknown and chaotic interactions between all of these and other unknown factors differing between mice and humans. For example, in a mouse model in which endogenous retroviruses trigger an SLE-like syndrome, the addition of raltegravir, a retroviral integrase inhibitor, caused worsening of the disease.[59] Raltegravir seemed to block processing of endogenous retroviral genomes, which then accumulated and caused increased immunostimulation via the endogenous retroviral coat protein superantigen.

However, if in fact herpes viruses such as EBV play a role in triggering autoimmunity, then anti-viral therapy might still be effective because in humans it could be suggested that there are many interacting factors that might alter the results of the mouse model.[17,60,61] Most important, the anti-herpes effects of raltegravir might be greater than the effects on endogenous retrovirus replication in humans as opposed to mice. The biology of endogenous retroviruses might be different in humans, the microbiome and other host factors of mice might differ from humans in the metabolism of raltegravir, and so on. Unlike linear models in which variables are additive, the chaos of actual human autoimmune diseases cannot be completely understood in model systems, although these systems are essential to clarify underlying disease mechanisms.

There are also no adequate animal models for EBV, because CD21 and other viral receptors are only present in humans, and even mouse/human bone marrow chimeras lack viral receptors on tissues such as epithelium that may play a role in viral replication and inflammation.[9] Mice age differently than humans, and age profoundly affects immune response.[11] As noted earlier, in humans, mutations in EBV proteins can dramatically alter viral tropism for epithelial cells, and mutations in viral transcription factors may alter viral replication. Variables in the biology of host MS cofactors such as development and metabolism of the neural crest, nutritional factors such as vitamin D and sodium intake, and host factors such as MHC are not independent of the biology of infectious agents such as herpes viruses (e.g. EBV) and endogenous retrovirus activated by EBV. Differences in neural crest development may alter herpes metabolism and replication because herpes viruses replicate in epithelial cells that are derived from the same epithelial layers as neuronal tissues during fetal development. Increased dietary sodium intake might alter herpes virus gene expression in some patients and not others, deficient dietary vitamin D might cause different replication and metabolism of herpes virus and retroviral genomes in diseased tissues, and so on.

6.2 Chaos: Implications of for Anti-viral Vaccines and Therapy and Personalized Medicine

Viral populations are genetic entities rather than single monoclonal species.[10,13] The EBV genome encodes approximately 100 genes with genetic polymorphisms similar to host gene polymorphisms, and any of these viral genes could differ between individuals and populations. Utilizing whole-genome sequencing – not only of the host genome but also of the microbiome, including herpes viruses – it may be possible in the future to identify particular markers suggesting a patient with an autoimmune disease may respond to a particular anti-viral drug, monoclonal antibody, or vaccine, as has been pioneered for therapy of HIV/AIDS. Catalytic antibodies have recently been identified that have intrinsic neutralizing properties against common pathogens, and if produced cheaply and in large quantities from plants or through other methods could be administered to provide immunity in the absence of an effective EBV vaccine.[62,63] Theoretically, synthetic or in vitro production of neutralizing antibodies may be preferable immunostimulatory vaccines in patients with autoimmunity because of the possibility of vaccine adjuvant-related inflammation and exacerbation rather than therapy.[64–68]

In the absence of a vaccine or neutralizing antibodies, pharmacologic anti-viral therapy remains an underused option, both for MS and for other autoimmune diseases.[17] Remarkably, two independent small studies demonstrated that a safe and effective anti-viral therapy active against EBV, acyclovir, prevented the progression of MS, as determined by CT scan, but did not affect symptom scores.[17] Acyclovir is only weakly effective against EBV, but other nucleoside analogues are in development.[69] A single case report suggests remission of MS related to anti-viral therapy in a patient with HIV.[70] These observations have apparently never been pursued in larger controlled studies, perhaps because acyclovir is not particularly potent against EBV and does not seem to have benefits in established disease (only in altering disease progression) and also possibly because "off-label" use of a generic medication such as acyclovir is not attractive to large pharmaceutical manufacturers, who would have to sponsor such a trial.

However, different classes of anti-viral therapy such as retroviral integrase inhibitors could be more effective against EBV because, unlike acyclovir and related nucleoside inhibitors, retroviral integrase inhibitors may interfere with herpes gene and protein expression in addition to viral genome replication.[17,44] A single case report demonstrated improvement in an autoimmune platelet syndrome in a patient treated with raltegravir, and another case report confirmed the safety and apparent efficacy of raltegravir in a patient with recurrent oral cold sores due to herpes simplex, although larger controlled studies obviously are necessary before any conclusions can be drawn.[60,70] Long-term use of retroviral integrase inhibitors, as with all anti-viral therapy, may also select for resistant viral strains.[71,72] Improved anti-viral immunity related to dietary modification, such as vitamin D supplementation, sodium reduction, and improved nutrition combined with stress reduction, may remain a cost-effective anti-viral strategy.

6.3 Chaos: Implications for Novel Therapies and Vaccines

Anti-viral therapy targeting HERV with an envelope-specific monoclonal antibody is also in clinical trials.[73] Evidence that activation of HERV by EBV is a critical factor in MS has been suggested based on experimental and clinical evidence that *HERV* gene expression is activated by EBV in memory B lymphocytes.[17,29,30,74–79] *HERV* polymorphisms are correlated with MS incidence, and response of MS to some therapies such as rituximab depletion of memory B lymphocytes may be related to reduced HERV superantigen expression. However, the effects of rituximab are variable in both MS and other autoimmune syndromes.

If the HERV hypothesis is correct, blocking or eliminating *HERV* gene expression may have major clinical implications not only for EBV-related diseases but also for autoimmune disease in general, because other types of autoimmunity that do not involve EBV as a cofactor, such as diabetes, may nonetheless involve HERV cofactors. However, HERV and herpes viruses have been coevolving with the immune system since the origins of immunity, and altering the intricate balance between viruses, HERV, and the immune system may have unexpected consequences.[7,8,43,80] As with all therapies of autoimmune disease, because of the multiple interactions and chaotic nature of the underlying disease process it is unlikely that a single therapy will be curative.

7 CONCLUSIONS: AUTOIMMUNITY AND THE BUTTERFLY EFFECT?

I suggest here that the role of EBV as a cofactor in autoimmune syndromes can best be modeled as a chaotic or non-linear system in which multiple factors, including the viral genome, the host genome, cytokines, the environment, and the microbiome, all interact with each other (Figure 6). The virus itself is almost certainly not constant over time; instead it changes in response to therapy through host mutational pathways shared with the host immune system. Chaos theory may provide a useful model to describe the multiple interacting cofactors between EBV and its human host that play a

Conclusions

- *Multiple factors influence autoimmune disease with non-linear or chaotic effects, termed the butterfly effect*
- *Small changes in viral replication, age of infection, host genetic factors may lead to large changes (non-linear) in host disease*
- *Other factors such as diet (vitamin D, sodium), environmental toxins, microbiome are also non-linear interactions*
- *Viral polymorphisms in key regulatory proteins such as BZLF-1 encoded ZEBRA may also be inherited in families and have strain differences that confound heritability studies*
- *Therapy must be personalized and monitored; consider multiple therapy targets rather than increase therapy directed at a single target i.e. combined anti-viral and anti-inflammatory agents, dietary modification*

Figure 6 Summary of implications of the chaos and the butterfly effect for autoimmune disease.

role in the onset and progression of autoimmune diseases because of the multiple interaction of cofactors influencing disease onset and progression, also termed the butterfly effect.

An important implication is that a non-linear or chaotic paradigm may be of use in understanding and caring for autoimmune diseases, in particular the role of anti-viral therapy and vaccines. If the viral cofactors such as EBV and HERV are "moving targets", constantly changing in response to therapy and the state of the host, this may be particularly important in characterizing viral resistance to therapy, as is noted, for example, in the response of HIV to multi-functional anti-retroviral drugs such as raltegravir. Of course, neutralizing antibodies, and vaccines are also subject to viral mutation and evasion.

Based on theoretical models of other chaotic systems, it is likely that therapies simultaneously targeting multiple interacting factors—including anti-viral therapies, virus-neutralizing antibodies and vaccines, host nutrition, inflammation, and the microbiome – may be more effective than any of these adopted as monotherapy in the absence of changes in other parameters. A better understanding of viral as well as host biology is required to model these interactions and to optimize personalized therapy.

REFERENCES

1. Gleick J, editor. *Chaos: making a new science*. Pantheon Press; 1987.
2. Lorenz EN, editor. *The essence of chaos*. University of Washington Press; 1993.
3. Peterson I, editor. *Newton's clock: chaos in the solar system*. W.H. Freeman; 1993.
4. Strogaz SH, editor. *Sync*. New York: Hyperion Press; 2003.
5. Mandelbaum BB, editor. *The fractal geometry of nature*. W.H. Freeman; 1982.

6. Stewart I, editor. *Does god play dice?*. Blackwell Press; 1990.
7. Dreyfus DH. Herpesviruses and the microbiome. *J Allergy Clin Immunol* 2013; **132**(6):1278–86.
8. Dreyfus DH. Paleo-immunology: evidence consistent with insertion of a primordial herpes virus-like element in the origins of acquired immunity. *PLoS One* 2009;**4**:e5778.
9. Dreyfus DH, Kelleher CA, Jones JF, Gelfand EW. Epstein–Barr virus infection of T cells: implications for altered T-lymphocyte activation, repertoire development and autoimmunity. *Immunol Rev* 1996;**152**:89–110.
10. Gupta S, Ferguson N, Anderson R. Chaos, persistence, and evolution of strain structure in antigenically diverse infectious agents. *Science* 1998;**280**:912–15.
11. Madi A, Kenett DY, Bransburg-Zabary S, et al. Analyses of antigen dependency networks unveil immune system reorganization between birth and adulthood. *Chaos* 2011;**21**:016109.
12. Mak TW. 'Order from disorder sprung': recognition and regulation in the immune system. *Philos Trans A: Math Phys Eng Sci* 2003;**361**:1235–50.
13. O'Connor DH, Burton DR. Immune responses and HIV: a little order from the chaos. *J Exp Med* 2006;**203**:501–3.
14. Shu H, Wang L, Watmough J. Sustained and transient oscillations and chaos induced by delayed antiviral immune response in an immunosuppressive infection model. *J Math Biol* 2014;**68**(1–2):477–503.
15. Ascherio A, Munger KL, Lunemann JD. The initiation and prevention of multiple sclerosis. *Nat Rev Neurol* 2012;**8**:602–12.
16. Comabella M, Kakalacheva K, Rio J, Munz C, Montalban X, Lunemann JD. EBV-specific immune responses in patients with multiple sclerosis responding to IFNbeta therapy. *Mult Scler* 2012;**18**:605–9.
17. Dreyfus DH. Autoimmune disease: a role for new anti-viral therapies? *Autoimmun Rev* 2012;**11**:88–97.
18. Lunemann JD, Munz C. EBV in MS: guilty by association? *Trends Immunol* 2009;**30**:243–8.
19. Munger KL, Levin LI, O'Reilly EJ, Falk KI, Ascherio A. Anti-Epstein–Barr virus antibodies as serological markers of multiple sclerosis: a prospective study among United States military personnel. *Mult Scler* 2011;**17**:1185–93.
20. Pender MP. CD8+ T-cell deficiency, Epstein–Barr virus infection, vitamin D deficiency, and steps to autoimmunity: a unifying hypothesis. *Autoimmune Dis* 2012;**2012**:189096.
21. Kleinewietfeld M, Manzel A, Titze J, et al. Sodium chloride drives autoimmune disease by the induction of pathogenic TH17 cells. *Nature* 2013;**496**:518–22.
22. Bruck W, Gold R, Lund BT, et al. Therapeutic decisions in multiple sclerosis: moving beyond efficacy. *JAMA Neurol* 2013;**70**:1315–24.
23. Zipp F, Gold R, Wiendl H. Identification of inflammatory neuronal injury and prevention of neuronal damage in multiple sclerosis: hope for novel therapies? *JAMA Neurol* 2013;**70**:1569–74.
24. Krone B, Grange JM. Is a hypothetical melanoma-like neuromelanin the underlying factor essential for the aetiopathogenesis and clinical manifestations of multiple sclerosis? *BMC Neurol* 2013;**13**:91.
25. Krone B, Grange JM. Paradigms in multiple sclerosis: time for a change, time for a unifying concept. *Inflammopharmacology* 2011;**19**:187–95.
26. Palacios N, Alonso A, Bronnum-Hansen H, Ascherio A. Smoking and increased risk of multiple sclerosis: parallel trends in the sex ratio reinforce the evidence. *Ann Epidemiol* 2011;**21**:536–42.
27. Riise T, Mohr DC, Munger KL, Rich-Edwards JW, Kawachi I, Ascherio A. Stress and the risk of multiple sclerosis. *Neurology* 2011;**76**:1866–71.

28. Hsiao FC, Tai AK, Deglon A, Sutkowski N, Longnecker R, Huber BT. EBV LMP-2A employs a novel mechanism to transactivate the HERV-K18 superantigen through its ITAM. *Virology* 2009;**385**:261–6.

29. Perron H, Germi R, Bernard C, et al. Human endogenous retrovirus type W envelope expression in blood and brain cells provides new insights into multiple sclerosis disease. *Mult Scler* 2012;**18**:1721–36.

30. Perron H, Hamdani N, Faucard R, et al. Molecular characteristics of Human End-ogenous Retrovirus type-W in schizophrenia and bipolar disorder. *Transl Psychiatry* 2012;**2**:e201.

31. Cavalcante P, Cufi P, Mantegazza R, Berrih-Aknin S, Bernasconi P, Le Panse R. Eti-ology of myasthenia gravis: innate immunity signature in pathological thymus. *Autoim-mun Rev* 2013;**12**:863–74.

32. Harley IT, Kaufman KM, Langefeld CD, Harley JB, Kelly JA. Genetic susceptibility to SLE: new insights from fine mapping and genome-wide association studies. *Nat Rev Genet* 2009;**10**:285–90.

33. Namjou B, Kilpatrick J, Harley JB. Genetics of clinical expression in SLE. *Autoimmunity* 2007;**40**:602–12.

34. Sestak AL, Nath SK, Kelly JA, Bruner GR, James JA, Harley JB. Patients with familial and sporadic onset SLE have similar clinical profiles but vary profoundly by race. *Lupus* 2008;**17**:1004–9.

35. Berrih-Aknin S, Ragheb S, Le Panse R, Lisak RP. Ectopic germinal centers, BAFF and anti-B-cell therapy in myasthenia gravis. *Autoimmun Rev* 2013;**12**:885–93.

36. Dreyfus DH. Role of T cells in EBV-infected systemic lupus erythematosus patients. *J Immunol* 2005;**175**:3460, author reply 1.

37. Gomez-Acevedo H, Li MY, Jacobson S. Multistability in a model for CTL response to HTLV-I infection and its implications to HAM/TSP development and prevention. *Bull Math Biol* 2010;**72**:681–96.

38. Tsai MH, Raykova A, Klinke O. Spontaneous lytic replication and epitheliotropism define an Epstein-Barr virus strain found in carcinomas. *Cell Reports* 2013;**5**:458–70.

39. Simon KC, Yang X, Munger KL, Ascherio A. EBNA1 and LMP1 variants in multiple sclerosis cases and controls. *Acta Neurol Scand* 2011;**124**:53–8.

40. Skalsky RL, Corcoran DL, Gottwein E, et al. The viral and cellular microRNA targe-tome in lymphoblastoid cell lines. *PLoS Pathog* 2012;**8**:e1002484.

41. Dreyfus DH, Liu Y, Ghoda LY, Chang JT. Analysis of an ankyrin-like region in Epstein Barr virus encoded (EBV) BZLF-1 (ZEBRA) protein: implications for interactions with NF-κB and p53. *Virol J* 2011;**8**:422.

42. Niller HH, Wolf H, Minarovits J. Viral hit and run-oncogenesis: genetic and epigenetic scenarios. *Cancer Lett* 2011;**305**:200–17.

43. Dreyfus DH. Immune system: success owed to a virus? *Science* 2009;**325**:392–3.

44. Bryant KF, Yan Z, Dreyfus DH, Knipe DM. Identification of a divalent metal cation binding site in herpes simplex virus 1 (HSV-1) ICP8 required for HSV replication. *J Virol* 2012;**86**:6825–34.

45. Chezar I, Lobel-Lavi L, Steinitz M, Laskov R. Ongoing somatic hypermutation of the rearranged VH but not of the V-lambda gene in EBV-transformed rheumatoid factor-producing lymphoblastoid cell line. *Mol Immunol* 2008;**46**:80–90.

46. Heath E, Begue-Pastor N, Chaganti S, et al. Epstein–Barr virus infection of naive B cells in vitro frequently selects clones with mutated immunoglobulin genotypes: implications for virus biology. *PLoS Pathog* 2012;**8**:e1002697.

47. Ponce RA, Gelzleichter T, Haggerty HG, et al. Immunomodulation and lymphoma in humans. *J Immunotoxicol* 2014;**11**:1–12.

48. Petersen T, Moller-Larsen A, Ellermann-Eriksen S, Thiel S, Christensen T. Effects of interferon-beta therapy on elements in the antiviral immune response towards the

human herpesviruses EBV, HSV, and VZV, and to the human endogenous retroviruses HERV-H and HERV-W in multiple sclerosis. *J Neuroimmunol* 2012;**249**:105–8.

49. Ascherio A, Marrie RA. Vitamin D in MS: a vitamin for 4 seasons. *Neurology* 2012;**79**:208–10.

50. Ben-Ami E, Miller A, Berrih-Aknin S. T cells from autoimmune patients display reduced sensitivity to immunoregulation by mesenchymal stem cells: role of IL-2. *Autoimmun Rev* 2014;**13**:187–96.

51. Cufi P, Dragin N, Weiss JM, et al. Implication of double-stranded RNA signaling in the etiology of autoimmune myasthenia gravis. *Ann Neurol* 2013;**73**:281–93.

52. Park J, Munagala I, Xu H, et al. Interferon signature in the blood in inflammatory common variable immune deficiency. *PLoS One* 2013;**8**:e74893.

53. Bayry J, Hermine O, Webster DA, Levy Y, Kaveri SV. Common variable immunodeficiency: the immune system in chaos. *Trends Mol Med* 2005;**11**:370–6.

54. Maglione PJ, Ko HM, Beasley MB, Strauchen JA, Cunningham-Rundles C. Tertiary lymphoid neogenesis is a component of pulmonary lymphoid hyperplasia in patients with common variable immunodeficiency. *J Allergy Clin Immunol* 2014;**133**:535–42.

55. Martinez-Gallo M, Radigan L, Almejun MB, Martinez-Pomar N, Matamoros N, Cunningham-Rundles C. TACI mutations and impaired B-cell function in subjects with CVID and healthy heterozygotes. *J Allergy Clin Immunol* 2013;**131**:468–76.

56. Romberg N, Chamberlain N, Saadoun D, et al. CVID-associated TACI mutations affect autoreactive B cell selection and activation. *J Clin Invest* 2013;**123**:4283–93.

57. Yong PF, Aslam L, Karim MY, Khamashta MA. Management of hypogammaglobulinaemia occurring in patients with systemic lupus erythematosus. *Rheumatology (Oxford)* 2008;**47**:1400–5.

58. Mirzaei F, Michels KB, Munger K, et al. Gestational vitamin D and the risk of multiple sclerosis in offspring. *Ann Neurol* 2011;**70**:30–40.

59. Beck-Engeser GB, Eilat D, Harrer T, Jack HM, Wabl M. Early onset of autoimmune disease by the retroviral integrase inhibitor raltegravir. *Proc Natl Acad Sci USA* 2009;**106**:20865–70.

60. Yan, Z, Bryant, KF, Gregory SM et al. HIV integrase inhibitors block replication of alpha-, beta-, and gamma herpes viruses. 2014 *mBio* vol 5 e01318–14 (mbio.asm.org).

61. Gentile I, Bonadies G, Buonomo AR, et al. Resolution of autoimmune thrombocytopenia associated with raltegravir use in an HIV-positive patient. *Platelets* 2013;**24**:574–7.

62. Brown EL, Nishiyama Y, Dunkle JW, et al. Constitutive production of catalytic antibodies to a *Staphylococcus aureus* virulence factor and effect of infection. *J Biol Chem* 2012;**287**:9940–51.

63. Paul S, Planque SA, Nishiyama Y, Hanson CV, Massey RJ. Nature and nurture of catalytic antibodies. *Adv Exp Med Biol* 2012;**750**:56–75.

64. Agmon-Levin N, Hughes GR, Shoenfeld Y. The spectrum of ASIA: 'Autoimmune (Auto-inflammatory) Syndrome induced by Adjuvants'. *Lupus* 2012;**21**:118–20.

65. Cruz-Tapias P, Agmon-Levin N, Israeli E, Anaya JM, Shoenfeld Y. Autoimmune (auto-inflammatory) syndrome induced by adjuvants (ASIA)—animal models as a proof of concept. *Curr Med Chem* 2013;**20**:4030–6.

66. Katzav A, Kivity S, Blank M, Shoenfeld Y, Chapman J. Adjuvant immunization induces high levels of pathogenic antiphospholipid antibodies in genetically prone mice: another facet of the ASIA syndrome. *Lupus* 2012;**21**:210–16.

67. Shoenfeld Y, Agmon-Levin N. 'ASIA'—autoimmune/inflammatory syndrome induced by adjuvants. *J Autoimmun* 2011;**36**:4–8.

68. Zafrir Y, Agmon-Levin N, Paz Z, Shilton T, Shoenfeld Y. Autoimmunity following hepatitis B vaccine as part of the spectrum of 'Autoimmune (Auto-inflammatory) Syndrome induced by Adjuvants' (ASIA): analysis of 93 cases. *Lupus* 2012;**21**:146–52.

69. Meng Q, Hagemeier SR, Fingeroth JD, Gershburg E, Pagano JS, Kenney SC. The Epstein–Barr virus (EBV)-encoded protein kinase, EBV-PK, but not the thymidine kinase (EBV-TK), is required for ganciclovir and acyclovir inhibition of lytic viral production. *J Virol* 2010;**84**:4534–42.

70. Maruszak H, Brew BJ, Giovannoni G, Gold J. Could antiretroviral drugs be effective in multiple sclerosis? A case report. *Eur J Neurol* 2011;**18**:e110–1.

71. Cooper DA, Steigbigel RT, Gatell JM, et al. Subgroup and resistance analyses of raltegravir for resistant HIV-1 infection. *N Engl J Med* 2008;**359**:355–65.

72. Steigbigel RT, Cooper DA, Kumar PN, et al. Raltegravir with optimized background therapy for resistant HIV-1 infection. *N Engl J Med* 2008;**359**:339–54.

73. Curtin F, Lang AB, Perron H, et al. GNbAC1, a humanized monoclonal antibody against the envelope protein of multiple sclerosis-associated endogenous retrovirus: a first-in-humans randomized clinical study. *Clin Ther* 2012;**34**:2268–78.

74. do Olival GS, Faria TS, Nali LH, et al. Genomic analysis of ERVWE2 locus in patients with multiple sclerosis: absence of genetic association but potential role of human endogenous retrovirus type W elements in molecular mimicry with myelin antigen. *Front Microbiol* 2013;**4**:172.

75. Garcia-Montojo M, Dominguez-Mozo M, Arias-Leal A, et al. The DNA copy number of human endogenous retrovirus-W (MSRV-type) is increased in multiple sclerosis patients and is influenced by gender and disease severity. *PLoS One* 2013;**8**:e53623.

76. Kremer D, Schichel T, Forster M, et al. Human endogenous retrovirus type W envelope protein inhibits oligodendroglial precursor cell differentiation. *Ann Neurol* 2013;**74**:721–32.

77. Leboyer M, Tamouza R, Charron D, Faucard R, Perron H. Human endogenous retrovirus type W (HERV-W) in schizophrenia: a new avenue of research at the gene–environment interface. *World J Biol Psychiatry* 2013;**14**:80–90.

78. Sutkowski N, Chen G, Calderon G, Huber BT. Epstein–Barr virus latent membrane protein LMP-2A is sufficient for transactivation of the human endogenous retrovirus HERV-K18 superantigen. *J Virol* 2004;**78**:7852–60.

79. Sutkowski N, Conrad B, Thorley-Lawson DA, Huber BT. Epstein–Barr virus transactivates the human endogenous retrovirus HERV-K18 that encodes a superantigen. *Immunity* 2001;**15**:579–89.

80. Dreyfus DH, Nagasawa M, Gelfand EW, Ghoda LY. Modulation of p53 activity by IkappaBalpha: evidence suggesting a common phylogeny between NF-kappaB and p53 transcription factors. *BMC Immunol* 2005;**6**:12.

CHAPTER 18

Roles for Cytomegalovirus in Infection, Inflammation, and Autoimmunity

Rodney P. Jones[*]
Healthcare Analysis & Forecasting, Camberley GU15 1RQ, UK
[*]Corresponding Author: hcaf_rod@yahoo.co.uk

1 INTRODUCTION

As the chapters in this book amply demonstrate, autoimmunity is a multi-factorial issue involving infection, inflammation and genetic and epigenetic factors interacting with the environment. In this respect there is now increasing evidence for a series of infectious-like outbreaks that are largely restricted to a cluster of medical diagnoses centered on immune impairment, namely infection and inflammation and with profound effects on health service providers.[1–24] The last three of these outbreaks center around the years 2002, 2007, and 2012; comprehensive reviews provide greater detail.[1,2] The ubiquitous herpes virus cytomegalovirus (CMV) has been tentatively implicated in these outbreaks,[1,2] and this adds a further dimension to the accumulating literature dedicated to the formidable array of immune evasive and modulatory effects exerted by this resourceful virus. The inflammatory and autoimmune effects of CMV have already been the topic of three comprehensive reviews,[25–27] and the aim of this chapter is to address issues not covered in those reviews.

2 ROLES FOR CMV

Infection with CMV increases with age, poverty, overcrowding, and multiple sexual partners.[28–32] Around 10% of Western populations may be resistant to infection; however, this is not the case in black African, Chinese, and Japanese populations, especially among females.[29–32] Until around 5 years ago this virus was considered largely innocuous except to the immune impaired, patients with HIV/AIDS, transplant recipients and developing

Infection and Autoimmunity
http://dx.doi.org/10.1016/B978-0-444-63269-2.00068-4

fetuses. This failed to explain the constant (and increasing) stream of hospital case reports where CMV was directly involved in hospital admission and death in the supposedly immunocompetent population. A study by Rafailidis et al.[33] uncovered some 273 such case studies up to 2007, and the online Cases Database resource reported a further 750 case studies between 2009 and 2013. CMV is now widely recognized as a serious risk factor in patients in intensive care and burns units[34–39] and in those with bacterial sepsis and septic shock.[40,41]

Around 2005 to 2008, several groups started publishing reviews of the evidence for the involvement of CMV in autoimmune disease,[25–27,42] and this has since been further augmented.[43,44] A number of population studies demonstrated that CMV is associated with a >20% increase in mortality and, when accompanied by high antibody levels or elevated markers of inflammation, such as C-reactive protein (CRP), there is possibly a >40% increase in mortality among the elderly.[45–48] Clearly, this virus is capable of causing a major infectious outbreak, and even if it is not the source of outbreaks of infectious immune impairment, it is capable of causing serious impairment to health in its own right.

As a focus for the wider discussion in this chapter, Table 1 presents a random sample of studies of CMV in the areas of infection, inflammation, and autoimmunity, with a particular emphasis on autoimmunity. Only confirmed autoimmune studies are included the Autoimmune section of Table 1, and it is likely that some of the other studies have an autoimmune component. The studies in Table 1 are by no means comprehensive; however, they give a rapid overview of the widespread effect of CMV as either a causative or opportunistic pathogen. The studies are grouped under section headings for the areas where CMV is most active, with a broad outline of the section supplemented by relevant cases. Points to note are widespread infection of multiple variants of endothelial tissue, diseases involving long-term inflammation, and the fact that it is sometimes difficult to draw a line between where inflammation ends and autoimmunity begins. Reference back to this table will be made throughout the text. The reader is advised to refer to other reviews covering wider CMV biology.[156–161,46,163–165]

3 KEY FEATURES OF CMV BIOLOGY

CMV biology has a number of key features that are central to understanding its powerful disease effects. These are outlined briefly here and are more fully explained elsewhere.[1,2]

Table 1 CMV in Infection, Inflammation, Disease, and Autoimmunity

Condition	Comments
Autoimmune diseases	
Amplification of autoimmune diseases	Review of the role of CMV in the amplification of autoimmune diseases[42]
Anti-phospholipid syndrome	Healthy young male developed anti-cardiolipin antibodies associated with CMV infection[49]
Autoantigen glutamic acid decarboxylase (GAD65)	GAD65 is a major autoantigen expressed in neurons and β-cells. GAD65-specific T cells cross-react with a peptide of the CMV major DNA-binding protein. Hence CMV may be involved in the loss of T-cell tolerance to autoantigen GAD65 by molecular mimicry, leading to autoimmunity[50]
Anti-40-kDa protein immune retinopathy	A case of autoimmune retinopathy in benign thymoma after CMV retinitis associates with Good syndrome[51]
Lymphopenia (<700/mL)	A risk factor in elevated blood CMV viral numbers (OR, 34.4)[52]
Polymyositis and dermatomyositis	Both are risk factors for having elevated levels of CMV viral cells in the blood (OR, 10.6)[52]
Pemphigus	In Indian patients CMV induces expansion in the CD4 + CD45RO + subset with increased IFN-γ. These changes are proposed to lead to hyperactivation of the immune system and aberrant cell-mediated and humoural responses, leading to antibody-mediated cantholytic disorder. CMV is likely to an occasional factor triggering both onset and exacerbation[43]
Rheumatoid arthritis/rheumatic disease	Those suffering from the disease have higher levels of CMV infection and re-activation plus aggravation of rheumatic disease[53]
Systemic lupus erythematosus (SLE)	CMV-induced autoimmunity is strongly implicated[54] and SLE is a risk factor for elevated levels of CMV in blood (OR, 6.7).[52] One study of Chinese patients admitted with febrile symptoms demonstrated that

Continued

Table 1 CMV in Infection, Inflammation, Disease, and Autoimmunity—cont'd

Condition	Comments
	the CMV group had received higher corticosteroid dosage (26.3 mg/day) and had a higher proportion of azathioprine before admission. Those who died had a higher number of infected polymorphonuclear neutrophils (>25 CMV per 5×10^5 PMNs) and a higher proportion of joint bacterial infection.[55,56] CMV leads to high proliferation of CD4 + CD45RO + and CD8 + CD45RO + T cells in Indian patients and a higher ratio of CD4 to CD8 in patients with SLE[43]
Childhood-onset SLE	A comprehensive review of the role of CMV in childhood-onset SLE. In SLE latent CMV infection is more frequent in those with anti-RNP antibodies, and lower levels of anti-snRNP are present in CMV IgM-positive patients with SLE. At the time of diagnosis of childhood-onset SLE, anti-RPN antibodies are more frequent in CMV-positive patients[44]
SLE, CMV viremia, and acute pericarditis with hemophagocytic syndrome	25-Year-old male with fever; all conditions developed concurrently with fever. The patient improved with antiviral medication[57]
Systemic sclerosis (scleroderma)	In Indian patients CMV induces expansion of CD4 + T cells while CD8 + T cells decrease. IFN-γ and IL-4 are elevated. These act as triggering factors for autoimmunity in predisposed individuals[43]
A "scleroderma-like" phenotype in dermal fibroblasts	The CMV-derived protein UL94 shows homology with the surface molecule NAG-2, which is found in endothelial cells. Anti-UL94 antibodies bind to fibroblasts and induce apoptosis, leading dermal fibroblasts to acquire a "scleroderma-like" phenotype[58]
Overlap syndrome of autoimmune hepatitis and primary biliary cirrhosis with CMV viremia	63-Year-old hepatitis-negative woman with severe jaundice and elevated conjugated bilirubin in the absence

Table 1 CMV in Infection, Inflammation, Disease, and Autoimmunity—cont'd

Condition	Comments
	of alcohol or drug use. Submassive lobar necrosis, inflammation with broad areas of collapse, and chronic nonsuppurative destructive cholangitis. Epithelial damage in interlobular bile duct. High levels of anti-nuclear antibody and anti-mitochondrial M2 antibody and slightly high levels of anti-RNP antibody. Active CMV infection progresses to severe viremia[59]
Autoimmune type 1 hepatitis triggered by CMV infection	Case report of a 17-year-old woman who developed autoimmune hepatitis triggered by a CMV infection. The patient improved with antiviral treatment[60]
Post-transplant new-onset diabetes mellitus (PTDM)	Case study and review of the literature on the involvement of CMV viremia in PTDM[61]
CMV viremia in simultaneous pancreas-kidney (SPK) transplant in patients with type 1 diabetes	Daclizumab (anti-CD25 that prolonged CMV-free survival) was safer than anti-thymocyte globulin. CMV viremia occurred earlier and was more severe in patients with an episode of rejection. CMV-specific T-cell counts were lower in those who went on to develop viremia[62]
Human pancreatic β-cell infection	B-Cells are susceptible to CMV infection, leading to increased production of major histocompatibility complex 1 and intracellular adhesion molecule-1 and release of pro-inflammatory cytokines (IL-6, IL-8, IL-15, and MCP-1). Binding of virus cells (including ultraviolet inactivated virus) was sufficient to increase cellular immunogenicity[63]
Type 2 diabetes in the elderly	CMV-seropositive patients were more likely to have type 2 diabetes (17% vs. 8%).[64] CMV nucleic acid sequences were detected in 44% of patients with type 2 diabetes but were absent in non-diabetic patients. The CMV was mainly located in the

Continued

Table 1 CMV in Infection, Inflammation, Disease, and Autoimmunity—cont'd

Condition	Comments
	islets of Langerhans, but no obvious signs of morphological injury or inflammation were apparent[65]
Stiff man syndrome (SMS)	SMS is thought to arise from impairment of GABAergic inhibition of α-motor neurons, presumably involving autoantibodies to GAD65 (see above).[66] Type 1 diabetes is developed by 35% of patients with SMS with GAD65 autoantibodies.[67] Clinical onset of SMS and type 1 diabetes have been reported following CMV viremia.[50] Increased admissions for CNS conditions occur after outbreaks of the infectious immune impairment[1]
Type 1 diabetes	CMV was present in the lymphocytes of 22% of type 1 diabetics but only 2.6% of non-diabetics. There was strong correlation between CMV in lymphocytes and islet cell antibodies[68]

Skin (including autoimmune)

Wegener's granulomatosis	IgM to CMV prevalent in patients with Wegener's. CMV IgG is associated with additional gastrointestinal and renal involvement[69]
Cutaneous inflammation	CMV increases cutaneous immunosuppression by action on dendritic cells and T-lymphocyte function, leading to sustained cutaneous inflammation[70]
Psoriasis	Persistent CMV infection is linked with disease activity and the phenotype of peripheral CD8+ T cells[71]
Cutaneous vasculitis	7-year-old girl with fever, arthralgia, and mild cutaneous vasculitis with papules, nodules, and livedo. Biopsy of a papule showed lymphocytic small-vessel vasculitis, with some atypical lymphocytic nuclei. Splenomegaly developed due to CMV infection, with atypical peripheral blood lymphocytes and a characteristic pattern of complement-

Table 1 CMV in Infection, Inflammation, Disease, and Autoimmunity—cont'd

Condition	Comments
	fixing antibodies to CMV antigen. CMV mononucleosis syndrome is rarely reported in children, and the cutaneous manifestations are usually rubelliform[72]
Erytheme multiforne	Case study of a 58-year-old female with CMV-induced EM.[73] Review of CMV-induced EM in non-immunosuppressed patients.[74]
Cutaneous CMV infection, severe burns	Histopathological findings.[75] CMV inclusion bodies are associated with poor wound healing.[76] High CMV seroconversion rates (18–22%) and 50% CMV re-activation rate in burn patients[36]
Drug-induced hypersensitivity syndrome	CMV present in 7 of 7 patients.[77] EBV can also play a role[78]
Atopic dermatitis	Patients with AD had higher CMV-positive peripheral blood mononuclear cells, higher incidence of CMV antigenemia and higher levels of TNF-α and IL-12[79]
Various skin conditions including autoimmune and infection	Reviews of CMV involvement[80,81]

Immunization, immunity and IFN-based therapy

Response of chronic hepatitis C virus-infected patients to interferon-based therapy	CMV DNA detected in 90% of IFN non-responders versus 35% of responders. Patients with reactivated CMV had higher fibrosis scores (73% vs. 24% for those with undetectable CMV DNA). Patients with high CMV DNA had higher rates of relapse (80% versus 19%)[82]
Response to influenza vaccination	Non-responders of any age had higher levels of CMV IgG, higher proportions of CD28 + CD57-lymphocytes, TNF-α, and IL-6. Vaccination induced increases in TNF-α and IL-10 in the non-responders[83]
Immune response to a dual CMV and EBV infection in the elderly	EBV is one of the main viruses in autoimmunity. CMV expansion of CD8 T cells occurs in the elderly,

Continued

Table 1 CMV in Infection, Inflammation, Disease, and Autoimmunity—cont'd

Condition	Comments
	with a reduction in effector function that is specific to EBV (but not influenza)[84]
Typical clinical CMV infection	
CMV pneumonitis induced by tocilizumab therapy, CMV mononucleosis, Granulomatous hepatitis (GH), CMV encephalitis and hepatitis due to CMV reactivation with development of secondary immunodeficiency, hepatitis and Guillain-barre syndrome (GBS)	CMV viremia and pneumonitis (fever, cough, white sputum, wheezing, nausea, mild diarrhea) induced by the IL-6 receptor antagonist therapy in a patient.[85] A 35-year-old with mononucleosis, arthralgia, vascular pharyngitis, and hepatitis. Initial CMV viremia in polymorphonuclear leucocytes followed by CMV in urine, throat and semen.[86] Case studies of CMV-induced GH.[87] A case of CMV encephalitis and hepatitis due to viral reactivation associated with development of secondary immunodeficiency in an HIV-negative patient.[88] A 19-year-old Chinese girl with fatigue, pain and numbness of the limbs with abnormal liver function, diagnosed as GBS. On day 13 of admission, her liver function was still abnormal. CMV hepatitis was diagnosed on positive serum anti-CMV IgG and IgM antibodies. Improved with only intravenous immunoglobulin therapy and without anti-viral therapy[89]
Eyes	
Lacrimal gland function, corneal endotheliitis, retinitis with arteriolar occlusions, anterior uveitis, immune recovery uveitis, neovascular age-related macular degeneration (AMD)	CMV infection can lead to lacrimal inflammation.[90] CMV-related corneal endotheliitis is an inflammation of the corneal endothelium that typically presents as coin-shaped keratic precipitates (KPs) with or without corneal edema. It may be associated with anterior uveitis and raised intraocular pressure (IOP). Making an accurate early diagnosis is crucial in preventing the loss of corneal endothelial cells

Table 1 CMV in Infection, Inflammation, Disease, and Autoimmunity—cont'd

Condition	Comments
	and unnecessary treatment resulting from misdiagnosis.[91] In elderly "immunocompetent" patients, 71% had CMV retinitis plus neovascularization. This was far higher than in the immunocompromised or younger HIV-infected groups.[92] CMV induced anterior uveitis and other ocular infections.[93] Development of CMV immune uveitis is associated with Th17 depletion and poor systemic CMV-specific CD4 T-cell response.[94] CMV IgG titer was higher in patients with wet and dry AMD. No major differences in antibody titer to *Chlamydia pneumonia* or *Helicobacter pylori* were observed[95]

Gastrointestinal

Condition	Comments
Jejunitis due to CMV vasculitis, colitis, superior mesenteric vein thrombosis in the small bowel, gastric foveolar hyperplasia, acute erosive esophagitis, inflammatory bowel disease	A 72-year-old admitted with diarrhea and abdominal pain due to CMV enteritis causing massive intestinal hemorrhage.[96] Colitis with megacolon due to CMV in an elderly man.[97] Case report of a small-bowel necrosis complicating a CMV-induced superior mesenteric vein thrombosis.[98] Ménétrier's disease-like process due to CMV in an elderly man.[99] Healthy young adult with active CMV infection 3 weeks after splenectomy.[100] A review of CMV infection in IBD[101]

Cardiovascular system

Condition	Comments
Thrombosis, coronary atherosclerosis, restenosis after coronary atherectomy, arterial and venous thrombosis, high blood pressure, thrombic vasculopathy in the fetus, ischemic heart disease (IHD), myocarditis (fatal)	6.4% Of patients with acute CMV infection had thrombosis. Immune impaired patients had DVT/PE as most common thrombosis (versus splanchnic in the immunocompetent).[102] In particular individuals CMV elicits a subclinical

Continued

Table 1 CMV in Infection, Inflammation, Disease, and Autoimmunity—cont'd

Condition	Comments
	inflammatory response leading to elevated CRP. The OR (4.3) for coronary artery disease in CMV seropositive with high CRP.[103] Another study demonstrated CMV in 93.3% of atherosclerotic tissue and CMV+EBV-1 in 43.3% of cases.[104] Prior infection with CMV was a risk factor in restenosis after atherectomy (OR, 12.9).[105] A 33-year-old with a factor V Leiden heterozygous mutation in which CMV active infection was a precipitator/causative factor in arterial and venous thrombosis.[106] Persistent MCMV infection in mice stimulates renin production and causes high arterial blood pressure.[107] CMV is frequently detected in stillbirths, especially those with thrombic vasculopathy.[108] Reviews of the role of CMV in angiogenesis and vasculopathy.[109,110] Risk of incident IHD increases 22% for those with high CMV antibodies.[111] Viral nucleic acids were detected in 43% of patients with fatal myocarditis. In 67% of these CMV DNA was detected in the cardiomyocytes[112]
Genitourinary	
Urinary retention, urinary infection with incomplete voiding, kidney infection, end-stage renal disease, (ESRD), cervical inflammation	If common causes of urinary retention are absent, CMV is highly likely.[113] Young laboratory workers all developed CMV urinary infection with common incomplete voiding. Typical symptoms of CMV infection not otherwise observed.[114] CMV causes active infection in renal tubular epithelial (RTE) cells and more limited infection in glomerular visceral epithelial cells.[115] All patients with ESRD showed profound naive T-cell lymphopenia at all ages. CMV seropositivity aggravated the

Table 1 CMV in Infection, Inflammation, Disease, and Autoimmunity—cont'd

Condition	Comments
	contraction of CD4 + naive T cells and increased the number of differentiated CD4 + and CD8 + memory T cells.[116] High prevalence of both EBV (20%) and CMV (26%) shedding (active infection) are seen in false-positive cancer screening associated with cervical inflammation[117]

Brain and nervous system

Acute transverse myelitis, cerebral venous sinus thrombosis, bilateral papillitis and Guillain barre syndrome, bilateral oophoritis, encephalitis with thymoma, Ross syndrome, Parkinson's disease, AD, psycho-geriatric patients (without cardiovascular disease)	CMV infection associated with CNS inflammation.[118] Migraine-like headache as the presenting symptom of cerebral venous sinus thrombosis due to CMV infection.[119] Healthy 40-year-old woman with a previous mild fever and cough presenting with CMV retinitis and GBS. Conduction blocks in median, ulnar, common peroneal, and anterior tibial nerves.[120] Bilateral CMV oophoritis in a 63-year-old woman that was mimicking a widely metastatic brain carcinoma.[121] Elderly woman with no circulating immunoglobulin-bearing lymphocytes, which were unresponsive to CMV antigen; she died within 6 months of onset of symptoms.[122] CMV induces apoptosis by generating mitochondrial and endoplasmic reticulum stress.[123] CMV-induced Ross syndrome case study.[124] CMV seropositive more likely to have Parkinson's disease (3% vs. 1%), although the study was too small to demonstrate statistical significance.[64] CMV antibody levels were associated with neurofibrillary tangles, and CNS interferon -γ was only detected in CMV-seropositive individuals.[125] The percentage of senescent T cells was higher in CMV-positive patients. In another

Continued

Table 1 CMV in Infection, Inflammation, Disease, and Autoimmunity—cont'd

Condition	Comments
	study patients with AD who were CMV seropositive had lower levels of naive CD8 and a higher proportion of effector CD8 T cells.[126] High CMV antibody levels were associated with frailty in psychogeriatric patients, whereas high IgG to HHV6 and EBV were associated with diabetes[127]
Hearing loss in congenitally infected infants (a murine model)	No significant inflammatory changes in the cochleae of the mice were observed. MCMV DNA signals were mainly detected in the spiral ganglion neurons and the endolymph area, but not in the perilymph area. The number of neurons decreased, and their ultrastructure changed. The number of neurons dramatically decreased with age, and the ultrastructural lesions of neurons became much more severe[128]

Infection of various tissues

Lymphoid nodules in bone marrow	38-Year-old patient with fever and fatigue for 2 weeks. Multiple lymphoid nodules caused by CMV confirmed by immunohistochemical analysis[129]
Telomere length in T cells	Active CMV infection leads to short telomeres in leucocytes and lymphocytes[130]
Endothelial tissue	Expression of the UL133–UL138 locus of CMV is required for efficient virus maturation in endothelial tissue[131]

Respiratory and mouth

Respiratory failure with fever, fulminant pneumonia, interstitial pneumonia, allergic asthma, viral respiratory infections in children, nasopharynx, endodontic abscesses, and cellulitis	A 75-year-old woman with chronic renal failure due to vasculitis was admitted with platypnea and orthodexia due to *Pneumocystis jirovecii* and CMV infection. Antibiotic treatment failed to halt a fatal decline.[132] Joint *Mycoplasma pneumonia* and CMV infection in a health young patient who had slow

Table 1 CMV in Infection, Inflammation, Disease, and Autoimmunity—cont'd

Condition	Comments
	recovery with joint antibiotic and antiviral therapy.[133] Interstitial pneumonia is a frequent manifestation of recurrent CMV infection.[134] Activated CD8+ T cells are significantly reduced in patients with allergic asthma who are CMV seropositive.[135] Infections with RSV, rhinovirus and enterovirus were more frequent in CMV-infected children.[136] Review of CMV infection in the nasopharynx.[137] CMV was the most common herpes virus associated with pain and bone destruction in endodontic abscesses and cellulitis[138]
Other	
Hemolytic anemia	Healthy adult developed hemolytic anemia due to CMV infection.[139]
Cirrhosis of the liver	Signs of acute or recent CMV infection are common.[140] Elderly mice overreact to herpes viral infection, leading to liver damage.[141] Serum IL-6 and CRP levels are higher in CMV-seropositive patients[142]
Cancer	
Gliomas, glioblastoma multiforme, B-cell lymphocytic leukemia, liver hepatocellular carcinoma, salivary duct cancer	CMV is confirmed to cause (oncogenic) mucoepidermoid carcinoma of the salivary glands.[143] CMV is oncomodulatory, and its presence enhances tumor development and decreases patient survival[144–148]
Breast ductal cancer and IBC	CMV is present in 97% of breast ductal carcinoma compared to 63% of normal breast glandular epithelia.[147] Elevation of CMV antibodies precedes the development of breast cancer in some women.[149] Patients with IBC are characterized by statistically higher levels of CMV IgG. CMV DNA was more prevalent in cancer tissue than adjacent tissue. Different CMV

Continued

Table 1 CMV in Infection, Inflammation, Disease, and Autoimmunity—cont'd

Condition	Comments
	strains were detected in IBC tissue compared to non-invasive ductal cancers. IBC tissue was enhanced in NF-κB/p65 signalling[150]
CMV in cancer therapy	
Children and adults receiving cancer therapy and risk of viremia and death. CMV antigenemia in cancer therapy. Effect of stem cell transplant (SCT) status	Primary infection and re-activation is common, with greatly enhanced risk of death in the absence of anti-viral treatment.[151–154] CMV antigenemia occurred in 9% of non-STC, 12% autologous SCT, and 39% allogeneic SCT cases. Patients with lymphoid tumors without SCT had a 14% incidence of antigenemia versus myeloid tumors 4%. Highest rate was with allogeneic SCT and multiple myeloma (57%). Highest rates of antigenemia were in Asians followed by blacks, Hispanics, then whites. Peak circulating CMV burden was highest for patients without SCT[155]

1. Action occurs via multiple strains with different infectious potential.
   a. Superinfection with multiple strains leads to the worst clinical outcomes.
   b. Joint infection with other pathogens leads to worse clinical outcomes.
2. These multiple strains exploit multiple immune impairments.
   a. So-called immunocompetent individuals have multiple (exploitable) temporary through to semi-permanent immune impairments.
   b. Trauma, wounds, surgery, and other infectious agents create a further layer of exploitable immune impairments.
   c. Nutritional deficiencies among institutionalized elderly people create further immune impairments, and this group is over-represented in hospital admissions.
3. Observable disease action occurs at two levels.
   a. Classical symptoms of CMV viremia (detected in the blood or lavage) such as influenza-like illness, fever, vomiting, diarrhea, lethargy, depression and CMV pneumonitis (misdiagnosed as pneumonia), which are often misdiagnosed in the elderly
   b. Infection of a wide range of specific tissues (mostly but not exclusively endothelial), which most often will *not* be detected in the blood.

Infection of certain tissues can lead to observable inflammation/auto-immunity. Individuals can accumulate (usually undiagnosed) multiple CMV-infected tissues/organs during the course of their life.

    c. Hence different assays for CMV seem to detect differential involvement for CMV.[166]

4. Active production of T cells by the thymus (even in old age) is necessary to prevent inflammation and maintain longevity.

    a. Active CMV infection of the thymus may be one cause of autoimmunity.

5. Vitamin D sufficiency seems to be central to modulating CMV's effects.

    a. In the United Kingdom, each outbreak initiates first in Scotland (furthest north, low sunlight, and known vitamin D sufficiency issues).

    b. In the south of England the outbreaks seem to initiate earlier among dark-skinned populations of Asians or Africans (unpublished data); however, these populations do not show the highest increase in emergency admissions. (These may be due to differences in genetic mutations and polymorphisms.)

6. The strong bi-directional relationship between immune function and mental health conditions (sickness behavior, depression, etc.) create a risk group and a set of behaviors, including self-harm, that seem to increase with each outbreak.

These points form the framework for interpreting the multiple diseases/conditions reported in Table 1.

3.1 Multiple CMV Strains

Not all CMV strains are of equal clinical importance, and certain strains may be associated with particular conditions.[1,2,167,168] Infection with multiple strains is of greater clinical significance.[2] Polymorphism in the *UL97* gene leads to different CMV strain populations being established in the host.[169] Mutations in the *UL133–UL138* section of the CMV genome show that these regulate the ability of CMV to replicate in endothelial cells.[131] This is important since somewhat ubiquitous endothelial tissue is one of the key loci for CMV infection; this is reflected in Table 1. An Australian study of congenital and perinatal CMV infections located four CMV types based on viral envelope glycoprotein B analysis – gB1 (39%) and gB3 (30%), plus gB6 and gB7 – which broke down to a further 22 conformational polymorphism subtypes. There was evidence for longitudinal infection over time, and these strains were different to those observed in adult patients with invasive HIV.[170] Since infants younger than 2 years have a negligible CD4 T-cell response,[171] these seem to indicate that CMV types and subtypes change over a person's lifetime, depending on the immune status of the patient[167,168] and environmental exposure to CMV strains.

3.2 All-Cause Mortality

The issue of all-cause mortality is central to understanding the profound impact of CMV on human health. The key observation from a number of studies in different countries and using different population groups is that a simple measure of whether an individual is CMV seropositive increases *all-cause* mortality by around 10–20%; this is increased by around 20–40% for those individuals who have elevated levels of CMV antibodies and/or high levels of inflammatory markers such as CRP and interleukin-6.[48] This all-cause mortality is a composite of those conditions in Table 1 that can lead to death as opposed to poor health; e.g. few people die from eye conditions, but the eye condition (possibly undiagnosed) may be the expression of wider infection and inflammation, leading to ultimate death from, say, pneumonia or one of various types of vasculopathy. Generally higher mortality has been noted for cardiovascular disease, respiratory conditions, cancer, gastrointestinal disease, and peripheral nervous system diseases,[45–48,111] which concurs with the range of diagnoses identified in hospital admissions by Rafalidis et al.[33] and in Table 1. CMV as the causative/modifying agent seems highly plausible.

In the relatively rural EPICK-Norfolk (England) study (including participants ages 40–79 at recruitment in 1993 to 1997), some 41% of participants were CMV seronegative and 20% of the population was considered to be in the group with high Ig G antibody, which was more prevalent in women (62% versus 50–53% in the low antibody or CMV-negative groups). The high antibody group had a higher prevalence of diabetes, myocardial infarction and cancer.[48] The higher prevalence of diabetes (3.9% in the high antibody group versus. 2.5% in the seronegative group) suggests higher levels of autoimmune processes, as reflected in Table 1.

In this respect an increase in all-cause mortality needs to be seen in view of the fact that there are over 100 inflammatory conditions/diseases and over 100 autoimmune conditions/diseases, and both sets have immune dysfunction as the cause. The observation that CMV is involved in increased mortality following hospital admission in patients with systemic lupus erythematosus is apposite.[56] Hence, any agent capable of causing widespread immune dysfunction will lead to a multitude of diseases/conditions in a seemingly indiscriminate way, as has been observed to occur during outbreaks of the new type of infectious immune impairment.[1,2]

3.3 Immune Modulation

CMV is the largest herpes virus, and the bulk of the genetic material is dedicated to immune evasion and modulation rather than simple replication.[27] The multiple mechanisms by which CMV exerts its effects against innate and adaptive immunity are covered by a huge number of research articles. Every conceivable nuance seems to have been documented, and several recent reviews and key studies cover many of these areas.[158,172–179] The key point is that the array of immune-modulating effects is so wide that any exploitable genetic, epigenetic, trauma, or lifestyle weakness will eventually be located by one or more CMV strains, perhaps in cooperation with other pathogens. Hence, individuals can accumulate an increasing number of CMV-infected tissues/organs over the course of their life. One study of eight deceased persons found CMV in the following tissues: nasal mucosa, trachea, thyroid, lung, mediastinal lymph nodes, large intestine, small intestine, liver, urinary bladder, and urethra.[180] It was noted that only the Epstein–Barr virus and human herpesvirus 6 were detected in all eight cases and across far more tissue types; however, these viruses do not have the sheer number of genes devoted to immune modulation as CMV. Interestingly, for those patients who are CMV seronegative but are infected with HHV-6 (variant A), it is the HHV-6 which often re-activates, leading to equally serious outcomes[181]; hence poor health and autoimmunity has much to do with exploitable weaknesses, interacting with whichever effector(s) are present at the time.

3.4 Inflammation

Controlled inflammation is required to heal sites of trauma in the body and respond to infection; however, its dysregulation leads to damage and the equivalent of accelerated ageing. For example, in the elderly, IL-6 (>2.71 pg/mL) or CRP (>3.14 mg/L) were both related with progressive loss of skeletal muscle.[182] Chronic inflammation can arise from multiple causes such as viral infection, malignancies, acute coronary syndrome, sleep, and lung disorders, autoimmune disease, poor diet, obesity, inactivity, and smoking.[159,183–185]

Table 2 Diagnoses and Deaths Showing Elevated Risk with High CRP[186]

Diagnosis/Condition	Odds Ratio
Respiratory cancer, death	2.32
Breast cancer, death	1.88
Myocardial infarction, death	1.84
All vascular system, deaths	1.82
Digestive system, deaths	1.72
Coronary heart disease, morbidity	1.68
Endocrine/metabolic/nutrition, death	1.64
Myocardial infarction, non-fatal	1.59
Miscellaneous, death	1.57
Blood cancer, death	1.57
Any non-vascular, death	1.55
Unclassified stroke, morbidity	1.41
Ischemic stroke, morbidity	1.27
Violence, suicide or trauma, death	1.26

Odds ratio is for a threefold higher CRP level than normal.

CMV tends to be less harmful in the absence of inflammation and more harmful as levels of inflammation and/or CMV antibodies increase.[48] Inflammatory markers such as CRP are known to be associated with a predisposition to disease and death. The results of a recent meta-analysis of the effects of CRP are given in Table 2. The range of conditions in Table 2 is highly reminiscent of the conditions in Table 1. Hence, CMV seems to act as an agent leading to inflammation, exacerbating inflammatory conditions and taking opportunistic advantage of inflammation, however it is caused.

Several elements of the innate immune system work in tandem against joint bacterial/CMV infections, several of which are detailed in Table 1. Two compounds are of importance, namely the potent chemotactic lipid leukotriene B4 (LTB4), which is a mediator of inflammation with antimicrobial activity, and the antimicrobial cathelicidin LL-37. Release of LTB4 against CMV is dependent on the activation of the high-affinity LBT4 receptor (BLT1), which then promotes neutrophil activation. LTB4 strongly promotes the release of LL-37 with feedback enhancement of LBT4.[187,188] LL-37 is produced in secondary neutrophilic granules, macrophages, NK cells and epithelial cells, the latter being a primary site of CMV infection, and a recent review has implicated LL-37 in elevated levels of inflammation and autoimmune disease, notably atopic dermatitis, psoriasis, systemic lupus erythematosus, and rheumatoid arthritis.[189]

Following allogenic bone marrow transplantation, LTB4 protects mice with a latent CMV infection against viral reactivation, whereas in 5-lipoxygenase-deficient mice, CMV viral load in the salivary gland is higher than in the 5-lipoxygenase-dependent LTB4-producing controls. LTB4 also protects mice against a lethal dose of CMV, whereas mice treated with LTB4 had far lower levels of CMV in the salivary gland after a sub-lethal dose of CMV.[190] 5-Lipoxygenase inhibitors and dual cyclooxygenase/5-lipoxygenase inhibitors are known to inhibit the production of LTB4,[191] whereas vitamin D plays a role in the expression of an array of the innate immune gene-expressed compounds discussed above.[192]

There is a strong bi-directional relationship between immune function, inflammation and mental health, including fatigue, depression, and sickness behavior.[159,183,193] Hence, in women newly diagnosed with breast cancer (before treatment), higher CMV antibody levels (but not for Epstein–Barr virus) were associated with fatigue, sleep problems and depression[194] as well as higher CRP levels.

With respect to outbreaks of the new type of infectious immune impairment, a cluster of 100 common diagnoses out of the 1300 diagnoses used at a large hospital in an area badly affected by the 2012 outbreak (mainly respiratory, cardiovascular, gastrointestinal, and autoimmune, including exacerbation of rheumatoid arthritis and other inflammatory conditions— reflecting the conditions in Table 1) showed a massive 50% increase (as a group) in admission and stayed at this high level for a 12-month period before beginning to abate[195]. This list has been cross-matched against diagnoses that showed a particular increase across the whole of England in the 2012/2013 fiscal year and during previous outbreaks.[1,6,20]

3.5 Autoimmunity

Figure 1 demonstrates how awareness of the roles of CMV in autoimmunity has expanded over the past two decades; 1996 and 2000 mark the onset of periods of rapid expansion. Comprehensive reviews of the role of CMV in autoimmunity and the exacerbation of autoimmunity demonstrate the clear potential of this virus in this area.[25–27,42,44] One study of treated patients with HIV showed that CMV induces chronic immune activation but that links with self-antigen-induced immune response are probably indirect.[166] Perhaps the best description is that CMV is one of many "agent provocateurs" capable of influencing the course of immune modulation and inflammation to the point of initiation of autoimmunity.[43] The evidence that

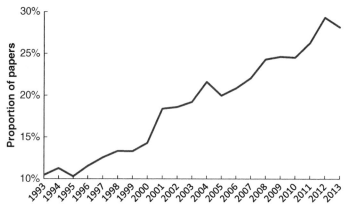

Figure 1 Proportion of articles that mention both *CMV* and *autoimmunity*. The counts show the articles from Google Scholar.

CMV would exacerbate existing autoimmunity is probably more convincing, and in this respect the long-term cycle arising from outbreaks of the new type of immune impairment should almost certainly be associated with a cycle in the number and severity of health service contacts (GP visits, outpatient and emergency department attendance and inpatient admission) with those who have an autoimmune disease. In this respect primary diagnosis codes for pyogenic arthritis, seropositive rheumatoid arthritis, other rheumatoid arthritis, other arthritis, other inflammatory spondylopathies, other spondylopathies, other joint disorders, synovitis, and tenosynovitis were among a group of over 100 conditions showing a sudden and large increase in admissions following the 2012 outbreak.[195] A similar cycle relating to the point of onset of autoimmune disease probably exists, although this will require accurate determination of the point at which symptoms commence. Research into autoimmunity therefore needs to be alert to this phenomena and especially to the recent 2012 outbreak (mid-2011 in parts of Scotland), which was characterized by higher numbers of deaths than in other outbreaks, and this could be reflected in clinical symptoms.[23]

A comprehensive review of the role of CMV in childhood-onset SLE has identified a number of ways in which CMV may specifically contribute to SLE.[44] SLE is characterized by multiple antibodies against nuclear proteins including chromatin, DNA, and RNA binding proteins. Anti-U1RNP and anti-Sm are commonly detected in sera of patients with childhood SLE; the anti-Sm antibodies are more frequent in CMV-positive patients, whereas lower anti-short nuclear RNP antibodies are observed in those who are CMV IgM positive compared to CMV IgG positive. Autoantibodies the Ro and La proteins, which are associated with hYRNA, are frequently found in SLE and Sjögren's syndrome (SS). *In vitro*, CMV infection can lead to the expression of the La protein on the cell surface, which can lead to the production of anti-La antibodies. There is additional molecular mimicry in the sequence homology of the epitopes in the La protein and CMV antigens.[44] Patients with SS and SLE have serum antibodies that cross-react with epitopes on CMV antigens. CMV IgG anti-pp65 antibodies are rarely detected in healthy individuals but are found in >60% of patients with SLE.

One further mechanism involves the main immune response directed against epitopes on the pp65 CMV viral antigen. Should one or more of these epitopes cross-react with nuclear proteins, then a self-antigen followed by autoreactive T and B cells may be produced.[44]

Two recent developments require discussion regarding CMV and auto-immune diseases, namely, the role of antigen-presenting γδ T cells in the pathogenesis of autoimmune diseases and the role of the immunosuppressive drug leflunomide (LEF) in the treatment of autoimmune conditions and its secondary role as an effective CMV anti-viral.

γδ T cells are a minor population of T cells that express TCR γδ chains. They are mainly distributed in epithelial and mucosal surfaces (a main target for CMV infection) and in the peripheral blood and lymphatic system. In the early stage of infection they may bridge innate and adaptive immunity through induction of DC maturation. Their mechanisms for possible of induction of rheumatoid arthritis and SLE have been recently reviewed,[196] and it is their presence in tissue favored by CMV that may provide insights into how CMV triggers autoimmunity in certain situations.

LEF is an immunomodulatory drug that inhibits protein kinase activity. It has been used in the treatment of rheumatoid arthritis (with *HLA-DRB1* gene mutation), SLE, transplant recipients, glomerular disease, and skin diseases,[197] all of which feature in Table 1. It should come as no surprise that this drug is also a potent CMV anti-viral that has been demonstrated to inhibit CMV apoptosis and proliferation in lung fibroblasts.[197] This drug is considerably cheaper than current CMV anti-virals and can be administered in tablet form. Wider clinical use of this drug will undoubtedly reveal which autoimmune diseases have a strong relationship with CMV.

In conclusion, CMV is associated with a disposition to high levels of inflammation-related diseases and mortality in approximately 20% of Western populations, and a subset of this population progresses to autoimmune disease. While Epstein–Barr virus seems to be implicated in more autoimmune diseases than CMV,[55] it is almost certain that CMV plays a far wider role in exacerbating autoimmune conditions. The development of LEF as a drug for autoimmune treatment may provide further insights.

4 RISK FACTORS

4.1 Nutrition and Deprivation

Those with less education, lower income, and non-white race/ethnicity have significantly higher anti-CMV antibody levels.[198] The levels of anti-CMV antibodies increased with age and their relationship with education and income was sex-dependent. Likewise, deprivation and nutrition are usually interlinked with nutritional deficiencies leading to inflammation[183] and involution of the thymus,[199] of which CMV is one of a number of agents infecting this autoimmune-sensitive organ (see Section 4.3).

4.2 Race and Genetic and Epigenetic Factors

Racial and ethnic differences in disease prevalence are best understood from the viewpoint of the prevalence of particular genetic variants.[200] Hence, diabetes prevalence is higher in Pakistani/Bangladeshi (6 times), Indian (3 times), black Caribbean (4 times among men and 2.5 times among women), and Chinese (2 times among men and 1.5 times among women).[201] Acquisition of CMV infection from sexual activity is lower in black (+8%) than white (+11%) American women, although this is the reverse of the incidence of sexually transmitted diseases.[29] In Mexican Americans (but not in whites and blacks), variants of three genes are associated with susceptibility to hepatitis A infection.[202] Cold urticarial, immunodeficiency, and aspects of autoimmunity seem to be related to PLCGZ deletions,[203] and uticaria (outpatient consultations) is one of a range of dermatological conditions that increased following the 2007 outbreak in England.[204] The risk of death due to influenza is inherited; a low-producing mannose-binding lectin gene (*MBL2*) increases the risk of co-infection with MRSA (OR 7.1) or bacteria (OR 3.0).[205] The same mannose-binding gene polymorphism has been implicated in pediatric CMV infection.[206]

The *KG2C* genotype influences steady-state numbers of NKG2C + NK-cells, which can contain CMV viral expansion in cases of T-cell deficiency. A homozygous deletion of the *NKG2C* gene exists in around 4% of the Dutch, Japanese, and Spanish populations. CMV seropositive individuals without the deletion have higher frequencies and absolute numbers of NKG2C+NK cells. It is suggested that the 4% of the population with the homozygous deletion may be more susceptible to active CMV infection.[207]

The development of neuroblastoma has recently been linked to the immunoglobulin GM (γ marker) specific to the GM genotype (GM 1/a, 3/f, 5/b). Interestingly, the allele GM3 in the uncommon genotype (GM 1, 3, 5) modulates the CMV viral strategy of encoding proteins with functional properties of the Fcγ receptor, which enables CMV to evade immunosurveillance by avoiding antibody-dependent cellular cytotoxicity, complement-dependent neutralization and phagocytosis.[208] Individuals with particular GM genotypes are proposed to be susceptible to both neuroblastoma and other CMV-mediated diseases.

Finally, HIV exposure does not guarantee HIV infection, and uninfected individuals are characterized by a specific CD4 and CD8 immune response.[209] In light of this, we probably need to view the apparent susceptibility of certain individuals to active CMV infection as due to an inflammatory response or autoimmunity.

Another interesting possibility arises from the observation of the increased frequency of locus mutation following the expression of CMV genes in infected cells.[210] CMV is also an agent of epigenetic reprogramming.[210] The presence of foreign DNA also is proposed to cause microcompetition to human DNA transcription, leading to chronic diseases.[211]

While particular genetic variants may predispose towards disease, a study of super-centenarians showed that they have a comparable number of known disease-associated variants but around 1% of variants are novel, and they have higher numbers of coding variants near other known longevity variants.[212] Epigenetic factors are also known to play a role in the expression of disease such that early life environment seems to influence both epigenetic modification[213] and the susceptibility to CMV infection.[214] The offspring of those with long lives have a lower CMV seroprevalence.[214]

In elderly Latinos, functional impairment has been shown to be clearly linked to levels of CRP, which is a marker for inflammation, and CMV also was implicated. However, the linkage with CMV becomes clearer when it is realized that the APOE-epsilon 4 genotype leads to alternative CRP responses. Those possessing this particular genotype have lower levels of CRP and exhibit higher levels of CMV antibodies. This disparity in the role of CRP explains why the role of CMV was difficult to discern in a study using just CPR levels as an inflammatory marker; i.e. specific immune impairments lead to particular pathways of CMV attack. The APOE-epsilon

4 genotype response was noted to be specific to CMV and not to HSV-1.[215] The whole area of the genetic and epigenetic sensitivity of individuals to CMV infection, inflammatory disease, and autoimmunity requires further investigation.

4.3 Vitamin D and the Thymus

Vitamin D is known to play a key role in the regulation of inflammation and autoimmunity,[216–218] and the hormonal form of the vitamin is a direct inducer of antimicrobial peptide and defensin gene expression,[192] which show antimicrobial activity against both bacteria and CMV (as discussed in 3.4 Section 3.4). Vitamin D also plays a role in the function of the thymus.[1,2] In elderly Western populations, vitamin D insufficiency is now considered to be of "epidemic" proportions.[216] It is of interest to note that each outbreak commences first in Scotland, with its more northern latitude, lower sunlight, and lower vitamin D sufficiency;[23] in the south of England earlier outbreak seems to occur in locations with higher numbers of Asian and black residents[195] and has a higher incidence of initiation at those times of the year when vitamin D sufficiency is low.[217]

For many years the thymus was considered only of functional importance in the young; however, recent research indicates continued thymic output is vital for survival in the elderly, including control of inflammation, and, along with levels of CRP, is an independent predictor of the likely number of years until death.[220,221] Thymic pathology has long been recognized in autoimmune disease, especially in the presence of thymic tumors.[222] CMV is capable of infecting the thymus and may therefore be a factor in diminished thymic output and perturbation in T-cell training, leading to autoimmunity.[1,2]

There is only one study to date regarding vitamin D concentrations and CMV, and this relates to pediatric-onset multiple sclerosis (MS). The MS group rather surprisingly had lower CMV antibody concentrations associated with vitamin D insufficiency and, conversely, vitamin D sufficiency was associated with higher CMV antibody concentrations; in the control group the reverse was true, and vitamin D sufficiency was associated with lower CMV antibody concentrations.[223] It seems that in the absence of MS vitamin D sufficiency is implicated in avoiding the deleterious effects of CMV, i.e. low CMV antibodies, suggesting controlled infection, but may interact with particular immune impairments in unexpected ways. See the previous section for a similar dichotomous response to CMV inflammation in the presence of a specific gene mutation.

4.4 Year-of-Birth Effects

Any disease generated by a recurring series of infectious outbreaks will lead to year-of-birth effects. When the disease has an immune-based component because of different strains of the infectious agent (as for influenza), the time series of outbreaks will create age-specific effects due to what is called "antigenic original sin".[224] Antigenic original sin is a term used to describe the effects that accrue when an individual's immune system is primed by exposure to a specific strain. The resulting specific immune response either benefit or limit the resulting immune response upon exposure to a different strain. The immune response to each strain is subject to the usual decay in the intensity of the response over time. Over a lifetime, each individual acquires multiple strain-specific responses of varying intensity, and these patterns lead to a specific single year-of-age saw-tooth pattern in the response to each outbreak. This saw-tooth pattern has been observed in the increase in emergency medical admissions following each outbreak[24] and in the deaths that accompany each outbreak.[24,195,219,225,226]

The key point is that antigenic original sin patterns create havoc for attempts to standardize particular diseases and populations by age. For example, each outbreak takes around 2–3 years to spread across the entire United Kingdom[227] and around 18 months to fully spread across countries with smaller county geographies.[219] In somewhere as large as the United States, the time pattern of emergency medical admissions suggests that the far larger geography and more dispersed population leads to an even longer spread.[8] Age standardization using traditional 5-year age bands breaks down under such conditions, and erroneous conclusions regarding the rates of disease in one location compared to another can be reached. Researchers need to be aware of this critical effect when attempting to analyze their data.

4.5 Disease Time Cascades

A curious feature of the outbreaks is that they seem to generate disease time cascades.[11,12,21,24] A study at a large acute hospital identified over 100 diagnoses with a cascade of distinct initiation dates during the 2012 outbreak.[195] Such time cascades are clinically feasible since different modes of immune function impairment lead to a time lag before the full expression of observable disease. At present only preliminary work is available, but the implication to interpreting time trends is apparent.

4.6 Role of Sex

Women are generally known to have higher rates of CMV infection.[29–31] This is partly because of contact with infants and children who are known to excrete CMV (principally in the urine) for extended periods of time up to around 5 years of age[228] and to sexual activity, which increases CMV acquisition in women (+8% in blacks, +11% in whites) but not in men.[28]

Outbreaks of the agent are associated with more deaths and higher rates of hospitalization among women.[8,11,18] Both return to a baseline position subsequent to the outbreak. Different roles for estrogen, progesterone, and testosterone in inflammatory responses[229] present an opportunity for any sex differences observed in the outbreaks.

It is well recognized that different autoimmune diseases have a characteristic sex ratio,[230] and the outbreaks of particular diagnoses/conditions seem to have a similar characteristic. Outbreaks are also characterized by a temporary reduction in the ratio of female to male live births.[22] This possibility was tested using the observation that the cycle of admissions created by recurring outbreaks leads to high year-to-year differences in admissions and hence high average year-to-year volatility over long time spans. This analysis yielded 106 female and 86 male ICD, 10th edition, primary diagnoses (three digits) that require further investigation.[231] Conditions specific to females included diseases of the peripheral nervous system, non-diabetic hypoglycemic coma, radio dermatitis, disorders of the choroid (the vascular layer of the eye), anemia due to enzyme disorders and viral conjunctivitis, all of which have a degree of resonance with Table 1.

A study of the role of CMV in coronary artery disease (CAD) exemplifies these differences. In men the effect of CMV seems to occur via CMV triggering an inflammatory response, leading to higher levels of CRP, which then are implicated in CAD. In women, however, the direct levels of CMV IgG lead to CAD in the absence of an increase in CRP.[232] The response in men was also more complex, and risk of CAD tended to be higher for those lacking a cellular response (T-lymphocyte proliferation) to CMV antigens.

5 CONCLUSIONS

This review has raised awareness of outbreaks of a new type of immune impairment, potential involvement of CMV and implications of both inflammation and autoimmunity. CMV has been demonstrated to be the ultimate opportunistic immune anarchist working alone or via the concerted efforts of multiple strains, as well as in cooperation with other pathogens, leading to inflammation, autoimmunity and, more specifically, to the exacerbation of particular autoimmune diseases. Its effects are profound and wide-reaching and have been greatly underestimated in clinical and population health contexts for the supposedly immunocompetent.

Either as direct cause or opportunistic bystander, CMV will undoubtedly be involved in the observed long-term cycle of outbreaks of the new type of immune impairment, creating year-of-birth cohorts via antigenic original sin-mediated effects and a long-term background cycle lying behind particular diseases involving inflammation and autoimmunity. The role of different CMV strains/subtypes in clinical manifestation of inflammation and autoimmunity requires far greater investigation, as does the immune specific role of sex.

Researchers in the field of autoimmunity need to be aware of the most recent outbreak, which occurred mainly in 2012 in the United Kingdom and Europe (where deaths were also high) and, judging by past outbreaks, more widely around the world. Indeed, initial analysis suggests that the increase in deaths that accompanies each outbreak is exclusively confined to a set of around 100 diagnoses that show increased admission as a result of the outbreak. This should allow retrospective analysis of new diagnoses of autoimmunity and its exacerbation to see whether it affords a further piece in the autoimmunity jigsaw. The new immunosuppressive and anti-CMV drug leflunomide seems to offer the potential for advances in exploring the links between CMV and autoimmunity.

ACKNOWLEDGMENTS

Comments and suggestions by the reviewers are gratefully acknowledged.

REFERENCES

1. Jones R. *Could cytomegalovirus be causing widespread outbreaks of chronic poor health?* In: Shoja MM, Agutta PS, Tubbs S, et al. *Hypotheses in clinical medicine.* New York: Nova Science Publishers Inc.; 2013. p. 37–79. Available from:*http://www.hcaf.biz/2013/CMV_Read.pdf*.
2. Jones R. Widespread outbreaks of a subtle condition leading to hospitalization and death. *Epidemiology* 2013;**3**:4[open access].
3. Jones R. *Emergency admissions in the UK: trend upward or fundamental shift?* Camberley: Healthcare Analysis & Forecasting; 1996. Available from:*http://www.hcaf.biz/Recent/Trend%20or%20step.pdf*.

4. Jones R. *Additional studies on the three to six year pattern in medical emergency admissions.* Camberley, UK: Healthcare Analysis & Forecasting; 2009. Available from: *http://www.hcaf.biz/Recent/Additional_Studies.pdf.*

5. Jones R. Unexpected, periodic and permanent increase in medical inpatient care: manmade or new disease. *Med Hypotheses* 2010;**74**(6):978–83.

6. Jones R. Can time-related patterns in diagnosis for hospital admission help identify common root causes for disease expression. *Med Hypotheses* 2010;**75**(2):148–54.

7. Jones R. The case for recurring outbreaks of a new type of infectious disease across all parts of the United Kingdom. *Med Hypotheses* 2010;**75**(5):452–7.

8. Jones R. Nature of health care costs and financial risk in commissioning. *Br J Healthcare Manage* 2010;**16**(9):424–30.

9. Jones R. Forecasting emergency department attendances. *Br J Healthcare Manage* 2010;**16**(10):495–6.

10. Jones R. Trends in programme budget expenditure. *Br J Healthcare Manage* 2010;**16**(11):518–26.

11. Jones R. Cycles in gender-related costs for long-term conditions. *Br J Healthcare Manage* 2011;**17**(3):124–5.

12. Jones R. Cycles in inpatient waiting time. *Br J Healthcare Manage* 2011;**17**(2):80–1.

13. Jones R. Time to re-evaluate financial risk in GP commissioning. *Br J Healthcare Manage* 2012;**18**(1):39–48.

14. Jones R. Increasing GP, referrals: collective jump or infectious push? *Br J Healthcare Manage* 2012;**18**(9):487–95.

15. Jones R. Diagnoses, deaths and infectious outbreaks. *Br J Healthcare Manage* 2012;**18**(10):539–48.

16. Jones R. End of life and financial risk in GP commissioning. *Br J Healthcare Manage* 2012;**18**(7):374–81.

17. Jones R. Excess deaths following a procedure in 2008. *Br J Healthcare Manage* 2012;**18**(10):554–5.

18. Jones R. An unexplained increase in deaths in England & Wales during 2012. *Br J Healthcare Manage* 2013;**19**(5):248–53.

19. Jones R. Is the demographic shift the real problem? *Br J Healthcare Manage* 2013;**19**(10):509–11.

20. Jones R. Trends in elderly diagnoses: links with multi-morbidity. *Br J Healthcare Manage* 2013;**19**(11):553–8.

21. Jones R. The funding dilemma: A lagged cycle in cancer costs. *Br J Healthcare Manage* 2013;**19**(12):606–7.

22. Jones R. Do recurring outbreaks of a type of infectious immune impairment trigger cyclic changes in the gender ratio at birth? *Biomed Int* 2013;**4**(1):26–39.

23. Jones R. A recurring series of infectious-like events leading to excess deaths, emergency department attendances and medical admissions in Scotland. *Biomed Int* 2013;**4**(2):72–86.

24. Jones R. Infectious-like spread of an agent leading to increased medical admission in the North East Essex area of the East of England. *Biomed Int* 2014;**5**(1)[in press].

25. Varani S, Landini M. Cytomegalovirus-induced immunopathology and its clinical consequences. *Herpesviridae* 2011;**2**:6.

26. Varani S, Frascaroli G, Landini M, Soderberg-Naucler C. Human cytomegalovirus targets different subsets of antigen-presenting cells with pathological consequences for host immunity: implications for immunosuppression, chronic inflammation and autoimmunity. *Rev Med Virol* 2009;**19**:131–45.

27. Varani S, Landini M, Soderberg-Naucler C. Cytomegalovirus-induced autoimmunity. In: Petrov ME, editor. *Autoimmune disorders: symptoms, diagnosis and treatment.* New York: Nova Science Publishers Inc.; 2010 Chapter 7.

28. Staras S, Flanders W, Dollard S, Pass R, McGowan J, Cannon M. Influence of sexual activity on cytomegalovirus seroprevalence in the United States, 1988–1994. *Sex Transm Dis* 2008;**35**(4):472–9.
29. Bate S, Dollard S, Cannon M. Cytomegalovirus seroprevalence in the United States: the national health and nutrition examination surveys, 1988-2004. *Clin Infect Dis* 2010;**50**(11):1439–47.
30. Hyde T, Schmid S, Cannon M. Cytomegalovirus seroconversion rates and risk factors: implications for congenital CMV. *Rev Med Virol* 2010;**20**:311–26.
31. Rubicz R, Leach C, Kraig E, Dhurandhar N, Grubbs B, Blangero J, et al. Seroprevalence of 13 common pathogens in a rapidly growing US minority population: Mexican Americans from San Antonio, TX. *BMC Res Notes* 2011;**4**:433.
32. Glanella S, Strain M, Rought S, Vargas M, Little S, Richman D. Association between virologic and immunologic dynamics in blood and in the male genital tract. *J Virol* 2012;**86**(3):1307–15.
33. Rafailidis P, Mourtzoukou E, Varbobitis I, Falagas M. Severe cytomegalovirus infection in apparently immunocompetent patients: a systematic review. *Virol J* 2008;**5**:47.
34. Heininger A, Vogel U, Aepinus C, Hauprecht K. Disseminated fatal human cytomegalovirus disease after severe trauma. *Crit Care Med* 2000;**28**(2):563–6.
35. Heininger A, Haeberle H, Fischer I, Beck R, Riessen R, et al. Cytomegalovirus reactivation and associated outcome for critically ill patients with severe sepsis. *Crit Care* 2011;**15**(2):R77.
36. Rennekampff H-O, Hamprecht K. Cytomegalovirus infections in burns: a review. *J Med Microbiol* 2006;**55**(5):483–7.
37. Limaye A, Kirby K, Rubenfeld G, Leisenring W, Bulger E, et al. Cytomegalovirus reactivation in critically-ill immunocompetent patients. *JAMA* 2008;**300**(4):413–22.
38. Limaye A, Boeckh M. CMV in critically ill patients: pathogen or bystander? *Rev Med Virol* 2010;**20**(6):372–9.
39. Clari M, Aguilar G, Benet I, Belda J, Gimenez E, Bravo B, et al. Evaluation of cytomegalovirus (CMV)-specific T-cell immunity for the assessment of the risk of active CMV infection in non-immunosuppressed surgical and trauma intensive care unit patients. *J Med Virol* 2013;**85**(10):1802–10.
40. Ho M. Cytomegalovirus infection in patients with bacterial sepsis. *Clin Infect Dis* 1998;**26**:1083–4.
41. Von Muller L, Klemm A, Weiss M, et al. Active cytomegalovirus infection in patients with severe septic shock. *Emerg Infect Dis* 2006;**12**(10):1517–22.
42. Posnett D, Yarilin D. Amplification of autoimmune disease by infection. *Arthritis Res Ther* 2005;**7**(2):74–84.
43. Dar S. *Molecular analysis of cytokine polymorphism in conjunction with the study of immune response to common recall antigens, superantigens and xenobiotic compounds in autoimmune skin disease.* PhD thesis, Department of Microbiology, University of Delhi; 2013. *http://shodhganga.inflibnet.ac.in/handle/10603/9032.*
44. Rozenblyum E, Allen U, Silverman E, Levy D. Cytomegalovirus infection in childhood-onset systemic lupus erythematosus. *Int Clin Rheum* 2013;**8**(1):137–46.
45. Savva G, Pachnio A, Kaul B, Morgan K, Huppert F, Brayne C, et al. Cytomegalovirus infection is associated with increased mortality in the older population. *Aging Cell* 2013;**12**(3):381–7.
46. Simanek A, Dowd J, Pawalec G, Melzer D, Dutta A, Aiello A. Seropositivity to cytomegalovirus, inflammation, all-cause and cardiovascular disease-related mortality in the United States. *PLoS One* 2011;**6**(2):e16103.
47. Roberts E, Haan M, Dowd J, Aiello A. Cytomegalovirus antibody levels, inflammation, and mortality among elderly Latinos over 9 years of follow-up. *Am J Epidemiol* 2010;**172**(4):363–71.

48. Gkrania-Klotsas E, Langenberg C, Sharp S, Luben R, et al. Seropositivity and higher IgG antibody levels against Cytomegalovirus are associated with mortality in the population based EPIC-Norfolk cohort. *Clin Infect Dis* 2012;**206**(12):1897–903.
49. Labarca J, Rabaggliati R, Radrigan F, Rojas P, et al. Antiphospholipid syndrome associated with cytomegalovirus infection: a case report and review. *Clin Infect Dis* 1997;**24**:197–200.
50. Hiemstra H, Schloot N, van Veelan P, Willemen S, Franklen K, van Rood J, et al. Cytomegalovirus in autoimmunity: T cell crossreactivity to viral antigen and autoantigen glutamic acid decarboxylase. *Proc Natl Acad Sci USA* 2001;**98**(7):3988–91.
51. Wan C, Teoh S. Autoimmune retinopathy in benign thyoma after Good syndrome-associated cytomegalovirus retinitis. *Ocular Immunol Inflamm* 2013;**21**(1):79–81[Abstr].
52. Fujimoto D, Matsushima A, Nago M, Takakura S, Ichiyama S. Risk factors associated with elevated blood cytomegalovirus pp 65 antigen levels in patients with autoimmune diseases. *Mod Rheumatol* 2013;**23**(2):345–50.
53. Einstein E, Wolf D. Cytomegalovirus infection in pediatric rheumatic diseases: a review. *Pediatric Rheum* 2010;**8**:17.
54. Soderberg-Naucler C. Autoimmunity induced by human cytomegalovirus in patients with systemic lupus erythematosis. *Arth Res Ther* 2012;**14**:101.
55. Barzilai O, Sherer Y, Ram M, Izhaky D, Anaya J, Shoenfeld Y. Epstein–Barr virus and cytomegalovirus in autoimmune diseases. *Ann NY Acad Sci* 2007;**1108**(4): 567–77.
56. Tsai W, Chen M, Lee M, Yu K, Nu M, Liou L. Cytomegalovirus infection causes morbidity and mortality in patients with autoimmune diseases, particularly systemic lupus: in a Chinese population in Taiwan. *Rheumatol Int* 2012;**32**(9):2901–8.
57. Kwon C, Jung Y, Yun D, Kim H, Cho H, et al. A case of acute pericarditis with hemophagocytic syndrome, cytomegalovirus infection and systemic lupus erythematosus. *Rheumatol Int* 2008;**28**(3):271–3. http://dx.doi.org/10.1007/s00296-007-0401-y.
58. Lunardi C, Dolcino M, Peterlana D, Bason C, Navone R, Tamassia N, et al. Autoantibodies against human cytomegalovirus in the pathogenesis of systemic sclerosis: a gene array approach. *PLoS Med* 2006;**3**(1):e2.
59. Toyoda-Akui M, Yokomori H, Kaneko F, Shimizu Y, Takeuchi H, Tahara K, et al. Association of an overlap syndrome of autoimmune hepatitis and primary biliary cirrhosis with cytomegalovirus infection. *Int J Gen Med* 2011;**4**:397–402.
60. Mouelhi L, Debbeche R, Salem M, Bouzaidi S, Mekki H, Houissa F, et al. Autoimmune hepatitis type 1 triggered by cytomegalovirus infection. One rare case report. *Tunis Med* 2010;**88**(9):674–7.
61. Hjelmesaeth J, Muller F, Jenssen T, Rollag H, Sagedal S, Hartmann A. Is there a link between cytomegalovirus infection and new-onset posttransplantation diabetes mellitus? Potential mechanisms of virus induced β-cell damage. *Nephrol Dial Transplant* 2005; **20**:2311–5.
62. Huurman V, Ringers J, Kalpoe J, Kroes A, van de Linde P, Roep B, et al. Choice of antibody immunotherapy influences cytomegalovirus viremia in simultaneous pancreas-kidney transplant recipients. *Diabetes Care* 2006;**29**(4):842–7.
63. Smelt M, Faas M, de Haan B, Draijer C, Hugenholz G, de Haan A, et al. Susceptibility of human pancreatic β cells for cytomegalovirus and the effects on cellular immunogenicity. *Pancreas* 2012;**41**:39–49.
64. Chen S, de Craen A, Raz Y, Derhovanessian E, Vossen A, et al. Cytomegalovirus seropositivity is associated with glucose regulation in the oldest old. Results from the Leiden 85-plus study. *Immun Ageing* 2012;**9**:8.
65. Lohr J, Oldstone M. Detection of cytomegalovirus nucleic acid sequences in pancreas in type 2 diabetes. *Lancet* 1990;**336**(8716):644–8.

66. Lorish T, Thorsteinsson G, Howard F. Stiff-man syndrome updated. *Mayo Clin Proc* 1989;**64**:629–36.
67. Solimena M, Folli F, Denis-Donini S, Comi G, Pozza G, DeCamilli P, et al. Autoantibodies to glutamic acid decarboxylase in a patient with stiff-man syndrome, epilepsy, and type I diabetes mellitus. *N Engl J Med* 1988;**318**:1012–20.
68. Pak C, Mcarthur R, Eun H-M, Yoon J-W. Association of cytomegalovirus infection with autoimmune type 1 diabetes. *Lancet* 1988;**332**(8601):1–4.
69. Lidar M, Lipschitz N, Langevitz P, Barzilai O, et al. Infectious serologies and auto antibodies in Wegener's granulomatosis and other vasculitides: novel associations disclosed using the RadBioplex 2200. *NY Acad Sci* 2009;**1173**:649–57.
70. Ballanger F, Bressollette C, Volteau C, Planche L, Dreno B. Cytomegalovirus: its potential role in development of cutaneous T-cell lymphoma. *Exper Dermatol* 2009;**18**:574–6.
71. Weitz M, Kiessling C, Friedrich M, et al. Persistent CMV infection correlates with disease activity and dominates the phenotype of peripheral CD8 + T-cells in psoriasis. *Exp Derm* 2011;**20**(7):561–7.
72. Weigand D, Burgdorf W, Tarpay M. Vasculitis in cytomegalovirus infection. *Arch Dermatol* 1980;**116**(10):1174–6.
73. Wanner M, Pol-Rodriguez M, Hinds G, Hutt C, et al. Persistent erythema multiforme and CMV infection. *J Drugs Dermatol* 2007;**6**(3):333–6.
74. Seishima M, Oyama Z, Yamamura M. Erythema multiforne associated with cytomegalovirus infection in nonimmunosuppressed patients. *Dermatology* 2001;**203**:299–302.
75. Resnik K, DiLeonardo M, Maillet M. Hiostopathologic findings in cutaneous cytomegalovirus infection. *Am J Dermatopathol* 2000;**22**(5):397–407.
76. Swanson J, Feldman P. Cytomegalovirus infection initially diagnosed by skin biopsy. *Am J Clin Pathol* 1987;**87**:113–36.
77. Seishima M, Yamanaka S, Fujisawa T, Tohyama M, Hashimoto K. Reactivation of human herpesvirus (HHV) family members other than HHV-6 in drug-induced hypersensitivity syndrome. *Br J Dermatoil* 2006;**155**(2):344–9.
78. Ozcan D, Seckin D, Bilezikci B, Arslan H. The role of human herpesvirus-6, Epstein–Barr virus and cytomegalovirus infections in the eitopathogenesis of different types of cutaneous drug reactions. *Int J Dermatol* 2010;**49**(11):1250–4.
79. Docke W, Kiessling C, Worm M, Friedrich M, Pruss A, et al. Subclinical activation of latent cytomegalovirus (CMV) infection and ant-CMV immune response in patients with atopic dermatitis. *Br J Dermatol* 2003;**148**(5):954–63.
80. Kano Y, Shiohara T. Current understanding of cytomegalovirus infection in immunocompetent individuals. *J Dermatol Sci* 2000;**22**(3):196–204.
81. Drago F, Aragone M, Lugani C, Rebora A. Cytomegalovirus infection in normal and immunocompromised humans: a review. *Dermatology* 2000;**200**(3):189–95.
82. Bader El Din N, El Meguid M, Tabil A, Anany M, Esmat G, Zayed N, et al. Human cytomegalovirus infection inhibits response of chronic hepatitis-C-virus-infected patients to interferon-based therapy. *J Gastro Hepatol* 2011;**26**:55–62.
83. Trzonkowski P, Mysliwska J, Szmit E, Wieckiewicz J, Lukaszuk K, Byrdak L, et al. Association between cytomegalovirus infection, enhanced proinflammatory response and low level of anti-hemagglutinins during anti-influenza vaccination—an impact of immunosenescence. *Vaccine* 2003;**21**:3826–36.
84. Khan N, Hislop A, Gudgeon N, Cobbold M, Khanna R, Nayak L, et al. Herpesvirus-specific CD8 T cell immunity in old age: cytomegalovirus impairs the response to a co-resident EBV infection. *J Immunity* 2004;**173**:7481–9.
85. Van Duin D, Miranda C, Husni E. Cytomegalovirus viremia, pneumonitis, and tocilizumab therapy. *Emerg Infect Dis* 2011;**17**(4):754–6.

86. Oill P, Fiala M, Sclofferman J, Byfield P, Guze L. Cytomegalovirus mononucleosis in a health adult: association with hepatitis, secondary Epstein–Barr virus antibody response and immunosuppression. *Am J Med* 1977;**62**(3):413–17.
87. Clarke J, Craig R, Saffro R, Murphy P, Yokoo H. Cytomegalovirus granulomatous hepatitis. *Am J Med* 1979;**66**(2):264–9.
88. Ferreira S, Delgado M, Simoes A, Nunes J, Pereira I, Gaspar O. Cytomegalovirus encephalitis in an HIV-negative patient. *Acta Med Port* 2013;**26**(5):608–13[Abstr].
89. Ma Y, Feng J, Qi Y, Dou XG. An immunocompetent adult patient with hepatitis and Guillain-Barre syndrome after cytomegalovirus infection. *Virol J* 2011;**8**:95.
90. Zoukhri D. Effect of inflammation on lacrimal gland function. *Exp Eye Res* 2006;**82**(5):885–98.
91. Alfawaz A. Cytomegalovirus-related corneal endotheliitis: a review article. *Saudi J Opthal* 2011;**27**(1):47–9.
92. Davis J, Haft P, Hartley K. Retinal arteriolar occlusions due to cytomegalovirus retinitis in elderly patients without HIV. *J Opthal Inflam Infect* 2013;**3**:17.
93. Pang C. Review of cytomegalovirus anterior uveitis. In: Khatami M, editor. *Inflammation, chronic diseases and cancer-cell and molecular biology, immunology and clinical basis.* Rijeka Croatia: InTech; 2012. p. 273–8.
94. Hartigan-O'Connor D, Jacobson M, Tan Q, Sinclair E. Development of cytomegalovirus (CMV) immune recovery Uveitis is associated with TH17 depletion and poor systemic CMV-specific T cell responses. *Clin Infect Dis* 2011;**52**(3):409–17.
95. Miller D, Legra J, Dubovy S, Suner I, Sedmark D, Dix R, et al. The association of prior cytomegalovirus infection with neovascular age-related macular degeneration. *Amer J Ophthalmol* 2004;**138**(3):323–8.
96. Morunglav M, Theate I, Bertin G, Hantson P. CMV enteritis causing massive intestinal hemorrhage in an elderly patient. *Case Rep Med* 2010; Article ID 385795, 4 pages. http://dx.doi.org/10.1155/2010/385795
97. Lin Y-H, Yeh C-J, Chen Y-J, et al. Recurrent cytomegalovirus colitis with megacolon in an immunocompetent elderly man. *J Med Virol* 2010;**82**(4):638–41.
98. Kalaitzis J, Basioukas P, Karzi E, Markakis C, Liarmakopoulos E, et al. Small-bowel necrosis complicating a cytomegalovirus-induced superior mesenteric vein thrombosis in an immunocompetent patient: a case report. *J Med Case Reports* 2012;**6**:118.
99. Xiao S, Hart J. Marked gastric foveolar hyperplasia associated with active cytomegalovirus infection. *Am J Gastroenterol* 2001;**96**(1):223–6.
100. Villar L, Massanari R, Mitros F. Cytomegalovirus infection with acute erosive esophagitis. *Am J Med* 1984;**76**(5):924–8.
101. Nakase H, Matsumura K, Yoshino T, Chiba T. Systematic review: cytomegalovirus infection in inflammatory bowel disease. *J Gastroenterol* 2008;**43**(10):735–40.
102. Justo D, Finn T, Atzmony L, Guy N, et al. Thrombosis associated with acute cytomegalovirus infection: a meta-analysis. *Eur J Intern Med* 2011;**22**(2):195–9.
103. Zhu J, Quyyumi A, Norman J, Csako G, Epstein S. Cytomegalovirus in the pathogenesis of atherosclerosis. *JACC* 1999;**34**(6):1738–43.
104. Imbronito A, Marcelino S, Grande S, Nunes F, Romito G. Detection of human cytomegalovirus and Epstein–Barr virus in coronary atherosclerotic tissue. *Braz J Microbiol* 2010;**41**(3):563–6.
105. Zhou Y, Leon M, Waclawiw M, Popina J, Yu Z, Finkel T, et al. Association between prior cytomegalovirus infection and the risk of restenosis after coronary atherectomy. *N Engl J Med* 1996;**335**:624–30.
106. Rovery C, Granel B, Parola P, Foucault C, Brouqui P. Acute cytomegalovirus infection complicated by venous thrombosis: a case report. *AnnClin Microbiol Antimicrob* 2005;**4**:11.
107. Cheng J, Ke Q, Jin Z, Wang H, Kocher O, Morgan J, et al. Cytomegalovirus infection causes an increase of arterial blood pressure. *PloS Pathog* 2009;**5**(5):e1000427.

108. Iwasenko J, Howard J, Arbuckle S, et al. Human cytomegovirus infection is detected frequently in stillbirths and is associated with fetal thrombic vasculopathy. *J Infrect Dis* 2011;**2003**(11):1526–33.
109. Caposio P, Orloff S, Strebbio D. The role of cytomegalovirus in angiogenesis. *Virus Res* 2011;**157**(2):204–11.
110. Botto S, Streblow D, DeFilippis V, et al. IL-6 in human secretome promotes angiogenesis and survival of endothelial cells through the stimulation of survivin. *Blood* 2011;**117** (1):352–61.
111. Gkrania-Klotsas E, Langenberg C, Sharp S, Luben R, Khaw K, Wareham N. Higher immunoglobulin G antibody levels against cytomegalovirus are associated with ischaemic heart disease in the population-based EPIC-Norfolk cohort. *J Infect Dis* 2012;**206** (12):1897–903.
112. Kyto V, Vuorinen T, Saukko P, Lautenschlager I, Lignitz E, Saraste A, et al. Cytomegalovirus infection of the heart is common in patients with fatal myocarditis. *Clin Infect Dis* 2005;**40**(5):683–8.
113. Michaelson R, Benson G, Friedman H. Urinary retention as the presenting symptom of acquired cytomegalovirus infection. *Am J Med* 1983;**74**(3):526–8.
114. Davies J, Taylor C, White R, George R, Purdham D. Cytomegalovirus infection associated with lower urinary tract symptoms. *BMJ* 1979;**1**(6171):1120.
115. Heieren M, Kim Y. Balfour H (1988) Human cytomegalovirus infection of kidney glomerular viscera epithelial and tubular epithelial cells in culture. *Transplantation* 1988;**46**(3):426–32.
116. Litjens N, Wit E, Betjes M. Differential effects of age, cytomegalovirus-seropositivity and end-stage renal disease (ESRD) on circulating T lymphocyte subsets. *Immun Ageing* 2011;**8**:2.
117. Silver M, Paul P, Soujana P, Ramakrishna G, Vedantham H, Kalpana B, et al. Shedding of Epstein–Barr virus and cytomegalovirus form the genital tract of women in a peri-urban community in Andhra Pradesh. *India J Clin Microbiol* 2011;**49**(7):2435–9.
118. Fux C, Pfister S, Nohl F, Zimmerli S. Cytomegalovirus-associated acute transverse myelitis in immunocompetent adults. *Clin Microbiol Infect* 2003;**9**(12):1187–90.
119. Slooter A, Ramos L, Kappelle L. Migraine-like headache as the presenting symptom of cerebral venous sinus thrombosis. *J Neurol* 2002;**249**(6):775–6.
120. Lamasal K, Agrawal J, Oli K. Cytomegalovirus infection in a patient causing bilateral papillitis and Gullain Barre syndrome. *Nepal J Neurosci* 2005;**2**:142–3.
121. Yu J, Solano F, Seethala R. Bilateral cytomegalovirus (CMV) oophoritis mimicking widely metastatic carcinoma: a case report and review of the literature. *Diagn Pathol* 2007;**2**:50.
122. Kauffman C, Linnemann C, Alvaria M. Cytomegalovirus encephalitis associated with thymoma and immunoglobulin deficiency. *Am J Med* 1979;**67**(4):724–8.
123. Nakamura H, Liao H, Minami K, Toyoda M, Akutsu H, Miyagawa Y, et al. Human cytomegalovirus induces apotosis in neural stem/progenitor cells derived from induced pluripotent stem cells by generating mitochondrial dysfunction and endoplasmic reticulum stress. *Herpesviridae* 2013;**4**:2.
124. Nagane Y, Utsugisawa K. Ross syndrome associated with cytomegalovirus infection. *Muscle Nerve* 2008;**38**(1):424–6.
125. Lurain N, Hanson B, Martinson J, Leurgans S, Landy A, et al. Virological and immunological characteristics of human cytomegalovirus infection associated with Alzheimer disease. *J Infect Dis* 2013;**208**(4):564–72. http://dx.doi.org/10.1093/infdis/jit210.
126. Westman G, Lidehall A, Ingelsson M, Lannfelt L, Korsgren O, Eriksson B. Decreased proportion of cytomegalovirus specific CD8 T-cells but no signs of general immunosenescence in Alzheimer's disease. *PLoS O* 2013;**8**(10):e77921.
127. Haeseker M, Piipers E, Dukers-Muijrers N, Nelemans P, Hoebe C, Bruggeman C, et al. Association of cytomegalovirus of cytomegalovirus and other pathogens with

frailty and diabetes mellitus, but not with cardiovascular disease and mortality in psycho-geriatric patients; a prospective cohort study. *Immun Ageing* 2013;**10**(1):30.

128. Juanjuan C, Yan F, Li C, Haizhi L, Ling W, Xinrong W, et al. Murine model for congenital hearing impairment. *Virol J* 2011;**8**:70.

129. Megalhaes S, Duarte F, Vassallo J, Costa S, Lorand-Metze I. *Multiple lymphoid nodules in bone marrow biopsy of immunocompetent patient with cytomegalovirus infection: an immunohistochemical analysis. Rev Soc Bras Med Trop* 2001;**34**(4):365–8. http://dx.doi.org/10.1590/S0037-86822000400009.

130. Van de Berg P, Griffiths S, Yong S, Macaulay R, Bemelman F, Jackson S, et al. Cytomegalovirus infection reduces telomere length in circulating T cell pool. *J Immunol* 2010;**184**(7):3417–23.

131. Bughio F, Elliott D, Goodrum F. An endothelial cell-specific requirement for the UL133-UL138 locus of human cytomegalovirus for efficient virus maturation. *J Virology* 2013;**87**(6):3062–75.

132. Katsoulis K, Minasidis I, Vainas A, Bikas C, Kontakiotis T, Vakianis P. Platypnea and orthodeoxia associated with Pneumocystis jiroveci and Cytomegalovirus pneumonia: a case report. *J Med Case Reports* 2009;**3**:9319.

133. Jacobi C, Riessen R, Schumacher U, Autenreith I, Jahn G, Gagor M, et al. Life-threatening pneumonia caused by human cytomegalovirus and Mycoplasma pneumonia coinfection in a young, immunocompetent patient. *J Med Microbiol* 2010;**59**(Pt8):980–3.

134. Balthesen M, Messerle M, Reddalase M. Lungs are a major organ site of cytomegalovirus latency and recurrence. *J Virol* 1993;**67**(9):5360–9.

135. Bratke K, Krieghoff L, Kuepper M, Lutlmann W, Virchow J. CD8 + T cell activation and differentiation in allergic asthma and the impact of cytomegalovirus serological status. *Clin Exp Immunol* 2007;**149**(2):311–16.

136. Chomel J, Allard J, Floret D, et al. Role of cytomegalovirus infection in the incidence of viral acute respiratory infections in children attending day-care centers. *Europ J Clin Microb Infect Dis* 2001;**20**(3):167–72.

137. Chan B, Woo J, Liew C. Cytomegalovirus infection of the nasopharynx. *J Clin Pathol* 2002;**55**(12):970–2.

138. Chen V, Chen Y, Hong L, Kent K, Baumgartner C, Machida C. Herpesviruses in abscesses and cellulitis of endodontic origin. *J Endod* 2009;**35**(2):182–8.

139. Taglietti F, Drapeau C, Grilli E, Capone A, et al. Hemolytic anemia due to acute cytomegalovirus infection in immunocompetent adult: a case report and review of the literature. *J Medical Case Rep* 2010;**4**:334.

140. Varani S, Lazzarotto T, Margotti M, Masi L, Gramantieri L, et al. Laboratory signs of acute or recent cytomegalovirus infection are common in cirrhosis of the liver. *J Med Virol* 2000;**62**(1):25–8.

141. Stout-Delgado H, Du W, Shirali A, Booth C, Goldstein D. Aging promotes neutrophil-induced mortality by augmenting 1 L-17 production during viral infection. *Cell Host Microbe* 2009;**6**(5):446–56.

142. Lepiller Q, Tripathy M, Martino V, Kantelip B, Herebein G. Increased HCMV seroprevalence in patients with hepatocellular cancer. *Virol J* 2011;**8**:485.

143. Melnick M, Sedghizadeh P, Allen C, Jaskoll T. Human cytomegalovirus and mucoepidermoid carcinoma of salivary glands: cell-specific localization of acute viral and oncogenic signaling proteins is confirmatory of casual relationship. *Exp Mol Pathol* 2011;**92**(1):118–25. http://dx.doi.org/10.1016/j.yexmp.2011.10.011.

144. Barami K. Oncomodulatory mechanisms of human cytomegalovirus in gliomas. *J Clin Neurosci* 2010;**17**(7):819–23.

145. Rahbar A, Stragillotto G, Orrego A, Peredo I, Taher C, Willems J, et al. Low levels of human cytomegalovirus infection in glioblastoma multiforme associates with patient survival; a-case-control study. *Herpesviridae* 2012;**3**:3.

146. Pourgheysari B, Brunton R, Parry H, Billingham L, et al. The number of cytomegalovirus-specific CD4+ cells is markedly expanded in patients with B-cell chronic lymphocytic leukaemia and determines the total CD4+ T-cell repertoire. *Blood* 2010;**116**(16):2968–74.

147. Lepiller Q, Khan K, DiMartinov V, Herbein G. Cytomegalovirus and tumors: two players for one goal—immune escape. *Open Virol* 2011;**5**:68–9.

148. Harkins L, Matlaf L, Soroceanu L, Klemm K, Britt W, et al. Detection of humancytomegalovirus in normal and neoplastic breast epithelium. *Herpesviridae* 2010;**1**:8. http://dx.doi.org/10.1186/2042-4280-1-8.

149. Cox B, Richardson A, Graham P, Gislefloss R, Jellum E, Rollag H. Breast cancer, cytomegalovirus and Epstein Barr virus: a nested case-control study. *Br J Cancer* 2010;**102**:1665–9.

150. El-Shinawi M, Mohamed H, El-Ghonaimy E, Tantawy M, Amal Y, Schneider R, et al. Human cytomegalovirus infection enhances NF-κB/p65 signaling in inflammatory breast cancer patients. *PLoS One* 2013;**8**(2):e55755.

151. Mera J, Whimbey E, Elting L, Preti A, Luna M, Bruner J, et al. Cytomegalovirus pneumonia in adult nontransplantation patients with cancer: review of 20 cases occurring from 1964 through 1990. *Clin Infect Dis* 1996;**22**:1046–50.

152. Michalek J, Horvath R. High incidence of Epstein–Barr virus, cytomegalovirus and human herpesvirus 6 infections in children with cancer. *BMC Pediatr* 2002;**2**:1.

153. Leach C, Pollock B, McClain K, Parmley R, et al. Human herpesvirus 6 and cytomegalovirus infections in children with human immunodeficiency virus infection and cancer. *Paed Infect Dis* 2002;**21**(2):125–32.

154. Wang Y-C, Wang N-C, Lin J-C, Perng C-L, et al. Risk factors and outcomes of cytomegalovirus viremia in cancer patients: a study from a medical centre in northern Taiwan. *J Microbiol Immunol Infect* 2011;**44**:442–8.

155. Han X. Epidemiologic analysis of reactivated cytomegalovirus antigenemia in patients with cancer. *J Clin Microbiol* 2007;**45**(4):1126–32.

156. Britt W. Manifestations of human cytomegalovirus infection: proposed mechanisms of acute and chronic disease. *Curr Top Microbiol Immunol* 2008;**325**:417–70.

157. Griffiths P. Burden of disease associated with human cytomegalovirus and prospects for elimination by universal immunisation. *Lancet Infect Dis* 2012;**12**:790–8.

158. Boeckh M, Geballe A. Cytomegalovirus: pathogen, paradigm, and puzzle. *J Clin Invest* 2011;**121**(5):1673–80.

159. Bosch J, Rector J, Turner J, Riddell N, O'Hartaigh B, Burns V. Psychoneuromicrobiology: cytomegalovirus infection as a putative link between stress, aging, and immunity. In: Bosch J, et al. editors. *Immunosenescence*. New York: Springer Science & Business Media; 2013. p. 81–100.

160. Bristow B, O'Keefe K, Shafir S, Sorvillo F. Congenital cytomegalovirus mortality in the United States, 1990-2006. *PLoS Negl Trop Dis* 2011;**54**(4):e1140.

161. Soderberg-Naucler C. Does cytomegalovirus play a causative role in the development of various inflammatory diseases and cancer? *J Intern Med* 2006;**259**(3):219–46.

163. Pawelec G, Akbar A, Caruso C, Solana R, Grubeck-Loebenstein B, Wikby A. Human immunoscenescence: is it infectious? *Immunol Rev* 2005;**205**(1):257–68.

164. Pawelec G, Derhovanessian E, Larbi A, Strindhall J, Wikby A. Cytomegalovirus and human immunoscenescence. *Rev Med Virol* 2009;**19**:47–56.

165. Pawelec G, McElhaney J, Aiello A, Derhovanessian E. The impact of CMV infection on survival in older humans. *Curr Opin Immunol* 2012;**24**(4):507–11.

166. Wittkop L, Bitard J, Lazaro E, Neau D, Bonnet F, Mercie P, et al. Effect of cytomegalovirus-induced immune response, self-antigen induced immune response, and microbial translocation on chronic immune activation in successfully treated HIV Type 1-infected patients: the ANRS CO3 Aquitaine cohort. *J Infect Dis* 2013; **207**:622–7.

167. Puchammer-Stockl E, Gorzer I, Zoufaly A, Jaksch P, Bauer C, et al. Emergency of multiple cytomegalovirus strains in blood and lung of lung transplant recipients. *Transplantation* 2006;**81**(2):187–94.
168. Puchammer-Stockl E, Gorzer I. Human cytomegalovirus: an enormous variety of strains and their possible clinical significance. *Future Virol* 2011;**6**(2):259–71.
169. Fang F, Wang X, Hu J, Zhang L, et al. The polymorphism disparity of cytomegalovirus UL97 gene in pediatric patients, renal-transplanted, and hematopoietic stem cell transplanted recipients. *Lab Med* 2010;**41**:601–6.
170. Trincado D, Scott G, White P, Hunt C, Rasmussen L, Rawlinson W. Human cytomegalovirus strains associated with congenital and perinatal infections. *J Med Virol* 2000;**61**(4):481–7.
171. Lidehall A, Engman M, Sund F, Malm G, Lewebgohn-Fuchs I, Ewald U, et al. Cytomegalovirus-specific CD4 and CD8 T-cell responses in infants and children. *Scand J Immunol* 2013;**77**(2):135–43.
172. Miller-Kittrell M, Sparer T. Feeling manipulated: cytomegalovirus immune manipulation. *Virol J* 2009;**6**:4.
173. Derhovanessian E, Larbi A, Pawelec G. Biomarkers of human immunoscenescence: impact of cytomegalovirus infection. *Curr Opin Immunol* 2009;**21**:1–6.
174. Derhovanessian E, Maier A, Hahnel K, Zelba H, de Craen A, et al. Lower proportion of naïve peripheral CD8+ T cells and an unopposed pro-inflammatory response to human cytomegalovirus proteins in vitro are associated with longer survival in very elderly people. *Age* 2013;**35**(4):1387–99.
175. Derhovanessian E, Maier A, Beck R, Jahn G, Hahnel K, Slagboom P, et al. Hallmark features of immunosenescence are absent in familial longevity. *J Immunol* 2010;**185**:4618–24.
176. Wang G, Kao W, Qian-Li Xue P, Chiou R, Detrick B, McDyer J, et al. Cytomegalovirus infection and the risk of mortality and frailty in older women: a prospective observational cohort study. *Am J Epidemiol* 2010;**171**(10):1144–52.
177. Arias R, Moro-Garcia M, Echeverria A, Solano-Jaurrieta J, Suarez-Garcia F, Lopez-Larrea C. Intensity of the humoral response to cytomegalovirus is associated with the phenotypic and functional status of the immune system. *J Virol* 2013;**87**(8):4486–95.
178. Mekker A, Tchang V, Haeberli L, Oxenius A, Trkola A, Karrer U. Immune scenescence: relative contributions of age and cytomegalovirus infection. *PLoS Pathog* 2012;**8**(8):e1002850.
179. Solana R, Tarazona R, Aiello A, Akbar A, Appay V, Beswick M, et al. CMV and immunoscenescence: from basics to clinics. *Immun Ageing* 2012;**9**:23.
180. Chen T, Hudnall S. Anatomical mapping of human herpesvirus reservoir of infection. *Mod Pathol* 2006;**19**:726–37.
181. Razonable R, Fanning C, Brown R, Espy M, Rivero A, Wilson J, et al. Selective reactivation of human herpesvirus 6 variant A occurs in critically ill immunocompetent hosts. *J Infect Dis* 2002;**185**:110–13.
182. Aleman H, Esparza J, Ramierez F, Astiazaram H, Payette H. Longitudinal evidence on the association between interleukin-6 and C-reactive protein with the loss of total appendicular skeletal muscle in free-living older men and women. *Age Ageing* 2011;**40**(4):469–75.
183. Berk M, Williams L, Jacka F, O'Neil A, Pasco J, Moylan S, et al. So depression is an inflammatory disease, but where does the inflammation come from? *BMC Med* 2013;**11**:200.
184. Leng S, Tian X, Matteini A, Li H, Hughes J, Jain A, et al. IL-6-independent association of elevated serum neopterin levels with prevalent frailty in community-dwelling older adults. *Age Ageing* 2011;**40**(4):475–81.

185. Alam I, Ng T, Larbi A. *Does inflammation determine whether obesity is metabolically healthy or unhealthy?* The Aging Perspective; Mediators of Inflammation: 2012, Article ID 456456, 14 pages. http://dx.doi.org/10.1155/2012/456456
186. Kaptoge S, DiAngelantonio E, Lowe G, Pepys M, Thompson S, Collins R, et al. C-reactive protein concentration and risk of coronary heart disease, stroke, and mortality: an individual participant meta-analysis. *Lancet* 2010;**375**(9709):132–40.
187. Gaudreault E, Gosselin J. Leukotriene B4-mediated release of antimicrobial peptides against cytomegalovirus is BLT1 dependent. *Viral Immunol* 2007;**20**(3):407–20.
188. Wan M, Sabirsh A, Wetterholm A, Agerberth B, Haeggstrom J. Leukotriene B4 triggers release of cathelicidin LL-37 from human neutrophils: novel lipid-peptide interatctions in innate immune responses. *FASEB J* 2007;**21**(11):2895–905.
189. Kahlenberg J, Kaplan M. Little peptide, big effects: the role of LL-37 in inflammation and autoimmune disease. *J Immunol* 2013;**191**:4895–901.
190. Gosselin J, Borgeat P, Flamand L. Leukotriene B4 protects latently infected mice against murine cytomegalovirus reactivation following allogenic transplantation. *J Immunol* 2005;**174**(3):1587–93.
191. Martel-Pelletier J, Lajeunesse D, Reboul P, Pelletier J-P. Therapeutic role of dual inhibitors of 5-LOX and COX, selective and non-selective non-steroidal anti-inflammatory drugs. *Ann Rheum Dis* 2003;**62**:501–9.
192. Wang T-T, Nestel F, Bourdeau V, Nagai Y, Wang Q, Liao J, et al. Dihydroxyvitamin D3 is a direct inducer of antimicrobial peptide gene expression. *J Immunol* 2004;**173**(5):2909–12.
193. Maes M, Berk M, Goehler L, Song C, Anderson G, et al. Depression and sickness behaviour are Janus-faced responses to shared inflammatory pathways. *BMC Med* 2012;**10**:66.
194. Fagundes C, Glaser R, Alfrano C, Bennett J, Povoski S, et al. Fatigue and herpesvirus latency in women newly diagnosed with breast cancer. *Brain Behav Immun* 2012;**26**(3):394–400.
195. Jones R. Unexpected and disruptive changes in admissions associated with an infectious-like event experienced at a hospital in Berkshire, England around May of 2012. *Brit J Med Medical Res* 2015;**5**:[in press].
196. Su D, Shen M, Li X, Sun L. *Roles of γδ T cells in the pathogenesis of autoimmune diseases.* Clin Develop Immunol 2013;985753. http://dx.doi.org/10.1155/2013/98753.
197. Qi R, Hua-Song Z, Xiao-Feng Z. Leflunomide inhibits the apotosis of human embryonic fibroblasts infected by human cytomegalovirus. *Eur J Med Res* 2013;**18**:3.
198. Dowd J, Aiello A. Socioeconomic differentials in immune response in the US. *Epidemiology* 2009;**20**(6):902–8.
199. Linder J. The thymus gland in secondary immunodeficiency. *Arch Pathol lab Med* 1987;**111**(12):1118–22.
200. Moonesinghe R, Ioannidis J, Flanders D, Yang Q, Truman B, Khoury M. Estimating the contribution of genetic variants to difference in incidence of disease between population groups. *Eur J Human Genetics* 2012;**20**(8):831–6.
201. Congdon P. Estimating diabetes prevalence by small area in England. *J Public Health* 2006;**28**(1):71–81.
202. Zhang L, Yesupriya A, Hu D, Chang M, Dowling N, et al. Variants in ABCB1, TGFB1, and XRCC1 genes and susceptibility to viral hepatitis A infection in Mexican Americans. *Hepatology* 2012;**55**(4):1008–18.
203. Ombrello M, Remmers E, Sun G, Freeman A, Datta S, Torabi-Parizi P, et al. Cold urticarial, immunodeficiency, and autoimmunity related to PLCGZ deletions. *N Engl Med* 2012;**366**:330–8.
204. Jones R. GP referral to dermatology: which conditions? *Br J Healthcare Manage* 2012;**18**(11):594–6.

205. Ferdinands J, Denison A, Dowling N, Jost H, et al. A pilot study of host genetic variants associated with influenza-associated deaths among children and young adults. *Emerg Infect Dis* 2011;**17**(12):2294–302.

206. Hu Y, Wu D, Tao R. Association between mannose-binding lectin gene polymorphism and pediatric cytomegalovirus infection. *Viral Immunol* 2010;**23**(4):443–7.

207. Muntasell A, Lopez-Montaries M, Vera A, Heredai G, Romo N, Penafiel J, et al. NKG2C zygosity influences CD94/NKG2C receptor function and the NK-cell compartment redistribution in response to human cytomegalovirus. *Eur J Immunol* 2013;**43** (12):3268–78. http://dx.doi.org/10.1002/eji.201343773.

208. Pandey J. Immunoglobulin GM, allotypes as effect modifiers of cytomegalovirus-spurred neuroblastoma. *Cancer Epidemiol Biomarkers Prev* 2013;**22**(11):1927–30.

209. Suy A, Castro P, Nomdedeu M, Garcia F, Lopez A, Fumero E, et al. Immunological profile of heterosexual highly HIV-exposed uninfected individuals: predominant role of CD4 and CD8 T-cell activation. *J Infect Dis* 2007;**196**(8):1191–201.

210. Allbrecht T, Fons M, Deng C, Boldogh I. Increased frequency of specific locus mutation following human cytomegalovirus infection. *Virology* 1997;**230**(1):48–61. http://dx.doi.org/10.1006/viro.1997.8467.

211. Polansky H. *Microcompetition with foreign DNA and the origin of chronic disease*. Rochester, New York, Centre for the Biology of Chronic DiseaseAvailable from: http://www.cbcd.net/Book%20by%20Hanan%20Polansky%20(Purple%20Book).pdf.

212. Sebastiani P, Riva A, Montano M, Pham P, Torkamani A, Scherba E, et al. *Whole genome sequences of a male and female supercentenarian, ages greater than 114 years*. Frontiers Genet 2012;**2**:90.Available from:http://www.frontiersin.org/genetics_of_aging/10.3389/fgene.2011.00090/full.

213. Klengel T, Mehta D, Anecker C, et al. Allele-specific FKBP5 DNA demethylation a molecular mediation of gene-childhood trauma interactions. *Nature Neurosci* 2013;**16**:33–41. http://dx.doi.org/10.1038/nn.3275.

214. Mortensen L, Maier A, Slagbom P, Pawalec G, Derhovanessian E, Petersen I, et al. Early-life environment influencing susceptibility to cytomegalovirus infection: evidence from the Leiden Longevity Study and the Longitudinal Study of Aging Danish Twins. *Epidemiol Infect* 2011;**140**(5):835–41. http://dx.doi.org/10.1017/S0950268811001397.

215. Aiello A, Nguyen H-O, Haan M. C-reactive protein mediates the effect of apolipoprotein E on cytomegalovirus infection. *J Infect Dis* 2008;**197**(1):34–41.

216. Holick M. The vitamin D epidemic and its health consequences. *J Nutr* 2005;**135** (11):2739S–2748S.

217. Yang C-Y, Leung P, Adamopoulos I, Gershwin M. The implication of vitamin D and autoimmunity: a comprehensive review. *Clin Rev Allerg Immunol* 2013;**45**:217–26 [Abstr].

218. Pludowski P, Holick M, Pilz S, Wagner C, Hollis B, Grant W, et al. Vitamin D effects on musculoskeletal health, immunity, autoimmunity, cardiovascular disease, cancer, fertility, pregnancy, dementia, and mortality—a review of recent evidence. *Autoimmunity Rev* 2013;**12**(10):976–89[Abstr].

219. Jones R, Beauchant S. Spread of a new type of infectious condition across Berkshire in England between June 2011 and March 2013: Effect on medical emergency admissions. *Brit J Med Medical Res* 2015;**5**:[in press].

220. Ferrando-Martinez S, Franco J, Hernandez A, Ordonez A, Gutierrez E, et al. Thymopoiesis in elderly human is associated with systemic inflammatory status. *Age* 2009;**31**:87–97.

221. Ferrando-Martinez S, Romario-Sanchez M, Solana R, Delgado J, de la Rossa R, et al. Thymic function failure and C-reactive protein levels are independent predictors of all-cause mortality in healthy elderly humans. *Age* 2013;**35**:251–9.

222. Irvine W. The thymus in autoimmune disease. *Proc Roy Soc Med* 1970;**63**:718–22.
223. Mowry E, James J, Krupp L, Waubant E. Vitamin D ststus and antibody levels to common viruses in paediatric-onset multiple sclerosis. *Mult Scler* 2011;**17**(6):666–71.
224. Francis T. On the doctrine of original antigenic sin. *Proc Amer Philosoph Soc* 1960;**104**(6):572–8.
225. Jones R. Infectious-like Spread of an Agent Leading to Increased Medical Admissions and Deaths in Wigan (England), During 2011 and 2012. *Brit J Med Medical Res* 2014;**4**(28):4723–41.
226. Jones R. Unexpected single-year-of-age changes in the elderly mortality rate in 2012 in England and Wales. *Brit J Med Medical Res* 2012;**4**(16):3196–207.
227. Jones R. A previously uncharacterized infectious-like event leading to spatial spread of deaths across England and Wales: Characteristics of the most recent event and a time series for past events. *Brit J Med Medical Res* 2015;**5**:[in press].
228. Cannon M, Hyde T, Schmid D. Review of cytomegalovirus shedding in body fluids, and relevance to congenital cytomegalovirus infection. *Rev Med Virol* 2011;**21**(4):240–55.
229. Tait A, Butts C, Sternberg E. The role of glucocorticoids and progestrins in inflammatory, autoimmune and infectious disease. *J Leukocyte Biol* 2008;**84**(4):924–31.
230. Fairweather D, Rose N. Women and autoimmune diseases. *Emerg Inf Dis* 2004;**10**(11):2005–11.
231. Jones R. Gender and financial risk in commissioning. *Br J Healthcare Manage* 2012;**18**(6):336–7.
232. Zhu J, Shearer G, Norman J, Pinto L, Marincola F, et al. Host response to cytomegalovirus infection as a determinant of susceptibility to coronary artery disease: sex-based differences in inflammation and type of immune response. *Circulation* 2000;**102**:2491–6.

CHAPTER 19

Hepatitis C and Mixed Cryoglobulinemia: An Update

A. Della Rossa[1], C. Stagnaro, S. Bombardieri

Dipartimento di Malattie Muscoloscheletriche e Cutanee, U.O. Reumatologia, Pisa, Italy
[1]Corresponding Author: a.dellarossa@ao-pisa.toscani.it

1 INTRODUCTION

Cryoglobulinemic vasculitis (CV), or cryoglobulinemic syndrome, is a chronic small-vessel vasculitis first described by Meltzer and Franklin in 1964. This disease is characterized by serum-positive cryoglobulins, namely immune complexes, which precipitate or form a gel at a temperature less than 37 °C and redissolve after rewarming.

Mixed cryoglobulinemia, which occurs in 30% to nearly 100% of cases, is triggered by chronic infection with the hepatitis C virus (HCV), but, less commonly, it may also complicate connective tissues diseases (Sjögren's syndrome, systemic lupus erythematosus and rheumatoid arthritis), lymphoproliferative disorders (Waldenstrom's macroglobulinemia, multiple myeloma or chronic lymphocytic leukemia) and other chronic infections (hepatitis B virus [HBV], cytomegalovirus and parvovirus B19). Nearly 10% of cases are regarded as idiopathic, or "essential", because an underlying cause cannot be identified.[1]

In the past four decades a number of steps forwards in the knowledge of this disorder have been made, and CV has changed from being considered solely an immune complex–mediated disease to a virally triggered condition. Nowadays we view this disease as a multifaceted condition with autoimmune features, triggered by HCV infection, coexisting with a chronic smouldering lymphoproliferative process that usually remains unmodified for years or even decades but can turn into a frank malignant lymphoma during long-term follow-up in a limited numbers of cases (<10%).[2]

Infection and Autoimmunity
http://dx.doi.org/10.1016/B978-0-444-63269-2.00061-1

2 ETIOPATHOGENESIS

The discovery of HCV in 1989 radically changed the focus of research from essential to HCV-related cryoglobulinemia.[1] HCV plays a central role in the pathogenesis of CV, based on a number of empirical observations such as the high prevalence of HCV antibodies and genome in the serum of patients with mixed cryoglobulemia (MC), the high concentration of viral particles in the cryoglobulins and the immunohistochemical localization of HCV or its markers in peripheral blood mononuclear cells and in tissue samples.[3] Moreover, the recent detection of HCV-negative stranded RNA in peripheral blood mononuclear cells of patients with CV lends new strength to the role of HCV in the pathogenesis of the disease.[4]

Cryoglobulins are generated by the clonal expansion of B-cells, which finds its first step in HCV lymphotropism. The HCV envelope protein E2 binds to CD81, a signaling molecule expressed by both hepatocytes and B and T lymphocytes; this interaction seems to trigger the chronic stimulation of B cells.[1] Rheumatoid factor activity seems to be an antigen-driven process, triggered by immune complexes containing HCV.[5] After the initial activation, the continuous exposure to antigen pressure may result in a positive selection of B cells, with the emergence of a B-cell population producing a monoclonal immunoglobulin M rheumatoid factor. These B-cell clones can be found within the peripheral blood, bone marrow and liver of patients with HCV infection; they are usually considered an indolent lymphoproliferative disorder evolving in a frank malignant lymphoma in a minority of cases.[2]

The monoclonal immunoglobulin M, secreted by B-cell clones, have the peculiarity to bear a cross-reacting idiotype called WA, which binds immunoglobulins directed to anti-HCV core proteins.[1] It has been demonstrated that WA B cells can be detected not only in all patients with CV but also in nearly 10% of asymptomatic patients with HCV infection. This discovery suggests that WA B cells may be a marker for the development of CV and for B-cell lymphomas in patients with HCV infection. Because antiviral therapy induces the decline of WA B cells in parallel with the decline in viremia, and because the duration of HCV infection required for CV to begin seems to be at least a decade, it may also be suggested that all asymptomatic patients with WA B cells infected with HCV should be treated with antiviral agents to prevent the development of all cases of CV and of a major portion of B-cell lymphomas.[6]

Although many steps forwards in the knowledge of CV have been made, several aspects of this disease's etiopathogenesis have to be clarified; for example, why do only a portion of HCV-infected patients (40–60%) develop cryoglobulinemic syndrome. Recent studies suggest that the host's genetic background plays an important role in determining the susceptibility to CV of some HCV-infected patients. Indeed, differences in the balance of immune complexes or in expression of a B-cell subset might be observed, depending on the expression and the severity of hepatic or extrahepatic features in subjects with chronic HCV infection.[7,8]

The host immune response against HCV is not always protective against infection; indeed, viral clearance is not associated with an immunisation against reinfection. Immune response in chronic HCV carriers seems to exert a selective pressure on the virus, favoring the emergence of viral strains more prone to escape from it. In particular, a substantial divergence between humoral and cell-mediated response to the virus has been unveiled; humoral response is responsible for extrahepatic manifestations and seems to have no effect in controlling infection. Cell-mediated immune response has greater importance in the production of antiviral cytokines but seems to also have a role in cytotoxic damage. In this regard, a substantial divergence in cytokine production between subjects with HCV infection not associated with CV and patients with HCV-related CV recently has been suggested. In particular, an emerging role for chemokines and type 1 cytokines has been claimed in the pathophysiology of this vasculitis. Serum concentrations of interleukin (IL) 1β are significantly higher in patients with MC and HCV compared with healthy controls and patients with HCV. Further, high serum concentrations of interferon-γ inducible chemokine (CXCL10) have been observed both in patients with HCV and patients with MC and HCV. Increased CXCL10 and IL-1β concentrations were associated with the presence of active vasculitis in patients with MC and HCV.[9] Furthermore, subjects with CV associated with autoimmune thyroiditis (AT) have a different serum expression of cytokines compared with subjects with only CV.[10,11]

3 CLINICAL FEATURES

MC can be found in up to 60% of HCV-infected patients; however, less that 5% of patients have clinical manifestations of CV. The two major mechanisms forming the basis for the development of CV are cryoglobulin precipitation in the microcirculation with consequent vascular occlusion and the more frequent immune complex–mediated inflammation of blood vessels. The tissue deposition of immunocomplexes is influenced by several factors such as blood viscosity, blood temperature and protein solubility, resulting from the primary structure of immune complexes and steric conformation, which, in turn, depend on temperature, pH and ionic strength.[1]

The most common presentation, first described by Meltzer and Franklin and observed in 80% of patients at disease onset, is the triad of purpura, arthralgia and weakness. The natural history of the disease generally shows a slow progression with a period of exacerbation and remission and rare emergencies. As we know, palpable purpura is the most characteristic manifestation of CV (54–82%); it is intermittent, orthostatic and usually localized to the lower extremities for physical reasons. Purpura is often complicated by perimalleolar chronic ulcers, and its histopathological pattern is leucocytoclastic vasculitis.[2] Cutaneous manifestations are usually associated with general symptoms such as fever, weakness, myalgia and arthralgia. Another common feature (17–60%) of the disease is a sensory peripheral polyneuropathy, which generally precedes motor involvement and is caused by immunologically mediated demyelinisation and by occlusion of the vasa nervorum by cryoglobulin precipitation.

In CV we less frequently can find renal involvement (in one-third of patients) with membranoproliferative glomerulonephritis, gastrointestinal involvement (2–6%) with abdominal vasculitis[12] and liver involvement (in two-thirds of patients) with signs of mild to moderate chronic hepatitis and central nervous system involvement (up to 6%); among the latter, the most common clinical presentation is stroke.

Finally, patients with CV seldom present signs of hyperviscosity syndrome, pulmonary involvement (<5%) with interstitial lung fibrosis, gynecologic involvement with vasculitis of the female genital tract[13] and cardiovascular involvement with coronary vasculitis complicated by myocardial infarction, heart failure and pericarditis.[2,14] Heart involvement, despite being a rare disease manifestation (4%), significantly affects disease outcome.[14]

The laboratory hallmarks of the disease are the presence of mixed cryoglobulinemia with rheumatoid factor activity and low levels of complement, primarily C4. In addition to the detection of serum cryoglobulin itself, other laboratory abnormalities may provide surrogate evidence of the presence of cryoglobulinemia, such as a small C4 serum complement fraction, decreased total hemolytic complement levels, presence of a serum monoclonal immunoglobulin or rheumatoid factor activity. Hypocomplementemia is a sensitive and important finding in CV found in 70–90% of patients with mixed cryoglobulinemia.[15]

A European task force recently developed preliminary classification criteria for CV through a study divided into two parts. In the first part, 17 experts in the diagnosis and treatment of CV from 12 centers had to formulate a dedicated questionnaire for patients with CV. First they proposed 83 questions, from which they then selected the most useful, including five questions on purpura, four on muscular symptoms and peripheral nerves, one each on HCV and leg skin ulcers and two each on weakness, ocular and oral dryness and articular involvement. These 17 questions were administered to 20 unselected patients with CV and to 30 unselected controls without CV from each of the 12 involved centres. Univariate analysis identified questions associated with CV and, using a logistic model, from among these the experts identified three questions that best contributed to the predictability of the disease (Figure 1). A positive response to at least two of the three questions showed a specificity of 83.5% and a sensitivity of 81.9% for CV. In the second part of the study, the engaged patients were divided into three groups: group A included 272 patients with CV (HCV related or HCV unrelated); group B included 228 controls with serum cryoglobulins but

---

Satisfied if at least two of the three items (questionnaire, clinical, laboratory) are positive the patient must be positive for serum cryos in at least 2 determinations at ≥ 12 week interval

(i) Questionnaire item: at least two out of the following

- Do you remember one or more episodes of small red spots on your skin, particularly involving the lower limbs?
- Have you ever had red spots on your lower extremities which leave a brownish color after their disappearance?
- Has a doctor ever told you that you have viral hepatitis?

(ii) Clinical item: at least three out of the following four (present or past)*

• Constitutional symptoms	Fatigue
	Low grade fever (37–37.9°C,>10 days, no cause)
	Fever (>38°C, no cause)
	Fibromyalgia
• Articular involvement	Arthralgias
	Arthritis
• Vascular involvement	Purpura
	Skin ulcers
	Necrotising vasculitis
	Hyperviscosity syndrome
	Raynaud's phenomenon
• Neurologic involvement	Peripheral neuropathy
	Cranial nerve involvement
	Vasculitic CNS involvement

III. Laboratory item: at least two out of the following three (present)

- Reduced serum C4
- Positive serum rheumatoid factor
- Positive serum M component

*See text for details

Figure 1 Preliminary classification criteria for the cryoglobulinemic vasculitis.

without CV and group C included 425 controls without serum cryoglobulins but with clinical or laboratory features that can be observed in CV.
Group C patients were further divided into two subgroups: C1 (173 controls
with systemic vasculitis other than CV) and C2 (250 controls with other
rheumatic disease). The preliminary classification criteria for CV were
developed by comparing data from group A with data from group B. An
initial analysis of data allowed De Vita et al.[16] to identify the set of questions
(the three questions chosen in the first part of the study); the set of clinical
features (constitutional symptoms, articular involvement, vascular and neurologic involvement); and the set of laboratory tests (reduced serum C4, positive RF and positive serum M component) associated with CV. Afterwards,
analysing the best combinations of the three items, the European experts
established the final classification criteria, which showed a sensitivity of
88.5% and a specificity of 93.6% for CV (Figure 1). The new criteria also
were applied for the comparison of group A with group C, and they were
useful in suspecting CV in patients with negative cryoglobulins on initial
testing but who had clinical and laboratory features characteristic of CV.
The main criticism of these criteria is that positive serum cryoglobulins
are considered an essential condition for CV classification. However, we
well know that there is a subset of patients with CV in whom cryoglobulins
may result negative at lab for low concentration or methodological issues
(i.e. collecting the blood sample without warming it at 37 degrees centigrade).
Finally, it is necessary to underline that these criteria have been elaborated
not for diagnostic purposes but for investigation and epidemiological purposes.[16] Quartuccio et al.[17] recently tested the new classification criteria
for CV in a cohort of 500 patients with positive cryoglobulins. The criteria
showed high sensitivity and specificity in both HCV-positive and HCV-
negative patients with CV.

4 TREATMENT

CV is a rheumatic disease in which a close interaction between a chronic
infection, autoimmunity and a non-neoplastic B-cell lymphoproliferation
can be found. The treatment of CV is still a challenge, and different specialists should ideally cooperate to get a better result. The three main aims of any
rational therapeutic approach are to eradicate HCV (etiologic therapy), to
limit or suppress the proliferation of B lymphocytes (pathogenetic therapy)
and to ameliorate symptoms and reduce the damage caused by circulating

immune complexes (symptomatic therapy).[2,18,19] Treatment should be tailored to the individual patient focusing on the clinical history, disease manifestations, possible comorbidities and previous therapies.[18,19]

In cryoglobulinemic patients with life-threatening manifestations (abdominal vasculitis, hemorrhagic alveolitis, hyperviscosity syndrome and sometimes acute motor neuropathy and rapidly progressing glomerulonephritis), the first-line intervention is represented by high doses of corticosteroids and plasmapheresis.[17] Concomitant immunosuppressive therapy with cyclophosphamide might be needed to prevent the postapheresis cryoglobulin rebound.[2] Rituximab (RTX) was recently used successfully in patients with CV and severe vasculitis refractory to conventional therapies.[18–20]

The common manifestations of severe CV are skin ulcers, peripheral neuropathy (motor or sensory refractory to symptomatic therapy) and active glomerulonephritis. In these cases the best therapeutic option is represented by RTX; it destroys CD20-positive cells that may harbor HCV and play an important pathogenetic role in cryoglobulin production. RTX decreases serum cryoglobulin and RF concentrations and increases C4 concentrations with the disappearance of bone marrow B–cell clonal expansion.[18,19] Glomerulonephritis responds to RTX within the first 3 months; skin ulcers usually improve within 3 months, but complete healing requires a longer time. Both sensitive and motor neuropathy improve within 1 to 5 months with stable or improved electromyography. RTX can increase HCV viral load without significant liver impairment; it has been given to patients with CV with liver cirrhosis and led to an improvement in both MC symptoms and liver function.[19] This effect on liver function may be due to the reduction of the hepatic B–cell infiltrates and to the improvement of Kupffer cell functions.[20] By contrast, it may induce the severe reactivation of HBV, so it should be used in patients positive for the HBV surface antigen and in occult HBV carriers (anti-HBc-positive patients) only when strictly needed and in combination with antiviral therapy.[19–21] The duration of the response to a single cycle of RTX is difficult to define because of the lack of long-term follow-up data; long-term responses (more than a year) have been most frequently observed, and re-treatment with RTX after relapses has proved to be effective in most cases.[18,22]

The possible persistence or onset of CV in patients with persistently negative serum HCV RNA suggests that the autoimmune process can become independent of viral triggering and play a predominant pathogenetic role in some disease stages. Therefore, antiviral therapy cannot be considered as a first option for severe cases. It has recently been suggested that patients with serious clinical manifestations may receive a combination therapy of RTX as a first step and, when its efficacy and safety have been demonstrated, antiviral therapy could be administered. This approach seems to reduce the time to clinical remission and to be more effective than the standard therapies.[23]

Antiviral therapy remains a cornerstone for the management of CV in HCV-related cases, and it should be used for more stable patients, particularly those with nonsevere CV manifestations, such as constitutional features, purpura or arthritis and very mild renal and neurologic features. The current standard antiviral treatment is a combination of pegylated interferon (Peg-INF)-α and ribavirin (RBV).[24]

However, one should be bear in mind that cryoglobulinemia might be an independent risk factor negatively associated with sustained virological response in patients with chronic hepatitis C.[25] The decision to treat patients with chronic hepatitis C depends on multiple parameters, including a precise assessment of the severity of liver disease, the presence of absolute or relative contraindications to therapy, its previous failure or intolerance. The HCV genotype is systematically determined before treatment because it determines the duration of treatment (up to 48 weeks for HCV genotypes 2 or 3 and 72 weeks for genotypes 1 or 4) and the dose of RBV. Peg-INF combined with RBV leads to 41–54% sustained viral response in the case of genotype 1 and approximately 80% in the case of genotypes 2 and 3.[19]

The use of combination treatment with Peg-IFN-α/RBV/protease inhibitor was highly effective in an open-label, 24-week study. However, considering the high rate of side effects, such therapeutic regimen should be administered cautiously.[24] When antiviral therapy is not effective, contraindicated or not tolerated it RTX should be considered to treat patients.[26]

Milder disease manifestations, such as joint involvement and purpura, might be treated with low doses of steroids. However, chronic treatment with low steroid doses should be avoided whenever possible and, in any case, carefully monitored. Alternative therapies (colchicines, a diet with low antigen content) should be considered for maintenance therapy.[19] Good results were obtained in one study in which HCV-related CV was treated with low doses of IL-2, a cytokine that promotes regulatory T-cell survival and function, without short-term detrimental effects on HCV infection.[27] Future treatment of patients with CV with anti-BAFF monoclonal antibody, a molecule that regulates B cell proliferation (Belimumab), can be supposed.[28]

5 OUTCOME

CV can cause significant morbidity and mortality. According to the literature, the worst prognostic factors are age >60 years and renal involvement, which is the main cause of death, followed by liver involvement, cardiovascular disease, infections and lymphomas. The current standard of care for patients with HCV-related vasculitis includes optimal antiviral therapy but no systematic use of immunosuppressive agents. The analysis of factors associated with outcome during follow-up showed that antiviral therapy is significantly associated with a good prognosis, whereas the use of immunosuppressive agents, most often in combination with high-dose corticosteroids, seems to have a negative impact on survival, regardless of the severity of the vasculitis.[15,29]

B-cell lymphoma has been reported in 5–22% of patients with CV. Hypogammaglobulinemia can be a marker for impending lymphomagenesis. B-cell lymphomas usually occur within 10 years of a diagnosis of MC. The most common types are diffuse, large, marginal zone, and lymphoplasmacytoid B-cell lymphomas.[1] The persistent stimulation of B-cells by viral antigens and/or the enhanced expression of lymphomagenesis-related genes could be responsible for leading to polyclonal and, later, to monoclonal expansion of B cells.[30]

REFERENCES

1. Ramos-Casals M, Stone JH, Cid MC, Bosch X. The cryoglobulinaemias. *Lancet* 2012;**379**:348–60.
2. Iannuzzella F, Vaglio A, Garini G. Management of hepatitis C virus-related mixed cryoglobulinemias. *Am J Med* 2010;**123**:400–8.
3. Della Rossa A, Baldini C, Tavoni A, Bombardieri S. How HCV has changed the approach to mixed cryoglobulinemia. *Clin Exp Rheumatol* 2009;**27**(Suppl 52):S115–23.
4. Jabłońska J, Ząbek J, Pawełczyk A, Kubisa N, Fic M, Laskus T, et al. Hepatitis C virus (HCV) infection of peripheral blood mononuclear cells in patients with type II cryoglobulinemia. *Hum Immunol* 2013;**74**:1559–62. http://dx.doi.org/10.1016/j.humimm.2013.08.273, pii: S0198-8859(13)00498-9.
5. Charles-Orloff ED, Nishiuchi E, Marukian S, Rice CM, Dustin LB. Somatic hypermutations confer rheumatoid factor activity in hepatitis C virus-associated mixed cryoglobulinemia. *Arthritis Rheum* 2013 Sep;**65**(9):2430–40.
6. Glenn B, Knight LG, Gragnani L, Elfahal MM, De Rosa FG, Frederic D, et al. Detection of WA B cells in hepatitis C virus infection. *Arthritis Rheum* July 2010;**62**(7):2152–9.
7. Gragnani L, Piluso A, Giannini C, Caini P, Fognani E, Monti M, et al. Genetic determinants in epatiti C virus-associated mixed cryoglobulinemia: role of polymorphic variants of BAFF promoter and Fcγ receptors. *Arthritis Rheum* May 2011;**63**(5):1446–51.
8. Santer DM, Ma MM, Hockman D, Landi A, Tyrrell DL, Houghton M. Enhanced activation of memory, but not naïve, B cells in chronic hepatitis C virus-infected patients with cryoglobulinemia and advanced liver fibrosis. *PLoS One* 2013 Jun 28;**8**(6):e68308.

9. Antonelli A, Ferri C, Ferrari SM, Ghiri E, Marchi S, Sebastiani M, et al. Serum concentrations of interleukin 1β, CXCL10, and interferon-γ in mixed cryoglobulinemia associated with epatiti C infection. *J Rheumatol* 2010;**37**:91–7.

10. Antonelli A, Ferri C, Ferrari SM, Di Domenicantonio A, Ferrari P, Pupilli C, et al. The presence of autoimmune thyroiditis in mixed cryoglobulinemia patients is associated with high levels of circulating interleukin-6, but not of tumour necrosis factor-alpha. *Clin Exp Rheumatol* 2011;**29**(Suppl. 64):S17–22.

11. Antonelli A, Fallahi P, Ferrari SM, Colaci M, Giuggioli D, Saraceno G, et al. Increased CXCL9 Serum Levels in Hepatitis C-Related Mixed Cryoglobulinemia, with Autoimmune Thyroiditis, Associated with High Levels of CXCL10. *J Interferon Cytokine Res* 2013;**33**:739–45.

12. Quartuccio L, Petrarca A, Mansutti E, Pieroni S, Calcabrini L, Avellini C, et al. Efficacy of rituximab in severe and mild abdominal vasculitis in the course of mixed cryoglobulinemia. *Clin Exp Rheumatol* 2010;**28**(Suppl. 57):S84–7.

13. Quartuccio L, Maset M, Di Loreto C, De Vita S. HCV-related cryoglobulinemic syndrome beginnig as isolated gynaecologic vasculitis. *Clin Exp Rheumatol* 2011;**29**(Suppl. 64):S136.

14. Terrier B, Karras A, Cluzel P, Collet JP, Sene D, Saadoun D, et al. Presentation and Prognosis of Cardiac Involvement in Hepatitis C Virus-Related Vasculitis. *Am J Cardiol* 2013;**111**:265–72.

15. Terrier B, Cacoub P. Cryoglobulinemia vasculitis: an update. *Curr Opin Rheumatol* 2013;**25**:10–8.

16. De Vita S, Soldano F, Isola M, Monti G, Gabrielli A, Tzioufas A, et al. Preliminary classification criteria for the cryoglobulinaemic vasculitis. *Ann Rheum Dis* 2011;**70**:1183–90.

17. Quartuccio L, Isola M, Corazza L, Maset M, Monti G, Gabrielli A, et al. Performance of the preliminary classification criteria for cryoglobulinaemic vasculitis and clinical manifestations in hepatitis C virus-unrelated cryoglobulinaemic vasculitis. *Clin Exp Rheumatol* 2012;**30**:S48–52.

18. De Vita S. Treatment of mixed cryoglobulinemia: a rheumatology perspective. *Clin Exp Rheumatol* 2011;**29**(Suppl. 64):S99–S103.

19. Pietrogrande M, De Vita S, Zignego AL, Pioltelli P, Sansonno D, Sollima S, et al. Recommendations for the management of mixed cryoglobulinemia syndrome in epatiti C virus-infected patients. *Autoimmun Rev* 2011;**10**:444–54.

20. Ferri C, Cacoub Mazzaro C, Roccatello D, Scaini P, Sebastiani M, et al. Treatment with rituximab in patients with mixed cryoglobulinemia syndrome: results of multi center color study and review of the literature. *Autoimmun Rev* 2011;**11**:48–55.

21. Petrarca A, Rigacci L, Caini P, Colagrande S, Romagnoli P, Vizzutti F, et al. Safety and efficacy of rituximab in patients with hepatitis C virus-related mixed cryoglobulinemia and severe liver disease. *Blood* 2010;**116**(3):335–42.

22. Talarico R, Baldini C, Della Rossa A, Ferrari C, Luciano N, Bombardieri S. Large- and small-vessel vasculitis: a critical digest of the 2010-2011 literature. *Clin Exp Rheumatol* 2012;**30**(1 suppl 70):130–8.

23. Saadoun P, Rigon M, Sene D, Terrier B, Karras A, Perard L, et al. Rituximab plus Peg-interferon-α/ribavirin compared with Peg-interferon-α/ribavirin in hepatitis C-related mixed cryoglobulinemia. *Blood* 2010;**116**(3):326–53.

24. Mazzaro C, Monti G, Saccardo F, Zignego AL, Ferri C, De Vita S, et al. Efficacy and safety of peginterferon alfa-2b plus ribavirin for HCV-positive mixed cryoglobulinemia: a multicentre open-label study. *Clin Exp Rheumatol* 2011;**29**:933–41.

25. Fan XH, Wu CH, Wang LF, Zheng YY, Yao Y, Lu HY, et al. Cryoglobulinemia is an independent factor negatively associated with sustained virological response in chronic hepatitis C patients. *Chin Med J (Engl)* 2012 Nov;**125**(22):4014–7.

26. Sneller MC, Hu Z, Langford CA. A randomized controlled trial of rituximab following failure of antiviral therapy for hepatitis C-associated cryoglobulinemic vasculitis. *Arthritis Rheum* 2012 Mar;**64**(3):835–42.
27. Saadoun D, Rosenzwaig M, Joly F, Six A, Carrat F, Thibault V, et al. Regulatory T-cell responses to low-dose interleukin-2 in HCV-induced vasculitis. *N Engl J Med* 2011 Dec 1;**365**(22):2067–77.
28. St Clair WE. Hepatitis C virus-related cryoglobulinemic vasculitis: emerging trends in therapy. *Arthritis Rheum* 2012 Mar;**64**(3):604–8.
29. Terrier B, Semoun O, Saadoun D, Sène D, Resche-Rigon M, Cacoub P. Prognostic factors in patients with hepatitis C virus infection and systemic vasculitis. *Arthritis Rheum* June 2011;**63**(6):1748–57.
30. Ito M, Kusonoki I, Mochida K, Yamaguchi K, Mizuochi T. HCV infection and B-cell lymphomagenesis. *Adv Hematol* 2011;**2011**:8, Article ID 835318.

CHAPTER 20

HIV Spectrum and Autoimmune Diseases

Alexander Abdurakhmanov, Gisele Zandman-Goddard[1]
Department of Medicine, C Wolfson Medical Center, Sackler Faculty of Medicine, Tel Aviv University, Tel Aviv, Israel
[1]Corresponding Author: goddard@wolfson.health.gov.il

1 INTRODUCTION

The diagnosis and treatment of autoimmune diseases in patients with human immunodeficiency virus (HIV) represents a challenging clinical scenario. This phenomenon has been increasing and evolving in patients with AIDS who receive highly active antiretroviral therapy (HAART) as a mainstay of treatment. A retrospective record review showed that 9% of patients with HIV suffer from rheumatic complications,[1] including arthritis, spondyloarthropathies, diffuse infiltrative lymphocytosis syndrome (DILS), vasculitides, systemic lupus erythematosus (SLE) and other autoimmune diseases. Although the rheumatic manifestations caused by initial infection with the HIV virus have decreased with the advent of HAART, the prevalence of autoimmune diseases caused by immune reconstitution inflammatory syndrome (IRIS) after treatment initiation has increased.[2] Before the breakthrough of HAART in 1995, spondyloarthropathies and DILS were the leading HIV-associated rheumatic findings; now, however, there is a resurgence of autoimmune diseases associated with IRIS.[3,4]

We previously proposed a staging system based on CD4 cell count and autoimmune manifestations to help identify autoimmune disease and establish therapy in patients with HIV.[5] During stage I, early in HIV infection, the immune system is still intact. Naturally, autoimmune diseases are present in this stage. In stage II there is a decreasing CD4 cell count, indicating some immunosuppression. However, autoimmunity is still possible. Stage III is described as full-blown AIDS with very low CD4 cell counts. Autoimmune disease does not typically occur in the profoundly immunosuppressed stage

Infection and Autoimmunity
http://dx.doi.org/10.1016/B978-0-444-63269-2.00067-2

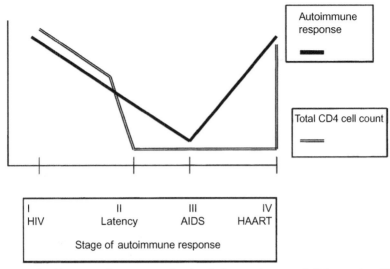

Figure 1 Autoimmune disease may develop in human immunodeficiency virus (HIV)-infected patients parallel to normal CD4 cell count (stages I and II). Once the CD4 cell count decreases past a threshold, autoimmune disease is not present (stage III). Following highly active antiretroviral therapy (HAART), an increase in the CD4 cell count above the threshold enables autoimmune disease to emerge (stage IV). AIDS, acquired immunodeficiency syndrome.

III. In stage IV immune competence is restored after antiretroviral therapy, and a resurgence of autoimmune disease is found (Figure 1). Using the PubMed database, we searched the English-language medical literature concerning various autoimmune diseases in patients with HIV and AIDS published from 2002 to 2013. This review summarizes the clinical findings of autoimmune disease in patients with HIV through the progression of infection from HIV to AIDS to IRIS.

2 MECHANISMS

Autoimmune inflammatory disorders in patients with HIV can occur de novo or as exacerbations. Proposed mechanisms include an infectious trigger for immune activation early in HIV infection and restoration of a dysregulated immune response after antiretroviral therapy. The immune system becomes dysfunctional because of the coexistence of immunodeficiency caused by the HIV virus and immune hyperactivity caused by the cell-mediated immune response, along with the dysregulated production or activity of cytokines.[6] Some of these mechanisms may explain the rheumatic manifestations found in patients with HIV. HAART therapy further changes the course of infection and rheumatic complications by increasing the immune response, introducing the immune reconstitution syndromes.

The effect of HAART on immune reconstruction and cytokine production was investigated in patients with HIV before treatment and after 6 and 12 months of treatment.[7] The study showed that all subtypes of helper T cells decreased rapidly in patients with HIV, whereas subtypes of cytotoxic T (Tc) cells increased compared with healthy controls, indicating an abnormal immune activation as well as immune deficiency. HAART affected the immune system by increasing Th cell counts and decreasing Tc cell counts, thus improving immunity and normalizing the overactivation of Tc cells. HAART also significantly improved interleukin (IL)-12 and interferon (IFN)-γ concentrations. Changes in IL-12 and IFN-γ correlated with changes in helper T cells. IL-12 is a key regulator of cellular immunity and inflammatory response, whereas both IL-12 and IFN-γ play a role in resistance against opportunistic infections in patients with HIV/AIDS. These changes may contribute to immune reconstitution syndromes and their associated autoimmune manifestations.

A minority of HIV-infected patients develop a neutralising antibody against the HIV envelope glycoprotein, from which monoclonal antibodies were isolated. Autoreactivity was demonstrated with the development of HIV broadly neutralizing antibodies (BNAbs) at both the cellular level and at the level of serum antibodies.[8] These monoclonal antibodies were found to exhibit autoreactivity and led to the development of autoimmune serum antibodies, which advanced the ideas of self-tolerance as an explanation of why these BNAbs against HIV are so rare and molecular mimicry as the mechanism of autoimmunity in HIV.

The role of molecular mimicry of HIV antibodies in HIV-associated immune thrombocytopenic purpura (ITP) was investigated.[9] In autoimmune thrombocytopenia, an antibody is directed against the GPIIIa integrin on platelets. To examine whether epitope are shared between host and parasite, the authors identified 14 phage–peptide clones. Ten of them were molecular mimics with sequence similarity to the HIV-1 proteins nef, gag, env and pol. Three antibodies raised against these peptides induced platelet oxidation/fragmentation in vitro and thrombocytopenia in vivo when transferred to mice. One of the peptides shared a known epitope region within a variant region of the HIV-1 nef protein. The data provide strong support for molecular mimicry in HIV-1-immunologic thrombocytopenia.

3 IMMUNE RESTORATION INFLAMMATORY SYNDROME

Following initiation of antiretroviral therapy, patients with HIV/AIDS are susceptible to immune reconstitution disorders as their CD4 cell count rises. The most common of these disorders is IRIS, a severe inflammatory process that results from a dysregulated immune response to pathogen-specific antigens.[10] Any pathogen that can cause an opportunistic infection in an immunodeficient state has the potential to cause IRIS after immune function is regained during HAART. These conditions are usually found in developing countries where patients are infected with an opportunistic pathogen when antiretroviral therapy is initiated. Autoimmune and other noninfectious conditions may occur or dramatically worsen after HAART is initiated, suggesting that inflammation induced by IRIS is responsible. IRIS presents with tissue inflammation or cellular proliferation after the restoration of pathogen-specific immune responses.

The restored immune response sometimes causes immunopathology while eradicating the infection. The inflammation that ensues can be misinterpreted for an opportunistic infection; however, it results from the restoration of pathogen-specific immune responses, not immune deficiency. The inflammation is atypical or more exaggerated than that found in opportunistic infection, with increased pain and suppuration. The HIV viral load is decreased and CD4 cell count is increased, also helping to distinguish IRIS from immunodeficiency. Examination of tissue samples reveals infiltrating lymphocytes, a scarcity of pathogens and granulomatous inflammation, where appropriate. Patients can present with only nonspecific findings such as fever, but usually there are worsening signs of the infection-affected tissue.

Up to 50% of patients with HIV responding to HAART suffer from IRIS within the first few months of therapy.[11] Patients are more at risk if they are starting HAART for the first time or if they have been recently diagnosed with an opportunistic infection. IRIS is most commonly associated with infection from *Mycobacterium tuberculosis* and *Cryptococcal meningitis*. Although the symptoms of IRIS may seem dangerous, they are a sign that the body is fighting the infection, and it may resolve without treatment. However, in severe cases, antibiotics are administered to help fight the infection and corticosteroids are needed to curtail the IRIS symptoms. It is important to remember that most of the time immune reconstitution is uneventful.

4 AUTOIMMUNE DISEASES

4.1 SLE

The unrestrained state of immune activation may contribute to chronic inflammatory and autoimmune conditions in HIV-infected individuals.[5] Several rheumatic entities, such as spondyloarthropathies, DILS, myopathy and HIV-related vasculitides, often are correlated with the severity of the HIV infection and improve with antiretroviral therapy. SLE and sarcoidosis, on the other hand, have lower incidences in the HIV-infected population than would be expected in the general population. This inconsistency suggests that the immunosuppressive effect of HIV may inhibit the development of these autoimmune diseases. However, now with immune reconstitution following HAART, a genetically predisposed host can develop autoimmunity.

Several BNAbs were found to exhibit autoreactivity, and autoimmune serum antibodies were observed in a minority of patients with HIV.[8] Researchers used the 9G4 anti-idiotype antibody system to examine the breakdown of self-tolerance in 90 HIV-infected patients. Compared with healthy controls, patients with HIV had significantly elevated 9G4+ serum immunoglobulin (Ig) G antibody concentrations and frequencies of 9G4+ B cells, a finding characteristic of patients with SLE, which positively correlated with HIV viral load. The results suggest that HIV viral replication may selectively promote the development of autoreactive 9G4+ B cells and 9G4+ serum antibodies. 9G4+ IgG serum antibody concentrations positively correlated ($r=0.403$; $P=0.0019$) with the serum HIV BNAbs. Interestingly, other serum autoantibodies commonly found in SLE (anti-double-stranded DNA [dsDNA] antibodies, antinuclear antibodies [ANAs] and anticardiolipin antibodies) did not correlate with serum HIV BNAbs. Compared with other SLE autoreactivities, 9G4-associated autoreactivity is preferentially expanded in chronic HIV infection. The 9G4 system provided an effective tool in examining autoreactivity in patients with HIV and showed some similarities with SLE. Both HIV infection and SLE disrupt B-cell homeostasis, reduce memory B cells and impair function of IgG and IgM antibodies. In addition, it was determined that patients with HIV and SLE have a reduced biodiversity in their *IGHM* gene transcriptome compared with healthy subjects mainly because of a decrease in unique allele combinations.[12] Antiretroviral therapy failed to increase the biodiversity of immunoglobulins in HIV-infected patients.

Proliferative lupus nephritis is rare in HIV-infected patients. SLE with nephritis in a patient with AIDS treated with HAART was described, along with a review of 18 cases of SLE in HIV-infected individuals.[13] An 18-year-old man with vertically transmitted HIV-1 infection presented with malaise, weight loss, malar rash, arthritis, proteinuria and hematuria. Kidney biopsy confirmed the diagnosis of lupus nephritis (class IV). The patient was treated successfully with high doses of corticosteroids and mycophenolate mofetil, along with HAART and *Pneumocystis pneumonia* prophylaxis. About 1 year after the onset of SLE, the patient was in remission, and both his SLE and AIDS were stable and controlled. Of the 18 reported cases of SLE in HIV-infected individuals, 11 patients had lupus nephritis; of those, only 5 had diffuse proliferative glomerulonephritis, 4 of whom improved with steroid treatment; 1 patient died. The stage of HIV infection in these patients is unclear in the literature. Including the case reported above, four of six patients had very elevated ANA titers, and all six patients had elevated titers of anti-dsDNA antibody. Low levels of C3 and C4 were found in four patients, and four of the six patients had CD4 cell counts >200 cells/μL. Extrarenal manifestations included arthritis, serositis, anemia, thrombocytopenia, ANAs, anti-dsDNA antibodies, anti-Smith antibodies and low complement levels and did not differ greatly from HIV-negative patients with lupus. Renal histopathology did not differ greatly between HIV-infected and HIV-negative patients.

Lupus-like glomerulonephritis is another form of glomerular disease in HIV-infected patients. It is defined by immunohistological and immunofluorescent features of lupus on biopsy (Ig and compliment deposition) without serologic evidence of SLE. A retrospective review of 77 total renal biopsies from patients with HIV found 14 samples to have lupus-like glomerulonephritis.[14] However, HIV-associated nephropathy (HIVAN), or focal segmental glomerulosclerosis, is still the leading nephropathy in patients with HIV.[15] SLE nephritis can be differentiated from HIVAN by immunofluorescence and biopsy. While both present with proteinuria, HIVAN is characterized by focal collapsing glomerulosclerosis and microcyst formation in the tubules. SLE nephritis is characterised by subendothelial IgG and C3 deposition on electron microscopy and immunofluorescence. Clinically, HIVAN typically has a faster downhill course than SLE nephritis. Although HIVAN is the leading nephropathy in HIV-infected patients, lupus-like glomerulonephritis and SLE nephritis are not uncommon in this patient population.

A case of an African woman living in the UK who was diagnosed with SLE in 2006 and HIV in 2007 was reported.[16] This patient was in stage I of her HIV infection, with normal CD4 cell counts. In 2006 she presented with a 9-month history of fever, rash, polyarthralgia, weight loss and Raynaud's phenomenon. Serology showed elevated titers of ANA (1:2560) and extractable nuclear antibody. Anti-dsDNA and rheumatoid factor antibody concentrations were negative. Although she was diagnosed with SLE at the time, she did not fulfill the American College of Rheumatology diagnostic criteria for the disease. The patient had a truncal rash that was not photosensitive, arthralgia but not arthritis and elevated ANA titers. Otherwise, she did not have serositis or oral ulcers and did not fulfill renal, neurological, hematological, or immunological criteria. Her CD4 cell count at presentation in December 2007, when she was diagnosed with HIV, was 1011 cells/µL, with an HIV viral load <50 copies/mL. When she was last seen in July 2009, she was clinically well, although her CD4 cell count had decreased to 836 cells/µL and her HIV viral load was detectable for the first time at 62 copies/mL. She remained ANA positive (>1:640) and anti-dsDNA negative. She had never received antiretroviral therapy. The multisystem manifestations of skin rash, weight loss, oral ulcers, arthralgia, myalgia, anemia, leucopenia and autoantibodies were consistent with both SLE and HIV infection. This patient's low-level HIV viremia in the absence of antiretroviral therapy may support the hypothesis that one disease may suppress the laboratory manifestations of the other.

A case of a man with tumid cutaneous lupus that was only unmasked during HAART therapy was described.[17] This patient fits stage IV because the immune reconstitution led to autoimmune disease. He started HAART in February 1999, and in November 1999 he developed a photosensitive facial rash. Examination demonstrated oedematous erythematous papules and plaques affecting the forehead, cheeks and ear lobes. A skin biopsy showed a superficial and deep perivascular and pariadnexal infiltrate mostly comprising Tc cells. The cutaneous and histological findings were characteristic of tumid lupus. The rash only improved when HAART was ceased and CD4 cell counts decreased below 200 cells/µL. The patient's ANA serology was negative, with no systemic findings, which is usually the case with tumid lupus. Once the correlation between flare-ups and immune reconstitution was made, the patient restarted HAART and the rash was treated with hydrochloroquine and improved. Although tumid cutaneous lupus is rare, it is its development only after HAART that is noteworthy in this patient.

Two female patients with HIV who were diagnosed with new-onset SLE and discoid lupus erythematosus a few months after the initiation of HAART were described.[18] A 39-year-old woman known to have AIDS for 3 years was admitted for persisting fever, arthralgia, myalgia, and malar rash of 2 weeks' duration. After 10 months of ongoing HAART, lupus symptoms surfaced (stage IV). Blood tests showed a Coomb's positive hemolytic anemia and leucopenia, elevated erythrocyte sedimentation rate, CD4 cell count of 291 cells/μL and viral load of <50 copies/mL. Chest x-ray and echocardiography revealed bilateral pleural effusions and pericardial effusion, respectively. Serology demonstrated elevated titers of ANAs and anti-dsDNA antibodies, negative rheumatoid factor and venereal disease research laboratory, and low serum C3 and C4 compliment levels. This patient met the American College of Rheumatology criteria for SLE, and treatment with prednisone and hydrochloroquine was initiated. After 21 days, the patient was in remission with the exception of mild anemia and leucopenia. Hydrochloroquine therapy was stopped and prednisone was tapered. The second case reported by the same authors was a 33-year-old woman known to have AIDS for 4 years who had been undergoing HAART for 16 months (stage IV) and who presented only with a discoid cutaneous rash. She had a CD4 cell count >500 cells/μL and an elevated HIV viral load at the time. Based on histopathological findings of the lesions on skin biopsy, a diagnosis of discoid lupus erythematosus was made. She improved following treatment with topical steroids and oral hydrochloroquine. These two cases are further examples of immune reconstitution after starting HAART as a cause of autoimmunity.

SLE symptoms generally improve with untreated HIV infection, and vice versa, because the two diseases are opposite in their immune involvement. Conversely, SLE flare-ups can occur after HAART. Reactivation of quiescent SLE during AIDS was reported in a 39-year-old female patient 6 months after initiating HAART (stage IV).[19] Differentiating between SLE and HIV can be difficult because the two diseases may share clinical (oral ulcers, alopecia, arthralgia, fever, neuropathy) and laboratory findings (leucopenia, thrombocytopenia, hypergammaglobulinemia, and transient ANA titers). Rheumatic signs and symptoms are common in HIV and many overlap with SLE.[20]

This overlap was evident in a case of HIV reported in a 32-year-old woman who was first diagnosed with SLE.[21] She had symptoms of joint pain, skin rash and alopecia and an intermittent low-grade fever for 8 months. She was diagnosed with SLE with elevated titers of ANAs and anti-dsDNA antibodies. She was treated conservatively with parenteral antibiotics and oral steroids. Her symptoms worsened; she was later found to have mycobacterial DNA in her sputum, as well as proteinuria. She was given the antitubercular regimen. Considering the proteinuria and elevated anti-dsDNA antibodies, the patient started cyclophosphamide therapy along with oral steroids for suspected worsening SLE. Her HIV antibody tests were negative at that point. Following three cycles of cyclophosphamide therapy, she complained of vision loss and was diagnosed with cytomegalovirus retinitis. Oral candidiasis also was found, and she was reevaluated with HIV testing, which was positive with a CD4 cell count of 114 cells/μL, leading to the diagnosis of AIDS. Just as HIV infection and HAART therapy can trigger the emergence of autoimmune disease, this case shows that SLE and its treatment (steroids and cyclophosphamide) can enhance retroviral replication, leading to a rapidly progressive course of HIV infection.

A possible protective role of autoantibodies against HIV infection in patients with SLE has been suggested.[22] The theory is that during the budding process, the HIV virus acquires several cellular proteins from the infected host cell. Antibodies against self-antigens found in sera of patients with autoimmune disorders may cross-react with host-derived proteins, or the HIV-specific proteins gp120 and gp41, on the viral envelope and help neutralize HIV infection. HIV-1 was directly recognized by 60% of sera taken from patients with SLE and other autoimmune diseases.

In total, 57 cases of SLE in patients with HIV have been reported up to March 2013.[23] De novo presentation of SLE after HAART initiation (stage IV) was reported in eight patients. SLE was diagnosed before HIV infection in six patients. Interestingly, 13 subjects had a CD4 cell count <200 cells/μL at the time of SLE manifestations (stage III), providing evidence that SLE is found in patients with AIDS as well. Common findings included the presence of ANAs, immunologic and hematologic disorders, hypocomplementemia and elevated titers of anti-dsDNA antibodies. Malar rash was more common among adults, whereas renal disorders were more common in the pediatric population. Fifty-four patients received treatment for SLE with steroids, immunosuppressants (cyclophosphamide, azathioprine, mycophenolate mofetil) or hydrochloroquine. Improvement in rheumatologic symptoms after treatment were reported in 75% of patients, whereas the remission of SLE due to the progression of HIV infection occurred in 11 patients. An SLE flair was reported in three patients after HAART was introduced, and a severe rebound spike in HIV RNA was detected in two patients following immune-suppressive therapy for SLE.

4.2 Antiphospholipid Syndrome

Antiphospholipid (aPL) antibodies often are found in patients with various viral infections. There is also a known association between anticardiolipin antibodies and HIV infection. A literature review showed that anticardiolipin antibodies occur frequently in infections with HIV (49.8%), hepatitis B virus (HBV) (24%) and hepatitis C virus (HCV) (20%), whereas the prevalence of anti-β2 glycoprotein I (GPI) antibodies is lower (HIV, 5.6%; HBV, 3.3%; HCV, 1.7%).[24] These antibodies are present in many nonsymptomatic patients without thrombotic events. Anticardiolipin and anti-beta2GPI antibody titers were elevated in a young male patient who, after acute HIV infection (stage I), presented with recurring fever, pleuritic chest pain and dyspnea due to pulmonary emboli.[25]

A case of a 25-year-old African American man with cutaneous necrotic lesions due to probable antiphospholipid syndrome (APS) as the initial presenting manifestation of HIV infection was reported.[26]

The patient had a 3-week history of severe left leg pain and multiple warm, erythematous, bullous, centrally necrotic skin lesions that were unresponsive to amoxicillin/clavulanic acid and accompanied by fever and night sweats. Initial differential diagnoses included a vasculitis or cellulitis. Further workup of a skin biopsy revealed capillary thrombosis with minimal inflammation and a high level of anticardiolipin IgG antibodies, suggesting APS. Enzyme-linked immunosorbant assay and Western blot confirmed HIV infection with a CD4 cell count of 351 cells/μL. This patient's autoimmune manifestations were found during the early stages of HIV infection (stage II). Another case of APS was reported in a patient with AIDS who had been receiving HAART for over a year (stage IV) and who presented with leg pain and coldness.[27]

The frequency of aPL antibodies in patients infected with HIV and their association with the presence of clinical manifestations of APS was studied.[28] Of 90 patients with HIV, 12 had clinical manifestations of APS (13.3%), and 40 were reactive for at least one type of aPL (44.4%). The frequency of anticardiolipin was 17.8%, and the frequency of anti-beta2GPI was 33.3%. No association between immunoreactivity to aPL antibodies and the presence of APS manifestations was observed. Similarly, no significant association between CD4 cell counts and APS or between HAART and APS was found. Although there is a prevalence of aPL antibodies in patients with HIV, the clinical picture of APS is rare. It is even more rare in children, but the first case of APS in an HIV-infected child has been reported (stage II).[29]

The clinical features related to APS in patients with chronic viral infection were analyzed.[30] Thrombotic or obstetric features of APS were found in 32 HIV-infected patients and 5 patients with HIV–HCV coinfection. The main APS features of HIV were avascular bone and cutaneous necrosis. Although no study has analyzed the prevalence of APS in HIV-infected patients, only 32 cases of APS in HIV-positive patients and 5 cases of APS in patients coinfected with HIV and HCV were reported up to August 2003, without any distinction between stages of HIV infection.

4.3 Autoimmune Thrombocytopenia

ITP was first recognized in association with AIDS in 1982. The incidence of ITP in the pre-HAART era was estimated between 10% and 30%; thrombocytopenia is the initial manifestation of HIV in 10% of cases. The rate of HIV-associated ITP after the advent of HAART was investigated and the clinical features, treatments and outcomes of patients with HIV-associated ITP were described.[31] Among 5290 patients with HIV found in the BC Centre for Excellence in HIV/AIDS database in the post-HAART era, the incidence of ITP was 0.6%. There were 31 patients, mostly men, who were diagnosed with HIV-associated ITP and had platelet counts $<20 \times 10^9$/L. Twenty-nine patients had a CD4 cell count taken at ITP diagnosis, and 21 of them had CD4 > 200 cells/μL, opposing the previous belief that ITP increases with severity of immune dysfunction. Ten patients were receiving HAART at the time of diagnosis and five had AIDS. Initial treatment at the first episode of a platelet count $<20 \times 10^9$/L included HAART (13 patients), intravenous immoglobulin (IVIG) (7 patients), anti-D (7 patients), prednisone (4 patients) and combinations of these. Overall, 25 patients achieved response in the median 14 days, with a median platelet count of 58×10^9/L. At a median follow-up of 48 months, 22 patients lost this response and required secondary ITP treatment, which included splenectomy in addition to the previously mentioned treatment options. Other than HAART therapy, there is no favored treatment for HIV-associated ITP. Those who acquired HIV via intravenous drug abuse responded more poorly to treatment, possibly because of coinfections with hepatitis.

4.4 Vasculitis

A wide range of vasculitides affecting patients in all stages of the HIV infection has been reported. Systemic necrotising vasculitis, cryoglobulinemia and central nervous system (CNS) vasculitis have been reported.

Polyarteritis nodosa, Henoch–Schonlein purpura and drug-induced hypersensitivity vasculitis are all found in patients with HIV, but the majority of findings are caused by an unspecific neutrophilic or monocytic inflammation.[32] In a study of rheumatic manifestations among 98 patients with HIV in China, vasculitis was the most common rheumatic manifestation (20 patients); 15 patients had a Behçet-like disease.[33]

A prospective study in Africa described 8 patients with AIDS with vasculitis.[34] Four men and four women with a mean age of 33 years and a mean CD4 cell count of 79 cells/μL were described (stage III). Five patients showed CNS involvement, and three patients had peripheral vasculitis. Two patients were coinfected with HBV. The authors concluded that vasculitis in patients with HIV occurs with severe immune suppression and often involves the CNS. Another case of vasculitis emerging in the advanced stage of HIV infection was described.[35] This patient suffered from a granulomatous necrotising vasculitis that was not restricted to the CNS. He was only diagnosed with HIV at presentation with a CD4 cell count of 175 cells/μL (stage III), and his autoimmune vasculitis drastically improved after starting antiretroviral therapy.

HIV does not play a significant role in circulating cryoglobulins, which are more associated with HCV infection.[36] Studies show no significant correlation between cryoglobulins and HIV infection or HIV–HCV coinfection. Circulating cryoglobulins were not associated with HIV viral load or CD4 cell counts.[37] However, another study showed that HAART decreases the prevalence of cryoglobulinemia in HIV-positive, HCV-negative patients, indirectly providing evidence for the role of HIV in the pathogenesis of cryoglobulins.[38] Vasculitis and hypercoagulability were found to be common mechanisms of stroke in patients with HIV.[39]

4.5 Polymyositis and Dermatomyositis

HIV-associated polymyositis occurs in 2–7% of patients and is indistinguishable from idiopathic polymyositis. It can be found in all stages of HIV infection. It responds well to immunosuppressive therapy and can even resolve spontaneously.[40] In a study of 64 patients with HIV referred with elevated creatine kinase concentrations, 13 patients had biopsy proven myositis. There was no correlation of the severity of weakness or stage of HIV infection with creatine kinase concentrations at presentation.

Dermatomyositis seems to be rare in patients with HIV but has been observed in five patients as of 2012.[41,42] A case of a woman who complained of proximal muscle weakness, arthralgias and rash was reported in Nigeria.[42] She tested positive for HIV (stage II) and started HAART. Her muscle pains subsided for the first few months of therapy and then returned after 1 year of HAART. Only then was she diagnosed with dermatomyositis. This patient follows the classical progression of autoimmune disease through the described stages of HIV infection.

4.6 Thyroid Disease

There is a suggested association between autoimmune thyroid disease (AITD) and HIV infection, especially after HAART therapy. AITD was studied in a cohort of patient with HIV and AIDS following HAART. Seventeen patients were diagnosed clinically with AITD (15 with Graves' disease, 1 with hashi thyrotoxicosis, and 1 with hypothyroidism). The mean baseline CD4 cell count before HAART was 67 cells/μL (stage IV), and the mean increase in CD4 cell count up until AITD detection was 355 cells/μL. This led researchers to believe that AITD may be a late complication of immune reconstitution, especially in those who respond well to HAART.[43] The frequency of AITD in female patients with AIDS in Brazil was evaluated. The frequency of AITD was 4.6%, and all were receiving HAART at the time of diagnosis (stage IV). The prevalence of AITD in patients with HIV not receiving HAART was 0% (non-stage IV).[44]

Graves' disease as a manifestation of IRIS in patients with HIV should be considered when patients present with clinical deterioration of hyperthyroidism despite favorable virological and immunological responses to HAART. Signs and symptoms of hyperthyroidism may be discrete or overt and develop 8–33 months after the initiation of antiretroviral therapy. Four more cases of Graves' disease after HAART were reported.[45] A case report of Graves' disease in a female patient with AIDS also supports the trend of autoimmune disease arising after HAART.[46] Another case of Graves' disease as a manifestation of IRIS in a patient with AIDS taking HAART was reported.[47] The patient had symptoms of hyperthyroidism 21 months after starting HAART; the symptoms vanished when HAART was discontinued. Five years after recommencing HAART, the patient had to begin antithyroid medication (thiamazole). No features of autoimmune disease were present before the initiation of HAART.

Similarly, a case of Hashimoto's thyroiditis as a complication of IRIS in a patient with AIDS was reported.[48] A painful acute thyroiditis occurred in a patient 10 months after beginning antiretroviral therapy. High titers of antithyroid peroxidase antibodies were discovered, leading to persistent hypothyroidism requiring thyroxine replacement.

4.7 Primary Biliary Cirrhosis

Primary biliary cirrhosis (PBC) is an autoimmune disease characterised by immune-mediated destruction of intrahepatic bile ducts and the serological marker antimitochondrial antibody. PBC is thought to have a viral etiology or association. The majority of patients with PBC were reported to have evidence of human betaretrovirus infection.[49] One year after untreated HIV infection (stage II), a patient was reported to have PBC.[50] After initiating antiretroviral therapy, along with ursodeoxycholic acid treatment, this patient's liver function tests improved dramatically. HAART is thought to improve PBC because a majority of these patients have evidence of retroviral infection; however, randomized controlled trials have failed to achieve significant results despite clinical improvements in liver and bile duct function tests.

5 INFLAMMATORY ARTHRITIS

The HIV virus itself causes arthralgia in 28–54% of acute cases, as well as a disposition toward infections and septic arthritis. Arthritis of any etiology is found in 10–12% of patients with HIV.[32] Whether the HIV virus causes the rheumatologic findings or simply creates an environment supportive of these conditions is unclear.[51]

A case of rheumatic immune reconstitution syndrome was reported in a patient with AIDS who previously only experienced mild joint pain with no limitations in work or exercise but experienced severely disabling polyarthritis after starting HAART (stage IV).[52] He had negative ANA, rheumatoid factor and cyclic citrullinated peptide antibody titers. Prednisone and hydrochloroquine therapy dramatically improved his symptoms. Rather than arising de novo, the arthritis seems to have surfaced as an exacerbation after HAART in this case.

Reviews of prospective and longitudinal studies, and the African experience, have provided support for a direct role of HIV infection in producing a spectrum of spondyloarthropathies and arthralgias.[53,54] A polyarticular presentation is seen frequently in patients. Reactive arthritis, psoriatic arthritis and undifferentiated spondyloarthropathy were uncommon in Africa before the HIV epidemic. Many patients responded to conventional symptomatic therapy, and disease-modifying agents were necessary for those with progressive arthritis. The lack of HAART in developing countries is attributed to the more severe manifestations seen in patients from these regions.

Psoriatic arthritis was found in 1.5% of new referrals to an HIV clinic. The average CD4 cell count at diagnosis was 160 cells/µL, indicating psoriatic arthritis occurs later in the course of HIV infection (stages III and IV). Patients typically presented with polyarthritis involving the knees, digits, hips and ankles.[53]

5.1 Diffuse Infiltrative Lymphocytosis Syndrome

DILS is characteristic of HIV infection. It is manifested by salivary and lacrimal gland swelling, circulating and visceral lymphocytic infiltration and varying sicca symptoms, which is why it is sometimes referred to as Sjögren–like syndrome. Before HAART, patients with DILS tended to have extraglandular manifestations such as interstitial pneumonitis and progressed more slowly to opportunistic infections. Since the start of HAART therapy, the prevalence of DILS has significantly decreased, leading to the belief that it is caused by the HIV virus itself.[55] In a retrospective study of 129 patients with DILS from 1994 to 2003, 111 patients (stages I and II) were diagnosed before or during 1998, and the remaining 18 were diagnosed after 1998 (stage IV), at the advent of HAART. The prevalence of lymphocytic interstitial pneumonitis also decreased significantly following HAART. The evidence suggests DILS is an antigen–driven response, and the treatment is antiretroviral therapy.

5.2 Sarcoidosis

Sarcoidosis is mostly seen in patients undergoing HAART therapy because of the role of CD4 cells in granuloma formation. The impact of HAART on sarcoidosis in patients with HIV was analyzed.[56] Sarcoidosis was diagnosed in 11 HIV-infected patients, of whom 8 were receiving HAART. Sarcoidosis occurred several months after the introduction of HAART, when CD4 cell counts increased and HIV viral load decreased. Clinical, radiological and laboratory characteristics of sarcoidosis did not differ between HIV-infected patients and HIV-negative patients. A case of a woman who was diagnosed with sarcoidosis and HIV in 1992 but only started HAART in 1996 was reported.[57] Her sarcoidosis was not severe before HAART and required only corticosteroid treatment in 2001, 5 years after initiating HAART. This is another example of autoimmune disease flaring up after HAART (stage IV). Before the HAART era, eight cases of sarcoidosis in patients with

HIV were reported; four of those patients did not require treatment. Of the 21 cases reported in the HAART era, most patients showed improvement in their sarcoidosis following immunosuppression.[57] Sarcoidosis is rarely observed in patients before HAART therapy and is associated with increasing CD4 cell counts (stage IV).[58]

5.3 Other Autoimmune Diseases

Autoimmune diabetes infrequently develops in patients with HIV as immune reconstitution after HAART (stage IV). Three HIV-infected patients were diagnosed with autoimmune diabetes based on their high anti-islet cell antibodies and requirement for insulin therapy.[59] To clarify the relationship between increasing CD4 cell counts and autoantibodies against pancreatic β-cells, the researchers stored plasma from these patients before HAART, and no antibodies were detected. The high magnitude of the CD4 cell increase during HAART, and the timing of the detection of autoantibodies, were similar to the magnitude and timing reported in HAART-associated AITD.

Adult-onset Still's disease was reported in an HIV-infected patient who presented with fever of unknown origin 10 weeks after initiating HAART (stage IV).[60] Giant-cell arteritis was reported in a patient with HIV receiving HAART for 15 years before the onset of severe headache, night sweats and fever with blurred vision and prominent scalp vessels.[61] Rheumatoid arthritis (RA) has been reported as well; however, it is difficult to determine reported numbers of true RA cases.[51]

6 TREATMENT

Treatment of autoimmune disorders in HIV-infected patients is a delicate situation. Although immunosuppressive agents help treat symptoms of autoimmune diseases, physicians often refrain from using them because of fear of the underlying viral infection progressing. Corticosteroid therapy has been shown to be effective in acute treatment of severe IRIS, regardless of the concerns about fighting the opportunistic infection. Treatment of autoimmune diseases in patients with HIV with cyclosporine A and anti-tumor necrosis factor-α may reduce HIV viral load while relieving autoimmune symptoms.[62] Researchers reviewed the safety and efficacy of these agents in autoimmune diseases such as RA, psoriasis and reactive arthritis in a number of studies, determining that cyclosporine A and anti-tumor necrosis factor-α are good alternative options for treating RA in patients with HIV.

7 DISCUSSION

Works reviewing all of the rheumatic manifestations found in patients with HIV have been published[1–4,32,33,51,63]; however, these include findings caused by the virus itself and side effects of antiretroviral medications. This review specifically covers autoimmune findings in patients with HIV and their relation to the progression of disease. There is a tendency for autoimmune manifestations to emerge either early in HIV infection or after immune reconstitution while receiving HAART (Table 1). HAART consists of three active antiretroviral medications in a combination of tenofovir and emtricitabine (nucleoside reverse transcriptase inhibitors) and efavirenz (a non-nucleoside reverse transcriptase inhibitor).

Inflammatory arthritis was the most common autoimmune manifestation in patients with HIV in the pre-HAART era. Although the incidence of reactive arthritis and DILS has decreased since the advent of HAART, they still remain the leading manifestations with a rheumatological component in this population, mostly found early in HIV infection (stages I and II). However, because DILS and reactive arthritis are directly related to the viral infection, and not of autoimmune nature, they were excluded from Figure 2. Figure 2, lists only known autoimmune diseases. Vasculitis is the

Table 1 Autoimmune Disease Breakdown in HIV-Infected Patients Through the Progression of the Spectrum

Disease	Patients with HIV (Stages I and II)	Patients with AIDS (Stage III)	Patients Receiving HAART (Stage IV)	Reported Cases*
SLE	36	9	12	57
APS	3	0	1	54
ITP	16	5	10	31
Vasculitis	4	9	7	36
Poly/dermatomyositis	3	2	10	18
Thyroid	0	0	30	30
Psoriatic arthritis	0	0	1	35
Sarcoidosis	11	0	30	41
Others (PBC, diabetes, Still's)	1	0	4	5
Totals	74	25	105	307

Data are numbers of patients. Patients with reactive arthritis and diffuse infiltrative lymphocytosis syndrome were not included.

APS, antiphospholipid syndrome; ITP, immune thrombocytopenic purpura; PBC, primary biliary cirrhosis; SLE, systemic lupus erythematosus.

*The discrepancy between reported cases and their disease stage breakdown is because of unavailable or unclear staging in the literature at the time of autoimmune manifestations.

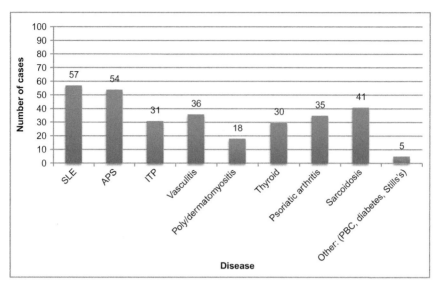

Figure 2 Autoimmune diseases in patients with human immunodeficiency virus/ acquired immunodeficiency syndrome. APS, antiphospholipid syndrome; ITP, immune thrombocytopenic purpura; PBC, primary biliary cirrhosis; SLE, systemic lupus erythematosus.

only autoimmune disease most prevalent in severe immune deficiency (AIDS) (stage III). The reason for this relationship is unclear. Possible theories include immunosuppression leading to other viral infections associated with vasculitides or immune dysregulation (few CD4 T cells, large numbers of CD8 T cells and B cells) associated with increasing severity of infection, resulting in auto-antibodies. After the initiation of HAART, autoimmune manifestations can arise de novo or as exacerbations. ITP, polymyositis, AITD and sarcoidosis show a tendency to emerge as CD4 cell counts increase during immune restoration (stage IV). Interestingly, AITD only surfaces as a result of IRIS. Symptoms of some autoimmune diseases such as SLE, RA and sarcoidosis can be alleviated after HIV infection suppresses the patient's immunity.

The distribution of autoimmune diseases in the stages of HIV infection (Table 1) confirms our original four-stage theory (Figure 1). Since our last review, the number of cases of HIV and autoimmunity has steadily increased. There are more than 300 patients with HIV/AIDS with reported autoimmune disease (Table 1). The diversity of disease also has grown, along with the number of patients with autoimmunity. Autoimmune diseases such as PBC, Still's disease, diabetes and different vasculitides are now being reported in the population of patients with HIV. These increases can be attributed to the superior knowledge and awareness of the matter gained over the past decade, leading clinicians to look for autoimmunity in patients with HIV, as well as to an increasing incidence of autoimmunity caused by IRIS. A caveat to consider is that data on autoimmune diseases in HIV-infected patients are scattered, and different diagnostic criteria are used. Patient records and studies that clearly indicate the stage of HIV infection at the time of autoimmune findings are necessary to further investigate the relationship between HIV, HAART, and autoimmunity.

REFERENCES

1. Yao Q, Frank M, Glynn M, Altman RD. Rheumatic manifestations in HIV-1 infected in-patients and literature review. *Clin Exp Rheumatol* 2008;**26**:799–806.
2. Louthrenoo W. Rheumatic manifestations of human immunodeficiency virus infection. *Curr Opin Rheumatol* 2008;**20**:92–9.
3. Maganti RM, Reveille JD, Williams FM. Therapy insight: the changing spectrum of rheumatic disease in HIV infection. *Nat Clin Pract Rheumatol* 2008;**4**:428–38.
4. Nguyen BY, Reveille JD. Rheumatic manifestations associated with HIV in the highly active antiretroviral therapy era. *Curr Opin Rheumotol* 2009;**21**:404–10.
5. Zandman-Goddard G, Shoenfeld Y. HIV and autoimmunity. *Autoimmun Rev* 2002;**1**:329–37.
6. Colmegna I, Koehler JW, Garry RF, Espinoza LR. Musculoskeletal and autoimmune manifestations of HIV, syphilis and tuberculosis. *Curr Opin Rheumatol* 2006;**18**:88–95.
7. Yao Y, Luo Y, He Y, et al. The effect of a year of highly active antiretroviral therapy on immune reconstruction and cytokines in HIV/AIDS patients. *AIDS Res Hum Retroviruses* 2013;**29**:691–7.
8. Kobie JJ, Alcena DC, Zheng B, et al. 9G4 Autoreactivity Is Increased in HIV-Infected Patients and Correlates with HIV Broadly Neutralizing Serum Activity. *PLoS One* 2012;**7**(e35356):1–11.
9. Li Z, Nardi MA, Karpatkin S. Role of molecular mimicry to HIV-1 peptides in HIV-1-related immunologic thrombocytopenia. *Blood* 2005;**15**(106):572–6.
10. French MA. Immune reconstitution inflammatory syndrome: A reappraisal. *Clin Infect Dis* 2009;**48**:101–7.
11. French MA. Disorders of immune reconstitution in patients with HIV infection responding to antiretroviral therapy. *Curr HIV/AIDS Rep* 2007;**4**:16–21.
12. Yin L, Hou W, Liu L, et al. IgM repertoire biodiversity is reduced in HIV-1 infection and systemic lupus erythematosus. *Front Immunol* November 2013, http://dx.doi.org/10.3389/fimmu.2013.00373.
13. Gindea S, Schwartzman J, Herlitz LC, Rosenberg M, Abadi J, Putterman C. Proliferative glomerulonephritis in lupus patients with human immunodeficiency virus infection: A difficult clinical challenge. *Semin Arthritis Rheum* 2010;**40**:201–9.
14. Haas M, Kaul S, Eustace JA. HIV-associated immune complex glomerulonephritis with "lupus-like" features: A clinicopathologic study of 14 cases. *Kidney Int* 2005;**67**:1381–90.
15. Berggren R, Batuman V. HIV-associated renal disorders: recent insights into pathogenesis and treatment. *Curr HIV/AIDS Rep* 2005;**2**:109–15.
16. Burton J, Vera JH, Kapembwa M. HIV and systemic lupus erythematosus: the clinical and diagnostic dilemmas of having dual diagnosis. *Int J STD AIDS* 2010;**21**:845–6.

17. Chamberlain AJ, Hollowood K, Turner RJ, Byren I. Tumid lupus erythematosus occurring following highly active antiretroviral therapy for HIV infection: A manifestation of immune restoration. *J Am Acad Dermatol* 2004;**51**:S161–5.
18. Calza L, Manfredi R, Colangeli V, D'Antuono A, Passarini B, Chiodo F. Systemic and discoid lupus erythematosus in HIV-infected patients treated with highly active antiretroviral therapy. *Int J STD AIDS* 2003;**14**:356–9.
19. Drake WP, Byrd VM, Olsen NJ. Reactivation of systemic lupus erythematosus after initiation of highly active antiretroviral therapy for acquired immunodeficiency syndrome. *J Clin Rheumatol* 2003;**9**:176–80.
20. Chowdhry IA, Tan IJ, Mian N, Mackay M, Keiser H, Davidson A. Systemic lupus erythematosus presenting with features suggestive of human immunodeficiency virus infection. *J Rheumatol* 2005;**32**:1365–8.
21. Hazarika I, Chakravarty BP, Dutta S, Mahanta N. Emergence of manifestations of HIV infection in a case of systemic lupus erythematosus following treatment with IV cyclophosphamide. *Clin Rheumatol* 2006;**25**:98–100.
22. Scherl M, Posch U, Obermoser G, et al. Targeting human immunodeficiency virus type 1 with antibodies derived from patients with connective tissue disease. *Lupus* 2006;**15**:865–72.
23. Carugati M, Franzetti M, Torre A, et al. Systemic lupus erythematosus and HIV infection: a whimsical relationship. Reports of two cases and review of the literature. *Clin Rheumatol* 2013;**32**:1399–405.
24. Sène D, Piette JC, Cacoub P. Antiphospholipid antibodies, antiphospholipid syndrome and infections. *Autoimmun Rev* 2008;**7**:272–7.
25. Diaz JS, Octavio JG, Fernandez-Guerrero ML. Antiphospholipid syndrome and acute HIV infection. *Emerg Infect Dis* 2010;**16**:360–1.
26. Hassoun A, Al-Kadhimi Z, Cervia J. HIV Infection and antiphospholipid antibody: Literature review and link to the antiphospholipid syndrome. *AIDS Patient Care STDS* 2004;**18**:333–40.
27. Konin C, Anzouan-Kacou JB, Essam N'loo A. Arterial thrombosis in patients with Human Immunodeficiency Virus: Two-case reports and review of the literature. *Case Rep Vasc Med* 2011;**2011**:847241.
28. Galrão L, Brites C, Atta ML, et al. Antiphospholipid antibodies in HIV-positive patients. *Clin Rheumatol* 2007;**26**:1825–30.
29. Shah I, Chudgar P. Antiphospholipid syndrome in a human immunodeficiency virus 1-infected child. *Pediatr Infect Dis J* 2006;**25**:185–6.
30. Ramos-Casals M, Cervera R, Lagrutta M, et al. Hispanoamerican Study Group of Autoimmune Manifestations of Chronic Viral Disease (HISPAMEC): Clinical features related to antiphospholipid syndrome in patients with chronic viral infections (hepatitis C virus/HIV infection): description of 82 cases. *Clin Infect Dis* 2004;**38**:1009–16.
31. Ambler KL, Vickars LM, Leger CS, et al. Clinical features, treatment, and outcome of HIV-Associated Immune Thrombocytopenia in the HAART era. *Adv Hematol* 2012;**2012**:910954.
32. Walker UA, Tyndall A, Daikeler T. Rheumatic conditions in human immunodeficiency virus infection. *Rheumatology* 2008;**47**:952–9.
33. Zhang X, Li H, Li T, Zhang F, Han Y. Distinctive rheumatic manifestations in 98 patients with Human Immunodeficiency Virus Infection in China. *J Rheumatol* 2007;**34**:1760–4.
34. Otedo AE, Oyoo GO, Obondi JO, Otieno CF. Vasculitis in HIV: report of eight cases. *East Afr Med J* 2005;**82**:656–9.
35. Garcia-Garcia JA, Macías J, Castellanos V, et al. Necrotizing granulomatous vasculitis in advanced HIV infection. *J Infect* 2003;**47**:333–5.

36. Fabris P, Tositti G, Giordani MT, et al. Prevalence and clinical significance of circulating cryoglobulins in HIV-positive patients with and without co-infection with hepatitis C virus. *J Med Virol* 2003;**69**:339–43.

37. Scotto G, Cibelli DC, Saracino A, et al. Cryoglobulinemia in subjects with HCV infection alone, HIV infection and HCV/HIV coinfection. *J Infect* 2006;**52**:294–9.

38. Kosmas N, Kontos A, Panayiotakopoulos G, Dimitrakopoulos A, Kordossis T. Decreased prevalence of mixed cryoglobulinemia in the HAART era among HIV-positive, HCV-negative patients. *J Med Virol* 2006;**78**:1257–61.

39. Ortiz G, Koch S, Romano JG, Forteza AM, Rabinstein AA. Mechanisms of ischemic stroke in HIV-infected patients. *Neurology* 2007;**68**:1257–61.

40. Johnson RW, Williams FM, Kazi S, Dimachkie MM, Reveille JD. Human immuno-deficiency virus-associated polymyositis: a longitudinal study of outcome. *Arthritis Rheum* 2003;**49**:172–8.

41. Carroll MB, Holmes R. Dermatomyositis and HIV infection: case report and review of the literature. *Rheumatol Int* 2011;**31**:673–9.

42. Ogoina D, Umar A, Obiako OR. Dermatomyositis associated with HIV-1 infection in a Nigerian adult female: a case report. *Afr Health Sci* 2012;**12**:74–6.

43. Chen F, Day SL, Metcalfe RA, et al. Characteristics of autoimmune thyroid disease occurring as a late complication of immune reconstitution in patients with advanced human immunodeficiency virus (HIV) disease. *Medicine (Baltimore)* 2005;**84**:98–106.

44. de Carvalho LG, Teixeira Pde F, Panico AL, et al. Evaluation of thyroid function and autoimmunity in HIV-infected women. *Arq Bras Endocrinol Metabol* 2013;**57**:450–6.

45. Rasul S, Delapenha R, Farhat F, Gajjala J, Zahra SM. Graves' disease as a manifestation of immune reconstitution in HIV-Infected individuals after initiation of highly active anti-retroviral aherapy. *AIDS Res Treat* 2011;**2011**:743597.

46. Knysz B, Bolanowski M, Klimczak M, Gladysz A, Zwolinska K. Graves' disease as an immune reconstitution syndrome in an HIV-1-positive patient commencing effective antiretroviral therapy: case report and literature review. *Viral Immunol* 2006;**19**:102–7.

47. Visković K, Stemberger L, Brnić Z, Begovac J. Repeated presentation of Graves' disease as a manifestation of immune reconstitution syndrome in an HIV-infected patient taking HAART: case report. *Acta Clin Croat* 2013;**52**:125–7.

48. Visser R, de Mast Q, Netea-Maier RT, van der Ven AJ. Hashimoto's thyroiditis presenting as acute painful thyroiditis and as a manifestation of an immune reconstitution inflammatory syndrome in a human immunodeficiency virus-seropositive patient. *Thyroid* 2012;**22**:853–5.

49. Ninomiya M, Ueno Y, Shimosegawa T. PBC: animal models of cholangiopathies and possible endogenous viral infections. *Int J Hepatol* 2012;**2012**:649290.

50. Schembri G, Schober P. Killing two birds with one stone. *Lancet* 2011;**377**:96.

51. Lawson E, Walker-Bone K. The changing spectrum of rheumatic disease in HIV infection. *Br Med Bull* 2012;**103**:203–21.

52. Calabrese LH, Kirchner E, Shrestha R. Rheumatic complications of human immuno-deficiency virus infection in the era of highly active antiretroviral therapy: Emergence of a new syndrome of immune reconstitution and changing patterns of disease. *Semin Arthritis Rheum* 2005;**35**:166–74.

53. Mody GM, Parke FA, Reveille JD. Articular manifestations of human immunodeficiency virus infection. *Best Pract Res Clin Rheumatol* 2003;**17**:265–87.

54. Chinniah K, Mody GM, Bhimma R, Adhikari M. Arthritis in association with human immunodeficiency virus infection in Black African children: causal or coincidental? *Rheumatology* 2005;**44**:915–20.

55. Basu D, Williams FM, Ahn CW, Reveille JD. Changing spectrum of the diffuse infiltrative lymphocytosis syndrome. *Arthritis Rheum* 2006;**55**:466–72.

56. Foulon G, Wislez M, Naccache JM, et al. Sarcoidosis in HIV-infected patients in the era of highly active antiretroviral therapy. *Clin Infect Dis* 2004;**38**:418–25.
57. Almeida Jr. FA, Sager JS, Eiger G. Coexistent sarcoidosis and HIV infection: an immunological paradox? *J Infect* 2006;**52**:195–201.
58. Morris DG, Jasmer RM, Huang L, Gotway MB, Nishimura S, King Jr. TE. Sarcoidosis following HIV infection: evidence for CD4fl lymphocyte dependence. *Chest* 2003;**124**:929–35.
59. Takarabe D, Rokukawa Y, Takahashi Y, et al. Autoimmune diabetes in HIV-infected patients on highly active antiretroviral therapy. *J Clin Endocrinol Metab* 2010;**95**:4056–60.
60. DelVecchio S, Skidmore P. Adult-onset Still's disease presenting as fever of unknown origin in a patient with HIV infection. *Clin Infect Dis* 2008;**46**:e41–3.
61. Dinesh KP, Owolabi A, Dwyer-Joyce L, Cronin PM, Schimmer BM, Mo GP. Temporal artery vasculitis in young: a report of two cases. *Rheumatol Int* 2010;**30**:1393–6.
62. Galeazzi M, Giannitti C, Manganelli S, et al. Treatment of rheumatic diseases in patients with HCV and HIV infection. *Autoimmun Rev* 2008;**8**:100–3.
63. Reveille JD, Williams FM. Rheumatologic complications of HIV infection. *Best Pract Res Clin Rheumatol* 2006;**20**:1159–79.

CHAPTER 21

Parvovirus Infection and Its Association with Autoimmune Diseases

Antonio Puccetti[*,†,1], **Dolcino Marzia**[*], **Tinazzi Elisa**[‡],
Patuzzo Giuseppe[‡], **Lunardi Claudio**[‡]
[*]Department of Immunology, Institute G. Gaslini, Genoa, Italy
[†]Department of Experimental Medicine, Unit of Histology, University of Genoa, Genoa, Italy
[‡]Department of Medicine, Unit of Internal Medicine, University of Verona, Verona, Italy
[1]Corresponding Author: antonio.puccetti@unige.it

1 INTRODUCTION

Human parvovirus B19 was identified in 1975 by Yvonne Cossart[1] and classified as a member of the *Parvoviridae* family in 1985. *Parvoviridae* is a large family of DNA viruses known to infect several animals and insects. This family is currently divided into two sub-families, *Parvoviridae* and *Densovirinae*, based on their ability to infect vertebrate or invertebrate cells, respectively. *Parvoviridae* includes three genera: *Parvovirus* (which autonomously replicates), *Dependovirus* (which requires a helper virus to replicate) and *Erythrovirus* (which preferentially replicates in erythroid cells), which included erythrovirus-parvovirus B19.[2]

Human parvovirus B19 is a small virus composed of a non–enveloped capsid 22–24 nm in diameter. Its genome consists of a single DNA strand of 5596 nucleotides and comprises a terminal palindromic sequence of 383 nucleotides. These palindromes can acquire a hairpin configuration and serve as primers for complementary strand synthesis. The proteins encoded include two structural proteins, VP1 (nucleotides 2444–4786) and VP2 (nucleotides 3125–4786), the major non-structural protein NS1 (nucleotides 436–2451)[3–5] and two small proteins of 7.5 and 11 kDa. Parvovirus B19 shows sequence variability; in particular the VP1 and VP2 regions exhibit a greater sequence variation in contrast to the highly conserved NS1 region.[6] The rate of such variation is high, and approximately $10(-4)$ nucleotide substitutions per site occur each year. A systematic

Infection and Autoimmunity
http://dx.doi.org/10.1016/B978-0-444-63269-2.00020-9

analysis of parvovirus variants of the NS1 and VP1 unique sequences[7] showed the presence of three distinct genotypes: genotype 1, corresponding to human parvovirus B19 (prototype strain Pvaua); genotype 2 (prototype Lali), comprising the recent identified strains A6 and K71; and genotype 3, with the V9 strain as the prototype.[8,9] A recent study based on phylogenetic analysis of human erythrovirus sequences from 11 countries in Europe, Asia and West Africa confirmed the worldwide predominance of genotype 1. Conversely, genotype 3 virus seems to be predominant in some parts of Africa and accounts for only 8.5% of infections. Pathogenetically, the three genotypes seem very similar.[10]

The icosahedral parvovirus B19 capsid consists of 60 capsomers, predominantly (95%) composed of the VP2 protein; the other structural protein VP1 makes up the remaining 5%.[11] The VP2 protein has a molecular weight of 58 kDa and is encoded by the sequence from nucleotide 3125 to 4786. The minor structural protein VP1, with a molecular mass of 84 kDa, is encoded by the sequence from nucleotide 2444 to 4786. VP1 is identical to the carboxyl terminus of VP2 with the addition of 227 amino acids at its amino terminus. This terminal domain, the VP1 "unique region", is located largely outside the virion and is therefore accessible to antibody binding.[12] The major non-structural protein NS1 has a molecular weight of 77 kDa and seems to be involved in several regulatory functions of the viral life cycle, such as the control of viral infectivity,[13] replication and packaging.[14] Moreover, the NS1 protein shows some properties that play a role in viral pathogenetic mechanisms such as cytotoxicity,[4,15,16] the arrest of target cell growth and induction of apoptosis.[17–19]

The two small proteins of 7.5 and 11 kDa are thought to play a critical role in the parvovirus B19 cell cycle or pathogenesis. The 11-kDa protein contains several proline-rich motifs that bind to the growth factor receptor-binding 2.[20] Moreover, the expression of this protein could be critical for viral pathogenetic activity because blocking the expression of the 11-kDa protein in recombinant virions significantly reduces viral infectivity.[13] In addition, the 11-kDa protein plays a key role in inducing apoptosis during B19 virus infection of primary erythroid progenitor cells.[21]

Parvovirus B19 infection is widespread, and the highest prevalence has been observed in developing countries, where it increases with age.[22,23] The virus is more frequently transmitted by inhaling infected aerosol droplets, but vertical transmission[24] and transmission after bone marrow and organ transplantation[25] and via transfused blood products[26] have also been described.

Replication of parvovirus B19 has been demonstrated only in human erythroid progenitor cells; its receptor, an antigen of the blood group P system, known as P antigen or globoside, is present on erythrocytes, erythroblasts, megakaryocytes, endothelial cells and fetal liver and heart cells.[27] Weigel-Kelley et al.,[28] however, demonstrated that the P antigen is necessary for the virus to bind to the cell surface but is not sufficient for the virus to enter human cells, suggesting the possible presence of a co-receptor. The cell surface co-receptor necessary for successful infection has been identified in $\alpha5\beta1$ integrin.[29] This finding may clarify the reason why virus replication is restricted to progenitor cells within the erythroid lineage, because these cells express high levels of both P antigen and co-receptor, whereas the P antigen-positive non-erythroid cells do not express the co-receptor and therefore are non-permissive to efficient infection.

Acute infection is characterized by the presence of anti-virus-specific immunoglobulin (Ig) M antibodies that are detectable late in the viremic stage (about 10–12 days after infection) and can persist for months, whereas specific IgG antibodies appear about 2 weeks after infection and last for years. The protective role of humoral response with the production of specific anti-virus antibodies is considered one of the major mechanisms of protection, as inferred from clinical studies of persistence of infection in cases of Ig defect[30] and by the efficacy of intravenous Ig therapy in these cases.[31,32] The humoral immune response during parvovirus B19 infection is directed against the two structural proteins, VP1 and VP2. Kurtzman et al.[30] demonstrated that the antibody response was primarily directed against the 83-kDa VP1 antigen both in late convalescent individuals and in an immune population routinely screened. In contrast, anti-parvovirus B19 antibodies directed against the VP2 protein were predominant in serum from patients with early infection. Moreover, antibodies against linear epitopes of the VP2 and, to same extent, VP1 proteins disappeared after acute infection, whereas antibodies against conformational VP2 and VP1 epitopes persisted.[33,34] It has been shown that antibodies directed against VP2 are maintained even when the response directed against the VP1 unique region is lost.[34] The cellular immune response to human parvovirus B19 also has been investigated, although it is not routinely used for detection of viral infection. Indeed, both a CD^{4+} response directed against the VP1 and VP2 capsid protein[35] and CD^{8+} T-lymphocyte response to an NS1 epitope in parvovirus B19-seropositive individuals has been reported.[36]

During acute infection increased concentrations of the pro-inflammatory cytokines interleukin (IL)-1β, IL-6 and interferon (IFN)-γ

have been described.[37] The cytokine profile may influence the symptoms and outcome of parvovirus B19 infection. Hsu et al.[38] reported that increased expression and secretion of IL-6 in B19 NS1 transfected epithelial cells may play a role in the pathogenesis of autoimmune diseases. That cytokine genetic polymorphisms may affect clinical symptoms during parvovirus B19 infection also has been suggested. This seems to be the case for the transforming growth factor-β1 +869 T allele, frequently associated with a high transcription level of the cytokine suppressing T-cell proliferation. Alteration of cell-mediated immunity during acute infection may modify parvovirus B19 virus replication in keratinocytes, with a consequential effect on the development of skin rash. Similarly, the IFN-γ +874 T allele resulting in increased IFN-γ expression is associated with the production of anti-NS1 antibodies and a more severe disease course in some individuals.[39]

Great effort has been put into the identification of serological and molecular biology tests able to discriminate between acute, past, and chronic infection.[40] Several studies showed that IgM and IgG antibodies directed against conformational VP1 and VP2 epitopes indicate an acute or past infection, respectively, whereas positive sera may show a negative result using linear epitopes alone.[33,34] The introduction of new molecular biology methods able to differentiate between the viral variants, such as real-time polymerase chain reaction, greatly helps clinicians in the identification of parvovirus B19 infection in some clinical conditions, such as in immunocompromised patients undergoing bone marrow transplant.

2 CLINICAL FEATURES OF PARVOVIRUS B19 INFECTION

Parvovirus B19 infection has been associated with a wide range of clinical disorders, although 25–50% of infected individuals may be asymptomatic. This pattern is influenced by the age and the hematological and immunological status of the host. The most common clinical manifestation of parvovirus B19 infection in children is the "fifth disease" or "erythema infectiosum", characterized by the typical "slapped cheek" rash.[41] This appearance is followed by the spread of a maculopapular rash on the trunk, back and extremities. The infection is normally self-limiting, and symptoms disappear within a week or two; however, the rash can be recurrent for some months following exposure to sunlight or exercise.[42] Joint symptoms (pain and swelling) are more common in adults, mainly women, but are rare in children, and the disease symmetrically affects wrists, knees and the small joints of the hands.[43]

These symptoms frequently resolve in a few weeks, but a persistent or recurrent arthropathy similar to rheumatoid arthritis (RA) has been described in 20% of affected subjects.[44] Interestingly, many patients with chronic disease meet the criteria for the diagnosis of RA, and the presence of parvovirus B19 infection should be considered when patients with symmetrical polyarthralgia/polyarthritis are seen for the first time.[45] The small percentage of patients with chronic polyarthritis that mimics RA raises the question of whether B19 virus may have a role as a concomitant or precipitating factor in the pathogenesis of autoimmune conditions.[46]

In children and adults, parvovirus B19 has been associated with a wide spectrum of diseases, such as transient anemia, leukocytopenia and thrombocytopenia, that usually go into remission without any therapy. In some patients, however, severe thrombocytopenia, pure red-cell aplasia or pancytopenia may occur.[47]

Parvovirus B19 replicates in erythroid cells, and during the viremic phase of infection it stops erythrocyte production, with a 1 g/dL decrease in the hemoglobin concentration of healthy subjects; it may lead to a dramatic decrease in hemoglobin concentration in hemolytic patients. Indeed, parvovirus B19 infection may cause a transient aplastic crisis in subjects who suffer from chronic hemolytic disorders (e.g. spherocytosis, sickle-cell disease).[48] This event usually terminates with the appearance of specific anti-parvovirus B19 antibodies. A direct cytotoxic effect on erythroid progenitors also has been clearly demonstrated for human parvovirus B19.[49]

During pregnancy, parvovirus B19 infection may result in fetal anemia, abortion and hydrops fetalis. In industrialized countries, about 40% of young women do not have anti-parvovirus B19 antibodies and are susceptible to the infection[50]; therefore screening for parvovirus B19 infection is mandatory for the diagnosis of acute infection during pregnancy when significant exposure to the virus has been documented or infection is suspected. Indeed, parvovirus B19 is a common cause of intrauterine fetal death in late gestation (third trimester) but without fetal hydrops in the majority of cases.[51]

Parvovirus B19 can also cause viral myocarditis, because it targets coronary endothelium, leading to myocardial ischemia and dysfunction.[52] In immunocompromised patients who are unable to mount a specific immune response and clear the virus, parvovirus B19 infection is followed by a persistent or recurrent viremia.[30,53] Such patients include those affected by congenital immunodeficiencies or acquired immunodeficiency syndrome (leukemia, lymphoma, myelodysplastic syndrome),[54–56] receiving high doses of chemotherapy[57] or receiving a bone marrow or solid organ transplantation.[58,59]

3 PARVOVIRUS B19 AND AUTOIMMUNITY

Some of the clinical features associated with parvovirus B19 infection are similar to those shown by systemic autoimmune diseases such as early RA, systemic lupus erythematosus and other connective tissue diseases, leading to the hypothesis that the virus might be involved in autoimmunity. Indeed, B19 infection has been associated with the appearance of rheumatoid factor and with antibodies directed against a vast array of auto-antigens including nuclear, mitochondrial, smooth muscle, gastric parietal cell and phospholipid antigens.[60–62] Even if extensively investigated, however, the relation between B19 infection and autoimmune disorders is still unclear. We demonstrated that chronic parvovirus B19 infection can induce antiviral antibodies with auto-antigen binding properties.[63] Anti-VP IgG antibodies were affinity-purified from the sera of patients with persistent parvovirus infection using a synthetic immunodominant VP peptide. Such anti-viral peptide antibodies reacted specifically with human keratin, collagen type II, single-stranded DNA and cardiolipin. The main reactivity was directed against keratin and collagen type II, and there was a correlation between the clinical features and the main auto-antigen specificity: Igs from patients with arthritis reacted preferentially with collagen II, whereas Igs affinity-purified from patients with skin rashes reacted preferentially with keratin. We hypothesized that the persistence of the virus might be responsible for the induction of autoimmunity through a mechanism of molecular mimicry. To confirm the role of the virus in inducing an autoimmune response, BALB/c mice were immunized with the viral peptide: auto-antibodies against keratin, collagen type II, cardiolipin and single-stranded DNA were detected in the majority of the mice which developed a strong anti-viral response.[63]

We also investigated whether the presence of viral DNA in the synovial tissue might be correlated with rheumatoid synovitis.[64] No differences were observed in rheumatoid and normal control synovial membranes in the presence of parvovirus B19 DNA. Therefore, the detection of viral DNA in synovial tissue is not sufficient to confirm a link between B19 virus and RA.[64]

In addition to RA, parvovirus B19 infection has been associated with a variety of autoimmune diseases including juvenile idiopathic arthritis, systemic lupus erythematosus,[65] progressive systemic sclerosis,[66–68] reactive arthritis, Sjögren's syndrome, primary biliary cirrhosis, polymyositis, dermatomyositis, autoimmune cytopenia and vasculitis.[69–71] Indeed, a significantly higher prevalence of parvovirus B19 DNA was observed in endothelial cells and fibroblasts from sclerodermic patients[72] and in the skin of patients with systemic sclerosis[73] compared with normal subjects.

Furthermore, the degree of viral transcript expression correlated with active endothelial cell injury and perivascular inflammation, features important in the initial phases of the disease. In conclusion, the authors suggested that tissue injury[72,73] may be a consequence of a direct viral cytotoxicity that eventually leads to autoimmune aggression in genetically predisposed individuals.

To further elucidate the relationship between parvovirus B19 infection and autoimmunity we used a random peptide library, a technique that has been successfully applied to study the link between infections and autoimmune disorders.[74–77] To test the role of molecular mimicry mechanisms in the induction of autoimmunity by parvovirus B19 infection, we screened a dodecamer random peptide library with pooled Igs obtained from the sera of patients with persistent parvovirus infection.[78] Using this approach we identified a peptide that shares homology with human cytokeratin (Figure 1), an auto-antigen target recognised by the anti-virus-derived peptides antibodies, as previously described.[63] Moreover, the same peptide 3 and another identified peptide (peptide 12) share similarities with two different sequences of overlapping regions of the viral structural proteins VP1 and VP2. The same VP regions are homologous to the transcription factor GATA1 (Figure 2), which is expressed in several hematopoietic lineages and plays an essential role in normal hematopoietic development during embryonic stages. Using mice, Gutierrez et al.[79] recently showed that GATA1 is necessary for adult megakaryopoiesis and for steady-state erythropoiesis and erythroid expansion in response to anemia, which play an essential role in megakaryopoiesis and erythropoiesis. Our data suggest that, in addition to the 'lytic' effect on erythroid cell precursors and the cytotoxicity of the NS1 protein proposed to explain anemia and

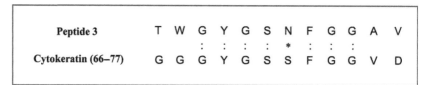

Figure 1 Homology between peptide 3 selected from sera immunoglobulins from patients with persistent parvovirus infection and human cytokeratin. ':'=identity; '*'=conservative substitution.

PEPTIDE 3	T	W	G	Y	G	S	N	F	G	G	A	V
			:			:	:	*		:	:	
VP 155–162	A	D	G	G	G	S	S	G	G	G	G	S

PEPTIDE 12	R	S	L	G	E	L	S	L	V	F	G	P
				:	*	:		*			:	:
VP 626–638	N	P	P	G	Q	L	F	V	H	L	G	P

VP 155–162	A	D	G	G	G	S	S	G	G	G	G	S
				:	:	:		:	:			
GATA-1 314–325	K	K	K	R	G	S	S	L	G	G	T	G

VP 626–638	N	P	P	G	Q	L	F	V	H	L	G	P
		*	:	*				:	:	:		
GATA-1 358–369	P	G	T	A	H	L	Y	Q	G	L	G	P

Figure 2 Sequence homology among peptides 3 and 12, selected using serum immunoglobulins from patients with persistent parvovirus infection and VP protein and GATA1. ':' = identity; '*' = conservative substitution.

thrombocytopenia, anti-viral antibodies cross-reacting with the transcription factor GATA1 may arrest the maturation of erythroblasts and megakaryoblasts (Figure 3).

It has recently been reported that, in a non-permissive cell line, NS1 induces the expression of apoptotic bodies, which are a source of altered self-antigens phagocytosed by antigen-presenting cells, eventually inducing an autoimmune response.[80] Another group previously showed that parvovirus B19 NS1 induces mitochondrial-dependent apoptosis in COS-7 cells and specific cleavage of 70-kDa U1 small nuclear ribonucleoprotein,[81] an auto-antigen against which auto-antibodies are found in particular autoimmune diseases.

In conclusion, several reports indicate that parvovirus B19 infection may play a role in the induction of not only an autoimmune response but also an autoimmune disorder, either by a mechanism of molecular mimicry or by altering the apoptotic process. Our data also suggest that anti-virus antibodies may have a pathogenetic role by interfering with erythropoiesis. In this light some typical clinical manifestations may be explained not only by the lytic effect of the virus on erythroid precursors but also by the anti-virus antibody response through a mechanism of molecular mimicry.

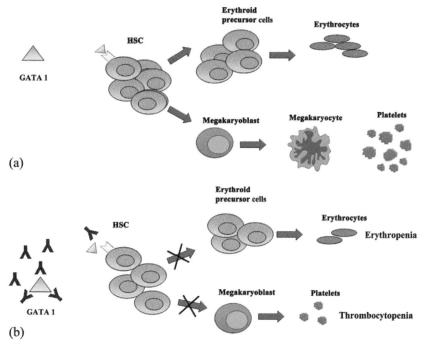

(a)

(b)

Figure 3 Suggested autoimmune mechanism in the pathogenesis of parvovirus B19-induced thrombocytopenia and anemia. (a) Normal erythromegakaryopoiesis. (b) Anti-viral VP antibodies cross-react with transcription factor GATA1, inhibiting its action and leading to defective erythroid differentiation and megakaryocyte proliferation and eventually to thrombocytopenia and anemia. HSC, hematopoietic stem cell.

REFERENCES

1. Cossart YE, Field AM, Cant B, Widdows D. Parvovirus-like particles in human sera. *Lancet* 1975;**1**:72–3.
2. Heegaard ED, Brown KE. Human parvovirus B19. *Clin Microbiol Rev* 2002;**15**:485–505.
3. Shade RO, Blundell MC, Cotmore SF, Tattersall P, Astell CR. Nucleotide sequence and genome organization of human parvovirus B19 isolated from the serum of a child during aplastic crisis. *J Virol* 1986;**58**:921–36.
4. Ozawa K, Ayub J, Hao YS, Kurtzman G, Shimada T, Young N. Novel transcription map for the B19 (human) pathogenic parvovirus. *J Virol* 1987;**61**:2395–406.
5. Ozawa K, Ayub J, Kajigaya S, Shimada T, Young N. The gene encoding the nonstructural protein of B19 (human) parvovirus may be lethal in transfected cells. *J Virol* 1988;**62**:2884–9.
6. Erdman DD, Durigon EL, Wang QY, Anderson LJ. Genetic diversity of human parvovirus B19: sequence analysis of the VP1/VP2 gene from multiple isolates. *J Gen Virol* 1996;**77**(Pt. 11):2767–74.
7. Servant A, Laperche S, Lallemand F, Marinho V, De Saint Maur G, Meritet JF, et al. Genetic diversity within human erythroviruses: identification of three genotypes. *J Virol* 2002;**76**:9124–34.

8. Nguyen QT, Wong S, Heegaard ED, Brown KE. Identification and characterization of a second novel human erythrovirus variant, A6. *Virology* 2002;**301**:374–80.

9. Hokynar K, Soderlund-Venermo M, Pesonen M, Ranki A, Kiviluoto O, Partio EK, et al. A new parvovirus genotype persistent in human skin. *Virology* 2002;**302**:224–8.

10. Hubschen JM, Mihneva Z, Mentis AF, Schneider F, Aboudy Y, Grossman Z, et al. Phylogenetic analysis of human parvovirus B19 sequences from eleven different countries confirms the predominance of genotype 1 and suggests the spread of genotype 3b. *J Clin Microbiol* 2009;**47**:3735–8.

11. Ozawa K, Young N. Characterization of capsid and noncapsid proteins of B19 parvovirus propagated in human erythroid bone marrow cell cultures. *J Virol* 1987;**61**:2627–30.

12. Kaufmann B, Chipman PR, Kostyuchenko VA, Modrow S, Rossmann MG. Visualization of the externalized VP2 n termini of infectious human parvovirus B19. *J Virol* 2008;**82**:7306–12.

13. Zhi N, Mills IP, Lu J, Wong S, Filippone C, Brown KE. Molecular and functional analyses of a human parvovirus B19 infectious clone demonstrates essential roles for NS1, VP1, and the 11-kilodalton protein in virus replication and infectivity. *J Virol* 2006;**80**:5941–50.

14. Momoeda M, Kawase M, Jane SM, Miyamura K, Young NS, Kajigaya S. The transcriptional regulator YY1 binds to the 5'-terminal region of B19 parvovirus and regulates P6 promoter activity. *J Virol* 1994;**68**:7159–68.

15. Li X, Rhode 3rd SL. Mutation of lysine 405 to serine in the parvovirus H-1 NS1 abolishes its functions for viral DNA replication, late promoter trans activation, and cytotoxicity. *J Virol* 1990;**64**:4654–60.

16. Momoeda M, Wong S, Kawase M, Young NS, Kajigaya S. A putative nucleoside triphosphate-binding domain in the nonstructural protein of B19 parvovirus is required for cytotoxicity. *J Virol* 1994;**68**:8443–6.

17. Poole BD, Zhou J, Grote A, Schiffenbauer A, Naides SJ. Apoptosis of liver-derived cells induced by parvovirus B19 nonstructural protein. *J Virol* 2006;**80**:4114–21.

18. Moffatt S, Yaegashi N, Tada K, Tanaka N, Sugamura K. Human parvovirus B19 nonstructural (NS1) protein induces apoptosis in erythroid lineage cells. *J Virol* 1998;**72**:3018–28.

19. Morita E, Nakashima A, Asao H, Sato H, Sugamura K. Human parvovirus B19 nonstructural protein (NS1) induces cell cycle arrest at G(1) phase. *J Virol* 2003;**77**:2915–21.

20. Fan MM, Tamburic L, Shippam-Brett C, Zagrodney DB, Astell CR. The small 11-kDa protein from B19 parvovirus binds growth factor receptor-binding protein 2 in vitro in a Src homology 3 domain/ligand-dependent manner. *Virology* 2001;**291**:285–91.

21. Chen AY, Zhang EY, Guan W, Cheng F, Kleiboeker S, Yankee TM, et al. The small 11 kDa nonstructural protein of human parvovirus B19 plays a key role in inducing apoptosis during B19 virus infection of primary erythroid progenitor cells. *Blood* 2010;**115**:1070–80.

22. Heegaard ED, Petersen BL, Heilmann CJ, Hornsleth A. Prevalence of parvovirus B19 and parvovirus V9 DNA and antibodies in paired bone marrow and serum samples from healthy individuals. *J Clin Microbiol* 2002;**40**:933–6.

23. Kerr JR. Parvovirus B19 infection. *Eur J Clin Microbiol Infect Dis* 1996;**15**:10–29.

24. Berry PJ, Gray ES, Porter HJ, Burton PA. Parvovirus infection of the human fetus and newborn. *Semin Diagn Pathol* 1992;**9**:4–12.

25. Heegaard ED, Laub PB. Parvovirus B19 transmitted by bone marrow. *Br J Haematol* 2000;**111**:659–61.

26. Koenigbauer UF, Eastlund T, Day JW. Clinical illness due to parvovirus B19 infection after infusion of solvent/detergent-treated pooled plasma. *Transfusion* 2000;**40**:1203–6.

27. Brown KE, Hibbs JR, Gallinella G, Anderson SM, Lehman ED, McCarthy P, et al. Resistance to parvovirus B19 infection due to lack of virus receptor (erythrocyte P antigen). *N Engl J Med* 1994;**330**:1192–6.

28. Weigel-Kelley KA, Yoder MC, Srivastava A. Recombinant human parvovirus B19 vectors: erythrocyte P antigen is necessary but not sufficient for successful transduction of human hematopoietic cells. *J Virol* 2001;**75**:4110–16.

29. Weigel-Kelley KA, Yoder MC, Srivastava A. Alpha5beta1 integrin as a cellular coreceptor for human parvovirus B19: requirement of functional activation of beta1 integrin for viral entry. *Blood* 2003;**102**:3927–33.

30. Kurtzman GJ, Cohen BJ, Field AM, Oseas R, Blaese RM, Young NS. Immune response to B19 parvovirus and an antibody defect in persistent viral infection. *J Clin Invest* 1989;**84**:1114–23.

31. Schwarz TF, Roggendorf M, Hottentrager B, Modrow S, Deinhardt F, Middeldorp J. Immunoglobulins in the prophylaxis of parvovirus B19 infection. *J Infect Dis* 1990;**162**:1214.

32. Keller MA, Stiehm ER. Passive immunity in prevention and treatment of infectious diseases. *Clin Microbiol Rev* 2000;**13**:602–14.

33. Corcoran A, Doyle S, Waldron D, Nicholson A, Mahon BP. Impaired gamma interferon responses against parvovirus B19 by recently infected children. *J Virol* 2000;**74**:9903–10.

34. Kerr S, O'Keeffe G, Kilty C, Doyle S. Undenatured parvovirus B19 antigens are essential for the accurate detection of parvovirus B19 IgG. *J Med Virol* 1999;**57**:179–85.

35. von Poblotzki A, Gerdes C, Reischl U, Wolf H, Modrow S. Lymphoproliferative responses after infection with human parvovirus B19. *J Virol* 1996;**70**:7327–30.

36. Tolfvenstam T, Oxenius A, Price DA, Shacklett BL, Spiegel HM, Hedman K, et al. Direct ex vivo measurement of CD8(+) T-lymphocyte responses to human parvovirus B19. *J Virol* 2001;**75**:540–3.

37. Wagner AD, Goronzy JJ, Matteson EL, Weyand CM. Systemic monocyte and T-cell activation in a patient with human parvovirus B19 infection. *Mayo Clin Proc* 1995;**70**:261–5.

38. Hsu TC, Tzang BS, Huang CN, Lee YJ, Liu GY, Chen MC, et al. Increased expression and secretion of interleukin-6 in human parvovirus B19 non-structural protein (NS1) transfected COS-7 epithelial cells. *Clin Exp Immunol* 2006;**144**:152–7.

39. Kerr JR, McCoy M, Burke B, Mattey DL, Pravica V, Hutchinson IV. Cytokine gene polymorphisms associated with symptomatic parvovirus B19 infection. *J Clin Pathol* 2003;**56**:725–7.

40. Peterlana D, Puccetti A, Corrocher R, Lunardi C. Serologic and molecular detection of human parvovirus B19 infection. *Clin Chim Acta* 2006;**372**:14–23.

41. Woolf AD, Campion GV, Chishick A, Wise S, Cohen BJ, Klouda PT, et al. Clinical manifestations of human parvovirus B19 in adults. *Arch Intern Med* 1989;**149**:1153–6.

42. Musiani M, Manaresi E, Gallinella G, Cricca M, Zerbini M. Recurrent erythema in patients with long-term parvovirus B19 infection. *Clin Infect Dis* 2005;**40**:e117–19.

43. White DG, Woolf AD, Mortimer PP, Cohen BJ, Blake DR, Bacon PA. Human parvovirus arthropathy. *Lancet* 1985;**1**:419–21.

44. Reid DM, Reid TM, Brown T, Rennie JA, Eastmond CJ. Human parvovirus-associated arthritis: a clinical and laboratory description. *Lancet* 1985;**1**:422–5.

45. Naides SJ, Scharosch LL, Foto F, Howard EJ. Rheumatologic manifestations of human parvovirus B19 infection in adults. Initial two-year clinical experience. *Arthritis Rheum* 1990;**33**:1297–309.

46. Colmegna I, Alberts-Grill N. Parvovirus B19: its role in chronic arthritis. *Rheum Dis Clin North Am* 2009;**35**:95–110.

47. Rogers BB, Rogers ZR, Timmons CF. Polymerase chain reaction amplification of archival material for parvovirus B19 in children with transient erythroblastopenia of childhood. *Pediatr Pathol Lab Med* 1996;**16**:471–8.

48. Serjeant BE, Hambleton IR, Kerr S, Kilty CG, Serjeant GR. Haematological response to parvovirus B19 infection in homozygous sickle-cell disease. *Lancet* 2001;**358**:1779–80.

49. Morinet F, Leruez-Ville M, Pillet S, Fichelson S. Concise review: anemia caused by viruses. *Stem Cells* 2011;**29**:1656–60.

50. Rodis JF. Parvovirus infection. *Clin Obstet Gynecol* 1999;**42**:107–20, quiz 74–5.

51. Norbeck O, Papadogiannakis N, Petersson K, Hirbod T, Broliden K, Tolfvenstam T. Revised clinical presentation of parvovirus B19-associated intrauterine fetal death. *Clin Infect Dis* 2002;**35**:1032–8.

52. Molina KM, Garcia X, Denfield SW, Fan Y, Morrow WR, Towbin JA, et al. Parvovirus B19 myocarditis causes significant morbidity and mortality in children. *Pediatr Cardiol* 2013;**34**:390–7.

53. Young NS. Parvovirus infection and its treatment. *Clin Exp Immunol* 1996;**104**(Suppl. 1):26–30.

54. Kurtzman GJ, Ozawa K, Cohen B, Hanson G, Oseas R, Young NS. Chronic bone marrow failure due to persistent B19 parvovirus infection. *N Engl J Med* 1987;**317**:287–94.

55. Kurtzman G, Frickhofen N, Kimball J, Jenkins DW, Nienhuis AW, Young NS. Pure red-cell aplasia of 10 years' duration due to persistent parvovirus B19 infection and its cure with immunoglobulin therapy. *N Engl J Med* 1989;**321**:519–23.

56. Frickhofen N, Abkowitz JL, Safford M, Berry JM, Antunez-de-Mayolo J, Astrow A, et al. Persistent B19 parvovirus infection in patients infected with human immunodeficiency virus type 1 (hHIV-1): a treatable cause of anemia in aids. *Ann Intern Med* 1990;**113**:926–33.

57. Graeve JL, de Alarcon PA, Naides SJ. Parvovirus B19 infection in patients receiving cancer chemotherapy: the expanding spectrum of disease. *Am J Pediatr Hematol Oncol* 1989;**11**:441–4.

58. Broliden K. Parvovirus B19 infection in pediatric solid-organ and bone marrow transplantation. *Pediatr Transplant* 2001;**5**:320–30.

59. Egbuna O, Zand MS, Arbini A, Menegus M, Taylor J. A cluster of parvovirus B19 infections in renal transplant recipients: a prospective case series and review of the literature. *Am J Transplant* 2006;**6**:225–31.

60. Meyer O. Parvovirus B19 and autoimmune diseases. *Joint Bone Spine* 2003;**70**:6–11.

61. von Landenberg P, Lehmann HW, Modrow S. Human parvovirus B19 infection and antiphospholipid antibodies. *Autoimmun Rev* 2007;**6**:278–85.

62. Lehmann HW, Plentz A, von Landenberg P, Kuster RM, Modrow S. Different patterns of disease manifestations of parvovirus B19-associated reactive juvenile arthritis and the induction of antiphospholipid-antibodies. *Clin Rheumatol* 2008;**27**:333–8.

63. Lunardi C, Tiso M, Borgato L, Nanni L, Millo R, De Sandre G, et al. Chronic parvovirus B19 infection induces the production of anti-virus antibodies with autoantigen binding properties. *Eur J Immunol* 1998;**28**:936–48.

64. Peterlana D, Puccetti A, Beri R, Ricci M, Simeoni S, Borgato L, et al. The presence of parvovirus B19 VP and NS1 genes in the synovium is not correlated with rheumatoid arthritis. *J Rheumatol* 2003;**30**:1907–10.

65. Rigante D, Mazzoni MB, Esposito S. The cryptic interplay between systemic lupus erythematosus and infections. *Autoimmun Rev* 2014;**13**:96–102.

66. Moroncini G, Mori S, Tonnini C, Gabrielli A. Role of viral infections in the etiopathogenesis of systemic sclerosis. *Clin Exp Rheumatol* 2013;**31**:3–7.

67. Zakrzewska K, Corcioli F, Carlsen KM, Giuggioli D, Fanci R, Rinieri A, et al. Human parvovirus B19 (B19V) infection in systemic sclerosis patients. *Intervirology* 2009;**52**:279–82.

68. Ferri C, Zakrzewska K, Longombardo G, Giuggioli D, Storino FA, Pasero G, et al. Parvovirus B19 infection of bone marrow in systemic sclerosis patients. *Clin Exp Rheumatol* 1999;**17**:718–20.

69. Kerr JR. Pathogenesis of human parvovirus B19 in rheumatic disease. *Ann Rheum Dis* 2000;**59**:672–83.

70. Tsay GJ, Zouali M. Unscrambling the role of human parvovirus B19 signaling in systemic autoimmunity. *Biochem Pharmacol* 2006;**72**:1453–9.

71. Lidar M, Lipschiz N, Langevitz P, Shoenfeld Y. The infectious etiology of vasculitis. *Autoimmunity* 2009;**42**:432–8.

72. Magro CM, Nuovo G, Ferri C, Crowson AN, Giuggioli D, Sebastiani M. Parvoviral infection of endothelial cells and stromal fibroblasts: a possible pathogenetic role in scleroderma. *J Cutan Pathol* 2004;**31**:43–50.

73. Ohtsuka T, Yamazaki S. Increased prevalence of human parvovirus B19 DNA in systemic sclerosis skin. *Br J Dermatol* 2004;**150**:1091–5.

74. Lunardi C, Bason C, Navone R, Millo E, Damonte G, Corrocher R, et al. Systemic sclerosis immunoglobulin G autoantibodies bind the human cytomegalovirus late protein UL94 and induce apoptosis in human endothelial cells. *Nat Med* 2000;**6**:1183–6.

75. Lunardi C, Bason C, Leandri M, Navone R, Lestani M, Millo E, et al. Autoantibodies to inner ear and endothelial antigens in Cogan's syndrome. *Lancet* 2002;**360**:915–21.

76. Zanoni G, Navone R, Lunardi C, Tridente G, Bason C, Sivori S, et al. In celiac disease, a subset of autoantibodies against transglutaminase binds toll-like receptor 4 and induces activation of monocytes. *PLoS Med* 2006;**3**:e358.

77. Frulloni L, Lunardi C, Simone R, Dolcino M, Scattolini C, Falconi M, et al. Identification of a novel antibody associated with autoimmune pancreatitis. *N Engl J Med* 2009;**361**:2135–42.

78. Lunardi C, Tinazzi E, Bason C, Dolcino M, Corrocher R, Puccetti A. Human parvovirus B19 infection and autoimmunity. *Autoimmun Rev* 2008;**8**:116–20.

79. Gutierrez L, Tsukamoto S, Suzuki M, Yamamoto-Mukai H, Yamamoto M, Philipsen S, et al. Ablation of GATA1 in adult mice results in aplastic crisis, revealing its essential role in steady-state and stress erythropoiesis. *Blood* 2008;**111**:4375–85.

80. Thammasri K, Rauhamaki S, Wang L, Filippou A, Kivovich V, Marjomaki V, et al. Human parvovirus B19 induced apoptotic bodies contain altered self-antigens that are phagocytosed by antigen presenting cells. *PLoS One* 2013;**8**:e67179.

81. Tzang BS, Chen DY, Tsai CC, Chiang SY, Lin TM, Hsu TC. Human parvovirus B19 nonstructural protein NS1 enhanced the expression of cleavage of 70 kDa U1-snRNP autoantigen. *J Biomed Sci* 2010;**17**:40.

CHAPTER 22

Human T-lymphotropic Virus Type 1 and Rheumatic Diseases: A Link Between Infection and Autoimmunity

Cezar Augusto Muniz Caldas[*,†,1], **Rita Catarina Medeiros Sousa**[‡],
Jozélio Freire de Carvalho[§]
[*]Department of Internal Medicine, Universidade Federal do Pará, Belém, PA, Brazil
[†]Curso de Medicina do Centro Universitário do Estado do Pará – CESUPA, Belém, PA, Brazil
[‡]Núcleo de Medicina Tropical, Universidade Federal do Pará, Belém, PA, Brazil
[§]Rheumatology Division, Aliança Medical Center, Salvador, Bahia, Brazil
[1]Corresponding Author: cezar_caldas@yahoo.com.br

1 HTLV, THE IMMUNE SYSTEM AND AUTOIMMUNITY

The human T-lymphotrophic virus (HTLV) belongs to the *Retroviridae* family, subfamily *Oncovirinae*, genus *Deltaretrovirus*. Four viral types have been described—HTLV-1, HTLV-2, HTLV-3, and HTLV-4—but only HTLV-1 is clearly associated with disease in humans.[1] Indeed, HTLV-1, described in 1980 as the first human retrovirus, is responsible for lymphoproliferative diseases, inflammation of central nervous system and increased susceptibility to certain infectious diseases and immunological changes. Among the most dramatic clinical expressions of HTLV-1 are the adult T-cell leukemia/lymphoma (ATL) and HTLV-1-associated myelopathy/tropical spastic paraparesis (HAM/TSP).[2–4] It is estimated that 10–20 million people worldwide are infected with the virus.[5,6] Most remain asymptomatic, but 0.3–4% develop HAM/TSP and 1–5% develop ATL.[7–9]

The transmission of HTLV can occur through sexual contact[10] or parenteral[11] or vertical transmission.[1] Breastfeeding for more than 6 months is associated with a 10.5–39.6% likelihood of viral transmission from mother to children.[12,13] This risk correlates with provirus load in breast milk, the concordance of human leukocyte antigen class I between mother and child, a high percentage of mononuclear cells present in contaminated milk and high titers of antibodies.[12–16] Intrauterine and perinatal transmission occur

Infection and Autoimmunity
http://dx.doi.org/10.1016/B978-0-444-63269-2.00022-2

in 4–14% of infants born to infected mothers.[12,13] The prevalence increases with age and is twice as common among women than men.[17,18]

The structure of HTLV-1 is similar to other retroviruses, with two molecules of single-stranded positive RNA. What differentiates HTLV-1 from other retroviruses is the pX region, which codes for two important regulatory proteins: Tax and Rex. HTLV-1 basic leucine zipper factor (HBZ) is another viral protein that needs to be mentioned because it plays a critical role in leukemogenesis of ATL.[19]

The target of HTLV-1 is CD4 + T cells, but other cells, such as CD8 + T cells and human dendritic cells, may be infected.[20,21] The mechanism of more efficient of viral spread is cell to cell through a virus-induced infection synapse.[8] Thus, different from human immunodeficiency virus (HIV) infection, there are few or no HTLV particles in the plasma, which measures the proviral load.[8] To be more exact, HTLV-1 might spread across the virological synapse, the specialized virus-induced area of contact, that is formed between a lymphocyte and another cell in which distinct protein microdomains mediate adhesion, antigen recognition, and secretion of cytokines or lytic granules; this resembled the immunological synapse, which promotes the directed transmission of the virus between cells.[8,22] This cell-to-cell transmission of HTLV-1 is $>10^4$ times more efficient than transmission of a cell-free virus.[23]

HTLV-1 infection is endemic in several regions of the world, especially in southern Japan,[18] the Caribbean,[24] sub-Saharan Africa,[25] South America,[26,27] Melanesia and Papua New Guinea.[28,29] In addition to ATL and HAM/TSP, HTLV-1 infection may result in other events involving the nervous system (peripheral neuropathy), muscles (polymyositis, myopathy), eyes (uveitis), lungs (alveolitis), skin (infective dermatitis), joints (arthritis/arthropathy) and thyroid (thyroiditis), or infection may be systemic (Sjögren's syndrome, sicca syndrome).[1,30,31] HTLV-1 infection also increases susceptibility to certain infectious diseases such as strongyloidiasis, crusted scabies, leprosy and tuberculosis.[1,32,33]

Although the mechanisms by which HTLV-1 infection leads to disease are not fully elucidated, complex virus–host interactions seem to play an important role in this process, involving the host's genetic characteristics and immune and viral factors.[1,34,35] The Tax protein is a critical transcriptional factor that interacts with cellular factors. Tax can upregulate the expression of cellular genes involved in T-cell growth and proliferation, in addition to other cellular genes such as IL-2, IL-2Rα, IL-15, tumor growth factor-β, and tumor necrosis factor (TNF)-α.[1,36,37] This viral protein also increases the expression of cellular proto-oncogenes and represses DNA repair and apoptosis.[1] Another important viral factor that may be involved in producing disease is the HBZ protein.[38,39] The HBZ messenger RNA load is correlated with the severity of ATL and neopterin concentration in cerebrospinal fluid in patients with HAM/TSP.[38,39] The expression of HBZ messenger RNA in infected cells reduces the response to treatment with immunomodulator agents in HAM/TSP.[38,39]

An efficient CD8+ T-cell response can protect people from disease, but the production of inflammatory factors can eventually result in HAM/TSP and other inflammatory diseases. In addition, the proliferation of infected cells can result in ATL.[1] Genetic factors, such as human leukocyte antigen class I and killer cell immunoglobulin-like receptor genes, as well viral factors such as HTLV-1 subgroup and proviral load, are implicated in determining the risk for HAM/TSP.[38,40] Several proinflammatory cytokines such as interferon-γ, TNF-α, interleukin (IL)-1 and IL-6 are increased in HAM/TSP.[6]

The autoimmunity observed in HTLV-1–associated diseases also can be induced by molecular mimicry.[41,42] Levin et al.[42] established a link between autoantibodies against HTLV-1 infection and the nervous system, resulting in HAM/TSP. They identified an immunoglobulin G from patients with HAM/TSP with heterogeneous nuclear ribonuclear protein-A1 as an autoantigen acting specifically against neurons of the corticospinal tract. This same immunoglobulin cross-reacts with the Tax protein. This suggests the importance of molecular mimicry in the development of HAM/TSP in patients with HTLV-1 infection.[42] It also was observed that an increase in the number of invariant natural killer T cells is associated with a decrease in HTLV-1 proviral load.[43]

2 HTLV AND ARTHROPATHY

HTLV-1 has been associated with the development of arthritis with proliferative synovitis.[44,45] Nishioka et al.[31] were the first researchers to describe the association of HTLV-1 and rheumatoid arthritis (RA). The arthropathy associated with HTLV-1 infection is chronic erosive oligoarthritis of large joints, with evidence of synovial proliferation and with a positive or negative rheumatoid factor.[31,46–49]

Arthritis in individuals carrying HTLV-1 is a very important model for studying the induction of autoimmunity. Ishihara et al.[50] demonstrated that HTLV-1 was a trigger inducing severe arthritis in mice with the appropriate genetic background (double-mutant mouse gp130/pX-Tg). The mechanism is uncertain, but it is possible that infected lymphocytes produce more cytokines, such as IL-1, IL-6, and TNF-α, leading to an inflammatory reaction within the joints and synovial proliferation, resulting in arthropathy.[31,44,51–53] The occurrence of HTLV-1 antibodies in the synovial fluid of affected joints, as well as the presence of ATL-like cells in fluid and synovial tissue, also have been described. Moreover, HTLV-1 proviral DNA integrated into the DNA of synovial fluid cells and synovial tissue cells has been detected.[54,55]

The role of the HTLV-1 proviral load has been studied in the development of arthropathy in patients infected with HTLV-1 as well as in HAM/TSP. Best et al.[6] found that proviral load was the only factor significantly associated with HAM/TSP in patients infected with HTLV-1. Likewise, Yakova et al.[56] found a high HTLV-1 proviral load in the synovial fluid and tissue cells in a patient with arthropathy; this patient had a higher percentage of memory and activated CD4+ T cells in the synovial compartment than in the peripheral blood.

Nakajima et al.[57] found that integration of HTLV-1 into synovial cells leads to the acquisition of a higher proliferative capacity. The HTLV-1 *tax* gene in particular seems to be responsible for synovial cell proliferation.[57] This fact, associated with overexpression of IL-1β and IL-6 in these cells, similar to that seen in RA, can induce, through a paracrine pathway, the proliferation of other synovial cells, perpetuating the process.[57,58]

These findings could influence the selection of appropriate therapy, suggesting that antiretroviral therapy could be useful in arthropathy associated with HTLV-1, but this point is unclear in the literature. Frenzel et al.,[59] however, reported a case of HTLV-1-associated arthropathy refractory to corticosteroids, disease-modifying antirheumatic drugs, and rituximab, that was treated successfully with etanercept, an anti-TNF-α agent.

Takahashi et al.[45] described a case of HTLV-1-associated arthropathy refractory to intra-articular injections of prednisolone and oral administration of a nonsteroidal anti-inflammatory drug. They achieved great results after arthroscopic synovectomy and treatment with oral prednisolone (5 mg/day). A biopsy specimen was obtained during the arthroscopy to investigate the effect of pirarubicin, bestatin, betamethasone, and hyaluronic acid on a synovial tissue culture. Bestatin was the only drug with a neutral effect. Pirarubicin induced synovial fibrosis and apoptosis; betamethasone slightly decreased cytotoxic T cells, and hyaluronic acid decreased the inflammation of the synovial tissue.[45]

An interesting observation was that HTLV-1 tax transgenic mice (a model used to study chronic arthritis similar to human RA) treated with intra-articular administration of anti-Fas monoclonal antibodies obtained improvement of oedema and histologic features of arthritis through the induction of apoptosis in synovial tissue, suggesting that this therapeutic modality can be an alternative for treating arthritis in humans.[60]

Although the possibility of an anti-TNF-α agent and anti-FAS monoclonal antibody administration in patients with arthropathy related to HTLV is interesting, nowadays the recommended first-line treatment is still the use of symptomatic drugs, such as nonsteroidal anti-inflammatory and analgesic drugs.[1]

3 HTLV AND SJÖGREN'S SYNDROME

Sjögren's syndrome (SS) is a systemic autoimmune disease characterized by lymphocytic infiltrates of exocrine glands. Retroviruses such as HIV and HTLV have clinical and histological features similar to those observed in SS.[61] In 1988, Vernant et al.[62] proposed the association between SS and HTLV-1.

The mechanism responsible for the glandular destruction may be similar to that occurring in the RA synovium, such as pseudolymphomatous lesions characterized by the infiltration of CD4+ T cells.[48] Green et al.[63] studied transgenic mice containing the HTLV-1 *tax* gene and observed that they developed an exocrinopathy of the salivary and lachrymal glands resembling SS.

Eguchi et al.[64] reported a high prevalence (36%) of the anti-HTLV-1 antibody in patients with SS in an endemic area of Japan. They described more extraglandular manifestations, such as uveitis and myopathy, in this population than in patients without antibodies to HTLV-1. In a population with HTLV-1 and myelopathy ($n = 20$), Nakamura et al.[65] found 13 (65%) with a diagnosis of primary SS.

In other studies there are controversies about the prevalence of clinical and laboratory manifestations in groups with SS with or without HTLV. For example, in a Japanese study, Hida et al.[66] found anti-SSA/Ro-positive antibodies in 42.2% and anti-SSB/La antibodies in 11.1% of patients with SS who were HTLV-1 positive. Ferraz-Chaoui et al.,[67] however, studying a Brazilian population, did not find anti-SSA/Ro- or anti-SSB/La-positive antibodies in patients with HTLV-1 and SS. These data suggest pathophysiological and geographic differences, and other studies are necessary to clarify these results.

In addition, Lee et al.[68] not only compared the clinical and laboratory findings of patients with SS with and without HTLV-1 but also studied whether there could be distinct features in the salivary glands. They did not identify clinical differences between the two groups of patients, but, among HTLV-1 patients, they found scarce autoantibodies. Lymphocyte count in the salivary glands was significantly higher than HTLV-1-negative patients.[68]

The treatment of manifestations resembling SS is uncertain; however, Pot et al.[69] described an interesting case of myelopathy in a patient with SS and HTLV-1 treated with prednisone, lamivudine, and tenofovir. The patient's evolution was quite favorable; spasticity and weakness improved, although dryness syndrome was unchanged. Pot et al. suggested that stronger immunosuppression could be dangerous and the use of antiretroviral therapy would be important in patients with SS and HTLV.[69] Perhaps the use of oral and ocular lubricants may be helpful in relieving xerostomia and keratoconjunctivitis sicca.

4 HTLV AND OTHER RHEUMATIC DISEASES

Some infectious agents have been associated with development of polymyositis, such as coxsackie and influenza, as well as HTLV-1 and HIV.[70] Studies of seroprevalence among patients with polymyositis showed more frequent HTLV-1 infection in these subjects compared with the general population.[71,72] Using polymerase chain reaction, Sherman et al.[73] amplified DNA detection, and immunohistochemical analysis reinforced the hypothesis that this association is true, but the pathophysiological mechanism is still unclear. Among the hypotheses are direct injury to myocytes caused by HTLV-1 or the expression of inflammatory cytokines induced by the virus.

Other studies based on weak evidence, such as case–control studies and case reports, have tried to involve HTLV-1 in the development of fibromyalgia and tenosynovial nodulosis, but these hypotheses still need to be elucidated.[74,75]

TAKE-HOME MESSAGES

- HTLV, especially type 1, has been continuously associated with the development of autoimmune diseases, particularly rheumatic diseases.

- The pattern of articular involvement related with HTLV-1 can resemble RA, but it can also be an oligoarthritis of large joints such as the shoulders, knees and wrists.
- HTLV-1 may produce clinical, laboratory, and histopathological findings quite similar to SS and so should be included among the differential diagnoses.
- The major difficulty in the clinical management of patients infected with HTLV-1 is the lack of accurate markers of disease. The measurement of proviral load, for example, has no established international parameters.
- The role of antiretroviral therapy or immunosuppressants in the treatment of autoimmune conditions related to HTLV should be further evaluated.

REFERENCES

1. Verdonck K, González E, Van Dooren S, Vandamme AM, Vanham G, Gotuzzo E. Human T-lymphotropic virus 1: recent knowledge about an ancient infection. *Lancet Infect Dis* 2007;**7**:266–81.
2. Poiesz BJ, Ruscetti FW, Gazdar AF, Bunn PA, Minna JD, Gallo RC. Detection and isolation of type C retrovirus particles from fresh and cultured lymphocytes of a patient with cutaneous T-cell lymphoma. *Proc Natl Acad Sci U S A* 1980;**77**:7415–19.
3. Kannagi M, Ohashi T, Harashima N, Hanabuchi S, Hasegawa A. Immunological risks of adult T-cell leukemia at primary HTLV-I infection. *Trends Microbiol* 2004;**12**:346–52.
4. Uchiyama T. Human T cell leukemia virus type I (HTLV-I) and human diseases. *Annu Rev Immunol* 1997;**15**:15–37.
5. de Thé G, Bomford R. An HTLV-I vaccine: why, how, for whom? *AIDS Res Hum Retroviruses* 1993;**9**:381–6.
6. Best I, Adaui V, Verdonck K, González E, Tipismana M, Clark D, et al. Proviral load and immune markers associated with human T-lymphotropic virus type 1 (HTLV-1)-associated myelopathy/tropical spastic paraparesis (HAM/TSP) in Peru. *Clin Exp Immunol* 2006;**146**:226–33.
7. Edlich RF, Arnette JA, Williams FM. Global epidemic of human T-cell lymphotropic virus type-I (HTLV-I). *J Emerg Med* 2000;**18**:109–19.
8. Nejmeddine M, Bangham CR. The HTLV-1 Virological Synapse. *Viruses* 2010;**2**:1427–47.
9. Sieczkarski SB, Whittaker GR. Differential requirements of Rab5 and Rab7 for endocytosis of influenza and other enveloped viruses. *Traffic* 2003;**4**:333–43.
10. Moriuchi M, Moriuchi H. Seminal fluid enhances replication of human T-cell leukemia virus type 1: implications for sexual transmission. *J Virol* 2004;**78**:12709–11.
11. Mahieux R, Gessain A. HTLV-1 and associated adult T-cell leukemia/lymphoma. *Rev Clin Exp Hematol* 2003;**7**:336–61.
12. Bittencourt AL, Sabino EC, Costa MC, Pedroso C, Moreira L. No evidence of vertical transmission of HTLV-I in bottle-fed children. *Rev Inst Med Trop Sao Paulo* 2002;**44**:63–5.
13. Maloney EM, Cleghorn FR, Morgan OS, Rodgers-Johson P, Cranston B, Jack N, et al. Incidence of HTLV-I-associated myelopathy/tropical spastic paraparesis (HAM/TSP) in Jamaica and Trinidad. *J Acquir Immune Defic Syndr Hum Retrovirol* 1998;**17**:167–70.

14. Li HC, Biggar RJ, Miley WJ, Maloney EM, Cranston B, Hanchard B, et al. Provirus load in breast milk and risk of mother-to-child transmission of human T lymphotropic virus type I. *J Infect Dis* 2004;**190**:1275–8.

15. Biggar RJ, Ng J, Kim N, Hisada M, Li HC, Cranston B, et al. Human leukocyte antigen concordance and the transmission risk via breast-feeding of human T cell lymphotropic virus type I. *J Infect Dis* 2006;**193**:277–82.

16. Fujino T, Nagata Y. HTLV-I transmission from mother to child. *J Reprod Immunol* 2000;**47**:197–206.

17. Larsen O, Andersson S, da Silva Z, Hedegaard K, Sandström A, Nauclér A, et al. Prevalences of HTLV-1 infection and associated risk determinants in an urban population in Guinea-Bissau, West Africa. *J Acquir Immune Defic Syndr* 2000;**25**:157–63.

18. Matsuzaki T, Otose H, Hashimoto K, Shibata Y, Arimura K, Osame M. Diseases among men living in human T-lymphotropic virus type I endemic areas in Japan. *Intern Med* 1993;**32**:623–8.

19. Yasunaga J, Matsuoka M. Human T-cell leukemia virus type I induces adult T-cell leukemia: from clinical aspects to molecular mechanisms. *Cancer Control* 2007;**14**:133–40.

20. Nagai M, Brennan MB, Sakai JA, Mora CA, Jacobson S. CD8(+) T cells are an in vivo reservoir for human T-cell lymphotropic virus type I. *Blood* 2001;**98**:1858–61.

21. Jones KS, Petrow-Sadowski C, Huang YK, Bertolette DC, Ruscetti FW. Cell-free HTLV-1 infects dendritic cells leading to transmission and transformation of CD4(+) T cells. *Nat Med* 2008;**14**:429–36.

22. Nejmeddine M, Barnard AL, Tanaka Y, Taylor GP, Bangham CR. Human T-lymphotropic virus, type 1, tax protein triggers microtubule reorientation in the virological synapse. *J Biol Chem* 2005;**280**:29653–60.

23. Mazurov D, Ilinskaya A, Heidecker G, Lloyd P, Derse D. Quantitative comparison of HTLV-1 and HIV-1 cell-to-cell infection with new replication dependent vectors. *PLoS Pathog* 2010;**6**:e1000788.

24. Gessain A, Cassar O. Epidemiological aspects and world distribution of HTLV-1 infection. *Front Microbiol* 2012;**3**:388.

25. Holmgren B, da Silva Z, Larsen O, Vastrup P, Andersson S, Aaby P. Dual infections with HIV-1, HIV-2 and HTLV-I are more common in older women than in men in Guinea-Bissau. *AIDS* 2003;**17**:241–53.

26. Bittencourt AL, Dourado I, Filho PB, Santos M, Valadão E, Alcantara LC, et al. Human T-cell lymphotropic virus type 1 infection among pregnant women in northeastern Brazil. *J Acquir Immune Defic Syndr* 2001;**26**:490–4.

27. Carneiro-Proietti AB, Catalan-Soares BC, Castro-Costa CM, Murphy EL, Sabino EC, Hisada M, et al. HTLV in the Americas: challenges and perspectives. *Rev Panam Salud Publica* 2006;**19**:44–53.

28. Cassar O, Capuano C, Meertens L, Chungue E, Gessain A. Human T-cellleukemiavirustype1 molecular variants, Vanuatu, Melanesia. *Emerg Infect Dis* 2005;**11**:706–10.

29. Takao S, Ishida T, Bhatia KK, Saha N, Soemantri A, Kayame OW. Seroprevalence of human T-lymphotropic virus type 1 in Papua New Guinea and Irian Jaya measured using different western blot criteria. *J Clin Virol* 2000;**16**:129–33.

30. Mochizuki M, Watanabe T, Yamaguchi K, Takatsuki K, Yoshimura K, Shirao M, et al. HTLV-I uveitis: a distinct clinicalentity caused by HTLV-I. *Jpn J Cancer Res* 1992;**83**:236–9.

31. Nishioka K, Maruyama I, Sato K, Kitajima I, Nakajima Y, Osame M. Chronic inflammatory arthropathy associated with HTLV-I. *Lancet* 1989;**1**:441.

32. Hirata T, Uchima N, Kishimoto K, Zaha O, Kinjo N, Hokama A, et al. Impairment of host immune response against strongyloides stercoralis by human T cell lymphotropic virus type 1 infection. *Am J Trop Med Hyg* 2006;**74**:246–9.

33. Marinho J, Galvão-Castro B, Rodrigues LC, Barreto ML. Increased risk of tuberculosis with human T-lymphotropic virus-1 infection: a case-control study. *J Acquir Immune Defic Syndr* 2005;**40**:625–8.

34. Bangham CR. The immune control and cell-to-cell spread of human-T cell lymphotropic virus type I. *J Gen Virol* 2003;**84**:3177–89.

35. Mosley AJ, Asquith B, Bangham C. Cell-mediated immune response to human T-lymphotropic virus type I. *Viral Immunol* 2005;**18**:293–305.

36. Carvalho EM, Bacellar O, Porto AF, Braga S, Galvao-Castro B, Neva F. Cytokine profile and immunomodulation in asymptomatic human T-lymphotropic virus type-I-infected blood donors. *J Acquir Immune Defic Syndr* 2001;**27**:1–6.

37. Santos SB, Porto AF, Muniz AL, de Jesus AR, Magalhães E, Melo A, et al. Exacerbated inflammatory cellular immune response characteristics of HAM/TSP is observed in a large proportion of HTLV-I asymptomatic carriers. *BMC Infect Dis* 2004;**4**:7.

38. Saito M. Immunogenetics and the pathological mechanisms of human T-cell leukemia virus type 1- (HTLV-1-) associated myelopathy/tropical spastic paraparesis (HAM/TSP). *Interdiscip Perspect Infect Dis* 2010;**2010**:478461.

39. Saito M, Matsuzaki T, Satou Y, Yasunaga J, Saito K, Arimura K, et al. In vivo expression of the HBZ gene of HTLV-1 correlates with proviral load, inflammatory markers and disease severity in HTLV-1 associated myelopathy/tropical spastic paraparesis (HAM/TSP). *Retrovirology* 2009;**6**:19.

40. Seich Al Basatena NK, Macnamara A, Vine AM, Thio CL, Astemborski J, et al. KIR2DL2 enhances protective and detrimental HLA class I-mediated immunity in chronic viral infection. *PLoS Pathog* 2011;**7**:e1002270.

41. García-Vallejo F, Domínguez MC, Tamayo O. Autoimmunity and molecular mimicry in tropical spastic paraparesis/human T-lymphotropic virus-associated myelopathy. *Braz J Med Biol Res* 2005;**38**:241–50.

42. Levin MC, Lee SM, Kalume F, Morcos Y, Dohan Jr. FC, Hasty KA, et al. Autoimmunity due to molecular mimicry as a cause of neurological disease. *Nat Med* 2002;**8**:509–13.

43. Azakami K, Sato T, Araya N, Utsunomiya A, Kubota R, Suzuki K, et al. Severe loss of invariant NKT cells exhibiting anti-HTLV-1 activity in patients with HTLV-1-associated disorders. *Blood* 2009;**114**:3208–15.

44. Kalden JR, Gay S. Retroviruses and autoimmune rheumatic diseases. *Clin Exp Immunol* 1994;**98**:1–5.

45. Takahashi T, Takemoto S, Kiyasu K, Yamamoto H, Tani T, Miyoshi I, et al. Treatment for HTLV-I associated arthropathy: a case study and synovial tissue culture analysis. *Rheumatol Int* 2005;**26**:74–9.

46. de Carvalho MMN, Novaes AE, de Carvalho EM, Araújo MI. Autoimmune rheumatic diseases in HTLV-1 infected individuals. *Rev Bras Reumatol* 2006;**46**:334–9.

47. Eguchi K, Origuchi T, Takashima H, Iwata K, Katamine S, Nagataki S. High seroprevalence of anti-HTLV-I antibody in rheumatoid arthritis. *Arthritis Rheum* 1996;**39**:463–6.

48. Nishioka K, Sumida T, Hasunuma T. Human T lymphotropic vírus type I in arthropathy and autoimmune disorders. *Arthritis Rheum* 1996;**39**:1410–18.

49. Mc Callum RM, Patel DD, Moore JO, Haynes BF. Arthritis syndromes associated with human T cell lymphotropic virus type I infection. *Med Clin North Am* 1997;**81**:261–76.

50. Ishihara K, Sawa S, Ikushima H, Hirota S, Atsumi T, Kamimura D, et al. The point mutation of tyrosine 759 of the IL-6 family cytokine receptor gp130 synergizes with HTLV-1 pX in promoting rheumatoid arthritis-like arthritis. *Int Immunol* 2004;**16**:455–65.

51. Salahuddin SZ, Markham PD, Lindner SG, Gootenberg J, Popovic M, Hemmi H, et al. Lymphokine production by cultured human T cells transformed by human T-cell leukemia-lymphoma virus-I. *Science* 1984;**223**:703–7.

52. Wano Y, Hattori T, Matsuoka M, Takatsuki K, Chua AO, Gubler U, et al. Interleukin 1 gene expression in adult T cell leukemia. *J Clin Invest* 1987;**80**:911–16.

53. de Carvalho MMN, Giozza SP, dos Santos ALMA, de Carvalho EM, Araújo MI. Frequency of rheumatic diseases in individuals infected with HTLV-1. *Rev Bras Reumatol* 2006;**46**:315–22.
54. Kitajima I, Yamamoto K, Sato K, Nakajima Y, Nakajima T, Maruyama I, et al. Detection of human T cell lymphotropic virus type I proviral DNA and its gene expression in synovial cells in chronic inflammatory arthropathy. *J Clin Invest* 1991;**88**:1315–22.
55. Sato K, Maruyama I, Maruyama Y, Kitajima I, Nakajima Y, Higaki M, et al. Arthritis in patients infected with human T lymphotropic virus type I, Clinical and immunopathologic features. *Arthritis Rheum* 1991;**34**:714–21.
56. Yakova M, Lézin A, Dantin F, Lagathu G, Olindo S, Jean-Baptiste G, et al. Increased proviral load in HTLV-1-infected patients with rheumatoid arthritis or connective tissue disease. *Retrovirology* 2005;**2**:4.
57. Nakajima T, Aono H, Hasunuma T, Yamamoto K, Maruyama I, Nosaka T, et al. Overgrowth of human synovial cells driven by the human T cell leukemia virus type I tax gene. *J Clin Invest* 1993;**92**:186–93.
58. Bucala R, Ritchlin C, Winchester R, Cerami A. Constitutive production of inflammatory and mitogenic cytokines by rheumatoid synovial fibroblasts. *J Exp Med* 1991;**173**:569–74.
59. Frenzel L, Moura B, Marcais A, Chapdelaine H, Hermine O. HTLV-1-associated arthropathy treated with anti-TNF-alpha agent. *Joint Bone Spine* 2013, pii:S1297-319.
60. Fujisawa K, Asahara H, Okamoto K, Aono H, Hasunuma T, Kobata T, et al. Therapeutic effect of the anti-Fas antibody on arthritis in HTLV-1 tax transgenic mice. *J Clin Invest* 1996;**98**:271–8.
61. Mariette X, Gottenberg JE, Theander E. Sjögren's syndrome and lymphoproliferations in autoimmune diseases. In: Bijlsma JWJ, editor. *EULAR compendium on rheumatic diseases*. London: Affinity; 2009. p. 314–28.
62. Vernant JC, Buisson G, Magdeleine J, De Thore J, Jouannelle A, et al. T-lymphocyte alveolitis, tropical spastic paresis, and Sjögren syndrome. *Lancet* 1988;**1**:177.
63. Green JE, Hinrichs SH, Vogel J, Jay G. Exocrinopathy resembling Sjögren's syndrome in HTLV-I transgenic mice. *Nature* 1989;**341**:72–4.
64. Eguchi K, Matsuoka N, Ida H, Nakashima M, Sakai M, Sakito S, et al. Primary Sjögren's syndrome with antibodies to HTLV-I: clinical and laboratory features. *Ann Rheum Dis* 1992;**51**:769–76.
65. Nakamura H, Kawakami A, Tominaga M, Hida A, Yamasaki S, Migita K, et al. Relationship between Sjögren's syndrome and human T-lymphotropic virus type I infection: follow-up study of 83 patients. *J Lab Clin Med* 2000;**135**:139–44.
66. Hida A, Kawabe Y, Kawakami A, Migita K, Tominaga M, Nakamura H, et al. HTLV-I associated Sjögren's syndrome is aetiologically distinct from anti-centromere antibodies positive Sjögren's syndrome. *Ann Rheum Dis* 1999;**58**:320–2.
67. Ferraz-Chaoui AK, Atta AM, Atta ML, Galvão-Castro B, Santiago MB. Study of autoantibodies in patients with keratoconjunctivitis sicca infected by the human T cell lymphotropic virus type 1. *Rheumatol Int* 2010;**30**:775–8.
68. Lee SJ, Lee JS, Shin MG, Tanaka Y, Park DJ, Kim TJ, et al. Detection of HTLV-1 in the labial salivary glands of patients with Sjögren's syndrome: a distinct clinical subgroup? *J Rheumatol* 2012;**39**:809–15.
69. Pot C, Chizzolini C, Vokatch N, Tiercy JM, Ribi C, Landis T, et al. Combined antiviral-immunosuppressive treatment in human T-lymphotrophic virus 1-Sjögren-associated myelopathy. *Arch Neurol* 2006;**63**:1318–20.
70. Lundberg IE, Vencovsky J, Dani L. Polymyositis, dermatomyositis, inflammatory diseases of muscle and other myopathies. In: Bijlsma JMJ, editor. *EULAR compendium on rheumatic diseases*. London: Affinity; 2009. p. 297–313.

71. Mora CA, Garruto RM, Brown P, Guiroy D, Morgan OS, Rodgers-Johnson P, et al. Seroprevalence of antibodies to HTLV-I in patients with chronic neurological disorders other than tropical spastic paraparesis. *Ann Neurol* 1988;**23**:S192–5.

72. Higuchi I, Nerenberg M, Yoshimine K, Yoshida M, Fukunaga H, Tajima K, et al. Failure to detect HTLV-I by in situ hybridization in the biopsied muscles of viral carriers with polymyositis. *Muscle Nerve* 1992;**15**:43–7.

73. Sherman MP, Amin RM, Rodgers-Johnson PE, Morgan OS, Char G, Mora CA, et al. Identification of human T cell leukemia/lymphoma virus type I antibodies, DNA, and protein in patients with polymyositis. *Arthritis Rheum* 1995;**38**:690–8.

74. Cruz BA, Catalan-Soares B, Proietti F. Higher prevalence of fibromyalgia in patients infected with human T cell lymphotropic virus type I. *J Rheumatol* 2006;**33**:2300–3.

75. Hasunuma T, Morimoto T, Tran TM, Müller-Ladner U, Aono H, Ogawa R, et al. Tenosynovial nodulosis in a patient infected with human T cell lymphotropic virus I. *Arthritis Rheum* 1997;**40**:578–82.

CHAPTER 23

Sjögren's Syndrome: Role of Viruses and Viral-Like Sequences

Clio P. Mavragani[*,1], Haralampos M. Moutsopoulos[†]

[*]Department of Physiology, School of Medicine, University of Athens, Athens, Greece
[†]Department of Pathophysiology, School of Medicine, University of Athens, Athens, Greece
[1]Corresponding Author: kmauragan@med.uoa.gr

1 INTRODUCTION

Sjögren's syndrome (SS), or autoimmune epithelitis, is a chronic autoimmune disorder characterized by lymphocytic infiltration of the salivary and lacrimal glands resulting in xerostomia and keratoconjunctivitis sicca. The disease can be seen as an entity alone (primary SS) or in association with other rheumatic autoimmune diseases. The prevalence of the syndrome is about 1–2% in the adult population; it primarily affects females (9:1 female-to-male ratio) in their fourth and fifth decade of life.[1] Symptoms of the disease may appear 6–8 years before the full-blown clinical development of the syndrome. Progression is slow and usually involves glandular tissues. About one third of patients can develop several extraglandular manifestations including interstitial renal disease, bronchitis sicca, autoimmune liver disorders and vasculitis.[2] Patients with SS have an 18-fold higher risk for developing lymphoma compared to the normal population, in association with increased mortality.[3,4]

2 CLINICAL PICTURE (REVIEWED IN REF. 5)

SS is characterized by dryness of the mouth (xerostomia) caused by decreased production of saliva. Unstimulated salivary flow rate is used to evaluate salivary gland function in clinical practice. Age, sex, medication and psychological factors may influence salivary flow. In patients with xerostomia, the

Infection and Autoimmunity
http://dx.doi.org/10.1016/B978-0-444-63269-2.00025-8

oral mucosa can be sticky, dry and erythematosus. Patients often report difficulties chewing and swallowing because of the dryness of the mouth. The tongue may be dry, with deep fissures and atrophic papillae. Dry mouth can lead to angular cheilitis and fungal overgrowth on the tongue. Recurrent caries is a problem that is often reported, as well as discomfort with dentures. Major salivary gland enlargement occurs in patients with primary SS, and although it may initially appear unilaterally, in most cases it develops bilaterally.

Chronic eye dryness leads to irritation and destruction of the corneal and conjunctival epithelium. Tear secretion rate is measured by the Schirmer's test, and staining of the corneal and conjunctival epithelial tissues with Rose Bengal and other stains reveals the extent of epithelium destruction.

About one third of patients with SS display some kind of extraglandular systemic manifestation at some point during the course of the disease. Raynaud's phenomenon precedes sicca manifestations in about one third of patients. Vasculitis of the skin presents with palpable purpuric or petechial lesions. Musculoskeletal involvement includes arthralgias, myalgias, fatigue and morning stiffness. Non-erosive arthritis and symmetric polyarthritis can also be observed. In patients with primary SS, respiratory tract involvement is mild but frequent. Dry cough is quite common and is mostly related to xerotrachea or bronchitis sicca. Dysphagia might also occur as a result of dryness of the pharynx and oesophagus. Liver involvement is quiet rare and presents either as primary biliary cirrhosis or chronic active hepatitis. About 4% of patients with SS have clinically significant renal involvement in the form of interstitial nephritis or glomerulonephritis. Peripheral sensory or sensorimotor polyneuropathy and mononeuritis multiplex occurs in 1–2% of patients. Furthermore, anxiety, depressed mood, personality structure disorders and defective coping strategies towards stressful life events are frequently observed.

In primary SS, malignant non-Hodgkin lymphoma occurs in about 5% of patients. Lymphoma usually develops later in the course of the disease; salivary glands are the most frequent site of involvement. The presence of parotid enlargement, palpable purpura, low levels of complement component 4 (C4) and mixed monoclonal cryoglobulinemia at first evaluation are adverse prognostic factors and adequately distinguish patients at high risk for developing lymphoproliferative disorders. At the level of salivary gland biopsy, germinal center formation, the presence of macrophages and elevated interleukin-12 concentrations also have been found to confer increased risk for lymphoma development. Patients with primary SS and adverse prognostic factors display increased mortality compared to the general population (mortality ratio, 1.15) and one to five deaths among patients with primary SS are attributed to lymphoma.[4] The presence of adverse prognostic factors is strongly associated with increased mortality.

3 IMMUNOPATHOLOGY (REVIEWED IN REF. 6)

The etiology of SS remains unknown. Even though environmental influences and different genetic factors are related to the disorder, no single factor can be identified as responsible for the pathogenesis of the syndrome. The presence of serum autoantibodies, focal lymphocytic infiltrations in the lesions and the association of SS with other autoimmune disorders strongly support the autoimmune nature of the disease. SS is characterized by B-cell reactivity and destruction of exocrine glands associated with dense lymphocytic infiltrations. B-cell activation is the most prominent immunologic feature associated with SS. B cells infiltrating the minor salivary glands are activated because they produce immunoglobulins with autoantibody reactivity. Rheumatoid factor and antinuclear antibodies are found with high frequency in patients with SS. The analysis of the specificity of antinuclear antibodies reveals the presence of antibodies against two ribonucleoproteins, Ro (SSA) and La (SSB). The component of the Ro/SSA Ro52—a major antigenic target in SS—has been shown to display E3 ligase activity and down-regulate pro-inflammatory responses.[7] La (SSB) is known to participate in the transcription termination of RNA polymerase III and in the translation of viral RNA.[8] Another SS-related autoantigen is the cytoskeletal protein a-fodrin.[9]

Oligoclonal B-cell expansion takes place early in the development of the disease. Monoclonal light chains are detected in higher frequencies in patients with systemic involvement compared to patients with glandular disease.[10,11] Furthermore, about one third of patients with primary SS display high concentrations of mixed monoclonal/polyclonal type II cryoglobulins with rheumatoid factor activity.[12] It is possible that B-cell neoplastic transformation takes place in the gland, possibly due to chronic immunologic stimulation. This transformation probably takes place along with immunoglobulin gene rearrangements and genetic variations in the p53 transcription factor and the B-cell activating factor (BAFF) gene.[13–15]

Pathological lesions in labial minor salivary gland tissues derived from patients with SS are characterized by the presence of round cell infiltrates surrounding ductal epithelial cells. The composition of cellular infiltrates in minor salivary gland tissues from patients with SS is highly dependent on the severity of the lesion. Thus, while CD4+ cells prevail in mild lesions, B cells are the major cellular types observed in advanced lesions. In addition, the incidence of inter-digitating dendritic cells (DCs) was found to be negatively associated with infiltration grade and biopsy focus score, whereas the opposite was observed with macrophage incidence. In contrast, the incidence of CD8(+) T cells, follicular DCs, and natural killer cells was not associated with lesion severity.[16]

Clinical and pathophysiologic findings reveal a central role of the epithelium in the pathogenesis of inflammatory lesions in the affected organs of patients with SS. The epithelium plays a central role in the initiation and perpetuation of immune response. This is attested by a series of immunopathologic findings showing the aberrant expression of various activation and immune response-associated molecules in epithelial cells of minor salivary gland biopsies. These cells express molecules implicated in antigen presentation, such as major histocompatibility complex class I (human leukocyte antigen ABC) and class II (human leukocyte antigen DR) and B7 costimulatory molecules. In addition, there is up-regulated expression of molecules that mediate B- and T-cell recruitment, as well as molecules that are involved in the expansion of the immune response. These molecules are adhesion molecules, lymphoattractant chemokines and pro-inflammatory cytokines. Furthermore, the activated state of epithelium is evidenced by the over-expression of apoptosis-related molecules (FAS, FAS ligand). Increased rates of epithelial apoptosis result in the release of intracellular antigens that are recognized by the immune system. These findings were substantiated by the detection of increased constitutive expression of the same molecules in non-neoplastic epithelial cells established from long-term cultures of cells from the salivary glands of patients with SS (Table 1). The establishment of long-term salivary gland epithelial cell cultures revealed the capacity of these cells to interact with immune cells through the expression of functional costimulatory molecules (B7 and CD40). Moreover, it has been shown that salivary gland epithelial cells can co-stimulate the growth of activated T cells, indicating that epithelial cells are able to participate in the antigen-mediated activation and proliferation of the immune response. It is therefore highly likely that there are intrinsic activation processes active in affected epithelial cells.[17] These data indicate that epithelial cells are suitably equipped to act as antigen-presenting cells and support their central role in SS pathogenesis.

Table 1 Aberrant Expression of Molecules Implicated in Epithelial Cell Activation in Sjögren's Syndrome

	Minor Salivary Gland Biopsies	Epithelial Cells from Salivary Gland Cultures
Activation markers	Proto-oncogenes	Not studied
Immune-reactive molecules	Major histocompatibility complex I and II	Major histocompatibility complex I and II
	B7 costimulatory molecules	B7 costimulatory molecules
	Adhesion molecules	Adhesion molecules
	Chemokines	Chemokines
	CD40	CD40
	Proinflammatory cytokines	Proinflammatory cytokines
Apoptosis–related molecules	FAS, FAS ligand	FAS, FAS ligand

4 VIRUSES AND SS (REVIEWED IN REF. 18)

Given the intrinsic activation of epithelial cells together with the presence of type I interferon (IFN) signature in patients with SS, the implication of viruses in the development and initiation of SS has long been suspected. However, several studies addressing the role of viruses such as cytomegalovirus, Epstein-Barr virus (EBV), human herpes virus type 6, human T-lymphotropic virus I (HTLV-1), retroviruses, hepatitis C virus (HCV) and enteroviruses were rather inconclusive.[19,20] EBV-associated antigens were found in the salivary glands of patients with SS displaying an increased content of EBV DNA in their saliva.[21,22] This, coupled with the fact that herpesviruses such as cytomegalovirus and EBV can replicate in the salivary glands, can be interpreted as an indication of viral involvement in the development of the disease. This hypothesis has been challenged by other groups that have demonstrated that the frequency of EBV detection in patients with SS is similar to the frequency observed in normal populations.[23,24] In a recent study, saliva from patients with SS was shown to transactivate target genes of the aryl hydrocarbon receptor, such as the *BZLF1* gene implicated in EBV reactivation, implying a novel contributory role of dioxins in the induction of autoimmunity.[25]

Another link between viruses and the disease comes from the fact that chronic lymphocytic sialadenitis that is linked to viral infection is histologically very similar to SS and can be found in 14–50% of patients infected with HCV.[26] Using in situ hybridization, HCV RNA was detected in the salivary glands of patients with chronic HCV infection.[27] Furthermore, sialadenitis was reported in transgenic animals carrying the HCV envelope genes.[28] HCV-related sialadenitis is characterized by the absence of specific SS autoantibodies such as anti-Ro/SSA and anti-La/SSB and a lesser degree of lymphocytic infiltration.[29,30]

Sialadenitis related to retroviruses also was described in patients infected with human immunodeficiency virus[31] and HTLV-1; salivary immunoglobulin A antibodies to HTLV-1 were described in sera of patients with SS with evidence of serum antibodies against HTLV-1.[32] Of interest, serum antibodies to the p24 capsid protein of the human immunodeficiency virus were reported in 30% of patients with SS compared to 1–4% of healthy controls.[33] Human intracisternal A-type retroviral particle and human retrovirus-5 also are implicated as factors triggering the development of SS.[34]

It is possible that viruses can act as the initiating factor in the activation of epithelial cells in the disease. Transient or persistent infection of epithelial cells by a putative virus may be the initiating event that leads to the accumulation of T and B cells. These cells could then prime a local autoimmune response using autoantigens provided by the epithelial cells as a result of the viral infection. Finally, monoclonal expansion of B cells under selective antigenic T-cell-induced pressure can lead to tissue destruction.

To further explore this activation of epithelial cells, it is essential to indentify the factors–possibly of viral origin–that trigger the immune response. The identity of gene products that play this activating role and their origin are essential information in the understanding of the pathogenesis of the disease. To identify genes that may contribute to primary SS pathogenesis, a differential display protocol was applied to minor salivary gland RNA samples of a patient with primary SS and a healthy individual used as a control. After sequencing several differentially expressed genes a 94-bp fragment homologous to the VP1 region of coxsackievirus B4, RNA expressed exclusively in the diseased sample was identified. The identification of this viral RNA suggests that this virus could have an active role in the pathogenesis of SS. The 5′ non-coding region (NCR) was amplified in 7 samples from patients with primary SS and in no samples from patients with secondary SS or controls. The 7 amplified products were sequenced; 4 of the sequences were found to be 98–99% identical to the 5′ NCR of coxsackievirus B4, and 3 were found to be 97–98% identical to the 5′ NCR of coxsackievirus A13. Immunohistochemistry of the enteroviral capsid protein VP1 revealed positive staining in epithelial cells and lymphocytic infiltrates in 11 primary SS samples, 1 secondary SS sample, and no control samples.[19]

5 ACTIVATION OF TYPE I INTERFERON PATHWAY IN SS: ROLE OF LONG INTERSPERSED NUCLEAR ELEMENT-1 RETROTRANSPOSABLE ELEMENTS

The type I IFN pathway—the main innate antiviral defensive mechanism in the human body—has been consistently found to be activated in patients with SS, as evidenced by the up-regulation of type I IFN-inducible genes in both peripheral blood and salivary gland tissues, elevated plasma/serum type I IFN activity and recruitment of plasmacytoid DCs (PDCs)—the 'professional' type I IFN producers—at the site of tissue injury. The identification of the primary inducers accounting for this activation remains a major challenge because no evidence to date suggests exogenous viruses as potential culprits.[35,36]

Endogenous nucleic acids—the major targets of autoimmune responses—are able to trigger type I IFN production by PDCs and other cell types through activation of Toll-like receptor-dependent or -independent pathways. Whether inappropriate expression of endogenous nucleic acids such as long interspersed nuclear element-1 (L1) retroelements at the level of affected tissues derived from patients with SS could account for the activation of type I IFNs in these patients was explored.[35,37]

L1 retroelements are an autonomous family of currently active retroelements comprising roughly 17% of the human genome. It contains two open reading frames (ORFs): ORF1, encoding p40, a 40-kDa RNA binding protein (ORF1/p40) that colocalizes with L1 RNA in cytoplasmic ribonucleoprotein particles, and ORF2, encoding a reverse transcriptase and endonuclease (approximately 150 kDa). While the majority of L1 inserts are truncated at the $5'$ end, around 80 members of the L1 families are full length and capable of transcription and translocation in another genome location (retrotransposition). L1 expression is rigorously regulated; methylation of the CpG-enriched promoter is the major suppressive mechanism.[37] While it was previously thought that L1 expression is mainly confined to germline, a growing body of evidence suggests its expression in several somatic tissues including rheumatoid arthritis synovial tissues and normal human brain.[38–40]

To investigate whether L1 over-expression from patients with SS could account for the increased expression of type I IFN, L1 and IFN-α were measured at both the messenger RNA and protein level in minor salivary gland tissues derived from patients with SS and controls with sicca symptoms. Two main observations were made: First, L1 messenger RNA and protein expression was increased in patients with benign SS (not complicated by lymphoma) compared to controls with sicca of a non-autoimmune origin. Second, a strong correlation between L1 and IFN-α transcripts was noted in salivary gland tissues. After L1 induction by human recombinant IFN-α was excluded in vitro, we showed that transfection of PDCs with a plasmid carrying L1 induced IFN-α production by those cells. Considering that methylation is a major controlling mechanism of L1 retroelements under physiological conditions, the transcript levels of a panel of methylating mediators previously shown to be implicated in methylation of repetitive elements was determined in minor salivary gland tissues derived from these patients. Coordinated expression of DNMT1, MeCP2 and DNMT3B, together with expression of L1, was observed, implying a compensating effort aimed at controlling inappropriate L1 responses in vivo.[35] Taken together, these findings highlight a significant role of epigenetic alterations in the induction of autoimmune processes, opening new avenues in our understanding of disease pathogenesis.

6 CONCLUSIONS

Over the past three decades, exogenous viruses or endogenous viral-like sequences have received continued attention as initiators and contributors of autoimmunity. Given the activation of the antiviral type I IFN pathway in systemic autoimmune disorders, the occurrence of disease exacerbations following viral infections and the presence of shared clinical manifestations between viral infections and autoimmune disease, the implication of viruses in the generation of autoimmunity has always been an attractive possibility. However, to date no single virus has been convincingly demonstrated to have a causal effect.

Because endogenous nucleic acids have been increasingly recognized as potent inducers of type I IFN responses through toll-like receptor-dependent or -independent pathways, impaired control of endogenous retrotransposable elements can provide a plausible explanation for the break of immune tolerance in patients with SS and other autoimmune diseases.

REFERENCES

1. Mavragani CP, Moutsopoulos HM. The geoepidemiology of Sjogren's syndrome. *Autoimmun Rev* 2010;**9**:A305–10.
2. Skopouli FN, Dafni U, Ioannidis JP, Moutsopoulos HM. Clinical evolution, and morbidity and mortality of primary Sjogren's syndrome. *Semin Arthritis Rheum* 2000;**29**:296–304.

3. Zintzaras E, Voulgarelis M, Moutsopoulos HM. The risk of lymphoma development in autoimmune diseases: a meta-analysis. *Arch Intern Med* 2005;**165**:2337–44.

4. Ioannidis JP, Vassiliou VA, Moutsopoulos HM. Long-term risk of mortality and lymphoproliferative disease and predictive classification of primary Sjogren's syndrome. *Arthritis Rheum* 2002;**46**:741–7.

5. Mavragani CP, Moutsopoulos HM. Sjogren's syndrome. *Can Med Assoc J* 2013;27.

6. Mavragani CP, Moutsopoulos HM. Sjogren's syndrome. *Annu Rev Pathol Mech Dis* 2014;**9**:273–85.

7. Yoshimi R, Ueda A, Ozato K, Ishigatsubo Y. Clinical and pathological roles of Ro/SSA autoantibody system. *Clin Dev Immunol* 2012;**2012**:606195.

8. Shiroki K, Isoyama T, Kuge S, Ishii T, Ohmi S, Hata S, et al. Intracellular redistribution of truncated La protein produced by poliovirus 3Cpro-mediated cleavage. *J Virol* 1999;**73**:2193–200.

9. Haneji N, Nakamura T, Takio K, Yanagi K, Higashiyama H, Saito I, et al. Identification of alpha-fodrin as a candidate autoantigen in primary Sjogren's syndrome. *Science* 1997;**276**:604–7.

10. Moutsopoulos HM, Steinberg AD, Fauci AS, Lane HC, Papadopoulos NM. High incidence of free monoclonal lambda light chains in the sera of patients with Sjogren's syndrome. *J Immunol* 1983;**130**:2663–5.

11. Moutsopoulos HM, Costello R, Drosos AA, Mavridis AK, Papadopoulos NM. Demonstration and identification of monoclonal proteins in the urine of patients with Sjogren's syndrome. *Ann Rheum Dis* 1985;**44**:109–12.

12. Tzioufas AG, Boumba DS, Skopouli FN, Moutsopoulos HM. Mixed monoclonal cryoglobulinemia and monoclonal rheumatoid factor cross-reactive idiotypes as predictive factors for the development of lymphoma in primary Sjogren's syndrome. *Arthritis Rheum* 1996;**39**:767–72.

13. Voulgarelis M, Skopouli FN. Clinical, immunologic, and molecular factors predicting lymphoma development in Sjogren's syndrome patients. *Clin Rev Allergy Immunol* 2007;**32**:265–74.

14. Tapinos NI, Polihronis M, Moutsopoulos HM. Lymphoma development in Sjogren's syndrome: novel p53 mutations. *Arthritis Rheum* 1999;**42**:1466–72.

15. Nezos A, Papageorgiou A, Fragoulis G, Ioakeimidis D, Koutsilieris M, Tzioufas AG, et al. B-cell activating factor genetic variants in lymphomagenesis associated with primary Sjogren's syndrome. *J Autoimmun* 2014;**51**:89–98.

16. Christodoulou MI, Kapsogeorgou EK, Moutsopoulos HM. Characteristics of the minor salivary gland infiltrates in Sjogren's syndrome. *J Autoimmun* 2010;**34**:400–7.

17. Tzioufas AG, Kapsogeorgou EK, Moutsopoulos HM. Pathogenesis of Sjogren's syndrome: what we know and what we should learn. *J Autoimmun* 2012;**39**:4–8.

18. Igoe A, Scofield RH. Autoimmunity and infection in Sjogren's syndrome. *Curr Opin Rheumatol* 2013;**25**:480–7.

19. Triantafyllopoulou A, Moutsopoulos H. Persistent viral infection in primary Sjogren's syndrome: review and perspectives. *Clin Rev Allergy Immunol* 2007;**32**:210–14.

20. Lee SJ, Lee JS, Shin MG, Tanaka Y, Park DJ, Kim TJ, et al. Detection of HTLV-1 in the labial salivary glands of patients with Sjogren's syndrome: a distinct clinical subgroup? *J Rheumatol* 2012;**39**:809–15.

21. Saito I, Servenius B, Compton T, Fox RI. Detection of Epstein-Barr virus DNA by polymerase chain reaction in blood and tissue biopsies from patients with Sjogren's syndrome. *J Exp Med* 1989;**169**:2191–8.

22. Fox RI, Pearson G, Vaughan JH. Detection of Epstein-Barr virus-associated antigens and DNA in salivary gland biopsies from patients with Sjogren's syndrome. *J Immunol* 1986;**137**:3162–8.

23. Venables PJ, Teo CG, Baboonian C, Griffin BE, Hughes RA. Persistence of Epstein-Barr virus in salivary gland biopsies from healthy individuals and patients with Sjogren's syndrome. *Clin Exp Immunol* 1989;**75**:359–64.

24. Merne ME, Syrjanen SM. Detection of Epstein-Barr virus in salivary gland specimens from Sjogren's syndrome patients. *Laryngoscope* 1996;**106**:1534–9.

25. Inoue H, Mishima K, Yamamoto-Yoshida S, Ushikoshi-Nakayama R, Nakagawa Y, Yamamoto K, et al. Aryl hydrocarbon receptor-mediated induction of EBV reactivation as a risk factor for Sjogren's syndrome. *J Immunol* 2012;**188**:4654–62.

26. Mariette X, Zerbib M, Jaccard A, Schenmetzler C, Danon F, Clauvel JP. Hepatitis C virus and Sjogren's syndrome. *Arthritis Rheum* 1993;**36**:280–1.

27. Arrieta JJ, Rodriguez-Inigo E, Ortiz-Movilla N, Bartolome J, Pardo M, Manzarbeitia F, et al. In situ detection of hepatitis C virus RNA in salivary glands. *Am J Pathol* 2001;**158**:259–64.

28. Koike K, Moriya K, Ishibashi K, Yotsuyanagi H, Shintani Y, Fujie H, et al. Sialadenitis histologically resembling Sjogren syndrome in mice transgenic for hepatitis C virus envelope genes. *Proc Natl Acad Sci USA* 1997;**94**:233–6.

29. Loustaud-Ratti V, Riche A, Liozon E, Labrousse F, Soria P, Rogez S, et al. Prevalence and characteristics of Sjogren's syndrome or Sicca syndrome in chronic hepatitis C virus infection: a prospective study. *J Rheumatol* 2001;**28**:2245–51.

30. Scott CA, Avellini C, Desinan L, Pirisi M, Ferraccioli GF, Bardus P, et al. Chronic lymphocytic sialoadenitis in HCV-related chronic liver disease: comparison of Sjogren's syndrome. *Histopathology* 1997;**30**:41–8.

31. Kordossis T, Paikos S, Aroni K, Kitsanta P, Dimitrakopoulos A, Kavouklis E, et al. Prevalence of Sjogren's-like syndrome in a cohort of HIV-1-positive patients: descriptive pathology and immunopathology. *Br J Rheumatol* 1998;**37**:691–5.

32. Terada K, Katamine S, Eguchi K, Moriuchi R, Kita M, Shimada H, et al. Prevalence of serum and salivary antibodies to HTLV-1 in Sjogren's syndrome. *Lancet* 1994;**344**:1116–19.

33. Talal N, Dauphinee MJ, Dang H, Alexander SS, Hart DJ, Garry RF. Detection of serum antibodies to retroviral proteins in patients with primary Sjogren's syndrome (autoimmune exocrinopathy). *Arthritis Rheum* 1990;**33**:774–81.

34. Sipsas NV, Gamaletsou MN, Moutsopoulos HM. Is Sjogren's syndrome a retroviral disease? *Arthritis Res Ther* 2011;**13**:212.

35. Mavragani CP, Crow MK. Activation of the type I interferon pathway in primary Sjogren's syndrome. *J Autoimmun* 2010;**35**:225–31.

36. Vakaloglou KM, Mavragani CP. Activation of the type I interferon pathway in primary Sjogren's syndrome: an update. *Curr Opin Rheumatol* 2011;**23**:459–64.

37. Crow MK. Long interspersed nuclear elements (LINE-1): potential triggers of systemic autoimmune disease. *Autoimmunity* 2010;**43**:7–16.

38. Babushok DV, Kazazian Jr HH. Progress in understanding the biology of the human mutagen LINE-1. *Hum Mutat* 2007;**28**:527–39.

39. Coufal NG, Garcia-Perez JL, Peng GE, Yeo GW, Mu Y, Lovci MT, et al. L1 retrotransposition in human neural progenitor cells. *Nature* 2009;**460**:1127–31.

40. Belancio VP, Roy-Engel AM, Pochampally RR, Deininger P. Somatic expression of LINE-1 elements in human tissues. *Nucleic Acids Res* 2010;**38**:3909–22.

CHAPTER 24

Viral Infection and Heart Disease: Autoimmune Mechanisms

Noel R. Rose[*,1], **Marina Afanasyeva**[†]
[*]Departments of Pathology and of Molecular Microbiology and Immunology, The Johns Hopkins Schools of Medicine and Public Health, Baltimore, Maryland, USA
[†]Department of Epidemiology and Community Medicine, Faculty of Medicine, University of Ottawa, Ottawa, Ontario, Canada
[1]Corresponding Author: nrrose@jhmi.edu

1 HUMAN MYOCARDITIS

1.1 Viral Etiology

According to the Dallas criteria, myocarditis is defined by the presence of an inflammatory infiltrate, as well as myocyte degeneration and necrosis of non-ischemic origin.[1] It was later suggested that the presence of myocardial necrosis was required for the diagnosis of acute, but not chronic, myocarditis.[2] Myocarditis is a major cause of sudden death in young adults.[3] In some individuals, myocarditis may evolve into chronic inflammatory dilated cardiomyopathy (DCM), which typically progresses to heart failure.[4] The 4-year case fatality rate of DCM is 46% in the absence of cardiac transplantation.[5] Although the etiology of myocarditis remains unknown in the majority of cases, clinical and epidemiologic evidence suggests an association with viral infection,[6] most often involving coxsackieviruses.[7] Other viruses reported to cause myocarditis include adenovirus, cytomegalovirus, human immunodeficiency virus, measles virus, mumps virus, hepatitis A and C viruses, Epstein-Barr virus, and human herpes virus 6. The role of parvovirus B19 has received considerable attention in recent years although recent evidence suggests it may serve as a bystander rather than an initiator of disease.[8]

Among coxsackieviruses, coxsackievirus B3 (CB3) has been frequently associated with myocarditis in the United States.[6] CB3, a small non-enveloped virus with a single-stranded positive-sense RNA, is an enterovirus within the *Picornaviridae* family. It is typically a cytolytic virus. Synthesis of negative-sense RNA is required for viral replication but not for viral protein synthesis. Most coxsackievirus infections are either subclinical or present with mild upper

Infection and Autoimmunity
http://dx.doi.org/10.1016/B978-0-444-63269-2.00026-X

429

respiratory or gastrointestinal symptoms.[6] A small percentage of infected individuals demonstrate signs and symptoms of acute myocarditis. Evidence supporting the role of coxsackieviruses in the development of myocarditis and DCM comes from epidemiologic, serologic, and viral studies demonstrating an association between recent coxsackievirus infection and subsequent cardiomyopathy.[9,10] Heart-reactive antibodies are found in many patients,[10,11] and viral RNA has been isolated from cardiac tissue of patients with myocarditis and DCM.[12] These studies have also demonstrated that a small proportion of patients with DCM have an actively replicating virus in the heart, as detected by the presence of minus-strand RNA. Many patients, however, have only positive-strand RNA, indicating the presence of a latent virus.

1.2 Evidence for Autoimmunity

A body of indirect evidence points to an important role for autoimmunity in myocarditis and DCM.[13] Although the mechanism for induction of cardiac-specific autoimmunity following infection by multiple viruses is still not completely understood, clinical and epidemiologic evidence suggests the involvement of both cardiac antigen-specific (e.g., through increased antigen expression by injured heart cells) and non–antigen-specific (adjuvant) effects. The latter could explain the fact that a number of widely different viruses can induce the same cardiac pathology. These non–antigen-specific effects are likely mediated by a set of alarmins, potent mediators of inflammation, released in response to infection and/or tissue injury.[14]

1.2.1 Autoantibodies

The presence of cardiac autoantibodies in patients with myocarditis provided the initial hint that an autoimmune response accompanied myocarditis. Some of the autoantibodies are specific for the α- and β-isoforms of cardiac myosin (CM) heavy chain.[15–17] Other autoantibodies described in patients with myocarditis are directed to mitochondrial antigens, such as adenine nucleotide translocator and the branched-chain α-ketoacid dehydrogenase,[18,19] as well to cardiac receptors such as β1-adrenoreceptor and M2 muscarinic receptor.[20,21] Of special interest is the recent finding of antibodies to troponin I, a cardiac-specific antigen, but not troponin T.[22,23]

An important question that arises from these reports is whether cardiac-specific antibodies mediate disease or represent a marker, or epiphenomenon, resulting from cardiac damage to cardiomyocytes. The findings that autoantibodies are detected in family members of patients with DCM years before the development of disease takes on special importance when one considers autoantibodies as predictors of oncoming autoimmune disease.[24] Myocardial infarction also leads to the production of cardiac–specific antibodies (Dressler syndrome).[25]

It has been shown that anti–receptor antibodies in the immunoglobulin (Ig) G3 subclass, particularly anti–β1 adrenoreceptor, either stimulate or block the receptor, thereby affecting cardiomyocyte contractility.[26] Striking beneficial effects of IgG3 immunoadsorption in patients with DCM with high titers of anti–β1 receptor have been reported.[27] Similarly, a randomized study by Felix et al.[28] showed a significant and long-lasting hemodynamic improvement in patients with DCM treated with immunoadsorption compared to controls.

1.2.2 Therapy

At present, most patients with myocarditis or DCM are treated with supportive therapy. If the disease does not remit spontaneously, cardiac transplantation is often indicated. Increasing effort is being directed towards developing treatment based on the etiology of the disease.[29] The pathway to appropriate treatment may depend upon the use of endomyocardial biopsy combined with polymerase chain reaction for viral genomes. Patients with evidence of viral infection may benefit from the use of antiviral treatments such as type 1 interferons (IFNs).[30] If an active viral infection has been ruled out by biopsy, immunosuppressive therapy may be considered.[31] Because biopsy is not widely used, the development of other non–invasive clinical markers to predict responses to immunosuppressive therapy is of paramount significance.

2 ANIMAL MODELS

2.1 CB3-Induced Myocarditis

To better understand the pathologic mechanisms of infection–associated autoimmune disease, we established an animal model of myocarditis. Following CB3 inoculation, mice develop an acute, inflammatory focal myocarditis with a mixed cellular infiltrate and cardiomyocyte damage, peaking in about 7 days after infection.[32] The severity of the acute disease varies widely among strains of mice and is associated with the appearance of neutralizing antibody in the serum.[33,34] Inflammation in the myocardium gradually subsides by day 21, when typically there is no histologic evidence of myocarditis. Some strains of mice, however, such as A/J and BALB/c, and their benchmark congenics, progress to the late chronic phase of myocarditis, peaking around day 35 after infection.[35–37] The course of CB3-induced myocarditis resembles human disease since the majority of humans recover from the acute viral disease without immunopathic sequelae, but a small fraction of predisposed individuals, similar to susceptible strains of mice, develop a late autoimmune disease.

Histologically, the late chronic phase of myocarditis in mice differs from the early acute disease. It is characterized by diffuse, rather than focal, leukocyte infiltration with signs of cardiomyocyte "drop out" and fibrosis. The acute viral phase is characterized by the presence of infectious virus in the heart, whereas during the chronic phase no infectious virus can be found, although viral RNA is often present. The two phases of myocarditis also differ in terms of the associated autoantibody profiles. Early after CB3 infection, there is a moderate increase in the natural IgM antibody that binds CM but cross-reacts with skeletal and brain myosin. Those mice that develop the autoimmune phase produce additional cardiac-specific, non-cross-reactive IgG antibody, with the α-isoform of CM heavy chain as the primary cardiac antigen.[38] This is the predominant CM heavy chain isoform in adult mouse ventricles. Adult human ventricles, on the other hand, predominantly express the β-isoform. In BALB/c mice, these antibodies are mainly of IgG1 subclass. The presence of CM-specific IgG in the serum represents another common feature of the disease in mice and humans.[38]

2.2 CM-Induced Experimental Autoimmune Myocarditis

The predominant autoantibody response to CM led to the hypothesis that an autoimmune response to CM is responsible for ongoing, chronic myocarditis. To test this hypothesis, we injected several strains of mice with either an emulsion of purified mouse CM in complete Freund adjuvant (CFA), or with mouse skeletal myosin in CFA, or with CFA alone.[39] CM, but not skeletal myosin or adjuvant alone, produced inflammation in the heart resembling that characteristic of the autoimmune phase of CB3-induced myocarditis. Remarkably, the same strains of mice that progressed to the chronic phase of myocarditis following CB3 infection developed myocarditis following injection with CM. Conversely, the strains of mice that were not susceptible to late-phase CB3-induced myocarditis did not develop disease following injection with CM. This finding suggested common genetic predisposing factors in the two models of myocarditis.

Both CB3- and CM-induced models have been extensively used to study the pathogenesis of autoimmune myocarditis. The CB3 model is irreplaceable for studies of viral virulence, viral entry and interaction between the virus and the cardiomyocyte. The CM-induced disease (the experimental autoimmune myocarditis [EAM] model) is valuable to investigate in depth the immunopathic phenomena in the absence of viral inflammation.

2.3 Other Models of Myocarditis

Similar to human myocarditis, which can be caused by viruses other than coxsackievirus, murine myocarditis can also be induced by murine cytomegalovirus (MCMV) and encephalomyocarditis virus (EMCB).[37–40] A/J and BALB/c mice, which are susceptible to CB3- and CM-induced autoimmune disease, develop both acute and chronic myocarditis following MCMV infection, whereas C57BL/6 mice, resistant to CB3-induced autoimmune disease, develop only the acute phase of MCMV myocarditis. The chronic phase of MCMV myocarditis is also characterized by the presence of CM-specific IgG in serum. EMCV infection produces myocarditis in susceptible mice (e.g. BALB/c and DBA/2) with distinct acute and chronic phases.

Kodama et al.[41] described a CM-induced model of myocarditis in Lewis rats. This model is characterized by the presence of giant cells in the myocardium, resembling human giant-cell myocarditis. Interestingly, A/J mice also develop giant cells and eosinophilic infiltrate in the heart upon CM immunization. The presence of giant cells and eosinophils correlates with disease severity.[42] In human disease, the presence of large numbers of giant cells and eosinophils is a dire diagnostic sign. In several strains of mice, disease-producing epitopes from CM heavy chain have been successfully used to reproduce EAM; one of them is a 19-amino acid peptide (myosin heavy chain $\alpha[334–352]$), which binds to I-A^k and produces severe myocarditis in A/J mice.[43] Immunization with troponin I induces myocarditis in A/J but not resistant C57BL/10-strains.[44]

2.4 Genetic Susceptibility to Myocarditis

2.4.1 Major Histocompatibility Complex Class II Association

The influence of the major histocompatibility complex (MHC) has been well established from studies of patients with DCM.[45] Several studies showed an association of DCM with MHC class II haplotypes, especially human leukocyte antigen DR4. The MHC haplotype association with DCM, however, varies depending on the ethnic background.

The role of the class II MHC haplotype is further supported by studies in mice. A/J, A.CA, and A.SW mice that share the same haplotype develop moderate to severe myocarditis following either CB3 infection or immunization with CM heavy chain peptide, whereas A.BY mice, which differ only in their *H-2* genes, develop mild or no disease.

2.4.2 Non-MHC Gene Associations

About 30% of DCM cases in humans are reported to be caused by mutations in non-MHC genes, suggesting that they may be due to deficiencies in immunoregulation. In experiments using mice that share the MHC haplotype, it was shown clearly that multiple non-MHC genes are pertinent to the expression of disease.[46,47] Two prominent non-MHC loci on murine chromosomes 1 and 6, referred to as *eam-11* and *eam-2*, respectively, influence the severity of autoimmune myocarditis.[48,49] These loci also are implicated in a number of other autoimmune disease models in mice, such as lupus, multiple sclerosis and type 1 diabetes, suggesting that similar immunoregulatory genes control multiple autoimmune diseases.

2.4.3 Sex-Based Differences

Unlike most autoimmune diseases, myocarditis is more prevalent and more severe in male patients.[50] Similarly, in mice, Frisancho-Kiss et al.[51] showed that the greater myocardial inflammation in male BALB/c mice was not related to increased viral replication in the heart but was associated with increased production of cytokines interleukin (IL)-1β, IL-18, and tumor necrosis factor (TNF)-α. Roberts et al.[52] studied sex differences in male and female C57BL/6 mice and reported that regulatory T cells were suppressed by Toll-like receptor (TLR) signaling in male but not female animals. Thus, sex-based differences in myocarditis induced by CB3 may be related to differences in immunoregulatory mechanisms.

3 DISEASE PROGRESSION: FROM VIRAL ENTRY TO HEART FAILURE

3.1 Early Events

Coxsackieviruses are known to enter cells via coxsackievirus–adenovirus receptor (CAR). As can be inferred from the name, this receptor is also important for cellular entry by adenoviruses, another group of viruses associated with myocarditis and DCM. It has been shown that the expression of CAR is low in normal hearts but is upregulated in the hearts of patients with

DCM.[53] Similarly, upregulation of CAR has been observed in rat models of EAM and myocardial infarction.[54,55] Decay accelerating factor, or CD55, represents a coreceptor for CB3 entry.[56]

Liu et al.[57] demonstrated in a mouse model that the sarcoma family kinase p56^{lck} is required for the effective CB3 replication, persistence and ability to cause myocarditis. The presence of p56^{lck} in T cells was sufficient to restore susceptibility to myocarditis in p56^{lck}-deficient mice. This study suggested the importance of T cells for CB3 delivery to the heart. Others showed that enteroviruses replicate in leukocytes, which may serve as carriers, promoting viral spread to different organs.[56]

Opavsky et al.[58] showed that activation of extracellular signal-regulated kinases 1 and 2 (ERK-1/2) downstream of p56^{lck} is important for viral replication in both T cells and cardiomyocytes. The authors suggested that ERK-1/2 activation might be linked to disease susceptibility based on the observation that such activation was more pronounced in the hearts of susceptible A/J mice compared to resistant C57BL/6. Luo et al.[59] also found that ERK-1/2 activation is important for CB3 replication and virulence.

3.2 Innate Immunity

The innate immune system protects the host against invading pathogens by prompt recognition of pathogen-associated molecular patterns. Sometimes the innate immune response eliminates a pathogen, but in most cases the adaptive immune response finishes the job. Innate immunity sets the stage for and determines the quality of the adaptive immune response. We found that there is a distinct difference in the innate immune response of susceptible and resistant strains of mice to CB3 infection and that this difference predicts the subsequent susceptibility of the mouse strain to autoimmune myocarditis. Susceptible animals develop earlier and significantly greater production of TNF-α and IL-1β in the heart. These differences were observed within 6 hours after infection.[60] The enhanced response in susceptible mice is reminiscent of the Dienes effect, which showed that the co-administration of *Mycobacterium tuberculosis* expanded the immune response, as demonstrated by increased delayed hypersensitivity reactions.[61] Thus, we found that induction of EAM with whole CM or cardiac myosin peptide requires co-administration with CFA containing a mycobacterial component. Although CM with incomplete adjuvant induces an antibody response, inflammatory lesions are not present in the heart. We suggest that infection itself can be considered an adjuvant for the induction of pathogenic autoimmunity. The decision of whether viral invasion proceeds to autoimmune disease depends upon the initial steps in activation of innate immunity involving activation through TLRs. As a single-stranded RNA virus, CB3 directly activates TLR3. Deficiency of TLR3 is associated with increased viral proliferation and higher mortality after infection.[62]

The critical role of early products of inflammation, TNF-α and IL-1β, is supported by the demonstration that blocking either one of these early cytokines prevents the development of autoimmune myocarditis, even in genetically susceptible strains. Furthermore, administration of recombinant TNF-α or recombinant IL-1β, along with CB3, induces myocarditis in normally resistant C57BL/10 mice. These findings show that a potent adjuvant can overcome relative genetic resistance to autoimmune disease.[63,64]

The mechanism by which IL-1β operates to determine an oncoming autoimmune response is not clearly understood. A recent study by Valaperti et al.[65] shows that the activation during innate immunity of IL-1 receptor-associated kinase 4 exacerbates CB3-induced myocarditis by impairing production of IFN regulatory factor and reducing macrophage localization. Monocytes and macrophages are key cells in directing the initiation of autoimmune heart disease.[66]

3.2.1 Lipopolysaccharide as Adjuvant

Lipopolysaccharide (LPS) of gram-negative bacteria represents another classic pathogen-associated molecular pattern that is recognized by TLR4 as well as CD14, which are expressed in the myocardium. LPS affects the susceptibility of mice to myocarditis since co-treatment with LPS makes typically resistant B10.A mice susceptible to CB3-induced autoimmune myocarditis with associated high titers of CM-specific IgG antibody.[63] Expression of TLR4 in the heart correlates with viral replication in human myocarditis.[67] In a mouse model, TLA4 deficiency resulted in reduced myocarditis and reduced viral multiplication in the heart on day 12 after infection despite significant CB3 replication in the heart on day 2 after infection, suggesting enhanced viral clearance or less proinflammatory environment in the absence of TLR4.[68] In support of the latter view, TLR4 activation increases IL-1β and IL-18. Abston et al.[69] showed that TLR3 deficient mice developed an IL-4-dominant T-cell response indicative of Th2 polarization, showing that the innate immune response qualitatively affects the adaptive response and subsequent autoimmune myocarditis.

3.2.2 Complement

Complement, a major component of the innate immune response, also affects the susceptibility of mice to developing myocarditis. Anderson et al.[70] showed that complement component C3 interacts with capsid proteins of CB3. This interaction triggers the alternative complement pathway. The authors proposed that C3 interaction with CB3 might be important for limiting viral load by retention of the virus in the spleen in an antibody-dependent fashion. Experiments using the CB3 model of myocarditis demonstrated a difference in response to C3 depletion with cobra venom factor between strains; decreased inflammation was found in DBA/2 mice, but not BALB/c mice, upon administration of cobra venom, as assessed on day 7 after infection.[71] Neither strain exhibited changes in viral load in the heart in response to cobra venom treatment. The authors suggested that the treatment mainly affected the antibody response and therefore had an effect in DBA/2 mice, which have mainly antibody-mediated disease, but not in BALB/c mice, which demonstrate a more pronounced cellular autoimmunity.

C3 has been shown to be critical for the development of autoimmune myocarditis in the A/J CM model. Administration of cobra venom factor to mice that were injected with CM resulted in impaired IgG antibody responses to CM and prevented myocarditis.[72] Depletion of C3 at the time of initiation, rather than progression of disease, was critical since multiple injections of cobra venom factor between days 1 and 9 after immunization, but not between days 10 and 18, prevented myocarditis. A major product generated during activation of the complement cascade is C3d, which acts mainly through two complement receptors: CR1 (or CD35) and CR2 (or CD21). The incidence and severity of disease are significantly reduced in CR1/CR2 double knockout (KO) mice compared with wild-type mice. Similarly, blockade of CR1 and CR2 during the time of CM immunization with a monoclonal antibody (mAb), which binds to the extracellular domain shared by the two receptors, abrogated disease, dramatically reduced the production of CM-specific IgG and was associated with decreased production of IL-1 and TNF-α by splenocytes cultured with CM. CR1 and CR2 have been shown to be present on a subset of activated/memory $CD44^{high}CD62L^{low}$ T cells and their engagement triggers T-cell responses, implicating complement as an important player not only in antibody-mediated but also in T-cell-mediated autoimmunity.[73]

3.2.3 Natural Killer Cells

Natural killer (NK) cells, another participant in the innate immune response, can directly kill their target cells and represent a rich source of cytokines, which in turn can influence the inflammatory milieu and affect the adaptive immune response. Godeny and Gauntt[74] showed that NK cells limit CB3 replication. Depletion of $NK1.1^{+}$ cells exacerbated acute myocarditis induced in mice with MCMV.[36] IL-18 augments NK cell activity, and its administration has been shown to improve survival, reduce viral load and decrease myocarditis in a murine model of EMCV-induced acute myocarditis.[75] The therapeutic effect of IL-18 was associated with increased NK cell activity in the spleen. The role of NK cells in the development of the autoimmune phase of myocarditis has been clarified in our recent experiments. Depletion of NK cells leads to enhancement of EAM, confirming their suppressor function. Moreover, the disease is marked by the presence of numerous eosinophils, pointing to activation of a Th2 response.

3.2.4 γδ T Cells

T cells expressing γ and δ chains of the T-cell receptor (TCR) have been shown to accumulate in the myocardium during fulminant myocarditis in humans.[76] Huber et al.[77,78] demonstrated that $\gamma\delta^{+}$ T cells comprise between 5% and 20%, and in some cases up to 50%, of the acute inflammatory cell infiltrate in the heart of CB3-infected mice. Upon CB3 infection of mice, depletion of $\gamma\delta^{+}$ T cells resulted in increased viral titers in the heart, indicating the importance of these cells in controlling viral replication.[79] $\gamma\delta^{+}$ T cells, particularly $\gamma4^{+}$ T cells, have been shown to be important in susceptibility to myocarditis induced by CB3. These cells can recognize MHC class I-like CD1d molecules, and this recognition has been proposed to mediate the susceptibility to CB3-induced myocarditis. CD1d-deficient mice developed minimal myocardial inflammation with no significant changes in the cardiac viral titers upon CB3 infection,[80] but this effect could not be explained by the lack of NK T-cell response, since mice deficient in invariant $J\alpha281$ gene, which is expressed in NK T cells, were highly susceptible to myocarditis. Therefore, it was suggested that the lack of $\gamma4^{+}$ T-cell response was responsible for the reduction in myocarditis.

3.2.5 Type 1 IFNs

Type 1 IFNs, α and β, are associated with early innate immune responses and represent a part of antiviral defence system. IFN-β treatment of patients with inflammatory cardiomyopathy associated with left ventricular (LV) dysfunction and the presence of either enteroviral or adenoviral genomes in the myocardium resulted in improvement of LV function and clearance of viral genomes.[81] In a small randomized clinical trial, Miric et al.[82] showed beneficial effects of IFN-α treatment in patients with idiopathic myocarditis and idiopathic DCM. There have been additional reports of successful treatment of enterovirus-induced myocarditis with IFN-α.[83] The importance of type 1 IFNs were demonstrated in a murine model of B3-induced myocarditis in which mice deficient for type 1 IFNs showed increased mortality within 2 to 4 days after infection.[84] Oral treatment with type 1 IFNs suppressed the inflammatory response in MCMV-induced myocarditis in mice.[85]

3.3 Adaptive Immunity
3.3.1 T Cells

Autoimmune myocarditis is primarily a T-cell-mediated disease. Endomyocardial biopsies from patients with myocarditis and idiopathic DCM show infiltration with $CD4^+$ and $CD8^+$ T cells. Transfer of peripheral blood leukocytes from patients with myocarditis and impaired LV function to mice with severe combined immunodeficiency (SCID) resulted in myocardial infiltration with human leukocytes and impaired LV function.[86,87] Omerovic et al.[88] found that transfer of peripheral blood lymphocytes from patients with DCM to SCID mice induced myocardial fibrosis and deterioration of LV function, as assessed by increased LV dimensions on echocardiography, 75 days after transfer.

Upon CB3 infection, CD4-deficient mice exhibited reduced myocardial infiltration and necrosis but the same survival as the control mice.[89] In the same study, CD8 deficiency increased the severity of disease in terms of both myocardial pathology and survival. However, CD4/CD8 double-deficient mice, as well as TCR-β-deficient mice, showed improved survival and decreased myocarditis as observed during 28 days after infection. None of these deficiencies affected cardiac viral titers on day 7 after infection. Other studies also demonstrated the effects of the absence of either $CD4^+$ or $CD8^+$ T cells on the survival, severity of myocarditis and viral titers after CB3 infection.[90] Overall, the results are rather confusing since it is difficult to dissect the effects on viral replication, viral tropism and inflammatory response in the heart. The possibility that lymphocytes can deliver CB3 to the heart further complicates the interpretation and underscores the complexity of the viral model.

Experiments by Smith and Allen[91] showed that CD4[+] T cells play a central role in the pathogenesis of CM-induced EAM. Depletion of CD4[+] T cells with mAb prevented the development of EAM, and transfer of CD4[+] T cells isolated from CM-immunized mice to immunologically deficient SCID mice reproduced the disease. The heart infiltrate in EAM has greater numbers of CD4[+] T cells compared to CD8[+] T cells.[92] The predominance of CD4[+] T cells persists to day 60 after immunization in BALB/c mice, but the ratio of CD4[+] to CD8[+] T cells in the myocardium decreases over time. During the chronic phase of EAM (around day 60 after immunization), the proportion of CD4[+] T cells within the total infiltrating leukocyte population correlates with systolic dysfunction and the development of large LV volumes, the hallmarks of DCM, suggesting the role of CD4[+] T cells in the development of cardiac dysfunction.[93]

The role of CD8[+] T cells in EAM is less well defined. It has been demonstrated that CD8 deficiency in mice leads to exacerbation of CM-induced myocarditis,[93] a finding similar to that in the CB3 model.[94] However, depletion of CD8[+] T cells with a mAb reduced the severity of EAM.[95] The ability of CD8[+] T cells to induce myocarditis was demonstrated in mice transgenically expressing an ovalbumin peptide in the heart under a cardiac-specific promoter.[96] These mice developed severe myocarditis upon the transfer of CD8[+] T cells from transgenic mice that expressed TCR specific for the ovalbumin peptide. In this system, IL-12 was thought to be crucial for pathogenicity of CD8[+] T cells.

3.3.2 B Cells and Antibody

The role of antibody in the development of myocarditis is less well characterized compared to the role of T cells. In both A/J and BALB/c mice, disease severity upon CM immunization correlates with CM-specific IgG1.[42] IgG1 is deposited in the heart, and clusters of IgG1-positive cells, which are most likely plasma cells, are found in the myocardial infiltrate on day 21 after immunization. While it is likely that antibody contributes to the pathogenesis of myocarditis, its role in disease initiation seems to vary among different strains of mice. Transfer of sera collected on day 21 after immunization in A. SW mice failed to induce myocarditis in A.SW recipients.[97] Liao et al.[98] demonstrated that the transfer of CM-specific mAb induced myocarditis in DBA/2 but not BALB/c mice. The authors found that DBA/2 mice, but not BALB/c mice, expressed myosin or myosin-like molecules in the extracellular matrix in the myocardium and offered this finding as a potential explanation for the strain difference. Furthermore, CM-specific IgM antibody failed to induce myocarditis in DBA/2 mice, and only CM-specific IgG was able to transfer the disease.[99] In another study using BALB/c mice deficient in B cells due to disruption in the IgM gene, B cells have been shown dispensable for the induction of CM-induced myocarditis.[100]

3.3.3 Monocytes/Macrophages

Macrophages are the most prominent cell in inflammatory myocarditis. Discerning their role in the disease process has proved difficult, however, because of the heterogeneity of these cells and the various roles they play in different stages of the disease process.[66] While usually considered part of the innate immune response, macrophages also are responsive to instruction from CD4 T cells and are major effectors in cell-mediated immunity.[101] Recent investigations distinguished at least two major subpopulations. Classically activated (M1) macrophages are induced during the innate immune response by TLR2 and TLR4 as well as IFN-δ, TNF-α, IL-1, and IL-6. They are involved in phagocytosis, antigen presentation, T-cell co-stimulation and production of reactive oxygen intermediates. By contrast, alternatively activated (M2) macrophages are induced by IL-4 and IL-13 and engage in wound healing, fibrosis and scavenger function. In addition, M2 macrophages or their subsets are engaged in T-cell suppression and the resolution of inflammation.

In EAM, myeloid lineage cells comprise the bulk of infiltrating leukocytes.[102] The majority express CDIIb, indicating their myeloid lineage, but do not express high levels of LY6C, excluding the possibility that they are neutrophils. During the course of EAM, however, influx of other inflammatory cells substantially diminishes the relative proportion of macrophages in the heart, with LYC6^{high} inflammatory macrophages peaking at day 14 after immunization, whereas LY6C^{low} resident macrophages are greatest on day 21. Macrophages and dendritic cells clearly orchestrate the activation of CD4$^+$ T cells and the selection of effector or suppressive mechanisms that determine both the course and severity of subsequent myocarditis.

3.4 Cytokine Regulation

Cytokines are the products of activation of both innate and adaptive immune cells and, therefore, can act early during disease initiation and later directing disease progression. For convenience, they often are classified as proinflammatory or anti-inflammatory, although the same cytokine can have vastly different functions, depending upon the prevailing cytokine profile.[103]

3.4.1 Th1 Cytokines

Our initial studies were carried out to determine the dependence of auto-immune myocarditis on the classical Th1 cytokines IL-12 and IFN-γ.[104] Mice deprived of the β1 chain of the major receptor for IL-12 signaling, IL-12R, were resistant to the development of myocarditis. The activation of signal transducer and activator of transcription (STAT) 4 is required for IL-12 signaling, and STAT4 KO mice also proved to be resistant to the disease. When it did occur in STAT4 KO mice, however, inflammation was marked by a shift to a predominantly Th2 profile. To confirm directly that IL-12 enhanced myocarditis of BALB/c mice (which are intermediate responders), these mice were treated with recombinant IL-12 during disease induction and developed enhanced myocarditis. These experiments show that autoimmune myocarditis can be initiated and enhanced by IL-12-induced Th1 T cells.

We next explored the role of IFN-γ in experimental autoimmune myo-carditis. Unexpectedly, blocking IFN-γ with an antibody or immunizing genetically IFN-γ-deprived mice resulted in a severe form of myocarditis and progression to DCM.[104] These experiments show that IFN-γ and IL-12, the classical Th1 cytokines, can have opposite effects in myocarditis.

There are a number of possible mechanisms by which IFN-γ can regu-late autoimmune myocarditis,[105] and the possibility considered initially is that diminution of a Th1 response enhances Th17 responses. This issue is discussed in section 3.4.3. Other possible factors are control of apoptosis of activated lymphocytes by IFN-γ. There is experimental evidence in both myocarditis studies as well as other autoimmune diseases that IFN-γ can directly regulate caspase-8 expression and promote apoptotic pathways. Finally, IFN-γ is produced by a number of cells known to be protective in EAM, including NK cells, as well as subsets of CD8$^+$ T cells, macrophages and dendritic cells.

3.4.2 Th2 Cytokines

In the CM model using A/J mice, the analysis of histopathological (presence of eosinophils and giant cells) and immunological (correlation of disease with CM-specific IgG1 and upregulation of total IgE responses) profiles has revealed a Th2-like phenotype, suggesting a pathogenic role for IL-4, which is important for eosinophil recruitment and IgG1 class switch.[44] In support of a disease-promoting role of IL-4, treatment with an anti-IL-4 mAb reduced the severity of EAM in A/J mice and induced a shift from a Th2-like to a Th1-like phenotype. Such a shift was demonstrated by suppressed IgE and IgG1 responses; upregulated IgG2a response; suppressed production of IL-4, IL-5, and IL-13 and increased production of IFN-γ by cultured splenocytes in response to in vitro stimulation with CM.[44] At the same time, IL-4Rα KO mice on a BALB/c background do not demonstrate reduced severity of EAM and seem to develop the disease earlier compared to the wild-type controls.[106]

Since IL-13, another Th2 cytokine, signals through the same receptor subunit,[107] we explored its role in the development of autoimmune myocarditis. IL-13 protects BALB/c mice from myocarditis induced either by CM peptide or CB3 viral infection.[108] The disease in IL-13 deficient animals is characterized by increased leukocyte infiltration, elevated CM autoantibodies and greater cardiac fibrosis. Many of the IL-13 KO mice developed severe cardiomyopathy with impaired cardiac function and heart failure. The hearts of the IL-13-deficient mice had increased concentrations of proinflammatory cytokines IL-1β and IL-18 but not IL-17.

IL-10, which often is classified as a Th2 cytokine, primarily exerts immunoregulatory effects by inhibiting the activation and effector functions of T cells and antigen-presenting cells.[109] IL-10 suppresses CM-induced murine myocarditis, since an anti-IL-10 mAb treatment enhanced disease.[110] This effect was observed when IL-10 was blocked relatively late (starting on day 10 after immunization) but not early (between days 0 and 12), suggesting that IL-10 is more important during the resolution rather than initiation of disease. IL-10 blockade also prevented suppression of EAM induced by nasal tolerance with intranasal administration of CM before immunization, implicating IL-10 as a mediator of mucosal tolerance.[110,111] Watanabe et al.[112] demonstrated the disease-suppressive effect of IL-10 in a rat model of EAM by delivering IL-10-expressing plasmid vector via electroporation into the tibialis anterior muscles. Treatment with recombinant IL-10 improved the outcomes in viral myocarditis induced by EMCV without any effects on the viral load in the myocardium.[113] These results suggest that IL-10, similar to IFN-γ, can be beneficial, regardless of whether the viral or autoimmune component predominates.

3.4.3 Th17 Cytokines

We previously pointed out that IL-12Rβ1 was essential for development of autoimmune myocarditis. The result initially suggested that Th1 responses were mainly responsible for autoimmune myocarditis. However, IFN-γ, the prototypic cytokine of Th1 response, actually down-regulated the severity of disease. In searching for an explanation for this paradox, we took into consideration the report that IL-23 also acted through the IL-12 receptor. The two cytokines share the same p40 subunit, but IL-12 has a p35 subunit, whereas IL-23 possesses a unique p19.[114] BALB/c mice deficient in the p40 subunit were completely protected from the disease, whereas p35-deficient mice were comparable to wild-type controls. Furthermore, when p40 KO mice were reconstituted with IL-23, they developed severe autoimmune myocarditis. On day 21, the peak time of myocarditis approximately equal number of cells producing IL-17A (the prototypic Th17 cytokine) and IFN-γ (the signature of Th1) were present in the heart, indicating that both lineages contributed to the histologic picture of disease. Functionally adoptive transfer experiments clearly showed that Th1 cells induced only mild myocarditis in recipients, whereas IL-17-polarized cells induced severe disease with extensive infiltration.

Since production of IL-17 is the hallmark of Th17 responses, we tested the effect of inhibiting IL-17A as well as other Th17 family members, IL-17 F and IL-22. Unexpectedly, injection of anti-IL-17A mAb produced little or no reduction in the incidence or severity of myocarditis.[114] Anti-IL-17 F mAb produced only a modest decrease in disease, whereas neutralization of IL-22 by mAb significantly enhanced the severity of myocarditis, showing that IL-22 had a protective effect.

Although inhibiting IL-17A did not significantly reduce the incidence and severity of inflammation, we found that IL-17A deficient animals did not develop DCM.[114] Thus, IL-17A is not required for development of the inflammatory phase of autoimmune myocarditis but is required for the later development of a life-threatening cardiac remodeling. In fact, administration of antibody to IL-17A during the inflammatory disease prevented the development of DCM in wild-type mice.

IL-17A is important mainly for the development of myocardial fibrosis evident as early as 18 days after immunization with CM. It facilitates production of matrix metalloproteinase (MMP)-2 and MMP-9,[114] the two MMPs that are primarily associated with cardiac remodeling.

Since IFN-γ-deficient mice develop unusually severe EAM, whereas IL-17A deficient mice are protected from later development of DCM, we tested BALB/c mice deficient in both cytokines. Unexpectedly, the double KO mice developed a rapidly fatal severe myocarditis in which eosinophils constituted about one third of the infiltrating leukocytes.[115] This eosinophilic disease represents the most severe phenotype of EAM reported to date. IL-17A signaling acts to increase the production of neutrophils and decrease production of IL-4 and IL-13 in IFN-γ-deficient mice. Eosinophils seem to play a primary role in the lethality of this disease since degranulated eosinophils are conspicuous in the inflammatory infiltrates. Eosinophil deficient double KO mice developed severe cardiac infiltration had improved survival.

4 MOLECULAR MIMICRY VERSUS MYOCYTE DAMAGE

The potential mechanisms of how CB3 or other cardiotropic viruses trigger the autoimmune response have been extensively reviewed in the literature.[116] Despite numerous attempts to study these mechanisms, they remain unclear. For some time, the molecular mimicry hypothesis attracted much attention, and investigators have sought evidence to support it. The concept of molecular mimicry implies that the infecting microorganisms share an epitope with the tissues of the host. For example, infection by β-hemolytic streptococci induces an antibody that cross-reacts with streptococcal M protein and CM.[117] It was shown that an antibody can cross-react with both CM and CB3.[118] However, the comparison of CB3 sequence with that of CM failed to demonstrate any significant sequence identity, suggesting a low likelihood for cross-reactivity at a T-cell level.[119] Massilamany et al.[120] recently pointed out that the peptide sequence of CM heavy chain α that induces autoimmune myocarditis in A/J mice is mimicked in a large number of natural sources, including many bacteria and even corn (*Zea mays*), which have no known relationship to myocarditis. Significantly, autoimmune myocarditis was not induced by immunizing A/J mice with most mimicry epitopes beyond the infiltrates expected with the injection of Freund adjuvant alone.

Horwitz et al.[121] demonstrated the pivotal role of direct viral damage to the heart in triggering myocarditis. In this study, non-obese diabetic mice with a pancreas-specific transgenic expression of IFN-γ were infected with CB3. They developed pancreatitis but no myocarditis, despite the production of heart-specific IgG. The authors concluded that myocarditis could occur only if the virus infected the heart and the presence of extensive viral infection elsewhere did not initiate the autoimmune process in the heart through molecular mimicry.

CB3 induction of autoimmune myocarditis provides us with the most complete model for understanding a mechanism by which a viral infection could induce autoimmune disease. The virus has the capability of providing the first antigen-specific signal either through molecular mimicry or as suggested originally by Gauntt et al.[122] by damage to the cardiomyocyte. Infection also produces the non-antigen-specific second signal in the form of alarmins. This topic is discussed more extensively in Chapter 1.

5 CONCLUSION

Despite a great deal of effort to understand the nature of virus-triggered inflammatory heart disease, the processes that underlie the progression from viral infection to an autoimmune disease and finally to cardiomyopathy and heart failure remain poorly understood. Animal models provide an opportunity to study the complex phenomena of viral entry and replication, immune response to the viral infection, autoimmune response to cardiac antigens, the role of individual inflammatory components in disease progression, the nature of cardiac remodeling in response to viral damage and inflammation and the development of cardiac dysfunction. A better knowledge of each of these stages of disease is needed to improve therapeutic interventions. Translation of the research findings into clinically meaningful data also requires an understanding of the advantages and limitations of individual animal models, formulation of hypotheses based on the basic research findings and careful design of clinical trials to address these hypotheses.

ACKNOWLEDGMENTS

We acknowledge the contributions of David Kass to the studies of cardiac function and of DeLisa Fairweather to the studies of CB3-induced myocarditis. This research was supported by National Institutes of Health research grants HL113008, HL077611, HL067290.

REFERENCES

1. Aretz HT, Billingham ME, Edwards WD, et al. Myocarditis: a histopathologic definition and classification. *Am J Cardiovasc Pathol* 1987;**1**:3–14.
2. Maisch B, Portig I, Ristic A, Hufnagel G, Pankuweit S. Definition of inflammatory cardiomyopathy (myocarditis): on the way to consensus: a status report. *Herz* 2000;**25**:200–9.
3. Maron BJ, Doerer JJ, Haas TS, Tierney DM, Mueller FO. Sudden deaths in Young competitive athletes: analysis of 1866 deaths in the United States, 1980-2006. *Circulation* 2009;**119**:1085–92.
4. Sagar S, Liu PP, Cooper LT. Myocarditis. *Lancet* 2012;**379**(9817):738–47.
5. Kawai C. From myocarditis to cardiomyopathy: mechanisms of inflammation and cell death: learning from the past for the future. *Circulation* 1999;**99**(8):1091–100.
6. Whitton JL. Immunopathology during coxsackievirus infection. *Springer Semin Immunopathol* 2002;**24**(2):201–13.
7. Riecansky I, Schreinerova Z, Egnerova A, Petrovicova A, Bzduchova O. Incidence of coxsackie virus infections in patients with dilated cardiomyopathy. *Cor Vasa* 1989;**31**(3):225–30.
8. Koepsell SA, Anderson DR, Radio SJ. Provovirus B19 is a bystander in adult myocarditis. *Cardiovasc Pathol* 2012;**21**:476–81.

9. Muir P, Nicholson F, Illavia SJ, McNeil TS, Ajetunmobi JF, Dunn H, et al. Serological and molecular evidence of enterovirus infection in patients with end-stage dilated cardiomyopathy. *Heart* 1996;**76**(3):243–9.

10. Deguchi H, Fujioka S, Terasaki F, Ukimura A, Hirasawa M, Kintaka T, et al. Enterovirus RNA replication in cases of dilated cardiomyopathy: light microscopic *in situ* hybridization and virological analyses of myocardial specimens obtained at partial left ventriculectomy. *J Card Surg* 2001;**16**(1):64–71.

11. Cambridge G, MacArthur CG, Waterson AP, Goodwin JF, Oakley CM. Antibodies to coxsackie B viruses in congestive cardiomyopathy. *Br Heart J* 1979;**41**(6):692–6.

12. Fujioka S, Kitaura Y, Ukimura A, Delguchi H, Kawamura K, Isomura T, et al. Evaluation of viral infection in the myocardium of patients with idiopathic dilated cardiomyopathy. *J Am Coll Cardiol* 2000;**36**(6):1920–6.

13. Reddy J, Massilamany C, Buskiewicz I, Huber SA. Autoimmunity in viral myocarditis. *Curr Opin Rev* 2013;**25**(4):502–8.

14. Chan JK, Roth J, Oppenheim JJ, Tracey KJ, Vogl T, Feldmann M, et al. Alarmins: awaiting a clinical response. *J Clin Invest* 2012;**122**(8):2711–19.

15. Latif N, Baker CS, Dunn MJ, Rose ML, Brady P, Yacoub MH. Frequency and specificity of antiheart antibodies in patients with dilated cardiomyopathy detected using SDS-PAGE and western blotting. *J Am Coll Cardiol* 1993;**22**(5):1378–84.

16. Goldman JH, Keeling PJ, Warraich RS, Baig MK, Redwood SR, Dalla LL, et al. Autoimmunity to alpha myosin in a subset of patients with idiopathic dilated cardiomyopathy. *Br Heart J* 1995;**74**(6):598–603.

17. Warraich RS, Dunn MJ, Yacoub MH. Subclass specificity of autoantibodies against myosin in patients with idiopathic dilated cardiomyopathy: pro-inflammatory antibodies in DCM patients. *Biochem Biophys Res Commun* 1999;**259**(2):255–61.

18. Schulze K, Schultheiss HP. The role of the ADP/ATP carrier in the pathogenesis of viral heart disease. *Eur Heart J* 1995;**16**(Suppl O):64–7.

19. Ansari AA, Neckelmann N, Villinger F, Leung P, Danner DJ, Brar SS, et al. Epitope mapping of the branched chain alpha-ketoacid dehydrogenase dihydrolipoyl transacylase (BCKD-E2) protein that reacts with sera from patients with idiopathic dilated cardiomyopathy. *J Immunol* 1994;**153**(10):4754–65.

20. Magnusson Y, Wallukat G, Waagstein F, Hjalmarson A, Hoebeke J. Autoimmunity in idiopathic dilated cardiomyopathy. Characterization of antibodies against the beta 1-adrenoceptor with positive chronotropic effect. *Circulation* 1994;**89**(6):2760–7.

21. Fu LX, Magnusson Y, Bergh CH, Liljeqvist JA, Waagstein F, Jhalmarson A, et al. Localization of a functional autoimmune epitope on the muscarinic acetylcholine receptor-2 in patients with idiopathic dilated cardiomyopathy. *J Clin Invest* 1993;**91**(5):1964–8.

22. Kaya Z, Goser S, Buss SJ, Leuschner F, Ottl R, Li J, et al. Identification of cardiac troponin 1 sequence motifs leading to heart failure by induction of myocardial inflammation and fibrosis. *Circulation* 2008;**118**(20):2063–72.

23. Kaya Z, Katus HA, Rose NR. Cardiac troponins and autoimmunity: their role in the pathogenesis of myocarditis and of heart failure. *Clin Immunol* 2010;**134**(1):80–8.

24. Caforio AL, Vinci A, Lliceto S. Anti-heart autoantibodies in familiar dilated cardiomyopathy. *Autoimmunity* 2008;**41**(6):462–9.

25. Bendjelid K, Pugin J. Is Dressler syndrome dead? *Chest* 2004;**126**(5):1680–2.

26. Limas CJ, Limas C. Beta-adrenoceptor antibodies and genetics in dilated cardiomyopathy – an overview and review. *Eur Heart J* 1991;**12**(Suppl D):175–7.

27. Muller J, Wallukat G, Dandel M, Bieda H, Brandes K, Spiegelsberger S, et al. Immunoglobulin adsorption in patients with idiopathic dilated cardiomyopathy. *Circulation* 2000;**101**(4):385–91.

28. Felix SB, Staudt A, Dorffel WV, Stangl V, Merkel K, Pohl M, et al. Hemodynamic effects of immunoadsorption and subsequent immunoglobulin substitution in dilated

cardiomyopathy: three-month results from a randomized study. *J Am Coll Cardiol* 2000;**35**(6):1590–8.

29. Frustaci A, Russo MA, Chimenti C. Randomized study on the efficacy of immunosuppressive therapy in patients with virus-negative inflammatory Cardiomyopathy: the TIMIC study. *Eur Heart J* 2009;**30**(16):1995–2002.

30. Schultheiss H-P, Kuhl U, Cooper LT. The management of myocarditis. *Eur Heart J* 2011;**32**:2616–25.

31. Caforio AL, Pankuweit S, Arbustini E, Basso C, Gimeno-Blanes J, Felix SB, et al. Current state of knowledge on aetiology, diagnosis, management, and therapy of myocarditis: a position statement of the European Society of Cardiology Working Group on Myocardial and Pericardial Diseases. *Eur Heart J* 2013;**34**(33):2636–48.

32. Rose NR, Wolfgram LJ, Herskowitz A, Beisel KW. Postinfectious autoimmunity: two distinct phases of coxsackievirus B3-induced myocarditis. *Ann NY Acad Sci* 1986;**475**:146–56.

33. Herskowitz A, Beisel KW, Wolfgram LJ, Rose NR. Coxsackievirus B3 muring myocarditis: wide pathologic spectrum in genetically defined inbred strains. *Hum Pathol* 1985;**16**(7):671–3.

34. Wolfgram LJ, Beisel KW, Herskowitz A, Rose NR. Variations in the susceptibility to coxsackievirus B3-induced myocarditis among different strains of mice. *J Immunol* 1986;**136**(5):1846–52.

35. Rose NR, Beisel KW, Herskowitz A, Neu N, Wolfgram LJ, Alvarez FL, et al. Cardiac myosin and autoimmune myocarditis. *Ciba Found Symp* 1987;**129**:3–24.

36. Fairweather D, Kaya Z, Shellam GR, Lawson CM, Rose NR. From infection to autoimmunity. *J Autoimmun* 2001;**16**(3):175–86.

37. Hill SL, Afanasyeva M, Rose NR. Autoimmune myocarditis. In: Bona CA, Theophilopoulos AN, editors. *The molecular pathology of autoimmune diseases*. Ann Arbor, MI: Taylor & Francis; 2002. p. 951–64.

38. Neu N, Beisel KW, Traystman MD, Rose NR, Craig SW. Autoantibodies specific for the cardiac myosin isoform are found in mice susceptible to coxsackievirus B_3-induced myocarditis. *J Immunol* 1987;**138**:2488–92.

39. Neu N, Rose NR, Beisel KW, Herskowitz A, Gurri-Glass G, Craig SW. Cardiac myosin induces myocarditis in genetically predisposed mice. *J Immunol* 1987;**139**(11):3630–6.

40. Lenzo JC, Fairweather D, Cull V, Shellam GR, James Lawson CM. Characterisation of murine cytomegalovirus myocarditis: cellular infiltration of the heart and virus persistence. *J Mol Cell Cardiol* 2002;**34**(6):629–40.

41. Kodama M, Matsumoto Y, Fujiwara M, Masani F, Izumi T, Shibata A. A novel experimental model of giant cell myocarditis induced in rats by immunization with cardiac myosin fraction. *Clin Immunol Immunopathol* 1990;**57**(2):250–62.

42. Afanasyeva M, Wang Y, Kaya Z, Park S, Zilliox MJ, Schofield BH, et al. Experimental autoimmuney myocarditis in A/J mice is an interleukin-4-dependent disease with a Th2 phenotype. *Am J Pathol* 2001;**159**(1):193–203.

43. Donermeyer DL, Beisel KW, Allen PM, Smith SC. Myocarditis-inducing epitope of myosin binds constitutively and stably to I-Ak on antigen-presenting cells in the heart. *J Exp Med* 1995;**182**(5):1291–300.

44. Goser A, Andrassy M, Buss SJ, Leuschner F, Volz CH, Ottl R, et al. Cardiac troponin I but Not cardiac troponin T induces severe autoimmune inflammation in the myocardium. *Circulation* 2006;**114**:1693–703.

45. Cihakova D, Rose NR. Pathogenesis of myocarditis and dilated cardiomyopathy. *Adv Immunol* 2008;**99**:95–114.

46. Guler ML, Ligons D, Rose NR. Genetics of autoimmune myocarditis. In: Oksenberg J, Brassat D, editors. *Immunogenetics of autoimmune disease* Berlin, Heidelberg: Landis Bioscience, Eurekah.com & Springer Science; 2005. p. 144–51.

47. Li HS, Ligons DL, Rose NR. Genetic complexity of autoimmune myocarditis. *Autoimmun Rev* 2008;**7**:168–73.

48. Guler ML, Ligons DL, Wang Y, Bianco M, Broman KW, Rose NR. Two autoimmune diabetes loci influencing T cell apoptosis control susceptibility to experimental autoimmune myocarditis. *J Immunol* 2005;**174**:2167–73.

49. Ligons DL, Guler J, Li HS, Rose NR. A locus on chromosome I promotes susceptibility of experimental autoimmune myocarditis and lymphocyte cell death. *Clin Immunol* 2009;**130**:74–82.

50. Fairweather D, Frisancho-Kiss S, Rose NR. Sex differences in autoimmune diseases from a pathological perspective. *Am J Pathol* 2008;**173**:600–9.

51. Frisancho-Kiss S, Nyland JF, Davis SE, Frisancho JA, Barrett MA, Rose NR, et al. Sex differences in coxsackievirus B3-induced myocarditis: IL-12Rβ1 signaling and IFN-γ increase inflammation in males dependent from STAT4. *Brain Res* 2006;**1126**:139–47.

52. Roberts BJ, Moussawi M, Huber SA. Sex differences in TLR2 and TLR4 expression and their effect on coxsackievirus-induced autoimmune myocarditis. *Exp Mol Pathol* 2013;**94**:58–64.

53. Noutsias M, Fechner H, de Jonge H, Wang H, Dekkers D, Houtsmuller AB, et al. Human coxsackie-adenovirus receptor is colocalized with integrins alpha(v)beta(3) and alpha(v)beta(5) on the cardiomyocyte sarcolemma and upregulated in dilated cardiomyopathy: implications for cardiotropic viral infections. *Circulation* 2001;**104**(3):275–80.

54. Ito M, Kodama M, Masuko M, Yamaura M, Fuse K, Uesugi Y, et al. Expression of coxsackievirus and adenovirus receptor in hearts of rats with experimental autoimmune myocarditis. *Circ Res* 2000;**86**(3):275–80.

55. Fechner H, Noutsias M, Tschoepe C, Hinze K, Wang X, Escher F, et al. Induction of coxsackievirus-adenovirus-receptor expression during myocardial tissue formation and remodeling: identification of a cell-to-cell contact-dependent regulatory mechanism. *Circulation* 2003;**107**(6):876–82.

56. Vuorinen T, Vainionpaa R, Heino J, Hyypia T. Enterovirus receptors and virus replication in human leukocytes. *J Gen Virol* 1999;**80**(Pt 4):921–7.

57. Liu P, Aitken K, Kong YY, Opavsky MA, Martino T, Dawood F, et al. The tyrosine kinase p56lck is essential in coxsackievirus B3-mediated heart disease. *Nat Med* 2000;**6**(4):429–34.

58. Opavsky MA, Martino T, Rabinovitch M, Penninger J, Richardson C, Petric M, et al. Enhanced ERK-1/2 activation in mice susceptible to coxsackievirus-induced myocarditis. *J Clin Invest* 2002;**109**(12):1561–9.

59. Luo H, Yanagawa B, Zhang J, Luo Z, Zhang M, Esfandiarei M, et al. Coxsackievirus B3 replication is reduced by inhibition of the extracellular signal-regulated kinase (ERK) signaling pathway. *J Virol* 2002;**76**(7):3365–73.

60. Fairweather D, Rose NR. Models of coxsackievirus-B3-induced myocarditis: recent advances. *Drug Discovery Today: Disease Models* 2004;**1**:381–6.

61. Rose NR. Autoimmunity, infection and adjuvants. *Lupus* 2010;**19**:354–8.

62. Antoniak S, Owens III P, Baunacke M, Williams JC, Lee RD, Weithauser A, et al. PAR-1 contributes to the innate immune response during viral infection. *J Clin Inves* 2013;**123**(3):1310–22.

63. Lane JR, Neumann DA, Lafond-Walter A, Herskowitz A, Rose NR. LPS promotes CB3-induced myocarditis in resistant B10.A mice. *Cell Immunol* 1991;**136**(1):219–33.

64. Lane JR, Neumann DA, Lafond-Walker A, Herskowitz A, Rose NR. Interleukin 1 or tumor necrosis factor can promote coxsackie B3-induced myocarditis in resistant B10.A mice. *J Exp Med* 1992;**175**:1123–9.

65. Valaperti A, Mototsugu N, Youan L, Naito K, Chan M, Zhang L, et al. Innate immune interleukin-1 receptor-associated kinase 4 exacerbates viral myocarditis by reducing

CCR5$^+$CD11b$^+$ monocyte migration and impairing interferon production. *Circulation* 2013;**128**:1542–54.

66. Barin JG, Rose NR, Cihakova D. Macrophage diversity in cardiac inflammation: a review. *Immunobiology* 2012;**217**:468–75.

67. Satoh M, Nakamura M, Akatsu T, Iwasaka J, Shimoda Y, Segawa I, et al. Expression of toll-like receptor 4 is associated with enteroviral replication in human myocarditis. *Clin Sci (Lond)* 2003;**104**(6):577–84.

68. Fairweather D, Yusung S, Frisancho S, Barrett M, Gatewood S, Steele R, et al. IL-12 receptor beta1 and toll-like receptor 4 increase IL-1beta- and IL-18-associated myocarditis and Coxsacki8evirus replication. *J Immunol* 2003;**179**(9):4731–7.

69. Abston ED, Coronado MJ, Bucek A, Bedja D, Shin J, Kim JB, et al. Th2 regulation of viral myocarditis in Mice: different roles for TLR3 versus TRIF in progression to chronic disease. *Clinical & Developmental Immunology* 2012;**2012**:129486.

70. Anderson DR, Carthy CM, Wilson JE, Yang D, Devine DV, McManus BM. Complement component 3 interactions with coxsackievirus B3 capsid proteins: innate immunity and the rapid formation of splenic antiviral germinal centers. *J Virol* 1997;**71**(11): 8841–5.

71. Huber SA, Lodge PA. Coxsackievirus B-3 myocarditis. Identification of different pathogenic mechanisms in DBA/2 and Balb/c mice. *Am J Pathol* 1986;**122**(2):284–91.

72. Kaya Z, Afanasyeva M, Wang Y, Dohmen KM, Schlichting J, Tretter T, et al. Contribution of the innate immune system to autoimmune myocarditis: a role for complement. *Nat Immunol* 2001;**2**(8):739–45.

73. Afanasyeva M, Rose NR. Cardiomyopathy is linked to complement activation. *Am J Pathol* 2002;**161**:351–7.

74. Godeny EK, Gauntt CJ. Murine natural killer cells limit coxsackievirus B3 replication. *J Immunol* 1987;**139**(3):913–18.

75. Kanda T, Tanaka T, Sekiguchi K, Seta Y, Kurimoto M, Wilson McManus JE, et al. Effect of interleukin-18 on viral myocarditis: enhancement of interferon-gamma and natural killer cell activity. *J Mol Cell Cardiol* 2000;**32**(12):2163–71.

76. Eck M, Greiner A, Kandolf R, Schmausser B, Marx A, Muller-Hermelink HK. Active fulminant myocarditis characterized by T-lymphocytes expressing the gamma-delta T-cell receptor: a new disease entity? *Am J Surg Pathol* 1997;**21**(9):1109–12.

77. Huber SA. Coxsackievirus-induced myocarditis is dependent on distinct immunopathogenic responses in different strains of mice. *Lab Invest* 1997;**76**(5):691–701.

78. Huber SA, Sartini D, Exley M. T cells promote autoimmune CD8(+) cytolytic T-lymphocyte activation in coxsackievirus B3-induced myocarditis in mice: role for CD4(+) Th1 cells. *J Virol* 2002;**76**(21):10785–90.

79. Huber SA, Gauntt CJ, Sakkinen P. Enteroviruses and myocarditis: viral pathogenesis through replication, cytokine induction, and immunopathogenicity. *Adv Virus Res* 1998;**51**:35–80.

80. Huber A, Sartini D, Exley M. Role of CD1d in coxsackievirus B3-induced myocarditis. *J Immunol* 2003;**170**(6):3147–53.

81. Kuhl U, Pauschinger M, Schwimmbeck PL, Seeberg B, Lober C, Noutsias M, et al. Interferon-beta treatment eliminates cardiotropic viruses and improves left ventricular function in patients with myocardial persistence of viral genomes and left ventricular dysfunction. *Circulation* 2003;**107**(22):2793–8.

82. Miric M, Vasiljevic J, Bojic M, Popovic Z, Keserovic N, Pesic M. Long-term follow Up of patients with dilated heart muscle disease treated with human leucocyte interferon alpha or thymic hormones initial results. *Heart* 1996;**75**(6):596–601.

83. Wessely R, Klingel K, Knowlton KU, Kanfold R. Cardioselective infection with coxsackievirus B3 requires intact type I interferon signaling: implications for mortality and early viral replication. *Circulation* 2001;**103**(5):756–61.

84. Daliento L, Calabrese F, Tona F, Caforio AL, Tarsia G, Angelini A, et al. Successful treatment of enterovirus-induced myocarditis with interferon-alpha. *J Heart KLung Transplant* 2003;**22**(2):214–17.
85. Lawson CM, Beilharz MW. Low-dose oral use of interferon inhibits virally induced myocarditis. *J Interferon Cytokine Res* 1999;**19**(8):863–7.
86. Schwimmbeck PL, Badorff C, Rohn G, Schulze K, Schultheiss HP. Impairment of left ventricular function in combined immune deficiency mice after transfer of peripheral blood leukocytes from patients with myocarditis. *Eur Heart J* 1995;**16**(Suppl O): 59–63.
87. Schwimmbeck PL, Rohn G, Wrusch A, Schulze K, Doerner A, Kuehl U, et al. Enteroviral and immune medicated myocarditis in SCID mice. *Herz* 2000;**25**(3):240–4.
88. Omerovic E, Bollano E, Andersson B, Kujacic V, Schulze W, Hjalmarson A, et al. Induction of cardiomyopathy in severe combined immunodeficiency mice by transfer of lymphocytes from patients with idiopathic dilated cardiomyopathy. *Autoimmunity* 2000;**32**(4):271–80.
89. Opavsky MA, Penninger J, Aitken K, Wen WH, Dawood F, Mak T, et al. Susceptibility to myocarditis is dependent on the response of alphabeta R lymphocytes to coxsackieviral infection. *Circ Res* 1999;**85**(6):551–8.
90. Henke A, Huber S, Stelner A, Whitton JL. The role of CD8+ T lymphocytes in coxsackievirus B3-induced myocarditis. *J Virol* 1995;**69**(11):6720–8.
91. Smith SC, Allen PM. Myosin-induced acute myocarditis is a T cell-mediated disease. *J Immunol* 1991;**147**:2141–7.
92. Afanasyeva M, Georgakopoulos D, Belardi DF, Ramsundar AC, Barin JG, Kass DA, et al. Quantitative analysis of myocardial inflammation by flow cytometry in murine autoimmune myocarditis. *Am J Pathol* 2004;**164**:807–15.
93. Penninger JM, Neu N, Timms E, Wallace VA, Koh DR, Kishihara K, et al. The induction of experimental autoimmune myocarditis in mice lacking CD4 or CD8 molecules. *J Exp Med* 1993;**178**(5):1837–42.
94. Pummerer C, Berger P, Fruhwirth M, Ofner C, Neu N. Cellular infiltrate, major histocompatibility antigen expression and immunopathogenic mechanisms in cardiac myosin-induced myocarditis. *Lab Invest* 1991;**65**(5):538–47.
95. Neu N, Pummerer C, Rieker T, Berger P. T cells in cardiac myosin-induced myocarditis. *Clin Immunol Immunopathol* 1993;**68**(2):107–10.
96. Grabie N, Delfs MW, Westrich JR, Love VA, Stavrakis G, Ahmad F, et al. IL-12 is required for differentiation of pathogenic CD8+ T cell effectors that cause myocarditis. *J Clin Invest* 2003;**111**(5):671–80.
97. Neu N, Polier B, Ofner C. Cardiac myosin-induced myocarditis. Heart autoantibodies are not involved in the induction of the disease. *J Immunol* 1990;**145**(12):4094–100.
98. Liao L, Sindhwani R, Rojkind M, Factor S, Leinwand L, Diamond B. Antibody-mediated autoimmune myocarditis depends on genetically determined target organ sensitivity. *J Exp Med* 1995;**181**:1123–31.
99. Kuan AP, Zuckier L, Liao L, Factor SM, Diamond B. Immunoglobulin isotype determines pathogenicity in antibody-medicated myocarditis in naïve mice. *Circ Res* 2000;**86** (3):281–5.
100. Malkiel S, Factor S, Diamond B. Autoimmune myocarditis does not require B cells for antigen presentation. *J Immunol* 1999;**163**(10):5265–8.
101. Fairweather D, Cihakova D. Alternatively activated macrophages in infection and autoimmunity. *J Autoimm* 2009;**33**(3–4):222–30.
102. Barin JG, Baldeviano GC, Talor MV, Wu L, Ong S, Quader F, et al. Macrophages participate in IL-17-mediated inflammation. *Eur J Immunol* 2012;**42**:726–36.
103. Rose NR. Critical cytokine pathways to cardiac inflammation. *J Interferon Cytokine Res* 2011;**31**:1–6.

104. Afanasyeva M, Wang Y, Kaya Z, Stafford EA, Dohmen KM, Sadigi Akha AA, et al. Interleukin-12 receptor/STAT4 signaling is required for the development of autoimmune myocarditis in mice by an interferon-γ-independent pathway. *Circulation* 2001;**104**:3145–51.

105. Barin JG, Talor MV, Baldeviano GB, Kimura M, Roe NR, Cihakova D. Mechanisms of IFNγ regulation of autoimmune myocarditis. *Exp Mol Pathol* 2010;**89**(2):83–91.

106. Eriksson U, Kurrer MO, Sebald W, Brombacher F, Kopf M. Dual role of the IL-12/ IFN-gamma axis in the development of autoimmune-myocarditis: induction by IL-12 and protection by IFN-gamma. *J Immunol* 2001;**167**(9):5464–9.

107. Chomarat P, Banchereau J. An update on interleukin-4 and its receptor. *Eur Cytokine Netw* 1997;**8**(4):333–44.

108. Cihakova D, Barin JG, Afanasyeva M, Kimura M, Fairweather D, Berg M, et al. Interleukin-13 protects against experimental autoimmune myocarditis by regulating macrophage differentiation. *Am J Pathol* 2008;**172**(5):1195–208.

109. Moore KW, de Waal MR, Coffman RL, O'Garra A. Interleukin-10 and the interleukin-10 receptor. *Annu Rev Immunol* 2001;**19**:683–765.

110. Kaya Z, Dohmen KM, Wang Y, Schlichting J, Afanasyeva M, Leuschner F, et al. Cutting edge: a critical role for IL-10 in induction of nasal tolerance in experimental autoimmune myocarditis. *J Immunol* 2002;**168**(4):1552–6.

111. Wang Y, Afanasyeva M, Hill SL, Kaya Z, Rose NR. Nasal administration of cardiac myosin suppresses autoimmune myocarditis in mice. *J Am Coll Cardiol* 2000;**36**(6):1992–9.

112. Watanabe K, Nakazawa M, Fuse K, Hanawa H, Kodama M, Aizawa Y, et al. Protection against autoimmune myocarditis by gene transfer of interleukin-10 by electroporation. *Circulation* 2001;**104**(10):1098–100.

113. Nishio R, Matsumori A, Shioi T, Ishida H, Sasayama S. Treatment of experimental viral myocarditis with interleukin-10. *Circulation* 1999;**100**(10):1102–8.

114. Baldeviano GC, Barin JG, Talor MV, Srinivasan S, Bedja D, Zheng D, et al. Interleukin-17A is dispensable for myocarditis but essential for the progression to dilated cardiomyopathy. *Circ Research* 2010;**106**:1646–55.

115. Barin JG, Baldeviano GC, Talor MV, Wu L, SuFey Ong, Fairweather D, et al. Fatal eosinophilic myocarditis develops in the absence of IFN-γ and IL-17A. *J Immunol* 2013;**191**:4038–47.

116. Rose NR, Herskowitz A, Neumann DA, Neu N. Coxsackie B₃ infection and autoimmune myocarditis. In: Lernmark A, Cyrberg T, Terenius L, Hokfelt B, editors. *Molecular mimicry in health and disease.* Amsterdam: Excerpta Medica; 1988. p. 273–84 (Discussion – pp. 287–300).

117. Krisher K, Cunningham MW. Myosin: a link between streptococci and heart. *Science* 1985;**227**(4685):413–15.

118. Gauntt CJ, Higdon AL, Arizpe HM, Tamayo MR, Crawley R, Henkel RD, et al. Epitopes shared between coxsacki8evirus B3 (CVB3) and normal heart tissues contribute to CVB3-induced murine myocarditis. *Clin Immunol Immunopathol* 1993;**68**(2):129–34.

119. Hill SL, Rose NR. The transition from viral to autoimmune myocarditis. *Autoimmunity* 2001;**34**:169–76.

120. Massilamany C, Gangaplara A, Steffen D, Reddy J. Identification of novel mimicry epitopes for cardiac myosin heavy chain-α that induce autoimmune myocarditis in A/J mice. *Cell Immunol* 2011;**271**(2):438–49.

121. Horwitz MS, La Cava A, Fine C, Rodriguez E, Ilic A, Sarvetnick N. Pancreative expression of interferon-gamma protects mice from lethal coxsackievirus B3 infection and subsequent myocarditis. *Nat Med* 2000;**6**(6):693–7.

122. Gauntt CJ, Trousdale MD, LaBadie DR, Paque RE, Nealon T. Properties of coxsackievirus B3 variants which Are amyocarditis or myocarditis for mice. *J Med Virol* 1979;**3**(3):207–20.

CHAPTER 25

Celiac Disease and Rotavirus Infection

Zanoni Giovanna[*,1], **Dolcino Marzia**[†], **Lunardi Claudio**[‡],
Antonio Puccetti[†,§]
[*]Department of Pathology and Diagnostics, Unit of Immunology, University of Verona, Verona, Italy
[†]Department of Immunology, Institute G. Gaslini, Genoa, Italy
[‡]Department of Medicine, Unit of Internal Medicine, University of Verona, Verona, Italy
[§]Department of Experimental Medicine, Unit of Histology, University of Genoa, Genoa, Italy
[1]Corresponding Author: giovanna.zanoni@univr.it

Celiac disease (CD) is a systemic autoimmune disorder[1,2] sustained by an inappropriate immune response to dietary gluten,[3] a protein contained in the majority of cereals. The disease may affect as many as 1–3% of the European and North American population.[4] Genetically susceptible individuals develop autoimmune injury in several organs and tissues including the gut, skin, joints, liver, brain, heart, and uterus. In addition, patients with CD have an increased prevalence of other autoimmune diseases, both systemic and organ specific. Similar to other autoimmune disorders, genetic and environmental factors play a role in the pathogenesis of CD.

The major genetic risk factor of CD is represented by human leukocyte antigen (HLA)-DQ genes: approximately 90–95% of patients with CD express the HLA-DQ2 heterodimers, whereas the remaining 5–10% of the patients carry the HLA-DQ8 allele.[5] Among individuals with such a genetic background, some develop CD very early in infancy and others develop the disease in adulthood; the reasons for the onset of disease at such different ages are still unknown. The HLA-DQ2/8 alleles are necessary but alone are not sufficient to cause the disease, and other factors are involved in disease development. Gluten, the main protein present in wheat, rye and barley, is the known environmental factor responsible for the signs and symptoms of the disease, but other exogenous (i.e. environmental) factors may also play a role in CD pathogenesis. When gluten is ingested by individuals expressing HLA-DQ2 and/or -DQ8 heterodimers, it provokes an altered T-cell immune response in the small intestine, where gluten is

Infection and Autoimmunity
http://dx.doi.org/10.1016/B978-0-444-63269-2.00028-3

absorbed; indeed, a strong T helper 1 cell–dominated inflammatory response has been described in the small intestine of patients with CD. This immune response leads to a series of histological changes resulting in lymphocytic infiltration of the lamina propria and epithelium, crypt hyperplasia and more or less severe villous atrophy. These histological abnormalities, documented by Marsh,[6] are characteristic of the disease and explain some of the clinical symptoms presented by patients with CD. A typical serological marker of CD is the presence of immunoglobulin (Ig) A directed against tissue trans-glutaminase (tTG) during the active phase of the disease. Treatment of CD consists of a gluten-free diet, resulting in clinical recovery, histological normalisation of the intestinal mucosa and disappearance of the anti-tTG antibodies.

In addition to the activation of adaptive immune responses typical of all autoimmune diseases, there is some evidence that innate immunity might be involved in the initial phases of CD.[7] Indeed, some gluten peptides have been shown to be able to activate the innate immune system.[8]

Another important aspect in the pathogenesis of CD is the potential involvement of infectious agents in the initiation of the disease; a role for rod-shaped bacteria of the intestinal epithelium has been hypothesised but never definitively proven.[9] Moreover, viral infections also have been associated with CD, and a possible link between viruses such as adenovirus and hepatitis C virus and the pathogenesis of CD has been suggested.[10] Indeed, infectious agents have been suggested as good candidate triggers in the pathogenesis of autoimmune responses. Infections may contribute to the onset of autoimmunity via different mechanisms: (1) promoting immune dysregulation and chronic inflammation and (2) triggering adaptive immune responses cross-reactive with self-antigens (antigenic mimicry). An autoimmune response and eventually an autoimmune disease may follow infection by a pathogen that exhibits some epitopes that are similar to the self-proteins of the host, a mechanism known as molecular mimicry.[11] An antigenic determinant on one of the infectious agent's proteins is structurally similar to a determinant on one of the proteins made by the host, although it is sufficiently different to be recognized as foreign by the host's immune system. The immune response (both humoral and cellular) to the exogenous determinant then cross-reacts with the host tissue and eventually lead to autoimmune aggression. Despite the huge progress made in understanding the pathogenesis of CD, there are still many unknowns, including the presence of autoaggression in different tissues and the role played by innate immunity and by infectious agents.

In an attempt to clarify some of these issues, we used a random peptide library approach that we had successfully applied to the study of different autoimmune diseases.[12–15] Using this strategy, we were able to identify a pathogenetically relevant peptide (called celiac peptide) recognized by serum Igs of patients with active disease[16] eating a diet containing gluten. This peptide shares homology with several autoantigens, including tTG, and with the rotavirus major neutralizing protein VP7 (Table 1). Human rotaviruses are the most frequent etiologic agents of gastroenteritis in infants and young children in most parts of the world[17] (see Box 1).

Antibodies directed against the celiac peptide, purified from the sera of patients with active CD, recognize rotavirus major neutralizing protein VP7; moreover, a subset of anti-tTG IgA antibodies cross-react with the VP7, suggesting the possible involvement of rotavirus infection in the pathogenesis of the disease and thus identifying a potential link between rotavirus infection and the onset of CD.

It is noteworthy that this subset of antirotavirus antibodies seems to be a hallmark of active disease and is not detectable in healthy controls. Antibodies affinity-purified against the rotavirus VP7 peptide are able to cross-react with the autoantigens desmoglein, expressed in intestinal epithelial cells, and Toll-like receptor (TLR) 4, expressed on monocytes. Upon binding with these molecules, such antibodies have important functional properties: they are able to increase epithelial permeability upon interaction with desmoglein and activate innate immune responses upon engagement of TLR4.

An antirotavirus antibody response is, therefore, present in patients with CD and is mainly directed against an epitope within the VP7 protein. The VP7 epitope could be important in determining an antivirus immune response that is able to cross-react with self-antigens and has functional consequences on TLR4 engagement and intestinal permeability, thus breaking self-tolerance and triggering the development of autoimmunity.[18,19] Therefore, it is likely that a molecular mimicry mechanism may be involved in CD pathogenesis. The link between rotavirus infection and CD was supported by an epidemiological study conducted using a large population of children carrying the risk allele for CD.[20] The authors found that frequent rotavirus infections predicted a higher risk of developing CD autoimmunity. Moreover, the potential involvement of rotavirus in CD was supported by the report of the onset of CD 2 months after rotavirus infection in two girls who were previously negative for CD markers.[21,22]

Table 1 Sequence Homology Between Celiac Peptide and Vp7 Rotavirus Protein and Between Celiac Peptide and Self-Antigens

Celiac peptide	V	V	K	V	G	G	S	S	S	L	G	W
	..	*	..	..	..	..	..	*	..	..	..	
Rotavirus VP7 (260–271)	V	I	Q	V	G	G	S	N	V	L	D	I
Celiac peptide	V	V	K	V	G	G	S	S	S	L	G	W
	..	*	..	*	..	..	*	..	..	*	..	
Heat shock protein 60 (403–414)	V	L	K	V	G	G	T	S	D	V	E	V
Celiac peptide	V	V	K	V	G	G	S	S	S	L	G	W
	*	*	..	*	..	..	*	..	..	*	..	
Myotubularin related protein 2 (135–146)	V	E	K	I	G	G	A	S	S	R	G	E
Celiac peptide	L	S	S	L	G	G	T	A	S	I	G	H
	..	*	*	*	..	..	..	*	*	*	..	
Desmoglein 1	V	S	K	L	G	G	T	S	S	L	G	W
Celiac peptide	R	I	R	V	G	G	S	M	N	M	G	S
	..	*	..	*	..	..	*	..	*	*	..	
Transglutaminase (476–487)	V	V	K	V	G	G	S	S	S	L	G	W
Toll-like receptor 4	V	L	K	M	A	G	N	S	F	Q	E	N

* = conservative substitution; : : = identity

BOX 1 Rotavirus

Rotaviruses are double-stranded RNA viruses comprising a genus within the family *Reoviridae*. The mature virus particles have three layers and have an approximate diameter of 70 nm and icosahedral symmetry. The rotavirus genome consists of 11 segments of double-stranded RNA, which encode for 6 structural viral proteins (VP1, VP2, VP3, VP4, VP6 and VP7) and 6 non-structural proteins (NSP1–NSP6)[1]; gene segment 11 encodes both NSP5 and 6. The genome is encompassed by an inner core consisting of VP2, VP1 and VP3 proteins. The intermediate layer, or inner capsid, is made of VP6, which determines group and subgroup specificities[2]. The outer capsid layer is composed of two proteins, VP7 and VP4, which elicit neutralizing antibody responses.

Rotaviruses are classified into seven different serogroups (A–G) on the basis of the antigenic specificity of the VP6 capsid proteins, as well as on the pattern of electrophoretic mobility of the 11 RNA segments of the viral genome. There are five species of these viruses, referred to as A, B, C, D and E. Groups A, B and C are known to infect humans. Rotavirus A, the most common species, causes more than 90% of infections in humans[3]. Severe, life-threatening disease among children worldwide is caused predominantly by group A rotaviruses.

Rotavirus is the most common cause of acute gastroenteritis in infants and young children worldwide, infecting nearly all children by the age of 5, often more than once. Most severe cases of rotavirus occur among children 6–24 months of age. Rotavirus infection can have a variable course, ranging from mild to severe disease. The classical symptoms at presentation are fever, vomiting and watery diarrhea. In severe cases, massive dehydration can occur. Each year rotavirus causes millions of cases of diarrhea in developing countries, with nearly 2 million resulting in hospitalisation[4]. More than 600,000 deaths due to rotavirus occur annually worldwide. The majority of these deaths (85%) are in developing countries. In industrialised countries, fatal outcomes are rare; however, rotavirus infection can cause serious morbidity and represents a severe burden in terms of resource use. Rotavirus infection is the leading single cause of severe diarrhea among infants and children, being responsible for about 20% of cases, and accounts for 50% of the cases requiring hospitalisation[5]. Rotavirus causes 37% of deaths attributable to diarrhea and 5% of all deaths in children younger than five[6].

Rotavirus is highly contagious and is transmitted from person to person via the fecal–oral route through contact with contaminated hands, surfaces and objects[7]. There is some evidence that the virus may also spread through respiratory droplets, which could complicate infection control. The incubation period is approximately 2 days, and rotavirus diarrhea episodes can last from 3 to 8 days. In tropical countries, transmission occurs year-round, whereas in countries with a temperate climate, rotavirus exhibits a marked seasonality, with annual winter epidemics.

The diarrhea is caused by multiple activities of the virus. Malabsorption occurs because of the destruction of enterocytes. The toxic rotavirus protein NSP4 induces

Continued

BOX 1 Rotavirus—cont'd

ion-dependent chloride secretion, disrupts transporter-mediated reabsorption of water, apparently reduces activity of brush-border membrane disaccharidases and possibly activates the calcium ion-dependent secretory reflexes of the enteric nervous system[8]. Healthy enterocytes secrete lactase into the small intestine; milk intolerance due to lactase deficiency is a symptom of rotavirus infection[9] that can persist for weeks[10]. A recurrence of mild diarrhea often follows the reintroduction of milk into the child's diet because of bacterial fermentation of the disaccharide lactose in the gut[11].

Because improved sanitation does not decrease the prevalence of rotaviral disease and the rate of hospitalisations remains high despite the use of oral rehydrating medicines, the primary public health intervention is vaccination.[2] Surveillance studies to exclude the risk of inducing autoimmune reactions by rotavirus vaccination in children genetically predisposed to CD are still expected.

1. Iturriza-Gomara M, Green J, Brown DW, Desselberger U, Gray JJ. Diversity within the VP4 gene of rotavirus P[8] strains: Implications for reverse transcription-pcr genotyping. *J Clin Microbiol* 2000;38:898-901.
2. Desselberger U. Rotaviruses: Basic facts. *Methods Mol Med* 2000;34:1-8.
3. Kirkwood CD. Genetic and antigenic diversity of human rotaviruses: Potential impact on vaccination programs. *J Infect Dis* 2010;202 Suppl:S43-S48.
4. Simpson E, Wittet S, Bonilla J, Gamazina K, Cooley L, Winkler JL. Use of formative research in developing a knowledge translation approach to rotavirus vaccine introduction in developing countries. *BMC Public Health* 2007;7:281.
5. Rheingans RD, Heylen J, Giaquinto C. Economics of rotavirus gastroenteritis and vaccination in europe: What makes sense? *Pediatr Infect Dis J* 2006;25: S48-S55.
6. Tate JE, Burton AH, Boschi-Pinto C, Steele AD, Duque J, Parashar UD, et al. 2008 estimate of worldwide rotavirus-associated mortality in children younger than 5 years before the introduction of universal rotavirus vaccination programmes: A systematic review and meta-analysis. *Lancet Infect Dis* 2012;12:136-41.
7. Butz AM, Fosarelli P, Dick J, Cusack T, Yolken R. Prevalence of rotavirus on high-risk fomites in day-care facilities. *Pediatrics* 1993;92:202-205.
8. Hyser JM, Estes MK. Rotavirus vaccines and pathogenesis: 2008. *Curr Opin Gastroenterol* 2009;25:36-43.
9. Farnworth ER. The evidence to support health claims for probiotics. *J Nutr* 2008;138:1250S-1254S.
10. Ouwehand A, Vesterlund S. Health aspects of probiotics. *IDrugs* 2003;6:573-580.
11. Arya SC. Rotaviral infection and intestinal lactase level. *J Infect Dis* 1984;150:791.

In light of these observations, we performed an additional study to further analyze the link between rotavirus infection and the pathogenesis of CD. To this aim we decided to investigate whether the presence of anti-VP7 peptide antibodies precedes the onset of CD and therefore whether the detection of such antibodies might be used as an early predictive marker, when anti-tTG and antiendomysium antibodies are not yet detectable. Moreover, we studied the effects of antiviral peptide antibodies on intestinal epithelial cells using a gene array analysis to confirm that such antibodies are able to induce in vitro some of the features observed in celiac epithelium in vivo.

For the first part of the study, we selected a cohort of 357 children affected by type 1 diabetes (T1DM), who were known to have a high risk of developing CD. Indeed, the prevalence of CD among children with T1DM is 5–10 times higher than in the general population[23] because the two diseases share a common genetic background that may be explained by the combined presence of the HLA-DQ transdimer, called HLA-DQ8 trans.[24] During the follow-up, 32 of 357 patients with T1DM developed CD. Statistically significantly higher concentrations of antirotavirus VP7 antibodies were detected in patients with T1DM and CD when compared to patients with T1DM without CD, suggesting that such antibodies are possibly related to the onset of CD.[25] Interestingly, anti-VP7 peptide antibodies were detectable before the onset of CD in the majority of the sera analyzed. In one patient in particular such antibodies appeared 120 months before humoral and histological evidence of disease (Table 2 and Figure 1). These findings further support a possible etiological link between rotavirus infection and the pathogenesis of CD.

In the second part of the work[25] we studied the effects of purified anti-rotavirus VP7 peptide antibodies on intestinal epithelial cells (T84) that are commonly used to study the intestinal barrier function. When we analyzed the gene expression profiles in T84 intestinal cells treated with antibodies against the rotavirus VP7 peptide, we observed that such treatment had a profound effect on the gene expression pattern by modulating a large number of genes. The vast majority of genes modulated by the anti-VP7 antibodies in T84 cells have been shown to be involved in the biological processes that lead to the most important features of the disease. Clusters of modulated genes included genes involved in triggering the apoptotic process and in the regulation of cell proliferation and differentiation.[26] Indeed, the classical gluten-induced lesions in the small intestine show mucosal villous atrophy with crypt hyperplasia, as well as decreased differentiation and

Table 2 Levels of Anti-VP7, Anticeliac Peptide and Antitransglutaminase Immunoglobulin A Antibodies Tested by Enzyme-Linked immunosorbent Assay in Sera of Patients with Celiac Disease Before and After Disease Onset

Patients	Months before onset	Before disease onset[a]			After disease onset		
		tTG (U/mL)	Celiac peptide	VP7 peptide	tTG (U/mL)	Celiac peptide	VP7 peptide
1	6	<7	0.123	0.517	69	0.126	0.511
2	28	<7	0.226	0.350	107	0.234	0.360
3	14	<7	0.097	0.170	27	0.102	0.172
4	120	<7	0.105	0.244	71	0.129	0.212
5	72	<7	0.111	0.340	97	0.205	0.460
6	16	<7	0.070	0.170	9	0.058	0.179
7	60	<7	0.114	0.215	7	0.228	0.326
8	16	<7	0.278	0.267	25	0.276	0.235

Cutoff: anti-tissue transglutaminase >7 U/mL; celiac peptide 0.105; VP7 peptide 0.160.
[a]Before disease onset: anti-tissue transglutaminase and EMA negativity at the screening test.

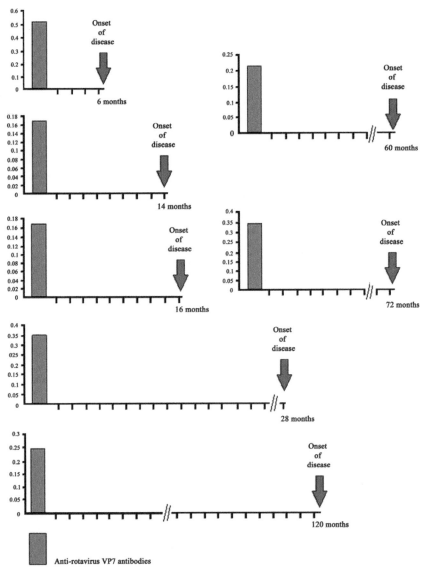

Figure 1 Detection of anti-VP7 rotavirus antibodies before the onset of celiac disease. In each graph the *y*-axis shows the mean absorbance at 405 nm and the *x*-axis shows the time (months) before the onset of the disease.

increased proliferation of epithelial cells. It has been proposed that dysregulated differentiation of epithelial cells in the small intestine plays a role in the generation of the celiac lesion. Diosdado et al.[26] suggested that stem cells in the villous crypt proliferate but do not receive the signal to differentiate, leading to the development of undifferentiated, hyperplastic crypts and sub-sequent villous atrophy. Moreover, increased apoptosis is considered an important mechanism in determining villous atrophy.

The treatment of T84 cells with antiviral peptide antibodies induces the typical alterations seen in CD because it up-regulates pro-apoptotic genes and down-regulates genes involved in the differentiation of epithelial cells. The gene expression profiles of the array analysis reported in this work also show the modulation of several genes involved in cytoskeleton organisation, and gliadin peptides were shown to exert a similar effect on epithelial cells.[27]

CD is associated with the dysregulation of cell–cell adhesion molecules, and genes encoding for tight junctions and gap junction proteins are over-expressed in our experiments, whereas desmosomes proteins are down-modulated by the treatment.[28] These alterations are associated with decreased transepithelial resistance and with increased permeability, both of which are typical features of the celiac intestinal epithelium. Another cluster of modulated genes included genes involved in cellular ion transport.[29]

In particular we found up-regulation of several ion channels and trans-porters and down-regulation of Na(+)/H(+) exchanger 3, which is present in celiac intestinal epithelial cells. Indeed, it has been supposed that the reduction in the expression of Na(+)/H(+) exchanger 3 may play a role in the onset of the celiac-associated diarrhea, one of the major clinical fea-tures of the disease.[30]

Similar to what was observed in the biopsies of patients with active dis-ease, we observed the up-regulation of genes coding for several matrix metalloproteases, in particular matrix metalloprotease-12, which is consid-ered crucial for the immunological mechanisms that lead to tissue injury.[31]

Anti-VP7 antibodies also show a pro-inflammatory effect on T84 intes-tinal cells, because they up-regulate many genes involved in inflammation. This effect is increased by the down-regulation of some anti-inflammatory molecules such as interleukin-10. The anti-VP7 antibodies up-regulated the expression of various receptors such as the galanin receptor, which is involved in inflammation-associated diarrhea,[32] epidermal growth factor receptor and its pathway-associated molecules, which regulate epithelial cell proliferation, and signal-transducing molecules such as ephrin-A2, a key regulator of developmental process in many epithelial cells.[33]

In conclusion, here we described two additional characteristics of the previously described antirotavirus VP7 antibodies that further support the link between rotavirus infection and CD. First, such antibodies identify sub-jects who will develop CD. Second, they modulate sets of genes in intestinal epithelial cells. These genes are involved in the induction of typical features of CD, such as apoptosis, alteration of the epithelial barrier integrity and inflammation.

An early diagnosis of CD is an important issue in medicine and is based on periodical autoantibody screening following the diagnosis of T1DM. In this context, the evaluation of anti-VP7 rotavirus antibodies may represent an additional marker with important predictive value. Further studies are required to confirm the predictive value of such antiviral antibodies by studying subjects with a family history of CD and with genetic predisposition. Another strategy to study the link between rotavirus infection and onset of CD would be the evaluation of the induction of this subset of anti-rotavirus antibodies and ultimately the incidence of the disease in children treated with rotavirus vaccines.

REFERENCES

1. Hadjivassiliou M, Williamson CA, Woodroofe N. The immunology of gluten sensitivity: beyond the gut. *Trends Immunol* 2004;**25**:578–82.
2. Dewar DH, Ciclitira PJ. Clinical features and diagnosis of celiac disease. *Gastroenterology* 2005;**128**:S19–24.
3. Macdonald TT, Monteleone G. Immunity, inflammation, and allergy in the gut. *Science* 2005;**307**:1920–5.
4. Rewers M. Epidemiology of celiac disease: what are the prevalence, incidence, and progression of celiac disease? *Gastroenterology* 2005;**128**:S47–51.
5. Trynka G, Wijmenga C, van Heel DA. A genetic perspective on coeliac disease. *Trends Mol Med* 2010;**16**:537–50.
6. Marsh MN. Gluten, major histocompatibility complex, and the small intestine. A molecular and immunobiologic approach to the spectrum of gluten sensitivity ('celiac sprue'). *Gastroenterology* 1992;**102**:330–54.
7. Maiuri L, Ciacci C, Ricciardelli I, Vacca L, Raia V, Auricchio S, et al. Association between innate response to gliadin and activation of pathogenic T cells in coeliac disease. *Lancet* 2003;**362**:30–7.
8. Londei M, Ciacci C, Ricciardelli I, Vacca L, Quaratino S, Maiuri L. Gliadin as a stimulator of innate responses in celiac disease. *Mol Immunol* 2005;**42**:913–18.
9. Sollid LM, Gray GM. A role for bacteria in celiac disease? *Am J Gastroenterol* 2004;**99**:905–6.
10. Plot L, Amital H. Infectious associations of celiac disease. *Autoimmun Rev* 2009;**8**:316–9.
11. Fierabracci A. Unravelling the role of infectious agents in the pathogenesis of human autoimmunity: the hypothesis of the retroviral involvement revisited. *Curr Mol Med* 2009;**9**:1024–33.
12. Lunardi C, Bason C, Navone R, Millo E, Damonte G, Corrocher R, et al. Systemic sclerosis immunoglobulin G autoantibodies bind the human cytomegalovirus late protein UL94 and induce apoptosis in human endothelial cells. *Nat Med* 2000;**6**:1183–6.
13. Lunardi C, Bason C, Leandri M, Navone R, Lestani M, Millo E, et al. Autoantibodies to inner ear and endothelial antigens in Cogan's syndrome. *Lancet* 2002;**360**:915–21.
14. Navone R, Lunardi C, Gerli R, Tinazzi E, Peterlana D, Bason C, et al. Identification of tear lipocalin as a novel autoantigen target in Sjogren's syndrome. *J Autoimmun* 2005;**25**:229–34.

15. Puccetti A, Bason C, Simeoni S, Millo E, Tinazzi E, Beri R, et al. In chronic idiopathic urticaria autoantibodies against Fc epsilonRII/CD23 induce histamine release via eosinophil activation. *Clin Exp Allergy* 2005;**35**:1599–607.

16. Zanoni G, Navone R, Lunardi C, Tridente G, Bason C, Sivori S, et al. In celiac disease, a subset of autoantibodies against transglutaminase binds toll-like receptor 4 and induces activation of monocytes. *PLoS Med* 2006;**3**:e358.

17. Clark B, McKendrick M. A review of viral gastroenteritis. *Curr Opin Infect Dis* 2004;**17**:461–9.

18. Waldner H, Collins M, Kuchroo VK. Activation of antigen-presenting cells by microbial products breaks self tolerance and induces autoimmune disease. *J Clin Invest* 2004;**113**:990–7.

19. Manfredi AA, Sabbadini MG, Rovere-Querini P. Dendritic cells and the shadow line between autoimmunity and disease. *Arthritis Rheum* 2005;**52**:11–15.

20. Stene LC, Honeyman MC, Hoffenberg EJ, Haas JE, Sokol RJ, Emery L, et al. Rotavirus infection frequency and risk of celiac disease autoimmunity in early childhood: a longitudinal study. *Am J Gastroenterol* 2006;**101**:2333–40.

21. Pavone P, Nicolini E, Taibi R, Ruggieri M. Rotavirus and celiac disease. *Am J Gastroenterol* 2007;**102**:1831.

22. Troncone R, Auricchio S. Rotavirus and celiac disease: clues to the pathogenesis and perspectives on prevention. *J Pediatr Gastroenterol Nutr* 2007;**44**:527–8.

23. Waisbourd-Zinman O, Hojsak I, Rosenbach Y, Mozer-Glassberg Y, Shalitin S, Phillip M, et al. Spontaneous normalization of anti-tissue transglutaminase antibody levels is common in children with type 1 diabetes mellitus. *Dig Dis Sci* 2012;**57**:1314–20.

24. Kooy-Winkelaar Y, van Lummel M, Moustakas AK, Schweizer J, Mearin ML, Mulder CJ, et al. Gluten-specific T cells cross-react between HLA-DQ8 and the HLA-DQ2alpha/DQ8beta transdimer. *J Immunol* 2011;**187**:5123–9.

25. Dolcino M, Zanoni G, Bason C, Tinazzi E, Boccola E, Valletta E, et al. A subset of anti-rotavirus antibodies directed against the viral protein VP7 predicts the onset of celiac disease and induces typical features of the disease in the intestinal epithelial cell lineT84. *Immunol Res* 2013;**56**:465–76.

26. Diosdado B, van Oort E, Wijmenga C. "Coelionomics": towards understanding the molecular pathology of coeliac disease. *Clin Chem Lab Med* 2005;**43**:685–95.

27. Barone MV, Gimigliano A, Castoria G, Paolella G, Maurano F, Paparo F, et al. Growth factor-like activity of gliadin, an alimentary protein: implications for coeliac disease. *Gut* 2007;**56**:480–8.

28. Bracken S, Byrne G, Kelly J, Jackson J, Feighery C. Altered gene expression in highly purified enterocytes from patients with active coeliac disease. *BMC Genomics* 2008;**9**:377.

29. Schulzke JD, Schulzke I, Fromm M, Riecken EO. Epithelial barrier and ion transport in coeliac sprue: electrical measurements on intestinal aspiration biopsy specimens. *Gut* 1995;**37**:777–82.

30. Gill RK, Saksena S, Tyagi S, Alrefai WA, Malakooti J, Sarwar Z, et al. Serotonin inhibits Na+/H+ exchange activity via 5-HT4 receptors and activation of PKC alpha in human intestinal epithelial cells. *Gastroenterology* 2005;**128**:962–74.

31. Ciccocioppo R, Di Sabatino A, Bauer M, Della Riccia DN, Bizzini F, Biagi F, et al. Matrix metalloproteinase pattern in celiac duodenal mucosa. *Lab Invest* 2005; **85**:397–407.

32. Benya RV, Matkowskyj KA, Danilkovich A, Hecht G. Galanin causes Cl- secretion in the human colon. Potential significance of inflammation-associated NF-kappa b activation on galanin-1 receptor expression and function. *Ann N Y Acad Sci* 1998;**863**:64–77.

33. Juuti-Uusitalo K, Maki M, Kainulainen H, Isola J, Kaukinen K. Gluten affects epithelial differentiation-associated genes in small intestinal mucosa of coeliac patients. *Clin Exp Immunol* 2007;**150**:294–305.

CHAPTER 26

Theiler's Murine Encephalomyelitis Virus-Induced Demyelinating Disease (TMEV-IDD) and Autoimmunity

Emily M.L. Chastain, Stephen D. Miller[1]
Department of Microbiology-Immunology and Interdepartmental Immunobiology Center, Feinberg School of Medicine, Northwestern University, Chicago, Illinois, USA
[1]Corresponding Author: s-d-miller@northwestern.edu

1 TMEV-IDD AS A MODEL OF MS

Theiler's murine encephalomyelitis virus (TMEV), belonging to the *Picornaviridae* family, is a natural enteric pathogen of mice.[1] Neurovirulence upon experimental intracerebral injection varies depending on the strain of TMEV and ranges from the rapidly fatal encephalitis of the GDVII strain to an ameliorated acute infection followed by chronic persistence, inflammation, and spinal cord demyelination after infection with the BeAn or Daniel's (DA) strains.[2,3] The acute disease phase in DA infection of SJL/J mice is characterized by microglial proliferation and necrosis of neuronal motor neurons, which results in flaccid paralysis (i.e. poliomyelitis).[4] Surviving mice develop TMEV-induced demyelinating disease (TMEV-IDD). In contrast, BeAn infection results in a very limited grey matter disease in the early acute phase, with no clinical signs. Chronic demyelinating disease in these mice appears later (after day 30) and is due to the immune response itself, not direct lysis of virally infected oligodendrocytes.[5,6]

Intracerebral injection of the BeAn strain of TMEV into SJL/J mice results in a chronic demyelinating disease, TMEV-IDD, which resembles multiple sclerosis (MS) in many ways. In addition to epidemiological data suggesting an infectious etiology of MS, histopathology indicating inflammatory infiltrates and focal areas of demyelination, as well as the clinical presentation of the disease, bear similarities to MS. Although no one virus has been shown to be consistently associated with MS, early infection may

Infection and Autoimmunity
http://dx.doi.org/10.1016/B978-0-444-63269-2.00023-4

trigger events, through molecular mimicry[7] or epitope spreading,[8] that eventually result in autoimmune disease. Like TMEV-IDD, MS is an immune-mediated demyelinating disease characterized by perivascular $CD4^+$ T-cell and mononuclear cell infiltration, with subsequent primary demyelination of axonal tracts, leading to progressive paralysis.[9] MS is generally considered to have an autoimmune component; however, a direct cause–effect relationship between myelin reactivity and disease has not been established. Interestingly, although TMEV-IDD is initially due to a persistent viral infection of the central nervous system (CNS), autoimmune antimyelin T helper (Th) 1 and Th17 responses are seen during the chronic phase of disease.[8,10,11]

2 PERSISTENT INFECTION AND CHRONIC DISEASE

Demyelination and the resulting clinical disease symptoms are not the consequence of viral lysis of oligodendrocytes, which construct the myelin sheath;[12] instead they are immune mediated, due to a $CD4^+$ T-cell inflammatory response in the CNS.[5,13] Supporting the major role of the immune response itself in this chronic phase of disease, nonspecific immunosuppression with cyclophosphamide, antithymocyte serum, or $CD4^+$ T cell (not $CD8^+$) depletion after the initial viremia reduces inflammatory mononuclear cell infiltration into the CNS and subsequent demyelination.[14–17] Although it is clear that the initial antivirus immune response is responsible for initiating the clinical symptoms of TMEV-IDD, viral persistence is required for chronic disease; mouse strains which clear the virus do not go on to develop TMEV-IDD.[18]

Viral persistence in different strains of mice has been an area of study for many years. The fact that mice with differing haplotypes are variously susceptible to viral persistence and thus TMEV-IDD harkens back to the notion of the similarity of this model to MS. The archetypal inbred mouse strains used to study viral persistence are C57BL/6 ($H-2D^b$) and SJL/J ($H-2D^s$). Both quantitatively and qualitatively differential antiviral cytotoxic T lymphocyte (CTL) responses have been observed in these strains.[19–22] Although SJL/J CTLs are fully functional and respond to three viral capsid epitopes, they do not possess polyfunctionality, that is, they do not both secrete interferon (IFN)-γ and lyse target cells.[20]

We also demonstrated limitation of CTL effector function in SJL/J mice by virally expanded natural T regulatory cells (nTregs). Although nTregs are expanded in both B6 and SJL/J mice after TMEV infection, the ratio of

Tregs to T effector cells was unfavorable in the SJL/J mice. When SJL/J mice were treated with an nTreg-depleting antibody, T effector cell responses increased and disease induction was delayed.[23] Thus, regulation of the effector response is a critical genetically determined element of disease susceptibility.

3 FROM VIRAL INFECTION TO AUTOIMMUNITY

3.1 Mechanisms for Inducing Autoimmunity During Infection

The mechanism(s) underlying the initiation and progression of MS and other autoimmune diseases are not well understood, but epidemiologic studies have provided strong evidence suggesting a role of virus infection(s) in the development and/or exacerbation of MS. The possible mechanisms by which virus infection can trigger an autoimmune response include bystander activation and molecular mimicry.[24] In the TMEV-IDD model of MS, we demonstrated bystander activation, the nonspecific activation of autoreactive T cells resulting from the virus-specific CD4$^+$ Th1 inflammatory response itself on tissue in the target organ, followed by epitope spreading, the activation of autoreactive T cells caused by the release of self-epitopes following tissue damage during that immune response.

Molecular mimicry, on the other hand, theoretically results following infection with a virus expressing a peptide determinant(s) that shares homology with a self-peptide. This can result in the activation of autoantigen-specific cross-reactive T cells. The discovery of T-cell receptor (TCR) degeneracy, the TCR's ability to recognize multiple peptides with only a few key amino acid positions in common, has led to the widespread belief that some microbial proteins probably contain peptide sequences that are able to activate self-reactive T cells.

3.2 Virus-Specific CD4$^+$ T Cell Responses Initiate Bystander Damage, Leading to Myelin Damage

The adaptive immune response is exquisitely specific in that T- and B-cell responses initiated against one pathogen usually do not target other pathogens or host tissue. Although CD8$^+$ cytotoxic lymphocytes kill in a very specific manner, CD4$^+$ T cells induce the influx and activation of "general effectors" such as inflammatory monocytes and macrophages, which carry out effector functions in a "nonspecific" manner. Macrophage influx and activation leads to bystander tissue destruction. During infection with TMEV, initiation of myelin damage is associated with the activation of monocyte/macrophages by pro-inflammatory cytokines[25–27] from TMEV-specific CD4[+] T cells responding to viral epitopes presented by CNS-resident antigen-presenting cells (APCs).[28]

Initial time course studies comparing the development of T-cell responses to both virus and myelin epitopes during TMEV-IDD showed that autoreactivity to myelin epitopes is not detected before disease onset (30–35 days after infection),[29,30] whereas immune responses to TMEV epitopes are clearly demonstrable by 5–7 days after infection.[31] Induction of peripheral tolerance to mouse spinal cord homogenate – which effectively prevents mouse spinal cord homogenate-induced experimental autoimmune encephalomyelitis (EAE)—at the time of TMEV infection does not affect the clinical onset or the development of virus-specific T-cell responses in TMEV-IDD.[32] These results demonstrate that virus-specific CD4[+] T-cell responses initiate bystander tissue destruction (demyelination) and the clinical signs of TMEV-IDD.

Infected animals exhibit a chronic progressive demyelinating disease characterized by low persistence of TMEV in CNS microglia/macrophages and/or astrocytes throughout the lifetime of the animals. CNS mononuclear infiltrates can be detected as early as 3 days after infection (E. Chastain, unpublished data) and are initially composed of peripheral inflammatory monocytes/macrophages, APCs and virus-specific T cells.[17,26,33,34] In the SJL/J mouse, CD4[+] T-cell reactivity to the dominant myelin epitope proteolipid protein (PLP139–151) can be detected in the periphery of these animals beginning 50–55 days after infection, indicating the initiation of an autoimmune component secondary to viral infection.[8] In contrast to molecular mimicry, these data suggest that myelin debris is being processed and presented to T cells specific for autoantigens (epitope spreading).

3.3 Myelin Damage Results in Endogenous Presentation of Myelin Epitopes and Epitope Spreading

Accumulating data demonstrate that chronic immune-mediated tissue damage can lead to de novo activation of autoreactivity via epitope spreading. Epitope spreading is the process whereby epitopes distinct from, and noncross-reactive with, an inducing epitope become major targets of an ongoing immune response. Two prominent examples of epitope spreading in CD4[+] T-cell-mediated autoimmune models are diabetes in nonobese diabetic mice[35–38] and relapsing EAE.[39–41] In addition, epitope spreading has been demonstrated following viral infections with picornaviruses, such as TMEV[8] and Coxsackie virus.[42]

Initiation of myelin damage in TMEV-infected SJL/J mice by TMEV-specific CD4$^+$ T cells targeting virus persisting in CNS-resident APCs leads to the up-regulation of pro-inflammatory cytokines in the CNS and is associated with the activation of CD4$^+$ myelin-specific T cells during the chronic phase of disease. These autoreactive T cells seem to be primed via epitope spreading, as determined by their late appearance in disease (≥ 50–60 days after infection) and by the fact that there are no apparent viral epitopes that are shared with the major encephalitogenic myelin epitopes on proteolipid protein, myelin basic protein (MBP) or myelin oligodendrocyte glycoprotein, that is, there is no evidence for molecular mimicry in this system.[8]

The spreading process was demonstrated in TMEV-IDD by observing temporal changes in the specificity of delayed-type hypersensitivity, T-cell proliferative, and IFN-γ responses to viral and myelin epitopes[43] in peripheral lymphoid tissues. Antiviral delayed-type hypersensitivity and in vitro antiviral T-cell responses appear within a few days after infection, and these responses continue throughout the course of the disease. In contrast, myelin-specific responses can be detected beginning only 40–60 days after infection, that is, 2–4 weeks after clinical disease onset. Most interestingly, T-cell responses against myelin epitopes arise in an ordered progression, initially targeting PLP139-151, the immunodominant myelin epitope in the SJL/J mouse. Reactivity towards this peptide then continues throughout disease. As disease progresses, T-cell responses to PLP178–191 followed by responses to MBP84–104 arise, paralleling the relative order of their appearance in PLP139–151-induced relapsing EAE in SJL/J mice.[44] Reactivity towards additional myelin epitopes also is observed.

3.4 Using TMEV to Investigate Molecular Mimicry, an Alternate Mechanism for Induction of Autoimmunity During Infection

Studies have shown degeneracy in the TCR specific for the human MBP85–99 peptide; the TCR requires only a few critical residues for recognition.[45] T-cell clones specific for MBP85–99 established from patients with MS were shown to cross-react with viral peptides expressed by a number of viruses, including herpes simplex virus, adenovirus, reovirus, and human papillomavirus.[45] Likewise, a few critical residues were shown to be necessary for recognition of PLP139–151 by its TCR.[46] PLP139–151-specific T-cell hybridomas derived from SJL/J mice also were shown to cross-react with peptides expressed by various mouse pathogens, demonstrating degeneracy in the PLP139–151 TCR.[46] Therefore, myelin-specific T cells have been shown by in vitro studies to have the potential to cross-react with viral epitopes, supporting the molecular mimicry model described in these studies.

To directly investigate molecular mimicry as a potential mechanism of CD4[+] T-cell-mediated autoimmunity, we developed an infectious model of molecular mimicry by inserting a sequence encompassing the immunodominant PLP139–151 epitope into the coding region of a nonpathogenic TMEV variant (PLP139-TMEV).[47,48] PLP139-TMEV-infected mice developed a rapid-onset paralytic, inflammatory, demyelinating disease paralleled by the activation of PLP139–151-specific CD4[+] Th1 responses within 10–14 days after infection. These data demonstrate that the early onset demyelinating disease induced by PLP139-TMEV is a direct result of autoreactive PLP139–151-specific CD4[+] T-cell responses. PLP139–151-specific CD4[+] T cells from PLP139-TMEV-infected mice transferred demyelinating disease to naive recipients, and infection with the mimic virus at sites peripheral to the CNS induced early demyelinating disease, suggesting that the PLP139–151-specific CD4[+] T cells could be activated in the periphery and traffic to the CNS. Importantly, PLP139–151 epitope-specific tolerance before infection with PLP139-TMEV resulted in the specific reduction of PLP139–151-specific CD4[+] Th1 responses that directly correlated with a significant reduction in the incidence and severity of the early onset demyelinating disease.

In addition, mimic PLP139–151 sequences in which amino acid substitutions were made at the primary (amino acid 144) or secondary (amino acid 147) TCR contact residues were constructed.[47,48] Infection with the virus carrying a substitution in the secondary TCR contact residue induced early onset demyelinating disease and activated cross-reactive PLP139–151-specific CD4[+] T cells. In contrast, infection with the virus substituted at the primary TCR contact residue (position 144) failed to induce early demyelinating disease or activation of cross-reactive PLP139–151-specific CD4[+] T cells. An additional mimic virus was constructed by inserting a sequence from *Hemophilus influenzae* that shared only 6 of 13 amino acids with the core PLP139–151 epitope.[47] More significant for a role for molecular mimicry in induction of autoimmune disease, infection with this mimic virus resulted in early onset demyelinating disease and activation of Th1 cells cross-reactive with the native PLP139–151 determinant. This model is the first to directly demonstrate that a virus encoding a mimic of an encephalitogenic self-myelin epitope could induce an autoreactive CD4[+] T cell response, leading to a CNS demyelinating disease.

4 APCs IN TMEV

A variety of cells within the normal CNS are capable of antigen presentation to T cells. Major histocompatibility complex (MHC) class II and costimulatory molecule-expressing cells can be found in MS lesions,[49–52] and human microglia have been shown to express costimulatory molecules required for activation of T cells.[53,54]

In vitro cultures of murine neonatal microglia are capable of being infected with TMEV; as a result of this infection, these cells are activated to function as competent APCs with the ability to process and present both virus and myelin epitopes to memory CD4[+] Th1 cells.[55] Concomitant with the acquisition of this capacity to present functional antigens, TMEV infection induced the up-regulation of cytokines involved in innate immune responses and of cytokines and costimulatory molecules required for the activation and differentiation of Th1 effector cells. Most significant is that direct TMEV infection of microglia was nearly as effective as stimulation with high levels of IFN-γ in conferring APC function.

We confirmed activation of microglia in vivo in TMEV-infected adult SJL/J mice. We showed that while microglial proliferate and upregulate both MHC class I and II after infection, up-regulation of the inhibitory molecule B7-H1 also occurs. Blockade of B7-H1 led to exacerbated disease, indicating that microglia, while able to initiate an immune response, can also act in a regulatory and protective manner.[56]

In TMEV-IDD, the inflammatory infiltrate is composed of T and B lymphocytes, activated microglia derived from the CNS-resident pool and macrophages infiltrating from the peripheral blood.[34,57,58] Macrophages/microglia within the demyelinated areas contain phagocytized myelin debris[59] and are capable of processing and presenting myelin epitopes. Indeed, we showed that naive PLP-specific CD4[+] T cells underwent activation and proliferation only within the CNS, indicating that APCs residing in the CNS were capable of activating naive autoreactive T cells.[60] Therefore, any myelin-specific T cells that enter the CNS during the antiviral inflammatory response, whether already primed in the periphery or naive, could potentially be induced to proliferate and/or secrete pro-inflammatory cytokines in response to myelin epitopes.

5 CONCLUSIONS

The epidemiology of MS strongly suggests a role for an infectious agent, most likely a virus, in disease initiation. Presentation of viral antigens within

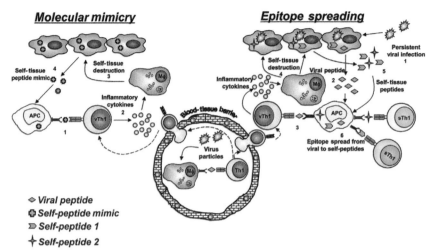

Figure 1 Possible mechanisms of virus-induced T-cell-mediated autoimmune disease. The figure illustrates induction of CD4$^+$ T-cell-mediated autoimmune tissue destruction via induction of a self antigen-specific cross-reactive T-cell response (i.e. molecular mimicry) following peripheral virus infection (*left*) and via epitope spreading to self-antigen-reactive T cells secondary to bystander tissue destruction and release of self-antigens initiated by a specific T-cell response to a virus persistent in the target tissue (*right*).

the CNS (leading to bystander demyelination), of neuroantigens cross-reactive with viral antigens (molecular mimicry) or of neuroantigens liberated by immune or virus-induced CNS damage (epitope spreading) are all potential mechanisms by which pathogenic immune reactions could be initiated by viruses within the CNS (Figure 1).

TMEV-IDD is a well-characterized CD4$^+$ T-cell-mediated model of MS. Life-long persistent viral infection of APCs and glial cells residing in the CNS is directly related to the development of chronic demyelinating disease. Initial myelin damage is mediated by a bystander mechanism whereby the primary effector cells are mononuclear phagocytes (microglia/macrophages) activated by inflammatory cytokines produced from TMEV-specific T cells responding to viral epitopes that persist in the CNS. Early myelin destruction leads to the de novo activation of myelin-specific T cells (epitope spreading). The initial myelin response is directed towards the immunodominant PLP139–151 epitope, and epitope spreading then leads to the ordered progression of T cell responses to multiple myelin autoepitopes, which seem to play a significant role in the chronic phase of the disease by escalating the demyelinating process. The continuous presence of the virus within the CNS perpetuates this chronic inflammatory process in which epitope spreading leads to the induction of autoreactive T cells.

These findings enhance our understanding of the pathogenesis of human MS. MHC class II-bearing macrophages, astrocytes, and endothelial cells, together with expression of B7 costimulatory molecules, have been observed in or near MS lesions. Therefore, multiple cells in MS lesions have the potential to fully activate both naive and memory T cells within the CNS. Although distinct from the mechanism of autoimmune disease induction in mice infected with native TMEV, mimic and natural pathogen peptide-engineered TMEV infection models demonstrate that molecular mimicry can also lead from viral infection to autoimmune disease.

ACKNOWLEDGMENT

Support: NIH Grant NS062365

REFERENCES

1. Theiler M. Spontaneous encephalomyelitis of mice, a new virus disease. *J Exp Med* 1937;**65**:705–19.
2. Lipton HL. Theiler's virus infection in mice: an unusual biphasic disease process leading to demyelination. *Infect Immun* 1975;**11**:1147–55.
3. Lipton HL, Dal Canto MC. Chronic neurologic disease in Theiler's virus infection of SJL/J mice. *J Neurol Sci* 1976;**30**:201–7.
4. Lehrich JR, Arnason BGW, Hochberg F. Demyelinative myelopathy in mice induced by the DA virus. *J Neurol Sci* 1976;**29**:149–60.
5. Dal Canto MC, Lipton HL. Primary demyelination in Theiler's virus infection. An ultrastructural study. *Lab Invest* 1975;**33**:626–37.
6. Clatch RJ, Melvold RW, Miller SD, Lipton HL. Theiler's murine encephalomyelitis virus (TMEV)-induced demyelinating disease in mice is influenced by the H-2D region: correlation with TMEV-specific delayed-type hypersensitivity. *J Immunol* 1985;**135**: 1408–14.
7. Miller SD, Olson JK, Croxford JL. Multiple pathways to induction of virus-induced autoimmune demyelination: lessons from Theiler's virus infection. *J Autoimmun* 2001;**16**:219–27.
8. Miller SD, Vanderlugt CL, Begolka WS, Pao W, Yauch RL, Neville KL, et al. Persistent infection with Theiler's virus leads to CNS autoimmunity via epitope spreading. *Nat Med* 1997;**3**:1133–6.
9. Wekerle H. Immunopathogenesis of multiple sclerosis. *Acta Neurologica* 1991;**13**: 197–204.
10. Katz-Levy Y, Neville KL, Girvin AM, Vanderlugt CL, Pope JG, Tan LJ, et al. Endogenous presentation of self myelin epitopes by CNS-resident APCs in Theiler's virus-infected mice. *J Clin Invest* 1999;**104**:599–610.
11. Miller SD, Katz-Levy Y, Neville KL, Vanderlugt CL. Virus-induced autoimmunity: epitope spreading to myelin autoepitopes in Theiler's virus infection of the central nervous system. *Adv Virus Res* 2001;**56**:199–217.

12. Lipton HL, Twaddle G, Jelachich ML. The predominant virus antigen burden is present in macrophages in Theiler's murine encephalomyelitis virus-induced demyelinating disease. *J Virol* 1995;**69**:2525–33.
13. Clatch RJ, Melvold RW, Dal Canto MC, Miller SD, Lipton HL. The Theiler's murine encephalomyelitis virus (TMEV) model for multiple sclerosis shows a strong influence of the murine equivalents of HLA-A, B, and C. *J Neuroimmunol* 1987;**15**:121–35.
14. Roos RP, Firestone S, Wollmann R, Variakojis D, Arnason BG. The effect of short-term and chronic immunosuppression on Theiler's virus demyelination. *J Neuroimmunol* 1982;**2**:223–34.
15. Lipton HL, Dal Canto MC. Theiler's virus-induced demyelination: prevention by immunosuppression. *Science* 1976;**192**:62–4.
16. Lipton HL, Dal Canto MC. Contrasting effects of immunosuppression on Theiler's virus infection in mice. *Infect Immun* 1977;**15**:903–9.
17. Gerety SJ, Karpus WJ, Cubbon AR, Goswami RG, Rundell MK, Peterson JD, et al. Class II-restricted T cell responses in Theiler's murine encephalomyelitis virus (TMEV)-induced demyelinating disease. V. Mapping of a dominant immunopathologic VP2 T cell epitope in susceptible SJL/J mice. *J Immunol* 1994;**152**:908–18.
18. Clatch RJ, Lipton HL, Miller SD. Class II-restricted T cell responses in Theiler's murine encephalomyelitis virus (TMEV)-induced demyelinating disease. II. Survey of host immune responses and central nervous system virus titers in inbred mouse strains. *Microb Pathog* 1987;**3**:327–37.
19. Lyman MA, Myoung J, Mohindru M, Kim BS. Quantitative, not qualitative, differences in CD8(+) T cell responses to Theiler's murine encephalomyelitis virus between resistant C57BL/6 and susceptible SJL/J mice. *Eur J Immunol* 2004;**34**:2730–9.
20. Lyman MA, Lee HG, Kang BS, Kang HK, Kim BS. Capsid-specific cytotoxic T lymphocytes recognize three distinct H-2D(b)-restricted regions of the BeAn strain of Theiler's virus and exhibit different cytokine profiles. *J Virol* 2002;**76**:3125–34.
21. Kang BS, Lyman MA, Kim BS. Differences in avidity and epitope recognition of CD8 (+) T cells infiltrating the central nervous systems of SJL/J mice infected with BeAn and DA strains of Theiler's murine encephalomyelitis virus. *J Virol* 2002;**76**:11780–4.
22. Kang BS, Lyman MA, Kim BS. The majority of infiltrating CD8+ T cells in the central nervous system of susceptible SJL/J mice infected with Theiler's virus are virus specific and fully functional. *J Virol* 2002;**76**:6577–85.
23. Richards MH, Getts MT, Podojil JR, Jin Y-H, Kim BS, Miller SD. Virus expanded regulatory T cells control disease severity in the Theiler's virus mouse model of MS. *J Autoimm* 2011;**36**:142–54.
24. Croxford JL, Olson JK, Miller SD. Epitope spreading and molecular mimicry as triggers of autoimmunity in the Theiler's virus induced demyelinating disease model of multiple sclerosis. *Autoimmun Rev* 2002;**1**:251–60.
25. Zavala F, Abad S, Ezine S, Taupin V, Masson A, Bach JF. G-CSF therapy of ongoing experimental allergic encephalomyelitis via chemokine- and cytokine-based immune deviation. *J Immunol* 2002;**168**:2011–19.
26. Whitney LW, Ludwin SK, McFarland HF, Biddison WE. Microarray analysis of gene expression in multiple sclerosis and EAE identifies 5-lipoxygenase as a component of inflammatory lesions. *J Neuroimmunol* 2001;**121**:40–8.
27. Ibrahim SM, Mix E, Bottcher T, Koczan D, Gold R, Rolfs A, et al. Gene expression profiling of the nervous system in murine experimental autoimmune encephalomyelitis. *Brain* 2001;**124**:1927–38.
28. Lipton HL, Kratochvil J, Sethi P, Dal Canto MC. Theiler's virus antigen detected in mouse spinal cord 2 1/2 years after infection. *Neurology* 1984;**34**:1117–19.
29. Miller SD, Clatch RJ, Pevear DC, Trotter JL, Lipton HL. Class II-restricted T cell responses in Theiler's murine encephalomyelitis virus (TMEV)-induced demyelinating

disease. I. Cross-specificity among TMEV substrains and related picornaviruses, but not myelin proteins. *J Immunol* 1987;**138**:3776–84.

30. Barbano RL, Dal Canto MC. Serum and cells from Theiler's virus-infected mice fail to injure myelinating cultures or to produce in vivo transfer of disease. The pathogenesis of Theiler's virus-induced demyelination appears to differ from that of EAE. *J Neurol Sci* 1984;**66**:283–93.

31. Clatch RJ, Lipton HL, Miller SD. Characterization of Theiler's murine encephalomyelitis virus (TMEV)-specific delayed-type hypersensitivity responses in TMEV-induced demyelinating disease: correlation with clinical signs. *J Immunol* 1986;**136**:920–7.

32. Miller SD, Gerety SJ, Kennedy MK, Peterson JD, Trotter JL, Tuohy VK, et al. Class II-restricted T cell responses in Theiler's murine encephalomyelitis virus (TMEV)-induced demyelinating disease. III. Failure of neuroantigen-specific immune tolerance to affect the clinical course of demyelination. *J Neuroimmunol* 1990;**26**:9–23.

33. Yauch RL, Kerekes K, Saujani K, Kim BS. Identification of a major T cell epitope within VP3(24-37) of Theiler's virus in demyelination-susceptible SJL/J mice. *J Virol* 1995;**69**:7315–18.

34. Pope JG, Vanderlugt CL, Lipton HL, Rahbe SM, Miller SD. Characterization of and functional antigen presentation by central nervous system mononuclear cells from mice infected with Theiler's murine encephalomyelitis virus. *J Virol* 1998;**72**:7762–71.

35. Tisch R, Yang XD, Singer SM, Liblau RS, Fugger L, McDevitt HO. Immune response to glutamic acid decarboxylase correlates with insulitis in non-obese diabetic mice. *Nature* 1993;**366**:72–5.

36. Kaufman DL, Clare-Salzler M, Tian J, Forsthuber T, Ting GS, Robinson P, et al. Spontaneous loss of T-cell tolerance to glutamic acid decarboxylase in murine insulin-dependent diabetes. *Nature* 1993;**366**:69–72.

37. Tian J, Atkinson MA, Clare-Salzler M, Herschenfeld A, Forsthuber T, Lehmann PV, et al. Nasal administration of glutamate decarboxylase (GAD65) peptides induces Th2 responses and prevents murine insulin-dependent diabetes. *J Exp Med* 1996;**183**:1561–7.

38. Prasad S, Kohm AP, McMahon JS, Luo X, Miller SD. Pathogenesis of NOD diabetes is initiated by reactivity to the insulin B chain 9-23 epitope and involves functional epitope spreading. *J Autoimm* 2012;**39**:347–53.

39. Lehmann PV, Forsthuber T, Miller A, Sercarz EE. Spreading of T-cell autoimmunity to cryptic determinants of an autoantigen. *Nature* 1992;**358**:155–7.

40. McRae BL, Vanderlugt CL, Dal Canto MC, Miller SD. Functional evidence for epitope spreading in the relapsing pathology of experimental autoimmune encephalomyelitis. *J Exp Med* 1995;**182**:75–85.

41. Yu M, Johnson JM, Tuohy VK. A predictable sequential determinant spreading cascade invariably accompanies progression of experimental autoimmune encephalomyelitis: a basis for peptide-specific therapy after onset of clinical disease. *J Exp Med* 1996;**183**:1777–88.

42. Horwitz MS, Bradley LM, Harbetson J, Krahl T, Lee J, Sarvetnick N. Diabetes induced by Coxsackie virus: initiation by bystander damage and not molecular mimicry. *Nat Med* 1998;**4**:781–6.

43. Katz-Levy Y, Neville KL, Padilla J, Rahbe SM, Begolka WS, Girvin AM, et al. Temporal development of autoreactive Th1 responses and endogenous antigen presentation of self myelin epitopes by CNS-resident APCs in Theiler's virus-infected mice. *J Immunol* 2000;**165**:5304–14.

44. Vanderlugt CL, Eagar TN, Neville KL, Nikcevich KM, Bluestone JA, Miller SD. Pathologic role and temporal appearance of newly emerging autoepitopes in relapsing experimental autoimmune encephalomyelitis. *J Immunol* 2000;**164**:670–8.

45. Wucherpfennig KW, Sette A, Southwood S, Oseroff C, Matsui M, Strominger JL, et al. Structural requirements for binding of an immunodominant myelin basic protein

peptide to DR2 isotypes and for its recognition by human T cell clones. *J Exp Med* 1994;**179**:279–90.

46. Carrizosa AM, Nicholson LB, Farzan M, Southwood S, Sette A, Sobel RA, et al. Expansion by self antigen is necessary for the induction of experimental autoimmune encephalomyelitis by T cells primed with a cross-reactive environmental antigen. *J Immunol* 1998;**161**:3307–14.

47. Olson JK, Croxford JL, Calenoff M, Dal Canto MC, Miller SD. A virus-induced molecular mimicry model of multiple sclerosis. *J Clin Invest* 2001;**108**:311–18.

48. Olson JK, Eagar TN, Miller SD. Functional activation of myelin-specific T cells by virus-induced molecular mimicry. *J Immunol* 2002;**169**:2719–26.

49. Hofman FM, von Hanwehr RI, Dinarello CA, Mizel SB, Hinton D, Merrill JE. Immunoregulatory molecules and IL 2 receptors identified in multiple sclerosis brain. *J Immunol* 1986;**136**:3239–45.

50. Traugott U, Reinherz EL, Raine CS. Multiple sclerosis: distribution of T cell subsets within active chronic lesions. *Science* 1983;**219**:308–10.

51. Traugott U. Multiple sclerosis: relevance of class I and class II MHC- expressing cells to lesion development. *J Neuroimmunol* 1987;**16**:283–302.

52. Windhagen A, Newcombe J, Dangond F, Strand C, Woodroofe MN, Cuzner ML, et al. Expression of costimulatory molecules B7-1 (CD80), B7-2 (CD80), and interleukin 12 cytokine in multiple sclerosis lesions. *J Exp Med* 1995;**182**:1985–96.

53. Desimone R, Giampaolo A, Giometto B, Gallo P, Levi G, Peschle C, et al. The costimulatory molecule B7 Is expressed on human microglia in culture and in multiple sclerosis acute lesions. *J Neuropathol Exp Neurol* 1995;**54**:175–87.

54. Williams K, Ulvestad E, Antel JP. B7/BB-1 antigen expression on adult human microglia studied in vitro and in situ. *Eur J Immunol* 1994;**24**:3031–7.

55. Olson JK, Girvin AM, Miller SD. Direct activation of innate and antigen presenting functions of microglia following infection with Theiler's virus. *J Virol* 2001;**75**:9780–9.

56. Duncan DS, Miller SD. CNS expression of B7-H1 regulates pro-inflammatory cytokine production and alters severity of Theiler's virus-induced demyelinating disease. *PLoS One* 2011;**6**:e18548.

57. Miller SD, Vanderlugt CL, Lenschow DJ, Pope JG, Karandikar NJ, Dal Canto MC, et al. Blockade of CD28/B7-1 interaction prevents epitope spreading and clinical relapses of murine EAE. *Immunity* 1995;**3**:739–45.

58. Karandikar NJ, Vanderlugt CL, Eagar TN, Tan L, Bluestone JA, Miller SD. Tissue-specific up-regulation of B7-1 expression and function during the course of murine relapsing experimental autoimmune encephalomyelitis. *J Immunol* 1998;**161**:192–9.

59. Dal Canto MC, Melvold RW, Kim BS, Miller SD. Two models of multiple sclerosis: experimental allergic encephalomyelitis (EAE) and Theiler's murine encephalomyelitis virus (TMEV) infection – a pathological and immunological comparison. *Microsc Res Tech* 1995;**32**:215–29.

60. McMahon EJ, Bailey SL, Castenada CV, Waldner H, Miller SD. Epitope spreading initiates in the CNS in two mouse models of multiple sclerosis. *Nat Med* 2005;**11**:335–9.

PART 3

Bacteria and Autoimmunity

CHAPTER 27

Rheumatic Fever: How Streptococcal Throat Infection Triggers an Autoimmune Disease

Luiza Guilherme[*,†,1], **Jorge Kalil**[*,†,‡]
[*]Heart Institute—InCor, University of São Paulo, School of Medicine, São Paulo, Brazil
[†]Institute for Immunology Investigation, National Institute for Science and Technology, São Paulo, Brazil
[‡]Clinical Immunology and Allergy, Department of Clinical Medicine University of São Paulo, School of Medicine, São Paulo, Brazil
[1]Corresponding Author: luizagui@usp.br

1 INTRODUCTION

Rheumatic fever (RF) is a sequel of throat infection by group A streptococci (GAS) affecting 3–4% of untreated children. Acute RF usually occurs 3 weeks after infection. Rheumatic heart disease (RHD) is the result of valvular damage caused by the abnormal immune response and develops 4–8 weeks or more after GAS infection in 30–45% of individuals with RF. It remains a major cause of morbidity and mortality in developing countries. Data from the World Health Organization showed that 25–40% of cardiovascular diseases in these countries are due to RF. In Brazil, the damage to heart valves as a consequence of RF is responsible for 90% of heart surgeries among children.

2 *STREPTOCOCCUS PYOGENES*

Studies by Rebecca Lancefield[1] in 1941 classified streptococci groups based on the cell wall polysaccharides (groups A, B, C, F, and G). The *S. pyogenes* (GAS) is characterized by carbohydrates composed of N-acetyl-β-D-glucosamine and rhamnose. The GAS contains the M, T, and R surface proteins and lipoteichoic acid involved in the adherence of bacteria to throat epithelial cells. The M protein extends from the cell wall and it is composed of approximately 450 amino acid residues, with antigenic variations but high homology on the amino terminal (N-terminal) portion, except for

Infection and Autoimmunity
http://dx.doi.org/10.1016/B978-0-444-63269-2.00029-5

479

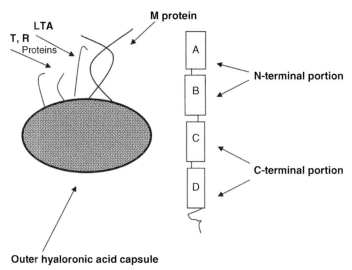

Figure 1 Schematic representation of *S. pyogenes*. The group A streptococcal cell is covered by an outer hyaluronic acid capsule and is characterized by the group A carbohydrates composed of *N*-acetyl-β-ᴅ-glucosamine and rhamnose. M, T, and R are surface proteins; lipoteichoic acid (LTA) is involved in the bacterial adherence to the throat epithelial cells; the N-terminal portion contains A and B regions (the A region defines the serotypes of streptococci strains); and the C-terminal portion contains C and D regions that are highly conserved among the streptococci strains.

the 11 first amino acid residues that define the different serotypes. The carboxy terminal end contains multiple repeat regions and is conserved.[2] Figure 1 provides a schematic representation of *S. pyogenes*.

Over 200 different serotypes of GAS have been described,[3] and studies have consistently found that some serotypes are more frequently associated with RF, whereas others are more often associated with acute glomerulonephritis. These serotypes or strains are called rheumatogenic and nephritogenic, respectively.[4,5] The emm1 type is one of the most frequent strains found in high-income countries, Asia, Latin America, and the Middle East[6] and is associated with both invasive and noninvasive infections worldwide. The M protein is the most important antigenic structure and shares structural homology with alpha helical coiled–coil human proteins such as cardiac myosin, tropomyosin, keratin, laminin, vimentin, and several valvular proteins.[7–10]

3 GENETIC MARKERS

A genetic pattern of susceptibility to RF and RHD was determined by Cheadle more than a century ago.[11] To define the pattern of inheritance of RF, some researchers have assumed an autosomic recessive model,[12] whereas others assume a Mendelian pattern of inheritance.[13] Observation of RF or RHD in identical twins suggested that if a Mendelian pattern is present, penetrance must be incomplete.[14] Patarroyo et al. described the presence of an alloantigen, designated 883, on the surface of B cells in more than 70% of patients with RF from Bogota and New York.[15] Indirect evidence, however, suggested that 883 alloantigen could be related to HLA class II molecules.[16,17] A monoclonal antibody called D8/17 was produced against the 883 alloantigen; this antibody identifies a B-cell antigen with enhanced expression in 90–100% of patients with RF.[18]

No consistent association with HLA class I antigens and RF/RHD was found; however, association with different HLA class II antigens has been indicated in several populations. The *HLA-DR7* allele seems to be most frequently associated with the disease (Table 1).[19–29]

HLA class II antigens play an important role in antigen presentation to the T-cell receptor (TCR). The divergence of HLA class II molecules associated with the disease in different countries is probably due to the capability of these molecules to present strain-specific streptococcal epitopes present in more than 250 streptococcal serotypes; some of them—including the rheumatogenic strains—have peculiar geographic distribution.

Using a molecular approach, several polymorphisms in genes related to both innate and adaptive immune response have recently been described.

Table 1 HLA Class II and Rheumatic Fever

HLA	Country	Population	References
DR4, DR9	The United	American Caucasian	19,20
DR2	States	American Black	
DR4	Saudi Arabia	Arabian	21
DR3, DQW2, D8/17	India	Indian	22
DR7, DR53	Brazil	Mulatto	23
Allogenotope TaqI DRβ, 13.81 kb	Brazil	Mulatto	24
DR7	Brazil	Caucasian	25
DR1	Brazil	Mulatto	26
DR7, DQ2	Egypt	Egyptian	27
DR1, DR6	South Africa	African	28
DR 11	Turkey	Turkish	29

Several HLA antigens are associated with RF/RHD in different countries. HLA-DR4, DR7, and DR9 were associated with HLA-DR53. HLA-DR4 and DR9 were found in American Caucasian and Arabian patients; DR7 was found in Brazilian (Caucasian and Mulatto) and Egyptian patients with RHD. HLA-DR1 was found in Brazilian patients with Sydenhams' chorea and South African patients with RF/RHD.

The *MBL2* and *FCN2* genes code for mannose-binding lectin and ficolin-2, respectively,[30–32] and act in the first line of infection defence because of their ability to opsonize pathogens, enhancing their phagocytosis and activating the complement cascade. Toll-like receptor 2 (*TLR2*) acts in pathogen recognition because of its ability to opsonize pathogens, enhancing their phagocytosis, and to activate the complement cascade via the lectin pathway.[33] The receptor for the Fc fragments of immunoglobulin G (*FCγRIIA*)[34] controls the ability to bind to human IgG2. Polymorphisms in genes that play a role in both innate and adaptive immunity, such as interleukin-1 receptor antagonist (*IL1RA*),[35,36] tumor necrosis factor-alpha (*TNFα*),[35,37–39] transforming growth factor-beta (*TGFβ*),[40,41] IL-10,[35] and cytotoxic T-cell lymphocyte antigen 4 (*CTLA4*),[42] also contribute to the pathogenesis of RF and RHD by acting as mediators of tissue inflammation later in the process. All these polymorphisms are described in Table 2.

4 PATHOGENESIS

The pathogenic mechanisms leading to RF/RHD involve the molecular mimicry mechanism responsible for the cross-reactions between streptococcal antigens and human tissue proteins, the epitope spreading of self-antigens, and the degeneracy of T-cell recognition in susceptible individuals. Nowadays it is clear that the disease is mediated by both humoral and cellular immune responses and that the cellular branch of the immune response is more involved with the development of RHD.

4.1 Humoral Immune Response

Streptococcal antibodies react with streptococcal antigens and several human tissues including heart, skin, brain, glomerular basement membrane, and striated and smooth muscles (reviewed by Cunningham).[43] Briefly, antibodies against *N*-acetyl-β-D-glucosamine, a polysaccharide present in both the streptococcal cell wall and heart valvular tissue, displayed cross-reactivity against laminin, an extracellular matrix alpha-helical coiled-coil protein that surrounds heart cells and is present in the valve. Among the human proteins, both cardiac myosin and vimentin, seem to be the major target antigens. Using affinity-purified antimyosin antibodies, a five-amino acid residue (Gln-Lys-Ser-Lys-Gln) epitope of the N-terminal M5 and M6 proteins was identified as cross-reactive with cardiac myosin.[43]

The analysis of humoral response against overlapping peptides of the N-terminal portion of M5 protein identified several immunodominant

Table 2 Other Genetic Polymorphisms Associated with RF/RHD

Gene	Chromosome localization	Polymorphism	Allele/genotype/haplotype associated with disease	Population studied	References
MBL2	10q11.2-q21	-221 X,Y	YA/YA, YA/XA	Brazilian	30
		A (52C, 54G, 57G) O (52T, 54A, 57A)	O, O/O	Brazilian	31
		A (52C, 54G, 57G) O (52T, 54A, 57A)			
FCN2	9q34	-986G/A, -602G/A, -4G/A	G/G/A	Brazilian	32
TLR2	4q32	2258A/G (753 Arg/Gln)	753Gln, Arg753Gln	Turkish	33
FCγRIIA	1q21-q23	494A/G (131H/R)	131R, R/R (high risk)	Turkish	34
			R/H (intermediate risk)		
IL1RA	2q14.2	A1,A2,A3,A4	A1/A1	Egyptian	35
TNFα	6p21.3	-308G/A	A1, A1/A1	Brazilian	36
			A	Mexican	37
			A/A, G/G	Egyptian	35
			A	Brazilian	38
			A	Turkish	39
		-238G/A	G, G/G	Mexican	37
			A	Brazilian	38
TGFβ	19q13.1	-509C/T	T	Egyptian	40
			C/C	Chinese	41
		869T/C	T, T/T	Egyptian	40
IL-10	1q31-q32	-1082G/A	G/G	Egyptian	35
			A/A	Egyptian	35
CTLA4		+49A/G	G/G	Turkish	42

TNF-α: tumor necrosis factor-α; *TGFβ*: transforming growth factor-β; *IL-1RA*: IL-1 receptor antagonist; *MBL2*: mannan binding lectin 2; *TLR2*: Toll-like receptor 2; *FCN2*: ficolin 2; *FCγRIIA*: IgG Fc receptor; *CTLA4*: cytotoxic T-cell lymphocyte antigen 4.

Residues	Peptide Sequences	Mild RHD/ Chorea Patients Antibodies	Severe RHD Patients	
			Antibodies	T Cells
11–25*	QRAKEALDKYELENH			
21–40	ELENHDLKTKNEGLKTENEG			
41–60	LKTENEGLKTENEGLKTEKK			
81–96*	DKLKQQRDTLSTQKET			
81–103*	LKQQRDTLSTQKETLEREVQN			
163–177*	ETIGTLKKILDETVK			
181–200	KILDETVKDKLAKEQKSKQN			
183–201*	LDETVKDKLAKEQKSKQNI			
191–210	LAKEQKSKQNIGALKQELAK			

Figure 2 Immunodominant epitopes of the streptococcal N-terminal region from the M5 protein recognized by antibodies and/or T cells of patients with severe and/or mild RHD. Humoral and cellular reactivity against overlapping peptides were tested by ELISA and T-cell proliferation assay. The immunodominant regions were determined by comparing the reactivity of sera and peripheral and/or heart tissue intralesional T cells from patients with RHD with sera and peripheral T cells from healthy individuals. P values <0.05 were considered significant. The peptides preferentially recognized by antibodies are represented as light grey for patients with mild RHD with or without Sydenham's chorea and medium grey for patients with severe RHD. T-cell reactivity (dark grey) was evaluated in patients with severe RHD. *The M5 peptide sequences were based on the sequence of the M5 protein published by Manjula et al.[44] The other M5 peptide sequences were based on the sequences of the M5 protein published by Robinson et al.[45] Overlapping peptides are aligned.

epitopes covering around 200 amino acid residues recognized by mild RHD patients, most of them with Sydenham's chorea associated. Antibodies from patients with severe RHD recognized some N-terminal epitopes (Figure 2).

Although the presence of antibodies against streptococcal antigens and human tissue proteins has been described for more than 50 years, their role in the development of the disease remains unclear. One possibility to explain the presence of antibodies in heart tissue was suggested by Roberts et al.,[46] who showed an increased expression of VCAM-1, an adhesion molecule, in the vascular endothelium that was activated after an inflammatory reaction started by antimyosin and N-acetyl-glucosamine. The VCAM-1 molecules interact with VLA-4, another adhesion molecule expressed on CD4+ T lymphocytes. We recently verified that ICAM and P-selectin, other integrins and several chemokines and their receptors also were up-regulated. Among the chemokines, CCL3/*MIP1α gene* expression was up-regulated in the myocardium, whereas CCL1/*I-309* and CXCL9/*Mig* were highly expressed in the valvular tissue of patients with RHD.[47] An *in vitro* assay demonstrated that valvular lesions infiltrating T cells migrated mainly towards a CXCL9/*Mig* gradient, suggesting that specific chemokine can mediate both the CD4$^+$ and CD8$^+$ T-cell infiltration to the site of inflammation in the heart.[47]

4.2 Cellular Immune Response

Studies of the cellular branch of the immune response began around 1970. In favor of the important role of T cells in RF, some studies of tonsils and human peripheral blood showed that CD4$^+$ T cells were increased.[48,49] It also was demonstrated that T cells were able to recognize streptococcal cell wall and tissue antigens.[50–55] Cytotoxic activity towards immortalized human heart cells also was described.[56,57]

The first evidence that CD4$^+$ T cells were involved in RHD lesions was described in 1983.[58] The isolation of T cells from heart valves led Yoshinaga et al.[59] to compare the reactivity of PHA-stimulated T-cell lines derived from heart valve specimens and peripheral blood lymphocytes of patients with RF. They showed that although these cells recognized cell wall and membrane streptococcal antigens, they failed to react with M protein, myosin, or other mammalian cytoskeletal proteins.

The functional activity of heart-infiltrating CD4$^+$ T-cell clones was directly demonstrated by our group. The presence of intralesional cross-reactive T-cell clones allowed us to establish the significance of T-cell molecular mimicry in the pathogenesis of RHD. We mapped the N-terminal reactivity of intralesional T-cell clones and identified three immunodominant regions—1–25, 81–103, and 163–177 residues—within the streptococcal M protein (Figure 2); these are cross-reactive with several heart tissue protein fractions, mainly those derived from valvular tissue with molecular mass of 95–150, 43–63, and 30–43 kDa, respectively.[10] A previous work described the recognition of 50- to 54-kDa myocardial-derived proteins by peripheral T lymphocytes from patients with RHD.[60] More recently, we identified several valve-derived proteins, such as vimentin, protein disulfide isomerase ER-60 precursor (PDIA3), 78-kDa glucose-regulated protein precursor (HSPA5), and other cytoskeleton proteins, that are recognized by peripheral blood and intralesional T-cell clones from patients with severe RHD; these proteins are probably targets of the valvular lesions in RHD.[61]

T cells from peripheral blood of patients with RF/RHD also recognized several M5 peptides. Interestingly, the immunodominant peptide M5(81–96) was preferentially recognized by DR7+DR53+ patients with severe RHD,[62] suggesting that HLA DR7 and DR53 molecules could be more involved with the selection of streptococcal peptides and their presentation to the TCR.

Our studies of TCR BV usage in the PBMCs of patients with severe RHD and infiltrating T-cell lines derived from myocardium and/or mitral valve showed expansion of several BV families with oligoclonal profiles, mainly in infiltrating T-cell lines. Some major oligoclonal BV expansions were shared between mitral valve and left atrium T-cell lines, but an in-depth analysis of the usage of BJ segments in these shared expansions, as well as the nucleotide sequencing of the CDR3 regions, suggested that different antigenic peptides could be predominantly recognized in the mitral valve and the myocardium.[63] The high frequency and the persistence of T-cell oligoclonal expansions in damaged heart valves seem to be associated with the progression of the disease;[64] this is probably related to the spreading of autoantigen epitope recognition. In agreement with these data, the possibility of detecting some T-cell expansions in damaged heart valves has been described, even 20 years after an episode of acute RF.[65]

The TCR analysis of intralesional T-cell clones showed a degenerate pattern of reactivity. Several mitral valve-derived T-cell clones recognizing different antigens presented the same TCR BVBJ and CDR3 sequences. They expressed two alpha chains at the RNA level with same AVAJ segments (Table 3), indicating that intralesional T-cell clones with common TCR usage can recognize several epitopes that probably amplify the deleterious immune reaction.[66]

4.3 Cytokine Profile

Cytokines are important secondary signals following an infection because they trigger effective immune responses in most individuals and probably deleterious responses in patients with autoimmune disease. Three subsets of T helper cytokines are currently described. Antigen-activated CD4+ T cells polarize to the Th1, Th2, or Th17 subsets, depending on the cytokine secreted. Th1 is involved with the cellular immune response and produces IL-2, IFN-γ, and TNF-α. Th2 cells mediate humoral and allergic immune

Table 3 Degeneracy of Antigen Recognition by Intralesional CD4$^+$ T-Cell Clones

T-cell Clone Identification	Antigens Recognized	BV Family	CDR3 (N-D-N) Sequences	BJ Family	AV Family	CDR3 (N-D-N) Sequences	AJ Family
Lu 3.1.8	35 kDa/pI 8.84 LMM 28 (1647–1664) LMM 28B (1660–1677) LMM 32 (1699–1716)	BV 13	SGRQGRYEQY (10 aa)	BJ 2S7	AV 2 AV 3	MRTPVTSSI (9 aa) TDPITGTASKLT (12 aa)	AJ–NT AJ 44
Lu 3. 1. 29	56–53 kDa/pI 6.76	BV 13	SGRQGRYEQY (10 aa)	BJ 2S7	AV 2 AV 3	MRTPVTSSI (9 aa) TDPITGTASKLT (12 aa)	AJ–NT AJ 44

NT, not tested; LMM, light meromyosin peptides: LMM28-SLQSLLKDTQIQLDDAVR; LMM28B-DDAVRANDDLKENIAIVE; LMM31-LEELRAVVEQTERSRKL; LMM32-RSRKLAEQELIETSERV (underlined, shared sequences).

Adapted from Faé et al.[66]

responses and produce IL-4, IL-5, and IL-13. Th17 has more recently been described as a type of proinflammatory response mediated by IL-17. The cytokines TGFβ, IL-6, and IL-23 are the factors that induce the Th17 lineage.

The evaluation of proinflammatory cytokines produced by peripheral blood and tonsillar mononuclear cells in after stimulation with streptococcal antigen and pokeweed mitogen in patients with RF/RHD without congestive heart failure showed a different pattern of PBMCs and tonsillar cells. TNF-α, IL-1, and IL-2 were overproduced by PBMCs and decreased by tonsillar mononuclear cells.[67] In patients with acute RF and active RHD, increased production of IL-2 and elevated numbers of $CD4^+CD25^+$ cells were observed, suggesting the expansion of activated $CD4^+$ T cells in the peripheral blood;[68] increased plasma concentrations of TNF-α also were described.[69–71] The Aschoff nodule, considered the pathognomonic lesion of RF, is composed of an agglomerate of cells having characteristics of monocytic and macrophage cells[72,73] and probably function as antigen-presenting cells to the T cells. In the valve lesions of patients with acute RF, the production of IL-1, TNF-α, and IL-2 correlated with progression of Aschoff nodules as follows: in stages 1 and 2, IL-1 and TNF-α were secreted by monocytes/macrophages; in stage 3, IL-2 was secreted by T lymphocytes.[74] We analyzed the cytokine pattern of infiltrating mononuclear cells in the mitral valve and myocardium tissue of patients with acute RF and chronic RHD. Our results showed that the infiltrating mononuclear cells in both myocardium and valvular tissue secrete the inflammatory cytokines interferon-γ and TNF-α. Mononuclear cells secreting IL-10 and IL-4 (regulatory cytokines) also were found in the myocardium tissue; however, in the valvular tissue, only a few cells secrete IL-4, suggesting that these low numbers of IL4-producing cells may contribute to the progression of valvular RHD lesions.[75] We recently identified large numbers of IL-17- and IL-23-producing cells in the valves, a Th17 subset of cytokines frequently involved in the development of autoimmune diseases.[76]

5 CONCLUSIONS

The knowledge acquired during the past 25 years favors the molecular mimicry mechanism as one of the most important mechanisms leading to autoimmune reactions in RHD. Altogether, the results presented here delineate RF/RHD as a complex autoimmune disease because of the role of several genes that regulate both innate and adaptive immune response as effectors of RF/RHD reactions. Both humoural and cellular immune responses are involved with the autoimmune reactions. $CD4^+$ T cells play a major role in the development of rheumatic heart lesions. The autoimmune reaction in the heart probably is mediated by a network of immune reactions involving the recognition of several autoantigens triggered on the periphery by an immunodominant streptococcal antigen that expands several T-cell clones by epitope spreading. Degeneracy of the TCR allowed several antigens to be recognized, and epitope spreading mechanisms are fundamental for the autoimmune process mediated by both T and B cells. T-cell clones, mainly $CD4^+$ cells, migrate to the heart, where the local production of inflammatory Th1 and Th17 cytokines trigger the activation of autoreactive infiltrating T cells. These cells recognize several autoantigens with conformational or sequence homologies. Both mechanisms – epitope spreading and degeneracy of antigen recognition by the TCR – amplify autoimmune reactions. Box 1 summarizes the major events leading to RF/RHD.

REFERENCES

1. Lancefield RC. Specific relationships of cell composition to biologic activity of hemolytic streptococci. *Harvey Lectures* 1941;**36**:251–65.
2. Fishetti V. Streptococcal M protein. *Sci Am* 1991;**264**(6):32–9.
3. McMillan DJ, Drèze PA, Vu T, Bessen DE, Guglielmini J, Steer AC, et al. Updated model of group A streptococcus M proteins based on a comprehensive worldwide study. *Clin Microbiol Infect* 2013;**19**:222–9.
4. Wannamaker LW. Differences between streptococcal infections of the throat and skin. (In two parts). *N Engl J Med* 1970;**282**(23–31):78–85.
5. Stollerman GH. The changing face of rheumatic fever in the 20th century. *J Med Microbiol* 1998;**47**:1–3.
6. Steer AC, Law I, Matatolu L, Beall BW, Carapetis JR. Global emm type distribution of group A streptococci: systematic review and implications for vaccine development. *Lancet Infect Dis* 2009;**9**:611–6.
7. Shikhman AR, Cunningham MW. Immunological mimicry between N-acetyl-β-D-glucosamine and cytokeratin peptides. *J Immunol* 1994;**152**:4375–87.
8. Manjula BN, Fischetti VA. Tropomyosin-like 7-residue periodicity in three immunologically distinct streptococcal M proteins and its implication for the antiphagocytic property of the molecule. *J Exp Med* 1980;**151**:695–708.
9. Manjula BN, Trus BL, Fischetti VA. Presence of two distinct regions in the coiled-coil structure of the streptococcal PepM5 protein: relationship to mammalian coiled-coil proteins and implications to its biological properties. *Proc Natl Acad Sci USA* 1985;**82**:1064–8.
10. Guilherme L, Cunha-Neto E, Coelho V, Snitcowsky R, Pomerantzeff PMA, Assis RV, et al. Human -infiltrating T cell clones from rheumatic heart disease patients recognize both streptococcal and cardiac proteins. *Circulation* 1995;**92**:415–20.

11. Cheadle WR. Harveian lectures on the various manifestations of the rheumatic state as exemplified in childhood and early life. *Lancet* 1889;**371**:821–7.
12. Wilson MG, Schweitzer M. Pattern of hereditary susceptibility in rheumatic fever. *Circulation* 1954;**10**:699–704.
13. Uchida IA. Possible genectic factors in the etiology of rheumatic fever. *Am J Hum Genet* 1953;**5**:61–9.
14. Taranta A, Torosdag S, Metrakos JD, Jegier W, Uchida I. Rheumatic fever in mono-zigotic and dizigotic twins (abstract). *Circulation* 1959;**20**:788.
15. Patarroyo ME, Winchester RJ, Vejerano A, Gibofsky A, Chalem F, Zabriskie JB, et al. Association of a B-cell alloantigen with susceptibility to rheumatic fever. *Nature* 1979;**278**:173–4.
16. Ayoub EM. The search for host determinants of susceptibility to rheumatic fever: the missing link. *Circulation* 1984;**69**:197–201.
17. Gibofsky A, Khanna A, Suh E, Zabriskie JB. The genetics of rheumatic fever: relation-ship to streptococcal infection and autoimmune disease. *J Rheumatol* 1991;**18** (suppl. 30):1–13.
18. Zabriskie JB, Lavenchy D, Willians Jr. RC, Fu SM, Yeadon CA, Fotino M, et al. Rheu-matic fever-associated B cell alloantigens as identified by monoclonal antibodies. *Arthritis Rheum* 1985;**28**(9):1047–51.
19. Ayoub EM, Barrett DJ, MacLaren NK, Krischen JP. Association of class II histocompat-ibility leukocyte antigens with rheumatic fever. *J Clin Invest* 1986;**77**:2019–26.
20. Anastasiou-Nana M, Anderson JL, Carquist JF, Nanas JN. HLA DR typing and lympho-cyte subset evaluation in rheumatic heart disease: a search for immune response factors. *Am Heart J* 1986;**112**(5):992–7.
21. Rajapakse CNA, Halim K, Al-Orainey L, Al-Nozha M, Al-Aska AK. A genetic marker for rheumatic heart disease. *Br Heart J* 1987;**58**:659–62.
22. Jhinghan B, Mehra NK, Reddy KS, Taneja V, Vaidya MC, Bhatia ML. HLA, blood groups and secretor status in patients with established rheumatic fever and rheumatic heart disease. *Tissue Antigens* 1986;**27**:172–8.
23. Guilherme L, Weidebach W, Kiss MH, Snitcowsky R, Kalil J. Association of human leukocyte class II antigens with rheumatic fever or rheumatic heart disease in a Brazilian population. *Circulation* 1991;**83**:1995–8.
24. Weidebach W, Goldberg AC, Chiarella J, Guilherme L, Snitcowsky R, Pileggi F, et al. HLA class II antigens in rheumatic fever: analysis of the DR locus by RFLP and oligo-typing. *Hum Immunol* 1994;**40**:253–8.
25. Guédez Y, Kotby A, El-Demellaway M, Galal A, Thomson G, Zaher S, et al. HLA class II associations with rheumatic heart disease are more evident and consistent among clinically homogeneous patients. *Circulation* 1999;**99**:2784–90.
26. Visentainer JE, Pereira FC, Dalalio MM, Tsuneto LT, Donadio PR, Moliterno RA. Association of HLA-DR7 with rheumatic fever in the Brazilian population. *J Rheumatol* 2002;**7**(6):1518–20.
27. Maharaj B, Hammond MG, Appadoo B, Leary WP, Pudifin DJ. HLA-A, B, DR and DQ antigens in black patients with severe chronic rheumatic heart disease. *Circulation* 1987;**76**:259–61.
28. Olmez U, Turgay M, Ozenirler S, Tutkak H, Duzgun N, Duman M, et al. Association of HLA class I and class II antigens with rheumatic fever in a Turkish population. *Rheu-matol* 1992;**22**(2):49–52.
29. Donadi EA, Smith AG, Louzada-Junior P, Voltarelli JC, Nepom GT. HLA class I and class II profiles of patients presenting RF with Sydenham's chorea. *J Neurol* 2000; **247**(2):122–8.
30. Messias Reason IJ, Schafranski MD, Jensenius JC, Steffensen R. The association between mannose-binding lectin gene polymorphism and rheumatic heart disease. *Hum Immunol* 2006;**67**:991–8.

31. Ramasawmy R, Spina G, Fae KC, Pereira AC, Nisihara R, Messias Reason IJ, et al. Association of mannose-binding lectin gene polymorphism but not of mannose-binding serine protease 2 with chronic severe aortic regurgitation of rheumatic etiology. *Clin Vaccine Immunol* 2008;**15**:932–6.

32. de Messias-Reason IJ, Schafranski MD, Kremsner PG, Kun JF. Ficolin 2 (FCN2) functional polymorphisms and the risk of rheumatic fever and rheumatic heart disease. *Clin Exp Immunol* 2009;**157**:395–9.

33. Berdeli A, Celik HA, Ozyürek R, Dogrusoz B. Aydin HH.TLR-2 gene Arg753Gln polymorphism is strongly associated with acute rheumatic fever in children. *J Mol Med* 2005;**83**:535–41.

34. Yee AM, Phan HM, Zuniga R, Salmon JE, Musher DM. Association between FcgammaRIIa-R131 allotype and bacteremic pneumococcal pneumonia. *Clin Infect Dis* 2000;**30**:25–8.

35. Settin A, Abdel-Hady H, El-Baz R, Saber I. Gene polymorphisms of TNFalpha(-308), IL-10(-1082), IL-6(-174), and IL-1Ra(VNTR) related to susceptibility and severity of rheumatic heart disease. *Pediatr Cardiol* 2007;**28**:363–71.

36. Azevedo PM, Bauer R, Vde Caparbo F, Silva CA, Bonfá E, Pereira RM. Interleukin-1 receptor antagonist gene (IL1RN) polymorphism possibly associated to severity of rheumatic carditis in a Brazilian cohort. *Cytokine* 2010;**49**:109–13.

37. Hernandez-Pacheco G, Flores-Domínguez C, Rodríguez-Pérez JM, Pérez-Hernández N, Fragoso JM, Saul A, et al. Tumor necrosis factor-alpha promoter polymorphisms in Mexican patients with rheumatic heart disease. *J Autoimmun* 2003;**21**:59–63.

38. Ramasawmy R, Fae KC, Spina G, Victora GD, Tanaka AC, Palácios SA, et al. Association of polymorphisms within the promoter region of the tumor necrosis factor alpha with clinical outcomes of rheumatic fever. *Mol Immunol* 2007;**44**:1873–8.

39. Sallakci N, Akcurin G, Köksoy S, Kardelen F, Uguz A, Coskun M, et al. TNFalpha G-308A polymorphism is associated with rheumatic fever and correlates with increased TNFalpha production. *J Autoimmun* 2005;**25**:50–4.

40. Kamal H, Hussein G, Hassoba H, Mosaad N, Gad A, Ismail M. Transforming growth factor-beta1 gene C-509T and T869C polymorphisms as possible risk factors in rheumatic heart disease in Egypt. *Acta Cardiol* 2010;**65**:177–83.

41. Chou HT, Chen CH, Tsai CH, Tsai FJ. Association between transforming growth factor-beta1 gene C-509T and T869C polymorphisms and rheumatic heart disease. *Am Heart J* 2004;**148**:181–6.

42. Düzgün N, Duman T, Haydardedeoðlu FE, Tutkak H. Cytotoxic T lymphocyte-associated antigen-4 polymorphism in patients with rheumatic heart disease. *Tissue Antigens* 2009;**74**:539–42.

43. Cunningham MW. Pathogenesis of group A streptococcal infections. *Clin Microbiol Rev* 2000;**13**:470–511.

44. Manjula BN, Acharya AS, Mische MS, Fairwell T, Fischetti VA. The complete amino acid sequence of a biologically active 197- residue fragment of M protein isolated from type 5 group A streptococci. *J Biol Chem* 1984;**259**:3686–93.

45. Robinson JH, Atherton MC, Goodacre JA, Pinkney M, Weightman H, Kehoe MA. Mapping T-cell epitopes in group A streptococcal type 5 M protein. *Infect Immun* 1991;**59**(12):4324–31.

46. Roberts S, Kosanke S, Terrence Dunn S, Jankelow D, Duran CM, Cunningham MW. Pathogenic mechanisms in rheumatic carditis: focus on valvular endothelium. *J Infect Dis* 2001;**183**:507–11.

47. Faé KC, Palacios SA, Nogueira LG, Oshiro SE, Demarchi LMF, Bilate AMB, et al. CXCL9/Mig mediates T cells recruitment to valvular tissue lesions of chronic rheumatic heart disease patients. *Inflammation* 2013;**36**(4):800–11.

48. Bathia R, Narula J, Reddy KS, Koicha M, Malaviya AN, Pothineni RB, et al. Lymphocyte subsets in acute rheumatic fever and rheumatic heart disease. *Clin Cardiol* 1989;**12**:34–8.

49. Bhatnagar PK, Nijhawan R, Prakash K. T cell subsets in acute rheumatic fever, rheumatic heart disease and acute glomerulonephritis cases. *Immunol Lett* 1987;**15**:217–19.

50. Mclaughin JF, Paterson PY, Hartz RS, Embury SH. Rheumatic carditis: in vitro responses of peripheral blood leukocytes to heart and streptococcal antigens. *Arthritis Rheum* 1972;**15**:600–8.

51. Read SE, Fischetti VA, Utermohlen V, Falk RE, Zabriskie JB. Cellular reactivity studies to streptococcal antigens. Migration inhibition studies in patients with streptococcal infections and rheumatic fever. *J Clin Invest* 1974;**54**:439–50.

52. Meric N, Berkel AI. Cellular immunity in children with acute rheumatic fever and rheumatic carditis. *Pediatr Res* 1979;**13**:16–20.

53. Read SE, Reid HFM, Fischetti VA, Poon-King T, Ramkissoon R, McDowell M, et al. Serial studies on the cellular immune response to streptococcal antigens in acute and convalescent rheumatic fever patients in Trinidad. *J Clin Immunol* 1986;**6**(6):433–41.

54. Gray ED, Wannamaker LW, Ayoub E, El Kholy A. Cellular immune responses to extracellular streptococcal products in rheumatic heart disease. *J Clin Invest* 1981;**68**:665–71.

55. Gross WL, Schlaak M. Modulation of human lymphocyte functions by group A streptococci. *Clin Immunol Immunopathol* 1984;**32**:234–47.

56. Dale JB, Simpson WA, Ofek I, Beachey E. Blastogenic responses of human lymphocytes to structurally defined polypeptide fragments of streptococcal M protein. *J Immunol* 1981;**126**:1499–505.

57. Kotb M, Courtney HS, Dale JB, Beachey EH. Cellular and biochemical responses of human T lymphocytes stimulated with streptococcal M proteins. *J Immunol* 1989;**142**:966–70.

58. Raizada V, Williams Jr. RC, Chopra P, Gopinath N, Prakash K, Sharma KB, et al. Tissue distribution of lymphocytes in rheumatic heart valves as defined by monoclonal anti-T cells antibodies. *Am J Med* 1983;**74**:90–6.

59. Yoshinaga M, Figueiroa F, Wahid MR, Marcus RH, Suh E, Zabriskie JB. Antigenic specificity of lymphocytes isolated from valvular specimens of rheumatic fever patients. *J Autoimmun* 1995;**8**:601–13.

60. El-Demellawy M, El-Ridi R, Guirguis NI, Alim MA, Kotby A, Kotb M. Preferential recognition of human myocardial antigens by T lymphocytes from rheumatic heart disease patients. *Infect Immun* 1997;**65**(6):2197–205.

61. Faé KC, Silva DD, Oshiro SE, Tanaka AC, Pomerantzeff PM, Douay C, et al. Mimicry in recognition of cardiac myosin peptides by heart-intralesional T cell clones from rheumatic heart disease. *J Immunol* 2006;**176**:5662–70.

62. Guilherme L, Oshiro SE, Fae KC, Cunha-Neto E, Renesto G, Goldberg AC, et al. T cell reactivty against streptococcal antigens in the periphery mirrors reactivity of heart infiltrating T lymphocytes in rheumatic heart disease patients. *Infect Immunity* 2001;**69**(9):5345–535.

63. Guilherme L, Dulphy N, Douay C, Coelho V, Cunha-Neto E, Oshiro SE, et al. Molecular evidence for antigen-driven immune responses in cardiac lesions of rheumatic heart disease patients. *Int Immunol* 2000;**12**:1063–74.

64. Guilherme L, Cunha-Neto E, Tanaka AC, Dulphy N, Toubert A, Kalil J. Heart-directed autoimmunity: the case of rheumatic fever. *J Autoimmun* 2001;**16**:363–7.

65. Figueroa F, Gonzalez M, Carrion F, Lobos C, Turner F, Lasagna N, et al. Restriction in the usage of variable beta regions in T-cells infiltrating valvular tissue from rheumatic heart disease patients. *J Autoimmun* 2002;**19**:233–40.

66. Faé K, Kalil J, Toubert A, Guilherme L. Heart infiltrating T-cell clones from a rheumatic heart disease patient display a common TCR usage and a degenerate antigen recognition pattern. *Mol Immunol* 2004;**40**:1129–35.

67. Miller LC, Gray ED, Mansour M, Abdin ZH, Kamel R, Zaher S, et al. Cytokines and immunoglobulin in rheumatic heart disease: production by blood and tonsillar mononuclear cells. *J Rheumatol* 1989;**16**:1436–42.

68. Morris K, Mohan C, Wahi PL, Anand IS, Ganguly NK. Enhancement of IL-1, IL-2 production and IL-2 receptor generation in patients with acute rheumatic fever and active rheumatic heart disease; a prospective study. *Clin Exp Immunol* 1993;**91**:429–36.

69. Narin N, Kütükçüler N, Özyürek R, Bakiler AR, Parlar A, Arcasoy M. Lymphocyte subsets and plasma IL-1 α, IL-2, and TNF- α concentrations in acute rheumatic fever and chronic rheumatic heart disease. *Clin Immunol Immunopathol* 1995;**77**:172–6.

70. Samsonov MY, Tilz GP, Pisklakov VP, Reibnegger G, Nassonov EL, Nassonova VA, et al. Serum-soluble receptors for tumor necrosis factor-α and interleukin-2 and neopterin in acute rheumatic fever. *Clin Immunol Immunopathol* 1995;**74**:31–4.

71. Yegin O, Coskun M, Ertug H. Cytokines in acute rheumatic fever. *Eur J Pediatr* 1997;**156**:25–9.

72. Kemeny E, Grieve T, Marcus R, Sareli P, Zabriskie JB. Identification of mononuclear cells and T cell subsets in rheumatic valvulitis. *Clin Immunol Immunopathol* 1989;**52**:225–37.

73. Chopra P, Narula J, Kumar SA, Sachdeva S, Bathia ML. Immunohistochemical characterization of Aschoff nodules and endomyocardial inflammatory infiltrates in left atrial appendages from patients with chronic rheumatic heart disease. *Int J Cardiol* 1988;**20**:99–105.

74. Fraser WJ, Haffejee Z, Jankelow D, Wadee A, Cooper K. Rheumatic Aschoff nodules revisited. II. Cytokine expression corroborates recently proposed sequential stages. *Histopathology* 1997;**31**:460–4.

75. Guilherme L, Cury P, Demarchi LM, Coelho V, Abel L, Lopez AP, et al. Rheumatic heart disease: proinflammatory cytokines play a role in the progression and maintenance of valvular lesions. *Am J Pathol* 2004;**165**:1583–91.

76. Guilherme L, Kalil J. Rheumatic heart disease; molecules involved in valve tissue inflammation leading to the autoimmune process and anti-*S. pyogenes* vaccine. *Frontiers Immunol* 2013;**4**:1–6. http://dx.doi.org/10.3389/fimmu.2013.00325.

CHAPTER 28

Helicobacter pylori Infection and Gastric Autoimmunity: Coincidence or a Cause and Effect Relationship?

Fabiola Atzeni[*,1], **Maurizio Benucci**[†], **Alberto Batticciotto**[*],
Piercarlo Sarzi-Puttini[*]
[*]Rheumatology Unit, L. Sacco University Hospital, Milan, Italy
[†]Unit of Rheumatology, Ospedale San Giovanni di Dio, Florence, Italy
[1]Corresponding Author: atzenifabiola@hotmail.com

1 INTRODUCTION

Helicobacter pylori is a Gram-negative gastrointestinal bacterium that has evolved together with its human hosts for at least 58,000 years, and it still infects 50% of the world's population.[1] It is usually acquired during childhood and, if left untreated, remains a life-long resident in its host's gastric ecosystem. *H. pylori* infection triggers a strong immune response that leads to high levels of *H. pylori*-specific antibodies, but it may require antibiotics to eradicate the pathogen and the associated gastritis. The infection causes chronic gastric mucosa inflammation that, although often clinically asymptomatic, systematically destroys the stomach, and as many as 15% of infected subjects subsequently develop serious diseases such as peptic ulcers, mucosa-associated lymphoid tissue (MALT) lymphoma, and gastric adenocarcinoma.[2–5]

The outcome of the infection depends on the severity and anatomical distribution of the gastritis induced by the bacterium. Almost 1% of infected subjects have corpus-predominant gastritis (the so-called gastric cancer phenotype), and they are more likely to develop hypochlorhydria, gastric atrophy and, eventually, gastric cancer. Up to 15% of infected individuals with antrum-predominant gastritis (the so-called duodenal ulcer phenotype) are affected by excessive acid secretion and are more likely to develop duodenal ulcer, whereas up to 5% of infected individuals experience mild, mixed

Infection and Autoimmunity
http://dx.doi.org/10.1016/B978-0-444-63269-2.00070-2

antrum and corpus gastritis (the so-called benign gastritis phenotype) with almost normal acid secretion, and they remain generally free of serious disease.[4,5]

Despite its declining incidence, gastric cancer (which kills >700,000 people each year) is still the fourth most common type of cancer, the second leading cause of cancer-related death, and the fourteenth most frequent cause of all-cause death. Furthermore, although worldwide rates of *H. pylori* infection are also decreasing, it is still a destructive and transmissible infectious disease that can lead to serious health consequences because antibiotic treatment reduces but does not necessarily eliminate the risk of a poor outcome.[5]

2 EPIDEMIOLOGY

The prevalence of *H. pylori* infection varies, and there are large differences between developed and developing countries.[6] In developing countries, such as India, Saudi Arabia and Vietnam, approximately 80% of the population is infected by the age of 20 years because the disease is most often acquired in childhood or in the presence of young children, and peak prevalence is observed in people aged 20–30 years. A study of 485 asymptomatic subjects aged 15–80 years in Houston, Texas (50% black and 50% white) found that prevalence increased at a rate of 1% per year, and other studies carried out in the United Kingdom, Australia, and France have also found that prevalence increases with age.[7,8] This age-related increase may be due to newly acquired infections or differences in childhood acquisition rates in different birth cohorts. The prevalence of *H. pylori* is also inversely related to socioeconomic status, particularly during childhood, when the risk is highest.[7,8]

3 TRANSMISSION ROUTES

H. pylori is a highly opportunistic bacterium that will do anything to gain access to the human stomach.[7] The primary routes of transmission appear to be gastro-oral (e.g., exposure to vomit) or fecal-oral, but it can also be transmitted as a result of exposure to contaminated food or water. Most of the published data indicate that transmission is mainly familial, although the main water supply may be a cause in developing countries.[7] Other risk factors seem to be smoking, population density and inadequate hygiene, but the infection does not seem to be gender related.[7] Ingested *H. pylori* survive in an acidic environment and do not seem to be controlled by the immune system.[9-11] Furthermore, the *H. pylori* genome encodes bacterial outer membrane proteins that facilitate gastric epithelial cell binding [10], and also encodes CagA, which acts as an intracellular growth factor and induces VacA-mediated apoptosis and cytokines production such as IL-1. Intracellular CagA also induces the production of IL-6, IL-10 and IL-8, whereas VacA interacts with B and T lymphocytes, and macrophages.[9-11] Finally, *H. pylori* induces a Th1 T cell response that leads to the production of IL-2 and interferon gamma, as well as the proliferation of B cells that produce autoreactive IgM and IgG3 antibodies, including the anti-H/K ATPase antibodies involved in the development of atrophic gastritis.[11]

4 GASTRITIS

There are two types of gastritis: type A involves the gastric corpus and fundus but not the antrum, and type B gastritis involves the antrum.[12-14] Type A, which is also known as autoimmune gastritis (AG), is an organ-specific inflammatory disease that is asymptomatic until the development of mucosal atrophy or pernicious anemia (PA). It is characterized by autoantibodies against gastric H^+/K^+ ATPase, high serum levels of gastrin, decreased acid secretion and a low pepsinogen I/II ratio, and it is frequently associated with endocrine autoimmune diseases.[13,14]

5 AUTOIMMUNE GASTRITIS

AG is mainly encountered in northern Europe and affects women three times as often as men.[7] The early stage is characterized by the focal or widespread lymphocytic infiltration of the oxyntic glands that eventually leads to gland destruction (active AG) and their partial or total replacement by metaplastic glands.[12-14] The mucosa become thinner and may resemble the small intestine. The chronic inflammatory infiltrate extends into the gastric mucosa, leads to the loss of acid-secreting parietal and zymogenic cells, and appearance of circulating parietal cell auto-antibodies directed against the α and β subunits of H+/K+ ATPase gastric proton pump.[12-14] Chronic proton pump autoaggression may decrease gastric acid secretion and give rise to hypergastrinemia and iron deficiency anemia.[14]

In the case of AG associated with reduced acid production,[13,14] the absorption of vitamin B12 is impaired, and the level of gastric intrinsic factor

(IF) falls, often followed by macrocytic anemia (PA). About 90% of patients with PA have parietal cell antibodies (PCAs), and 50–70% have antibodies against IF.[14] The later stages of this type of atrophic gastritis are associated with the disappearance of *H. pylori* from the gastric mucosa. Although it is associated with antral intestinal metaplasia, this and the PCAs also disappear in some patients, thus resembling classic AG.[13,14]

6 PATHOGENESIS

Autoimmunity may be triggered by many environmental factors, but its clinical progression is due to impaired personal immunotolerance resuling from molecular mimicry, antigen secretion, or the ability of environmental factors to serve as superagents.[14]

However, there is a lack of consistent evidence that molecular mimicry contributes to autoreactivity, and researchers must identify the epitopes recognized by antigastric autoantibodies. Some studies have observed molecular mimicry between *H. pylori*, hydrogen and potassium receptors and ATPase, which suggests that the infection may stimulate a T cell response.[15–18] Other mechanisms involve IgG4 (plasma IgG4 cells have been found in gastric biopsies),[14,19] the inflammatory setting, and the paracrine secretion of T cell growth factors that induce the activation of autoreactive T cells (bystander activation).[12–14,19]

7 *H. PYLORI* AND IMMUNE MECHANISMS

H. pylori infection induces an influx of T and B lymphocytes and macrophages into the gastric mucosa. Influenced by the predominantly Th1 cytokine milieu created by the infection, the gastric epithelial cells seem to acquire the properties that are essential for antigen presentation.[19] The presentation of bacterial antigens by gastric epithelial or parietal cells and professional antigen-presenting cells (APCs) may lead to the activation of *H. pylori*-specific FasL$^+$ gastric T cells, which kill antigen-presenting epithelial cells by means of *H. pylori* antigen-dependent mechanisms (e.g., perforin-mediated lysis) or apoptosis.[15–17] Surrounding Fas$^+$ parietal cells may also be killed as a result of antigen-independent T cell-mediated bystander lysis. In addition, professional APCs and epithelial cells can present gastric H$^+$K$^+$ ATPase to specific autoreactive T cells that have avoided negative selection in the thymus and thus induce T cell activation.[15–18] This leads to the expansion of H$^+$K$^+$ ATPase-specific Th1 cells that can assist

B cell autoantibody production and kill Fas$^+$ parietal cells. It is generally agreed that *H. pylori* infection provokes a Th1-dominant response and that gastric inflammation largely depends on increased Th1 cell production of IL-1β, TNF-α and IL-8, but not IL-4 or IL-10 and interferon γ (IF γ).[20–23] Moreover, IFN γ and TNF-α can increse the expression of MHC class II molecules by gastric cells, which would allow these cells act as APCs.

Furthermore, a subset of effector T cells that can be identified by their secretion of IL-17 (Th17 cells) are distinct from Th1 and Th2 cells in terms of differentiation and function[21]: TNF-α and IL-6 from activated macrophages/dendritic cells (DCs) are required for Th17 cell differentiation, but IL-12 and interferon-γ promote Th1 cell development, and Il-4 primes Th2 cell differentiation. It has recently been suggested that *H. pylori* infection mainly leads to a specific Th17/Th1 immune response that plays a major role, insofar as the bacterial burden and inflammation are both reduced by blocking IL-17 in vivo or in IL-17$^{-/-}$ mice.[22] On the basis of their dynamics, Th cell immune responses to *H. pylori* seem to be induced earlier than Th1 cell responses, which suggests that Th17 and Th1 cells promote inflammation at different stages. The Th17/Il-17 pathway likely modulates Th1 cell responses, and Th17 and Th1 cells probably act synergistically to induce gastritis by triggering the recruitment of inflammatory cells into the gastric mucosa as a result of the induction of chemokines.[22–24] The activated Th17/Th1 pathway may also destroy gastric tissue by inducing the production of matrix metalloproteinases (MMPs), thus favoring the spread of the pathogen and persistent infection.[25,26]

8 ANTIBODIES AND *H. PYLORI*

Studies have shown that patients with autoimmune gastritis have PCAs and intrinsic factor antibodies (IFAs).

8.1 Parietal Cell Antibodies

The target antigen of PCAs is the gastric enzyme H$^+$/K$^+$ ATPase, which consists of a catalytic 100-kDa α subunit and a 60–90-kDa β subunit. It is the main protein of the secretory canaliculi of gastric parietal cells, and it produces acid by secreting H$^+$ ions in exchange for K$^+$ ions.[15–18] PCAs are frequent in autoimmune gastritis, especially in early stages of the disease, and they bind to both the α and β subunits of gastric H$^+$/K$^+$ ATPase. Antibody reactivity to the α subunit includes epitopes on the cytosolic side of the secretory membrane, whereas antibody reactivity to the β subunit requires the antigen to be in a disulfide-bond and glycosylated, thus suggesting that autoepitopes are located in the luminal domain of the glycoprotein.[17,18] Circulating PCAs are IgG, IgA and IgM isotypes, although the antibody isotypes in gastric juices are mainly IgA and IgG.[27] In later disease stages, the incidence of PCAs decreases because of the progression of autoimmune gastritis and the loss of gastric parietal cell mass. However, PCAs are not specific and may be infrequently found in patients with other autoimmune diseases such as Hashimoto's thyroiditis or type 1 diabetes.[1]

8.2 Intrinsic Factor Autoantibodies

IF is a 60-kDa glycoprotein secreted by gastric parietal cells that is responsible for the high-affinity binding and transport of vitamin B_{12}. The IF/vitamin B_{12} complex reaches the terminal ileum, where it is absorbed after binding to specific receptors in ileal lumen cell membranes. IgA IFAs interfere with this absorption and are considered specific markers for a diagnosis of PA.[28,29] Recent studies have found that 40–60% of PA patients are positive for IFAs, and the proportion increases to 60–80% of those with long-lasting disease.[27]

9 DOES *H. PILORI* REALLY INDUCE AUTOIMMUNE GASTRITIS?

The existence of an autoimmune pathway in at least some patients with *H. pylori* gastritis is supported by the increased influx of B cells and/or T cells around the glands and in the epithelium of the corpus mucosa, the marked severity of the inflammatory and atrophic changes in the oxyntic compartment, increased apoptosis in oxyntic glands, and the coexistence of decreased gastric acid secretion and increased gastrin levels.[13,14,30]

Various studies have investigated the relationship between *H. pylori* and autoimmune gastritis.[2,13,14] These studies have found that subjects with atrophic corpus gastritis have a high prevalence of *H. pylori* seropositivity and a low prevalence of positive *H. pylori* staining, that 20–50% of *H. pylori*-infected patients have gastric autoantibodies, and that there is a positive correlation between gastric autoantibodies and *H. pylori* antibodies in patients with autoimmune gastritis/pernicious anemia.[31] Furthermore, a recently published meta-analysis of cross-sectional data found that *H. pylori* infection is strongly associated with autoimmune gastritis, and another meta-analysis showed that *H. pylori*-positive subjects consistently had substantially higher incidence rates than their *H. pylori*-negative counterparts. The first of these meta-analyses made a summary estimate of 5.0 (95% confidence interval 3.1–8.3), noting that the patients who had undergone proximal gastric vagotomy, those with reflux esophagitis, and those who were receiving long-term omeprazole treatment had a remarkably high incidence of autoimmune gastritis.[32] Furthermore, autoimmune gastritis has been associated with other autoimmune diseases, particularly thyroiditis, diabetes, vitiligo, and Addison's disease.[14]

Not all studies have found a correlation between *H. pylori* and PCAs or a positive relationship between *H. pylori* and atrophic corpus gastritis,[33] but the fact that the eradication of *H. pylori* in some patients with gastric antibodies leads to the loss of the antibodies supports the possibility of a causal relationship between *H. pylori* and gastric autoimmunity.

10 DIAGNOSIS AND MANAGEMENT

Noninvasive methods of diagnosis include a urea breath test, serological tests for antibodies against *H. pylori*, and the stool antigen test; however, the diagnosis needs to be confirmed by means of urease testing a biopsy specimen.[14] Patients with symptoms should undergo endoscopy and an antral biopsy.

The treatment consists of antibiotics and either a proton pump inhibitor or an H2 receptor antagonist for 7–14 days, with a stool test carried out 8 weeks later in order to confirm eradication.[14]

11 CONCLUSION

H. pylori can induce gastritis and other serious complications, but this can be avoided by early diagnosis and aggressive treatment. However, some patients have genetic and environmental risk factors that can lead to a form of gastritis characterized by autoantibody markers.

REFERENCES

1. Marshall BJ, Warren JR. Unidentified curved bacilli in the stomach of patients with gastritis and peptic ulceration. *Lancet* 1984;**1**:1311–15.
2. Lee EL, Feldman M. Gastritis and other gastropathies. In: Feldman M, Friedman LS, Sleisenger MH, editors. *Sleisenger & Fordtran's gastrointestinal and liver disease.* 7th ed. Philadelphia: Saunders; 2002. p. 810–27.
3. Topal D, Göral V, Yilmaz F, Kara IH. The relation of Helicobacter pylori with intestinal metaplasia, gastric atrophy and BCL-2. *Turk J Gastroenterol* 2004;**15**:149–55.
4. Kuipers EJ. Review article: exploring the link between Helicobacter pylori and gastric cancer. *Aliment Pharmacol Ther* 1999;**13**(Suppl 1):3–11.

5. Weck MN, Brenner H. Prevalence of chronic atrophic gastritis in different parts of the world. *Cancer Epidemiol Biomarkers Prev* 2006;**15**:1083–94.
6. McColl KE. Clinical practice. Helicobacter pylori infection. *N Engl J Med* 2010;**362**:1597–604.
7. Brown LM. Helicobacter pylori: epidemiology and routes of transmission. *Epidemiol Rev* 2000;**22**:283–97.
8. Bruce MG, Maaroos HI. Epidemiology of Helicobacter pylori infection. *Helicobacter* 2008;**13**(Suppl 1):1–6.
9. Suerbaum S, Michetti P. Helicobacter pylori infection. *N Engl J Med* 2002;**347**:1175–86.
10. Blaser MJ. Ecology of Helicobacter pylori in the human stomach. *J Clin Invest* 1997;**100**:759–62.
11. Peek Jr. RM, Fiske C, Wilson KT. Role of innate immunity in Helicobacter pylori-induced gastric malignancy. *Physiol Rev* 2010;**90**:831–58.
12. Bergman MP, Vandenbroucke-Grauls CM, Appelmelk BJ, et al. The story so far: Helicobacter pylori and gastric autoimmunity. *Int Rev Immunol* 2005;**24**:63–91.
13. Bergman MP, Faller G, D'Elios MM, Del Prete G, Vandenbroucke-Grauls CMJE, Appelmelk BJ. Gastric autoimmunity. In: Mobley HLT, Mendz GL, Hazell SL, editors. *Helicobacter pylori: physiology and genetics*. Washington (DC): ASM Press; 2001 Chapter 36.
14. Neumann WL, Coss E, Rugge M, Genta RM. Autoimmune atrophic gastritis—pathogenesis, pathology and management. *Nat Rev Gastroenterol Hepatol* 2013;**10**:529–41.
15. Amedei A, Bergman MP, Appelmelk BJ, et al. Molecular mimicry between Helicobacter pylori antigens and H+, K+: adenosine triphosphatase in human gastric autoimmunity. *J Exp Med* 2003;**198**:1147–56.
16. Toh BH, Sentry JW, Alderuccio F. The causative H^+/K^+ ATPase antigen in the pathogenesis of autoimmune gastritis. *Immunol Today* 2000;**21**:348–54.
17. D'Elios MM, Bergman MP, Azzurri A, Amedei A, Benagiano M, De Pont JJ, et al. H(+), K(+)-ATPase (proton pump) is the target autoantigen of Th1-type cytotoxic T cells in autoimmune gastritis. *Gastroenterology* 2001;**120**:377–86.
18. Callaghan JM, Khan MA, Alderuccio F, van Driel IR, Gleeson PA, Toh BH. Alpha and beta subunits of the gastric H+/K+-ATPase are concordantly targeted by parietal cell autoantibodies associated with autoimmune gastritis. *Autoimmunity* 1993;**16**:289–95.
19. Robinson K, Argent RH, Atherton JC. The inflammatory and immune response to Helicobacter pylori infection. *Best Pract Res Clin Gastroenterol* 2007;**21**:237–59.
20. Veijola LI, Oksanen AM, Sipponen PI, Rautelin HIK. Association of autoimmune type atrophic corpus gastritis with Helicobacter pylori infection. *World J Gastroenterol* 2010;**16**:83–8.
21. Bergman MP, D'Elios MM. Cytotoxic T cells in H. pylori-related gastric autoimmunity and gastric lymphoma. *J Biomed Biotechnol* 2010;**2010**:104918.
22. Toh BH, Chan J, Kyaw T, Alderuccio F. Cutting edge issues in autoimmune gastritis. *Clin Rev Allergy Immunol* 2012;**42**:269–78.
23. Gray BM, Fontaine CA, Poe SA, Eaton KA. Complex T cell interactions contribute to Helicobacter pylori gastritis in mice. *Infect Immun* 2013;**81**:740–52.
24. Eaton KA, Meffird M, Thevenot T. The role of T cell subsets and cytokinese in the pathogenesis of Helicobacter pylori gastritis in mice. *J Immunol* 2011;**166**:7456–61.
25. Bergin PJ, Anders E, Sicheng W, et al. Increased production of matrix metalloproteinases in Helicobacter pylori-associated human gastritis. *Helicobacter* 2004;**9**:201–10.
26. Sampieri CL. Helicobacter pylori and gastritis: the role of extracellular matrix metalloproteases, their inhibitors, and the disintegrins and metalloproteases—a systematic literature review. *Dig Dis Sci* 2013;**58**:2777–83.
27. Bizzaro N, Antico A. Diagnosis and classification of pernicious anemia. *Autoimmun Rev* 2014;**13**:565–8.

28. Carmel R. Reassessment of the relative prevalences of antibodies to gastric parietal cell and to intrinsic factor in patients with pernicious anaemia: influence of patient age and race. *Clin Exp Immunol* 1992;**89**:74–7.

29. Parente F, Negrini R, Imbesi V, Maconi G, Cucino C, Bianchi Porro G. The presence of gastric autoantibodies impairs gastric secretory function in patients with *H. pylori*-positive duodenal ulcer. *Gut* 1999;**45**:A40.

30. Ohata H, Kitauchi S, Yoshimura N, Mugitani K, Iwane M, Nakamura H, et al. Progression of chronic atrophic gastritis associated with Helicobacter pylori infection increases risk of gastric cancer. *Int J Cancer* 2004;**109**:138–43.

31. Weck MN, Brenner H. Association of Helicobacter pylori infection with chronic atrophic gastritis: meta-analyses according to type of disease definition. *Int J Cancer* 2008;**123**:874–81.

32. Adamu MA, Weck MN, Gao L, Brenner H. Incidence of chronic atrophic gastritis: systematic review and meta-analysis of follow-up studies. *Eur J Epidemiol* 2010;**25**:439–48.

33. Annibale B, Lahner E, Negrini R, et al. Lack of specific association between gastric autoimmunity hallmarks and clinical presentations of atrophic body gastritis. *World J Gastroenterol* 2005;**11**:5351–7.

34. Toh BH, Alderuccio F. Parietal cell and intrinsic factor autoantibodies. In: Shoenfeld Y, Gershwin ME, Meroni PL, editors. *Autoantibodies*. 2nd ed. Amsterdam: Elsevier; 2007. p. 479–86.

CHAPTER 29

Multiple Sclerosis and Creutzfeldt–Jakob Disease are Autoimmune Diseases Probably Caused by Exposure to the Nasal Microbe *Acinetobacter*

Alan Ebringer[*,1], Taha Rashid[*], Clyde Wilson[†]
[*]Analytical Sciences Group, King's College, London, UK
[†]Departments of Microbiology and Pathology, King Edward VII Memorial Hospital, Hamilton, Bermuda
[1]Corresponding Author: alan.ebringer@kcl.ac.uk

1 THE YEHUDA SHOENFELD CONJECTURE

At the Autoimmune Symposium held in Dresden, Germany, in 2009, Professor Yehuda Shoenfeld publicly proposed his now famous conjecture about autoimmune diseases. The conjecture states: "All autoimmune diseases are caused by external agents (viruses, bacteria, parasites, drugs) until proved otherwise." The conjecture has proven to be a potent stimulus to look for external causes in the etiology of many autoimmune diseases, and it is essentially a challenge to the Burnettian hypotheses that autoimmune diseases arise by mutations. So far, no such mutations have been discovered.

The first edition of "Infection and Autoimmunity" by Shoenfeld and Rose is a testimonial to the productive influence of this conjecture in finding external agents that are triggering factors in the etiology of many autoimmune diseases.

2 RHEUMATIC FEVER, SYDENHAM'S CHOREA, RHEUMATOID ARTHRITIS, AND ANKYLOSIS SPONDYLITIS AS EXAMPLES OF AUTOIMMUNE DISEASES EVOKED BY INFECTION

Autoimmune diseases are characterized by the presence of antibodies that bind to self-antigens and therefore are known as autoantibodies. Many human diseases, such as juvenile diabetes or rheumatoid arthritis, are considered examples of autoimmune diseases.

Infection and Autoimmunity
http://dx.doi.org/10.1016/B978-0-444-63269-2.00071-4

Two main theories of the origin of such autoantibodies have been proposed: either the immune system spontaneously starts producing tissue-damaging immune cells, or infection occurs by a microbial agent that possesses antigens exhibiting molecular similarity, or "molecular mimicry" with some tissues of the host. There is scant evidence for the "lymphocyte mutation" hypothesis. The "infection hypothesis" seems to have greater merit in providing an explanation for the origin of autoimmune diseases. Following infection, an immune response occurs, and antibodies against the invading microbe are produced. A portion of these antibodies bind to self-tissues of the host and therefore act as autoantibodies. When present in high concentrations, such autoantibodies can activate the complement cascade and cause tissue damage. Cytotoxic autoantibodies have been demonstrated in rheumatoid arthritis and ankylosing spondylitis.[1]

The classical model of an autoimmune disease evoked by an infection is "rheumatic fever". The microbe *Streptococcus* possesses molecular sequences that resemble the human heart; it produces cross-reactive antibodies that can bind cardiac tissues.[2,3] Sydenham's chorea occurs in patients with rheumatic fever who have a high titer of antistreptococcal antibodies. Some of these immunoglobulin (Ig) G antibodies cross the blood–brain barrier and bind to the basal ganglia of the brain, producing ataxia and the choreiform movements characteristic of the disease.[4] Sydenham's chorea usually wanes following treatment with high doses of antibiotics, such as penicillin, and is an example of a neurological autoimmune disease evoked by an infection and where IgG autoantibodies are produced at an extrathecal site.

Clearly, the demonstration of four different autoimmune diseases evoked by an infection through the mechanism of "molecular mimicry" raises the question of whether a similar approach might be relevant in studying bovine spongiform encephalopathy (BSE), experimental allergic encephalomyelitis (EAE), and multiple sclerosis (MS). Lower limb ataxia occurs in MS, which resembles hindquarter paralysis in BSE, leading to the question of whether some environmental agents might possess antigens resembling or cross-reacting with brain tissues.[5]

3 EAE AS AN ANIMAL MODEL OF MS

An experiment that showed that EAE could be considered an animal model of MS was discovered almost by accident in 1880 by Pasteur and his colleagues in Paris. Pasteur was trying to immunize patients who had been bitten by rabid dogs and wolves. To produce antirabies immunity, he had available the brains of only two rabid animals: one from a rabid dog and the other from a rabid wolf. In an endeavor to increase the quantity of rabies material, he injected the brains of the two animals into 60 rabbits. He then injected patients who had been bitten by rabid dogs or wolves with the rabbit brain homogenates to immunize them. As expected, some patients developed immunity to rabies, but a small number of injected subjects developed a neurological disease that was characterized by ataxia and in some cases led to a fatal outcome. Extensive literature is present in European medical journals describing these serious complications, and by the 1940s, the World Health Organization in Geneva had reported between 200 and 300 cases of patients who had died from a disease known as "post-rabies vaccination allergic encephalomyelitis". The cause for this unexpected and lethal response was not explained until the 1930s, when it was shown that injection of foreign brain homogenates evokes an immune response in the immunized individual or animal by the production of antibrain autoantibodies that damage the brain tissues of the host.[6] In the 1950s it became apparent that this was a general observation in immunology: immunization with any organ homogenate would produce an autoimmune disease in the target organ. The classical work of Rose and Witebsky[7] demonstrated that peripheral injection of thyroid tissue homogenates produced an experimental disease in animals that was similar to the human autoimmune disease Hashimoto's thyroiditis.

4 SPONGIFORM CHANGES IN EAE, BOVINE MYELIN, AND *ACINETOBACTER*

In acute EAE, observed 1 to 3 weeks following immunization with brain homogenates, there is perivascular infiltration of inflammatory cells that eventually leads to the formation of fibrotic plaques resembling those observed in patients with MS. This is one of the main reasons why EAE is considered to be an animal model of MS. Antimyelin antibodies are produced in an extrathecal site, as occurs in Sydenham's chorea. In chronic EAE, observed 3 to 6 months following immunization, characteristic spongiform changes were described in rabbits in 1969[8] and in guinea pigs in 1974.[9] It seems that spongiform changes occur not only in BSE but also in EAE.

One of the main components of the central nervous system responsible for the production of EAE is a basic protein present in the white matter of the brain. In 1970, Eylar et al.,[10] from San Diego, identified a highly active peptide from bovine myelin that, when injected in microgram quantities into guinea pigs, produced hind leg paralysis, tremors, weight loss, and eventually death. These features also were described in cattle affected by BSE. Furthermore, the biological activity of this peptide was retained when it was heated to 100°C for 1 hour or treated with 8 M urea; these are properties also described for prions.[11]

Computer analysis of proteins in the SwissProt database, using the Eylar sequence as a probe, revealed that the microbe *Acinetobacter*, which is present in soil, on skin and in contaminated waters and fecal material, has such a sequence (Figure 1). The sequence is present in the 4-carboxy-muconolactone decarboxylase molecule of *Acinetobacter*;[5] a similar sequence was subsequently found in γ-carboxy-mucono-lactone decarboxylase of *Pseudomonas*.[12] Both groups of microbes—*Acinetobacter* and *Pseudomonas*—belong to the same family of Gram-negative bacteria and share many antigens.

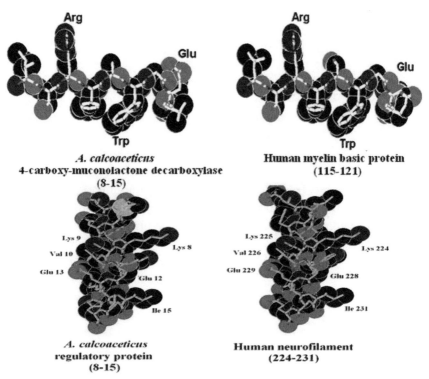

Figure 1 Molecular similarity between neuronal self-antigens (myelin basic protein and neurofilament) and *Acinetobacter calcoaceticus* bacterial antigens.

The discovery that the common environmental microbe *Acinetobacter* had a sequence showing molecular mimicry with bovine brain antigens suggested a possible mechanism for how cattle could have developed BSE. Offal material from abattoirs was used in the preparation of the meat and bone material (MBM) foodstuffs given to cattle, which could have become inadvertently contaminated by *Acinetobacter*. Although heat treatment was applied, albeit at a lower temperature, during the preparation of the MBM, the demonstration by Eylar and coworkers that the myelin peptides were highly resistant to heat denaturation meant that these bacterial fragments retained their biological activity in being able to induce EAE in experimental animals. The presence of such biologically active fragments in MBM meant that the cows would not only make antibodies against them but, because of the molecular similarity between brain tissues and *Acinetobacter*, any antibodies produced, especially of the IgG isotype, which can cross the blood–brain barrier, could also attack the brain and cause a neurological disease.

5 ANTIBODIES TO *ACINETOBACTER* AND AUTOANTIBODIES TO BRAIN ANTIGENS IN BSE

The demonstration that *Acinetobacter*, which is a common environmental microbe, had antigens cross-reacting with mammalian brain tissue raised the question of whether animals with BSE had been exposed to it or to fragments of the bacterium. Antibodies to *Acinetobacter calcoaceticus* were significantly elevated in the 29 BSE-positive animals when compared to 18 BSE-negative animals ($P < 0.001$), 30 organically raised cows aged <30 months ($P < 0.001$) and 28 organically raised cows aged >30 months ($P < 0.001$), but no such elevations were found against two control bacteria, *Escherichia coli* and *Agrobacterium*.[13] High concentrations of autoantibodies against bovine neurofilaments, which are components of the white matter of the brain, also were found. This was the first report of autoantibodies to brain components being present in animals affected by BSE. The highest relatively increased concentrations of antibodies, in comparison to controls, were found in the IgA isotype. This suggested that they had been produced by the immune system in the gut following the transit of *Acinetobacter* antigens present in the MBM feed across the gut mucosa and not as a result of brain damage by prions.

In another coded study, antibody responses to seven different bacteria—*Klebsiella*, *Proteus*, *Serratia*, *Escherichia*, *Bacillus*, *Pseudomonas*, and

Acinetobacter—were measured in 128 BSE-positive animals, 63 BSE-negative animals and 64 healthy control animals. Significantly elevated concentrations of antibodies to *Acinetobacter* were found in the BSE-affected animals when compared with the BSE-negative animals ($P < 0.001$) and healthy controls ($P < 0.001$). Antibodies to *Pseudomonas* also were elevated, although these titers were not as high as those found against *Acinetobacter* bacteria.[14] This is not surprising because *Pseudomonas* species belong to the same family as *Acinetobacter* bacteria. The important observation of specificity is that BSE-affected animals did not have antibody elevations against the six other bacteria. The conclusion that arises from these investigations is that BSE-affected cattle were exposed to *Acinetobacter* antigens that probably were present in the MBM supplements they were fed. The use of MBM supplements was legally banned in 1988, and no residual MBM material has been available for further analysis.

The demonstration of specific antibodies to a microbe bearing antigens cross-reacting with brain tissue, as well as the presence of autoantibodies to brain components, in a disease showing clinical features resembling those found in EAE and MS would tend to suggest that BSE could at least be considered an autoimmune disease that is evoked by *Acinetobacter* bacteria, similar to situation of antistreptococcal antibodies causing a neurological autoimmune disease such as Sydenham's chorea.

6 IMPLICATIONS OF ANTI-*ACINETOBACTER* ANTIBODIES IN BSE TO HUMAN DISEASES

In humans, *Acinetobacter* species usually produce respiratory chest infections, especially in patients in intensive care units. More than 50% of patients with MS in England suffer from sinusitis,[15] and similar results have been reported in Scotland.[16] Furthermore, investigation of American patients with sinusitis by antral tap and endoscopically directed nasal cultures show that they grow predominantly *Acinetobacter* and *Pseudomonas* bacteria.[17] If these results can be confirmed and patients with MS are shown to suffer from sinusitis with *Acinetobacter* and *Pseudomonas* bacteria, then entirely new therapeutic possibilities can be opened up. The use of anti-*Acinetobacter* therapy such as antibiotics, drainage of sinuses, immunosuppressive drugs, and other measures could be evaluated in the earliest stages of MS, before irreversible neurological changes occur in such patients. After all, rheumatic fever and Sydenham's chorea have disappeared in the Western World because of the use of proper courses of antibiotics in the early stages of the disease.

7 FROM EAE TO MS VIA AUTOIMMUNITY

Neuroparalytic complications resulting from the injection of brain tissues of rabies-infected animals indicated that an autoimmune reaction could be produced through the introduction of heterologous or even homologous antigens.[18] These heterologous antigens most likely possess amino acid sequences that are shared with those of the recipient animal. More than 20 years later, Eylar and coworkers[19] discovered that the most active myelin constituent in the induction of EAE is myelin basic protein (MBP). Furthermore, EAE can be induced in a variety of animals by inoculation of myelin components that give rise to a spongiform appearance.[20] EAE is the most extensively studied animal model of immune-mediated demyelinating disease.[21] The extrapolation of EAE to its human counterpart, MS, was mainly based on the involvement of common targeted antigens, mainly MBP, as well as the associated clinical and pathological similarities between these conditions.[22,23]

More than 60 years ago, the humoral immune response was suggested to have a pivotal role in MS pathogenesis, where elevated concentrations of Igs were observed in the cerebrospinal fluid (CSF) of >90% of patients with MS.[24] Moreover, intrathecal synthesis of IgM, as detected by CSF oligoclonal bands, was reported as a useful parameter in monitoring disease relapse activity in MS.[25] A recent study found that there is no elevation and binding of high-affinity anti-*Acinetobacter* or anti-*Pseudomonas* antibodies in the CSF of patients with MS,[26] thereby suggesting that these autoantibodies are extrathecal in origin, similar to the situation of EAE and Sydenham's chorea.

8 ROLE OF IMMUNITY IN TRANSMISSIBLE ENCEPHALOPATHY

Transmissible spongiform encephalopathy (TSE) is a group of potentially fatal neurodegenerative diseases that comprise BSE in cattle, scrapie in sheep and goats, chronic wasting disease in mule deer and elk, as well as kuru and CJD in humans. Unlike MS, the search for the involvement of autoimmunity in the pathogenesis of these diseases is surprisingly lacking, despite a long history in the discovery of some of these conditions, such as scrapie, which dates back to the 17th century.

How can devastating lesions such as those occurring in the CNS of animals affected by a TSE such as scrapie develop without evidence of immune-mediated or inflammatory reactions? In spite of the failure of some groups to find signs of enhanced immunity in TSE-affected animals,[27,28] others have shown some evidence of humoral immune responses and inflammatory activity in a number of TSE diseases. Toh et al.[29] from Boston found that sera from scrapie-affected sheep were reactive mainly to the 62-kDa neurofilament protein preparations obtained from mouse brain. Intraperitoneal inoculation of immune-deficient mice with 1% homogenate of brain tissues prepared from mice infected with the Rocky Mountain Laboratory scrapie strain failed to produce clinical disease when B cells were absent.[30] BSE animals were shown to have elevated concentrations of antibodies to bovine MBP and neurofilaments[13] as well as to prion antigens.[31]

In addition, significantly increased values of the total IgG, IgA, and C3 complement component in the CSF, and IgA in the serum, of patients with CJD have been detected when compared with healthy controls.[32] Patients with sporadic CJD have elevated concentrations of MBP autoantibodies.[33] Patients with CJD and kuru were observed to have high titers of anti-neurofilament antibodies;[34] patients with CJD might occasionally present increased concentrations of other autoantibodies, such as those targeted against thyroid antigens.[35]

The accumulation and activation of microglial cells, which are the brain's macrophages, have been observed in and around the brain lesions of animals with TSE[36] and patients with CJD.[37] Patients with CJD have elevated plasma concentrations of C-reactive proteins and interleukin-6 cytokines,[38] which are indicative of ongoing inflammation somewhere in the body. In a study from California, brain tissues from five of six patients with sporadic CJD, as well as from scrapie-infected mice, were found to be infiltrated with increased concentrations of lymphocytes.[39] Finally, the antibody-triggered active components C1q and C3b of the complement proteins have been detected in the pathological lesions of patients with sporadic and variant CJD.[40]

9 THE PROBLEM WITH THE VARIANT CJD EPIDEMIC

The link between CJD, a fatal neurological disease in humans, particularly the variant or new variant type (vCJD), with BSE epidemics was a source of considerable concern to the government and public in the UK and throughout the world. This led to banning British beef on the bone, with a subsequent decline in meat consumption in mid 1990s.[41] Although the maximum incubation period of more than 20 years has passed since the entrance of infected beef into the human food chain in the 1980s, the expected vCJD epidemic never occurred. Moreover, the number of patients with vCJD has declined significantly and is still decreasing.[42] It should also be emphasized that the incidence of CJD is fairly similar in many other European countries,[43] and the distribution of vCJD in the UK[44] shows the highest incidence in Scotland, which does not tally with the distribution of BSE-affected cattle, which was highest in the south of England.[45,46] Moreover, contrary to the British surveillance data on the increased frequency of CJD among individuals with occupational exposure to cattle products, such as farmers, butchers, and veterinary workers,[47] a meta-analysis of three case-control studies conducted in UK, Japan, and the USA failed to confirm such observations.[48] Furthermore, there are no accurate data showing how long subclinical BSE or vCJD existed in the UK before the BSE epidemic.

10 A POSSIBLE LINK BETWEEN BSE, CJD, AND MS INVOLVING IMMUNE RESPONSES TO *ACINETOBACTER*

10.1 Acinetobacter and CJD

Antibodies against four microbial agents were determined in serum samples from 2 patients with sporadic CJD, 53 patients with MS, 20 patients with rheumatoid arthritis, 20 patients with ankylosing spondylitis, 18 patients with cerebrovascular accident (CVA) and 20 patients with viral encephalitis, as well as from 29 healthy controls. The results showed significantly elevated concentrations of IgA antibodies to *Acinetobacter* ($P < 0.001$) in patients with MS and CJD compared with healthy controls. No such antibody elevations were detected in these patients when tested against *Proteus mirabilis, Klebsiella pneumoniae*, and *E. coli* bacteria.[33]

10.2 Acinetobacter and MS

Antibody levels against 5 strains of *Acinetobacter* sp., *Pseudomonas aeruginosa,* and *E. coli* were measured by enzyme-linked immunosorbant assay in 26 English patients with MS, 20 patients with CVA and 25 corresponding healthy controls. There were highly significant elevations of IgA and IgG antibodies to at least three strains of *Acinetobacter* in patients with MS when compared with patients with CVA ($P < 0.0001$) and healthy controls ($P < 0.0001$).[12] A less significant increase in the levels of antibodies against *P. aeruginosa* were observed in patients with MS ($P < 0.001$) compared with patients with CVA or healthy subjects. However, no such elevation in antibodies to *E. coli* was observed in patients with MS. Furthermore, all patients with MS had values exceeding the 99.9% confidence limits of the healthy controls when the myelin–*Acinetobacter*–neurofilament antibody index was calculated using the 5 *Acinetobacter* strains, but only 88.5% of the patients with MS had such elevated values when antibodies were targeted against *P. aeruginosa*.

Molecular similarity was previously identified between a number of amino acid sequences from *Acinetobacter* and/or *Pseudomonas* bacteria and each of the brain components: MBP, myelin oligodendrocyte glycoprotein and neurofilaments[49] (Figure 1). In another study, concentrations of antibodies against synthetic peptides from *Acinetobacter* ($P < 0.001$) and *Pseudomonas* ($P < 0.001$) microbes were elevated in patients with MS compared with patients with CVA or healthy controls.[50] However, no such antibodies were observed when an irrelevant human papillomavirus peptide was used.

11 CONCLUSIONS

- Extensive studies involving more than 200 cows affected by BSE indicate that they have elevated concentrations of antibodies to the soil and the nasal microbe *Acinetobacter* and, to a lesser extent, the related microbe *Pseudomonas*.
- *Acinetobacter* microbes possess amino acid sequences that resemble or cross-react with MBP and neurofilament tissues in the nervous system.
- Antibodies to *Acinetobacter* bind to brain components such as MBP, myelin oligodendrocyte glycoprotein and neurofilaments and therefore act as autoantibodies. These antibodies are produced outside the nervous system in an extrathecal space, but IgG1 and IgG3 antibodies cross the blood–brain barrier and, if present in high enough concentrations, activate the complement cascade and cause tissue damage.
- A similar situation occurs with antibodies in EAE and Sydenham's chorea; the autoantibodies are produced outside the nervous system but upon crossing the blood–brain barrier initiate a neurological disease.
- It is suggested that EAE and BSE are animal models of MS and that MS is caused by an infection by the nasal microbe *Acinetobacter*.
- It is proposed that CJD is a severe form of MS caused by *Acinetobacter* infection; therefore multicentre studies are required to examine this hypothesis.

ACKNOWLEDGMENTS

We thank the Trustees of the Middlesex Hospital, the Arthritis Research Campaign (Grant EO514) and "American Friends of King's College London" for their support.

REFERENCES

1. Wilson C, Rashid T, Tiwana H, Beyan H, Hughes L, Bensal S, et al. Cytotoxicity responses to peptide antigens in rheumatoid arthritis and ankylosing spondylitis. *J Rheumatol* 2003;**30**:972–8.
2. Cunningham MW. Streptococcus and rheumatic fever. *Curr Opin Rheumatol* 2012;**24**:408–16.
3. Delunardo F, Scalzi V, Capozzi A, Camerini S, Misasi R, Pierdominici M, et al. Streptococall-vimentin cross-reactive antibodies induce microvascular cardiac endothelial proinflammatory phenotype in rheumatic heart disease. *Clin Exp Immunolo* 2013;**173**:419–29.
4. Church AJ, Cordoso F, Dale RC, Lees AJ, Thompson EJ, Giovannoni G. Anti-basal ganglia antibodies in acute and persistent Sydenham's chorea. *Neurology* 2002;**59**:227–31.
5. Ebringer A, Thorpe C, Pirt J, Wilson C, Cunningham P, Ettelaie C. Bovine spongiform encephalopathy: is it an autoimmune disease due to bacteria showing molecular mimicry with brain antigens? *Environ Health Perspect* 1997;**105**:1172–4.
6. Westonhurst E. The effects of the injection of normal brain emulsion into rabbit with specific reference to the aetiology of the paralytic accidents of the anti-rabic treatment. *J Hyg* 1932;**32**:33–44.
7. Rose NR, Witebsky E. Studies on organ specificity. V. Changes in the thyroid glands of rabbits following active immunization with rabbit thyroid extracts. *J Immunol* 1956;**76**:417–27.
8. Prineas J, Raine CS, Wisniewski H. An ultrastructural study of experimental demyelination. III. Chronic experimental allergic encephalomyelitis in the central nervous system. *Lab Invest* 1969;**21**:472–83.
9. Raine CS, Synder DH, Valsamis MP, Stone SH. Chronic experimental allergic encephalomyelitis in inbred guinea pigs. An ultrastructural study. *Lab Invest* 1974;**31**:369–80.
10. Eylar EH, Caccam J, Jackson JJ, Westall FC, Robinson AB. Experimental allergic encephalomyelitis: synthesis of disease-inducing site of the basic protein. *Science* 1970;**168**:1220–3.
11. Sang JC, Lee CY, Luh FY, Huang YW, Chiang YW, Chen RP. Slow spontenuous α-t-β structural conversion in a non-denaturing neutral condition reveals the intrinsically disordered property of the disulfide-reduced recombinant mouse prion protein. *Prion* 2012;**6**:489–97.
12. Hughes LE, Bonell S, Natt RS, Wilson C, Tiwana H, Ebringer A, et al. Antibody responses to *Acinetobacter* spp. and *Pseudomonas aeruginosa* in multiple sclerosis: prospects for diagnosis using the myelin-*Acinetobacter*-neurofilament antibody index. *Clin Diagn Lab Immunol* 2001;**8**:1181–8.
13. Tiwana H, Wilson C, Pirt J, Cartmell W, Ebringer A. Autoantibodies to brain components and antibodies to *Acinetobacter calcoaceticus* are present in bovine spongiform encephalopathy. *Infect Immun* 1999;**67**:6591–5.
14. Wilson C, Hughes LE, Rashid T, Ebringer A, Bansal S. Antibodies to *Acinetobacter* bacteria and brain peptides, measured in bovine spongiform encephalopathy (BSE) in an attempt to develop an ante-mortem test. *J Clin Lab Immunol* 2003;**52**:23–40.
15. Gay D, Dick G, Upton G. Multiple sclerosis associated with sinusitis: case-controlled study in general practice. *Lancet* 1986;**1**(8485):815–19.
16. Callaghan TS. Multiple sclerosis and sinusitis. *Lancet* 1986;**2**(8499):160–1.
17. Casiano RR, Cohn S, Villasuso 3rd. E, Brown M, Memari F, Barquist E, et al. Comparison of antral tap with endoscopically directed nasal culture. *Laryngoscope* 2001;**111**:1333–7.

18. Kabat EA, Wolf A, Bezer AE. The rapid production of acute disseminated encephalomyelitis in rhesus monkey by injection of heterologous and homologous brain tissue with adjuvants. *J Exp Med* 1947;**85**:117–30.

19. Eylar EH, Salk J, Beveridge GC, Brown LW. Experimental allergic encephalomyelitis: an encephalitogenic basic protein from bovine myelin. *Arch Biochem Biophys* 1969;**132**:34–48.

20. Raine CS. Analysis of autoimmune demyelination: its impact upon multiple sclerosis. *Lab Invest* 1984;**50**:608–35.

21. Rao P, Segal BM. Experimental autoimmune encephalomyelitis. *Methods Mol Biol* 2012;**900**:363–80.

22. Lassmann H, Winiewski HM. Chronic relapsing experimental allergic encephalomyelitis: clinicopathological comparison with multiple sclerosis. *Arch Neurol* 1979;**36**:490–7.

23. Storch MK, Stefferl A, Brehm U, Weissert R, Wallstrom E, Kerschensteiner M, et al. Autoimmunity to myelin oligodendrocyte glycoprotein in rats mimics the spectrum of multiple sclerosis pathology. *Brain Pathol* 1998;**8**:681–94.

24. Kabat EA, Glusman M, Knaub V. Quantitative estimation of the albumin and gamma globulin in normal and pathologic cerebrospinal fluid by immunochemical methods. *Am J Med* 1948;**4**:653–62.

25. Sharief MK, Thompson EJ. Intrathecal immunoglobulin M synthesis in multiple sclerosis. Relationship with clinical and cerebrospinal fluid parameters. *Brain* 1991;**114**:181–95.

26. Chapman MD, Hughes LE, Wilson CD, Namnyak S, Thompson EJ, Giovannoni G. No evidence for production of intrathecal immunoglobulin G against Acinetobacter or Pseudomonas in multiple sclerosis. *Eur Neurol* 2005;**53**:27–31.

27. Kaspar KC, Stites DP, Bowman KA, Panitch H, Prusiner SB. Immunological studies of scrapie infection. *J Neuroimmunol* 1982;**3**:187–201.

28. Mabbott NA, Bruce ME. The immunobiology of TSE diseases. *J Gen Virol* 2001;**82**:2307–18.

29. Toh DH, Gibbs CJ, Gajdusek DC, Tuthill DD, Dahl D. The 200- and 150-kDa neurofilament proteins react with IgG autoantibodies from chimpanzees with kuru or Creutzfeldt–Jakob disease; a 62-kDa neurofilament-associated protein reacts with sera from sheep with natural scrapie. *Proc Natl Acad Sci USA* 1985;**82**:3894–6.

30. Klein MA, Frigg R, Flechsig E, Raeber AJ, Kalinke U, Bluethmann H, et al. A crucial role of B cells in neuroinvasive scrapie. *Nature* 1997;**390**:687–90.

31. Wilson C, Hughes L, Rashid T, Cunningham P, Bansal S, Ebringer A, et al. Antibodies to prion and *Acinetobacter* peptide sequences in bovine spongiform encephalopathy. *Vet Immunol Immunopathol* 2004;**98**:1–7.

32. Galvez S, Farcas A, Monari M. Cerebrospinal fluid and serum immunoglobulins and C3 in Creutzfeldt–Jakob disease. *Neurology* 1979;**29**:1610–12.

33. Ebringer A, Rashid T, Wilson C, Tiwana H, Green AJ, Thompson EJ, et al. Multiple sclerosis, sporadic Creutzfeldt–Jakob disease and bovine spongiform encephalopathy: are they autoimmune diseases evoked by *Acinetobacter* microbes showing molecular mimicry to brain antigens? *J Nutr Environ Med* 2004;**14**:293–302.

34. Sotelo J, Gibbs CJ, Gajdusek DC. Autoantibodies against axonal neurofilaments in patients with kuru and Creutzfeldt–Jakob disease. *Science* 1980;**210**:190–3.

35. Cossu G, Melis M, Molari A, Pinna L, Ferrigno P, Melis G, et al. Creutzfeldt–Jakob disease associated with high titre of antithyroid autoantibodies: case report and literature review. *Neurol Sci* 2003;**24**:138–40.

36. Giese A, Brown DR, Groschup MH, Feldmann C, Haist I, Kretzschmar HA. Role of microglia in neuronal cell death in prion disease. *Brain Pathol* 1998;**8**:449–57.

37. Van Everbroeck B, Dewulf E, Pals P, Lubke U, Martin JJ, Cras P. The role of cytokines, astrocytes, microglia and apoptosis in Creutzfeldt–Jakob disease. *Neurobiol Aging* 2002;**23**:59–64.
38. Volkel D, Zimmermann K, Zerr I, Lindner T, Bodemer M, Poser S, et al. C-reactive protein and IL-6: new marker proteins for the diagnosis of CJD in plasma? *Transfusion* 2001;**41**:1509–14.
39. Lewicki H, Tishon A, Homann D, Mazarguil H, Laval F, Asensio VC, et al. T cells infiltrate the brain in murine and human transmissible spongiform encephalopathies. *J Virol* 2003;**77**:3799–808.
40. Kovacs GG, Gasque P, Strobel T, Lindeck-Pozza E, Strohschneider M, Ironside JW, et al. Complement activation in human prion disease. *Neurobiol Dis* 2004;**15**:21–8.
41. Will RG, Ironside JW, Zeidler M, Cousens SN, Estibeiro K, Alperovitch K, et al. A new variant of Creutzfeldt–Jakob disease in the UK. *Lancet* 1996;**347**:921–5.
42. The National Creutzfeldt–Jakob Disease Surveillance Unit, University of Edinburgh. http://www.cjd.ed.ac.uk/figures.htm.
43. Will RG, Alperovitch A, Poser S, Pocchiari M, Hofman A, Mitrova E, et al. Descriptive epidemiology of Creutzfeldt–Jakob disease in six European countries, 1993–1995. *Ann Neurol* 1998;**43**:763–7.
44. Cousens SN, Linsell L, Smith PG, Chandrakumar M, Wilesmith JW, Knight RS, et al. Geographical distribution of variant CJD in the UK (excluding Northern Ireland). *Lancet* 1999;**353**:18–21.
45. Anderson RM, Donnelly CA, Ferguson NM, Woolhouse ME, Watt CJ, Udy HJ, et al. Transmission dynamics and epidemiology of BSE in British cattle. *Nature* 1996;**382**:779–88.
46. Scholz R, Lorenzen S. *Phantom BSE-Gefahr*. Innsbruck: Berenkamp; 2005.
47. Cousens SN, Zeidler M, Esmonde TF, De Silva R, Wilesmith JW, Smith PG, et al. Sporadic Creutzfeldt–Jakob disease in the United Kingdom: analysis of epidemiological surveillance data for 1970–96. *Br Med J* 1997;**315**:389–95.
48. Wientjens DPW, Davanipour Z, Hofman A, Kondo K, Matthews WB, Will RG, et al. Risk factors for Creutzfeldt–Jakob disease: a reanalysis of case–control studies. *Neurology* 1996;**46**:1287–91.
49. Ebringer A, Hughes L, Rashid T, Wilson C. *Acinetobacter* immune responses in multiple sclerosis: etiopathogenetic role and its possible use as a diagnostic marker. *Arch Neurol* 2005;**62**:33–6.
50. Hughes L, Smith PA, Bonell S, Natt RS, Wilson C, Rashid T, et al. Cross-reactivity between related sequences found in *Acinetobacter* sp., *Pseudomonas aeruginosa*, myelin basic protein and myelin oligodendrocyte glycoprotein in multiple sclerosis. *J Neuroimmunol* 2003;**144**:105–15.

CHAPTER 30

Infection and Autoimmunity in Antibiotic-Refractory Lyme Arthritis

Allen C. Steere[1], Klemen Strle, Elise E. Drouin
The Center for Immunology and Inflammatory Diseases, Massachusetts General Hospital, Harvard Medical School, Boston, Massachusetts, USA
[1]Corresponding Author: ASTEERE@mgh.harvard.edu

1 INTRODUCTION

Lyme disease, which is caused by tick-borne spirochetes of the *Borrelia burgdorferi* sensu lato complex, occurs in the United States, Europe, and Asia.[1] In the United States, the infection is caused exclusively by *B. burgdorferi* sensu stricto strains (*B. burgdorferi* in the strict sense, hereafter referred to as *B. burgdorferi*), whereas in Europe and Asia, the illness is caused primarily by *Borrelia afzelii* and *Borrelia garinii* strains.[2]

In all geographic locations, the infection usually begins with an expanding skin lesion (stage 1), called erythema migrans, which occurs at the site of the tick bite.[1,3] However, there are regional variations in the disease. For example, in the northeastern United States, *B. burgdorferi* often disseminates, primarily to the nervous system, heart or joints.[3] Within weeks (stage 2), about 15% of untreated patients develop neurologic abnormalities, including lymphocytic meningitis, cranial neuropathy (primarily facial palsy), or radiculoneuropathy,[3] and about 5% of patients develop cardiac involvement, most commonly AV nodal block. Months later (stage 3), approximately 60% of untreated patients in the northeastern United States develop intermittent or persistent attacks of arthritis, especially affecting knees. In Europe, *B. afzelii* may cause chronic infection of the skin, called acrodermatitis chronica atrophicans,[4] but the organism disseminates less often, and arthritis is an unusual manifestation of the disease.[1] *B. garinii* is especially neurotropic and may cause Bannwarth's syndrome, a syndrome of painful radiculopathy followed by meningitis or cranial neuropathy or, rarely, borrelial encephalomyelitis.[1]

Infection and Autoimmunity
http://dx.doi.org/10.1016/B978-0-444-63269-2.00032-5

All stages of Lyme disease can usually be treated successfully with oral or intravenous antibiotic therapy.[5] However, certain signs and symptoms may persist after apparent spirochetal killing with antibiotics. In both the United States and Europe, about 10% of patients with erythema migrans have persistent subjective symptoms after antibiotic treatment, such as headache, arthralgias, or fatigue, which usually resolve within months.[6] In addition, a small percentage of patients with Lyme arthritis in the northeastern United States have persistent, proliferative synovitis lasting months or years after 2–3 months of both oral and intravenous (IV) antibiotics, called antibiotic-refractory Lyme arthritis.[7] After antibiotic therapy, these patients are usually treated with disease-modifying antirheumatic drugs (DMARDs) or sometimes with arthroscopic synovectomy.[7]

2 HYPOTHESES TO EXPLAIN ANTIBIOTIC-REFRACTORY LYME ARTHRITIS

Antibiotic-refractory Lyme arthritis has been hypothesized to result from persistent infection, immune reactivity with retained spirochetal antigens or infection-induced autoimmunity. An antibiotic-refractory outcome is associated with infection with highly inflammatory strains for *B. burgdorferi*,[8] which are found primarily in the northeastern United States. However, in antibiotic-refractory patients, culture and PCR results of *B. burgdorferi* in synovial tissue have been uniformly negative after antibiotic therapy,[9] and treatment with immunosuppressive DMARD therapy, which is usually effective in resolving synovitis, has not led to reactivation of infection.[7] Thus, persistent infection seems not to be the explanation for persistent synovitis after oral and IV antibiotic therapy.

In MyD88$^{-/-}$ mice, which have high pathogen loads, *B. burgdorferi* antigens are retained near cartilage surfaces after antibiotic therapy, and patellar homogenates containing these antigens induce macrophages to secrete TNF-α.[10] However, patients with Lyme arthritis have low pathogen loads,[9] and the extensive synovitis found in patients with antibiotic-refractory arthritis[11] is not replicated in mice. Moreover, T- and B-cell responses to *B. burgdorferi* decline similarly in patients with either antibiotic-refractory or antibiotic-responsive arthritis,[12,13] whereas levels of inflammatory mediators in synovial fluid remain high or even increase in patients with refractory arthritis in the period after antibiotics. Thus, the role of spirochetal remnants in post-infectious immune responses in human disease remains unclear.

In support of the infection-induced autoimmunity hypothesis, specific HLA-DR alleles, including the DRB1*0101, 0401, and 1501 alleles, are the greatest known genetic risk factor for antibiotic-refractory arthritis,[14] a risk factor commonly associated with autoimmune diseases.[15] As in other chronic inflammatory arthritides, HLA-DR molecules in antibiotic-refractory Lyme arthritis are intensely expressed in synovial tissue.[11] In addition, current data suggest that excessive inflammation likely triggered by the initial infection,[16,17] elevated presentation of pathogenic autoantigens,[18] and difficulty in down-regulating inflammation after spirochetal killing[19,20] set the stage for infection-induced autoimmunity in patients with antibiotic-refractory Lyme arthritis.

3 INFECTION-INDUCED AUTOIMMUNITY IN LYME DISEASE

Initial efforts to study the autoimmunity hypothesis focused on a search for molecular mimics between spirochetal and host proteins. Partial sequence homology was found between the human peptide LFA-1$\alpha_{L332-340}$ and an epitope of B. burgdorferi outer-surface protein A (OspA$_{163-175}$),[21] which binds HLA-DR molecules associated with refractory arthritis.[14] Our chapter in the previous edition of this textbook focused on this finding and its possible role in antibiotic-refractory Lyme arthritis.

A second human peptide was subsequently identified, MAWD-BP$_{280-288}$, which had greater sequence homology with OspA$_{163-175}$ than LFA-1 $\alpha_{L332-340}$.[22,23] However, only a minority of patients had low-level T-cell reactivity with either the LFA-1 or MAWD-BP self-peptide, and none had autoantibody responses to these self-proteins. In a later study, Ghosh et al. identified human cytokeratin 10 as a cross-reactive target ligand recognized by anti-OspA antibodies in a small group of patients with refractory arthritis (3 of 15 patients) but not in those with responsive arthritis.[24] Finally, several neural proteins have been reported to induce T- or B-cell responses in patients with neuroborreliosis[25-27] or post-Lyme syndrome.[28] However, responses against neural proteins would be unlikely to explain antibiotic-refractory arthritis. We concluded that a new approach was needed for the identification of potential autoantigens in Lyme disease.

4 NEW PROTOCOL FOR IDENTIFYING AUTOANTIGENS

Several years ago we developed an unbiased protocol for the identification of autoantigens in synovial tissue, the target tissue of immune attack in antibiotic-refractory Lyme arthritis. This method used discovery-based proteomics coupled with translational research. In the proteomics portion

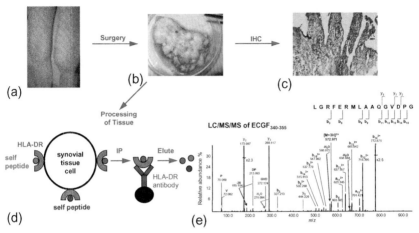

Figure 1 An overview of the isolation and identification of *in vivo* HLA-DR presented peptides from patients' synovial tissue. Antibiotic-refractory Lyme arthritis usually manifests as one swollen knee (a). In those cases in which therapeutic arthroscopic synovectomies are performed, 20–60 g of inflamed synovial tissue and subcutaneous fat are removed (b). Immunohistologic staining of the synovial tissue shows marked exogenous expression of HLA-DR molecules (c). HLA-DR complexes are immunoprecipitated from synovial cell lysates (d). HLA-DR presented peptides are eluted and identified by tandem mass spectrometry (e). In this figure, the LC/MS/MS spectrum of the ECGF$_{340-355}$ peptide is shown. *Reprinted with permission from Drouin EE et al., Arthritis & Rheumatism, 2013;65:186–96.*

of the protocol, naturally presented HLA-DR self-peptides from patients' synovium were identified using tandem mass spectrometry (Figure 1). As reported in our first article using this methodology, we identified ~100 nonredundant HLA-DR-presented peptides from the synovial tissue sample of each of four patients: two with antibiotic-refractory Lyme arthritis and, for comparison, two with rheumatoid arthritis.[29]

5 IDENTIFICATION OF ENDOTHELIAL CELL GROWTH FACTOR AS AN AUTOANTIGEN

In the translational research part of the protocol, the peptides from each patient were synthesized and reacted with the matching patient's PBMC. Of 120 HLA-DR-presented self-peptides identified from the first Lyme patient tested, one peptide, derived from endothelial cell growth factor (ECGF), induced the proliferation of this patient's PBMCs.[18] ECGF, which is also called thymidine phosphorylase, has a proliferative effect of endothelial cells, is a chemotactic factor, and induces angiogenesis.[30] However, it was not previously known to be an autoantigen in any disease. To validate ECGF as a Lyme disease-associated autoantigen, all available PBMCs and serum samples collected over a 25-year period from patients with erythema migrans (the initial skin lesion of Lyme disease) and from those with Lyme arthritis were tested for T- and B-cell reactivity with ECGF.

6 T-CELL RESPONSES TO ECGF

Because ECGF was known to inhibit the readout of the ^{3}H-thymidine proliferation assay and because ECGF nonspecifically induced PBMCs to secrete IFN-γ, we instead tested ECGF peptides predicted to be promiscuous HLA-binders using three HLA-DR T-cell epitope prediction algorithms.[31,32] In total, seven peptides were identified and synthesized, including the peptide initially isolated from the patient's synovial tissue sample (ECGF$_{340-355}$). IFN-γ ELISpot assays were used for testing because they have greater sensitivity than proliferation assays.

As shown in Figure 2, healthy control subjects and patients with RA had only minimal responses to a few of the seven ECGF peptides tested. Of the patients with erythema migrans, 16% had low-level T-cell responses.

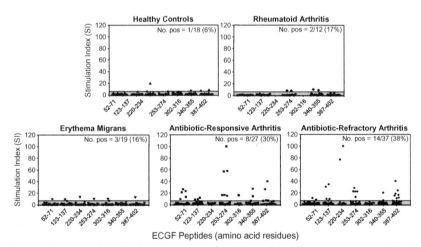

Figure 2 Testing of PBMC from patients with EM, antibiotic-responsive or antibiotic-refractory Lyme arthritis, RA, or healthy control subjects for T cell recognition of ECGF peptides. PBMC were incubated with individual ECGF and assayed by IFN-γ ELISpot assay. The results were quantified using a stimulation index (SI) that was defined as >3 standard deviation above the mean in healthy control subjects (the area above the shaded region) *Reprinted with permission from Drouin EE et al., Arthritis & Rheumatism, 2013;65:186–96.*

In contrast, 30% of patients with antibiotic-responsive arthritis and 38% of those with antibiotic-refractory arthritis had robust responses, often to multiple ECGF peptides. Overall, patients with Lyme arthritis had substantially greater T-cell responses to ECGF peptides than patients in the other groups; their T cells recognized all 7 peptides tested; and 10 patients had responses to 2 to 4 ECGF peptides, suggesting epitope spreading. Of the 21 patients with refractory or responsive Lyme arthritis who were tested and had T-cell reactivity with ECGF peptides, 20 (95%) had known refractory arthritis-associated HLA-DR alleles.[14] Therefore, T-cell responses to ECGF may begin to develop early in the illness; they may occur in patients with either antibiotic-responsive or antibiotic-refractory arthritis, and they are found primarily in patients with antibiotic-refractory risk alleles.

7 B-CELL RESPONSES TO ECGF

ECGF-reactive CD4+ T cells likely contribute to pathogenicity by providing help to B cells to produce anti-ECGF autoantibodies. Therefore, we tested patients' serum samples for IgG anti-ECGF antibodies. When ECGF antibody responses were determined by ELISA, none of the 74 healthy control subjects had a positive response (defined as >3 SD above the mean value of healthy subjects) (Figure 3). In comparison, 15% of patients with erythema migrans ($P=0.001$), 8% of patients with responsive arthritis

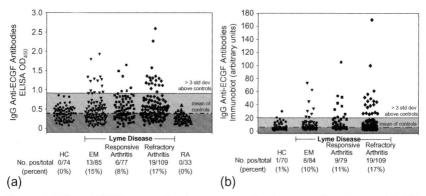

Figure 3 IgG anti-ECGF autoantibody responses in the sera of patients with EM, antibiotic-responsive or antibiotic-refractory Lyme arthritis, RA or healthy control subjects as determined by ELISA. *Reprinted with permission from Drouin EE et al., Arthritis & Rheumatism, 2013;65:186–96.*

($P=0.04$), and 17% patients with refractory arthritis ($P<0.0001$) had positive responses. In addition, patients with antibiotic-refractory arthritis tended to have ECGF autoantibodies more frequently than those with antibiotic-responsive arthritis (17% vs. 8%; $P=0.09$). In contrast, none of the 33 patients with RA had a positive response. Thus, as with T-cell responses, antibody reactivity with ECGF may be found early and late in the disease, particularly in patients with antibiotic-refractory arthritis.

8 ANTIBODY RESPONSES TO ECGF IN NON-ANTIBIOTIC-TREATED PATIENTS

Archival serum samples were tested from 42 non-antibiotic-treated patients with Lyme disease who were followed longitudinally throughout the illness in the 1970s for a median duration of 6 years before the cause of the illness was known.[33] Of the 15 patients who did not develop arthritis, 2 (13%) had ECGF antibody responses 2 to 3 weeks after the onset of erythema migrans. In contrast, 7 of the 27 patients (26%) who later developed arthritis had positive ECGF antibody responses, although this trend was not statistically significant. In six of the seven patients with ECGF-positive arthritis, reactivity developed weeks to months after disease onset, before joint inflammation. Moreover, the duration of active arthritis was significantly longer in the 7 patients who had ECGF responses than in the 20 patients who did not (median value, 67 versus 17 weeks, respectively; $P=0.004$). Thus, non-antibiotic-treated patients usually developed ECGF antibody responses early in the illness, before the onset of arthritis; in those who subsequently developed arthritis, this response was associated with a significantly longer duration of joint inflammation.

9 ECGF IN JOINT FLUID AND SYNOVIAL TISSUE

For ECGF to have pathogenic relevance as an autoantigen in antibiotic-refractory Lyme arthritis, one would predict that this protein would be present in high concentrations in patients' inflamed synovial fluid and tissue. As determined by sandwich ELISA, patients with antibiotic-refractory arthritis often had very high concentrations of ECGF in synovial fluid (mean value, 448 ng/mL) (Figure 4), which were significantly greater than those in patients with antibiotic-responsive arthritis (154 ng/mL) ($P<0.0001$). Patients with RA also often had high concentrations of ECGF (313 ng/mL), which is consistent with the findings of other investigators,[34] but ECGF is rarely, if ever, an autoantigen in RA. Finally, patients with osteoarthritis

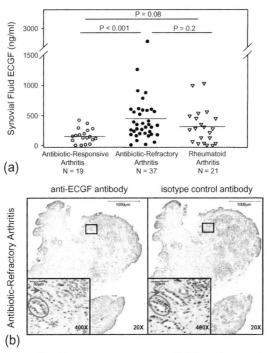

Figure 4 Detection of ECGF protein in joint fluid and synovial tissue. ECGF concentrations in joint fluid of patients with antibiotic-responsive or antibiotic-refractory Lyme arthritis, or RA were measured by sandwich ELISA (a). Representative serial synovial tissue sections from a patient with antibiotic-refractory Lyme arthritis stained with anti-ECGF or isotype control antibodies. Both slides were counterstained with Mayer's hematoxylin. Circles indicate the sublining area around blood vessels; arrows indicate large cells, most likely synoviocytes (b). *Reprinted with permission from Drouin EE et al., Arthritis & Rheumatism, 2013;65:186–96.*

(OA), a minimally inflammatory form of arthritis, had much lower concentrations (8.7 ng/mL).[34]

When synovial tissue samples, obtained by synovectomy, were examined for the presence of ECGF, 10 of 16 patients (63%) with antibiotic-refractory Lyme arthritis had moderate to intense staining for this protein in the lining and sub-lining of the tissue; 4 (25%) had mild staining and 2 (12%) had no staining in these areas. Synovial tissue was not available from patients with antibiotic-responsive arthritis because therapeutic synovectomies are never necessary in this patient group. Thus, the majority of patients with antibiotic-refractory arthritis had large amounts of ECGF in synovial fluid and intense staining in synovial tissue, where the protein could act as an autoantigen.

10 AUTOANTIBODIES TO ECGF AND OBLITERATIVE MICROVASCULAR LESIONS

We next addressed the question of whether anti-ECGF autoantibodies have specific pathologic consequences in synovial tissue in patients with antibiotic-refractory Lyme arthritis ($N=14$) and, for comparison, from patients with other forms of chronic inflammatory arthritis ($N=6$), primarily rheumatoid arthritis.[35] Synovial tissue from all 20 patients showed synovial hypertrophy, vascular proliferation, immune cell infiltrates, and fibrosis. However, among the 14 patients with antibiotic-refractory arthritis, 8 (57%) also had obliterative microvascular lesions in the tissue compared with none of the control patients ($P=0.04$). Of the patients with obliterative microvascular lesions, 5 of 14 (36%) also had anti-ECGF antibody responses; and the magnitude of ECGF antibody reactivity correlated directly with the extent of obliterative lesions ($P=0.02$). This correlation implies that ECGF autoantibodies are involved in the obliterative process and have specific pathologic consequences in patients with antibiotic-refractory Lyme arthritis.

Autoantibodies to ECGF also are found in a subset of patients with neurologic or cardiac involvement of Lyme disease (unpublished data), and obliterative microvascular lesions have been seen in these tissues.[36,37] In several patients with fatal pancarditis due to Lyme disease, obliterative microvascular lesions were noted in myocardial tissue.[37,38] Although affected tissue from patients with neuroborreliosis is rarely available, obliterative microvascular lesions were found in neurologic tissue, heart, and skeletal muscle in nonhuman primates experimentally infected with *B. burgdorferi*.[39-41] Thus, obliteration of small blood vessels would seem to be a more general consequence of *B. burgdorferi* infection in susceptible individuals.

11 ELEVATED INTERLEUKIN-23 LEVELS, ECGF AUTOANTIBODIES, AND POST-LYME DISEASE SYMPTOMS

B. burgdorferi is a large extracellular pathogen, and Th17 cells are important in host defence against such pathogens.[42] In addition, aberrant Th17 responses have been implicated as playing a key role in a number of autoimmune diseases, including rheumatoid arthritis, psoriatic arthritis, lupus, inflammatory bowel disease, and type 1 diabetes.[43] Interestingly, mice and hamsters vaccinated with killed *B. burgdorferi* and then infected with live spirochetes developed severe destructive arthritis,[44] which was ameliorated by neutralizing antibodies against IL-17[45] or IL-23,[46] a cytokine that promotes the survival and proliferation of Th17 cells. These results imply that Th17 responses have a role in more severe and prolonged *B. burgdorferi*-induced arthritis in mice.

Although the frequency of Th17 cells is usually low in human patients with antibiotic-refractory Lyme arthritis,[19] we hypothesized that Th17 cells may have a role during early infection. Thus, we addressed the potential role of Th17 in Lyme disease using a unique collection of serum samples from an antibiotic treatment study of 510 European patients who had erythema migrans,[6] the initial skin lesion of Lyme disease. The patients were assessed at baseline, treated with antibiotics for 2 weeks, and evaluated 2, 6, and 12 months later regarding health-related difficulties. At the initial evaluation and before antibiotic treatment, 159 of the 510 patients (31%) with erythema migrans had one or more associated symptom such as fatigue, arthralgias, myalgias, headache, or paresthesias. Following antibiotic therapy, 62 patients (12%) had post-Lyme disease symptoms at 2 months, and 18 (4%) still had symptoms after 12 months.[6]

In our study, the levels of 23 cytokines and chemokines, representative of innate and adaptive immune responses, were assessed in sera from 86 patients, including 45 patients with post-Lyme disease symptoms and 41 randomly selected patients who did not have such symptoms.[47] Of the 23 cytokines and chemokines measured, significant differences between the groups were found only with the Th1-associated chemokines CXCL9 and CXCL10 and the Th17-associated cytokine, IL-23.[47] Importantly, within the subgroup of the 41 patients with detectable levels of IL-23, the values were significantly higher in the 25 patients (61%) who developed post-Lyme disease symptoms than in the 16 patients who did not ($P=0.003$), and all 7 patients with the highest levels of IL-23 (>230 ng/mL) had such symptoms. Furthermore, antibody responses to the ECGF autoantigen correlated directly with IL-23 levels ($P=0.02$) (Figure 5), and anti-ECGF autoantibodies were more common in patients with post-Lyme disease symptoms ($P=0.07$). These observations suggested that the key factor in the correlation between IL-23 and post-Lyme disease symptoms was the magnitude of the Th17 immune response.

We concluded that a subgroup of patients with erythema migrans has an immune response to *B. burgdorferi* tilted towards a Th17 response. Patients with low levels of IL-23 may not have an increased frequency of untoward events. In contrast, in patients with high levels of IL-23, Th17 immune responses early in the illness may have disadvantageous aspects, including the development of autoimmune phenomena or post-Lyme disease symptoms. In patients with antibiotic-refractory Lyme arthritis, Th17 responses early in the illness, before the development of arthritis, may be one—but not

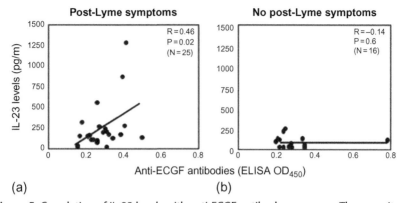

Figure 5 Correlation of IL-23 levels with anti-ECGF antibody responses. The magnitude of the anti-ECGF antibody response correlated with IL-23 levels in patients with post-Lyme symptoms (a), but not in patients without post-Lyme symptoms (b). *Reprinted with permission from Strle et al., Clin Infect Dis, 2014;58:372–80.*

the only—route leading to infection-induced autoimmunity and persistent synovitis after antibiotic therapy.

12 PATHOGENETIC HYPOTHESIS TO EXPLAIN THE ROLE OF ECGF IN LYME DISEASE

We postulate the following sequence of events related to ECGF immunity in the pathogenesis of antibiotic-refractory Lyme arthritis. After transmission of *B. burgdorferi* by the tick, spirochetes spread in the skin, invade blood vessels, and often home in on joints;[48] in each of these sites, the spirochetes are targeted by the immune system.[37,49] In patients genetically prone to greater inflammation, such as those with a particular TLR1 polymorphism[17] who are infected with highly inflammatory strains of *B. burgdorferi*,[8] exceptionally strong innate and adaptive immune responses develop, resulting in markedly elevated levels of TNF-α, IL-1β, and IFN-γ.[16,17]

IFN-γ in particular stimulates ECGF production by macrophages[50] and possibly other cells, resulting in vascular proliferation. In patients who subsequently develop refractory arthritis, very high concentrations of ECGF protein in joint fluid and synovial tissue likely lead to increased HLA-DR presentation of ECGF epitopes.[18] The presentation of these epitopes within the context of a strong pro-inflammatory environment likely alters the threshold of T-cell activation, triggering a break in tolerance. A similar process may occur in patients with antibiotic-responsive arthritis, but the lower concentrations of IFN-γ[16] and ECGF seem not to cross the threshold necessary to induce pathogenic autoimmunity.[18]

After 2–3 months of oral and IV antibiotic therapy, live spirochetes are no longer detectable.[9] However, because patients with refractory arthritis have difficulty down-regulating their immune response,[19,20] the concentrations of pro-inflammatory cytokines and ECGF protein remain significantly higher in these patients than those with antibiotic-responsive arthritis.[16–18] In refractory patients, it is likely that anti-ECGF immune complexes form in and around endothelial cells, leading to complement activation and eventually to obliteration of these vessels.

Antibiotic-refractory Lyme arthritis eventually resolves in all patients.[7,33] Why might infection-induced autoimmunity resolve? First, we postulate that spirochetal killing either by the immune system or with the assistance of antibiotic therapy removes the "danger" signals that alert the innate immune system to infection. Second, any remaining spirochetal remnants may eventually be phagocytosed. Finally, an increase in the number and function of T regulatory (Treg) cells likely increases over time, which eventually allows the immune system to regain homeostasis.[19,20] This hypothesis is supported by a murine model of Ova-induced autoimmune dermatitis in which persistent expression of this "self" antigen in skin results in the activation, proliferation and differentiation of memory Treg cells that possess enhanced suppressive activity.[51] These site-specific memory Treg cells re-establish immune homeostasis, and pathogenic autoimmunity resolves.

Similarly, in human antibiotic-refractory Lyme arthritis, the duration of arthritis after antibiotic treatment correlates with the ratio of Treg to T effector cells.[20] Patients with higher Treg-to-T effector ratios at the conclusion of antibiotic therapy had a shorter duration of subsequent arthritis, whereas lower ratios were associated with a longer duration of arthritis. Thus, in the absence of innate immune danger signals and with an increase in the numbers and function of Treg cells, we postulate that the immune system regains homeostasis, leading to the resolution of arthritis.

13 MULTI-FACTORIAL NATURE OF AUTOIMMUNE DISEASE

It is unlikely that autoimmunity to ECGF alone accounts for antibiotic-refractory Lyme arthritis. In human autoimmune diseases, multiple factors are usually required for clinical expression of autoimmunity.[15] First, in antibiotic-refractory Lyme arthritis, excessive inflammation, immune dysregulation, and particular HLA-DR alleles may be necessary for infection-induced autoimmunity to develop. Furthermore, immune reactivity with multiple autoantigens is probably required for an antibiotic-refractory course. Thus, we are continuing to use discovery-based proteomics and translational research in an effort to identify additional pathogenic autoantigens in Lyme disease. Furthermore, we believe that this method is applicable for the identification of currently unknown pathogenic autoantigens in other immune-mediated diseases.

ACKNOWLEDGMENTS

This work was supported by National Institutes of Health Grant AI-101175, the English, Bonter, Mitchell Foundation, the Lyme/Arthritis Research Fund at Massachusetts General Hospital, The Mathers Foundation, and the Eshe Fund.

REFERENCES

1. Steere AC. Lyme disease. *N Engl J Med* 2001;**345**:115–25.
2. Baranton G, Postic D, Saint Girons I, Boerlin P, Piffaretti JC, Assous M, et al. Delineation of *Borrelia burgdorferi* sensu stricto, *Borrelia garinii* sp. nov., and group VS461 associated with Lyme borreliosis. *Int J Syst Bacteriol* 1992;**42**:378–83.
3. Steere AC. Lyme disease. *N Engl J Med* 1989;**321**:586–96.
4. Mullegger RR. Dermatological manifestations of Lyme borreliosis. *Eur J Dermatol* 2004;**14**:296–309.
5. Wormser GP, Dattwyler RJ, Shapiro ED, Halperin JJ, Steere AC, Klempner MS, et al. The clinical assessment, treatment, and prevention of Lyme disease, human granulocytic anaplasmosis, and babesiosis: clinical practice guidelines by the Infectious Diseases Society of America. *Clin Infect Dis* 2006;**43**:1089–134.
6. Stupica D, Lusa L, Ruzic-Sabljic E, Cerar T, Strle F. Treatment of erythema migrans with doxycycline for 10 days versus 15 days. *Clin Infect Dis* 2012;**55**:343–50.
7. Steere AC, Angelis SM. Therapy for Lyme arthritis: strategies for the treatment of antibiotic-refractory arthritis. *Arthritis Rheum* 2006;**54**:3079–86.
8. Jones KL, McHugh GA, Glickstein LJ, Steere AC. Analysis of *Borrelia burgdorferi* genotypes in patients with Lyme arthritis: high frequency of ribosomal RNA intergenic spacer type 1 strains in antibiotic-refractory arthritis. *Arthritis Rheum* 2009;**60**:2174–82.
9. Li X, McHugh GA, Damle N, Sikand VK, Glickstein L, Steere AC. Burden and viability of *Borrelia burgdorferi* in skin and joints of patients with erythema migrans or Lyme arthritis. *Arthritis Rheum* 2011;**63**:2238–47.
10. Bockenstedt LK, Gonzalez DG, Haberman AM, Belperron AA. Spirochete antigens persist near cartilage after murine Lyme borreliosis therapy. *J Clin Invest* 2012;**122**:2652–60.
11. Steere AC, Glickstein L. Elucidation of Lyme arthritis. *Nat Rev Immunol* 2004;**4**:143–52.
12. Kannian P, Drouin EE, Glickstein L, Kwok WW, Nepom GT, Steere AC. Decline in the frequencies of *Borrelia burgdorferi* OspA$_{161-175}$-specific T cells after antibiotic therapy in HLA-DRB1*0401-positive patients with antibiotic-responsive or antibiotic-refractory Lyme arthritis. *J Immunol* 2007;**179**:6336–42.
13. Kannian P, McHugh G, Johnson BJ, Bacon RM, Glickstein LJ, Steere AC. Antibody responses to *Borrelia burgdorferi* in patients with antibiotic-refractory, antibiotic-responsive, or non-antibiotic-treated Lyme arthritis. *Arthritis Rheum* 2007;**56**:4216–25.

14. Steere AC, Klitz W, Drouin EE, Falk BA, Kwok WW, Nepom GT, et al. Antibiotic-refractory Lyme arthritis is associated with HLA-DR molecules that bind a *Borrelia burgdorferi* peptide. *J Exp Med* 2006;**203**:961–71.

15. Cho JH, Gregersen PK. Genomics and the multifactorial nature of human autoimmune disease. *N Engl J Med* 2011;**365**:1612–23.

16. Shin JJ, Glickstein L, Steere AC. High levels of inflammatory chemokines and cytokines in joint fluid and synovial tissue throughout the course of antibiotic-refractory Lyme arthritis. *Arthritis Rheum* 2007;**56**:1325–35.

17. Strle K, Shin JJ, Glickstein LJ, Steere AC. Association of a toll-like receptor 1 polymorphism with heightened Th1 inflammatory responses and antibiotic-refractory Lyme arthritis. *Arthritis Rheum* 2012;**64**:1497–507.

18. Drouin EE, Seward RJ, Strle K, McHugh G, Katchar K, Londono D, et al. A novel human autoantigen, endothelial cell growth factor, is a target of T and B cell responses in patients with Lyme disease. *Arthritis Rheum* 2013;**65**:186–96.

19. Shen S, Shin JJ, Strle K, McHugh G, Li X, Glickstein LJ, et al. Treg cell numbers and function in patients with antibiotic-refractory or antibiotic-responsive Lyme arthritis. *Arthritis Rheum* 2010;**62**:2127–37.

20. Vudattu NK, Strle K, Steere AC, Drouin EE. Dysregulation of CD4+CD25hi+ T cells in the synovial fluid of patients with antibiotic-refractory Lyme arthritis. *Arthritis Rheum* 2013;**65**:1643–54.

21. Gross DM, Forsthuber T, Tary-Lehmann M, Etling C, Ito K, Nagy ZA, et al. Identification of LFA-1 as a candidate autoantigen in treatment-resistant Lyme arthritis. *Science* 1998;**281**:703–6.

22. Drouin EE, Glickstein L, Kwok WW, Nepom GT, Steere AC. Human homologues of a *Borrelia* T cell epitope associated with antibiotic-refractory Lyme arthritis. *Mol Immunol* 2008;**45**:180–9.

23. Drouin EE, Glickstein L, Kwok WW, Nepom GT, Steere AC. Searching for borrelial T cell epitopes associated with antibiotic-refractory Lyme arthritis. *Mol Immunol* 2008;**45**:2323–32.

24. Ghosh S, Seward R, Costello CE, Stollar BD, Huber BT. Autoantibodies from synovial lesions in chronic, antibiotic treatment-resistant Lyme arthritis bind cytokeratin-10. *J Immunol* 2006;**177**:2486–94.

25. Martin R, Ortlauf J, Sticht-Groh V, Bogdahn U, Goldmann SF, Mertens HG. *Borrelia burgdorferi*–specific and autoreactive T-cell lines from cerebrospinal fluid in Lyme radiculomyelitis. *Ann Neurol* 1988;**24**:509–16.

26. Kuenzle S, von Budingen HC, Meier M, Harrer MD, Urich E, Becher B, et al. Pathogen specificity and autoimmunity are distinct features of antigen-driven immune responses in neuroborreliosis. *Infect Immun* 2007;**75**:3842–7.

27. Lunemann JD, Gelderblom H, Sospedra M, Quandt JA, Pinilla C, Marques A, et al. Cerebrospinal fluid-infiltrating CD4+ T cells recognize *Borrelia burgdorferi* lysine-enriched protein domains and central nervous system autoantigens in early Lyme encephalitis. *Infect Immun* 2007;**75**:243–51.

28. Chandra A, Wormser GP, Klempner MS, Trevino RP, Crow MK, Latov N, et al. Anti-neural antibody reactivity in patients with a history of Lyme borreliosis and persistent symptoms. *Brain Behav Immun* 2010;**24**:1018–24.

29. Seward RJ, Drouin EE, Steere AC, Costello CE. Peptides presented by HLA-DR molecules in synovia of patients with rheumatoid arthritis or antibiotic-refractory Lyme arthritis. *Mol Cell Proteomics* 2011;**10**, M110 002477.

30. Ishikawa F, Miyazono K, Hellman U, Drexler H, Wernstedt C, Hagiwara K, et al. Identification of angiogenic activity and the cloning and expression of platelet-derived endothelial cell growth factor. *Nature* 1989;**338**:557–62.

31. Sturniolo T, Bono E, Ding J, Raddrizzani L, Tuereci O, Sahin U, et al. Generation of tissue-specific and promiscuous HLA ligand databases using DNA microarrays and virtual HLA class II matrices. *Nat Biotechnol* 1999;**17**:555–61.

32. Wang P, Sidney J, Dow C, Mothe B, Sette A, Peters B. A systematic assessment of MHC class II peptide binding predictions and evaluation of a consensus approach. *PLoS Comput Biol* 2008;**4**:e1000048.

33. Steere AC, Schoen RT, Taylor E. The clinical evolution of Lyme arthritis. *Ann Intern Med* 1987;**107**:725–31.

34. Takeuchi M, Otsuka T, Matsui N, Asai K, Hirano T, Moriyama A, et al. Aberrant production of gliostatin/platelet-derived endothelial cell growth factor in rheumatoid synovium. *Arthritis Rheum* 1994;**37**:662–72.

35. Londono D, Cadavid D, Drouin EE, Strle K, McHugh G, Aversa J, et al. Antibodies to endothelial cell growth factor and obliterative microvascular lesions in synovia of patients with antibiotic-refractory Lyme arthritis. *Arthritis Rheumatol* 2014;**66**:2124–33.

36. de Koning J, Hoogkamp-Korstanje JA, van der Linde MR, Crijns HJ. Demonstration of spirochetes in cardiac biopsies of patients with Lyme disease. *J Infect Dis* 1989;**160**:150–3.

37. Duray PH. Histopathology of clinical phases of human Lyme disease. *Rheum Dis Clin North Am* 1989;**15**:691–710.

38. Marcus LC, Steere AC, Duray PH, Anderson AE, Mahoney EB. Fatal pancarditis in a patient with coexistent Lyme disease and babesiosis. Demonstration of spirochetes in the myocardium. *Ann Intern Med* 1985;**103**:374–6.

39. Cadavid D, Bai Y, Dail D, Hurd M, Narayan K, Hodzic E, et al. Infection and inflammation in skeletal muscle from nonhuman primates infected with different genospecies of the Lyme disease spirochete *Borrelia burgdorferi*. *Infect Immun* 2003;**71**:7087–98.

40. Cadavid D, Bai Y, Hodzic E, Narayan K, Barthold SW, Pachner AR. Cardiac involvement in non-human primates infected with the Lyme disease spirochete *Borrelia burgdorferi*. *Lab Invest* 2004;**84**:1439–50.

41. Cadavid D. The mammalian host response to *borrelia* infection. *Wien Klin Wochenschr* 2006;**118**:653–8.

42. Kolls JK, Linden A. Interleukin-17 family members and inflammation. *Immunity* 2004;**21**:467–76.

43. Maddur MS, Miossec P, Kaveri SV, Bayry J. Th17 cells: biology, pathogenesis of autoimmune and inflammatory diseases, and therapeutic strategies. *Am J Pathol* 2012;**181**:8–18.

44. Munson E, Nardelli DT, Du Chateau BK, Callister SM, Schell RF. Hamster and murine models of severe destructive Lyme arthritis. *Clin Dev Immunol* 2012;**2012**:504215.

45. Burchill MA, Nardelli DT, England DM, DeCoster DJ, Christopherson JA, Callister SM, et al. Inhibition of interleukin-17 prevents the development of arthritis in vaccinated mice challenged with *Borrelia burgdorferi*. *Infect Immun* 2003;**71**:3437–42.

46. Kotloski NJ, Nardelli DT, Peterson SH, Torrealba JR, Warner TF, Callister SM, et al. Interleukin-23 is required for development of arthritis in mice vaccinated and challenged with *Borrelia* species. *Clin Vaccine Immunol* 2008;**15**:1199–207.

47. Strle K, Stupica D, Drouin EE, Steere AC, Strle F. Elevated levels of IL-23 in a subset of patients with post-Lyme disease symptoms following erythema migrans. *Clin Infect Dis* 2014;**58**:372–80.

48. Coburn J, Medrano M, Cugini C. *Borrelia burgdorferi* and its tropisms for adhesion molecules in the joint. *Curr Opin Rheumatol* 2002;**14**:394–8.

49. Duray PH. The surgical pathology of human Lyme disease. An enlarging picture. *Am J Surg Pathol* 1987;**11**(Suppl. 1):47–60.

50. Goto H, Kohno K, Sone S, Akiyama S, Kuwano M, Ono M. Interferon gamma-dependent induction of thymidine phosphorylase/platelet-derived endothelial growth factor through gamma-activated sequence-like element in human macrophages. *Cancer Res* 2001;**61**:469–73.
51. Rosenblum MD, Gratz IK, Paw JS, Lee K, Marshak-Rothstein A, Abbas AK. Response to self antigen imprints regulatory memory in tissues. *Nature* 2011;**480**:538–42.

CHAPTER 31

Streptococcus Pneumoniae and Autoimmunity: A Systematic Review of the Literature

How Pneumococcal Infection Might Be Related to Rheumatic Diseases

E. Borella, M. Domeneghetti, L. Palma, A. Doria[1]
Division of Rheumatology, Department of Medicine, University of Padova, Padova, Italy
[1]Corresponding Author: adoria@unipd.it

1 INTRODUCTION

Infection and autoimmunity are two closely linked pathological conditions. People with autoimmune diseases are more predisposed to develop infection because of both the immune alterations occurring in their disease and their immunosuppressive drug intake.[1–5] Moreover, although the etiopathogenetic mechanism of rheumatic diseases (RDs) is still elusive, nowadays it is clear that genetic and environmental factors both are involved in the onset of RDs.[6] Indeed, people with a decreased self-immune tolerance may develop an autoimmune reaction when exposed to external triggers such as infections and drugs.[6] Epstein–Barr virus (EBV), hepatitis C virus (HCV), and parvovirus B-19 are just few examples of infectious agents involved in the development of RDs.[7–9]

Thus, the aim of this systematic review was to clarify the relationship between *Streptococcus pneumoniae*, a widely diffuse infectious agent, and autoimmunity. In particular, we focused on[1] *Pneumococcus* as a trigger of RDs and[2] RDs as risk factors of pneumococcal infection.

2 SEARCH STRATEGIES

We performed a systematic review of the literature using the PubMed database. Moreover, we hand-searched for the relevant articles referenced in other publications and not available in the database. Randomized controlled

Infection and Autoimmunity
http://dx.doi.org/10.1016/B978-0-444-63269-2.00034-9

trials, controlled studies, prospective studies, retrospective studies, case series, and case reports were considered in the analysis.

We used the following search terms: *Streptococcus pneumoniae*, *Pneumococcus*, *infections*, *autoimmunity*, *rheumatic disease*, *systemic lupus erythematosus*, and *rheumatoid arthritis*. We included only articles written in the English language in our research. The initial search, based on the search terms, returned 11,013 titles. Among these, 231 titles pertained to the search. By reading the abstracts, 59 articles were selected.[10–68] We found 31 case reports,[10,12,14–16,18–20,22,23,28,29,31–34,38–52] 11 case series,[11,13,17,21,25–27,30,35–37] 14 retrospective studies,[24,55–67] 2 prospective studies,[53,68] and 1 case-control study.[54]

3 *PNEUMOCOCCUS* AS A TRIGGER OF RDs

We found one case describing the onset of an RD after pneumococcal infection:[25] SLE was diagnosed 1 month after the infection. Given that we found just one case in the literature reporting pneumococcal infection before the onset of an RD and we did not find epidemiological studies supporting the role of *Pneumococcus* as a trigger of autoimmune diseases, it is likely that *S. pneumoniae* does not play a major role in triggering RDs. Interestingly, *Pneumococcus* might have a protective function on autoimmunity. It has been recently suggested that ES-62 is the molecule responsible for the beneficial effect of parasites and their ova in RDs; the important epitope in this compound is phosphorylcholine (PC).[69] PC is expressed not only in helminths but also in the pneumococcal capsule. Moreover, it is exposed on apoptotic cells as well as on oxidized low-density lipoproteins. PC can both promote and protect against diseases.[69] In fact, it drives the maturation of dendritic cells, promotes the differentiation of CD4+ T cells with a Th2 phenotype, and suppresses the production of some cytokines such as IL-12, IL-6, and TNF-α.[69] Thus, it plays an immunomodulating role that delays the control of the infection but, at the same time, protects from the onset of RDs.

S. pneumoniae is the main cause of bacterial community-acquired pneumonia and meningitis in Western countries and leads to thousands of deaths in developing countries.[70] Since the late '70s, several anti-pneumococcal vaccines have been created, and nowadays three vaccines are available, all of them containing different PC capsular antigens of the main pathogenic strains.[71,72] The safety profile of pneumococcal vaccines is reassuring,[73] and their use has been proved safe in rheumatic patients.[74–80] Therefore, it could be of interest to investigate whether immunization with pneumococcal vaccines is protective against the development or the relapse of RDs.

4 RDs AS RISK FACTORS FOR PNEUMOCOCCAL INFECTION

We found 17 epidemiological studies[24,53–68] (Table 1) and 65 case reports[10–23,25–52] from between 1969 and 2013 (Tables 2 and 3) describing pneumococcal infection in rheumatic patients. The prevalence of *Pneumococcus* among other infections in patients with SLE is 9.01% (Table 1). There were 47 cases of SLE[10–23,25–37] (Table 2) and 18 of rheumatoid arthritis (RA)[39–52] (Table 3). There were 12 men: 5 with SLE (10.6%) and 7 with RA (38.9%), and 51 women: 40 with SLE (85.1%) and 11 with RA (61.1%). The mean age was 31 years among patients with SLE (range, 10–56 years) and 57 years among patients with RA (range, 37–81 years). Forty patients (61.5%) were

Table 1 Epidemiological Studies About Pneumococcal Infections and SLE Reported in the Literature Between 1969 and 2013

Author	Cases of SP, *n* (%)	Cases of Infection, *n* (%)	Patients (*n*)	Study Design
General population				
Bosch[53]	3 (4.76)	63 (57.3)	110	Controlled, prospective study
Ruiz-Irastorza[54]	5 (6.02)	83 (29.2)	284	Case-control study
Costa-Reis[55]	2 (4.55)	44 (37)	120	Retrospective study
Zonana-Nacach[56]	1 (1.54)	65 (32)	200	Retrospective study
Noël[57]	4 (11.43)	35 (40)	87	Retrospective study
Lee[58]	1 (2.13)	61 (129.8)	47	Retrospective study
Staples[59]	1 (7)	14 (60.9)	23	Retrospective study
Pryor[60]	2 (2)	45 (45)	100	Retrospective study
Andonopoulos[61]	2 (17.65)	17 (36.2)	47	Retrospective study
Al-Mayouf[62]	4 (13.79)	29 (41)	70	Retrospective study
Goldblatt[24]	3 (18.75)	16 (15.4)	104	Retrospective study
Jeong[63]	5 (11.9)	42 (38.2)	110	Retrospective study
Infected patients				
Marcos[64]	1 (2)	50 (100)	50	Retrospective study
Han[65]	1 (4)	25 (100)	25	Retrospective study
Patients who died				
Harisdangkul[66]	1 (7)	14 (28)	50	Retrospective study
Jacobsen[67]	4 (16)	25 (20.5)	122	Retrospective study
Ward[68]	5 (22.72)	32 (22.2)	144	Prospective study

CF, cyclophosphamide.

Table 2 Cases of Pneumococcal Infection in SLE Patients Reported in the Literature Between 1969 and 2013

Author	Sex, Age	Area	Immunosuppressive Drugs	Amount of C3, C4	Blood Culture	Site Culture	Antibiotics	Outcome
Sabio[10]	F, 37	Face	PRD 7.5 mg/day MMF 500 mg	Low	Negative	Positive	Ceftriaxone	Alive
Patel[11]	F, 14	Face, neck fasciitis	PRD, AZA	ND	Positive	ND	Penicillin	Alive
	F, 49	Glossitis	No	ND	ND	ND	Cefazolin	Alive
Page[12]	F, 23	Pharynx, neck cellulitis	PRD, high dose	Low	Positive	ND	Vanco, ampic, sulbactam	Alive
DiNubile[13]	F, 18	Chest, breast	ND	ND	Positive	Positive	Penicillin	Alive
	F, 22	Septic arthritis	PRD 5 mg/day	ND	Positive	Positive	Penicillin	Alive
	F, 23	Breast	Alternate–day PRD	Low	Positive	Positive	Cefazolin	Alive
	M, 38	Epiglottitis	PRD	Normal	Positive	ND	ND	Alive
	F, 35	Epiglottitis	PRD 10 mg/day	ND	Positive	Positive	Penicillin	Alive
Hill[14]	F, 30	Neck, pharynx fasciitis, epiglottitis	PRD, CF (100 mg)	Low	Positive	ND	Penicillin	Alive
McDonald[15]	F, 22	Neck fasciitis, glottitis	PRD 5 mg/day	Low	Positive	ND	Penicillin	Alive
Karsh[16]	F, ND	Epiglottits	PDN, CF	ND	ND	ND	ND	Died
Naveau[17]	F, 32	Meningoencephalitis, pneumonia	PRD, 20 mg/day	ND	Positive	Positive	Penicillin	Alive
	F, 54	Bilateral pneumonia	PRD 12.5 mg/day, AZA	ND	Positive	Positive	Cetriaxone	Alive
	F, 12	Meningitis, pneumonia, acute otitis media	PRD 5 mg/day	ND	Positive	Positive	Ampicillin	Alive
	F, 39	Meningitis, sinusitis	No	ND	Positive	Positive	Ceftriaxone	Alive
	F, 13	Septic arthritis	PRD 20 mg/day	ND	Positive	Positive	Penicillin	Alive

Matsumura[18]	F, 53	Bronchitis, osteomielitis, psoas abscess	PRD 8 mg/day	Low	Positive	Positive	Vancomycin	Alive
Chiu[19]	F, 13	Necrotizing pneumonia	PRD, AZA	ND	Positive	ND	ND	Alive
Isik[20]	F, 46	Necrotizing fasciitis	No	ND	ND	Positive	Metranidaziole, sulbactam, cefoperazone	Died
Lipsky[21]	F, 14	Peritonitis	PRD 30 mg/day, AZA 50 mg/day	ND	Positive	Positive	Penicillin	Alive
Shalit[22]	F, 35	Peritonitis	PRD 60 mg/day	ND	Positive	Positive	Penicillin	Alive
	M, 21	Epiglottitis	PRD 20 mg/day	Normal	Positive	Negative	Penicillin	Alive
Kamran[23]	M, 12	Necrotizing fasciitis	ND	ND	Positive	ND	ND	Alive
Yee[25]	F, 24	Pneumonia, siusitis, periorbital cellulitis	PRD 15 mg/day	Normal	Positive	Positive	ND	ND
	F, 34	Peritonitis	PRD 10 mg/day	Low	ND	ND	ND	ND
	F, 30	Pneumonia	PRD 2 mg/day	Low	Positive	ND	ND	ND
	F, 27	Pneumonia	PRD 10 mg/day	Low	Positive	ND	ND	ND
Vargas[26]	F, 56	Meningitis in splenectomized patient	ND	ND	Positive	Positive	Penicillin	Alive
Hung[27]	F, 38	Meningitis	ND	ND	Positive	Positive	Penicillin	Alive
	M,11	Meningitis	PRD	ND	Negative	Positive	ND	Alive
	F, 30	Meningitis	PRD	ND	Positive	Negative	ND	Alive
Dillon[28]	F, 17	Sepsis in functional asplenia	ND	Low	Positive	ND	ND	Died

Continued

Table 2 Cases of Pneumococcal Infection in SLE Patients Reported in the Literature Between 1969 and 2013—cont'd

Author	Sex, Age	Area	Immunosuppressive Drugs	Amount of C3, C4	Blood Culture	Site Culture	Antibiotics	Outcome
Wachtel[29]	F, 56	Sepsis in functional asplenia	ND	ND	Positive	ND	ND	Died
Van Der Straeten[30]	F, 31	Sepsis in functional asplenia	ND	ND	Positive	ND	ND	Died
Malleson[31]	F, 10	Sepsis in functional asplenia	ND	Low	Positive	ND	ND	Died
Piliero[32]	F, 44	Sepsis in functional asplenia	ND	Low	Positive	ND	ND	Alive
Scerpella[33]	F, 22	Sepsis in functional asplenia	ND	Low	Positive	ND	ND	Alive
Petros[34]	F, 18	Sepsis, pneumonia, arthritis	No	Low	Positive	Negative	Penicillin + cefotaxime	Died
ter Borg[35]	ND	Pneumonia, sepsis	PRD 60 mg/day	ND	Positive	ND	ND	ND
	ND	Pneumonia, sepsis	PRD 22.5 mg/day	ND	Positive	ND	ND	ND
Van Der Straeten[30]	M, 31	Sepsis in asplenic patient	PRD, CF	ND	Positive	ND	Gentamicin	Died
	F, 31	Sepsis	PRD	ND	Positive	ND	Tobramycin, fefotaxin	Died
	F, 56	Sepsis	PRD 10 mg on alternate days	ND	Positive	Positive	Chloramphenicol, cafazolin, decadron	Died
Perez[36]	F, 50	Pneumonia	No	Normal	Positive	ND	ND	Alive
	F, 41	Pneumonia	PRD 20 mg/day	Normal	Positive	ND	ND	Alive
Epstein[37]	F, 50	Meningitis	ND	ND	Positive	Positive	ND	Died

F, female; M, male; PRD, prednisone; AZA, azathioprine; MMF, micofenolato mofetile; CF, cyclophosphamide; ND, not determined/ not known; pos, positive; neg, negative.

Table 3 Cases of Pneumococcal Infection in Patients with Rheumatoid Arthritis Reported in the Literature Between 1969 and 2013

Author	Sex, Age	Area	Immunosuppressive Drugs	Blood Culture	Site Culture	Antibiotics	Outcome
Rowe[38]	M, 60	Rigour, septic arthritis, pneumonia	PRD	Positive	Positive	ND	Alive
Lohse[39]	M, 64	Polyarticular septic arthritis	PRD	ND	Positive	ND	Died
Good[40]	M, 77	Polyarticular septic arthritis	No	ND	Positive	Penicillin	Died
	M, 54	Polyarticular septic arthritis	PRD	ND	Positive	Penicillin	Alive
Litwin[41]	F, 40	Polyarticular septic arthritis	ND	ND	Positive	Penicillin, floxacillin	Alive
Wilkins[42]	F, 51	peripheral corneal thinning	ND, local PRD	ND	Positive	Vancomycin	Allive
Altman[43]	F, 81	Scleritis	ND, Local PRD	ND	Positive	Tobramycin, bacitracin ophtalmic solution	Alive
Baghai[44]	F, 37	Sepsis, necrotizing fasciitis	Etanercept 25 mg twice/week, PRD 5 mg/day	Positive	ND	Clindamycin, vancomycin, levofloxacin	Died
Killingley[45]	F, 52	Meningitis, otitis media	Etanercept 25 mg twice/week, PRD 4 mg/day	Positive	ND	ceftriaxone	Alive

Continued

Table 3 Cases of Pneumococcal Infection in Patients with Rheumatoid Arthritis Reported in the Literature Between 1969 and 2013—cont'd

Author	Sex, Age	Area	Immunosuppressive Drugs	Blood Culture	Site Culture	Antibiotics	Outcome
Manolios[46]	M, ND	Sepsis, septic arthritis	IFN inhibitor	Positive	Positive	ND	Alive
Hayashi[47]	M, 38	Septic arthritis	IFX 3 mg/kg, MTX 10 mg/wk PRD 5 mg/day	Positive	Positive	Ceftriaxone	Alive
Yanagawa[48]	F, 78	Pneumonia	Tocilizumab, PRD	Positive	ND	ND	Alive
Raad[49]	F, 47	Meningitis, septic arthritis	ND	ND	Positive	Vacomycin and ceftriaxone	Alive
Morley[50]	F, 48	Pneumonia, septic arthritis	ACTH 20 U/wk	ND	Positive	Penicillin	Alive
	F, 60	Pneumonia, septic arthritis	ND	ND	Positive	Penicillin	Alive
	M, 70	Pneumonia, septic arthritis	ND	ND	Positive	Erythromycin	Alive
Myers[51]	F, 61	Pneumonia, septic arthritis	No	ND	Positive	Penicillin	Alive
Peters[52]	F, old	Cellulitis	No	Positive	ND	Penicillin	Alive

F, female; M, male; PRD, prednisone; ND, not determined/not known; pos, positive; neg, negative; MTX, metotrexate; wk, week; IFN, interferon; IFX, infliximab; ACTH, adreno cortico tropic hormone.

taking immunosuppressant drugs when infected, and the therapy of 14 patients (21.5%) was not specified. In only five SLE cases, the complement was found to be normal (10.6%), whereas in the others it was low or not detected (89.4%). Seven patients with SLE who developed pneumococcal infection (14.9%) were asplenic. Notably, patients with SLE are at risk of asplenia due to autosplenectomy (functional asplenia)[81] or as a consequence of surgical treatment for severe thrombocytopenia.[82] Because of the high risk of infection with capsulated bacteria, especially *Pneumococcus*, asplenic patients are usually immunized with a pneumococcal vaccine.[71,72]

Intriguingly, the infection occurred more frequently in the joints in patients with RA and in the soft tissues in patients with SLE. Septic arthritis (SA) is a debilitating condition that may cause disruption of synovial joints and death.[83,84] Therefore, it requires early diagnosis and treatment. Increasing age, joint prosthesis, skin infection, and pre-existing joint damage are important risk factors for SA.[4,85] Patients with RA are more susceptible to SA because they may have many of these risk factors combined with the use of immunosuppressive medications. Approximately 40% of SAs occur in patients with RA,[86] and the risk of SA is increased by 4- to 15-fold in patients with RA, irrespective of therapy.[5,85] It has been shown that several gram-positive cocci stimulate macrophage production of interferon, enhancing immune defence.[87] Immunosuppressive drugs, especially anti-tumor necrosis factor monoclonal antibodies, expose patients with RA to a higher risk of infection.[3] Moreover, it has been observed that immunosuppressive drugs decrease the number of synovial leukocytes, increasing the risk of SA.[4]

Pneumococcus is a common cause of sepsis, meningitis, sinusitis, otitis media, and pneumonia[88]; it less frequently infects soft tissues. Nevertheless, in SLE cases reported in literature, pneumococcal infection frequently occurred in soft tissues. This may suggest a possible association between pneumococcal soft-tissue infection and connective tissue diseases.

5 INFECTIONS IN DEVELOPING COUNTRIES

As for RA, patients with SLE are more susceptible to infections, which remain a major cause of disease morbidity and mortality.[89–92] Long-term prognosis is poor in patients with severe SLE, whereas short- and medium-term prognoses seem to have improved in the last 30 years: the survival rates at 5, 10, and 15 years after diagnosis are 96%, 93%, and 76%, respectively.[93] The survival curve of patients with severe disease coincides with that of patients with mild disease until 15 years from diagnosis;

thereafter, the survival rate of patients with severe disease shows a remarkable decline.[93] It has been shown that the use of immunosuppressants, as well as organ damage and a high SLE disease activity index,[94,56,95] expose patients to a higher risk of infection.

Moreover, recent studies support the notion that intrinsic factors increase the risk of infection in patients with SLE, for example, mannose-binding lectin (MBL) deficiency associated with homozygous MBL variant alleles and complement deficiency.[96–99] Thus, patients with an RD have a higher risk of mortality in part because of their disease and in part because of their therapy.

Bacterial, viral, fungal, and parasitic infections have been reported in patients with SLE,[100] with a prevalence of respiratory and urinary tract infections. In developing countries, food- and water-borne infections are largely diffused; *Salmonella* spp. and endemic pathogens are the infections described most frequently.[101–103] Notably, there are no clinical data supporting a significant difference in the incidence of pneumococcal infection between patients with SLE living in developing countries and in Western countries.

Infections play a leading role in the lifetime of patients with SLE in developing countries, strongly affecting morbidity and mortality rates.[93,104] On the other hand, in Western countries a bimodal pattern of mortality has been observed: infectious diseases and active lupus account for deaths within 5 years of onset of SLE, whereas cardiovascular diseases and malignancies account for late deaths.[93,104] US and UK studies[105–107] demonstrated that these differences are determined by ethnic and social differences. African and Asian people have higher mortality rates than Caucasians because of racial differences, overall standard of living[108] and the availability of medical technologies such as autoantibodies tests and the use of immunosuppressive drugs. Thus, the prevention of infections, their early recognition and their proper management should be considered an important strategy to reduce the mortality rate of patients with SLE, especially in developing countries.

6 CONCLUSION

No clinical data support the hypothesis that *Pneumococcus* promotes the onset of RDs; thus, its pathogenic role in RDs is still to be proved. On the other hand, several data indicate the possibility of an immunoprotective effect of PC in RDs.[68,109–112]

Patients with an RD are more susceptible to infections, in part because of the disease itself and in part because of their therapy. In particular, it seems that patients with RA have a high risk of pneumococcal septic arthritis and patients with SLE have a high risk of pneumococcal soft-tissue infection.[4,86]

Pneumococcal infection is still a frequent cause of death in developing countries. The vaccines available are recommended for children up to 2 years old, for old people ($\geq$ 65 years) and in cases of immunodepression, immuno-deficiency, and chronic diseases.[71,72] Pneumococcal vaccines are mainly composed of the pneumococcal capsule of different strains, exposing people to the PC molecule and leading to the production of protective anti-PC antibodies. According to the current notion that PC plays an immunomodulant role against RDs, and considering the fact that pneumococcal vaccines are believed to be safe in patients with autoimmune diseases, the administration of the pneumococcal vaccine might be a protective weapon against RDs.

REFERENCES

1. Navarra SV, Leynes MS. Infections in systemic lupus erythematosus. *Lupus* 2010;**19** (12):1419–24.
2. Zandman-Goddard G, Shoenfeld Y. Infections and SLE. *Autoimmunity* 2005;**38** (7):473–85.
3. Galloway JB, Hyrich KL, Mercer LK, Dixon WG, Ustianowski AP, Helbert M, et al. Risk of septic arthritis in patients with rheumatoid arthritis and the effect of anti-TNF therapy: results from the British Society for Rheumatology Biologics Register. *Ann Rheum Dis* 2011;**70**(10):1810–14.
4. Favero M, Schiavon F, Riato L, Carraro V, Punzi L. Rheumatoid arthritis is the major risk factor for septic arthritis in rheumatological settings. *Autoimmun Rev* 2008;**8** (1):59–61.
5. Doran MF, Crowson CS, Pond GR, O'Fallon WM, Gabriel SE. Frequency of infection in patients with rheumatoid arthritis compared with controls: a population-based study. *Arthritis Rheum* 2002;**46**(9):2287–93.
6. Selmi C. Autoimmunity in 2011. *Clin Rev Allergy Immunol* 2012;**43**(1–2):194–206.
7. Draborg AH, Duus K, Houen G. Epstein-Barr virus in systemic autoimmune diseases. *Clin Dev Immunol* 2013;**2013**:1–9. http://dx.doi.org/10.1155/2013/535738, Article ID. 535738.
8. Ferrari SM, Fallahi P, Mancusi C, Colaci M, Manfredi A, Ferri C, et al. HCV-related autoimmune disorders in HCV chronic infection. *Clin Ter* 2013;**164**(4):e305–12.
9. Severin MC, Levy Y, Shoenfeld Y. Systemic lupus erythematosus and parvovirus B-19: casual coincidence or causative culprit? *Clin Rev Allergy Immunol* 2003;**25**(1):41–8.
10. Sabio JM, Vargas JA, Jiménez-Alonso J. Pneumococcal cellulitis in a patient with systemic lupus erythematosus: a case report and review. *Lupus* 2006;**15**(1):54–7.
11. Patel M, Ahrens JC, Moyer DV, DiNubile MJ. Pneumococcal soft-tissue infections: a problem deserving more recognition. *Clin Infect Dis* 1994;**19**(1):149–51.
12. Page KR, Karakousis PC, Maslow JN. Postoperative pneumococcal cellulitis in systemic lupus erythematosus. *Scand J Infect Dis* 2003;**35**(2):141–3.
13. DiNubile MJ, Albornoz MA, Stumacher RJ, Van Uitert BL, Paluzzi SA, Bush LM, et al. Pneumococcal soft-tissue infections possible association with connective tissue diseases. *J Infect Dis* 1991;**163**(4):897–900.
14. Hill MD, Karsh J. Invasive soft tissue infections with Streptococcus pneumoniae in patients with systemic lupus erythematosus: case report and review of the literature. *Arthritis Rheum* 1997;**40**(9):1716–19.
15. McDonald E, Marino C. Swelling in two patients with lupus. *Hosp Pract (Off Ed)* 1993;**28** (3):42–4.
16. Karsh J, Klippel JH, Balow JE, Decker JL. Mortality in lupus nephritis. *Arthritis Rheum* 1979;**22**(7):764–9.

17. Naveau C, Houssiau FA. Pneumococcal sepsis in patients with systemic lupus erythematosus. *Lupus* 2005;**14**(11):903–6.

18. Matsumura M, Ito K, Kawamura R, Fujii H, Inoue R, Yamada K, et al. Pneumococcal vertebral osteomyelitis and psoas abscess in a patient with systemic lupus erythematosus disclosing positivity of pneumococcal urinary antigen assay. *Intern Med* 2011;**50**(20):2357–60.

19. Chiu WJ, Kao HT, Huang JL. Necrotizing pneumonia caused by Streptococcus pneumoniae in a child with systemic lupus erythematosus. *Acta Paediatr Taiwan* 2002;**43**(5):291–4.

20. Isik A, Koca SS. Necrotizing fasciitis resulting from Streptococcus pneumoniae in recently diagnosed systemic lupus erythematosus case: a case report. *Clin Rheumatol* 2007;**26**(6):999–1001.

21. Lipsky PE, Hardin JA, Schour L, Plotz PH. Spontaneous peritonitis and systemic lupus erythematosus. Importance of accurate diagnosis of gram-positive bacterial infections. *JAMA* 1975;**232**(9):929–31.

22. Shalit M, Gross DJ, Levo Y. Pneumococcal epiglottitis in systemic lupus erythematosus on high-dose corticosteroids. *Ann Rheum Dis* 1982;**41**(6):615–16.

23. Kamran M, Wachs J, Putterman C. Necrotizing fasciitis in systemic lupus erythematosus. *Semi Arthritis Rheum* 2008;**27**(4):236–42.

24. Goldblatt F, Chambers S, Rahman A, Isenberg DA. Serious infections in British patients with systemic lupus erythematosus: hospitalisations and mortality. *Lupus* 2009;**18**(8):682–9.

25. Yee AMF, Ng SC, Sobel RE, Salmon JE. FcγRIIA polymorphism as a risk factor for invasive pneumococcal infections in systemic lupus erythematosus. *Arthritis Rheum* 1997;**40**(6):1180–2.

26. Vargas PJ, King G, Navarra SV. Central nervous system infections in Filipino patients with systemic lupus erythematosus. *Int J Rheum Dis* 2009;**12**(3):234–8.

27. Hung JJ, Ou LS, Lee WI, Huang JL. Central nervous system infections in patients with systemic lupus erythematosus. *J Rheumatol* 2005;**32**(1):40–3.

28. Dillon AM, Stein HB, Kassen BO, Ibbott JW. Hyposplenia in a patient with systemic lupus erythematosus. *J Rheumatol* 1980;**7**(2):196–8.

29. Wachtel TJ, Meissner GF, Williams DO. Case record: Rhode Island Hospital. *R I Med J* 1986;**69**(2):75–8.

30. Van Der Straeten C, Wei N, Rothschild J, Goozh JL, Klippel JH. Rapidly fatal pneumococcal septicemia in systemic lupus erythematosus. *J Rheumatol* 1987;**14**(6):1177–80.

31. Malleson P, Petty RE, Nadel H, Dimmick JE. Functional asplenia in childhood onset systemic lupus erythematosus. *J Rheumatol* 1988;**15**(11):1648–52.

32. Piliero P, Furie R. Functional asplenia in systemic lupus erythematosus. *Semin Arthritis Rheum* 1990;**20**(3):185–9.

33. Scerpella EG. Functional asplenia and pneumococcal sepsis in patients with systemic lupus erythematosus. *Clin Infect Dis* 1995;**20**(1):194–5.

34. Petros D, West S. Overwhelming pneumococcal bacteremia in systemic lupus erythematosus. *Ann Rheum Dis* 1989;**48**(4):333–5.

35. ter Borg EJ, Horst G, Limburg PC, van Rijswijk MH, Kallenberg CG. Observational studies of infections in rheumatoid arthritis: a metaanalysis of tumor necrosis factor antagonists. *J Rheumatol* 2010;**37**(5):928–31.

36. Perez HD, Andron RI, Goldstein IM. Infection in patients with systemic lupus erythematosus. Association with a serum inhibitor of complement-derived chemotactic activity. *Arthritis Rheum* 1979;**22**(12):1326–33.

37. Epstein JH, Zimmermann 3rd B, Ho Jr G. Polyarticular septic arthritis. *J Rheumatol* 1986;**13**(6):1105–7.

38. Rowe IF, Deans AC, Keat AC. Pyogenic infection and rheumatoid arthritis. *Postgrad Med J* 1987;**63**(735):19–22.

39. Lohse A, Despaux J, Auge B, Toussirot E, Wendling D. Pneumococcal polyarticular septic arthritis in a patient with rheumatoid arthritis. *Rev Rhum Engl Ed* 1999;**66**(6):344–6.
40. Good AE, Gayes JM, Kauffman CA, Archer GL. Multiple pneumococcal pyarthrosis complicating rheumatoid arthritis. *South Med J* 1978;**71**(5):502–4.
41. Litwin MS, Kirkham BW. Polyarticular pneumococcal sepsis in rheumatoid arthritis. *Aust N Z J Med* 1994;**24**(2):218–19.
42. Wilkins J, Whitcher JP, Margolis TP. Penicillin-resistant Streptococcus pneumoniae keratitis. *Cornea* 1996;**15**(1):99–100.
43. Altman AJ, Cohen EJ, Berger ST, Mondino BJ. Scleritis and *Streptococcus pneumoniae*. *Cornea* 1991;**10**(4):341–5.
44. Baghai M, Osmon DR, Wolk DM, Wold LE, Haidukewych GJ, Matteson EL. Fatal sepsis in a patient with rheumatoid arthritis treated with etanercept. *Mayo Clin Proc* 2001;**76**(6):653–6.
45. Killingley B, Carpenter V, Flanagan K, Pasvol G. Pneumococcal meningitis and etanercept—chance or association? *J Infect* 2005;**51**(2):E49–51.
46. Manolios N, Burneikis A, Spencer D, Howe G. Failure of anti-TNF therapy to reactivate previously septic prosthetic joints. *BMJ Case Rep* 2013;**2013**:1–3. http://dx.doi.org/10.1136/bcr-2013-009827.
47. Hayashi M, Kojima T, Funahashi K, Kato D, Matsubara H, Shioura T, et al. Pneumococcal polyarticular septic arthritis after a single infusion of infliximab in a rheumatoid arthritis patient: a case report. *J Med Case Rep* 2012;**6**(1):81.
48. Yanagawa Y, Hirano Y, Kato H, Iba T. The absence of typical pneumonia symptoms in a patient with rheumatoid arthritis during tocilizumab and steroid treatment. *BMJ Case Rep* 2012;**2012**:1–2. http://dx.doi.org/10.1136/bcr.02.2012.5835, pii: bcr0220125835.
49. Raad J, Peacock Jr JE. Septic arthritis in the adult caused by Streptococcus pneumoniae: a report of 4 cases and review of the literature. *Semin Arthritis Rheum* 2004;**34**(2):559–69.
50. Morley PK, Hull RG, Hall MA. Pneumococcal septic arthritis in rheumatoid arthritis. *Ann Rheum Dis* 1987;**46**(6):482–4.
51. Myers AR, Miller LM, Pinals RS. Pyarthrosis complicating rheumatoid arthritis. *Lancet* 1969;**2**(7623):714–16.
52. Peters NS, Eykyn SJ, Rudd AG. Pneumococcal cellulitis: a rare manifestation of pneumococcaemia in adults. *J Infect* 1989;**19**(1):57–9.
53. Bosch X, Guilabert A, Pallarés L, Cervera R, Ramos-Casals M, Bové A, et al. Infections in systemic lupus erythematosus: a prospective and controlled study of 110 patients. *Lupus* 2006;**15**(9):584–9.
54. Ruiz-Irastorza G, Olivares N, Ruiz-Arruza I, Martinez-Berriotxoa A, Egurbide MV, Aguirre C. Predictors of major infections in systhemic lupus erythematosus. *Arthritis Res Ther* 2009;**11**(4):R109. http://dx.doi.org/10.1186/ar2764.
55. Costa-Reisa P, Nativ S, Isgro J, Rodrigues T, Yildirim-Toruner C, Starr A, et al. Major infections in a cohort of 120 patients with juvenile-onset systemic lupus erythematosus. *Clin Immunol* 2013;**149**(3):442–9.
56. Zonana-Nacach A, Camargo-Coronel A, Yañez P, Sánchez L, Jimenez-Balderas FJ, Fraga A. Infections in outpatients with systemic lupus erythematosus:a prospective study. *Lupus* 2001;**10**(7):505–10.
57. Noël V, Lortholary O, Casassus P, Cohen P, Généreau T, André MH, et al. Risk factors and prognostic influence of infection in a single cohort of 87 adults with systemic lupus erythematosus. *Ann Rheum Dis* 2001;**60**(12):1141–4.
58. Lee PP, Lee TL, Ho MH, Wong WH, Lau YL. Recurrent major infections in juvenile-onset systemic lupus erythematosus-a close link with long-term disease damage. *Rheumatology* 2007;**46**(8):1290–6.
59. Staples PJ, Gerding DN, Decker JL, Gordon Jr RS. Incidence of infection in systemic lupus erythematosus. *Arthritis Rheum* 1974;**17**(1):1–10.

60. Pryor BD, Bologna SG, Kahl LE. Risk factors for serious infection during treatment with cyclophosphamide and high-dose corticosteroids for systemic lupus erythematosus. *Arthritis Rheum* 1996;**39**(9):1475–82.

61. Andonopoulos AP. Adult respiratory distress syndrome: an unrecognized premortem event in systemic lupus erythematosus. *Br J Rheumatol* 1991;**30**(5):346–8.

62. Al-Mayouf SM, Al-Jumaah S, Bahabri S, Al-Eid W. Infections associated with juvenile systemic lupus erythematosus. *Clin Exp Rheumatol* 2001;**19**(6):748–50.

63. Jeong SJ, Choi H, Lee HS, Han SH, Chin BS, Baek JH, et al. Incidence and risk factors of infection in a single cohort of 110 adults with systemic lupus erythematosus. *Scand J Infect Dis* 2009;**41**(4):268–74.

64. Marcos M, Fernández C, Soriano A, Marco A, Martínez JA, Almela M, et al. Epidemiology and clinical outcomes of bloodstream infections among lupus patients. *Lupus* 2011;**20**(9):965–71.

65. Han BK, Bhatia R, Trainsak P, Hunter K, Milcarek B, Schorr C, et al. Clinical presentations and outcomes of systemic lupus erythematosus patients with infection admitted to the intensive care unit. *Lupus* 2013;**22**(7):690–6.

66. Harisdangkul V, Nilganuwonge S, Rockhold L. Cause of death in systemic lupus erythematosus: a pattern based on age at onset. *South Med J* 1987;**80**(10):1249–53.

67. Jacobsen S, Petersen J, Ullman S, Junker P, Voss A, Rasmussen JM, et al. Mortality and causes of death of 513 Danish patients with systemic lupus erythematosus. *Scand J Rheumatol* 1999;**28**(2):75–80.

68. Ward MM, Pyun E, Studenski S. Causes of death in systemic lupus erythematosus. Long-term followup of an inception cohort. *Arthritis Rheum* 1995;**38**(10):1492–9.

69. Goodridge HS, McGuiness S, Houston KM, Henkle E, Deloria-Knoll M, McCall N, et al. Phosphorylcholine mimics the effects of ES-62 on macrophages and dendritoc cells. *Parasite Immunol* 2007;**29**(3):127–37.

70. O'Brien KL, Wolfson LJ, Watt JP, Egan CA, Al-Riyami L, Alcocer MJ, et al. Burden of disease caused by streptococcus pneumoniae in children younger than 5 years: global estimates. *Lancet* 2009;**374**(9693):893–902.

71. *Advisory Committee on Immunization Practices (ACIP) Recommended Immunization Schedule for Adults Aged 19 Years and Older—United States, 2013*. http://www.cdc.gov/mmwr/preview/mmwrhtml/su6201a3.htm; 2013 [accessed 20.10.13].

72. *Advisory Committee on Immunization Practices (ACIP) Recommended Immunization Schedule for Persons Aged 0 Through 18 Years—United States, 2013*. http://www.cdc.gov/mmwr/preview/mmwrhtml/su6201a2.htm; 2013 [accessed 20.10.13].

73. Paradiso PR. Advances in pneumococcal disease prevention: 13-valent pneumococcal conjugate vaccine for infants and children. *Clin Infect Dis* 2011;**52**(10):1241–7.

74. Black S, Shinefield H, Fireman B, Lewis E, Ray P, Hansen JR, et al. Efficacy, safety and immunogenicity of heptavalent pneumococcal conjugate vaccine in children. Northern California Kaiser Permanente Vaccine Study Center Group. *Pediatr Infect Dis J* 2000;**19**(3):187–95.

75. Elkayam O, Paran D, Caspi D, Litinsky I, Yaron M, Charboneau D, et al. Immunogenicity and safety of pneumococcal vaccination in patients with rheumatoid arthritis and systemic lupus erythematosus. *Clin Infect Dis* 2002;**34**(2):147–53.

76. Tarján P, Sipka S, Maródi L, Nemes E, Lakos G, Gyimesi E, et al. No short term immunological effects of pneumococcus vaccination in patients with systemic lupus erythematosus. *Scand J Rheumatol* 2002;**31**(4):211–15.

77. Elkayam O, Ablin J, Caspi D. Safety and efficacy of vaccination against streptococcus pneumonia in patients with rheumatic diseases. *Autoimmun Rev* 2007;**6**(5):312–4.

78. Pisoni C, Sarano J, Benchetrit G, Rodríguez D, Suárez L, Perrota C, et al. Antipneumococcal vaccination in patient with systemic lupus erythematosus. *Medicina (Buenos Aires)* 2003;**63**(5):388–92.

79. Mori S, Ueki Y, Akeda Y, Hirakata N, Oribe M, Shiohira Y, et al. Pneumococcal polysaccharide vaccination in rheumatoid arthritis patients receiving tocilizumab therapy. *Ann Rheum Dis* 2013;**72**(8):1362–6.

80. Heijstek MW, Ott de Bruin LM, Bijl M, Borrow R, van der Klis F, Koné-Paut I, et al. EULAR recommendation for vaccination in paediatric patients with reumatic diseases. *Ann Rheum Dis* 2011;**70**(10):1704–12.

81. Santilli D, Govoni M, Prandini N, Rizzo N, Trotta F. Autosplenectomy and antiphospholipid antibodies in systemic lupus erythematosus: a pathogenetic relationship? *Semin Arthritis Rheum* 2003;**33**(2):125–33.

82. Li R, Liu G, Wang K, Liu Y, Xie Q, Liu Y, et al. Splenectomy for thrombocytopenia associated with systemic lupus erythematosus in 11 Chinese patients. *Rheumatol Int* 2011;**31**(1):9–15.

83. Mitchell WS, Brooks PM, Stevenson RD, Buchanan WW. Septic arthritis in patients with rheumatoid disease: a still underdiagnosed complication. *J Rheumatol* 1976;**3**(2):124–33.

84. Doran MF, Crowson CS, O'Fallon WM, Hunder GG, Gabriel SE. Trends in the incidence of polymyalgia rheumatica over a 30 year period in Olmsted County, Minnesota, USA. *J Rheumatol* 2002;**29**(8):1694–7.

85. Kaandorp CJ, Van Schaardenburg D, Krijnen P, Habbema JD, van de Laar MA. Risk factors for septic arthritis in patients with joint disease. A prospective study. *Arthritis Rheum* 1995;**38**(12):1819–25.

86. Goldenberg DL. Septic arthritis. *Lancet* 1998;**351**(9097):197–202.

87. Keller R, Fischer W, Keist R, Bassetti S. Macrophage response to bacteria: induction of marked secretory and cellular activities by lipoteichoic acids. *Infect Immun* 1992;**60**(9):3664–72.

88. Burman LA, Norrby R, Trollfors B. Invasive pneumococcal infections: incidence, predisposing factors, and prognosis. *Rev Infect Dis* 1985;**7**(2):133–42.

89. Petri M. Infection in systemic lupus erythematosus. *Rheum Dis Clin North Am* 1998;**24**(2):423–56.

90. Zandman-Goddard G, Shoenfeld Y. SLE and infections. *Clin Rev Allergy Immunol* 2003;**25**(1):29–40.

91. Fessler BJ. Infectious diseases in systemic lupus erythematosus: risk factors, management and prophylaxis. *Best Pract Res Clin Rheumatol* 2002;**16**(2):281–91.

92. Bouza E, Moya JG, Munoz P. Infections in systemic lupus erythematosus and rheumatoid arthritis. *Infect Dis Clin North Am* 2001;**15**(2):335–61.

93. Doria A, Iaccarino L, Ghirardello A, Zampieri S, Arienti S, Sarzi-Puttini P, et al. Long-term prognosis and causes of death in systemic lupus erythematosus. *Am J Med* 2006;**119**(8):700–6.

94. Gladman DD, Hussain F, Ibanez D, Urowitz MB. The nature and outcome of infection in systemic lupus erythematosus. *Lupus* 2002;**11**(4):234–9.

95. Li Z, Chen L, Tao R, Fan X. Clinical and bacteriologic study of eighty-six patients with systemic lupus erythematosus complicated by infections. *Chin Med J (Engl)* 1998;**111**(10):913–16.

96. Garred P, Voss A, Madsen HO, Junker P. Association of mannose-binding lectin gene variation with disease severity and infections in a population-based cohort of systemic lupus erythematosus patients. *Genes Immun* 2001;**2**(8):442–50.

97. Takahashi R, Tsutsumi A, Ohtani K, Muraki Y, Goto D, Matsumoto I, et al. Association of mannose binding lectin (MBL) gene polymorphism and serum MBL concentration with characteristics and progression of systemic lupus erythematosus. *Ann Rheum Dis* 2005;**64**(2):311–14.

98. Holers VM. Complement deficiency states, disease susceptibility, and infection risk in systemic lupus erythematosus. *Arthritis Rheum* 1999;**42**(10):2023–5.

99. Amadei N, Baracho GV, Nudelman V, Bastos W, Florido MP, Isaac L. Inherited complete factor I deficiency associated with systemic lupus erythematosus, higher susceptibility to infection and low levels of factor H. *Scand J Immunol* 2001;**53**(6):615–21.
100. Woon-Leung NG. Infections in patients with systemic lupus erythematosus. *APLAR J Rheumatol* 2006;**9**(1):89–97.
101. Kasitanon N, Louthrenoo W, Sukitawut W, Vichainun R. Causes of death and prognostic factors in Thai patients with systemic lupus erythematosus. *Asian Pac J Allergy Immunol* 2002;**20**(2):85–91.
102. Li EK, Cohen MG, Ho AK, Cheng AF. Salmonella bacteraemia occurring concurrently with the first presentation of systemic lupus erythematosus. *Br J Rheumatol* 1993;**32**(1):66–7.
103. Lin YC, Liang SJ, Liu YH, Hsu WH, Shih CM, Sung FC, et al. Tuberculosis as a risk factor for systemic lupus erythematosus: results of a nationwide study in Taiwan. *Rheumatol Int* 2012;**32**(6):1669–73.
104. Moss KE, Ioannou Y, Sultan SM, Haq I, Isenberg DA. Outcome of a cohort of 300 patients with systemic lupus erythematosus attending a dedicated clinic for over two decades. *Ann Rheum Dis* 2002;**61**(5):409–13.
105. Walsh SJ, Algert C, Gregorio DI, et al. Divergent racial trends in mortality from systemic lupus erythematosus. *J Rheumatol* 1995;**22**(9):1663–8.
106. Samanta A, Feehally J, Roy S, Reisine ST, Rothfield NF. High prevalence of systemic disease and mortality in Asian subjects with systemic lupus erythematosus. *Ann Rheum Dis* 1991;**50**(7):490–2.
107. Alarcon GS, Friedman AW, Straaton KV, Moulds JM, Lisse J, Bastian HM, et al. Systemic lupus erythematosus in three ethnic groups: III. A comparison of characteristics early in the natural history of the LUMINA cohort LUpus in Minority populations: nature vs nurture. *Lupus* 1999;**8**(3):197–209.
108. Pons-Estel BA, Catoggio LJ, Cardiel MH, Soriano ER, Gentiletti S, Villa AR, et al. The GLADEL multinational Latin American prospective inception cohort of 1,214 patients with systemic lupus erythematosus: ethnic and disease heterogeneity among 'Hispanics'. *Medicine (Baltimore)* 2004;**83**(1):1–17.
109. Binder CJ, Hörkkö S, Dewan A, Chang MK, Kieu EP, Goodyear CS, et al. Pneumococcal vaccination decreases atherosclerotic lesion formation: molecular mimicry between Streptococcus pneumoniae and oxidized LDL. *Nat Med* 2003;**9**(6):736–43.
110. Caligiuri G, Khallou-Laschet J, Vandaele M, Gaston AT, Delignat S, Mandet C, et al. Phosphorylcholine-targeting immunization reduces atherosclerosis. *J Am Coll Cardiol* 2007;**50**(6):540–6.
111. Peng Y, Martin DA, Kenkel J, Zhang K, Ogden CA, Elkon KB. Innate and adaptive immune response to apoptotic cells. *J Autoimmun* 2007;**29**(4):303–9.
112. Kooyman FN, de Vries E, Ploeger HW, van Putten JP. Antibodies elicited by the bovine lungworm, Dictyocaulus viviparus, cross-react with platelet-activating factor. *Infect Immun* 2007;**75**(9):4456–62.

CHAPTER 32

Mycobacteria and Autoimmunity

Anna Dubaniewicz[1]
Department of Pneumology, Medical University of Gdansk, Gdansk, Poland
[1]Corresponding Author: aduban@gumed.edu.pl

ABBREVIATIONS

AIA	adjuvant-induced arthritis
APC	antigen-presenting cells
BAG1	family molecular chaperone regulator 1
BCL2	is a membrane protein that blocks a step in a pathway leading to apoptosis
CIs	circulating immune complexes
CRs	complement receptor
DAMPs	tissue damage-associated molecular patterns
ESAT6	the 6-kDa early secretory antigenic target of *Mycobacterium tuberculosis*
FcγR	receptor for fragment of immunoglobulin G
HLA	human leukocyte antigens
HSP	heat shock proteins
IBD	inflammatory bowel disease
IL	interleukin
INF	interferon
mkatG	mycobacterial catalase-peroxidase
MS	multiple sclerosis
Mtb-HSP	*M. tuberculosis* HSP
NO	nitric oxide
NRAMP1	Natural-resistance-associated macrophage protein 1
PAMPs	pathogen-associated molecular patterns
PRR	pattern recognition receptors
RA	reumathoid arthritis
SA	sarcoidosis
SLC11A1	gene *Solute Carrier 11A1*
SLE	systemic lupus erythematosus
SOD	superoxide dismutase A
T1DM	type 1 diabetes mellitus type
TLR	toll-like receptor

Autoimmunity occurs when the immune system recognizes and attacks host tissue. The autoimmune disorders develop due to a combination of genetic, immunologic, hormonal and environmental factors, comprising what is known as 'the mosaic of autoimmunity'[1–5] (Figure 1).

Infection and Autoimmunity
http://dx.doi.org/10.1016/B978-0-444-63269-2.00069-6

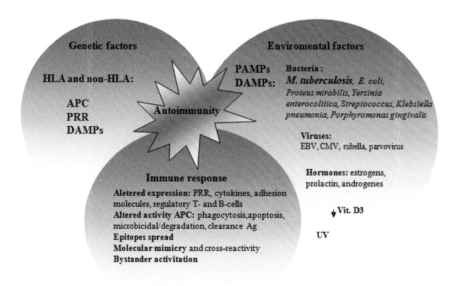

Figure 1 Etiopathogenesis of autoimmune disorders. Ag, antigen; APC, antigen-presenting cell; CMV, cytomegalovirus; DAMP, tissue damage-associated molecular patterns; EBV, Epstein-Barr virus; PAMP, pathogen-associated molecular pattern; PRR, pattern recognition receptor; UV, ultraviolet; Vit, vitamin.

1 THE PRESENCE OF MYCOBACTERIA IN TISSUES OF PATIENTS WITH AUTOIMMUNE DISORDERS

Association between the immune response against mycobacterial infections and autoimmune disease has long been suspected, especially in rheumatoid arthritis (RA), systemic lupus erythematosus (SLE), type 1 diabetes mellitus type (T1DM), multiple sclerosis (MS), microscopic polyangiitis, inflammatory bowel disease (IBD), adjuvant-induced arthritis and sarcoidosis (SA).[6–18]

One-third of the world's population is believed to be latently infected with *Mycobacterium tuberculosis*, and in 5–10% of individuals, bacilli reactivate and cause active disease at some point during their lives.[19] It has been reported that low-virulence strains of *Mycobacteria* with the capacity to persist in host macrophages for prolonged periods may generate evolutionary conserved host heat shock proteins (HSP) as well as mycobacterial HSP (Mtb-HSP).[20]

A study of genomic and proteomic expression of *M. tuberculosis* under stress conditions, especially a low level of nitric oxide (NO), showed an increased expression of RNA polymerase çF unit following the accumulation of Mtb-HSP16 in the cell wall during the dormant stage of the bacteria (reviewed in Refs. 8 and 19). The *M. tuberculosis* genetic dormancy program leads to a non-replicating persistent state characterized by bacteriostasis and metabolic, structural and chromosomal changes in bacteria (reviewed by Dubaniewicz et al.[8]). In addition, persistent mycobacterial HSP stimulation may decrease inducible NO synthase expression with a resulting low NO concentration and reduce phagocytes apoptosis and microbicidal activity, causing persistent antigenemia (reviewed by Dubaniewicz et al.[12]). In the persistent stage of phagocytosed *M. tuberculosis*, the involvement of other mycobacterial antigens, such as the 6-kDa early secretory antigenic target of *M. tuberculosis* (ESAT6), superoxide dismutase A and catalase-peroxidase (mKatG), is proposed in the formation of sarcoid tissue.[21]

An immunohistochemical analysis of lymph nodes revealed that, in contrast to TB, a higher expression of Mtb-HSP16 than Mtb-HSP70 and Mtb-HSP65 was detected in sarcoid tissue.[11] In sera from the same patients with SA and TB, higher levels of Mtb-HSP70 than Mtb-HSP65 and Mtb-HSP16 were found only in SA; this was caused by a sequestration of the bound form of Mtb-HSP16 and Mtb-HSP65 in immune complexes (CIs).[8,12] Recent evidence showed that Mtb-HSP16 may be more important than Mtb-HSP70 and Mtb-HSP65 in the formation of CIs in SA and may initiate autoimmune response in SA related to the stationary phase of mycobacteria.[8] Lower nitrate/nitrite production after Mtb-HSP stimulation in SA than in TB could explain the reduced microbicidal abilities of monocytes followed by persistent phagocytosed mycobacteria with chronic release of Mtb-HSP, persistent antigenemia and immunocomplexemia.[8,9] In addition, low NO production after Mtb-HSP stimulation could be the result of increased synthesis of peroxynitrite, which may reveal cryptic epitopes of several autoantigens; this establishes a potential role for iron in the development of autoimmunity in SA (reviewed in Refs. 8 and 9).

Mycobacterial HSP70, HSP65 and HSP40 were revealed in tissues of patients with RA, and Mtb-HSP65 and Mtb-HSP70 were revealed in MS, SLE and IBD.[13–18]

2 MYCOBACTERIA AND THE IMMUNE RESPONSE

Human HSPs as the main group of 'danger signals' (tissue damage-associated molecular patterns [DAMPs]) and/or microbial HSP pathogen-associated molecular patterns (PAMPs) recognized by pattern recognition receptors

(PRRs) on/in antigen–presenting cells (APCs) may induce autoimmunity in genetically different predisposed hosts.[7,22–24] Moreover, both endogenous DAMPs and exogenous PAMPs via the same PRR often initiate the same signaling cascades and elicit similar responses; many DAMPs and PAMPs can be expressed on host cells and on microbes.[22–24]

2.1 Mycobacterial and Human HSP as PAMP/DAMPs, PRRs, and Autoimmunity

Both microbial and human HSPs as PAMPs/DAMPs recognized by PRRs (e.g. receptors for advanced glycation end products, fragments Fc for immunoglobulin G in immune complexes FcγRI [CD64], FcγRII [CD32], FcγRIII [CD16]; complements CR1 [CD35], CR3 [CD11b], CR4 [CD11c]; and Toll-like receptors [TLRs] 2, 4, 9, CD14, CD40) on/in APCs, transmitting signals into the cell, initiating the autoimmune response. HSP signaling through the Toll/interleukin (IL)-1 homology domain, trigger nuclear factor-κB with secretion of pro-inflammatory tumor necrosis factor (TNF)-α, IL-6 and IL-1β as well as the anti-inflammatory cytokines IL-10 or IL-4.[7,25,26] In macrophages, HSPs, for example, HSP65, induce the production of NO and TNF-α via TLR4, which is also critical for HSP70 induction of IL-12 release and for HSP16 activation of dendritic cells.[23] Activation of aberrant TLRs, especially TLR2, 4 and 9, is also thought to contribute to SA and RA, SLE, IBD and MS.[25,26] TLR9, the polymorphism that was detected in some chronic disorders, recognizes, for example, fragments of mycobacterial wall and *M. tuberculosis* DNA. It strongly activates dendritic cells and macrophages to increase the release of pro-inflammatory cytokines, increase expression of human leukocytes antigens (HLAs) and co-stimulatory molecules (CD40, CD80 and CD86) developing the T helper (Th)1/Th2 immune response and/or autoimmunity, which is considered in SA and other autoimmune diseases (reviewed in Refs. 7 and 26). Mycobacterial and human HSPs may bind and activate another PRR, the nucleotide-binding oligomerization domain receptors, especially NLRP3, with the subsequent release of IL-1β and IL-18, playing an important role in the regulation of host immune response against inflammation and the in induction of autoimmunity (reviewed by Dubaniewicz[7]). It is known that IL-1β, which plays a critical role in promoting IL-17 production by γδ and CD4+ T cells, may induce autoimmunity.[27] It was recently revealed that *Mycobacterium leprae* HSP65 and Mtb-HSP65 may induce Th17, developing a chronic autoinflammatory process in experimental autoimmune uveitis or adjuvant-induced arthritis.[28]

2.1.1 Activity of APCs in the Induction of Autoimmunity

Polymorphisms of Fcγ receptors, especially CD32, CD16 and CR1 on APCs, detected in autoimmune disorders and in SA may associate with altered phagocytic ability, and decreased elimination of antigens caused persistent antigenemia and immunocomplexemia.[7,8,29–33]

2.1.1.1 Phagocytosis, Microbicidal Activity of APCs, and Clearance of Antigens

Insignificantly higher phagocytic activity of blood monocytes and significantly lower levels of NO-stable metabolites, nitrate/nitrite, were detected in patients with SA in contrast to patients with tuberculosis (TB).[8,31,32] Increased frequencies of receptors $CD64^+$ and $CD32^+$ on surface of monocytes were found in both patients with SA and patients with TB, but in contrast to TB, sarcoid monocytes had increased CD16 occurrence with CD35 and CD11c deficiency.[31] It might explain the elevated phagocytosis of mycobacteria in both diseases, but in contrast to TB, decreased antimicrobial/degrading system of monocytes/macrophages, with their resistance to apoptosis, may be the cause of chronic mycobacterial infection, persistent antigenemia/epitope spread, immunocomplexemia and sarcoid granuloma formation.[8,12,31,32] In addition, in contrast to TB, the CD35 and CD11c deficiency on sarcoid phagocytes causes decreased clearance of CIs with subsequent elevated immunocomplexemia, inducing the chronic immune response in SA and SLE.[8,26,33] Moreover in patients with SA and SLE, a polymorphic gene-encoded receptor, CD11c, was found.[30] Therefore, in contrast to TB, sarcoid mononuclear phagocytes with decreased apoptosis and microbicidal activity cannot damage and remove mycobacteria, which persist and release both mycobacterial and human HSPs with subsequent antigenemia and immunocomplexemia.

2.1.1.2 Mycobacterial Antigen-Induced Release of Cytokines and Autoimmunity

Despite higher phagocytic activity, $CD16^+$ monocytes occurred in our patients with SA and SLE but not in those with TB; they produced huge amounts of pro-inflammatory cytokines, mostly TNF-α, IL-1, IL-6, IL-12 and IL-17, and expressed higher levels of HLA-promoting persistent inflammation and/or autoimmunity[26] (reviewed by Dubaniewicz et al.[31]). The heavier antigenic/epitope load with Mtb-HSP in CIs, which causes the chronic inflammation, was connected with the highest levels of TNF-α and IL-6 in both SA and TB.[8,34] In contrast to TB, the increased levels of IL-10 and low levels of IL-4 observed in our patients with SA and in SLE may be the results of activation by pathogens of regulatory T cells cross-reactive with self-antigens.[9,26,34] It is possible that a shift to Th1 in affected organs, caused by an IL-4 deficiency due to the reduced number or function of the CD8$^+\gamma\delta^+$IL-4$^+$ T-cell subset in our patients with SA may facilitate an efficient response to Mtb-HSP and induce autoimmunity.[34] Presumably, this kind of regulation may be able to cause the peripheral anergy characteristic of SA and could trigger autoimmune reactions in the most susceptible individuals.

It is well known that Mtb-HSP70, Mtb-HSP65 and Mtb-HSP16 induce APC and T cells to proliferate and secrete DAMPs, for example, chemokines and IL-1, IL-3, IL-6, IL-8, IL-12, IL-10, granulocyte-monocyte colony-stimulating factor, low amounts of interferon-γ, and TNF-α but not IL-2, IL-4, IL-5 or transforming growth factor (TGF)-β (reviewed in Refs. 7, 8, 20 and 34). In turn, pro-inflammatory mediators are up-regulated and trigger further tissue damage, leading to increasing DAMPs. Hence a vicious cycle is continued and may cause the chronic inflammation and autoimmunity (reviewed by Dubaniewicz[7]).

2.1.1.3 Mycobacterial Antigen-Induced Apoptosis and Autoimmunity

Studies of monocytes/macrophages infected with intracellular pathogens have shown the involvement of host and mycobacterial HSP70, HSP65 and HSP16 in the prevention of apoptosis in phagocytes (reviewed in Refs. 12 and 20). HSP65 and HSP70 protect cells from apoptosis by maintaining the integrity of the cell mitochondria and/or binding to the apoptotic protease-activating factors BAG-1 and Bcl-2. An over-expression of HSP70 also reduces Fas-, TNF-α- and NO-induced apoptosis. Mtb-HSP70 and Mtb-HSP65 induced the release of pro-apoptotic cytokines IL-1β, IL-6, IL-8, TNF-α and anti-apoptotic IL-10 from human mononuclear cells (reviewed in Refs. 12, 20 and 34). The expression of HSP16 was shown to be essential for preventing cells from undergoing apoptosis by decreasing the intracellular level of reactive oxygen species (e.g. NO), which also was found in patients with SA (reviewed in Refs. 8 and 9). In the same group of patients with TB and with SA, analysis of early apoptotic peripheral blood mononuclear cells before and after stimulation revealed that sarcoid monocytes were resistant to Mtb-HSP-induced apoptosis, in contrast to TB; Mtb-HSP-induced CD4[+] T-cell apoptosis was significantly lower in TB versus SA. CD8[+] T-cell apoptosis before and after Mtb-HSP stimulation was significantly increased in all tested groups. It seems likely that dysregulated apoptosis of CD4[+] T lymphocytes increased the apoptosis of CD8[+] T cells; resistant apoptosis of monocytes may be involved in the pathogenesis of not only SA but also other autoimmune diseases.[12,35] Activated CD8[+] T cells can directly recognize and kill antigen-expressing cell types by releasing cytolytic granules at the effector/target cell binding; this occurs via tissue damage by secreting high levels of DAMPs (e.g. pro-inflammatory cytokines) in T1DM, EAE and demyelinating central nervous system diseases and through the Fas/Fas ligand pathway with subsequent apoptosis.[35]

Apoptosis is considered a factor in the pathogenesis of autoimmune diseases as well as in TB (reviewed in Refs. 12 and 36–38). It was recently revealed that the induction of serine protease inhibitor 9 by mycobacteria inhibits apoptosis and promotes the survival of infected macrophages.[36,38] Also, a defect in the recognition and phagocytosis of apoptotic cells contributes to the development of chronic inflammation and autoimmune disorders.[33] The clustering and concentration of autoantigens at the surface of apoptotic cells, along with the striking tolerance-inducing function of apoptotic cells, have focused attention on abnormalities in apoptotic cell execution and clearance as potential susceptibility and initiating factors in systemic autoimmunity. Structural changes that occur during cell death may influence the immunogenicity of self-antigens.[37]

Increased phagocytosis, low apoptosis of APCs, neutrophils and low NO product concentration with a decrease of microbicidal/degradal activity may cause a persistent mycobacterial antigen load and immunocomplexemia and/or increased local proliferation of CD4[+] T cells.[7,8,12,31–33]

2.1.2 Mycobacterial Antigens, HLA, and Autoimmunity

Mycobacterial antigens expressed on the surface of APCs can be also presented effectively to CD4[+] and CD8[+] T cells in the context of HLA class I and II antigens and B lymphocytes to induce specific exaggerated immunity.[20,39–41] The specific antigens which cause CD8[+] T cells to respond to mycobacteria are poorly characterized.[42–47] At present, only four human CD8[+] T-cell-reactive epitopes have been identified: two in ESAT-6, present in SA, one in the 19-kDa antigen, and one in the 38-kDa protein of *M. tuberculosis*, which occurs in tuberculous tissue.[43–47] Strong cytolytic CD8$^+$ T-cell activity against peptide p242–250 was found in antigen 85A and peptide p48–56 in antigens 85B and 85C of *M. tuberculosis* in HLA-A*0201-positive monocytes.[42,46,48] Others revealed that Mtb-HSP65-specific epitopes were able to recognize and lyse macrophages infected with *M. tuberculosis*.[40,47]

In agreement with most studies, analysis of the occurrence of HLA class I antigens in patients with SA and TB revealed a higher occurrence of HLA-B5 and B8 antigens in SA compared with a healthy group.[40] The correlation of B5 and B15 has been previously detected for patients with TB in different ethnic groups (reviewed in Refs. 40 and 48). Analysis of the haplotypes of patients with SA and TB revealed an opposite occurrence of HLA-B:5, 8, 13, 15 and Cw4. Antigens B5 and B8 were significantly more frequent and B13, B15 and Cw4 antigens were significantly less present in SA when we compared with TB and healthy controls. The presence of the remaining antigens were comparable in both populations studied. An important role for position 116 of the HLA-B15 class I heavy chain also was revealed in an immune response against mycobacteria.[49]

Other data suggest that multiple antigens or mycobacterial epitopes are recognized by T-cell clones that are paired with different HLA class II molecules. It was revealed that DRB1:*01, *02, *04, *06, *08, *11, *15 and DQB1:*02 and *03 alleles interact with T lymphocytes with mycobacterial ESAT-6 antigen recognition.[21,40,47] Despite ESAT-6, Oswald-Richter et al.[21] showed a correlation between immunological responses to mkatG and DRB1*1101, with different capacities to bind in SA. In contrast to active SA, the occurrence of DRB1*11 and DQB1*02 alleles with a decreased probability of developing of TB have been connected (reviewed by Dubaniewicz et al.[41]). Furthermore, several epitopes of *M. tuberculosis* antigens, for example, the HSP65 p2-12 peptide binding specifically to HLA encoded by the DRB1*03 allele (characteristic of acute SA) and peptides p61-75 and p141-155, interacting mostly with DRB1*16 and DRB1*07, as well as p501-515, also interacting with DRB1*16, were shown to affect the immunoregulation of an individual during mycobacterial infection (reviewed in Refs. 7 and 41). The immunoreactivity of an organism to mycobacterial infection also is regulated by Mtb-HSP, which epitopes bind selectively to DRB1:*01, *03, *04, *07, *08, *11, *15 and *16, DQB1*03 and DQA1*03 (reviewed in Refs. 9 and 48). In addition, DQB1*05, linked with higher susceptibility to tuberculosis and lower risk of developing SA, was shown to influence the charge in the putative peptide binding pocket P9 of the DQ molecule and down-regulate the immune response. In Americans, susceptibility to SA has been associated with pocket 7 on DRB1:*1101, *1201 and *1501. The amino acid residue on DQB1*0602 is likely to affect the pocket, whereas the amino acid residue on DRB1*01 and *04 alleles can affect pocket 6 in European individuals, which may be important in protection from SA. Peptide-binding studies have demonstrated that these changes in the P4 pocket have a significant effect on the repertoire of self-peptides that can be presented particularly by the haplotype A1/B8/DR2/DR3/DQ2(DQB1*0201/DQA1*0501)/ DQ8(DQB1*0302/DQA1*0301) (reviewed in Refs. 40, 41 and 50).

Some authors observed a strong association of the DQB1*03 allele and no association of HLA-DR with immunosuppression in advanced TB.[48,51] Others noticed that DRB1*03-positive patients with TB have decreased Th1 lymphocyte reaction when compared to DRB1*03-negative patients.[40,52] It was found that this allele is associated with decreased interferon-γ and TNF-α as well as increased TGF-β production, and thus with reduced Th1 response in patients with SA.[9,40,53,54] Furthermore, the high presence of DRB1*03 and DQB1*02 is associated with acute SA, whereas the DRB1*15 and DQB1*05 alleles correlated with a chronic course of SA and not with good prognosis (reviewed in Refs. 41 and 55). Hence there is a possibility that the low Th1 lymphocyte response connected with this particular haplotype, together with a higher presence of HLA alleles predisposing to the development of TB, could have induced TB. Conversely, other authors showed that the DRB1*03 and DQB1*03 alleles increase the efficiency of the immune reaction to *M. tuberculosis* while presenting Mtb-HSP65 epitopes to T cells. The DRB1:*03, *07, *15 and *16 alleles also were found to enhance Th1 activity because of the presentation of *M. tuberculosis* MPB70 p8, p12 and p13 peptides (reviewed in Refs. 9 and 40). In addition, the DRB1*16 allele, connected with a high risk of the development of TB, was proved to elevate the level of circulating antibodies against the 38-kDa protein of mycobacteria and thus to increase the immune response during TB.[40,41] This is in agreement with a study in which patients with TB with the DRB1:*15 and *16 alleles and a decreased occurrence of DRB1*03 had elevated levels of immunoglobulin G after the PPD skin test (reviewed by Dubaniewicz et al.[48]).

Some HLA alleles also are linked with the development of either the acute or chronic form of SA. For example, the DRB1*15- and *16-positive and TNF-A2-negative haplotype is associated with a chronic course of SA and worse prognosis (reviewed by Dubaniewicz et al.[40]). A correlation between the DRB1:*11 and *15 alleles and the presence of *M. tuberculosis* DNA also was revealed in a chronic course of SA, whereas the DRB1:*03,*04 alleles combined with the absence of mycobacterial DNA was found in an acute stage of disease.[21,40,41,55,56] Furthermore, some of the HLA alleles (e.g. A*01, B*08, DRB1*03, DQB1*02, DQB1*03 and DQA1*05) in an acute SA and Löfgren's syndrome can be linked with the high risk of developing autoimmune disorders. Moreover, the contribution of the DQB1*05 allele in the development of SA and autoimmune manifestations was revealed (reviewed in Refs. 9, 40, 41 and 55).

The frequency of the HLA-DR1 (DRB1*0101/DRB1*0102) and HLA-DR4 (DRB1*0401/DRB1*0404) alleles is elevated among Caucasian patients with RA and in SA (reviewed by Kapitány et al.[57]). The HLA-DRB1:*03, *04, *0402 and *0405; the DQA1:*0301 and *0501; the DQB1*0201; and the DQB1*0302 alleles are associated with an increase in the development of T1DM, whereas the DRB1:*1501 and *1503 and DQB1*06 alleles were characteristic of increased occurrence of MS, as well as in TB in different ethnic groups (reviewed by Dubaniewicz et al.[41]). In SLE, the DR2 (DRB1*1501/DQB1*0602) and DR3 (DRB1*0301/DQB1*0201) and DRB1*1101 alleles were more frequent, as in SA and other autoimmune disorders, as well as TB.[41,58,59] Increased risk of the developing celiac disease is connected with the DQ2 alleles.[60]

2.1.2.1 Mycobacterial Antigens, non-HLA genes, and Autoimmunity

According to a study performed among African Americans by Maliarik et al., in patients with SA and TB, allele 3 of the functional (GT)n promoter region repeat of the solute carrier 11A1 (*SLC11A1*, formerly natural–resistance–associated macrophage protein 1 [*NRAMP1*]) gene was related to SA, whereas there was a decrease in the occurrence of allele 2, connected with TB in different ethnic groups worldwide.[61] In various populations of patients with SA, an increase in the presence of allele 3, in accordance with previous analyses of Crohn's disease, RA, juvenile RA, MS and T1DM, may stand for the link with susceptibility to develop SA (reviewed in Ref. 62).[62,63]

Previous functional studies showed that allele 3 of the *SLC11A1* (GT)n promoter polymorphism causes increased activity of the reporter gene without any exogenous stimulation. Thus, this allele might be linked with the increased expression of the NRAMP1 protein and inducible NO synthase, high activation of macrophages (e.g., HLA, NO) and the enhancement of pro–inflammatory reactions through TNF-α, IL-1β and chemokines. The above-mentioned actions are the features of immunopathology connected with chronic inflammation, characteristic of SA and other autoimmune disorders as well as TB.[61,62] In addition, studies of the innate response of macrophages during mycobacterial infection suggested that SLC11A1-mediated deficiency of divalent cations might change the phagosomal microenvironment that impairs the pathogenesis of intracellular pathogens.[62] Moreover, a study recently revealed a function of *SLC11A1* in the processing and presentation of islet cell self-antigens to dendritic cells in the pathogenesis of T1DM, where *Mycobacterium avium* subspecies *paratuberculosis* was detected in blood from these patients. Thus, non-HLA genes could affect the HLA-restricted T-cell response through altered antigen processing and presentation (reviewed by Paccagnini et al.[63]).

According to our results, Maertzdorf et al.[64] showed highly similar patterns with common up-regulation of Fcγ receptor-mediated phagocytosis and signaling pro-inflammatory pathways in both SA and TB.[31,32] Previously published comparative analyses of the immunogenetics of patients with SA and TB and the study conducted by Maertzdorf et al. indicated several differences in the gene expression metabolic activity and significantly higher antimicrobial defence responses in TB, such as the microbicidal defensins α-3 and α-4, the hypoxia–activated genes lactotransferrin and lipocalin 2 and the serine protease cathepsin G.[7] Some of these, with altered expression, have been detected in autoimmune disorders.[29,65,66]

2.1.3 Mycobacterial Antigens and the Loss of Self-Tolerance

It has been reported that mycobacterial HSP70 delayed maturation of bone marrow-derived murine APCs, which are known not only to drive differentiation into Th1 or Th2 profiles but also to ensue T-cell tolerance or activation of regulatory CD4$^+$CD25$^+$ T lymphocytes.[6,9,20,39,67,68] The mycobacterial HSP70 or HSP65 modulating of the expression costimulatory and adhesion molecules (e.g. ICAM-1, CD80/86, BTNL2) may also participate in the initiation and maintenance of autoimmune responses.[7,9,20,68] In addition to the abnormal expression of co-stimulatory molecules and regulatory cells, clonal deletion, epitope spreading, polyclonal activation, bystander activation and molecular mimicry between human and microbial HSPs also are responsible for the loss of self-tolerance and the development of autoimmunity (reviewed in Refs. 3, 7, 9, 13, 14, 20, 23, 24, 39, 40, 69).

2.1.3.1 Molecular Mimicry Among Microbial HSPs and Between Mycobacterial and Human HSPs

HSPs may provide a link between the immune reaction to infection and autoimmunity caused by T lymphocyte cross-reactivity, not only between microbial and human HSPs but also between pathogens.[3,6,7,9,20,70,71] Moreover, Mtb-HSP-responsive $\gamma\delta^+$ T-cell clones also respond to homologous human HSPs, suggesting a possible link between infection and autoimmunity.[71] Mycobacterial HSP16, HSP65 and HSP70 demonstrate 18–60% identity to their human homologs (reviewed in Refs. 8, 9 and 72).

HLA class I and II restricted T-cell epitopes from host proteins that share similarities with *M. tuberculosis* antigens were identified.[69] Epitopes of mycobacterial and homologous human HSP60, especially KPLVIIAEDVD-GEALSTLVLN, binds to many alleles, including HLA-DRB1:*0101, *0301, *0401, *0701, *0802, *1101 and *1501, with high affinity in both MS and RA. It worth noting that, in contrast to RA, the epitope KPLVIIAEDVDGEALSTLVLN also binds to HLA-DRB1*1301 in MS.[69]

Moreover, because the phylogenetically closely related genera of *Mycobacterium*, *Corynebacterium* and *Streptomyces* share an extended set of genes with *Propionibacterium*, the homology among bacterial HSPs is greater, with an 78% similar identity between propionibacterial and Mtb-HSP60; the identity of Mtb-HSP70 is 67% similar.[72] It is worth noting that HSP70, HSP65 and HSP16 of *M. tuberculosis* or *Mycobacterium leprae* are identical to HSPs of *Mycobacterium bovis* bacillus Calmette-Guerin (BCG).[73]

The data regarding a connection between the BCG vaccination and autoimmune diseases is conflicting (reviewed by Dubaniewicz et al.[10]). Some studies[1,3,74,75] showed that BCG vaccination protects (via, e.g. down-regulation of adhesion molecules, induction of Th2 CD4$^+$ T cells to produce IL-10 and induction of $\gamma\delta^+$ T cells to produce TGF-β) from autoimmunity, whereas results (reviewed in Refs. 10 and 76) revealed the possible immune mechanisms (e.g. lack of regulatory T cells, up-regulation of co-stimulation, polyclonal activation, Th1 CD4$^+$ T cells, CD8$^+$ T cells, molecular mimicry) by which BCG can trigger autoimmune diseases. Other studies have suggested that regulatory polymorphisms at the IL-4 locus and the region encoding the DNA binding protein interferon-regulating factor 1 may directly regulate this difference in Th1 or Th2 immune response to mycobacterial antigens and BCG.[2,77] It has been suggested that polymorphism at *SLC11A1* also influences immune response to exposures to *Mycobacteria* via priming/BCG vaccination. Blackwell et al.[77] and others[2,5,74,75] suggested that the prevalence of autoimmune diseases can also be modulated by immune response to mycobacterial antigens after BCG vaccination.

2.1.3.2 *M. tuberculosis* and Human Cross-Reactive T-Cell Epitopes Restricted to Predominant HLA Class I and II

Some autoreactive CD4 and CD8 T-cell epitopes that may act as molecular mimics and result in autoimmune response during *M. tuberculosis* infection were recently identified.[69] The study showed mycobacterial and human cross-reactive T-cell epitopes restricted to predominant HLA class I (A:*0201, *1101, *0301, *2402 and *0101 and B:*0702 and *0801) and class alleles II (DRB1:*0101, *0701, *1101, *04:01, *1302, *0301, *0801), some of which occur in RA, SLE and SA. It was revealed that the total number of antigenic epitopes and secretory, structural, and metabolic proteins binding to HLA class I alleles was significantly smaller than those binding to HLA class II alleles.[69] The largest number of CD4$^+$ T-cell structural epitopes were restricted to DRB1*0101, *0701 and *1501; the latter is also a susceptibility allele for TB, RA, SLE and chronic SA. CD8 epitopes indicated the maximum number of peptides binding to allele A*0201, *1101 and *0301. The highest number of epitopes homologous to antigenic, structural, secretory and metabolic proteins was restricted to DRB1*0101, *0301 and *1302. Babu Chodisetti et al.[69] also revealed putative CD4 T-cell epitopes of established antigens involved in autoimmune disease, such as GLPHYGHIL of mycobacterial and human isoleucyl transfer RNA synthase bound to HLA-DRB1*0101 and DRB1*1501 in arthritis/SLE and interstitial lung disease, or the epitope LNLILTTGGTG of mycobacterial molybdopterin, similar to human gephyrin bound to HLA-DRB1:*0101, *0401, *0701, *1101, *1301 and *1501 in stiff man's syndrome, as well as the epitope HRDLKPENLLL of mycobacterial serine/threonine protein kinase-pknD and human of BR serine/threonine-protein kinase-2 bound to DRB1:*0101, *0701 and *1301. Thus, there are some mechanisms through which particular antigens from *Mycobacteria* can provoke an autoimmune response.

REFERENCES

1. Molina V, Shoenfeld Y. Infection, vaccines and other environmental triggers of autoimmunity. *Autoimmunity* 2005;**38**:235–45.
2. Shoenfeld Y, Zandman-Goddard G, Stojanovich L, et al. The mosaic of autoimmunity: hormonal and environmental factors involved in autoimmune diseases-2008. *Isr Med Assoc J* 2008;**10**:8–12.
3. Blank M, Barzilai O, Shoenfeld Y. Molecular mimicry and autoimmunity. *Clin Rev Allergy Immunol* 2007;**32**:111–18.
4. Shoenfeld Y, Gilburd B, Abu-Shakra M, Amital H, Barzilai O, Berkun Y, et al. The mosaic of autoimmunity: genetic factors involved in autoimmune diseases-2008. *Isr Med Assoc J* 2008;**10**:3–7.

5. Kivity S, Agmon-Levin N, Blank M, Shoenfeld Y. Infections and autoimmunity—friends or foes? *Trends Immunol* 2009;**30**:409–14.

6. Tishler M, Shoenfeld Y. Anti-heat-shock protein antibodies in rheumatic and autoimmune diseases. *Semin Arthritis Rheum* 1996;**26**:558–63.

7. Dubaniewicz A. Microbial and human heat shock proteins as 'danger signals' in sarcoidosis. *Hum Immunol* 2013;**74**:1550–8.

8. Dubaniewicz A, Holownia A, Kalinowski L, Wybieralska M, Dobrucki IT, Singh M. Is mycobacterial heat shock protein 16 kDa, a marker of the dormant stage of *Mycobacterium tuberculosis*, a sarcoid antigen? *Hum Immunol* 2013;**74**:45–51.

9. Dubaniewicz A. *Mycobacterium tuberculosis* heat shock proteins and autoimmunity in sarcoidosis. *Autoimmun Rev* 2010;**9**:419–24.

10. Dubaniewicz A, Kämpfer S, Singh M. Serum anti-mycobacterial heat shock proteins antibodies in sarcoidosis and tuberculosis. *Tuberculosis (Edinb)* 2006;**86**:60–7.

11. Dubaniewicz A, Dubaniewicz-Wybieralska M, Sternau A, Zwolska Z, Izycka-Swieszewska E, Augustynowicz-Kopec E, et al. *Mycobacterium tuberculosis* complex and mycobacterial heat shock proteins in lymph node tissue from patients with pulmonary sarcoidosis. *J Clin Microbiol* 2006;**44**:3448–51.

12. Dubaniewicz A, Trzonkowski P, Dubaniewicz-Wybieralska M, Dubaniewicz A, Singh M, Myśliwski A. Comparative analysis of mycobacterial heat shock proteins-induced apoptosis of peripheral blood mononuclear cells in sarcoidosis and tuberculosis. *J Clin Immunol* 2006;**26**:243–50.

13. Cossu D, Masala S, Frau J, Mameli G, Marrosu MG, Cocco E, et al. Antigenic epitopes of MAP2694 homologous to T-cell receptor gamma-chain are highly recognized in multiple sclerosis Sardinian patients. *Mol Immunol* 2014;**57**:138–40.

14. Tasneem S, islam N, Ali R. Crossreactivity of SLE autoantibodies with 70 kDa heat shock proteins of *Mycobacterium tuberculosis*. *Microbiol Immunol* 2001;**45**:841–6.

15. Sheikhi A, Nazarian M, Khadem-Al-Melleh A, et al. In-vitro effects of *Mycobacterium bovis* BCG-lysate and its derived heat shock proteins on cytokines secretion by blood mononuclear cells of rheumatoid arthritis patients in comparison with healthy controls. *Int Immunopharmacol* 2008;**8**:887–92.

16. Komiya I, Arimura Y, Nakabayashi K, Yamada A, Osaki T, Yamaguchi H, et al. Increased concentrations of antibody against heat shock protein in patients with myeloperoxidase anti-neutrophil cytoplasmic autoantibody positive microscopic polyangiitis. *Microbiol Immunol* 2011;**55**:531–8.

17. Panchapakesan J, Daglis M, Gatenby P. Antibodies to 65 kDa and 70 kDa heat shock proteins in rheumatoid arthritis and systemic lupus erythematosus. *Immunol Cell Biol* 1992;**70**:295–300.

18. Huszti Z, Bene L, Kovács A, Fekete B, Füst G, Romics L, et al. Low levels of antibodies against *E. coli* and mycobacterial 65kDa heat shock proteins in patients with inflammatory bowel disease. *Inflamm Res* 2004;**53**:551–5.

19. Walzl G, Ronacher K, Hanekom W, Scriba TJ, Zumla A. Immunological biomarkers of tuberculosis. *Nat Rev Immunol* 2011;**11**:343–54.

20. Pockley AG, Muthana M, Calderwood SK. The dual immunoregulatory roles of stress proteins. *Trends Biochem Sci* 2008;**33**:71–9.

21. Oswald-Richter KA, Beachboard DC, Zhan X, Gaskill CF, Abraham S, Jenkins C, et al. Multiple mycobacterial antigens are targets of the adaptive immune response in pulmonary sarcoidosis. *Respir Res* 2010;**11**:161.

22. Matzinger P. Tolerance, danger, and the extended family. *Annu Rev Immunol* 1994;**12**:991.

23. Bianchi ME. DAMPs, PAMPs and alarmins: all we need to know about danger. *J Leukoc Biol* 2007;**81**:1–5.

24. Zhang X, Mosser DM. Macrophage activation by endogenous danger signals. *J Pathol* 2008;**214**:161–78.
25. Marshak-Rothstein A. Toll-like receptors in systemic autoimmune disease. *Nat Rev Immunol* 2006;**6**:823–35.
26. Byrne JC, Ní Gabhann J, Lazzari E, Mahony R, Smith S, Stacey K, et al. Genetics of SLE: functional relevance for monocytes/macrophages in disease. *Clin Dev Immunol* 2012;**2012**:1–15.
27. Lalor SJ, Dungan LS, Sutton CE, Basdeo SA, Fletcher JM, Mills KH. Caspase-1-processed cytokines IL-1beta and IL-18 promote IL-17 production by gammadelta and CD4T-cells that mediate autoimmunity. *J Immunol* 2011;**186**:5738–48.
28. Marengo EB, Commodaro AG, Peron JP, de Moraes LV, Portaro FC, Belfort R Jr, et al. Administration of *Mycobacterium leprae* rHsp65 aggravates experimental autoimmune uveitis in mice. *PLoS One* 2009;**4**:e7912.
29. Bournazos S, Woof JM, Hart SP, Dransfield I. Functional and clinical consequences of Fc receptor polymorphic and copy number variants. *Clin Exp Immunol* 2009;**157**:244–54.
30. Zorzetto M, Bombieri C, Ferrarotti I, Medaglia S, Agostini C, Tinelli C, et al. Complement receptor 1 gene polymorphisms in sarcoidosis. *Am J Respir Cell Mol Biol* 2002;**27**:17–23.
31. Dubaniewicz A, Typiak M, Wybieralska M, Szadurska M, Nowakowski S, Staniewicz-Panasik A, et al. Changed phagocytic activity and pattern of Fcγ and complement receptors on blood monocytes in sarcoidosis. *Hum Immunol* 2012;**73**:788–94.
32. Klimont P, Typiak M, Rebala K, Dubaniewicz A, Rekawiecki B. Are there differences in the functional polymorphism of FCGR3A gene between sarcoidosis and tuberculosis? Preliminary study. *Eur Respir J* 2013;**42**(Suppl. 57):s644.
33. Majai G, Kiss E, Tarr T, Zahuczky G, Hartman Z, Szegedi G, et al. Decreased apopto-phagocytic gene expression in the macrophages of systemic lupus erythematosus patients. *Lupus* 2014;**23**(2):133–45.
34. Dubaniewicz A, Trzonkowski P, Dubaniewicz-Wybieralska M, Dubaniewicz A, Singh M, Myśliwski A. Mycobacterial heat shock protein-induced blood T lymphocytes subsets and cytokine pattern: comparison of sarcoidosis with tuberculosis and healthy controls. *Respirology* 2007;**12**:346–54.
35. Gravano DM, Hoyer KK. Promotion and prevention of autoimmune disease by CD8$^+$T cells. *J Autoimmun* 2013;**45**:68–79.
36. Gatto M, Iaccarino L, Ghirardello A, Bassi N, Pontisso P, Punzi L, et al. Serpins, immunity and autoimmunity: old molecules, new functions. *Clin Rev Allergy Immunol* 2013;**45**:267–80.
37. Nagata S, Hanayama R, Kawane K. Autoimmunity and the clearance of dead cells. *Cell* 2010;**140**:619–30.
38. Toossi Z, Wu M, Rojas R, Kalsdorf B, Aung H, Hirsch CS, et al. Induction of serine protease inhibitor 9 by *Mycobacterium tuberculosis* inhibits apoptosis and promotes survival of infected macrophages. *J Infect Dis* 2012;**205**:144–51.
39. Rajaiah R, Moudgil KD. Heat shock proteins can promote as well as regulate autoimmunity. *Autoimmun Rev* 2009;**8**:388–93.
40. Dubaniewicz A, Zimmermann A, Smigielska M, Dubaniewicz-Wybieralska M, Moszkowska G, Wysocka J, et al. Sarcoidosis and tuberculosis: a connection to the human leukocyte antigen system. *Adv Exp Med Biol* 2013;**756**:229–37.
41. Dubaniewicz A, Dubaniewicz-Wybieralska M, Moszkowska G, Sternau A, Dubaniewicz A. Comparative analysis of DR and DQ alleles occurrence in sarcoidosis and tuberculosis in the same ethnic group: preliminary study. *Sarcoidosis Vasc Diffuse Lung Dis* 2006;**23**:180–9.

42. Smith SM, Brookes R, Klein MR, Malin AS, Lukey PT, King AS, et al. Human CD8[+]CTL specific for the mycobacterial major secreted antigen 85A. *J Immunol* 2000;**165**:7088–95.

43. Lalvani A, Brookes R, Wilkinson RJ, Malin AS, Pathan AA, Andersen P, et al. Human cytolytic and interferon γ-secreting CD8[+] T lymphocytes specific for *Mycobacterium tuberculosis*. *Proc Natl Acad Sci USA* 1998;**95**:270.

44. Mohagheghpour N, Gammon D, Kawamura LM, van Vollenhoven A, Benike CJ, Engleman EG. CTL response to *Mycobacterium tuberculosis*: identification of an immunogenic epitope in the 19-kDa lipoprotein. *J Immunol* 1998;**161**:2400.

45. Wilkinson RJ, Zhu X, Wilkinson KA, Lalvani A, Ivanyi J, Pasvol G, et al. 38 000 MW antigen-specific major histocompatibility complex class I restricted interferon-γ-secreting CD8[+]T cells in healthy contacts of tuberculosis. *Immunology* 1998;**95**:58.

46. Smith SM, Malin AS, Lukey PT, Atkinson SE, Content J, et al. Characterisation of human *Mycobacterium bovis* bacille Calmette-Guérin-reactive CD8[+]T cells. *Infect Immun* 1999;**67**:5223.

47. Arlehamn CS, Sidney J, Henderson R, Greenbaum JA, James EA, Moutaftsi M, et al. Dissecting mechanisms of immunodominance to the common tuberculosis antigens ESAT-6, CFP10, Rv2031c (hspX), Rv2654c (TB7.7), and Rv1038c (EsxJ). *J Immunol* 2012;**188**:5020–31.

48. Dubaniewicz A, Moszkowska G, Szczerkowska Z. Frequency of DRB1-DQB1 two-locus haplotypes in tuberculosis: preliminary report. *Tuberculosis (Edinb)* 2005;**85**:259–67.

49. Hildebrand WH, Turnquist HR, Prilliman KR, Hickman HD, Schenk EL, McIlhaney MM, et al. HLA class I polymorphism has a dual impact on ligand binding and chaperone interaction. *Hum Immunol* 2002;**63**:248–55.

50. Plesner A, Greenbaum CJ, Gaur LK, Ernst RK, Lernmark A. Macrophages from high-risk HLA-DQB1*0201/*0302 type 1 diabetes mellitus patients are hypersensitive to lipopolysacharide stimulation. *Scand J Immunol* 2002;**56**:522–9.

51. Yim JJ, Selvaraj P. Genetic susceptibility in tuberculosis. *Respirology* 2010;**15**:241–56.

52. Kurian SM, Selvaraj P, Reetha AM, et al. HLA-DR phenotypes and lymphocyte response to *M. tuberculosis* antigens in cures spinal tuberculosis patients and their contacts. India. *Indian J Tuberc* 2004;**51**:71–5.

53. Idali F, Wikén M, Wahlström J, Mellstedt H, Eklund A, Rabbani H, et al. Reduced Th1 response in the lungs of HLA-DRB1*0301 patients with pulmonary sarcoidosis. *Eur Respir J* 2006;**27**:451–9.

54. Mrazek F, Holla LI, Hutyrova B, Znojil V, Vasku A, Kolek V, et al. Association of tumor necrosis factor-α, lymphotoxin-α and HLA-DRB1 gene poymorhisms with Löfgren's syndrome in Czech patients with sarcoidosis. *Tissue Antigens* 2005;**65**:163–71.

55. Morgenthau AS, Iannuzzi MC. Recent advances in sarcoidosis. *Chest* 2011;**139**:174–82.

56. Grosser M, Luther T, Fuessel M, Bickhardt J, Magdolen V, et al. Clinical course of sarcoidosis in dependence on HLA-DRB1 allele frequencies, inflammatory markers, and the presence of *M. tuberculosis* DNA fragments. *Sarcoidosis Vasc Lung Dis* 2005;**22**:66–74.

57. Kapitány A, Zilahi E, Szántó S, Szücs G, Szabó Z, Végvári A, et al. Association of rheumatoid arthritis with HLA-DR1 and HLA-DR4 in Hungary. *Ann N Y Acad Sci* 2005;**1051**:263–70.

58. Cruz-Tapias P, Pérez-Fernández OM, Rojas-Villarraga A, Rodríguez-Rodríguez A, Arango MT, Anaya JM. Shared HLA class II in six autoimmune diseases in Latin America: a meta-analysis. *Autoimmune Dis* 2012;**2012**:569728. http://dx.doi.org/10.1155/2012/569728.

59. Graham RR, Ortmann W, Rodine P, Espe K, Langefeld C, Lange E, et al. Specific combinations of HLA-DR2 and DR3 class II haplotypes contribute graded risk for disease susceptibility and autoantibodies in human SLE. *Eur J Hum Genet* 2007;**15**:823–30.

60. van Heel DA, Hunt K, Greco L, Wijmenga C. Genetics in coeliac disease. *Best Pract Res Clin Gastroenterol* 2005;**19**:323–39.
61. Dubaniewicz A, Jamieson SE, Dubaniewicz-Wybieralska M, Fakiola M, Nancy Miller E, Blackwell JM. Association between SLC11A1 (formerly NRAMP1) and the risk of sarcoidosis in Poland. *Eur J Hum Genet* 2005;**13**:829–34.
62. Searle S, Blackwell JM. Evidence for a functional repeat polymorphism in the promoter of the human NRAMP1 gene that correlates with autoimmune versus infectious disease susceptibility. *J Med Genet* 1999;**36**:295–9.
63. Paccagnini D, Sieswerda L, Rosu V, Masala S, Pacifico A, Gazouli M, et al. Linking chronic infection and autoimmune diseases: *Mycobacterium avium subspecies paratuberculosis, SLC11A1* polymorphisms and type-1 diabetes mellitus. *PLoS One* 2009;**4**:e7109.
64. Maertzdorf J, Weiner J 3rd., Mollenkopf HJ, Bornot TB, Bauer T, Prasse A, et al. Common patterns and disease-related signatures in tuberculosis and sarcoidosis. *Proc Natl Acad Sci USA* 2012;**109**:7853–8.
65. Neuwirth A, Dobeš J, Oujezdská J, Ballek O, Benešová M, Sumník Z, et al. Eosinophils from patients with type 1 diabetes mellitus express high level of myeloid alpha-defensins and myeloperoxidase. *Cell Immunol* 2012;**273**:158–63.
66. Sharifipour F, Zeraati A, Sahebari M, Hatef M, Naghibi M, Rezaieyazdi Z, et al. Association of urinary lipocalin-2 with lupus nephritis. *Iran J Basic Med Sci* 2013;**16**:1011–5.
67. Salvetti M, Ristori G, Buttinelli C, Fiori P, Falcone M, Britton W, et al. The immune response to mycobacterial 70-kDa heat shock proteins frequently involves autoreactive T cells and is quantitatively disregulated in multiple sclerosis. *J Neuroimmunol* 1996;**65**:143–53.
68. Osterloh A, Breloer M. Heat shock proteins: linking danger and pathogen recognition. *Med Microbiol Immunol* 2008;**197**:1–8.
69. Chodisetti SB, Rai PK, Gowthaman U, Pahari S, Agrewala JN. Potential T cell epitopes of *Mycobacterium tuberculosis* that can instigate molecular mimicry against host: implications in autoimmune pathogenesis. *BMC Immunol* 2012;**13**:13.
70. Valdez MM, Clark JI, Wu GJ, Muchowski PJ. Functional similarities between the small heat shock proteins *Mycobacterium tuberculosis* HSP 16.3 and human α B-crystallin. *Eur J Biochem* 2002;**269**:1806–13.
71. Haregowoin A, Singh B, Gupta RS, Finberg RW. A mycobacterial heat-shock protein – responsive gamma delta T cell clone also responds to the homologous human heat-shock protein: a possible link between infection and autoimmunity. *J Infect Dis* 1991;**163**:156–60.
72. Jee B, Katoch VM, Awasthi SK. Dissection of relationship between small heat shock proteins and mycobacterial diseases. *Indian J Lepr* 2008;**80**:231–45.
73. Ottenhoff TH, Ab BK, Van Embden JD, Thole JE, Kiessling R. The recombinant 65-kD heat shock protein of *Mycobacterium bovis* bacillus Calmette-Guerin/*M. tuberculosis* is a target molecule for CD4$^+$ cytotoxic T lymphocytes that lyse human monocytes. *J Exp Med* 1988;**168**:1947–52.
74. Aron-Maor A, Shoenfeld Y. BCG immunisation and the "Trojan Horse" phenomenon of vaccination. *Clin Rheumatol* 2003;**22**:6–7.
75. Shoenfeld Y, Aron-Maor A, Tanai A, Ehrenfeld M. BCG and autoimmunity: another two-edged sword. *Autoimmunity* 2001;**16**:235–40.
76. Sewell DL, Reinke EK, Co DO, Hogan LH, Fritz RB, Sandor M, et al. Infection with *Mycobacterium bovis* BCG diverts traffic of myelin oligodendroglial glycoprotein autoantigen-specific T cells away from the central nervous system and ameliorates experimental autoimmune encephalomyelitis. *Clin Diagn Lab Immunol* 2003;**10**:564–72.
77. Blackwell JM, Black GF, Sharples C, Soo SS, Peacock CS, Miller N. Roles of Nramp1, HLA, and a gene(s) in allelic association with IL-4, in determining T helper subset differentiation. *Microbes Infect* 1999;**1**:95–102.

CHAPTER 33

Mycobacterium avium Subspecies *Paratuberculosis* and Human Disease: Bridging Infection and Autoimmunity

Coad Thomas Dow[1]

McPherson Eye Research Institute, University of Wisconsin-Madison, Madison, WI, United States, Chippewa Valley Eye Clinic, Eau Claire, WI, United States. [1]Corresponding Author: ctdow@me.com

1 INTRODUCTION

It has been determined that the three main pathogenic mycobacteria—those microbes responsible for tuberculosis, leprosy and paratuberculosis—went through an 'evolutionary bottleneck' about 10,000 years ago. It is speculated that this was due in part to the domestication of and living closely with animals.[1] Two of these mycobacteria species are well known and studied: tuberculosis has claimed more lives than any other disease caused by a bacterium, and a third of the world population is latently infected with *Mycobacterium tuberculosis*.[2] *Mycobacterium leprae*, responsible for leprosy, is literally biblical in presence and continues to infect people today. Official figures show that almost 182,000 people, mainly in Asia and Africa, were affected by leprosy at the beginning of 2012, with approximately 219,000 new cases reported during 2011.[3]

The third bacterial agent, *Mycobacterium avium* subspecies *paratuberculosis* (MAP), has long been known as the cause of Johne's disease (paratuberculosis), an enteric inflammatory infectious disease mostly studied in ruminant animals such as cattle, sheep and goats. MAP is the suspected cause of Crohn's disease in humans and may be involved in many other human diseases.[4]

2 MAP AND CROHN'S DISEASE: THE HUNDRED-YEAR WAR

To accept that MAP is a zoonotic agent that may be responsible for one or more human diseases, one needs to understand the controversy surrounding

Infection and Autoimmunity
http://dx.doi.org/10.1016/B978-0-444-63269-2.00037-4

MAP. The first several sections of this chapter explain the current thinking (of this author) surrounding the controversies.

In 1913 a clear description of what today is known as Crohn's disease was given by Scottish surgeon Kennedy Dalziel.[5] About two decades earlier, in 1895, German veterinary doctor H. A. Johne was the first to describe the cause of a disease in cattle characterized by chronic, profuse, intractable diarrhea. He noted acid-fast bacteria (most often indicating the organism that causes tuberculosis) that, when transferred to a guinea pig, did not cause tuberculosis.[6] Johne first labelled the disease 'pseudotuberculosis' and it eventually became known as 'paratuberculosis'.

The gross pathology of the infected cow's intestines had the same cobblestone appearance as those of Dalziel's patient; the patient's diseased intestines and the diseased cattle intestines were so alike microscopically that Dalziel wrote that the tissue characteristics were

. . .so similar as to justify a proposition that the diseases may be the same'.[5]

He theorised that the disease in cattle and the disease in people were the same entity. The disease in humans was later named after Dr. Crohn, who described a series of patients in 1932.[7]

The crux of this 100-year controversy revolves around the fact that the usual methods of detecting bacteria, stain and culture, are largely ineffective in identifying MAP in humans. A short explanation is that it is very difficult to grow MAP from humans; in addition, MAP drops its cell wall—the component of the bacterium that takes up the characteristic acid stain. Without the cell wall the bacterium is no longer 'acid fast' and cannot be detected microscopically. Recent work identified the capacity of MAP to undergo a morphologic change to become spore-like. The spore morphotype survives heat and other stressors and may lead to increased persistence in hosts and the environment.[8]

3 NEW DIRECTION IN DETECTION

The DNA of MAP is found in 92% of colon biopsies from patients with Crohn's disease.[9] Sceptics of the role of MAP in human disease discount the presence of MAP DNA in various human samples, saying that a positive polymerase chain reaction, which detects dead bacteria, is incidental and that dead MAP has no place in triggering human disease. Two new technologies will likely have a definitive role in identifying *viable* MAP in human samples. One is hybridizing magnetic relaxation nanosensors; these are designed to bind to unique genome sequences of MAP, causing changes in the sample's magnetic resonance signal. Clinically relevant samples can be tested in an hour instead of a 12-week (or more) culture.[10] A second technology uses a phage-mediated immunoassay. This too permits the sensitive and relatively fast detection of viable MAP in various samples.[11]

4 M. AVIUM SS. PARATUBERCULOSIS

MAP is a Gram-positive, acid-fast staining, small, rod-shaped bacterium. Like other members of the *Mycobacteriaceae* genus, it has a unique cell wall structure rich in complex lipids (Figure 1). The thick and chemically distinctive cell wall of mycobacteria is largely responsible for the robust nature of these bacteria, both within the host cell and in the environment. The pathogenic potential of mycobacteria is correlated with their growth rate. Paradoxically, slow-growing mycobacteria are more virulent than fast-growing mycobacteria. With the exception of *M. leprae* (the cause of leprosy in humans), which cannot be cultured in vitro, MAP has the slowest growth rate of pathogenic mycobacteria. After isolation from infected animals and growth under optimal conditions, colonies of MAP are typically not visible for 3 months or more.[12]

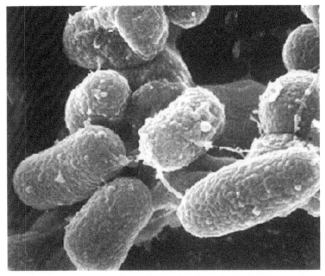

Figure 1 *Mycobacterium avium* subspecies *paratuberculosis. Image courtesy of Dr. Mike Collins, University of Wisconsin—Madison.*

5 MAP AND HUMAN EXPOSURE

MAP is present in pasteurized milk,[13,14] infant formula made from pasteurised milk,[15] surface water,[16–18] soil,[16] cow manure, 'lagoons' that can leach into surface water, cow manure in both solid and liquid forms that is applied as fertilizer to agricultural land[19] and municipal tap water;[20] these sources provide multiple routes of transmission to humans. In a recent study in Ohio, the DNA of MAP was detected in >80% of domestic water samples.[21] Normal water treatment processes such as filtration and chlorination amplify rather than eliminate mycobacteria organisms by killing off their competitors.[22] In addition, mycobacteria organisms grow on tap water pipes,[23] in biofilms[24] and on plastic water bottles.[25] One estimate is that mycobacteria may be present in drinking water in 'massive Numbers', on the level of up to 700,000 (7×10^5) organisms per litre of water.[23] If humans are so readily exposed to MAP, why are Crohn's disease and the other diseases featured in this chapter not pervasive? The answer is genetics.

6 GENETIC LESSONS FROM TUBERCULOSIS

A frequently cited tragic account demonstrating the inherent spectrum of resistance/susceptibility to mycobacterial infection is the accidental exposure of infants to a Bacille-Calmette-Guerin vaccine contaminated with virulent *M. tuberculosis* in Lubeck, Germany, in 1929–1930. Of 251 vaccinated children, 72 children died from tuberculosis, 61 had severe tuberculosis, 95 had mild tuberculosis, and 17 were infected (positive tuberculin test) but asymptomatic, demonstrating the large range of responses among humans to a deadly infectious disease.[26]

7 GENETIC LESSONS FROM LEPROSY

The results of genome-wide analyses (linkage and association) and candidate gene studies suggest independent genetic control over both the susceptibility to leprosy and the development of a clinical subtype. Also, the recognition of a shared genetic susceptibility between leprosy and several inflammatory/autoimmune diseases suggests that leprosy is a model for studying the genetic predisposition and pathogenesis of both infectious and inflammatory/autoimmune diseases.[27] *NOD2* (now *CARD15*) is an example of a gene causing susceptibility for both Crohn's disease and leprosy. Interestingly, the phenotype of *CARD15* related to Crohn's disease is that of aggressive disease. Loss-of-function defects associated with the *CARD15* defects result in the inability of the innate immune system to detect the presence of pathogens.[28]

8 GENETIC LESSONS FROM BLAU SYNDROME: CARD15

Insights into genetic susceptibility and MAP infection can be found in Blau syndrome, a rare inflammatory disease. This syndrome is an inherited granulomatous inflammatory disorder with clinical findings of uveitis, arthritis and dermatitis.[29] Although rare, Blau syndrome has been of interest in current medical literature because of the discovery that places its genetic defect on the *CARD15* gene,[30,31] the same gene imparting susceptibility to Crohn's disease. Linkage studies have placed the gene on chromosome 16; it was originally referred to as the *NOD2* gene.[32] The Blau syndrome susceptibility component of the *CARD15* gene is at the nucleotide binding site domain,[30,33] whereas the Crohn's susceptibility component is at the N-terminal leucine-rich repeat domain.[32,34] The *CARD15* gene is part of the ancestral innate immune system that senses and eliminates bacteria.[28,35]

The clinical findings of Blau syndrome are the same as juvenile sarcoidosis; indeed, de novo *CARD15* defects are consistently found in cases of sporadic juvenile sarcoidosis and Blau syndrome.[36,37] For these reasons – the clinical appearance of sarcoidosis and a shared genetic susceptibility with Crohn's disease – it was proposed that MAP could have a role in Blau syndrome. A series of Blau tissues comprised of skin, synovial samples as well as Blau granulomas of the liver and kidney were tested for the presence of MAP. Six tissues from five patients representing three different families were found to have MAP present in the tissue granulomas. These results were presented at the 2005 Colloquium on Paratuberculosis (Dow) and published in 2010.[38]

The complexity of genetic susceptibility and microbial infection can be reflected in these two diseases (Crohn's and Blau), both of which have polymorphisms of the *CARD15* gene. The proposed etiopathology is that with adequate exposure to MAP, an individual with single nucleotide polymorphisms within one *CARD15* location (nucleotide binding domain) will exhibit Blau syndrome, and if the single nucleotide polymorphisms are within another location of the same gene (leucine-rich repeat domain), they exhibit Crohn's disease. *CARD15* defects of the leucine-rich repeat domain result in an aggressive phenotype of Crohn's disease.[39] Adding to the complexity is that there are several susceptibility genes associated with Crohn's disease.[40]

9 SLC11A1

An additional gene associated with susceptibility to Crohn's disease is the *SLC11A1* gene.[41] Natural resistance-associated macrophage protein 1 (NRAMP1) is now strictly referred to as SLC11A1 (solute carrier 11a1).

The gene that encodes for this protein is recognized as having a role in the susceptibility of humans and animals to a number of infections, including mycobacterial infections, and is associated with a number of autoimmune diseases as well. In humans, the *SLC11A1* gene is located on chromosome 2q35. It encodes an integral membrane protein of 550 amino acids that is expressed exclusively in the lysosomal compartment of monocytes and macrophages.[42]

The product of the *SLC11A1* gene modulates the cellular environment in response to activation by intracellular pathogens by acidifying the phagosome, thus killing the pathogen.[43] As such, it plays a role in host innate immunity.[44] Mutation of *SLC11A1* impairs phagosome acidification, yielding a permissive environment for the persistence of intracellular bacteria.[45]

10 SLC11A1 IN INFECTIOUS AND AUTOIMMUNE DISEASE

Sarcoidosis, the previously mentioned systemic disease associated with MAP, also is associated with polymorphisms of the *SLC11A1* gene.[46] Susceptibility to mycobacterial diseases such as tuberculosis, leprosy and Buruli's ulcers are associated with polymorphisms of the *SLC11A1* gene.[47] Similar polymorphisms are associated with Johne's disease (paratuberculosis) in cattle,[48] goats[49] and sheep.[50] When researchers at the Pasteur Institute in Belgium developed a murine model for MAP infection, they created a mouse with an *SLC11A1* defect.[51]

Given the pivotal roles that *SLC11A1* plays in innate immunity, it is not surprising that the relationship between polymorphisms in *SLC11A1* and a number of mycobacterial as well as autoimmune diseases has been explored.[52] Associations have been found with leprosy,[53] tuberculosis,[54] rheumatoid arthritis,[55] multiple sclerosis,[56,57] inflammatory bowel disease[57,58,41] and type 1 diabetes mellitus (TIDM).[59,60]

11 MAP AND TYPE 1 DIABETES

T1DM is an autoimmune disease manifest by progressive T-cell-mediated autoimmune destruction of insulin-producing β cells in the pancreatic islets of Langherans.[61] Dow in 2005 postulated a causative role for MAP in T1DM, and in 2007 Rosu et al.[62] and Sechi et al.[63] found the DNA of MAP in the blood of autoimmune (type 1) but not non-autoimmune (type 2) diabetics. Paccagnini[64] also found an association of polymorphisms of the *SLC11a1* gene and MAP in patients with T1DM.

While it may be intuitive to envision an occult presence of MAP as an infective agent producing a granulomatous lesion of Crohn's or sarcoidosis, it is broader divide to assign a role for MAP in T1DM. The link connecting MAP and T1DM comes from the concept of molecular mimicry: protein elements of the pathogen 'look like' elements of the host to such a degree that immune responses directed at the pathogen also attack the host. One of the proposed links is the mimicry of mycobacterial heat shock protein (HSP) of MAP (HSP65) and pancreatic glutamic acid decarboxylase[65] (Figure 2).

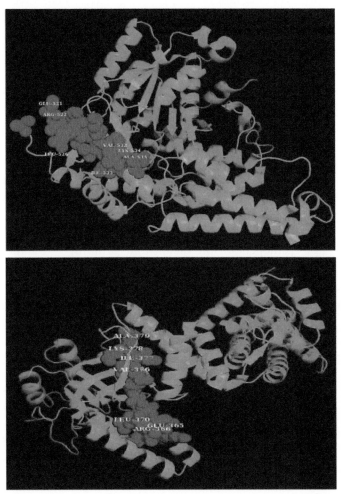

Figure 2 Sequential and conformational molecular mimicry between MAP heat shock protein 65 (HSP65) and pancreatic glutamic acid decarboxylase (GAD). *Image from Naser SA, Thanigachalam S, Dow CT, Collins MT. Exploring the role of Mycobacterium avium subspecies paratuberculosis in the pathogenesis of type 1 diabetes mellitus: a pilot study. Gut Pathog 2013;5:14.*

12 MOLECULAR MIMICRY/HEAT SHOCK PROTEINS: HSP65

Molecular mimicry has long been implicated as a mechanism by which microbes can induce autoimmunity.[66,67] Rheumatic fever is the classical example of molecular mimicry between an infecting agent—*Streptococcus pyogenes* (group A streptococcus)—and a related autoimmune disease in humans.[68–70] The disease is characterized by damage to the heart, joints and the central nervous system (Sydenham's chorea). The activity of the host's immune system against the *S. pyogenes* generates a cross-recognition to human tissue, causing an autoimmune reaction. Heart damage is the most serious consequence and is present in 30–45% of the cases; it mostly causes damage to heart valves.

HSPs are produced in response to environmental stress. They act in a protective capacity, helping cells survive stressful conditions and promoting recovery.[71] During an active immune response to infection, both the host and the micro-organisms synthesize HSPs. The increased expression of both self- and infective stress proteins and the extensive sequence homology between microbial and human HSP (50–80% amino acid homology of mycobacterial HSP65 vs. human HSP60) led to the concept that HSPs are involved in the etiology and pathogenesis of many immune-mediated disorders.[72] Mycobacterial HSPs have been found in a myriad of autoimmune diseases.[73] For example, the mycobacterial 65-kDa HSP was implicated in the pathogenesis of rheumatoid arthritis,[74,75] autoimmune hepatitis,[76] primary biliary cirrhosis[77] and scleroderma.[78] HSP65 is implicated in multiple vasculitis-associated systemic autoimmune diseases, such as Kawasaki disease,[79] Behçet's disease[80] and Takayasu's arteritis.[81]

13 MAP AND OTHER AUTOIMMUNE DISEASES: THYROIDITIS AND MULTIPLE SCLEROSIS

Two articles link MAP to autoimmune (Hashimoto's) thyroiditis. The same molecular mimicry principle is suggested as in the link between MAP (HSP65) and the organ-specific autoantigens of thyroiditis.[82,83] Cossu et al.[84,85] published articles implicating MAP in multiple sclerosis. Molecular mimicry and *SLC11A1* associations are central to this association as well.

14 THE FUTURE: MAP AND HUMAN DISEASE

As the MAP/Crohn's debate resolves and as more diseases are linked to MAP, there will likely be seismic shift in the public health approach to

MAP and human disease. Early indictions of such a shift are two clinical trials including anti-mycobacterial drugs: one for Crohn's disease[86] and another for multiple sclerosis.[87] Positive results from efforts like these will further solidify the role of MAP as a zoonotic agent in human disease.

REFERENCES

1. Frothingham R. Evolutionary bottlenecks in the agents of tuberculosis, leprosy, and paratuberculosis. *Med Hypotheses* 1999;**52**(2):95–9.
2. *World Health Organization Tuberculosis Fact Sheet.* http://www.who.int/mediacentre/factsheets/fs104/en/; [accessed 10.15.13].
3. *WHO Leprosy Sheet.* http://www.who.int/mediacentre/factsheets/fs101/en/.
4. Dow CT. *M. paratuberculosis* heat shock protein 65 and human diseases: bridging infection and autoimmunity. *Autoimmune Dis* 2012;**2012**:150824. http://dx.doi.org/10.1155/2012/150824.
5. Dalziel TK. Chronic interstitial enteritis. *British J Med* 1913;**2**:2756.
6. *From History of Johne's Disease, Johne's Information Center.* http://www.johnes.org/history/index.html; [accessed 10.15.13].
7. Crohn BB, Ginzburg L, Oppenheimer GD. Regional ileitis – a pathologic and clinical entity. *JAMA* 1932;**99**(16):1323–9.
8. Lamont EA, Bannantine JP, Armién A, Ariyakumar DS, Sreevatsan S. Identification and characterization of a spore-like morphotype in chronically starved *Mycobacterium avium* subsp. paratuberculosis cultures. *PLoS One* 2012;**7**(1):e30648.
9. Bull TJ, McMinn EJ, Sidi-Boumedine K, Skull A, Durkin D, Neild P, et al. Detection and verification of *Mycobacterium avium* subsp. paratuberculosis in fresh ileocolonic mucosal biopsy specimens from individuals with and without Crohn's disease. *J Clin Microbiol* 2003;**41**(7):2915–23.
10. Kaittanis C, Boukhriss H, Santra S, Naser SA, Perez JM. Rapid and sensitive detection of an intracellular pathogen in human peripheral leukocytes with hybridizing magnetic relaxation nanosensors. *PLoS One* 2012;**7**(4):e35326. http://dx.doi.org/10.1371/journal.pone.0035326.
11. Stewart LD, Foddai A, Elliott CT, Grant IR. Development of a novel phage-mediated immunoassay for the rapid detection of viable *Mycobacterium avium* subsp. paratuberculosis. *J Appl Microbiol* 2013;**115**(3):808–17. http://dx.doi.org/10.1111/jam.12275.
12. Collins MT. Paratuberculosis: review of present knowledge. *Acta Vet Scand* 2003;**44**:217–21.
13. Millar D, Ford J, Sanderson J, Withey S, Tizard M, et al. IS900 PCR to detect Mycobacterium paratuberculosis in retail supplies of whole pasteurized cows' milk in England and Wales. *Appl Environ Microbiol* 1996;**62**:3446–52.
14. Ellingson JL, Anderson JL, Koziczkowski JJ, Radcliff RP, Sloan SJ, Allen SE, et al. Detection of viable Mycobacterium avium subsp. paratuberculosis in retail pasteurized whole milk by two culture methods and PCR. *J Food Prot* 2005;**68**(5):966–72.
15. Hruska K, Bartos M, Kralik P, Pavlik I. Mycobacterium avium subsp. paratuberculosis in powdered infant milk: paratuberculosis in cattle—the public health problem to be solved. *Vet Med* 2005;**50**(8):327–35.
16. Pickup RW, Rhodes G, Arnott S, Sidi-Boumedine K, Bull TJ, et al. Mycobacterium avium subsp. paratuberculosis in the catchment area and water of the River Taff in South Wales, United Kingdom, and its potential relationship to clustering of Crohn's disease cases in the city of Cardiff. *Appl Environ Microbiol* 2005;**71**:2130–9.

17. Whan L, Ball HJ, Grant IR, Rowe MT. Occurrence of *Mycobacterium avium* subsp. paratuberculosis in untreated water in Northern Ireland. *Appl Environ Microbiol* 2006;**71**:7107–12.

18. Pickup RW, Rhodes G, Bull TJ, Arnott S, Sidi-Boumedine K, et al. *Mycobacterium avium* subsp. paratuberculosis in lake catchments, in river water abstracted for domestic use, and in effluent from domestic sewage treatment works: diverse opportunities for environmental cycling and human exposure. *Appl Environ Microbiol* 2006;**72**: 4067–77.

19. Grewal SK, Rajeev S, Sreevatsan S, Michel Jr. FC. Persistence of *Mycobacterium avium* subsp. paratuberculosis and other zoonotic pathogens during simulated composting, manure packing, and liquid storage of dairy manure. *Appl Environ Microbiol* 2006;**72**:565–74.

20. Collins MT. Miliotis MD, Bier JW, editors. *International handbook of foodborne pathogens.* London: CRC Press; 2003.

21. Beumer A, King D, Donohue M, Mistry J, Covert T, Pfaller S. Detection of *Mycobacterium avium* subsp. paratuberculosis in drinking water and biofilms by quantitative PCR. *Appl Environ Microbiol* 2010;**76**(21):7367–70.

22. Falkinham III JO. Factors influencing the chlorine susceptibility of *Mycobacterium avium*, *Mycobacterium intracellulare*, and *Mycobacterium scrofulaceum*. *Appl Environ Microbiol* 2003;**69**:5685–9.

23. Falkinham III JO, Norton CD, LeChevallier MW. Factors influencing numbers of *Mycobacterium avium*, *Mycobacterium intracellulare*, and other Mycobacteria in drinking water distribution systems. *Appl Environ Microbiol* 2001;**67**:1225–31.

24. Vaerewijck MJ, Huys G, Palomino JC, Swings J, Portaels F. Mycobacteria in drinking water distribution systems: ecology and significance for human health. *FEMS Microbiol Rev* 2005;**29**:911–34.

25. Tatchou-Nyamsi-Konig JA, Dailloux M, Block JC. Survival of Mycobacterium avium attached to polyethylene terephtalate (PET) water bottles. *J Appl Microbiol* 2009;**106**:825–32.

26. Moegling A. Die Epidemiologie der Lubecker Sa–uglingstuberkulose. *Arbeiten ad Reichsges-Amt* 1935;**69**:1–24.

27. Alter A, Grant A, Abel L, Alcaïs A, Schurr E. Leprosy as a genetic disease. *Mamm Genome* 2011;**22**(1–2):19–31.

28. Girardin SE, Hugot J-P, Sansonetti PJ. Lessons from Nod2 studies: towards a link between Crohn's disease and bacterial sensing. *Trends Immunol* 2003;**24**(12):652–8.

29. Blau B. Familial granulomatous arthritis, iritis, and rash. *J Pediatr* 1985;**107**(5):689–93.

30. Hampe J, Grebe J, Nikolaus S, et al. Association of NOD2 (CARD 15) genotype with clinical course of Crohn's disease: a cohort study. *Lancet* 2002;**359**(9318):1661–5.

31. Miceli-Richard C, Lesage S, Rybojad M, et al. CARD15 mutations in Blau syndrome. *Nat Genet* 2001;**29**(1):19–20.

32. Hugot J-P, Chamaillard M, Zouali H, et al. Association of NOD2 leucine-rich repeat variants with susceptibility to Crohn's disease. *Nature* 2001;**411**(6837):599–603.

33. Wang X, Kuivaniemi H, Bonavita G, et al. CARD15 mutations in familial granulomatosis syndromes: a study of the original Blau syndrome kindred and other families with large-vessel arteritis and cranial neuropathy. *Arthritis Rheum* 2002;**46** (11):3041–5.

34. Lesage S, Zouali H, C´ezard JP, et al. CARD15/NOD2 mutational analysis and genotype-phenotype correlation in 612 patients with inflammatory bowel disease. *Am J Hum Genet* 2002;**70**(4):845–57.

35. Inohara N, Ogura Y, Fontalba A, et al. Host recognition of bacterial muramyl dipeptide mediated through NOD2: implications for Crohn's disease. *J Biol Chem* 2003;**278** (8):5509–12.

36. Kanazawa N, Okafuji I, Kambe N, et al. Early-onset sarcoidosis and CARD15 mutations with constitutive nuclear factor-κB activation: common genetic etiology with Blau syndrome. *Blood* 2005;**105**(3):1195–7.

37. Rose CD, Doyle TM, McIlvain-Simpson G, et al. Blau syndrome mutation of CARD15/NOD2 in sporadic early onset granulomatous arthritis. *J Rheumatol* 2005;**32**(2):373–5.

38. Dow CT, Ellingson JL. Detection of Mycobacterium avium ss. Paratuberculosis in Blau syndrome tissues. *Autoimmune Dis* 2010;**2011**:127692.

39. Lacher M, Helmbrecht J, Schroepf S, Koletzko S, Ballauff A, Classen M, et al. NOD2 mutations predict the risk for surgery in pediatric-onset Crohn's disease. *J Pediatr Surg* 2010;**45**(8):1591–7.

40. Franke A, McGovern DP, Barrett JC, Wang K, Radford-Smith GL, Ahmad T, et al. Genome-wide meta-analysis increases to 71 the number of confirmed Crohn's disease susceptibility loci. *Nat Genet* 2010;**42**(12):1118–25.

41. Sechi LA, Gazouli M, Sieswerda LE, Molicotti P, Ahmed N, Ikonomopoulos J, et al. Relationship between Crohn's disease, infection with Mycobacterium avium subspecies paratuberculosis and SLC11A1 gene polymorphisms in Sardinian patients. *World J Gastroenterol* 2006;**12**(44):7161–4.

42. Canonne-Hergaux F, Gruenheid S, Govoni G, Gros P. The Nramp1 protein and its role in resistance to infection and macrophage function. *Proc Assoc Am Physicians* 1999;**111**:283–9.

43. Lapham AS, Phillips ES, Barton CH. Transcriptional control of Nramp1: a paradigm for the repressive action of c-Myc. *Biochem Soc Trans* 2004;**32**(Pt 6):1084–6.

44. Wyllie S, Seu P, Goss JA. The natural resistance-associatedmacrophage protein 1 Slc11a1 (formerly Nramp1) and iron metabolism in macrophages. *Microbes Infect* 2002;**4**(3):351–9.

45. Hackam DJ, Rotstein OD, Zhang W, Gruenheid S, Gros P, Grinstein S. Host resistance to intracellular infection: mutation of natural resistance-associated macrophage protein 1 (Nramp1) impairs phagosomal acidification. *J Exp Med* 1998;**188**(2):351–64.

46. Dubaniewicz A, Jamieson SE, Dubaniewicz-Wybieralska M, Fakiola M, Nancy Miller E, Blackwell JM. Association between SLC11A1 (formerly NRAMP1) and the risk of sarcoidosis in Poland. *Eur J Hum Genet* 2005;**13**(7):829–34.

47. Stienstra Y, van der Werf TS, Oosterom E, Nolte IM, van der Graaf WT, Etuaful S, et al. Susceptibility to Buruli ulcer is associated with the SLC11A1 (NRAMP1) D543N polymorphism. *Genes Immun* 2006;**7**(3):185–9.

48. Ruiz-Larrañaga O, Garrido JM, Manzano C, Iriondo M, Molina E, Gil A, et al. Identification of single nucleotide polymorphisms in the bovine solute carrier family 11 member 1 (SLC11A1) gene and their association with infection by Mycobacterium avium subspecies paratuberculosis. *J Dairy Sci* 2010;**93**(4):1713–21.

49. Korou LM, Liandris E, Gazouli M, Ikonomopoulos J. Investigation of the association of the SLC11A1 gene with resistance/sensitivity of goats (Capra hircus) to paratuberculosis. *Vet Microbiol* 2010;**144**(3-4):353–8.

50. Purdie AC, Plain KM, Begg DJ, de Silva K, Whittington RJ. Candidate gene and genome-wide association studies of *Mycobacterium avium* subsp. paratuberculosis infection in cattle and sheep: a review. *Comp Immunol Microbiol Infect Dis* 2011;**34**(3):197–208.

51. Roupie V, Rosseels V, Piersoel V, Zinniel DK, Barletta RG, Huygen K. Genetic resistance of mice to Mycobacterium paratuberculosis is influenced by Slc11a1 at the early but not at the late stage of infection. *Infect Immun* 2008;**76**(5):2099–105.

52. Blackwell JM, Searle S, Mohamed H, White JK. Divalentcation transport and susceptibility to infectious and autoimmune disease: continuation of the Ity/Lsh/Bcg/Nramp1/Slc11a1 gene story. *Immunol Lett* 2003;**85**(2):197–203.

53. Hatta M, Ratnawati, Tanaka M, Ito J, Shirakawa T, Kawabata M. NRAMP1/SLC11A1 gene polymorphisms and host susceptibility to Mycobacterium tuberculosis and *M. leprae* in South Sulawesi, Indonesia. *Southeast Asian J Trop Med Public Health* 2010;**41**(2): 386–94.

54. Bellamy R, Ruwende C, Corrah T, McAdam KP, Whittle HC, Hill AV. Variations in the NRAMP1 gene and susceptibility to tuberculosis in West Africans. *N Engl J Med* 1998;**338**:640–4.

55. Ates O, Dalyan L, Musellim B, Hatemi G, Turker H, Ongen G, et al. NRAMP1 (SLC11A1) gene polymorphisms that correlate with autoimmune versus infectious disease susceptibility in tuberculosis and rheumatoid arthritis. *Int J Immunogenet* 2009;**36**:15–19.

56. Kotze MJ, de Villiers JN, Rooney RN, Grobbelaar JJ, Mansvelt EP, Bouwens CS, et al. Analysis of the NRAMP1 gene implicated in iron transport: association with multiple sclerosis and age effects. *Blood Cells Mol Dis* 2001;**27**:44–53.

57. Gazouli M, Atsaves V, Mantzaris G, Economou M, Nasioulas G, Evangelou K, et al. Role of functional polymorphisms of NRAMP1 gene for the development of Crohn's disease. *Inflamm Bowel Dis* 2008;**14**:1323–30.

58. Kotlowski R, Bernstein CN, Silverberg MS, Krause DO. Population-based case-control study of alpha 1-antitrypsin and SLC11A1 in Crohn's disease and ulcerative colitis. *Inflamm Bowel Dis* 2008;**14**:1112–17.

59. Paccagnini D, Sieswerda L, Rosu V, Masala S, Pacifico A, Gazouli M, et al. Linking chronic infection and autoimmune diseases: Mycobacterium avium subspecies par atuberculosis, SLC11A1 polymorphisms and type-1 diabetes mellitus. *PLoS One* 2009;**214** (9):e7109.

60. Takahashi K, Satoh J, Kojima Y, Negoro K, Hirai M, Hinokio Y, et al. Promoter polymorphism of SLC11A1 (formerly NRAMP1) confers susceptibility to autoimmune type 1 diabetes mellitus in Japanese. *Tissue Antigens* 2004;**63**(3):231–6.

61. Eisenbarth GS. Type I diabetes mellitus. A chronic autoimmune disease. *N Engl J Med* 1986;**314**(21):1360–8.

62. Rosu V, Ahmed N, Paccagnini D, Gerlach G, Fadda G, Hasnain SE, et al. Specific immunoassays confirm association of *Mycobacterium avium* Subsp. paratuberculosis with type-1 but not type-2 diabetes mellitus. *PLoS One* 2009;**4**(2):e4386.

63. Sechi LA, Rosu V, Pacifico A, Fadda G, Ahmed N, Zanetti S. Humoral immune responses of type 1 diabetes patients to Mycobacterium avium subsp. paratuberculosis lend support to the infectious trigger hypothesis. *Clin Vaccine Immunol* 2008;**15**(2):320–6.

64. Paccagnini D, Sieswerda L, Rosu V, Masala S, Pacifico A, Gazouli M, et al. Linking chronic infection and autoimmune diseases: *Mycobacterium avium* subspecies paratuberculosis, SLC11A1 polymorphisms and type-1 diabetes mellitus. *PLoS One* 2009;**214**(9): e7109.

65. Dow CT. Paratuberculosis and type I diabetes: is this the trigger? *Med Hypotheses* 2006;**67** (4):782–5.

66. Oldstone MB. Molecular mimicry and autoimmune disease. *Cell* 1987;**50**(6):819–20.

67. Raska M, Weigl E. Heat shock proteins in autoimmune diseases. *Biomed Pap Med Fac Univ Palacky Olomouc Czech Repub* 2005;**149**(2):243–9.

68. Guilherme L, Faé K, Oshiro SE, Kalil J. Molecular pathogenesis of rheumatic fever and rheumatic heart disease. *Expert Rev Mol Med* 2005;**7**(28):1–15.

69. Kaplan MH, SVEC KH. Immunologic relation of streptococcal and tissue antigens. III. Presence in human sera of streptococcal antibody cross-reactive with heart tissue. Association with streptococcal infection, rheumatic fever, and glomerulonephritis. *J Exp Med* 1964;**119**:65166.

70. Kirvan CA, Swedo SE, Heuser JS, Cunningham MW. Mimicry and autoantibody-mediated neuronal cell signaling in Sydenham chorea. *Nat Med* 2003;**9**(7):914–20.

71. Parsell DA, Lindquist S. The function of heat shock proteins in stress tolerance: degradation and reactivation of damaged proteins. *Annu Rev Genet* 1993;**27**:437–96.
72. Lamb JR, Young DB. T cell recognition of stress proteins. A link between infectious and autoimmune disease. *Mol Biol Med* 1990;**7**(4):311–21.
73. Jarjour WN, Jeffries BD, Davis 4th JS, et al. Autoantibodies to human stress proteins A survey of various rheumatic and other inflammatory diseases. *Arthritis Rheum* 1991;**34**(9):1133–8.
74. Moudgil KD, Chang TT, Eradat H, et al. Diversification of T cell responses to carboxy-terminal determinants within the 65 kD heat-shock protein is involved in regulation of autoimmune arthritis. *J Exp Med* 1997;**185**(7):1307–16.
75. Quayle AJ, Wilson KB, Li SG, et al. Peptide recognition, T cell receptor usage and HLA restriction elements of human heat-shock protein (hsp) 60 and mycobacterial 65 kDa hspreactive T cell clones from rheumatoid synovial fluid. *Eur J Immunol* 1992;**22**(5):1315–22.
76. Miyata M, Kogure A, Sato H, et al. Detection of antibodies to 65 KD heat shock protein and to human superoxide dismutase in autoimmune hepatitis-molecular mimicry between 65 KD heat shock protein and superoxide dismutase. *Clin Rheumatol* 1995;**14**(6):673–7.
77. Vilagut L, Pares A, Vinas O, et al. Antibodies to mycobacterial 65 kD heat shock protein cross-react with the main mitochondrial antigens in patients with primary biliary cirrhosis. *Eur J Clin Invest* 1997;**27**(8):667–72.
78. Danieli MG, Candela M, Ricciatti AM, et al. Antibodies to mycobacterial 65 kDa heat shock protein in systemic sclerosis (scleroderma). *J Autoimmun* 1992;**5**(4):443–5.
79. Yokota S, Tsubaki S, Kuriyama T, et al. Presence in Kawasaki disease of antibodies to mycobacterial heatshock protein HSP65 and autoantibodies to epitopes of human HSP65 cognate antigen. *Clin Immunol Immunopathol* 1993;**67**:163–70.
80. Direskeneli H, Saruhan-Direskeneli G. The role of heat shock proteins in Behcet's disease. *Clin Exp Rheumatol* 2003;**21**(Suppl. 30):S44–8.
81. Aggarwal A, Chag M, Sinha N, Naik S. Takayasu's arteritis: role of Mycobacterium tuberculosis and its 65 kDa heat shock protein. *Int J Cardiol* 1996;**55**(1):49–55.
82. D'Amore M, Lisi S, Sisto M, Cucci L, Dow CT. Molecular identification of Mycobacterium avium subspecies paratuberculosis in an Italian patient with Hashimoto's thyroiditis and Melkersson-Rosenthal syndrome. *J Med Microbiol* 2010;**59**(Pt. 1):137–9.
83. Sisto M, Cucci L, D'Amore M, Dow TC, Mitolo V, Lisi S. Proposing a relationship between Mycobacterium avium subspecies paratuberculosis infection and Hashimoto's thyroiditis. *Scand J Infect Dis* 2010;**42**(10):787–90.
84. Cossu D, Cocco E, Paccagnini D, Masala S, Ahmed N, et al. Association of Mycobacterium avium subsp. paratuberculosis with multiple sclerosis in Sardinian Patients. *PLoS One* 2011;**6**(4):e18482.
85. Cossu D, Masala S, Cocco E, Paccagnini D, Tranquilli S, Frau J, et al. Association of Mycobacterium avium subsp. paratuberculosis and SLC11A1 polymorphisms in Sardinian multiple sclerosis patients. *J Infect Dev Ctries* 2013;**7**(3):203–7.
86. *Crohn's disease clinical trial with anti-mycobacterial drugs.* www.clinicaltrials.gov/ct2/show/NCT0195132; [accessed 10.14.13].
87. *Multiple sclerosis clinical trial with anit-mycobacterial drugs.* www.clinicaltrials.gov/ct2/show/NCT017176641; [accessed 10.14.13].

CHAPTER 34

Leprosy and Autoimmunity

Francinne Machado Ribeiro[*,1], **Yehuda Shoenfeld**[†,‡]
*Rheumatologist; Department of Rheumatology. Universidade do Estado do Rio de Janeiro, RJ, Brazil
†MD, FRCP (hon), MaACR Head of Zabludowicz Center for Autoimmune Diseases, Sheba Medical Center (Affiliated to Tel-Aviv University)
‡Incumbent of the Laura Schwarz-Kipp Chair for Research of Autoimmune Diseases, Tel-Aviv University, Israel
1Corresponding Author: fran.machadoribeiro@gmail.com

> ... all individuals called lepers were subjected to total ostracism from society...[1]

1 INTRODUCTION

Leprosy, or Hansen's disease, is a chronic mycobacterial infection that affects the skin and peripheral nerves.[2] It is caused by *Mycobacterium leprae*, an acid-alcohol-fast, obligate intracellular bacillus. The prevalence of infection is variable, and the majority of cases occur in tropical countries. According to a WHO report, the countries with the highest number of new cases are India, Brazil, Indonesia, Bangladesh, and Nepal.[3] However, the increasing amount of international travel requires clinical suspicion worldwide. In the region of the Americas the proportion of new multi-bacillary (MB) infections and new infections in children ranges from 0.6% to 7.8% and from 34.8% to 94.3%, respectively.[3]

This disease remains poorly understood and feared by the general population, although it is curable. The reason for this is its capacity to cause life-long disability that is frequently irreversible. In addition, the means of transmission is not entirely known. No relationship between the bacillus and a vector has been established, although exposure to armadillos has been associated with human leprosy in the United States.[4,5] The respiratory tract plays a role in transmission, with the evidence of large numbers of bacilli in nasal discharge of patients with the MB form of the disease.[6,7] Prolonged contact with infected patients, overcrowding and type of leprosy index are risk factors.[7,8] The mycobacterial load is extremely high in the lepromatous form (MB disease) and much lower in others; subjects in close contact with this form carry a higher risk of contamination.[9,10]

Infection and Autoimmunity
http://dx.doi.org/10.1016/B978-0-444-63269-2.00038-6

Table 1 Prevalence of Autoantibodies in Patients with Leprosy

Antibody	Prevalence (%)
Rheumatoid factor	13–60
Anti-CCP	0–3.1
ANA	0–30
Anticardiolipin, IgG and IgM	37–98
Anti-β2-GPI	2.9–89
ANCA	5–62.5

ANA, antinuclear antibody; Anti-β2-GPI, anti-β2-glycoprotein I; ANCA, antineutrophil cytoplasmic antibody.

M. leprae has a special tropism for reticuloendothelial and peripheral nerve cells. The bacilli are collected in groups, called globi, within macrophages, and the replication time is around 11–13 days—longer than that of *Mycobacterium tuberculosis;*[2] this makes their growth in culture media impossible. A propensity to affect cold areas of the body such as the nasal mucosa and peripheral nerves and skin correlates with a predilection for growth at lower temperatures (27–30 °C).[11,12]

The clinical manifestations are variable and encompass a wide spectrum determined by the host immune response. The leprosy spectrum ranges from an intense, organized cellular response with few bacilli at the tuberculoid leprosy (TT) to an absence of specific immune response and a high burden of microorganisms at the opposite pole in lepromatous leprosy (LL).[2,11,13]

The Ridley–Jopling classification reflects the entire clinical and pathological spectrum and correlates with the number of acid-fast bacilli present in the skin biopsy (Table 1). Borderline forms (tuberculoid [BT], mid-borderline [BB], and lepromatous [BL]) are intermediate states that eventually move towards one of the poles. Indeterminate forms represent the initial stage after contamination.[14,15]

2 PATHOGENESIS

The development of clinical disease in the minority of exposed individuals relates to the low virulence of the bacillus and an effective innate immune response. Dendritic cells (DCs) play a central role in the early response to *M. leprae*. After uptake of the bacilli at the site of invasion, DCs modulate inflammation through local production of cytokines and chemokines and regulate the adaptive cell-mediated immunity into a Th1 or Th2 response.[12,16] The ability of *M. leprae* to regulate cytokine production and to drive Th1 or Th2 responses may contribute to mycobacterial survival and clinical relevant infection.[17]

It has been shown that the numbers of Langerhans cells, a subset of DCs, are substantially increased in the lesions of the TT pole in comparison with uninfected controls and LL forms.[18] DCs are considered to be effective presenters of *M. leprae* antigens. Insofar as major histocompatibility complex (MHC) class I and II expression is down-regulated in monocyte-derived DCs infected with bacilli, DCs stimulated with *M. leprae* membrane antigens up-regulate MHC class II and CD40 ligand-associated interleukin (IL)-12 production.[11,12,19,20] This suggests that the whole live bacilli may suppress the interaction of DCs and T cells.[19]

The cytokine profile present in the lesion site seems to be related to toll-like receptor (TLR) function. Biopsy samples of TT leprosy revealed that monocytes and DCs expressed TLR1 and TLR2 much more strongly than samples of LL forms. Activation of TLR1 and TLR2 correlates with a Th1-pattern cytokine. On the other hand, inhibition of activation is associated with a Th2-pattern cytokine.[21] Both IL-12 and IL-10 are produced by DCs and inhibit the lymphoproliferative response after bacilli presentation.[22] In vivo studies demonstrated that monocytes and monocyte-derived DCs could be activated by *M. leprae* 19- and 33-kDa lipoproteins through TLR2.[21]

A susceptibility locus at chromosome 10p13 near the mannose receptor 1 gene exerts a role of genetics in the development of leprosy. These receptors are an important tool in phagocytosis.[23] Moreover, class II MHC genes have been involved with the clinical expression of this infection: *DR2* and *DR3* genes correlate with TT leprosy, and *DQ1* is most often related to the LL pole.[2] A recent study reinforces the role of *M. leprae* in the negative regulation of the immune response through decrease of the expression of various genes and mitochondrial metabolism related to the bacilli infection.[24]

Many other immune system components, such as neutrophils, have been implicated in the clinical phenotype and course of the disease. Analyses of erythema nodosum leprosum (ENL) show massive neutrophil migration and TLR2 and Fc receptor activation. This pathway includes IL-1b secretion, endothelial activation, neutrophil attachment, and up-regulation of inflammatory mediators.[11,25] It has been suggested that acetylated FoxP3 containing Treg cells may influence immune suppression in leprosy.[26]

3 ACUTE REACTIONS

Reactions are immunological complications that occur either before, during or after treatment and affect 30–50% of patients with leprosy.[12,27,28] The mechanisms of these reactions remain an enigma. These reactions seem to have different immunological mechanisms and trigger events, although they are poorly understood. There are two types of leprosy reactions: type 1, also known as T1R, reversal reaction (RR); and type 2, also referred as T2R, ENL. Both reactions may occur spontaneously, may be recurrent and persistent and are not exclusive.[29]

3.1 Reversal Reaction

Clinical manifestations of T1R include worsening of previous lesions with red and swollen patches, reactions that may result in severe nerve injury, dactylitis and arthralgia with puffy hands and feet, skin ulceration, and pain or tenderness in nerves with loss of function. These manifestations typically occur in patients with borderline (BT, BB, or BL) disease and may be associated with hormonal changes, such as during puerperium, or with antileprosy therapy.[2,30,31] T1R is also known as RR because it is caused by the upgrading of a patients' immune reactions, moving towards paucibacillary poles of the spectrum, or by down-grading and moving to the lepromatous pole, as suggested by clinical and histopathological evidence.[12,31] An infiltration of interferon-γ and tumor necrosis factor (TNF)-α-secreting CD4-positive lymphocytes can be demonstrated in the tissues.[32] It may be caused by increased cell-mediated immunity to the bacilli, even in the absence of therapy. The natural course may last for many weeks and result in neural irreversible damage.

3.2 Erythema Nodosum Leprosum

ENL is accompanied by systemic symptoms such as fever, arthralgia, weight loss and malaise, and affects patients with MB forms of the disease (BL and LL). They present with acute onset of disseminated erythematous nodules that may ulcerate and discharge sterile material that contains degenerating acid-fast bacilli and polymorphonuclear neutrophils. These findings are useful for diagnosis since they are rare in all other types of leprosy lesions. Some patients may have recurrences over several months. Other manifestations, such as episcleritis, anterior uveitis, orchitis, lymphadenopathy, myositis, and arthritis, may occur.[12] The pathogenesis may be related to immune complex deposition, although high circulating concentrations of TNF-α and other pro-inflammatory cytokines are seen in T2R and lead to neutrophil infiltration with activation of complement.[32] However, their role in the pathogenesis of the reaction remains unknown (Figure 1).[12]

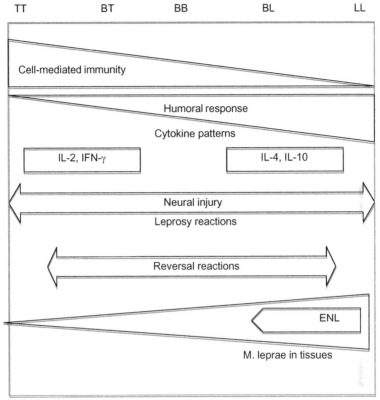

Figure 1   Clinical and immunological spectrum of leprosy. Adapted from Britton and Lockwood[32].

4 LUCIO'S PHEMOMENON

Lucio's phenomenon, also considered a variant of T2R, is a severe manifestation that occurs primarily in patients with Mexican ancestry.[33] This manifestation is associated with high morbidity and mortality. It is an acute necrotizing vasculopathy in untreated patients with longstanding LL. Patients presented with extensive and life-threatening ulcers that were related to high levels of cryoglobulins, but the real significance of these immune complexes in the pathogenesis remains unclear.[12,13,34] Moreover, the lesions are similar to those that occur in the antiphospholipid syndrome (APS).

Some of these manifestations resemble those of immune reconstitution inflammatory syndrome (IRIS). IRIS gained notoriety with the advent of highly active antiretroviral therapy (HAART) for HIV infection. It is an exacerbated immune response to a previous pathogen that occurs after the beginning of the treatment, with appearance of new symptoms or worsening of pre-existing manifestations. As *M. leprae* infection improves under specific therapy, the host immune system reacts against quiescent antigens in a severe manner,[35] showing the dynamic nature of the immune response to the bacilli. Excessive cytokine production and good response to immunosuppressive therapy reinforce this concept.[32] Curiously, patients infected with both HIV and leprosy experience rates of response to treatment similar to HIV-negative patients with leprosy,[35] and most patients co-infected with IRIS presented with preserved histological features, including granuloma formation, even in advanced disease. This fact suggests that local cell-mediated immunity may be intact in these patients.[35–39]

5 LEPROSY AND AUTOANTIBODIES

Although the presence of autoantibodies is considered to be a hallmark of autoimmune diseases, many chronic infections share these immunological abnormalities. Aberrant changes in the humoral immune system of patients with leprosy can be expressed by positive rheumatoid factor (RF) test and antinuclear antibodies (ANAs). The prevalence of autoantibodies varies widely among different studies (Table 1). Positive RF and ANA have been described in the LL pole, since MB status could act as a potent stimulus for immune complex generation. The different prevalence rates may reflect heterogeneous patients, the effects of antibiotics and differences in disease duration.[40] Kroumpouzos et al.[41] described a similar prevalence of anti-ssDNA between patients with systemic lupus erythematosus (SLE), LL leprosy, and tuberculosis. In most studies ANA prevalence varies from 0% to 30%, always in the LL pole. However ANA have been classified only as positive or negative, with little data about titration and patterns.[42–44] The appearance of ANAs may relate to weak cross-reactivity between mycobacterial antigens and human DNA. Also, chronic cell destruction and continuous exposition of hidden antigens perpetuate B-cell stimulation.[40]

RF is positive in erosive rheumatoid arthritis (RA) but its specificity is low; it has been positive in healthy individuals and many other neoplastic, autoimmune and infectious diseases, including leprosy. Antibodies against citrullinated peptides residues (anti-CCP) were described in the sera of patients with RA with higher specificity than RF. It was recently described in active lung tuberculosis, as well.[45] Other authors showed low prevalence of anti-CCP antibodies among patients with leprosy.[46,47] Furthermore, higher RF and anti–CCP titers in patients with the LL than TT pole have been described.[47,48] Zavala-Cerna et al.[48] did not find an association between high titers of these autoantibodies and rheumatic manifestations such as arthritis. Interestingly, a Brazilian study reported a positive association between autoimmune manifestations (arthritis and antibodies) and low serum concentrations of vitamin D, reinforcing the hypothesis that vitamin D deficiency could have a pathogenic role in the immune response in many chronic diseases.[49]

Antineutrophil cytoplasmic antibodies (ANCAs) are autoantibodies associated with systemic vasculitic syndromes, chiefly granulomatosis with polyangiitis, and have two immunofluorescence patterns: cytoplasmic (c-ANCA) and perinuclear (p-ANCA). Nonetheless, the spectrum of ANCA-positive diseases includes RA, SLE, ulcerative colitis, infective endocarditis, tuberculosis, HIV infection and leprosy. The use of some drugs, like propylthiouracil, can also induce ANCA positivity. A high prevalence of ANCA positivity has been shown in the LL pole. Medina et al.[50] detected MPO-related ANCA (p-ANCA) in patients with LL. Moreover, Pradhan et al.[51] found c-ANCA in 62.5% of patients, especially those in the LL pole. These findings were not replicated in a Brazilian study in which ANCA was tested in 20 patients but p-ANCA was found in only one patient.[52] Reactivity to heat shock proteins could be implicated in the origin of ANCA in leprosy and other infectious diseases.[50,53] Although still obscure, polyclonal B-cell activation by bacterial components may rely on the participation of T cells.[50]

Antiphospholipid antibodies (aPLs) are a group of autoantibodies implicated in the APS. In this setting they cause arterial or venous thrombosis, gestational complications, and many other manifestations. These antibodies have been reported in association with a variety of malignancies, drugs, and infectious diseases (syphilis, hepatitis C, parvovirus B19 and HIV infection, and leprosy). During the course of primary and secondary APS, these antibodies are directly implicated in the thrombotic phenomena in a β2-glycoprotein I (β2-GPI) dependent way. By contrast, in other disorders they are β2-GPI independent and may decline or even disappear after treatment.[54–58] aPLs are reported to be positive in 3–98% of patients with leprosy,[54,57,59–61] especially in MB forms. However, recent studies reported heterogeneity of β2-GPI dependent aPLs in leprosy, as demonstrated by Hojnik et al.[56] Histopathological findings in Lucio's phenomenon show microangiopathic thrombosis in the absence of inflammatory infiltration of the vessel walls, and Levy et al.[62] confirmed the β2-GPI dependence of aPLs in this condition. Anti-β2-GPI antibodies also were described in serum of patients with leprosy. In a Brazilian cohort of patients with leprosy, the prevalence of anti-cardiolipin (aCL) and anti-β2-GPI was higher in patients with LL than in healthy controls (15.8% vs. 3.1% [$p < 0.01$] and 46.2% vs. 9.4% [$p < 0.01$], respectively). Although the aPL positivity was β2-GPI dependent, there was no association with APS manifestations.[63] Genetic factors involved in the production of these antibodies include some polymorphisms at human chromosome 17q23-24.[64,65]

Some patients with infectious diseases have presented with thrombotic complications. Indeed, it has been shown that infection may trigger, as a "second hit", catastrophic APS in about 30% of cases. A probable explanation is the molecular mimicry phenomenon that is supported by the evidence of shared sequence homology of peptides between bacteria and viruses and β2-GPI binding site of aCL.[66] Moreover, gangrene of the extremities, a rare manifestation of the leprosy spectrum, has been associated with aPLs. In this setting intimal thickening and medial infiltration, as well as embolization of Virchow cell and vascular entrapment by nerve trunk hypertrophy, may contribute to arterial occlusion.[67–69]

Anti-mitochondrial,[57] anti-actin and anti-myosin,[41] and anti-endothelial cell antibodies[70] are other autoantibodies described in patients with leprosy. These antibodies activate endothelial cells, inducing apoptosis, and may be implicated in the pathogenesis of leprosy.[70]

6 LEPROSY AND OTHER DISEASES

HIV infection caused a profound effect on the incidence and clinicopathological features of tuberculosis. However, in contrast to *M. tuberculosis* infection, the incidence of leprosy is not higher among HIV-infected individuals. The clinical, immunological and pathological features are not influenced by *M. leprae*, even in advanced HIV. The decrease in CD4+ T cells would result in decreased ability to contain bacilli. Recent reviews showed that patients infected with both HIV and leprosy and who have a low CD4 count have borderline forms with well-formed granuloma; patients in the LL pole show diffuse macrophage infiltrates and CD8 lymphocytes,[71,72] the so called "granuloma paradox".[73] Nevertheless, there is a possible increase in the frequency of acute leprosy reactions, but the exact immunopathological mechanism underlying these is not clear. Impaired phagocytic function of macrophages with decreased clearance of *M. leprae* and an enhanced state of immune activation in HIV infection may be responsible.[74] Although epidemiological data suggest that tuberculosis accelerates a decline in immune function in HIV-infected patients, the natural course of both HIV infection and leprosy does not seem to be influenced by each other since marked pro-inflammatory cytokine drive is present only during severe acute reactions.[75] Furthermore, there is no evidence that co-infection decreases the efficacy of multi-drug therapy for leprosy. These individuals respond equally, with no indication for a prolonged treatment course.[74,75] Another paradox concerns the introduction of HAART for HIV infection. Co-infected patients may experience severe deterioration in clinical features after starting HAART, also known as IRIS, as described earlier.[74,75]

Several similarities exist between SLE and MB leprosy (LL).[76] Application of the American College of Rheumatology criteria for SLE in 100 patients with LL showed an elevated prevalence of clinical and even immunological criteria, as demonstrated by a Brazilian study.[77] However, more specific autoantibodies, such as anti-dsDNA, anti-Sm, anti-P, are infrequently found in leprosy sera.[78] After demonstrating monoclonal IgM autoantibodies in patients with the LL pole, some studies reported that idiotypes derived from 8E7 and TH9 antibodies share some epitopes with monoclonal antibodies from patients with SLE.[79–81] These data may suggest that a subset of B cells in both diseases encoded Ig-variable region genes and may explain several similarities between them.

TNF-α-blocking (anti-TNF) agents are effective therapy for chronic inflammatory conditions, especially RA and spondyloarthritis, but they also are associated with many adverse effects. In this regard this group of drugs causes disorganization of granulomas, high risk of neoplasms, and reactivation of latent granulomatous infections, such as mycobacterial infections. Pharmacological characteristics of anti-TNF may explain differences among them regarding efficacy and safety.[82,83] Some anti-TNF agents, for example, promote more apoptosis and reduce the serum concentrations of INF-γ, which may be crucial for inhibiting mycobacterial growth.[84] Infections caused by pathogens that require organized granuloma formation are associated with anti-TNF use, especially tuberculosis. There are few reported cases of leprosy in patients treated with anti-TNF therapy.[83,85–88] In a study based on the Brazilian Biological Registry (Brazil is an endemic area for leprosy), only one case of TT leprosy was reported.[89] Surprisingly, some patients developed acute leprosy reactions after discontinuing anti-TNF therapy.[85,90] This event could be explained by the restoration of cell-mediated immunity that was suppressed by TNF-blocking therapy,[85] similar to IRIS after HAART treatment in HIV-infected individuals. Indeed, severe polyarthritis, peripheral neuropathy, fever, and other systemic features may be misinterpreted as rheumatic manifestations.

Zhang et al.[91] scanned genetic markers of MB and paucibacillary leprosy among Chinese patients; a total of 93 single nucleotide polymorphisms were shown to have a significant association with leprosy. The data implicate many loci where several proteins are involved in microbial detection and in the innate immune response, such as *NOD2*, which recognizes a component of the mycobacterial wall. Interestingly, some of these genes also are associated with inflammatory bowel diseases. The authors report a link between susceptibility to leprosy and Crohn's disease.[91] Another study reviewed the negative association between psoriasis and leprosy.[92,93] The data reinforce the concept that enhanced innate immune response in psoriasis protects against many infections, including leprosy. The possible mechanisms involved include an elevated IL-12, IL-23, and IFN-γ cytokine pattern and reduced Treg cell activity that increase Th1 and Th17 immune response; heightened expression of antimicrobial peptides in sera of patients with psoriasis; up-regulation of TLR2 in dermal DCs, which is involved in the recognition of bacilli lipoproteins; and the absence of mutations in genes encoding the activation of the type 1 cytokine axis.[92] The small genomic variability of *M. leprae* may explain the reduced influence on host susceptibility.[94]

7 CONCLUSION

Leprosy remains a great challenge. Although most aspects of its pathophysiology and clinical behavior have been well known, our level of knowledge is not enough to eradicate this disease. It is important to keep in mind that great efforts are necessary to diagnose, treat precociously, prevent disability and contagion.

REFERENCES

1. Petrucelli RJ. The middle ages. In: Lyons AS, Petrucelli RJ, editors. *Medicine: an illustrated history*. New York: Abradale Press; 1987. p. 337–68.
2. Eichelmann K, González González SE, Salas-Alanis JC, Ocampo-Candiani J. Leprosy. An update: definition, pathogenesis, classification, diagnosis, and treatment. *Actas Dermosifiliogr* 2013;**104**:554–63.
3. Global leprosy situation, 2010. *Wkly Epidemiol Rec* 2010; 85:337–48.
4. Truman RW, Singh P, Sharma R, Busso P, Rougemont J, Paniz-Mondolfi A, et al. Probable zoonotic leprosy in the southern United States. *N Engl J Med* 2011;**364**:1626–33.
5. Moet FJ, Pahan D, Schuring RP, Oskam L, Richardus JH. Physical distance, genetic relationship, age, and leprosy classification are independent risk factors for leprosy in contacts of patients with leprosy. *J Infect Dis* 2006;**193**:346–53.

6. Davey TF, Rees RJ. The nasal discharge in leprosy: clinical and bacteriological aspects. *Lepr Rev* 1974;**25**:121–34.

7. Abraham S, Mozhi NM, Joseph GA, Kurian N, Rao PS, Job CK. Epidemiological significance of first skin lesion in leprosy. *Int J Lepr Other Mycobact Dis* 1998;**66**:131–9.

8. Bakker M, Hatta M, Kwenang A. Population survey to determine risk factors for *Mycobacterium leprae* transmission and infection. *Int J Epidemiol* 2004;**33**:1329–36.

9. van Beers SM, Hatta M, Klatser PR. Patient contact is the major determinant in incident leprosy; implications for future control. *Int J Lepr Other Mycobact Dis* 1999;**67**:119–28.

10. Eiglmeier K, Parkhill J, Honoré N, Garnier T, Tekaia F, Telenti A, et al. The decaying genome of *Mycobacterium leprae*. *Lepr Rev* 2001;**72**:387–98.

11. Gulia A, Fried I, Massone C. New insights in the pathogenesis and genetics of leprosy. *F1000 Med Rep* 2010;**2**:30(doi:10.3410/M2-30).

12. Scollard DM, Adams LB, Gillis TP, Krahenbuhl JL, Truman RW, Williams DL. The continuing challenges of leprosy. *Clin Microbiol Rev* 2006;**19**:338–81.

13. Sansonetti P, Lagrange PH. The immunology of leprosy: speculations on the leprosy spectrum. *Rev Infect Dis* 1981;**3**:422–69.

14. Ridley DS, Jopling WH. Classification of leprosy according to immunity. A five-group system. *Int J Lepr Other Mycobact Dis* 1966;**34**:255–73.

15. Pardillo FE, Fajardo TT, Abalos RM, Scollard D, Gelber RH. Methods for the classification of leprosy for treatment purposes. *Clin Infect Dis* 2007;**44**:1096–9.

16. Demangel C, Britton WJ. Interaction of dendritic cells with mycobacteria: where the action starts. *Immunol Cell Biol* 2000;**78**:318–24.

17. Rodrigues LS, da Silva ME, Moreira ME, Tempone AJ, Lobato LS, Ribeiro-Resende VT, et al. *Mycobacterium leprae* induces insulin-like growth factor and promotes survival of Schwann cells upon serum withdrawal. *Cell Microbiol* 2010;**12**:42–54.

18. Gimenez MF, Gigli I, Tausk FA. Differential expression of Langerhans cells in the epidermis of patients with leprosy. *Br J Dermatol* 1989;**121**:19–26.

19. Maeda Y, Gidoh M, Ishii N, Mukai C, Makino M. Assessment of cell mediated immunogenicity of *Mycobacterium leprae*-derived antigens. *Cell Immunol* 2003;**222**:69–77.

20. Mittal A, Mishra RS, Nath I. Accessory cell heterogeneity in lepromatous leprosy: dendritic cells and not monocytes support T cell responses. *Clin Exp Immunol* 1989;**76**:233–9.

21. Krutzik SR, Ochoa MT, Sieling PA, Uematsu S, Ng YW, Legaspi A, et al. Activation and regulation of toll-like receptors 2 and 1 in human leprosy. *Nat Med* 2003;**9**:525–32.

22. Santos AR, Suffys PN, Vanderborght PR, Moraes MO, Vieira LM, Cabello PH, et al. Role of tumor necrosis factor-alpha and interleukin-10 promoter gene polymorphisms in leprosy. *J Infect Dis* 2002;**186**:1687–91.

23. Alter A, Grant A, Abel L, Alcaïs A, Schurr E. Leprosy as a genetic disease. *Mamm Genome* 2011;**22**:19–31.

24. Saini C, Ramesh V, Nath I. CD4+ Th17 cells discriminate clinical types and constitute a third subset of non Th1, Th2 cells in human leprosy. *PLoS Negl Trop Dis* 2013;**9**:e2338.

25. Lee DJ, Li H, Ochoa MT, Tanaka M, Carbone RJ, Damoiseaux R, et al. Integrated pathways for neutrophil recruitment and inflammation in leprosy. *J Infect Dis* 2010;**201**:558–69.

26. Kumar S, Naqvi RA, Ali R, Rani R, Khanna N, Rao DN. CD4(+)CD25(+) T regs with acetylated FoxP3 are associated with immune suppression in human leprosy. *Mol Immunol* 2013;**56**:513–20.

27. Scollard DM, Smith T, Bhoopat L, Theetranont C, Rangdaeng S, Morens DM. Epidemiologic characteristics of leprosy reactions. *Int J Lepr Other Mycobact Dis* 1994;**62**:559–67.

28. Kumar B, Dogra S, Kaur I. Epidemiological characteristics of leprosy reactions: 15 years experience from North India. *Int J Lepr Other Mycobact Dis* 2004;**72**:125–33.

29. Gibson T. Bacterial infections: the arthritis of leprosy. *Baillieres Clin Rheumatol* 1995;**9**:179–91.

30. Rodríguez-Pazos L, Gómez-Bernal S, Sánchez-Aguilar D, Toribio J. Leprorreacción tipo 1 y embarazo. *Actas Dermosifiliogr* 2010;**101**:190–1.
31. Ridley DS, Radia KB. The histological course of reactions in borderline leprosy and their outcome. *Int J Lepr Other Mycobat Dis* 1981;**49**:383–92.
32. Britton WJ, Lockwood DN. Leprosy. *Lancet* 2004;**363**:1209–19.
33. Donner RS, Shively JA. The "Lucio phenomenon" in diffuse leprosy. *Ann Intern Med* 1967;**67**:831–6.
34. Quismorio Jr. FP, Rea T, Chandor S, Levan N, Friou GJ. Lucio's phenomenon: an immune complex deposition syndrome in lepromatous leprosy. *Clin Immunol Immunopathol* 1978;**9**:184–93.
35. Amerson EH, Maurer TA. Immune reconstitution inflammatory syndrome and tropical dermatoses. *Dermatol Clin* 2011;**29**:39–43.
36. Ustiantowski AP, Lawn SD, Lockwood DN. Interactions between HIV and leprosy: a paradox. *Lancet Infect Dis* 2006;**6**:350–60.
37. Couppié P, Abel S, Voinchet H, Roussel M, Hélénon R, Huerre M, et al. Immune reconstitution inflammatory syndrome associated with HIV and leprosy. *Arch Dermatol* 2004;**140**:997–1000.
38. Lawn SD, Wood C, Lockwood DN. Borderline tuberculoid leprosy: an immune reconstitution phenomenon in a human immunodeficiency virus-infected person. *Clin Infect Dis* 2003;**36**:e5–6.
39. Menezes VM, Sales AM, Illarramendi X, Miranda A, Gonçalves Morgado M, Gutierrez-Galhardo MC, et al. Leprosy reaction as a manifestation of immune reconstitution inflammatory syndrome: a case series of a Brazilian cohort. *AIDS* 2009;**23**:641–3.
40. Garcia-de la Torre I. Autoimmune phenomena in leprosy, particularly antinuclear antibodies and rheumatoid factor. *J Rheumatol* 1993;**20**:900–3.
41. Kroumpouzos G, Vareltzidis A, Konstadoulakis MM, Avgerinou G, Anastasiadis G, Kroubouzou H, et al. Evaluation of the autoimmune response in leprosy. *Lepr Rev* 1993;**64**:199–207.
42. Masala C, Amendolea MA, Nuti M, Riccarducci R, Tarabini CGL, Tarabini CG. Autoantibodies in leprosy. *Int J Lepr Other Mycobac Dis* 1979;**47**:171–5.
43. Miller RA, Wener MH, Harnisch JP, Gilliland BC. The limited spectrum of antinuclear antibodies in leprosy. *J Rheumatol* 1987;**14**:108–10.
44. Sharma VK, Saha K, Sehgal VN. Serum immunoglobulins and autoantibodies during and after erythema nodosum leprosum (ENL). *Int J Lepr Other Mycobact Dis* 1982;**50**:159–63.
45. Elkayam O, Segal R, Lidgi M, Caspi D. Positive anti-cyclic citrullinated proteins and rheumatoid factor during active lung tuberculosis. *Ann Rheum Dis* 2006;**65**:1110–2.
46. Guedes-Barbosa LS, Mangueira C, Scheinberg M. Anticitrulline peptide antibodies (CCP3) in leprosy sera: a negative association. *Clin Rheumatol* 2008;**27**:515–6.
47. Ribeiro SLE, Pereira HLA, Silva NP, Neves RMS, Sato EI. Anti-cyclic citrullinated peptide antibodies and rheumatoid factor in leprosy patients with articular involvement. *Braz J Med Biol Res* 2008;**41**:1005–10.
48. Zavala-Cerna MG, Fafutis-Morris M, Guille-Vargas C, Salazar-Páramo M, García-Cruz DE, Riebeling C, et al. Anti-cyclic citrullinated peptide antibodies and rheumatoid factor sera titers in leprosy patients from Mexico. *Rheumatol Int* 2012;**32**:3531–6.
49. Ribeiro SLE, Pereira HAL, Mangueira CM, Ferreira CES, Rosseto E, Scheinberg M. The development of arthritis and antinuclear antibodies correlate with serum 25-hydroxyvitamin D levels in patients with leprosy. *Ann Rheum Dis* 2012;**71**:2062–3.
50. Medina F, Camargo A, Moreno J, Zonana-Nacach A, Aceves-Avila J, Fraga A. Antineutrophil cytoplasmic autoantibodies in leprosy. *Br J Rheumatol* 1998;**37**:270–3.

51. Pradhan V, Badakere SS, Shankar Kumar U. Increased incidence of cytoplasmic ANCA (cANCA) and other autoantibodies in leprosy patients from western India. *Lepr Rev* 2004;**75**:50–6.
52. Edington FLB, Bacellar MOAR, Machado PR, Barbosa L, Reis E, Reis M, et al. Anti-neutrophil cytoplasmic antibodies in leprosy. *Clin Rheumatol* 2007;**26**:208–10.
53. Esaguy N, Águas AP, van Embden JDA, Silva MT. Mycobacteria and human autoimmune disease: direct evidence of cross-reactivity between human lactoferrin and the 65-kilodalton protein of tubercle and leprosy bacilli. *Infect Immun* 1991;**59**:1117–25.
54. Loizou S, Singh S, Wypkema E, Asherson RA. Anticardiolipin anti-beta2-glycoprotein I and antiprothrombin antibodies in black South African patients with infectious disease. *Ann Rheum Dis* 2003;**62**:1106–11.
55. Sammaritano LR, Gharavi AE, Lockshin MD. Antiphospholipid antibody: immunologic and clinical aspects. *Semin Arthritis Rheum* 1990;**20**:81–96.
56. Hojnik M, Gilburd B, Ziporen L, Blank M, Tomer Y, Scheinberg MA, et al. Anticardiolipin antibodies in infections are heterogeneous in their dependence on beta2-glycoprotein I: analysis of anticardiolipin antibodies in leprosy. *Lupus* 1994;**3**:515–21.
57. Guedes-Barbosa LS, Gilbrut B, Shoenfeld Y, Scheinberg MA. Autoantibodies in leprosy sera. *Clin Rheumatol* 1996;**15**:26–8.
58. de Laranaga GF, Forastieiro RR, Carreras LO, Alonso BS. Different types of antiphospholipid antibodies in AIDS: a comparison with syphilis and the antiphospholipid syndrome. *Thromb Res* 1999;**96**:19–25.
59. Zandman-Goddard G, Blank M, Shoenfeld Y. Antiphospholipid antibodies and infections-drugs. In: Asherson RA, Cervera R, Piette JC, Shoenfeld Y, editors. *The antiphospholipid syndrome II*. Amsterdam: Elsevier Science; 2002. p. 343–60.
60. Elbeialy A, Strassburger-Lorna K, Altsumi T, Bertolaccini ML, Amengual O, Hanafi M, et al. Antiphospholipid antibodies in leprotic patients: a correlation with disease manifestation. *Clin Exp Rheumatol* 2000;**18**:492–4.
61. de Laranaga GF, Forastiero RR, Martinuzzo ME, Carreras LO, Tsariktsian G, Sturno MM, et al. High prevalence of antiphospholipid antibodies in leprosy: evaluation of antigen reactivity. *Lupus* 2000;**9**:594–600.
62. Levy RA, Pierangeli SA, Espinola RG. Antiphospholipid beta-2 glycoprotein I dependency assay to determine antibody pathogenicity. *Arthritis Rheum* 2000;**43**(Suppl.):1476.
63. Ribeiro SLE, Pereira HLA, Silva NP, Souza AWS, Sato EI. Anti-ß2 glycoprotein I antibodies are highly prevalent in a large number of Brazilian leprosy patients. *Acta Reumatol Port* 2011;**36**:30–7.
64. Brochado MJF, Figueiredo JFC, Mendes-Junior CT, Louzada-Junior P, Kim OM, Roselino AM. Correlation between beta-2-glycoprotein I gene polymorphism and anti-beta-2 glycoprotein I antibodies in patients with multibacillary leprosy. *Arch Dermatol Res* 2010;**302**:583–91.
65. Brochado MJF, Louzada-Junior P, Roselino AM, Nascimento MMP, Figueiredo JFC. Val24Leu polymorphism of ß2 glycoprotein I gene may justify the genesis of antiß2GPI antibodies and antiphospholipid syndrome in multibacillary leprosy. *An Bras Dermatol* 2009;**84**:355–9.
66. Asherson RA, Shoenfeld Y. The role of infections in the pathogenesis of catastrophic antiphospholipid syndrome—molecular mimicry? *J Rheumatol* 2000;**27**:12–14.
67. Kaur S, Wahi PL, Chakravarti RN, Sodhi JS, Vadhwa MB, Khera AS. Peripheral vascular deficit in leprosy. *Int J Lepr Other Mycobact Dis* 1976;**44**:332–9.
68. Bakos L, Correa CC, Bergmann L, Bonamigo RR, Muller LF. Antiphospholipid antibodies thrombotic syndrome misdiagnosed as Lucio's phenomenon. *Int J Lepr Other Mycobact Dis* 1996;**64**:320–3.
69. Akerkar SM, Bichile LS. Leprosy and gangrene: a rare association; role of antiphospholipid antibodies. *BMC Infectious Dis* 2005;**5**:74–6.

70. Dugué C, Perraut R, Youinou P, Renaudineau Y. Effects of anti-endothelial cell anti-bodies in leprosy and malaria. *Infect Immun* 2004;**72**:301–9.
71. Sampaio EP, Caneshi JRT, Nery JA, Duppre NC, Pereira GM, Vieira LM, et al. Cellular immune response to *Mycobacterium leprae* infection in human immunodeficiency virus-infected individuals. *Infect Immun* 1995;**63**:1848–54.
72. Carvalho KL, Maeda S, Marti L, Yamashita J, Haslett PAJ, Kallas EG. Immune cellular parameters of leprosy and human immunodeficiency virus-1 coinfected subjects. *Immunology* 2008;**124**:206–14.
73. Adya KA, Inamadar AC, Palit A. Paradoxes in dermatology. *Indian Dermatol J* 2013;**4**:133–42.
74. Lockwood DNJ, Lambert SM. Human immunodeficiency virus and leprosy: an update. *Dermatol Clin* 2011;**29**:125–8.
75. Ustianowski AP, Lawn SD, Lockwood DNJ. Interactions between HIV infection and leprosy: a paradox. *Lancet Infect Dis* 2006;**6**:350–60.
76. Paira SO, Roverano S. The rheumatic manifestations of leprosy. *Clin Rheumatol* 1991;**10**:274–6.
77. Teixeira Júnior GJ, Silva CEF, Magalhães V. Application of the diagnostic criteria for systemic lupus erythematosus to patients with multibacillary leprosy. *Rev Soc Bras Med Trop* 2011;**44**:85–90.
78. Bonfá E, Llovet R, Scheinberg M, de Souza JM, Elkon KB. Comparison between auto-antibodies in malaria and leprosy with lupus. *Clin Exp Immunol* 1987;**70**:529–37.
79. Mackworth-Young CG, Sabbaga J, Schwartz RS. Idiotypic markers of polyclonal B cell activation. Public idiotypes shared by monoclonal antibodies derived from patients with systemic lupus erythematosus or leprosy. *J Clin Invest* 1987;**79**:572–81.
80. Mackworth-Young CG. Cross-reactive idiotypes in sera from patients with leprosy, lupus and Lyme disease and from healthy individuals. *Clin Exp Immunol* 1990;**79**:78–82.
81. Mackworth-Young CG, Cairns E, Sabbaga J, Massicotte H, Diamond B, Bell DA, et al. Comparative study of idiotypes on monoclonal antibodies derived from patients with lupus and leprosy and from normal individuals. *J Autoimmunity* 1990;**3**:415–19.
82. Wallis RS, Broder MS, Wong JY, Hanson ME, Beenhouwer DO. Granulomatous infectious diseases associated with tumor necrosis factor antagonists. *Clin Infect Dis* 2004;**38**:1261–5.
83. Freitas DS, Machado N, Andrigueti FV, Reis Neto ET, Pinheiro MM. Lepromatous leprosy associated with the use of anti-TNFα therapy: case report. *Bras J Rheumatol* 2010;**50**:333–9.
84. Furst DE, Wallis R, Broder M, Beenhouwer DO. Tumor necrosis factor antagonists: different kinetics and/or mechanisms of action may explain differences in the risk for developing granulomatous infection. *Semin Arthritis Rheum* 2006;**36**:159–67.
85. Scollard DM, Joyce MP, Gillis TP. Development of leprosy and type 1 leprosy reactions after treatment with infliximab: a report of 2 cases. *Clin Infect Dis* 2006;**43**:e19–22.
86. Oberstein EM, Kromo O, Tozman EC. Type I reaction of Hansen's disease with expo-sure to adalimumab: a case report. *Arthritis Rheum* 2008;**59**:1040–3.
87. Vilela Lopes R, Barros Ohashi C, Helena Cavaleiro L, de Britto Pereira Cruz R, da Veiga RR, Fernando Ribeiro Miranda M, et al. Development of leprosy in a patient with ankylosing spondylitis during the infliximab treatment: reactivation of a latent infection? *Clin Rheumatol* 2009;**28**:615–17.
88. Lluch P, Urruticoechea A, Lluch J, Moll MC, Matos M, Benet JM, et al. Development of leprosy in a patient with rheumatoid arthritis during treatment with etanercept: a case report. *Sem Arthritis Rheum* 2012;**42**:127–30.
89. Titton DC, Silveira IG, Louzada-Júnior P, Hayata AL, Carvalho HM, Ranza R, et al. Brazilian biological registry: BiobadaBrasil implementation process and preliminary results. *Bras J Rheumatol* 2011;**51**:145–60.
90. Camacho ID, Valencia I, Rivas MP, Burdick AE. Type 1 leprosy reaction manifesting after discontinuation of adalimumab therapy. *Arch Dermatol* 2009;**145**:349–51.

91. Zhang F-R, Huang W, Chen S-M, Sun LD, Liu H, Li Y, et al. Genomewide association study of leprosy. *N Engl J Med* 2009;**361**:2609–18.
92. Bassukas ID, Gaitanis G, Hundeiker M. Leprosy and the natural selection for psoriasis. *Med Hypot* 2012;**78**:183–90.
93. Kumar B, Raychaudhuri SP, Vossough S, Farber EM. The rare co-existence of leprosy and psoriasis. *Int J Dermatol* 1992;**31**:551–4.
94. Schurr E, Gros P. A common genetic fingerprint in leprosy and Crohn's disease? *N Engl J Med* 2009;**361**:2666–8.

CHAPTER 35

Screening Strategies for the Identification of Latent Tuberculosis

E. Záňová[1], D. Kozáková, J. Rovenský
National Institute of Rheumatic Disease, Piešťany, Slovakia
[1]Corresponding Author: rovensky.jozef@nurch.sk

1 INTRODUCTION

Nowadays, many different therapeutics are prescribed for the treatment of systemic autoimmune disorders, including novel biological treatments, than before.[1] In the last 10 years, many TNF-α inhibitors played a crucial role in the treatment of autoimmune inflammatory diseases, namely rheumatoid arthritis (RA), psoriatic arthritis (PsA), ankylosing spondylitis (AS), juvenile idiopathic arthritis (JIA), idiopathic inflammatory bowel diseases, psoriasis, and others. The number of diagnoses successfully treated in clinical trials is increasing.[2] TNF-α inhibitors have been used for more than 15 years in clinical settings. The key role of TNF-α in the pathogenesis of RA was discovered by the work group of Sir R. Maini in 1992.[3] TNF-α exerts both local and systemic effects and plays a role in many autoimmune and protective mechanisms in organisms.[4–6] Inhibiting TNF-α by administering anti-TNF-α antibody suppresses pathological inflammatory processes on several levels and hence is currently the most effective tool for the treatment of the aforementioned rheumatic diseases. The basic aim of the treatment is to induce remission and suppress the activity of the disease.[1,7–9] The treatment's effectiveness in, for example, RA is measured according to the ACR improvement criteria (20, 50, 70). Alternatively, a positive response to the treatment may be measured as a change of DAS (>1.2). The functional stage is evaluated by the HAQ.[3,10]

TNF-α is a part of the human immune response to an infection.[11,12] Prescriptions containing the TNF-α inhibitors inhibit the immune response and thus contribute to imbalance of the immune system. The long-term inhibition of TNF-α, a key cytokine crucially involved in the pathogenesis of

Infection and Autoimmunity
http://dx.doi.org/10.1016/B978-0-444-63269-2.00039-8

RA,[13] is accompanied by the increased risk of infectious complications,[14–16,74] mainly activation of chronic latent tuberculosis (TB) infection (LTBI),[17] sepsis or mycotic and other opportunistic infections. In case of a minor active infection (urinary and respiratory tract, sinusitis), the anti-TNF-α treatment has to be interrupted and the infection cured.[18] In case of a more severe infection, approved therapeutic approaches are followed. Some patients undergoing the treatment with TNF-α blockers may develop cancer, congestive heart failure, demyelination and other neurological disorders, pancytopenia (infliximab, etanercept), and lupus-like syndrome. A negative reaction to the site of treatment administration (injection, infusion) may also appear.[6,11]

The long-term safety of anti-TNF-α treatment is unknown.[19] A meta-analysis of clinical studies using infliximab (after 4 or 5 doses) and adalimumab showed increased risk of infectious complications and tumor growths.[19] However, it should be mentioned that complete information about patients who suffer infectious complications associated with treatment with immunosuppressants and corticosteroids is lacking. A possible reactivation of TB during an anti-TNF-α treatment, resulting from the addition of another immunomodulator (immunosuppressant) into an already immunosuppressive environment, should be considered.[19]

TB knows no borders. The incidence of TB is twice as high in men as in women[20], and its incidence among patients treated with biological treatment is closely related to the overall incidence of TB in the human population.

The worldwide incidence of TB is a warning. It is estimated that 32% of the population (1.86 billion people) is infected with TB. Eight million new cases develop annually, of which 3.52 million are confirmed positive by microscopy, and 2.8 million people die of diseases directly or indirectly related to TB.[21] The WHO estimates that without improvement in health care, another billion of people will become infected, 200 million will develop TB, and 35 million will die by the year 2020.[22]

The majority of TB cases occur in developing countries. In developed countries, TB occurs mainly among immigrants from developing countries with a high incidence of TB.[75] The risk factors for TB persistence vary: poverty, few health care providers, living in overcrowded regions, stress, smoking (increases the risk by three), gastrectomy (increases the risk by five) and contact with people with active infection (increases the risk by five). The US Centers for Disease Control and Prevention (CDC) reported the incidence as 5.8–6.6 per 100,000 people in the common population (non-Hispanic population, 2.2 per 100,000) between 1999 and 2000 and did not find an increased amount of TB infection among patients with RA.[23] In Spain, the incidence of TB was 21 per 100,000 people in 2000.

In patients with RA without any anti-TNF-α treatment, the incidence was 95 per 100,000 patients in 1990–2000 (the EMECAR cohort). The risk of TB in patients with RA is 4.13 times higher than in the rest of the population.[19] However, it should be mentioned that complete information about patients who suffer infectious complications associated with immunosuppressant and corticosteroid treatment is lacking. Pulmonary TB was observed after treatment with methotrexate[24] and after systemic and pulse corticosteroid therapy.[25] Differential diagnosis of TB is usually challenging.[26,27] Decreased cellular immunity in patients with RA is substantial and increases the risk of pulmonary TB in these patients. Because of this, RA is treated with infliximab and TB is treated with the addition of methotrexate (etanercept was not combined with methotrexate in the period of the highest reactivation of LTBI). It is likely that methotrexate may have a synergistic effect with the immunosuppressive and antigranulomatous effects of infliximab.[24]

2 THE ROLE OF TNF-α IN THE FORMATION OF GRANULOMAS

The basic mechanism by which the organism protects itself against *Mycobacterium tuberculosis* infection is the formation of granulomas, inside which the microorganisms are localized. The first line of defence consists of alveolar macrophages that engulf inhaled *M. tuberculosis* bacteria. Such activated macrophages produce large amounts of cytokines,[28] chemokines and antimicrobial effector molecules, which influence the activation of specific immune responses, such as the maturation of antigen-presenting cells and their transport to lymphatic nodes or the activation of T lymphocytes and their transport to the site of infection. In the case of positive infection, the result is a formation of granulomas[29] with centrally positioned infected macrophages surrounded by activated T lymphocytes. Such granulomas represent a reliable physical and immunological barrier against the further spread of the pathogen. Production of TNF-α is required for the formation and maintenance of the granulomas, which isolate the bacteria.[30] This manifestation is consistent with the primary TB infection. In the case of unsuccessful granuloma production by the infected organism, a massive TB infection may occur. On the other hand, if there is a successful immune response, the infection evolves into a dormant or latent form, where it may stay undetected for several years. Under certain conditions (e.g. long-term decreased concentrations of TNF-α), the infection may be reactivated – this is known as a postprimary infection. TNF-α is an important cytokine in several steps of the formation and stabilization of the granulomas.[31]

TNF-α produced by macrophages is necessary for the activation of apoptosis in the activated macrophages (destroying mycobacteria) and maturation of dendritic cells (DCs) (antigen-presenting cells), which then activate T lymphocytes. DCs are present in the epithelial layers and react with mycobacteria through interaction of bacterial lipoarabinomannan and DC-specific lectin C. Disruption of this bond leads to incorrect presentation of the antigens by macrophages.[32,33] TNF-α enhances the transfer of monocytes and activated T lymphocytes through the vascular endothelium (TNF-α upregulates the expression of vascular cell adhesion molecules and influences the secretion of chemokines and their receptors) to enhance the expression of other adhesive molecules, which ensure spatial organization of T lymphocytes and macrophages within the granulomas. TNF-α influences cell death and granuloma reorganization and contributes to pulmonary necrosis and disease persistence.[34,35]

3 LATENT TUBERCULOSIS INFECTION

Patients with LTBI[10] are not contagious, their tuberculin skin test (TST) is positive and alive but inactive *M. tuberculosis* bacteria reside within them. The bacteria are present in a so-called dormant form. Such patients do not feel ill and are not contagious until their immune system becomes weakened. The TB bacteria may profit from that weakness and activate.[36] Not all patients diagnosed with TB bacteria develop active tuberculosis. In most infected people the infection stays in the dormant form. It is estimated that active disease develops only in 10–12% of infected people.[37] Only 10–30% of people exposed to mycobacteria develop LTBI, and 10% of them develop active disease. This leads to the development of a reservoir of noncured LTBI, which represents the major source of active TB disease.

The highest risk for disease activation is present within 2 years after infection and decreases over time.[38] The LTBI complicates the diagnostics. The risk of the active disease developing among *M. tuberculosis*-infected patients varies. The screening for LTBI is desirable in all examined subjects as well as health care providers. Immigrants comprise an important group in which active TB often develops within 2 years after immigration.[39] Another huge group consists of patients with a risk of immunosuppression and patients prepared for immunosuppressive and biological treatment.

According to adverse effect classification, the disease develops as an immunodeficient reaction type γ. LTBI usually progresses quickly, with no tendency for marginalization of infectious foci, and hence spreads quickly within the pulmonary parenchyma and its proximity. It is well known that extra-pulmonary localizations are prevalent. The standard diagnostic approach becomes limited. After the reactivation of LTBI in patients treated with an anti-TNF-α treatment, more than 50% of TB represents the extra-pulmonary form (lymphatic node, complex liver and spleen affection, urogenital tract) and more than 25% is present as the disseminated form.[40] In comparison to the healthy, immunocompetent population, the extra-pulmonary form is manifested in 15% and disseminated in 1% of cases.

An increased risk of TB infection also was documented after administration of the TNF-α receptor antagonist etanercept, as well as the fully humanized antibody adalimumab. During treatment with infliximab, development of active TB disease is described as fast, occurring in a median of 12 weeks. In 98% of cases, the disease develops within 6 months after beginning anti-TNF-α treatment. The prevalent extra-pulmonary and disseminated forms of the disease may have severe progression in and become life-threatening for immunocompromised patients.[41] This trend was found to be increased during treatment with monoclonal antibodies, mainly infliximab,[42] in comparison to other anti-TNF-α treatments. It is caused by the mechanism of action of the antibody (stable bond with TNF-α). The bond of etanercept to membranous TNF-α creates unstable complexes; the majority binds to soluble TNF-α and lymphotoxin. TNF-α, which is released, renders its biological activity. Thus, complete neutralization of TNF-α by infliximab may lead to the disruption of granulomas and possible TB reactivation. On the other hand, etanercept renders a part of TNF-α active,[43] which could possibly contribute to the preservation of the structures of the granulomas. Patients with LTBI have a 4.5 times higher risk of disease reactivation after beginning anti-TNF-α (infliximab) treatment.[44]

In a group of patients assigned to a "biological treatment register" in Slovakia (fulfilled until December 2008) who were treated by anti-TNF-α treatment, low prevalence of LTBI reactivation was found – 0.55% – with an incidence of 0.27 per 100 patients per year. According to data obtained from this register, 4 of 734 patients developed TB: 3 women with RA and 1 man with AS. Three of these four cases were extra-pulmonary (one peritonitis, one urogenital infection and one pleuritis) and one was pulmonary (miliary TB). The median time to develop active disease from LTBI was 11.5 months (range, 3.5–22 months). Until the end of 2008, we noted extra-pulmonary TB in 75% of patients subjected to anti-TNF-α treatment.[45] The last reported case was a 55-year-old man with RA and extra-pulmonary affection of the knee with fistula.

Thorough screening for LTBI before beginning a biological treatment significantly reduces the incidence of active TB by 85%. The standard diagnostic approaches of LTBI are medical history and clinical examination, chest radiography, TST and examination of interferon (IFN)-γ levels (interferon-γ release assay [IGRA] tests).

The medical history evaluation is an important part of the examination. Especially during screening for LTBI, it is important to document the history of exposure. An unrecognized LTBI may progress to active TB. When collecting the history, one must bear in mind that a person with acute TB is a threat to everyone he or she is in contact with and thus "enlivens" the TB cycle.[46] After the discovery of any new TB case, fast monitoring of all family members and co-workers with repeated TST is required. The examination is performed within 2–3 months after the exposition to the disease and repeated after 1 year.

Indications of LTBI on a chest radiograph are signs of either surpassed massive TB infection (healed caverns, thickened apical areas, pleura, apicalization, and calcifications) or minor alterations.[46] Minor alterations can be seen, but are not inevitable, upon examination of the radiograph. These findings are usually clinically silent and detected only coincidentally. Small shadows of calcifications typical for post-primary TB are included here. CT examination is the best way to detect small granulomas in pulmonary parenchyma.[47] In a study published in May 2009, the authors investigated the possibility of using CT examination to improve LTBI diagnostics; they correlated the CT results with those obtained from a quantiferon-gold test (QFT-G). The study was performed to investigate the contacts after the spread of TB at a university (a cohort of 1044 employees and students). The authors performed CT examination of lungs and mediastinum, which, together with a positive QFT-G test and negative chest radiographs in patients with active TB, showed possible TB-associated alterations in 52% of the patients.[47] Evans et al.[48] described 4 of 16 patients with negative IGRA tests who had older post-tubercular alterations on their chest radiographs. The majority of cases of primary TB infection progresses without clinical symptoms and hence are not diagnosed and treated. In the chest radiographs of untreated patients, various foci of primary TB may be seen as foci with deposits of calcium salts. These deposits are the source of clinically manifested TB, which either directly follows the primary disease or may evolve later after the bacteria multiply within these foci or within macrophages.[49]

TST in patients with RA is often accompanied by anergy (43% of patients with RA compared to 2% of the healthy population). A drawback of this method is its inability to distinguish between non-pathogenic mycobacteria (NTM) and BCG vaccination against *M. tuberculosis*. A smaller study showed smaller diameter of TST induration in patients with RA compared to healthy immunocompetent controls;[20] this way the amount of false-negative results in patients with RA increases (median TST induration is 4.5–11.5 mm [$p < 0.01$]; 79 of 112 (70.6%) vs. 5 of 69 (26%) [$p < 0.01$]). Laffitte et al. documented that 20% of false-negative results obtained by TST were diagnosed as positive by IGRA.[20] By combining both tests, the possibility of false-negative results was excluded.[45] False-negative results obtained by TST in non-diagnosed LTBI may lead to flare-up of active TB disease.[38]

Several high-risk groups in the United States are recognized. In most non-vaccinated people with induration >10 mm in combination with HIV infection or with proof of old, healed TB, the lifelong risk of the reactivation of LTBI is higher than 20%. The lifelong risk of TB flare-up in 10–20% in people with recent TST conversion and in people younger than 35 years treated with infliximab and with TST induration >15 mm.[49] Children younger than the age of 5 with a TST induration ≥ 10 mm are at high risk of TB flare-up, with a lifelong risk from 10% to 20%.

Nowadays, alternative testing strategies to TST are the IGRA tests QuantiFERON TB Gold and T.SPOT.TB. These tests enable significantly more exact and faster diagnosis of infections caused by *M. tuberculosis*. Tests are based on the ability of effector T lymphocytes stimulated by specific TB antigens to produce the cytokine IFN-γ. The key role of IFN-γ in the defence against infection with mycobacteria, and its elevation in patients with TB showed that the cytokine is a promising biomarker of protective immunity.[50]

The QFT-G test is a breakthrough in the diagnosis of *M. tuberculosis* infection. The first tests were performed in 1990 in cattle (marked as Bovigam), with *Mycobacterium bovis* as the tested antigen. The first human study was published in 1997, followed by a large study by the CDC in 2001 and approval by the US FDA. QFT-G is a novel, more exact, indirect *in vitro* diagnostic test that is useful in uncovering *M. tuberculosis* infection (including active disease). The test is based on the principle of so-called bulk method. The principle is in the measurement of the concentration of IFN-γ produced by effector T lymphocytes in heparinized blood stimulated by specific mycobacterial antigens (ESAT-6, CFP-10, and TB-7 = p4). These antigens are not present in any of the strains included in the BCG vaccine or non-tuberculous mycobacteria, with exception of *M. kansasi*, *M. szulgai*, and *M. marinum*. The production of specific IFN-γ is then quantified by ELISA. It is appropriate to correlate QFT-G with other methods for examination of LTBI (risk assessment, radiography and other medical and diagnostic approaches).[51] The test is not recommended for the diagnostics of the active TB.[52] For fast detection of acute TB infection, the molecular biology methods are recommended (PCR).

The result of the test may be negative, positive, or uncertain. A positive result means the presence of LTBI; negative means the opposite. The positive result should not be the only diagnostic criterion for *M. tuberculosis* infection and should be combined with other medical and diagnostic examinations. A negative test result does not exclude the possibility of *M. tuberculosis* infection or TB disease.[41]

The possibility of obtaining false-positive or false-negative results is linked with this test. A false-positive result may be caused by not following the 48-h interval between the TST application and the collection of a blood sample to measure the level of the specific IFN-γ (the IFN-γ level oscillates during the 1–6 weeks after TST application), by technical mistakes (incorrect blood collection, sample transport and storage), by the presence of cytomegalovirus or the persistence of repeated positivity of quantiferon after an anti-TB treatment.[45,53]

False-negative results may occur if, for example, the blood sample was collected before a cellular immune reaction developed, during anti-TB treatment, immune function disruptions and other diseases, by incorrectly manipulating the blood collecting tubes after blood collection (incorrect mixing, incorrect amount of blood collected), incorrectly performing the testing procedure or other immunological variables.[54]

Indeterminate results may occur in immunocompromised patients, suggesting that it is impossible to determine the state of the infection caused by *M. tuberculosis* in these patients and that whether this infection really exists cannot be determined. In healthy immunocompetent people (those with low risk of TB infection, e.g. health care providers) the incidence of uncertain results obtained from QFT-G tests is very low (0–0.35%).

4 THE TEST FOR ESTABLISING THE NUMBER OF CELLS PRODUCING IFN-γ T.SPOT

T.SPOT.TB is a breakthrough *in vitro* diagnostic test based on the principles of the so-called single-cell method, or ELISpot, which enables the overall number of IFN-γ-producing T lymphocytes to be established. In contrast with QFT-G, there is no need for special collecting tubes during T.SPOT.TB (collection into lithium–heparin tubes) because the specific antigens ESAT-6 and CFP-10 are added to the sample later in the laboratory. This method uses an exactly defined and equal number of isolated mononuclear cells; because of this there is no bias from IFN-γ produced by other cell populations. T.SPOT.TB is a novel, sensitive standard used mainly in immunocompromised patients; the false-negative result bias is very low among patients taking corticosteroids with this test in comparison to TST.[55] The test is appropriate for diagnosing LTBI as well as TB. No uncertain results are mentioned in the test description, and increased laboratory intensity is declared. The product has been approved for use in the European Union in 2004 and by the US FDA in 2008. It is expected that this product will set a new tone in TB diagnosing, especially in patients with negative TST results.[56] Six or more positive "spots" on the T.SPOT.TB test indicate a positive result.[57] The use of T.SPOT.TB alone or in combination with TST in LTBI screening is highly financially favorable in light of the financial costs of TB outbursts and disease prevention.[58]

5 QFT-G TEST VERSUS T.SPOT.TB

Clinical studies showed that T.SPOT.TB is more sensitive in children aged younger than 5 years. In immunocompromised patients, small deviations between the tests may appear. QFT-G is more automated; T.SPOT.TB can be read faster (8 h after blood collection). This can cause problems when the samples need to be transported long distances. QFT-G enables transport for 16 h, or the material can be incubated at the site of collection, and the time of transport may be elongated for up to 3 days.[59] For T.SPOT.TB, the number of uncertain results is described by an incidence of 0–5.4%; for QFT-G, the incidence of uncertain results is 10–12%. It seems that uncertain results are connected to immunosuppression and very young or very old age (less than 5 or more than 80 years).[60]

The specificity of QFT-G (95% CI) in the BCG-vaccinated healthy population ranges between 0.94 and 0.98, whereas the specificity of the TST is between 0.43 and 0.73. In the non–BCG-vaccinated population, the specificity of QFT-G and TST are equal.[47] In LTBI, the sensitivity of the QFT-G test (67%) is lower compared to the T.SPOT.TB (99.4%), but the ratio of specificity is inverted (QFT-G, 99.4% vs. T.SPOT.TB, 98%).

The importance of using both IGRA tests for diagnostics has recently increased, mainly in relation to biological treatments, especially anti-TNF-α therapies. Using our own observations, we aimed to evaluate the benefit of the QFT-G test in diagnosing LTBI in comparison to the standard diagnostic approaches (medical history, clinical examination, radiography, TST) in patients before beginning anti-TNF-α treatment. The studied group consisted of 328 patients (132 men and 196 women). The average age of the patients in the cohort was 46.79 years (women, 47.357 years; men, 45.95 years). The average age of patients with RA was 49.31 years; patients with AS were on average 39.79 years old and patients with PsA were 50.74 years old. The results often showed low positivity or anergy in TST. The disagreement between TST positivity and IGRA negativity may be present in BCG-vaccinated patients; TST negativity and IGRA positivity may be present in patients treated with corticosteroids. The positive results of IGRA tests, in contrast to TST, are closely related to the presence of risk factors for LTBI.[61] We found that none of the standard diagnostic methods (medical history, chest radiograph, TST) proved successful in detecting 32.25% of the QFT-G-positive patients with the dormant form of LTBI. Medical history collection in the main group correlated with LTBI presence only in 3.20% of the cases (31 patients). Chest radiography was successful in diagnosing LTBI in only 32% of cases. Positive TST results were in line with LTBI in 29%. The combination of these methods in comparison to QFT-G decreased the overall diagnostic compliance of LTBI. A positive chest radiography combined with TST detected 21% of QFT-G-positive patients with LTBI. A combination of medical history collection, chest radiography and TST compared to QFT-G alone showed compliance of 3.20%. Overall, we found 13 positive TST results, of which 69% were diagnosed with LTBI. False-positive results were found in 31% of the cases. Those were saved from an unnecessary chemoprophylactic treatment. In 22 patients with LTBI, the TST test result was negative, meaning that 71% of the patients showed false-negative results. Hypoergy and anergy of TST could be related to the well-known immunosuppressive variables (treatment, disease itself) present in rheumatic patients.

In our study we also emphasized examination of uncertain results. They showed two different groups of IFN-γ levels (NIL, mitogen, TB antigens).

The low level significantly correlated with male sex ($p < 0.005$). In women, both high and low levels were found. High level of IFN-γ significantly correlated with female sex when compared to males ($p < 0.005$). The lowest p value (0.00038) that was obtained by comparing men to women was from IFN-γ measurement in mitogen, followed by NIL ($p = 0.0089$) and TB antigen ($p = 0.019$). The influence of male and female hormones on the levels of IFN-γ have been known for some time. It has been proved that testosterone is involved in the decrease of IFN-γ levels. On the contrary, physiological levels of estrogens increase the bond between IFN-γ and lymphocytes. After stimulation with 17-β-estradiol,[62] the number of cells that express IFN-γ and IFN-γ levels increase.[63-66] By contrast, testosterone decreases[67] or tends to decrease the stimulated secretion of cytokines (IFN-γ, TNF-α).

It is surprising that the uncertain results obtained from QFT-G significantly correlate with the season in which the test is performed. The majority of the uncertain results were measured in the spring ($n = 10$) and in the winter ($n = 12$; $p < 0.005$). The values were calculated for the measurements performed in May and February. Bongartz and co-workers[68] showed that transport of samples in the winter and spring is more often followed by uncertain results in comparison to samples collected in the summer or autumn ($p = 0.0007$). The distance between the site of sample collection and the laboratory is not important.

Repeat QFT-G testing (3 months after the first test) of 31 patients who yielded uncertain results yielded 8 patients who again showed uncertain results (25.80%), 1 positive sample (3.23%) and 22 patients with negative results (70.97%).

With the progression of time and the increasing number of patients undergoing biological treatment, the conversion of QFT-G results from formerly negative (before the treatment) to positive (after the onset of treatment) has become the key issue. We screened 924 patients examined in 2011 (Zanova, E. et al. The conversion of Quantiferon TB Gold Test during biological Treatment by anti-TNF preparation - poster session 08.06.2012). Negative results were found in 807 patients (87.34%); results were positive in 117 patients (12.66%). Of these, the conversion of the QFT-G test during anti-TNF-α treatment appeared in 23 patients who tested negative in the first test. The majority were women (87%). This was not congruent with the percentage of women (60%) from the overall anti-TNF-α-treated patients. The group of patients in whom conversion was recognized was aged between 60 and 69 years. The highest number of anti-TNF-α treatment-related QFT-G negative-to-positive conversions was found in patients treated with adalimumab (9 of 23) and etanercept (8 of 23). The number of conversions, documented for the individual anti-TNF-α drugs, corresponded with the prescribed dosage of the drug. Surprisingly, a higher number of conversions were discovered after treatment with certolizumab—13.4% of all conversions—when compared to the overall anti-TNF-α treatment (5%). In search of the causes of this observation, we followed the testing in 2012 and focused on IFN-γ levels. The results from QFT-G tests are obtained from QFT software through mutual evaluation of IFN-γ levels in mitogen, TB antigen, and NIL tube.

We included 930 patients in the study group. The NIL parameter showed 14.4 times higher levels of IFN-γ in the patients treated with IL-6 blockade, and the levels were 91.1 times higher in patients receiving anti-TNF-α treatment. The mitogen–NIL parameter showed almost the same increase of IFN-γ levels in the patients undergoing all treatments. These results suggested the possible usefulness of examining IFN-γ levels in patients with the conversion of the QFT-G test while receiving biological treatment or for evaluating the effects of the individual biological treatments on the patient's IFN-γ levels. Because this is the first observation of these relationships, there is a need for further investigations and confirmation in a larger number of patients.

Based on the aforementioned results, the question of the causality of the conversion of the QFT-G test during biological treatment arises. There are several different possibilities, varying from LTBI reactivation due to an anti-TNF-α biological treatment (as a consequence of the disruption of the stability of the granulomas filled with mycobacteria) to exposure to a patient with the active TB while receiving a biological treatment (newly diagnosed TB infection). Several other factors cannot be excluded, namely the effects of contaminants elevating IFN-γ in plasma and alternative pathways of their production (interleukins, chemokines), the presence of heterophilic antibodies and the influence of sex hormones on IFN-γ levels. It is also noteworthy mentioning the influence of cells with the potential of releasing IFN-γ in the peripheral blood (helper (Th1) and cytotoxic [Tc1] T cells) – acquired immune response (effectors, memory, NK cells) and natural early immune response (effector and NKT cells) – and the connection between natural and acquired immune response (effector and memory cells). A positive result obtained from a QFT-G test may in fact be a false-positive result because of mistakes in the pre-analytical phase after chemoprophylaxis (the test is negative ranging from 6 months to 2 years after the treatment, afterwards positivity persists until the end of the life, and no repeated prophylactic treatment is recommended).

Mistakes made during the analytical phase of the QFT-G test often are discovered during closer analyses of the conversions. They are caused mainly by incorrect blood collection methods or manipulation of the collection tube (shaking too vigorously), collection of too small a volume of blood, incorrect incubation time or incorrect performance of the QFT-G test (ELISA method).

6 TREATMENT OF LTBI

The treatment of LTBI reduces the risk of progression to active TB disease by 20 times. This treatment is much cheaper and easier than the treatment of active TB disease. In case of low risk of TB exposition, the best diagnostic strategy is to perform TST, and positive results should be confirmed by IGRA.[20] Thus, the treatment is performed only when indicated. A patient affected by LTBI is treated by a chemoprophylactic anti-tubercular treatment based on age and the established clinical praxis. The treatment of LTBI is necessary to prevent the spread of novel, active, manifested TB diseases. The basic chemoprophylactic treatments are isoniazid and rifampicin. Isoniazid is considered the more effective and less toxic option for the treatment of LTBI compared to rifampicin. It is administered orally once per day. A possible side effect is hepatopathy, with a 0.5–1% risk of liver damage in the patients aged 20–50 years and a 2.5% risk of liver damage in patients older than 50 years.[45] The chemoprophylactic treatment (according to the methodological guidelines from 27 September 2005) is the anti-tubercular treatment administered at a dosage of 300 mg/day (Nidrazid 5 mg/kg/day + pyridoxin) for no longer than 6 months. These include children who are in contact with active TB, patients with high conversion of tubercular reaction, patients with a high tubercular reaction who simultaneously suffer from another disease or condition that leads to a decrease in immunity (silicosis, diabetes mellitus, gastroduodenal ulceration, HIV-positive patients exposed to active TB and therapy with corticosteroids). Patients undergoing the anti-TNF-α treatment also have been added to this group.

Patients receiving LTBI treatment are regularly controlled and followed in risk group RII, as people in contact with active TB and ongoing chemoprophylactic treatment. These patients are eliminated from the RII risk group 1 year after the end of treatment of the person affected with active TB that they contacted or after his or her death. The predicted duration of follow-up is 1.5 years. Although the length of follow-up is not exactly determined, the risk of LTBI reactivation or novel-specific infection is present during biological or any other immunosuppressive treatment, including long-term or repeated use of systemic corticosteroids. These aspects should be considered in the clinical praxis, and the patients should receive long-term follow-up.

The flare-up of LTBI in patients on anti-TNF-α treatment became such serious problem that several countries recently accepted national guidelines for the prevention of LTBI reactivation. They are not uniform, however, and more guidelines can be found within some states or a government might institute one uniform guideline. University hospitals and professional societies create their own guidelines.

According to the conclusions drawn by a panel of experts (Use of interferon-gamma release assays in support of TB diagnosis, Stockholm, ECDC, March 2011), IGRA is useful for diagnosing LTBI, identifying people who could prosper from prophylactic treatment, and among the BCG-vaccinated population and in cases where the probability of repeated TST evaluation is low. In 2005, the CDC recommended IGRA tests in all cases with indicated TST, including an examination of the history of exposure, immigrant status, and health care providers.[69]

Canada has a low incidence of TB, and mass BCG vaccination is not performed. There is high immigration from countries with a high incidence of TB and BCG vaccination. The country follows the control guidelines accepted in Great Britain. The Canadian Tuberculosis Committee carefully evaluated the recommendations for the use of quantiferon test published up to October 2006. They focused on objective comparison of the methods used as alternatives to TST and IGRA. The experiences with TST were long-lasting, and the interpretation of IGRA test results was not definitively established until then. The recommendations suggested by the committee to Public Health Agency of Canada are useful for us as well.[76] The following implications were identified:

- Performance of repeated LTBI examination in combination with TST
- For diagnosis of LTBI and active TB in children, the group of experts did not recommend performing ab IGRA test until the results were confirmed in a sufficiently high number of people
- Testing of immigrants will be performed by TST only in people born outside of Canada, where the conditions that predispose one to the development of TB disease may be evaluated: HIV, transplantation (associated with immunosuppressive treatment), TNF-α inhibitors, diabetes mellitus, silicosis, chronic renal failure with the need for hemodialysis, treatment with glucocorticoids and others
- Testing with both TST and IGRA was recommended for people exposed to patients with active TB disease. Screening for fresh active TB disease was recommended in those in contact with people with a massive active TB infection. The positivity of any of the test means LTBI.

- After occasional contacts, where no intensive exposition to mycobacteria was expected, and in those who have none of the predisposing conditions mentioned above, the IGRA test should be performed following a positive TST test. LTBI was characterized only by a positive IGRA test. There is a need for blood collection shortly after or simultaneously with PPD microsensibilization.
- Immunocompromised people should be tested first with a TST test; after negative results, the IGRA test should follow. If the test comes out positive (LTBI), prophylactic treatment should follow. In the case of uncertain IGRA results, it should be repeated to rule out any mistake caused by the laboratory. In the case of repeated uncertain results, anergy should be considered. The question regarding the diagnosis of LTBI in this group is still open.
- A person with a low risk of TB infection should be tested with the IGRA to rule out false positivity of the TST and to prevent unnecessary chemoprophylactic treatment.
- IGRAs should not be used for diagnosing active TB; microbiological examination should guide this diagnosis.
- Uncertain results: the test should be repeated and in the case of repeated uncertain results, the patient should be evaluated in congruence with a TST test and clinical evaluation.

The BCG vaccine is not applied collectively in the United States (a difference from the LTBI diagnostic approach), and thus in 2006 in Great Britain, guidelines were made recommending a hybrid, two-step protocol based on long-term experiences with using the TST test. The tuberculin test is a basic one and its positivity (LTBI diagnosis) should be confirmed by a positive IGRA. The aim is to exclude a "false-positive" LTBI diagnosis and make the chemoprophylactic indication more exact. Similar approaches were established in Germany and Switzerland in 2007.[69]

In Slovakia[70] there is valid methodical guidance from the main expert in pneumology and tuberculosis from the Ministry of Health of the Slovak Republic, which unifies the rules of diagnosis, follow-up and treatment of LTBI before and after biological treatment with the use of standard diagnostic IGRA (QFT-G was used from April 2007 and T-SPOT.TB from July 2011). QFT-G is performed before beginning biological treatment and then regularly once per year during the treatment. In the case of suspected TB flare-up or novel infection, the test is performed at any time during the treatment. Pneumological controls are performed before beginning biological treatment, every 3 months within the first year of the treatment and then once per year during the treatment. In the last supplementary material of the methodical guidance of the Ministry of Health of Slovak Republic from 1 July 2011, providing chemoprophylactic treatment even if the TST is hyperreactive (>18 mm) and the QFT-G is negative was recommended before the onset of standard treatment. Biological treatment should start after 2 months of chemoprophylactic treatment, whereas chemoprophylactic treatment is continued according to the standard application procedure: 6 months for isoniazid or 4 months for isoniazid plus rifampicin. In the case of a change from a QFT-G negative result to a positive result during the treatment, continuing the biological treatment without interruption and simultaneously applying chemoprophylactic treatment according to the standard procedure was recommended.

In 2011 in Slovakia, the mass BCG vaccination was terminated. We are now a mixed population with both BCG-vaccinated and non-vaccinated people. Thus, from 2013, the first children who were not vaccinated may start to be indicated.

7 CONCLUSION

The screening strategies for identifying LTBI developed in Europe and North America are able to decrease the incidence of TB reactivation during anti-TNF-α treatment.[49] The exclusion of active TB and the treatment of LTBI are crucial for the onset of an anti-TNF-α treatment.

Screening for LTBI and active TB before beginning a biological treatment is very important.[52] The examination of IFN-γ levels is more sensitive and specific[71] in comparison to TST, both in immunocompromised and BCG-vaccinated patients. However, the results should be evaluated in congruence with the patient's epidemiological history, actual health state and other diagnostic evaluations. To increase the benefit and decrease the risk of anti-TNF-α treatment,[72,73] good interdisciplinary cooperation between rheumatologists, pneumologists, and immunologists must occur.

REFERENCES

1. Pavelka K, Rovensky J, Szilasiova A. a spol. Rheumatoid arthritis. In: Pavelka K, Rovensky J, editors. *Klinicka revmatologie.* Praha: Galen; 2003. p. 181–215, ISBN:80-7262-174-2.
2. Pavelkova A. The biologic treatment. In: Pavelkova A, editor. *Rheumatoid arthritis and biologic therapy (in Czech).* Prague: Maxdorf Jesenius; 2009. p. 42–83, ISBN:978-80-7345-192-9 sv. 40.
3. American College of Rheumatology Subcommittee on Rheumatoid Arthritis Guidelines. Guidelines for the management of rheumatoid arthritis, 2002 update. *Arthritis Rheum* 2002;**46**:328–46.

4. Bucova M. The role of cytokines in develop of local and systemic inflammatory a septic shock. *Vnitrni lekarstvi* 2002;**48**(8):755–62.
5. Pavelka K, Vencovsky J, Tegzova D. TNF blocking drugs. In: Pavelka K, et al., editor. *Pharmacotherapy of rheumatic diseases (in Czech)*. Grada; 2005. p. 147–162, ISBN:80-247-0459-5.
6. Vilcek J. First demonstration of the role of TNF in the pathogenesis of disease. *J Immunol* 2008;**181**(1):5–6.
7. Pavelka K. TNF treatment of rheumatoid arthritis. In: Pavelka K, et al., editor. *Pharmacotherapy of rheumatic diseases (in Czech)*. Grada; 2005. p. 215–227, ISBN:80-247-0459-5.
8. Pavelka K. Disease modifying antirheumatic drugs in a rheumatoid arthritis. In: Pavelka K, et al., editor. *Pharmacotherapy of rheumatic diseases (in Czech)*. Grada; 2005. p. 63–65, ISBN:80-247-0459-5.
9. Goekoop-Ruiterman YP, de Vries-Bouwstra JK, Allaart CF, et al. Clinical and radiographic outcomes of four different treatment strategies in patients with early rheumatoid arthritis (the BeSt Study). *Arthritis Rheum* 2005;**52**:3381–90.
10. *Medinfo—The clinical view of tuberculosis, differential diagnosis.* http://www.medinfo.sk/%3Fs%3Dheslo%26id%3D673; 2002.
11. Pichler WJ. Adverse side-effects to biological agents. *Allergy* 2006;**61**(8):912–20.
12. Ellerin T, Rubin RH, Weinblatt ME. Infections and anti-tumor necrosis factor alpha therapy. *Arthritis Rheum* 2003;**48**:3013–22.
13. *The Health Protection Agency. Position statement on the use of interferon gamma assay (IGRA) test for tuberculosis (TB).* http://www.hpa.org.uk/Topics/InfectionsDiseases/InfectionsAZ/Tuberculosis; [accessed October, 2007].
14. Vourlekis JS., Brown KK. *Poststudy questions review the pulmonary complications of common antirheumatic drugs. Thoracis complication of rheumatoid arthritis.* 14; 1998, Lesson 17.
15. Libby D, White DA. Pulmonary toxicity of drugs used to treat systemic autoimmune diseases. *Clin Chest Med* 1998;**19**:809–21.
16. Carmona L, Hernandez-Garcia C, Vadillo C, Pato E, Balsa A, Gonzalez-Alvaro I, et al. Increased risk of tuberculosis in patients with rheumatoid arthritis. *J Rheumatol* 2003;**30**:1436–9.
17. Scheinfeld N. A comprehensive review and evaluation of the side effects of the tumor necrosis factor alpha blockers etanercept, infliximab and adalimumab. *J Dermatolog Treat* 2004;**15**(5):280–94.
18. *Research Projects: tuberculosis. about tuberculosis.* http://www.stoptb.org./events/partners_forum/2004/assets/flash/default.html; [accessed 2006].
19. Gomez-Reino JJ, Carmona L, Valverde VR, Mola EM, Montero MD, BIOBADASER Group. Treatment of rheumatoid arthritis with tumor necrosis factor inhibitors may predispose to significant increase in tuberculosis risk: a multicenter active-surveillance report. *Arthritis Rheum* 2003;**48**(8):2122–7.
20. Laffitte E, Janssens JP, Roux-Lombard R, Thielen AM, Barde C, Marazza G, et al. Tuberculosis screening in patients with psoriasis before antitumour necrosis factor therapy: comparison of an interferon-γ release assay vs. tuberculin skin test. *Brit J Dermatol* 2009;**161**(4):797–800.
21. Kim EY, Lim JE, Jung JY. et al., Performance of the tuberculin skin test and interferon-γ release assay for detection of tuberculosis infection in immunocompromised patients in a BCG-vaccinated population. *BMC Infect Dis* 2009;**9**:207.
22. Lalvani A, Millington KA. Screeening for tuberculosis infection prior to initiation of anti-TNF therapy. *Autoimmun Rev* 2008;**8**:147–52.
23. Wolfe F, Michaud K, Anderson J, Urbansky K. Tuberculosis infection in patients with rheumatoid arthritis and the effect of infliximab therapy. *Arthritis Rheum* 2004;**50**:372–9.
24. di Girolamo C, Pappone N, Mellilo R, et al., et al. Cavitary lung tuberculosis in a rheumatoid arthritis patient treated with low dose methotrexate and steroid pulse therapy. *Br J Rheumatol* 1998;**37**(10):1136–7.

25. Kim HA, Yoo CD, Back HJ, et al. Mycobacterium tuberculosis infection in a cortico-steroid treatment rheumatic disease patient population. *Clin Exp Rheumatol* 1998;**16**(1):9–13.
26. Mariandyshey AO, Martiushov SI, Gagarin BP, et al. Trudnosti diagnostiki legochno—vistseralnych form revmatoidnovo artrita v klinike tuberkuloza. *Probl Tuberk* 1998;**1**:21–3.
27. Terao I, Hagiwara T, Iijima S. Analysis factor for the development of pulmonary tuber-culosis in persons with collagenosis. *Kekkaku* 1991;**69**(2):65–9.
28. Engele M, Stossel E, Castiglione K, Schwerdtner N, Wagner M, Bolcskei P, et al. Induc-tion of TNF in human alveolar macrophages as a potential evasion mechanism of virulent *Mycobacterium tuberculosis*. *J Immunol* 2002;**168**:1328–37.
29. Keane J, Remold HG, Kornfeld H. Virulent *Mycobacterium tuberculosis* strains evade apoptosis of infected alveolar macrophages. *J Immunol* 2000;**164**:2016–20.
30. Stenger S. Adverse events with biologics immunological control of tuberculosis: role of tumour necrosis factor and more. *Ann Rheum Dis* 2005;**64**:iv24–8.
31. Carmona L, Gomez-Reino JJ, Rodrguez-Valverde V, Montero D, Pascual-Gomez E, Mola EM, et al. Effectiveness of recommendations to prevent reactivation of latent tuberculosis infection in patients treated with tumor necrosis factor antagonists. *Arthritis Rheum* 2005;**52**(6):1766–72.
32. Geijtenbeek TB, Van Vliet SJ, Koppel EA, Sanchez-Hernandez M, Vandenbroucke-Grauls CM, Appelmelk B, et al. Mycobacteria target DC-SIGN to suppress dendritic cell function. *J Exp Med* 2003;**197**:7–17.
33. Tailleux L, Schwartz O, Herrmann JL, Pivert E, Jackson M, Amara A, et al. DC-SIGN Is the major mycobacterium tuberculosis receptor on human dendritic cells. *J Exp Med* 2003;**197**:121–7.
34. Clay H, Volkman HE, Ramakrishnan L. Tumor necrosis factor signaling mediates resis-tance to mycobacteria by inhibiting bacterial growth and macrophage death. *Immunity* 2008;**29**:283–94.
35. Spira A, Carroll JD, Liu G, Aziz Z, Shah V, Kornfeld H, et al. Apoptosis genes in human alveolar macrophages infected with virulent or attenuated Mycobacterium tuberculosis: a pivotal role for tumor necrosis factor. *Am J Respir Cell Mol Biol* 2003;**29**:545–51.
36. *Tuberculosis—GlaxoSmithKline. Project—tuberculosis*. http://www.gsk.sk/verejnost_svet_tuberkuloza.html; [accessed 13.05.10].
37. Anonymous. *Global tuberculosis control: surveillance, planning, financing*. Geneva, Switzerland: WHO; 2008.
38. *Cellestis developed QuantiFERON Gold*. http://www.cellestis.com//; [accessed 04.03.07].
39. Greenberg JD, Reddy SM, Schloss SG, Kurucz OS, Bartlett SJ, Abramson SB, et al. Comparison of an in vitro tuberculosis interferon-gamma assay with delayed-type hypersensitivity testing for detection of latent *Mycobacterium tuberculosis*: a pilot study in rheumatoid arthritis. *J Rheumatol* 2008;**35**(5):770–5, Erratum in: J Rheumatol. 2008 May, 35(5): 943.
40. Mayordomo L, Marenco JL, Gomez-Mateos J, Rejon E. Pulmonary military tubercu-losis in a patient with anti-TNF-alpha treatment. *Scand J Rheumatol* 2002;**31**:44.
41. Chen DY, Shen GH, Hsieh TY, Hsieh CW, Lan JL. Effectiveness of the combination of a whole-blood interferon-gamma assay and the tuberculin skin test in detecting latent tuberculosis infection in rheumatoid arthritis patients receiving adalimumab therapy. *Arthritis Rheum* 2008;**59**(6):800–6.
42. Keane J, Gershon S, Wise RP, et al. Tuberculosis associated with infliximab, a tumor necrosis factor-alpha neutralizing agent. *N Engl J Med* 2001;**345**:1098–104.
43. Roach DR, Bean AG, Demangel C, France MP, Briscoe H, Britton WJ. TNF regulates chemokine induction essential for cell recruitment, granuloma formation, and clearance of mycobacterial infection. *J Immunol* 2002;**168**:4620–7.

44. Scallon B, Cai A, Solowski N, Rosenberg A, Song XY, Shealy D, et al. Binding and functional comparisons of two types of tumor necrosis factor antagonists. *J Pharmacol Exp Ther* 2002;**301**:418–26.

45. Kharbanda P, Dagaonkar R, Balakrishnan C, Udwadia ZF. Tumor necrosis factor—α blocker induced tuberculosis. *J Rheumatol* 2010;**37**:7–11.

46. Solovic I, Polanova M. Diagnosis and differential diagnosis of tuberculosis. In: Solovic I, editor. *a kolektív: Tuberkuloza—vybrané kapitoly*. Poprad: NUTPCHaHCH Vysne Hagy; 2008. p. 25–26, ISBN:978-80-970024-4-2.

47. Lew WJ, Jung YJ, Song JW, Jang YM, et al. Combined use of QuantiFERON((R))-TB gold assay and chest computed tomography in a tuberculosis outbreak. *Int J Tuberc Lung Dis* 2009;**13**(5):633–9.

48. Evans LC, Chapman T, Linstead S, Cootauco M, Groth J, Chua FJ. INF-gamma release assays improve detection of latent tuberculosis infection in Tuberculin-Anergic candidates for anti-TNF-alpha blocade. *Am J Respir Crit Care Med* 2009;**179**:5927.

49. Brock I, Weldingh K, Lillebaek T, Follmann F, Andersen P. Comparison of tuberculin skin test and new specific blood test in tuberculosis contacts. *Am J Respir Crit Care Med* 2004;**170**(1):65–9.

50. Doherty AM, Wallisb ES, Zumlac A. WHO-tropical Disease Research/European Commission Biomarkers in relationship to status and diagnosis of tuberculosis. *Curr Opin Pulm Med* 2009;**6**:49–55.

51. Solovic I, Svecova J. Epidemiology of tuberculosis. In: Solovic I, et al. editors. *Tuberkuloza—vybrane kapitoly*. Poprad: NUTPCHaHCH Vysne Hagy; 2008. p. 25–26, ISBN:978-80970024-4-2.

52. British Thoracic Society Standards of Care Committee. BTS recommendations for assessing risk and for managing Mycobacterium tuberculosis infection and disease in patients due to start anti-TNF-alpha treatment. *Thorax* 2005;**60**(10):800–5.

53. Higuchi K, Harada N, Fukazawa K, Mori T. Relationship between whole blood interferon gamma responses and the risk of active tuberculosis. *Tuberculosis (Edinb)* 2008;**88**:244 8.

54. Dheda K, Pooran A, Pai M, et al. Interpretation of Mycobacterium tuberculosis antigen-specific IFN-gamma release assaya (T-SPOT.TB) and factors that may modulate test results. *J Infect* 2007;**55**:169–73.

55. Arend SM, Breedveld FC, Van Dissel JT. TNF-Alpha blockade and tuberculosis: better look before you leap. *Neth J Med* 2003;**61**(4):111–19.

56. Berlinger Ch, Dudler J, Mottet Ch, Nicod L, Seibold F, Villiger PM, et al. Screening for tuberculosis infection before initiation of anti-TNF-α therapy. *Swiss Med WKLY* 2007;**137**:621–2.

57. *Center of Disease Control and Prevention, Guidelines for using the QuantiFERON TB Gold test for detecting Mycobacterium tuberculosis infection, United States.* http://www.cdc.gov/mmwr/preview/mmwrhtml/rr5415a4.htm; [accessed 03.08.07].

58. Diel E, Wrighton-Smith P, Zellweger J-P. Cost-effectiveness of IGRA testing for the treatment of latent tuberculosis in Switzerland. *Eur Respir J* 2007;**30**:321–32.

59. Pratt A, Nicholl K, Kay L. Use of the QuantiFERON TB Gold test as part of a screening programme in patients with RA under consideration for treatment with anti-TNF-alpha agents: the Newcastle (UK) experience. *Rheumatology (Oxford)* 2007;**46**:1035–6.

60. Bocchino M, Bellofiore B, Matarese A, Galati D, Sanduzzi A. IFN-γ release assays in tuberculosis management in selected high-risk populations. *Expert Rev Mol Diagn* 2009;**9**(2):165–77.

61. Takahashi H, Shigehara K, Yamamoto M, Suzuki C, Naishiro Y, Tamura Y, et al. Interferon gamma assay for detecting latent tuberculosis infection in rheumatoid arthritis patients during infliximab administration. *Rheumatol Int* 2007;**27**(12):1143–8.

62. Panchanathan R, Shen H, Zhang X, Ho SM, Choubey D. Mutually positive regulatory feedback loop between interferons and estrogen receptor-alpha in mice: implications for sex bias in autoimmunity. *PLoS One* 2010;**5**:e10868.

63. Nakaya M, Tachibana H, Yamada K. Effect of estrogens on the interferon-gamma producing cell population of mouse splenocytes. *Biosci Biotechnol Biochem* 2006;**70**(1):47–53.

64. Fox HS, Bond BL, Parslow TG. Estrogen regulates the IFN-gamma promoter. *J Immunol* 1991;**146**(12):4362–7.

65. Maret A, Coudert JD, Garidou L, et al. Estradiol enhances primary antigen-specific CD4 T cell responses and Th1 development in vivo. Essential role of estrogen receptor alpha expression in hematopoietic cells. *Eur J Immunol* 2003;**33**:512–21.

66. Siracusa MC, Overstreet MG, Housseau F, Scott AL, Klein SL. 17beta-estradiol alters the activity of conventional and IFN-producing killer dendritic cells. *J Immunol* 2008;**180**(3):1423–31.

67. Janele D, Lang T, Capellino S, Cutolo M, Pereira da Silva JA, Straub RH. Effects of testosterone, 17beta-estradiol, and downstream estrogens on cytokine secretion from human leukocytes in the presence and absence of cortisol. *Ann NY Acad Sci* 2006;**1069**:168–82.

68. Bongartz T, Sutton AJ, Sweeting MJ, Buchan I, Matteson EL, Montori V. Anti-TNF antibody therapy in rheumatoid arthritis and the risk of serious infections and malignancies. Systematic review and meta-analysis of rare harmful effects in randomized controlled trials. *JAMA* 2006;**295**:2275–85.

69. Trnka L. Wallenfels: diagnosis of latent tuberculosis infection with IGRA tests. Actual guideline. *Stud Pneumol Phthiseol* 2009;**69**(1):26–8.

70. Rybar I, Kriska M, Miceková D, Kristanova M, Rovensky J, Zlnay D, et al. The failure of anti-TNF treatment in patients with inflammatory rheumatic diseases in Sloval republic 2001-2008. *Reumatologia* 2010;**26**:1–6.

71. Lee JY, Choi HJ, Park IN, et al. Comparison of two commercial interferon gamma assays for diagnosing mycobacterium tuberculosis infection. *Eur Respir J* 2006;**28**:24–30.

72. Zanova E, Solovic I, Polanová M, Rovensky J, Rybar I, Raffayova H. Diagnosis of latent form of tuberculosis in patients with rheumatoid arthritis before the biologic (anti-TNF) treatment. *Respiro* 2007;**3**:15–19.

73. Rybar I, Rozborilova E, Zanová E, Micekova D, Solovic I, Rovensky J. Effectiveness of prevention of tuberculosis by patients with inflammatory rheumatic diseases in anti-TNF treatment. *Bratisl Lek Listy* 2008;**109**(4):164–7.

74. Imperato AK, Bingham CO, Abramson SB. Overview of benefit/risk of biological agents. *Clin Exp Rheumatol* 2004;**22**(Suppl. 35):108–14.

75. Ponce de Len D, Acevedo-Vasquez E, Sanchez-Torres A, Cucho M, Alfaro J, Perich R, et al. Attenuated response to purified protein derivative in patients with rheumatoid arthritis: study in a population with a high prevalence of tuberculosis. *Ann Rheum Dis* 2005;**64**(9):1360–1.

76. An Advisory Committee Statement, Canadian Tuberculosis Committee. *Updated recommendations on interferon gamma release assaya for latent tuberculosis infection.* Canada Communicable Disease Report; 2008, 34,ACS-6.

CHAPTER 36

Parasitic Infection and Autoimmunity

Mahmoud Abu-Shakra[*,1], **Eduard Ling**[†], **Yehuda Shoenfeld**[‡]

[*]Rheumatic Diseases Unit, Soroka Medical Center and Ben-Gurion University, Beer-Sheva, Israel
[†]Pediatric Rheumatic Diseases Unit, Soroka Medical Center and Ben-Gurion University, Beer-Sheva, Israel
[‡]Zabludowicz Center for Autoimmune Diseases, Sheba Medical Center and Sackler Faculty of Medicine, Tel-Hashomer, Israel
[1]Corresponding Author: Mahmoud@bgu.ac.il

During the last five decades it has become understood that microbial antigens play a significant role in the pathogenesis of the immune dysregulation leading to autoimmune disorders. Viral, bacterial, or parasitic infection of subjects with specific genetic backgrounds, immune abnormalities, or hormonal constellations may trigger autoimmunity that leads to the development of an overt autoimmune disease.[1–3]

Activation of autoimmune mechanisms has been associated with infection with various parasites. Observations that link autoimmunity and parasitic infections include the presence of pathogenic autoantibodies and autoreactive cytotoxic T cells to heart and nerve cells in mice and in patients with Chagas disease,[4,5] the detection of antibodies directed against self-antigens of the inner retina in the sera of patients with onchocerciasis,[6] and the development of complement-mediated hemolytic anemia associated with autoantibodies reacting with triosephosphate isomerase (TPI) in patients with long-standing malaria.[7]

Autoantibodies associated with parasitic infections are polyreactive, thus binding various foreign- and self-antigens.[8] Autoantibodies to nuclear antigens detected in the sera of *Schistosoma*-infected mice bind DNA, polynucleotides, and malaria and cercarial antigens.[9] This pattern of autoantibody binding is similar to that of human monoclonal anti-DNA antibodies derived from patients with systemic lupus erythematosus (SLE).[10]

The clinical significance of autoimmune activity in patients with chronic infections is not clear. Autoimmunity-related clinical manifestations occur in chronic parasitic infections.[11] Furthermore, despite earlier controversies,

Infection and Autoimmunity
http://dx.doi.org/10.1016/B978-0-444-63269-2.00040-4

621

current thinking attributes to autoimmune mechanisms a significant role in the pathogenesis of cardiac manifestations in Chagas disease.[12] In addition, a protective role of autoimmune mechanisms has been proposed. Autoantibodies in malaria may protect against infection by inhibiting the growth of *Plasmodium* spp., destroying infected cells, or blocking receptors for *Plasmodium* on the surface of red blood cells (RBCs).[13,14]

Parasitic antigens may induce autoimmune activity and immune-mediated damage to self-antigens by several mechanisms, including molecular mimicry between host and parasites, induction of pathogenic autoantibodies, polyclonal activation of B cells, and manipulation of the idiotypic network.[1–3]

This chapter summarizes the link between parasitic infections, autoimmunity, and autoimmune diseases. The association between autoimmunity and malaria, leishmania, schistosomiasis, and onchocerciasis is detailed. Autoimmunity and Chagas disease is discussed in the next chapter.

1 MALARIA AND AUTOIMMUNITY

Malaria is a protozoan disease transmitted to humans by the bite of *Anopheles* mosquitoes. It remains among the main causes of human sickness and death in the world. Over 1 billion people reside in malaria-endemic regions of the world; in 2010 the WHO reported 219 million new cases of malaria, with 660,000 deaths annually. Malaria is characterized by fever, rigors, splenomegaly, hemolytic anemia, and hyperglobulinemia.

Autoantibodies are detected in patients with acute malaria and chronic malaria and in the sera of healthy subjects living in endemic malarious areas.[13] Various autoantibodies were detected in the sera of patients with malaria. In a seminal paper published in 1968, Shaper et al.[15] were the first to detect anti-nuclear antibodies (ANAs) and antibodies reacting with heart tissue in the sera of patients with malaria. Subsequent studies found the sera of patients with malaria to bind single-stranded[16] and double-stranded DNA, as well as ribonucleoproteins (RNPs), smooth muscle and parietal cells,[17] cationic phospholipids,[18] RBCs,[19] lymphocytes,[20] rheumatoid factor (RF),[21] and neutrophil cytoplasmic enzymes.[22] Anti-dendrite and functional IgE autoantibodies that recognize brain 14-3-3 ε protein have been described.[23,24] In should also be noted that the clearance of immune complexes (ICs) containing self- and non-self-antigens is impaired in malaria.[25]

Autoantibodies are seen in all ethnic groups. The frequency of ANAs and anti-smooth muscle was similar in the sera of Caucasians, Asians, and Africans with acute malaria, chronic malaria and chronic exposure to malaria.[26] A correlation was found between the presence of autoantibodies and high titers of anti-malarial antibodies, suggesting that acute malaria might trigger the generation of ANAs and possibly other autoantibodies. However, the persistence of these autoantibodies did not correlate with the level of parasitemia once the acute infection was treated, indicating that autoantibodies are associated with chronic infection.[27]

The clinical significance of autoantibodies in the sera of patients with malaria is not clear. Autoantibodies derived from splenocytes of a *Plasmodium chabaudi*-infected BALB/c mice exhibited characteristics similar to those of natural autoantibodies, suggesting that the generation of autoantibodies in the sera of patients with malaria has no clinical significance.[8] In addition, various evidence suggests that malaria has a protective effect against autoimmune disease, as judged by the lower prevalence of classic autoimmune diseases such as SLE in endemic malarious areas compared with the Caucasian population.[28] Furthermore, the incidence of rheumatoid arthritis (RA) is increased in urban compared to rural areas of Senegal, clearly suggesting an environmental influence.[29] In a challenging review, Daniel-Ribeiro and Zanini[13] proposed that malaria may prevent the development of autoimmune diseases or diminish their severity. Pattern of activation of toll-like receptors (TLRs) determines Th1 or Th2 polarization and extent of immune or autoimmune response.[30] One may entertain the possibility of activation of different (compared to those seen in SLE) TLRs by *Plasmodium* spp. with resultant protection from autoimmune diseases. That activation of both TLR4[31] and TLR9[32] occurs in malaria and is required for protection from this disease is well established, whereas in SLE, TLR4 is down-regulated[33] and TLR9 is activated and governs the development of autoimmune response.[34] Another explanation for the protective effect of malaria on the development of autoimmune disorders stems from the ability of certain *Plasmodium* spp. to induce CD4+CD25+ T regulatory cells (Tregs) that interfere with the development of autoimmune encephalitis.[35] This phenomenon was accompanied by a decreased expression of IL-17 and IFNγ and an increased expression of IL-10 and TGFβ.

A current concept proposes that autoantibodies in malaria participate in the immune protection against malaria. The generation of autoantibodies reacting with cryptic or neo-antigens[36] or anti-idiotypic antibodies against plasmodial antigens may have a role in destroying infected cells or by blocking RBC invasion. Negative correlation between IgE autoantibodies that recognize brain 14-3-3 ε protein (a protein of a family of CD81 binding proteins) and severity of parasitemia suggests the protective role of these antibodies, probably by interfering with the development of liver-stage parasites.[24] In addition, the autoantibodies may bind parasitic antigens and inhibit their activity. This notion was confirmed by Brahimi et al.,[14] who demonstrated the ability of the sera of autoimmune patients to inhibit the growth of *Plasmodium* spp. All of these plausible mechanisms need further research.

However, the association between malaria, hemolytic anemia, thrombocytopenia, and nephritis indicates an autoimmune mechanism and a pathogenic role for malaria-associated autoantibodies. The appearance or persistence of hemolysis or nephritis in the chronic phase of the malaria, which is associated with a low load of parasitic antigens, indicates that pathogenic autoantibodies may have a role in nephritis and hemolysis in patients with malaria.

Anti-RBC antibodies that bind RBCs are present in the sera of patients with malaria.[19] The origin of these antibodies is not clear. Two main hypotheses have been suggested. Sayles and Wassom[36] reported that anti-RBC antibodies are anti-idiotypic antibodies of anti-plasmodial antibodies. Molecular mimicry between the anti-idiotypic antibodies and plasmodial peptides leads to the binding of the anti-idiotypic antibodies to RBC (reviewed by Daniel-Ribeiro and Zanini[13]) and prevents infection of RBC. Others have suggested that parasite-induced mechanical hemolysis of RBCs leads to the development of autoantibodies against the cytoplasmatic enzyme TPI. Anti-TPI is found in the sera of patients with malaria and is associated with persistent hemolysis.[7]

Renal disease, manifested mainly by nephritic syndrome, contributes significantly to the morbidity and mortality of malaria. Deposition of ICs composed of plasmodium antigens and their antibodies is the main mechanism of this sequela of malaria. Induction of anti-DNA antibodies and impaired clearance of ICs during malaria infection are well known.[16,17,25] The latter is probably due to the inhibition of surface expression of complement receptor 1 in monocytes/macrophages by *Plasmodium* spp.[37] These phenomena are of utmost importance for pathogenesis of SLE as well. Likewise, anti-DNA antibodies and possibly their idiotypes may have a role in the development of nephritic syndrome, as judged by the detection of these antibodies in the glomeruli of mice with malaria and renal damage.[38,39]

2 *LEISHMANIA* AND AUTOIMMUNITY

Leishmania is an intracellular protozoon that resides within mononuclear phagocytes of the host. Depending on the *Leishmania* species, the infected host develops localized or disseminated disease. The localized form of leishmaniasis is characterized by cutaneous or mucocutaneous lesions which are caused by *Leishmania tropica*, *Leishmania major*, *Leishmania aethiopica*, *Leishmania mexicana*, and *Leishmania braziliensis*. Visceral leishmaniasis or kala-azar is caused primarily by *Leishmania donovani*. Leishmaniasis is a public health problem in tropical areas and most countries bordering the Mediterranean basin.

Autoimmune phenomena in leishmaniasis are well known: Argov et al.[40] detected anti-Sm, RNP, SS-A, and SS-B in high titers in 83, 86, 36, and 73%, respectively, of the sera of patients with visceral leishmaniasis compared with 7, 14, 25, and 25%, respectively, in the sera of patients with cutaneous leishmaniasis. The binding of visceral leishmaniasis sera to RNPs was inhibited by prior incubation of the sera with either leishmanial membrane antigens from four different species of *Leishmania* or with intact cells of *L. donovani*, suggesting a similarity between host and *Leishmania* antigens. In later studies, sera of animals and humans with cutaneous leishmaniasis and visceral leishmaniasis was shown to recognize various autoantibodies including ANAs, native DNA, cyclic citrulinated peptide and RF, Sm, RNP, SS-A, SS-B, cardiolipin, β2-glycoprotein I, actin, smooth muscle, and hemoglobin.[41–46] It should be noted that a particularly high prevalence (53%) of anti-β2-glycoprotein I antibodies has been demonstrated in patients with kala-azar.[47] Anti-IgE autoantibodies in sera of patients with visceral leishmaniasis also have been detected;[48] however, their significance in disease pathogenesis is not yet clear.

A pathogenic role for autoimmunity in leishmaniasis was reported. Three cases of pancytopenia in patients with kala-azar were described. In all three cases, anti-platelet, anti-neutrophil, and anti-RBC IgG antibodies were documented on the cell surface of platelets, RBCs, and neutrophils. Bone marrow suppression was not found, suggesting that pancytopenia resulted from the rapid destruction of antibody-coated blood cells.[49] Visceral leishmaniasis presents a diagnostic challenge in the context of autoimmune disease since it is a well-known mimicker of SLE.[50,51] Furthermore, Liberopoulos et al.[41] demonstrated asymptomatic hypocomplementemia in the sera of patients with visceral leischmaniasis. In addition, cases of visceral leishmaniasis were found to be associated with cryoglobulinemia,[52] SLE, autoimmune hepatitis, and primary biliary cirrhosis.[53] This is in accordance with an earlier case report of a patient who developed concurrent SLE and leishmaniasis.[54] The SLE was characterized by thrombocytopenia, nephritis, skin lesions, and positive ANAs and anti-cardiolipin. Renal biopsy showed lupus nephritis without evidence of infection with leishmania. Complete and prolonged remission of SLE and disappearance of ANAs were observed after treating the leishmanial infection.

Renal involvement in leishmaniasis is manifested by acute glomerulonephritis, nephritic syndrome, and interstitial nephritis.[55] Pathological studies of canine leishmaniasis demonstrated a wide spectrum of renal injuries,[56] including membranous and membranoproliferative glomerulonephritis (18% each), focal segmental glomerulosclerosis (14%), tubular and fibrosis hypertrophy, periglomerular inflammatory infiltrate, and multifocal and diffuse peritubular inflammatory infiltrate. In other studies, renal biopsies showed leishmanial antigens in some cases and deposition of immunoglobulins, complement, and fibrinogen without direct infection of the kidneys in others.[57,58] Circulating ICs that induce the proinflammatory cytokines GM-CSF and IL-6, as well as the immunosuppressive or anti-inflammatory cytokines IL-10 and IL-1RA, but with a more general proinflammatory effect, were detected in the sera of patients with leishmaniasis. The role of these ICs in disease pathogenesis is being elucidated.[59]

3 SCHISTOSOMIASIS AND AUTOIMMUNITY

Three main schistosome species infect humans: *Schistosoma mansoni* and *Schistosoma japanicum* mostly infect the liver, and *Schistosoma hematobium* infects the venules of the urinary tract, mainly the ureters and bladder. Schistosomiasis is a granulomatous disease characterized by the development of granulomas surrounding helminths' eggs.

Autoantibodies, including anti-DNA, ANAs, RF, anti-Sm, anti-sperm, anti-lymphocytic, anti-thyroid, anti-tubulin, and anti-parietal cells, were detected in the sera of humans and animals infected with various *Schistosoma* species.[9,60–65] The sera of 234 patients with chronic *S. mansoni* infection were screened for a wide range of autoantigens;[65] 15% were positive for ANAs or smooth muscle or gastric parietal cell antibodies, and 27% had antibodies against the hepatic asialoglycoprotein receptor (ASGP-R). Anti-ASGP-R antibodies occurred more commonly in patients with hepatosplenic involvement than in patients with hepatointestinal disease or in patients who underwent splenectomies (33, 4.5, and 5.8%, respectively). The data suggest that anti-ASGP-R may have a role in the pathogenesis of hepatosplenic schistosomiasis.

Similarly, mice infected with *S. mansoni* generated autoantibodies and T cells responsive to collagen.[66] Anti-collagen antibodies have been identified in a variety of autoimmune rheumatic diseases, including scleroderma, RA, and relapsing polychondritis. A role for anti-collagen activity in hepatic and other visceral fibroses of patients with schistosomiasis has been reported, and it has been postulated that the anti-collagen activity may result in the secretion of proinflammatory cytokines that stimulate fibroblasts to migrate and synthesize collagen.[66]

In a subsequent study,[9] various autoantibodies to nuclear antigens, including anti-dsDNA, anti-poly (I), anti-Sm, and anti-SS-B were detected in the sera of 15 mice 9 weeks after infection with *Schistosoma*. The binding of the sera of the mice with schistosomiasis to cercarial extract was inhibited by incubation of the sera with DNA, polynucleotides, and cercarial extract.

A possible link between SLE and schistosomiasis has been suggested. High levels of a pathogenic anti-DNA idiotype (16/6 Id) and anti-cardiolipin antibodies were reported in the sera of patients with schistosomiasis.[67] In addition, sera of mice with experimental SLE and patients with SLE reacted with the schistosomal extract. Immunoblot analyses showed that the sera of mice and patients with SLE reacted with 60-, 85-, and 94-kDa cercarial proteins, whereas the sera of patients with SLE also reacted with 10- to 18-, 29-, and 52-kDa cercarial proteins.[9] The significance of this binding of SLE sera to schistosoma extracts is not clear. It may indicate that antigens with homology to schistosoma may trigger SLE. However, inverse correlation between schistosoma infection and ANA titer was demonstrated, with significant elevation of the latter following anti-parasitic treatment.[68] One is tempted to consider the possibility of protective effects of schistosomiasis against autoimmune disorders acting in a similar manner to the protective effects of malaria infection.

4 ONCHOCERCIASIS AND AUTOIMMUNITY

Onchocerciasis, or river blindness, is a tropical infection caused by the filarial nematode *Onchocerca volvulus*. In endemic areas, an estimate of 50% of adults older than 40 years may become blind as a result of corneal or retinal lesions induced by *O. volvulus*. Two forms of corneal disease occur in onchocerciasis. Punctate keratitis occurs within the first 10 years of infection and is characterized by acute inflammation and oedema around dead microfilaria. A complete resolution of the infection without residual damage may occur. Sclerosing keratitis is associated with prolonged infection and consists of a fibrovascular pannus, which may affect the entire cornea. Some patients infected with *O. volvulus* develop chronic hyperreactive onchodermatitis (sowda) along with corneal and retinal disease.

Autoimmune mechanisms have been associated with onchocerciasis. Autoantibody activity was observed in the sera of patients with onchocerciasis and includes anti-tubulin, RF, and anti-laminin antibodies[64,69,70] and antibody activity directed against corneal and retinal antigens.[6] Anti-tubulin was found in 89% of the patients, and it is also seen in patients various parasitic infections, including visceral leishmaniasis (67%), cutaneous leishmaniasis (60%), and all patients with schistosomiasis.[64]

Autoantibodies that bind retinal extract were generated in the sera of guinea pigs after subconjunctival or subcutaneous injections of microfilaria over 4–14 weeks.[71] Severe corneal inflammation was induced by autoimmunization with the corneal extract followed by intraocular injections of cytokines, suggesting that exposure to microfilaria may induce pathogenic anti-corneal autoantibodies.[72] In another study, 10 of 12 sera and ocular fluid from patients with onchocerciasis reacted with autoantigens of the inner retinal, including nerve fibre, ganglion, and Müller cells. Antibodies against the outer segment of the photoreceptor were noted in 7 of the 12 patients.[73] Another study identified the presence of autoantibodies directed against human S-antigen and interphotoreceptor retinoid binding protein in the sera of patients with onchocerciasis.[74] The frequency of all autoantibodies was significantly higher in patients with onchocerciasis compared with controls living in the same area; however, no correlation was found between their presence and the clinical features of the disease.

Subsequent studies identified autoantibody reactivity against five major cytoplasmic non-RNA-associated autoantigens with molecular weights of 35, 51, 64, 83, and 110 kDa.[75] In addition, anti-calreticulin reactivity,[75] the human homologue of the onchocercal Ag RAL-1, anti-retinal pigment epithelial and neural retinal cells[6] and antibody reactivity against the 65-kDa arthritis–associated mycobacterial heat shock protein also were seen in onchocerciasis.[75]

Chronic hyperreactive onchodermatitis (sowda) caused by *O. volvulus* infection is characterized by the development of autoantibodies to defensins 1–3, neutrophil proteins important for defence against bacterial, fungal, and certain viral infections.[76]

Of particular interest is the development of autoantibodies to calreticulin during *Onchocerca* infection.[75] Calreticulin is a molecular chaperone also involved in the control of Ca^{2+} homeostasis.[77] Recent evidence suggest that calreticulin can function as a potent B cells and macrophages stimulatory molecule via the TLR-4/CD14 pathway and plays important roles in the pathogenesis of autoimmune diseases.[78] Arthritis is a well-described feature of onchocerciasis.[79] In spite of this fact, particular interest is given to the findings of Ling et al.,[80] who demonstrated the presence of an RA shared epitope binding site on calreticulin. In addition, calreticulin binds to the Ro/SS-A antigen complex and forms a common target for autoimmune responses.[81,82] Calreticulin participates in the clearance of apoptotic bodies;[83] however, anti-calreticulin antibodies can interfere with this process, with implications in the development of autoimmune diseases such as SLE. Indeed, anti-calreticulin antibodies are present in sera from patients with SLE and celiac disease.[84,85]

5 HELMINTHS AND AUTOIMMUNITY

Intestinal carriage of parasitic worms is virtually concurrent with human existence. Intestinal helminths are multi-cellular organisms that belong to two distinct phyla: nematodes and flatworms. Helminths invade different organs (lungs, intestine, liver) via different routes. Helminthic infections of humans usually lead to malnutrient, growth, and cognitive disturbances. Description of the biology and pathological effects of helminthic infestation is beyond the scope of this chapter. Instead, we concentrate on the immunomodulatory effects of helminths on their human host.

Helminths are long-lived parasites that usually do not replicate within human host. Therefore, the helminths' survival strategy is based on immunomodulation. Immunomodulation by helminths is thought to be mutually beneficial for host and parasite, since it protects the host from the severe consequences of inflammatory response and it prevents the elimination of helminths.

The helminths' immunomodulatory effects are multi-tiered: first, they are able to interfere with the maturation of dendritic cells, thus affecting the presentation of antigen and changing the direction of immune response with preference to Th2 or Th3 pathways.[86,87] Tregs play a critical role in maintaining immune homeostasis and in the suppression of autoimmunity.[88] Therefore, of particular interest is the ability of helminths to induce $CD4^+CD25^+Foxp3^+$ Tregs[89] since it contributes not only to the longevity of hookworm survival in infected people but also can explain the protective effects of helminthic infection against certain autoimmune diseases such as multiple sclerosis[90] and inflammatory bowel disease.[91]

It should be noted that similar immunomodulatory phenomena were observed in infection with protozoan parasites such as *Schistosoma* and *Leishmania*.[92,93] One should keep in mind that the immunomodulatory ability of helminths is a double-edged sword since it also stipulates a decreased efficacy of both oral and parenteral immunizations in infected humans.[94,95]

6 MECHANISMS OF AUTOIMMUNITY IN PATIENTS WITH PARASITIC INFECTIONS

Parasites may induce autoimmune activity by several mechanisms (Table 1), including molecular mimicry between parasitic polypeptides and host antigens, alteration of host antigens, polyclonal activation of B cells, and manipulation of the idiotypic network.[1–3] All of these mechanisms are detailed in other chapters of this book.

The host immune system responds to parasitic infections by recruiting and activating inflammatory cells and by secreting various inflammatory mediators. This process may be associated with the damage and alteration of the structure of host antigens, triggering the release of sequestered antigens, or the exposure of cryptic antigen. Those modified host antigens may no longer be recognized as self and may induce the secretion of autoantibodies and the generation of autoreactive T cells.[1–3,13] *Plasmodium falciparum* infection of RBCs results in the exposure of band 3-related neoantigens to the immune system and the subsequent development of autoantibodies reacting with those antigens.[96] *Plasmodium* spp. are able to modify certain host determinants, and this process might also result in the generation of autoantigens.[97]

Table 1 Possible Mechanisms for Parasite-Induced Autoimmunity

Polyclonal activation of B cells
Modified self-antigens
Release of sequestered antigens
Alteration of host cell proteins
Neoantigens
Idiotypic network
Molecular mimicry
Linear-sequence homology
Three-dimensional structural similarity
Over-representation of specific motifs

Parasites can trigger autoimmunity by polyclonal activation and the expansion of B-cell clones that produce a large number of natural autoantibodies.[98] *Plasmodium* strains were shown to release mitogens that activate B cells.[99,100] *Trypanosoma cruzi* infection leads to the abnormal release of immature $CD4^+CD8^+$ cells to peripheral lymphoid organs, where they acquire an activated phenotype similar to that of activated effector or memory T cells. These cells apparently bypass the negative selection process, and some of them are potentially autoimmune.[101] Furthermore, the ability of *T. cruzi* to induce massive extrafollicular and follicular splenic B-cell response with enhanced production on non-parasite-specific antibodies is well documented.[8,102] This phenomenon is probably mediated by *T. cruzi* malate dehydrogenase[103] and trans-sialidase, which upon administration to wild-type mice mediated B-cell proliferation in a T-cell-independent mechanism with non-specific Ig secretion.[104]

A possibility of manipulation of the idiotypic network in patients with parasitic infection has been considered.[105] The idiotypic network indicates that idiotypes and their anti-idiotype antibodies have a major role in regulating the immune response to self- and foreign-antigens. Auto-anti-idiotypes are a normal component of the immune system, and their role is to down-regulate autoreactive clones.[105] In people susceptible to autoimmune diseases (those with the appropriate genetic, hormonal, immunological, and environmental backgrounds), the parasite-induced activation of the idiotypic cascade may proceed from anti-idiotypes (anti-anti-parasite) to the generation of anti-anti-idiotypes (Ab3) that may be pathogenic. This process may be the result of exposure of cryptic antigens by Ab2, or as a result of epitope spreading, based on molecular mimicry existing between the idiotype structure and intracellular or intranuclear antigens.[105]

In malaria, anti-merozoite ligand for RBC receptors triggers the production of anti-idiotypic antibodies mirroring the merozoite ligand. Those autoantibodies bind the RBC receptor and induce hemolysis.[13,36] Unfortunately, experimental data that might further confirm this intriguing hypothesis are scarce.

7 MOLECULAR MIMICRY BETWEEN HOST AND PARASITES

The molecular mimicry theory is based on the antigenic similarity between host tissue and infectious agents. Antigenic cross-reactivity occurs between host and bacterial, viral, or parasitic antigens. The similarity between host and microbial antigens may suppress the immune system and protect invading parasites and other infectious agents from being eliminated by the immune system. A salient example is molecular mimicry between peptides of *Plasmodium knowlesi* and human CD99.[106] Given the immunosuppressive role of the latter, the parasites' homologous peptides might induce apoptosis of double-positive T cells and escape immune surveillance.

The presence of common epitopes shared by pathogen and host antigens may lead to the expansion of self-reacting lymphocytes and to the induction of autoimmune phenomena. This is supported by the following observations: binding of autoantibodies to parasitic antigens, inhibition of binding of autoantibodies to their respective autoantigens by parasitic determinants and sequence homology between various parasitic antigens and self-antigens and genetic studies showing that parasite genomes contain genomic sequences that encode proteins close to self-antigens.[107] Indeed, molecular mimicry is of the utmost importance for the pathogenesis of heart involvement in Chagas disease, where T cells cross-reactive with trypanosomal B13 protein also recognize the host's cardiac myosin with resultant damage of myocard.[108]

8 HOMOLOGY BETWEEN SELF AND PARASITIC ANTIGENS

The following are observations that suggest molecular mimicry between parasitic and human antigens.

1. The binding of the monoclonal anti-circulating cathodic antigen (CCA) antibodies from patients with schistosomiasis to the repeating Lewis-x units on the surface of human granulocytes. The CCA, a glycoprotein which contains polysaccharide side chains repeating tri-saccharide Lewis-x units.[109] This autoactivity was associated with granulocyte lysis in a complement-dependent cytotoxic assay, suggesting that autoimmune mechanisms may be associated with the development of moderate neutropenia seen in patients with schistosomiasis.

2. Amino acids sequence homology between a 2.5-kDa *O. volvulus* antigen and human defensins 1–3 of neutrophils. The titer of anti-2.5-kDa antibody is directly related to disease activity and it has an anti-defensin activity.[76]

3. An immunogenic TbDIP13 protein of *Trypanosoma brucei* was found to be homologous to human Sjögren's syndrome nuclear autoantigen 1 (also known as NA14), a major specific target for autoantibodies in Sjögren's syndrome. The pathogenetic role of this homology is yet unclear.[110]

9 GENETIC SIMILARITY BETWEEN PARASITES AND HUMANS

The following studies point to a sequence homology between genes encoding parasitic and human antigens.

1. Homology between human thrombospondin-related anonymous protein (TRAP) of *P. falciparum* is well known.[111] The current concept proposes that TRAP plays a key role in the sporozoite invasion of hepatocytes.[112]

2. A novel (Epidermal Growth Factor) EGF-like domain-containing protein of *P. falciparum* that encodes a polypeptide of 597 amino acids was recently identified. This protein is proposed to play a role in the process of RBC invasion.[113]

3. *FL-160-1* is a gene encoding the COOH terminus of a protein associated with the flagellum of *T. cruzi* trypomastigotes. The COOH terminus of FL-160 has an epitope of 12 amino acids, which molecularly mimics a nervous tissue antigen of 48 kDa present in the myenteric plexus, sciatic nerve, and a subset of cells in the central nervous system. Homology also was found between an epitope located on the NH2 terminus of FL-160 and nervous tissues. The *FL-160* genes belong to a family of highly related genes. More than 750 copies of FL-160 are present in the DNA of the parasite. Sequence analysis of genes revealed that all members of the *FL-160* gene family retain the 12-amino acid molecular mimicry epitope. Antibodies directed against this epitope also were found to bind the epineurium.[114]

4. A high sequence homology between the *O. volvulus* RAL-1 antigen, one of the subunits of human and mouse Ro antigen and calreticulin, a high-affinity calcium binding protein, is well established.[115] These findings shed light on one of possible mechanisms of autoantibody development to nuclear antigens in patients with parasitic infections.

5. In patients with malaria, cloning of a *P. falciparum* gene related to the human 60-kDa heat shock protein revealed more than 50% homology to heat shock protein 60 from human and other eukaryotes.[116]

6. The *in silico* comparison of broken down into overlapping fragments predicted proteome of *P. falciparum* with human proteome revealed a 14-amino acid motif in several of the PfEMP1 variants identical to part of the heparin-binding domain in the immunosuppressive serum protein vitronectin.[117]

10 SIGNIFICANCE OF MOLECULAR MIMICRY

The biologically significant homology between parasitic, microbial or viral, and self-antigens may result from linear-sequence homology of amino acid motifs, over-representation of a specific motif, and/or three-dimensional structural similarity between the pathogenic peptide and (Major Histocompatibility Complex) MHC antigens. This homology results in an interaction of the T-cell receptor with specific MHC–peptide ligands of parasites that leads to proliferation and clonal expansion of autoreactive cells.[118,119]

A similarity between peptides located on the β-chain of human MHC and viral and bacterial peptides has been identified. In patients with RA, the QKRAA/QRRAA motif of the β-chain of HLA-DR4 is located on peptides from HIV, EBV gp110, and *Escherichia coli* dnaJ.[120,121] This motif is highly associated with RA, suggesting that linear molecular mimicry (shared epitopes) between MHC antigens and microbial and self-antigens is associated with the activation of T cells and the induction of autoimmunity in patients with RA.

Others have indicated that the activation of T cells and the induction of cross-reactive immunity require homology between the three-dimensional structure of epitopes of MHC and pathogenic antigens but not necessarily linear-sequence homology. In a model of experimental autoimmune uveitis, a strong three-dimensional similarity was found between peptides of three antigens (retinal S-antigen, HLA-B27, and B7), although the linear structure of the S and HLA peptides revealed homology in only 5 of 14 amino acids.[122]

Roudier et al.[123] performed statistical and mathematical analyses of the amino acids of proteins using the SWISS-PROT database and suggested that over-representation of certain amino acids motifs in patients with autoimmunity may result in overt clinical disease. The QKRAA motif, associated with RA, was found to be 37 times more common than the expected number of matches for QKRAA on theoretical calculations in the database. Their analyses revealed that it is easy to identify a five to seven amino acids match between unrelated proteins because of the large size of the protein databases, and molecular mimicry between proteins is a common finding and not necessarily associated with pathogenic significance.

While similarity between parasitic and self-antigens has been long suggested, the reports showing the biologic significance of specific parasitic epitopes in generating autoimmunity at the level of T-cell recognition are scarce.[124,125]

11 SUMMARY

The studies summarized in this chapter suggest that parasites may trigger the activation of autoimmune mechanisms. The association between parasites and autoimmunity could be manifested by the development of pathogenic anti-parasitic antibodies and cytotoxic T cells that attack and damage self-tissues as a result of molecular mimicry between host and parasites. On the other hand, the homology between parasitic and self-antigens may enable parasites to protect themselves from the immune system and to induce a state of immunosuppression.

REFERENCES

1. Abu-Shakra M, Buskila D, Shoenfeld Y. Molecular mimicry between host and pathogens: examples from parasites implication. *Immunol Lett* 1999;**67**:147–52.
2. Abu-shakra M, Shoenfeld Y. Parasitic infections and autoimmunity. *Autoimmunity* 1991;**9**:337–44.
3. Abu-Shakra M, Shoenfeld Y. Chronic infections and autoimmunity: molecular immunobiology of self reactivity. *Immunol Ser* 1991;**55**:285–313.
4. Cunha-Neto E, Bilate AM, Hyland KV, Fonseca SG, Kalil J, Engman DM. Induction of cardiac autoimmunity in Chagas heart disease: a case for molecular mimicry. *Autoimmunity* 2006;**39**:41–54.
5. Teixeira A, Hecht M, Guimaro M, Sousa A, Nitz N. Pathogenesis of Chagas' disease: parasite persistence and autoimmunity. *Clin Microbiol Rev* 2011;**3**:592–630.
6. Zhou Y, Dziak E, Unnasch TR, Opas M. Major retinal cell components recognized by onchocerciasis sera are associated with the cell surface and nucleoli. *Invest Ophthalmol Vis Sci* 1994;**35**:1089–99.
7. Ritter K, Kuhlenecord A, Thomssen R, Bommer W. Prolonged hemolytic anemia in malaria and autoantibodies against triosephosphate isomerase. *Lancet* 1993;**342**:1333–4.
8. Adib-Conquy M, Avrameas S, Ternynck T. Monoclonal IgG and IgM autoantibodies obtained after polyclonal activation, show reactivities similar to those of polyclonal natural autoantibodies. *Mol Immunol* 1993;**30**:119–27.
9. Rahima D, Tarrab-Hazdai R, Blank M, Arnon R, Shoenfeld Y. Anti-nuclear antibodies associated with schistosomiasis and anti-schistosomal antibodies associated with SLE. *Autoimmunity* 1994;**17**:127–41.
10. Shoenfeld Y, Rauch J, Massictte H, Datta SK, Stollar BD, Schwartz RS. Polyspecifity of monoclonal lupus autoantibodies produced by human-human hybridomas. *N Engl J Med* 1983;**308**:414–20.
11. Gironès N, Cueryp H, Fresno M. *Trypanosoma cruzi*-induced molecular mimicry and Chagas' disease. *Curr Top Microbiol Immunol* 2005;**296**:89–123.
12. Bonney KM, Taylor JM, Daniels MD, Epting CL, Engman DM. Heat-killed *Trypanosoma cruzi* induces acute cardiac damage and polyantigenic autoimmunity. *PLoS One* 2011;**6**:e14571.
13. Daniel-Ribeiro C, Zanini G. Autoimmunity and malaria: what are they doing together? *Acta Trop* 2000;**76**:205–21.
14. Brahimi K, Martin Y, Zanini G, Ferreira-sa-Cruz M, Daniel-Ribeiro C. Monoclonal auto-antibodies and sera of autoimmune patients react with *Plasmodium falciparum* and inhibit its in vitro growth. *Mem Inst Oswaldo Cruz* 2011;**106**(Suppl. I):44–51.
15. Shaper AG, Kaplan MH, Mody NJ, McIntyre PA. Malaria antibodies and autoantibodies to heart and other tissues in immigrant and indigenous people of Uganda. *Lancet* 1968;**1**:1342–7.

16. Mannoor K, Li C, Inafuku M, Taniguchi T, Abo T, Sato Y, et al. Induction of ssDNA-binding autoantibody secreting B cell immunity during murine malaria infection is a critical part of the protective immune responses. *Immunobiol* 2013;**218**:10–20.
17. Boonpucknavig S, Ekapanyakul G. Autoantibodies in sera of Thai patients with *Plasmodium falciparum* infection. *Clin Exp Immunol* 1984;**58**:77–82.
18. Skouri H, Gandouz R, Kraiem I, Harrabi I, Said MB. Antibodies to anionic phospholipids and cofactors in kala-azar. Comparative study with malaria, toxoplasmosis and "autoimmune diseases" *Clin Exp Rheumatol* 2008;**26**:894–902.
19. Lefrancois G, Bouvet E, Le Bras J, Vroklans M, Simonneau M, Vachon F. Anti-erythrocyte autoimmunization during chronic falciparum malaria. *Lancet* 1981;**2** (8248):661–4.
20. De Souza JB, Playfair JHL. Anti-lymphocyte autoantibody in lethal malaria and its suppression by non lethal malaria. *Parasite Immunol* 1983;**5**:257–65.
21. Greenwood BM, Muller AS, Valkenburg HA. Rheumatoid factor in Nigerian sera. *Clin Exp Immunol* 1971;**8**:161–73.
22. Pradhan V, Badakere SS, Shankarkumar U, Iyer YS, Ghosh K, Karnad D. Anti-neutrophil cytoplasmic antibodies (ANCA) in malaria. *Indian J Malariol* 2002;**39**:51–9.
23. Gallien S, Roussilhon C, Blanc C, Pérignon JL, Druilhe P. Autoantibody against dendrite in *Plasmodium falciparum* infection: a singular auto-immune phenomenon preferentially in cerebral malaria. *Acta Trop* 2011;**118**:67–70.
24. Duarte J, Herbert F, Guiyedi V, Franevich J, Roland J, Cazenave PA, et al. High levels of immunoglobulin E autoantibody to 14-3-3 epsilon protein correlate with protection against sever *Plasmodium falciparum* malaria. *J Infect Dis* 2012;**206**:1781–9.
25. Thomas BN, Diallo DA, Noumsi GT, Moulds JM. Circulating immune complex levels are associated with disease severity and seasonality in children with malaria from Mali. *Biomark Insights* 2012;**7**:81–6.
26. Daniel-Ribeiro C, Ben Slama L, Gentiline M. Anti-nuclear and anti-smooth muscle antibodies in Caucasians, Africans and Asians with acute malaria. *J Clin Lab Immunol* 1991;**35**:109–12.
27. Phanuphak P, Tirwatpong S, Hanvanich M, Panmuong W, Mollar P, Vejjajiva S. Autoantibodies in falciparum malaria: a sequential study in 183 Thai patients. *Clin Exp Immunol* 1983;**53**:627–33.
28. Gilkeson G, James J, Kamen D, Knackstedt T, Maggi D, Meyer A, et al. The United States to Africa lupus prevalence revisited. *Lupus* 2011;**20**:1095–103.
29. Lekpa F, Ndongo S, Tiendrebeogo J, Ndao A, Daher A, Pouye A, et al. Rheumatoid arthritis in Senegal: a comparison between patients coming from rural and urban areas, in an urban tertiary health care center in Senegal. *Clin Rheumatol* 2012;**31**:1617–20.
30. Krieg AM, Vollmer J. Toll-like receptors 7, 8, and 9: linking innate immunity to autoimmunity. *Immunol Rev* 2007;**220**:251–69.
31. Basu M, Maji A, Chakraborty A, Banerjee R, Mullick S, Saha P, et al. Genetic association of toll-like-receptor 4 and tumor necrosis factor-alpha polymorphisms with *Plasmodium falciparum* blood infection levels. *Infect Genet Evol* 2010;**10**:686–96.
32. Gowda N, Wu X, Gowda D. TLR9 and MyD88 are crucial for the development of protective immunity to malaria. *J Immunol* 2012;**188**:5073–85.
33. Kirchner M, Soonenschein A, Schoofs S, Schmidtke P, Umlauf V, Mannhardt-Laakman W. Surface expression and genotypes of toll-like receptors 2 and 4 in patients with juvenile idiopathic arthritis and systemic lupus erythematosus. *Pediatr Rheumatol Online J* 2013;**11**:9.
34. Nickerson N, Christensen S, Shupe J, Kashagarian M, Kim D, Elkon K, et al. TLR9 regulates TLR7- and MyD88-dependent autoantibody production in a murine model of lupus. *J Immunol* 2010;**184**:1840–8.

35. Farias A, Talaisys R, Blanco Y, Lopes S, Longhini A, Prdella F, et al. Regulatory T cell induction during *Plasmodium chabaudi* infection modifies the clinical course of experimental autoimmune encephalomyelitis. *PLoS One* 2011;**6**:e17849.
36. Sayles PC, Wassom DL. Are antibodies important in mice infected with *Plasmodium yoelii*? *Parasitol Today* 1992;**8**:368–70.
37. Fernandez-Arias C, Lopez JP, Hernandez-Perez JN, Bautista-Ojeda MD, Branch O, Rodriguez A. Malaria inhibits surface expression of complement receptor 1 in monocytes/macrophages, causing decreased immune complex internalization. *J Immunol* 2013;**190**:3363–72.
38. Wozencraft AO, Lloyd CM, Staines NA, Griffiths VJ. Role of DNA binding antibodies in kidney pathology associated with murine malaria infectious. *Infec Immun* 1990;**58**:2156–64.
39. Lloyd CM, Collins I, Belcher AJ, Manuelpillai N, Wozencraft AO, Staines NA. Characterization and pathological significance of monoclonal DNA-binding antibodies from mice with experimental malaria infection. *Infect Immun* 1994;**62**:1982–8.
40. Argov S, Jaffe CL, Krupp M, Slor H, Shoenfeld Y. Autoantibody production by patients infected with leishmania. *Clin Exp Immunol* 1989;**76**:190–7.
41. Liberopoulos E, Kei A, Apostolou F, Elisaf M. Autoimmune manifestations in patients with visceral leishmaniasis. *J Microbiol Immunol Infect* 2013;**46**:302–5.
42. Ahlin E, Elshafei A, Nur M, El Safi S, Johan R, Elghazali G. Anti-citrullinated peptide antibodies and rheumatoid factor in Sudanese patients with *Leishmania donovani* infection. *Rev Bras Reumatol* 2011;**51**:579–86.
43. Atta AM, Carvalho EM, Jerônimo SM, Sousa Atta ML. Serum markers of rheumatoid arthritis in visceral leishmaniasis: rheumatoid factor and anti-cyclic citrullinated peptide antibody. *J Autoimmun* 2007;**28**:55–8.
44. Makaritisis K, Gatselis N, Ioannou M, Petinaki E, Dalekos G. Polyclonal hypergammaglobulinemia and high smooth-muscle autoantibody titers with specificity against filamentous actin: consider visceral leishmaniasis, not just autoimmune hepatitis. *Int J Infect Dis* 2009;**13**:e157 60.
45. Bhatnagar H, Kala S, Sharma L, Jain S, Kim K, Pal R. Serum and organ-associated anti-hemoglobin humoral autoreactivity: association with anti-Sm responses and inflammation. *Eur J Immunol* 2011;**41**:537–48.
46. Karagianni AE, Solano-Gallego L, Breitschwerdt EB, Gaschen FP, Day MJ, Trotta M, et al. Perinuclear antineutrophil cytoplasmic autoantibodies in dogs infected with various vector-borne pathogens and in dogs with immune-mediated hemolytic anemia. *Am J Vet Res* 2012;**73**:1403–9.
47. Santiago M, Martinelli R, Ko A, Reis EA, Fontes RD, Nascimento EG, et al. Anti-beta2 glycoprotein I and anticardiolipin antibodies in leptospirosis, syphilis and Kala-azar. *Clin Exp Rheumatol* 2001;**19**:425–30.
48. Atta A, Sousa-Atta M, D'Oliveira A, Almeida R, Araujo M, Carvalho E. IgG anti-IgE autoantibodies in visceral leishmaniasis. *Mem Inst Oswaldo Cruz* 2002;**97**:101–3.
49. Pollack S, Nagler A, Liberman D, Oren I, Alroy G, Katz R, et al. Immunological studies of pancytopenia in visceral leishmaniasis. *Isr J Med Sci* 1988;**24**(2):70–4.
50. Braun J, Sieper J, Schulte KL, Thiel E, Janitschke K. Visceral leishmaniasis mimicking a flare of systemic lupus erythematosus. *Clin Rheumatol* 1991;**10**:445–8.
51. Ossandon A, Bompane D, Alessandri C, Marocchi E, Conti F, Valesini G. Leishmania in SLE mimicking an exacerbation. *Clin Exp Rheumatol* 2006;**24**:186–90.
52. Casato M, de Rosa F, Pucillo L, Ilardi I, diVico B, Zorzin L, et al. Mixed cryoglobulinemia secondary to visceral leishmaniasis. *Arthritis Rheum* 1999;**42**:2007–11.
53. Tunccan OG, Tufan A, Telli G, Akyürek N, Pamukçuoğlu M, Yılmaz G, et al. Visceral leishmaniasis mimicking autoimmune hepatitis, primary biliary cirrhosis, and systemic lupus erythematosus overlap. *Korean J Parasitol* 2012;**50**:133–6.

54. Granel B, Serratrice J, Swiader L, Gambarelli F, Daniel L, Fossat C, et al. Crossing of antinuclear antibodies and anti-leishmania antibodies. *Lupus* 2000;**9**:548–50.
55. Dutra M, Martinelli R, de Carvalho EM, Rodrigues LE, Brito E, Rocha H. Renal involvement in visceral leishmaniasis. *Am J Kidney Dis* 1985;**198**(6):22–7.
56. Rigo R, Carvalho C, Honer M, de Andrade G, Silva I, Rigo L, et al. Renal histopathological findings in dogs with visceral leishmaniasis. *Rev Inst Med Trop Sao Paulo* 2013;**55**:113–16.
57. Mary C, Ange G, Dunan S, Lamouroux D, Quilici M. Characterization of a circulating antigen involved in immune complexes in visceral leishmaniasis patients. *Am J Trop Med Hyg* 1993;**49**(4):492–501.
58. Desjeux P, Santoro F, Afchain D, Loyens M, Capron A. Circulating immune complexes and anti-IgG antibodies in mucocutaneous leishmaniasis. *Am J Trop Med Hyg* 1980;**29** (2):195–8.
59. Elshafie A, Ahlin E, Mathsson L, ElGhazali G, Rönnelid J. Circulating immune complexes (IC) and IC-induced levels of GM-CSF are increased in Sudanese patients with acute visceral *Leishmania donovani* infection undergoing sodium stibogluconate treatment: implications for disease pathogenesis. *J Immunol* 2007;**178**:5383–9.
60. Shamma AH, Ali AJ, el-Shawi NN. Auto-antibodies in *Schistosoma haematobium* infections. *J Pathol Bacteriol* 1965;**90**(2):659–61.
61. Abdel Aal H, el Atribi A, Abdel Hafiz A, Aidaros M. Azoospermia in bilharziasis and the presence of sperm antibodies. *J Reprod Fertil* 1975;**42**:403–6.
62. Kawabata M, Hosaka Y, Kumada M, Matsui N, Kobayakawa T. Thymocytotoxic autoantibodies found in mice infected with *Schistosoma japonicum*. *Infect Immun* 1981;**32** (2):438–42.
63. Bendixen G, Hadidi T, Manthorpe R, Permin H, Struckmann J, Wilk A, et al. Antibodies against nuclear components in schistosomiasis. Results compared to values in patients with rheumatoid arthritis, systemic lupus erythematosus, and osteoarthrosis. *Allergy* 1984;**39**(2):107–13.
64. Howard MK, Gull K, Miles MA. Antibodies to tubulin in patients with parasitic infections. *Clin Exp Immunol* 1987;**68**:78–85.
65. Pereira LM, McFarlane BM, Massarolo P, Saleh MG, Bridger C, Spinelli V, et al. Specific liver autoreactivity in *Schistosomiasis mansoni*. *Trans R Soc Trop Med Hyg* 1997;**91**:310–14.
66. Wyler DJ, Lammie PJ, Michael AI, Rosenwasser LJ, Philips SM. In vitro and in vivo evidence that autoimmune reactivity to collagen develops spontaneously in *Schistosoma mansoni*-infected mice. *Clin Immunol Immunopath* 1987;**44**:140–8.
67. Thomas MA, Frampton G, Isenberg DA, Shoenfeld Y, Akinsola A, Ramsay M. A common anti-DNA antibody idiotype and anti-phospholipid antibodies in sera from patients with schistosomiasis and filariasis with and without nephritis. *J Autoimmunity* 1990;**2**:803–12.
68. Mutapi F, Imai N, Nausch N, Bourke C, Rujeni N, Mitchell K, et al. Schistosome infection intensity is inversely related to auto-reactive antibody levels. *PLoS One* 2011;**6**(5): e19149.
69. Kawabata M, Flores GZ, Izui S, Kobayakawa T. IgM rheumatoid factors in Guatemalan onchocerciasis. *Trans R Soc Trop Med Hyg* 1984;**78**(3):356–8.
70. Petralanda I, Piessens WF. Pathogenesis of onchocercal dermatitis: possible role of parasite proteases and autoantibodies to extracellular matrix proteins. *Exp Parasitol* 1994;**79** (2):177–86.
71. Donnelly JJ, Xi MS, Holdar JP, Hill DE, Lok JB, Khatami M, et al. Autoantibody induced by experimental Onchocerca infection. Effect of different routes of administration of microfilariae and of treatment with diethylcarbamazine citrate and ivermectin. *Invest Ophthalmol Vis Sci* 1988;**29**:827–31.

72. Liu SH. Experimental model of autoimmune keratitis. *Invest Opthalmol Vis Sci* 1983;**24**:100.

73. Chan CC, Nussenblatt RB, Kim MK, Palestine AG, Awadzi K, Ottesen EA. Immunopathology of ocular onchocerciasis. II. Anti-retina autoantibodies in serum and ocular fluids. *Opthalmology* 1987;**94**:439–43.

74. Van-der-Lelij A, Doekes G, Hwan BS, Vetter JC, Stilma JS, Kijlstra A. Humoral autoimmune response against S-antigen and IRBP in ocular onchocerciasis. *Invest Ophthalmol Vis Sci* 1990;**31**:1374–80.

75. Meilof JF, Van der Lelij A, Rokeach LA, Hoch SO, Smeenk RJ. Autoimmunity and filariasis. Autoantibodies against cytoplasmic cellular proteins in sera of patients with onchocerciasis. *J Immunol* 1993;**151**:5800–9.

76. Gallin M, Jacobi A, Büttner D, Schönberger O, Marti T, Erttmann K. Human autoantibody to defensin: disease association with hyperreactive onchocerciasis (sowda). *J Exp Med* 1995;**182**:41–7.

77. Gelebart P, Opas M, Michalak M. Calreticulin, a Ca2 + -binding chaperone of the endoplasmic reticulum. *Int J Biochem Cell Biol* 2005;**37**:260–6.

78. Hong C, Qiu X, Li Y, Huang Q, Zhong Z, Zhang Y, et al. Functional analysis of recombinant calreticulin fragment 39-272: implications for immunobiological activities of calreticulin in health and disease. *J Immunol* 2010;**185**:4561–9.

79. Thomson I. Onchocerciasis in an oil palm estate. *Trans R Soc Trop Med Hyg* 1971;**65**:484–9.

80. Ling S, Cheng A, Pumpens P, Michalak M, Holoshitz J. Identification of the rheumatoid arthritis shared epitope binding site on calreticulin. *PLoS One* 2010;**5**:e11703.

81. Kinoshita G, Purcell A, Keech C, Farris A, McCluskey J, Gordon T. Molecular chaperones are targets of autoimmunity in Ro(SS-A) immune mice. *Clin Exp Immunol* 1999;**115**:268–74.

82. Kinoshita G, Keech CL, Sontheimer RD, Purcell A, McCluskey J, Gordon TP. Spreading of the immune response from 52 kDaRo and 60 kDaRo to calreticulin in experimental autoimmunity. *Lupus* 1998;**7**.7–11.

83. Takemura Y, Ouchi N, Shibata R, Aprahamian T, Kirber MT, Summer RS, et al. Adiponectin modulates inflammatory reactions via calreticulin receptor-dependent clearance of early apoptotic bodies. *J Clin Invest* 2007;**117**:375–86.

84. Scofield R, Racila D, Gordon T, Kurien B, Sontheimer R. Anti-calreticulin segregates anti-Ro sera in systemic lupus erythematosus: anti-calreticulin is present in sera with anti-Ro alone but not in anti-Ro sera with anti-La or anti-ribonucleoprotein. *J Rheumatol* 2000;**27**:128–34.

85. Sánchez D, Palová-Jelínková L, Felsberg J, Simsová M, Pekáriková A, Pecharová B, et al. Anti-calreticulin immunoglobulin A (IgA) antibodies in refractory coeliac disease. *Clin Exp Immunol* 2008;**153**:351–9.

86. Terrazas CA, Alcántara-Hernández M, Bonifaz L, Terrazas L, Satoskar A. Helminth-excreted/secreted products are recognized by multiple receptors on DCs to block the TLR response and bias Th2 polarization in a cRAF dependent pathway. *FASEB J* 2013;**27**(11):4547–60.

87. Imai S, Fujita K. Molecules of parasites as immunomodulatory drugs. *Curr Top Med Chem* 2004;**4**:539–52.

88. Lourenco E, La Cava A. Natural regulatory T cells in autoimmunity. *Autoimmunity* 2011;**44**:33–42.

89. Ricci N, Fiúza J, Bueno L, Cançado G, Gazzinelli-Guimarães P, Martins V, et al. Induction of CD4 + CD25 + FOXP3 + regulatory T cells during human hookworm infection modulates antigen-mediated lymphocyte proliferation. *PLoS Negl Trop Dis* 2011;**5**: e1383.

90. Fleming J. Helminth therapy and multiple sclerosis. *Int J Parasitol* 2013;**43**:259–74.

91. Ashour D, Othman A, Shareef M, Gaballah H, Mayah W. Interactions between *Trichinella spiralis* infection and induced colitis in mice. *J Helminthol* 2013;**12**:1–9.

92. Zaccone P, Fehérvári Z, Jones FM, Sidobre S, Kronenberg M, Dunne DW, et al. *Schistosoma mansoni* antigens modulate the activity of innate immune response and prevent onset of type 1 diabetes. *Eur J Immunol* 2003;**33**:1439–49.

93. Srivastava S, Pandey S, Jha M, Chandel H, Saha B. Leishmania expressed lipophosphoglycan interacts with toll-like receptor (TLR)-2 to decrease TLR-9 expression and reduce anti-leishmanial responses. *Clin Exp Immunol* 2013;**172**:403–9.

94. Cooper P, Chico M, Losonski G, Sandoval C, Espinel I, Guevara A, et al. Human infection with Ascaris lumbricoides is associated with suppression of the interleukin-2 response to recombinant cholera toxin B subunit following vaccination with the live cholera vaccine CVD 103-HgR. *Infect Immun* 2001;**69**:1574–80.

95. Elias D, Wolday D, Akuffo H, Petros B, Bronner U, Britton S. Effect of deworming on human T cell responses to mycobacterial antigens in helminth-exposed individuals before and after bacilli Calmette-Guerin (BCG) vaccination. *Clin Exp Immunol* 2001;**123**:1326–34.

96. Winograd E, Prudhomme J, Sherman I. Band 3 clustering promotes the exposure of neoantigens in *Plasmodium falciparum*-infected erythrocytes. *Mol Biochem Parasitol* 2005;**142**:98–105.

97. Kumar K, Singh S, Babu P. Studies on the glycoprotein modification in erythrocyte membrane during experimental cerebral malaria. *Exp Parasitol* 2006;**114**:173–9.

98. Ternynck T, Falanga PB, Unterkirscher C, Gregoire J, da Silva LP, Avrameas S. Induction of high levels of IgG autoantibodies in mice infected with *Plasmodium chabaudi*. *Int Immunol* 1991;**3**:29–37.

99. Donati D, Zhang L, Chêne A, Chen Q, Flick K, Nyström M, et al. Identification of a polyclonal B-cell activator in *Plasmodium falciparum*. *Infect Immun* 2004;**72**:5412–18.

100. Pinzón-Charry A, Vernot JP, Rodríguez R, Patarroyo ME. Proliferative response of peripheral blood lymphocytes to mitogens in the owl monkey Aotus nancymae. *J Med Primatol* 2003;**32**:31–8.

101. Morrot A, Barreto de Albuquerque J, Berbert L, de Carvalho Pinto C, de Meis J, Savino W. Dynamics of lymphocyte populations during *Trypanosoma cruzi* infection: from thymocyte depletion to differential cell expansion/contraction in peripheral lymphoid organs. *J Trop Med* 2012;http://dx.doi.org/10.1155/2012/747185 Article ID 747185, Epub February 12, 2012.

102. Bermejo D, Amezcua Vesely M, Khan M, Acosta Rodríguez E, Montes C, Merino M, et al. *Trypanosoma cruzi* infection induces a massive extrafollicular and follicular splenic B-cell response which is a high source of non-parasite-specific antibodies. *Immunology* 2011;**132**:123–33.

103. Montes CL, Zuniga EI, Vazquez J, Arce C, Gruppi A. *Trypanosoma cruzi* mitochondrial malate dehydrogenase triggers polyclonal B-cell activation. *Clin Exp Immunol* 2002;**127**:27–36.

104. Gao W, Wortis HH, Pereira MA. The *Trypanosoma cruzi* trans-sialidase is a T cell-independent B cell mitogen and an inducer of non-specific Ig secretion. *Int Immunol* 2002;**14**:299–308.

105. Shoenfeld Y. Idiotypic induction of autoimmunity: a new aspect of autoimmunity. *FASEB J* 1994;**8**:1296–301.

106. Pain A, Böhme U, Berry AE, Mungall K, Finn RD, Jackson AP, et al. The genome of the simian and human malaria parasite *Plasmodium knowlesi*. *Nature* 2008;**455**:799–803.

107. Cusick MF, Libbey JE, Fujinami RS. Molecular mimicry as a mechanism of autoimmune disease. *Clin Rev Allergy Immunol* 2012;**42**:102–11.

108. Iwai LK, Juliano MA, Juliano L, Kalil J, Cunha-Neto E. T-cell molecular mimicry in Chagas disease: identification and partial structural analysis of multiple cross-reactive

epitopes between *Trypanosoma cruzi* B13 and cardiac myosin heavy chain. *J Autoimmun* 2005;**24**:111–17.

109. Van Dam GJ, Claas FH, Yazdanbakhsh M, Kruize YC, Van Keulen AC, Ferreira ST, et al. *Schistosoma mansoni* excretory circulating cathodic antigen shares Lewis × epitopes with a human granulocyte surface antigen and evokes host antibodies mediating complement dependent lysis of granulocytes. *Blood* 1996;**88**:4246–51.

110. Price HP, Hodgkinson MR, Curwen RS, MacLean LM, Brannigan JA, Carrington M, et al. The orthologue of Sjögren's syndrome nuclear autoantigen 1 (SSNA1) in *Trypanosoma brucei* is an immunogenic self-assembling molecule. *PLoS One* 2012;**7**:e31842.

111. Robson K, Hall J, Jennings M, Harris T, Marsh K, Newbold C, et al. A highly conserved amino-acid sequence in thrombospondin, properdin and in proteins from sporozoites and blood stages of a human malaria parasite. *Nature* 1988;**335**:79–82.

112. Morahan B, Wang L, Coppel R. No TRAP, no invasion. *Trends Parasitol* 2009;**25**:77–84.

113. Black CG, Wu T, Wang L, Hibbs AR, Coppel RL. Merozoite surface protein 8 of *Plasmodium falciparum* contains two epidermal growth factor-like domains. *Mol Biochem Parasitol* 2001;**114**:217–26.

114. Van-Voorhis WC, Barrett L, Koelling R, Farr AG. Fl-160 proteins of *Trypanosoma cruzi* are expressed from a multigene family and contain two distinct epitopes that mimic nervous tissues. *J Exp Med* 1993;**178**:681–94.

115. McCauliffe DP, Zappi E, Lieu TS, Michalak M, Capra JD. A human Ro autoantigen is the homologue of calreticulin and is highly homologous with onchocercal RAL-1 antigen and an aplysia "memory molecule" *J Clin Invest* 1990;**86**:332–5.

116. Syin C, Goldman ND. Cloning of a *Plasmodium falciparum* gene related to the human 60-kDa heat shock protein. *Mol Biochem Parasitol* 1996;**79**:13–19.

117. Ludin P, Nilsson D, Mäser P. Genome-wide identification of molecular mimicry candidates in parasites. *PLoS One* 2011;**6**:e17546.

118. Hernandez HJ, Stadecker MJ. Elucidation and role of critical residues of immunodominant peptide associated with T cell-mediated parasitic disease. *J Immunol* 1999;**163**:3877–82.

119. Joshi S, Suresh P, Chauhan V. Flexibility in MHC and TCR recognition: degenerate specificity at the T cell level in the recognition of promiscuous Th epitopes exhibiting no primary sequence homology. *J Immunol* 2001;**166**:6693–9703.

120. Auger I, Lepecuchel L, Roudier J. Interaction between heat-shock protein 73 and HLA-DRB alleles associated or not with rheumatoid arthritis. *Arthritis Rheum* 2002;**46**:929–33.

121. Roudier J, Peterson J, Rhodes G, Luka J, Carson DA. Susceptibility to RA maps to a T cell epitope shared by the HLA-DW4 DR beta 1 chain and the EBV glycoprotein. *Proc Natl Acad Sci U S A* 1989;**86**:5104–8.

122. Wildner G, Thurau SR. Database screening for molecular mimicry. *Immunol Today* 1997;**18**:252.

123. Roudier C, Auger I, Roudier J. Molecular mimicry reflected through database screening: serendipity or survival strategy? *Immunol Today* 1996;**17**:357–8.

124. Cunha-Neto E, Moliterno R, Coelho V, Guilherme L, Bocchi E, Higuchi Mde L, et al. Restricted heterogeneity of T cell receptor variable alpha chain transcripts in hearts of Chagas' disease cardiomyopathy patients. *Parasite Immunol* 1994;**16**:171–9.

125. Champange E. γδ T cell receptor ligands and model of antigen recognition. *Arch Immunol Ther Exp* 2011;**59**:117–37.

CHAPTER 37

Toxoplasma and Autoimmunity

Jana Petríková[1], Peter Jarčuška, Daniel Pella

1st Department of Internal Medicine, Medical Faculty of P. J. Šafárik University Košice, Slovakia
[1]Corresponding Author: jana.petrikova@upjs.sk

1 INTRODUCTION

The possible link between infectious diseases, mainly caused by viruses and bacteria, and autoimmune diseases (AIDs) has been repeatedly suggested based mostly on epidemiological and experimental data.[1,2] The role of parasitic infections has been largely overlooked, but parasites elicit a complex immunomodulatory effect in the host.[3,4] On one hand, geoepidemiological as well as experimental evidence may well support the protective effect of specific parasitic infections in the susceptibility to autoimmunity.[4] In addition, helminths were shown to be protective in several experimental models, including type 1 diabetes, autoimmune encephalitis, and ulcerative colitis, most likely via a Th2 environment; helminths were also shown to induce regulatory responses.[4] Conversely, some parasites have been implicated in the evolution of autoimmunity.[5,6]

Toxoplasma gondii (TG) is an obligate intracellular parasitic protozoan that infects most genera of warm-blooded animals, including humans, but the primary host is the felid (cat) family. Sexual stages of the parasite occur within gut epithelial cells of the cat, and the products of gamete fusion, the oocysts, are shed in feces. Once in contact with the atmosphere, the oocysts sporulate and become infective to other definitive or intermediate hosts. Nevertheless, in contrast to other coccidia, *Toxoplasma* has evolved to infect a wide variety of vertebrate species, including humans. Indeed, this asexual stage of the parasite's life cycle, unlike the sexual phase in cats, is notable for its lack of both host and tissue specificity. In the intermediate host, after infecting intestinal epithelial cells, the infective stages (oocysts or bradyzoites) transform into tachyzoites, which display rapid multiplication within an intracellular parasitophorous vacuole. If not controlled by the immune system, tachyzoites are highly virulent and cause a generalized toxoplasmosis that is always fatal.[7] Therefore, induction of T–cell-mediated

Infection and Autoimmunity
http://dx.doi.org/10.1016/B978-0-444-63269-2.00044-1

immune responses and resistance to the tachyzoite stage is a key step in the TG life cycle, determining the survival of the intermediate host and the parasite itself. After development of immunity, the tachyzoite stage is cleared from host tissues, and bradyzoites—the slowly multiplying, essentially dormant and harmless form of the parasite—persist. Moreover, it is probable that strain- or isolate-specific variation exerts an effect on host control of infection.[8]

Humans become infected with TG mainly by eating uncooked meat or by ingesting food or water contaminated with the feces of infected cats. During the first few weeks, the infection typically causes no illness or only a mild flu-like illness. It is estimated that worldwide infection rates are extremely high, around 30%.[9] However, there is a quite large geographical difference in prevalence: in the United States prevalence of TG infection is estimated around 10.8%,[10] and the rate in South Korea is only 4.3%. In countries with high consumption of uncooked raw meat, such as France, Germany, Netherlands, and Brazil, the prevalence is over 60%.[11]

2 FROM ANIMALS TO HUMANS THROUGH THE IMMUNE SYSTEM

The host immune response to toxoplasmosis combines a strong cell-mediated response with a Th1 cytokine profile and a humoral response, which results in the production of specific anti-*Toxoplasma* antibodies (ATA). The induction of a type 1 inflammatory cytokine response is a key event in the initiation of immunity to TG. Because polymorphonuclear leukocytes rapidly respond to infection by exiting the peripheral blood and accumulating at the site of infection, some groups sought to determine whether these cells produce cytokines in response to TG. When human peripheral blood neutrophils were stimulated with *Toxoplasma* parasite antigen, they produced both IL-12 and TNF-α. Similarly, up-regulated expression of macrophage-inflammatory protein 1α and 1β gene transcripts was induced. These results establish that TG possesses the ability to drive the production of neutrophil pro-inflammatory cytokines.[12] Much progress in determining how early innate responses, namely the production of cytokines such as IL-12 and TNF-α, drive the development of a strong Th1 response to TG was made recently. While this response is crucial in controlling infection, it is becoming increasingly appreciated that an excessively vigorous response induced by the parasite can lead to pathologic changes in the host. Therefore, it is important for the host and parasite to maintain tight control of the inflammatory response. Within the context of the host–parasite relationship, *Toxoplasma* may seek to induce strong protective host immunity because without such a response, the parasite rapidly overcomes the host, resulting in the death of the host and as a consequence a minimal chance for the parasite to transmit itself to a new host.[13] Neutrophils have recently been shown to release DNA-based extracellular traps that contribute to microbicidal killing and have been implicated in autoimmunity. The role of neutrophil extracellular trap (NET) formation in the host response to nonbacterial pathogens has received much less attention. Abi Abdallah et al. showed that TG elicits the production of NETs from human and mouse neutrophils. Tachyzoites of each of the three major parasite strains were efficiently entrapped within NETs, resulting in decreased viability of the parasite. This group also demonstrated that *Toxoplasma* activates a MEK–extracellular signal-regulated kinase pathway in neutrophils and that the inhibition of this pathway leads to decreased NET formation. These data indicate a role for NETs in the host's innate response to protozoan infection. They propose that NET formation limits infection through direct microbicidal effects on *Toxoplasma* as well as by interfering with the ability of the parasite to invade target host cells.[14]

TG infects over one billion people worldwide. Host resistance to this protozoan parasite depends on a Th1 immune response with potent production of the cytokines IL-12 and interferon (IFN)-γ. Toll-like receptors (TLRs) play an important role in host defence against a variety of microbial pathogens. The mechanism by which TLRs contribute to host defense against the lethal parasite TG was addressed using mice with targeted inactivation of a TLR adaptor protein—myeloid differentiation primary response gene 88 (MyD88)—in different innate cell types. Lack of MyD88 in dendritic cells (DCs), but not in macrophages or neutrophils, resulted in high susceptibility to TG infection. In the mice deficient in MyD88 in DCs, the early IL-12 response by DCs was ablated, the IFN-γ response by natural killer cells was delayed and the recruited inflammatory monocytes were incapable of killing the TG parasites. The T-cell response, although attenuated in these mice, was sufficient to eradicate the parasite during the chronic stage, provided that defects in DC activation were compensated for by IL-12 treatment soon after infection. These results demonstrate a central role for DCs in orchestrating the innate immune response to an intracellular pathogen and establish that defects in pathogen recognition by DCs can predetermine sensitivity to infection.[15] Although TLR11 plays a major role in controlling Th1 immunity to this pathogen in mice, this innate immune receptor is nonfunctional in humans, and essentially the entire human population is at risk for infection. The mechanisms of TLR11-independent sensing of TG remain elusive. Benson et al. showed that oral infection by TG triggers a TLR11-independent but MyD88-dependent Th1 response that is impaired in TLR2xTLR4 double knockout and TLR9 single knockout mice. Signaling through the TLR adaptor protein MyD88 is indispensable for activating early innate immune responses and inducing production of IL-12. These mucosal innate and adaptive immune responses to TG rely on the indirect stimulation of DCs by normal gut microflora. Thus, these results reveal that gut commensal bacteria can serve as molecular adjuvants during parasitic infection, providing indirect immunostimulation that protects against TG in the absence of TLR11.[16]

Moreover, the chemokine receptor CCR7 is a well-established homing receptor for DCs and T cells. Interactions with its ligands, CCL19 and CCL21, facilitate priming of immune responses in lymphoid tissue, yet CCR7-independent immune responses can be generated in the presence of sufficient antigen. A study by Noor et al. investigated the role of CCR7 signaling in the generation of protective immune responses TG. The results demonstrated a significant increase in the expression of CCL19, CCL21, and CCR7 in peripheral and central nervous system tissues over the course of infection. Unexpectedly, despite the presence of abundant antigen, CCR7 was an absolute requirement for protective immunity to TG: CCR7$-/-$ mice succumbed to the parasite early in the acute phase of infection. Although serum concentrations of IL-12, IL-6, TNF-α and IL-10 remained unchanged, there was a significant decrease in CCL2/monocyte chemoattractant protein 1 and inflammatory monocyte recruitment to the site of infection. In addition, CCR7$-/-$ mice failed to produce sufficient IFN-γ, a critical Th1-associated effector cytokine required to control parasite replication. As a result, there was increased dissemination of the parasite and a significant increase in parasite burden in the lungs, livers, and brains of infected mice. Adoptive transfer experiments revealed that expression of CCR7 on the T-cell compartment alone is sufficient to enable T-cell priming, increase IFN-γ production and allow the survival of CCR7$-/-$ mice. These data demonstrate an absolute requirement for T-cell expression of CCR7 for the generation of protective immune responses to *Toxoplasma* infection.[17]

Chronic helminthic infections are characterized by skewing the immune reaction towards a Th2-type response (which typically include IL-4, IL-5, and IL-13, which induce B lymphocytes to switch to producing IgE antibody) as well as to regulatory responses.[4] Indeed, many studies showed that normally avirulent strains of TG are highly virulent in T-lymphocyte-deficient animals.[18,19] Therefore, induction of T-cell-mediated immune responses and resistance to the tachyzoite stage is a key step in the TG life cycle, determining the survival of the intermediate host and the parasite itself.

A cohort study showed that leukocyte, natural killer cell and monocyte counts were increased in male patients with latent toxoplasmosis and were increased in *Toxoplasma*-positive women in comparison with controls. B-cell counts were reduced in both *Toxoplasma*-positive men and women. The difference between *Toxoplasma*-positive and *Toxoplasma*-negative subjects diminished with the decline of the specific *Toxoplasma* antibody titer (a proxy for the length of infection).[20] Furthermore, during chronic infection TG cysts are well controlled by the host immune response, mainly because of CD8$^+$ effector lymphocytes[21] and TG antigen-elicited production of IFN-γ.[13]

3 THE EVIDENCE OF AUTOIMMUNITY

A link between TG and infections was demonstrated in a rat model in which infection with TG in proximity to the thymus was able to inhibit the suppression of response to an autoantigen of rat male accessory glands selectively impairing the influence of thymic suppression. Furthermore, another study demonstrated that subcutaneous injection of viable TG trophozoites into the footpad of Wistar rats was able to induce a localized inflammatory arthritic process that was accompanied by iridocyclitis and immune response against articular and ocular antigens.[22,23]

In another study, the lupus experimental model of NZB/NZWXF1 mice was used to investigate the protective effect of parasitic infection with TG. Mice were found to develop milder renal disease and live longer compared to non-infected mice. Down-regulation of IL-10 and IFN-γ was shown in spleen cells of the infected mice. A marked decrease in the levels of IgM and IgG anti-DNA antibodies, especially pathogenic IgG2a and IgG3 subclasses, was observed in mice at 9 months of age in this study.[24] Regarding the observations of the role of TG infection in the diseased human population, significantly lower levels of ATAs were found in patients with type 1 diabetes mellitus.[25] The lower level of antibodies against infectious agents in diabetic patients may be related to their younger ages but may also point to a protective role of those infections in the development of type 1 diabetes mellitus in susceptible individuals.

Studies of experimental models of AID and TG infection reported conflicting results.[26–28] Previous case reports and case–control studies linked ATAs with polymyositis,[29] rheumatoid arthritis (RA),[30–32] autoimmune thyroid diseases,[33,34] Crohn's disease,[35] anti-phospholipid syndrome (APS),[36] Wegener's granulomatosis[37] and autoimmune bullous diseases.[38] While ATAs have been previously associated with SLE,[39] subsequent studies challenged this association.[40,41]

Results of another study showed a higher seroprevalence of ATAs in patients with RA compared with patients with SLE. ATA seropositivity was associated with older age in patients with RA, although it did not correlate with RA disease activity or other manifestations of the disease. These data suggest a possible link between exposure to TG infection and RA.[42] On the other hand, infection with TG was capable of ameliorating the spontaneous development of arthritis in IL-1 receptor antagonist-deficient BALB/c mice developing spontaneous arthritis resembling human RA. The onset of arthritis development was delayed, and the severity score of arthritis was significantly suppressed in TG-infected mice. The severity of arthritis was related to Th1 cell polarization accompanied by Th17 cell reduction, demonstrating the protective role of the TG-derived Th1 response against Th17 cell-mediated arthritis in IL-1Ra-deficient mice.[43]

A contributing role for TG in inducing bullous pemphigoid has been suggested.[44] Patients with ocular toxoplasmosis develop autoreactivity to several retinal antigens, including retinal S-antigen. But in a study by Garweg et al., the data afford no evidence of similarities between toxoplasmic and retinal antigens nor of infection-induced humoral autoimmunity. Their data indicate, rather, that retinal autoantigens are liberated in the context of inflammatory tissue destruction due to ocular toxoplasmosis.[45]

In a large populational study of a Latin American and European population of patients with AID and healthy controls, a higher prevalence of ATA IgG was found in European patients with APS, cryoglobulinemia, ANCA-associated vasculitides, AIT, and systemic sclerosis (SSc) compared to matched controls. The association between ATA IgG positivity and RA was observed only among the patients and controls from Europe, whereas the Latin American group failed to achieve significant differences. Among Europeans, ATA IgM was more prevalent in patients with APS, SSc, and IBD when compared with geographically matched controls. ATA IgG antibodies also were associated with specific AIDs; this is, in some cases, consistent with previous reports.[33,35–38] Nevertheless, the association between APS and SSc with ATAs of both Ig subclasses is novel and further supported by the significant association of this serum reactivity with serum autoantibodies specific for APS (anti-CL, B2GPI, CL-B2, PT, PE), and SSc (anti-centromere, Scl-70).[46] There is a broader interpretation of these data when considering the novel evidence of a geoepidemiology of AID worldwide.[47-49] Geoepidemiology demonstrates that individual genetic susceptibility interacts with lifestyle and environmental factors, which include socioeconomic status, nutritional habits, environmental pollutants, ultraviolet radiation exposure, and infections (in each case acting as triggering or protective agents) to determine the risk of developing autoimmunity.[47,48]

According to the hygiene hypothesis, a lower exposure to infection is associated with increased prevalence of allergic diseases. Thus, a study aimed to investigate the association between atopy and TG infection by analyzing the antibody and cytokine responses to house dust mite allergens and TG antigens in Brazilian subjects. A total of 275 individuals were assessed and divided into atopics and non-atopics based on allergy markers (positive skin prick test and ELISA-IgE to mite allergens) or TG-seropositive and TG-seronegative groups according to infection markers (positive ELISA-IgG to TG). TG-seropositive individuals presented lower allergenic sensitization to mite allergens than TG-seronegative subjects. A significant association was found between atopy and negative serology to TG. Hence, a negative association between atopy and infection by TG was demonstrated for the first time in Brazilian subjects, indicating that the immunomodulation induced by the parasite may play a protective role in the development of allergic diseases.[50] A brief summary of autoimmune conditions in relation to TG infection is provided in Table 1.

4 DISCUSSION

TG infection is generally initiated by ingesting the parasite during either its tissue cyst stage, found in the meat of infected animals, or its oocyst stage, released in the feces of infected cats.[51] Adult-acquired toxoplasmosis is normally mild to asymptomatic, but disease can be severe in the immunosuppressed.[52,53] In addition, the ability of sex- and pregnancy-associated hormones to influence the severity of TG infection is of particular interest.[52] There is currently considerable evidence that steroid hormones affect the course of toxoplasmosis in humans and mice. Henry and Beverley were the first to demonstrate that female mice developed more severe brain inflammation than male mice following infection.[54] Moreover, a direct role for sex hormones was demonstrated in experiments that found that

Table 1 Autoimmune Conditions and Their Relevance to Toxoplasmosis

Autoimmune Condition	Protective Role	Possible Causal Agent	References
Toxoplasmosis	Lupus mouse model		24
	Type 1 diabetes mellitus		25
		RA (in Europe)	42,46
	RA mouse model		43
		Bullous pemphigoid	44
		APS	46
		Cryoglobulinemia	46
		ANCA vasculitidies	46
		AIT	46
		SSc	46
	Atopy		50

gonadectomy increased resistance, whereas estrogen administration exacerbated disease in mice.[55,56] Similarly, lymphadenopathy as a possible disease manifestation varies. In those younger than 15 years old, lymphadenopathy was more frequently observed in males than females. However, in sexually mature adults (>25 years old), lymphadenopathy was more frequently observed in females.[57] TG infection can also be an opportunistic infection. A frequent manifestation in those infected with human immunodeficiency virus is encephalitis. Toxoplasmic encephalitis was found to be a more frequent AIDS-defining disease in females than in males.[58] These observations support a detrimental role for female hormones during the course of TG infection that also occurs in AIDs.

The protozoan parasite TG specifically influences the behavior of intermediate hosts[59] and has been linked to several non-infectious conditions such as deteriorated psychomotor performance,[60] and higher risk of traffic accidents[61] and schizophrenia[62] as well as Parkinson's disease.[63] Modified reactivity of the immune system has been suggested to play a key role in many of these effects. For example, the immunosuppression hypothesis explains the higher probability of the birth of male offspring observed in *Toxoplasma*-positive humans and mice by the protection of the (more immunogenic) male embryos against abortion.[20] In a study of >10,000 patients, Chen et al. demonstrated a positive association between inpatients with schizophrenia and several AIDs and confirmed the long-recognized negative association of schizophrenia with RA. When compared with the control group, the inpatients with schizophrenia had an increased risk of

Graves' disease, psoriasis, pernicious anemia, celiac disease, and hypersensitivity vasculitis, whereas a reverse association with RA was observed. The latter observation is now thought to be the result of two alleles of the same gene, one of which confers a predisposition to schizophrenia and the other to RA, thus becoming mutually exclusive. Sex-specific variation was found for Sjögren's syndrome, hereditary hemolytic anemia, myasthenia gravis, polymyalgia rheumatica and dermatomyositis. Schizophrenia seems to be associated with a greater variety of AIDs than initially anticipated.[64] These results are similar, albeit from an Asian perspective, to an analysis from the Danish National Registers by Eaton et al., who observed that a personal history of any AID was associated with a 45% increase in risk for schizophrenia. In addition, 9 AIDs were more prevalent among patients with schizophrenia, and 12 had a higher prevalence among parents of people with schizophrenia than parents of controls.[65] These observations are, of course, indirect evidence of autoimmune involvement in the pathogenesis of schizophrenia. Efforts to find cerebral antibodies and other immunological abnormalities specific to schizophrenia have produced inconsistent and contradictory results. The recent recognition of autoimmune limbic encephalitis, however, has directed attention to autoantibodies that antagonize proteins involved in synaptic function, with positive findings in some patients with first-episode schizophrenia.[66] Of course, further investigation is needed to gain a better understanding of the etiology of schizophrenia and AIDs. But if toxoplasmosis has been linked to schizophrenia and schizophrenia showed an association with AID, the connecting factor in between might be the toxoplasmosis.

Based on reported data we may hypothesize the mechanisms by which IgG ATAs may be correlated with AID. First, we should note that it is not uncommon for adult sera to manifest naturally occurring antibodies against TG,[67] and the presence of these natural antibodies could reflect the cross-reactivity of parasitic antigens with antigens from the host.[68] This is well supported by the observation that ATAs from healthy individuals cross-react with malignant cervical tissue antigens.[69] Second, an association between IgG antibodies and ATAs was observed in sera from 1591 pregnant women,[34] thus supporting, along with data on AIT, the hypothesis that *Toxoplasma* can initiate a pathogenic process that may eventually result in clinically overt autoimmunity. Similarly, researchers previously suggested mimicry between TG antigens and phospholipids based on a strong homology found between B2-GPI-related peptides (i.e. target epitope for anti-B2-GPI Abs) and the parasite.[27] The present data support this view of APS pathogenesis by demonstrating an association of ATAs with aPL antibodies and the APS. Third, we may hypothesize that TG infection induces a bystander effect via activation of TLRs,[34] as previously demonstrated for multiple TLRs,[70] and may thus lead to the expansion of autoantibodies under aberrant conditions (e.g. excessive and/or chronic TLR activation).[34,71] In addition, a direct inflammatory insult may be caused by TG infection, as illustrated by a mouse model of IBD. TG induced massive necrosis of the villi and digestive mucosal cells in the ileum of C57BL/6 mice, with a CD4+ T-cell immunopathology characterized by a robust Th1-mediated increase in pro-inflammatory mediators.[26,72]

5 CONCLUSION

Although it would be intriguing to postulate a link between past infection by TG and several AIDs, further studies are needed. There are, however, interesting associations between parasitic response and specific autoantibodies and autoimmune conditions. We propose that further comparative immunology be performed to identify the mechanisms involved in this relationship and whether the data herein are primarily an epiphenomenon or whether they reflect a direct association of either *Toxoplasma* or a related infection with either the initiation or exacerbation of AID.

REFERENCES

1. Kivity S, Agmon-Levin N, Blank M, Shoenfeld Y. Infections and autoimmunity—friends or foes? *Trends Immunol* 2009;**30**(8):409–14.
2. Shoenfeld Y, Zandman-Goddard G, Stojanovich L, Cutolo M, Amital H, Levy Y, et al. The mosaic of autoimmunity: hormonal and environmental factors involved in autoimmune diseases–2008. *Isr Med Assoc J* 2008;**10**(1):8–12.
3. van Riet E, Hartgers FC, Yazdanbakhsh M. Chronic helminth infections induce immunomodulation: consequences and mechanisms. *Immunobiology* 2007;**212**:475–90.
4. Zandman-Goddard G, Shoenfeld Y. Parasitic infection and autoimmunity. *Lupus* 2009;**18**:1144–8.
5. Girones N, Cuervo H, Fresno M. Trypanosoma cruzi-induced molecular mimicry and Chagas' disease. *Curr Top Microbiol Immunol* 2005;**296**:89–123.
6. Abu-Shakra M, Shoenfeld Y. Chronic infections and autoimmunity. *Immunol Ser* 1991;**55**:285–313.
7. Frenkel JK. Pathophysiology of toxoplasmosis. *Parasitol Today* 1988;**4**:273–8.
8. Suzuki Y, Joh K. Effect of the strain of *Toxoplasma gondii* on the development of toxoplasmic encephalitis in mice treated with antibody to interferon-gamma. *Parasitol Res* 1994;**80**:125–30.
9. Tenter AM, Heckeroth AR, Weiss LM. *Toxoplasma gondii*: from animals to humans. *Int J Parasitol* 2000;**30**(12–13):1217–58.

10. Jones JL, Kruszon-Moran D, Sanders-Lewis K, Wilson M. *Toxoplasma gondii* infection in the United States, 1999-2004, decline from the prior decade. *Am J Trop Med Hyg* 2007;**77**(3):405–10.

11. Kortbeek LM. Toxoplasmose in Nederland. *Ned Tijdschr Klin Chem* 1999;**24**:65–70.

12. Bliss SK, Marshall AJ, Zhang Y, Denkers EY. Human polymorphonuclear leukocytes produce IL-12, TNF-α, and the chemokines macrophage-inflammatory protein-1α and -1β in response to *Toxoplasma gondii* antigens. *J Immunol* 1999;**162**:7369–75.

13. Denkers EY, Gazzinelli RT. Regulation and function of T-cell-mediated immunity during *Toxoplasma gondii* infection. *Clin Microbiol* 1998;**11**:569–88.

14. Abi Abdallah DS, Lin C, Ball CJ, King MR, Duhamel GE, Denkers EY. *Toxoplasma gondii* triggers release of human and mouse neutrophil extracellular traps. *Infect Immun* 2012;**80**(2):768–77.

15. Hou B, Benson A, Kuzmich L, DeFranco AL, Yarovinsky F. Critical coordination of innate immune defense against *Toxoplasma gondii* by dendritic cells responding via their toll-like receptors. *Proc Natl Acad Sci USA* 2011;**108**(1):278–83.

16. Benson A, Pifer R, Behrendt CL, Hooper LV, Yarovinsky F. Gut commensal bacteria direct a protective immune response against *Toxoplasma gondii*. *Cell Host Microbe* 2009;**6** (2):187–96.

17. Noor S, Habashy AS, Nance JP, Clark RT, Nemati K, Carson MJ, et al. CCR7-dependent immunity during acute *Toxoplasma gondii* infection. *Infect Immun* 2010;**78**(5):2257–63.

18. Gazzinelli RT, Hieny S, Wynn TA, Wolf S, Sher A. IL-12 is required for the T cell independent induction of IFN-g by an intracellular parasite and induces resistance in T-cell-deficient hosts. *Proc Natl Acad Sci USA* 1993;**90**:6115–19.

19. Lindberg RE, Frenkel JK. Toxoplasmosis in nude mice. *J Parasitol* 1977;**63**:219–21.

20. Flegr J, Stříž I. Potential immunomodulatory effects of latent toxoplasmosis in humans. *BMC Infect Dis* 2011;**11**:274.

21. Brown CR, Mcleod R. Class I MHC and CD8+ T cells determine cyst number in *T. gondii* infection. *J Immunol* 1990;**145**:3438–41.

22. Romero-Piffiguer MD, Ferro ME, Riera CM. Potentiation of autoimmune response in rats infected with *Toxoplasma gondii*. Inhibition of suppressor system and impairment of thymic cellular populations. *Autoimmunity* 1990;**6**:161–72.

23. Romero-Piffiguer M, Ferro ME, Riera CM. Potentiation of autoimmune response in rats infected with *Toxoplasma gondii*. Effect of the infection route. *Jpn J Med Sci Biol* 1987;**40**:175–85.

24. Chen M, Aosai F, Norose K, Mun HS, Ishikura H, Hirose S, et al. *Toxoplasma gondii* infection inhibits the development of lupus-like syndrome in autoimmune (New Zealand black X New Zealand white) F1 mice. *Int Immunol* 2004;**16**:937–46.

25. Krause I, Anaya JM, Fraser A, Barzilai O, Ram M, Abad V, et al. Anti-infectious antibodies and autoimmune-associated autoantibodies in patients with type I diabetes mellitus and their close family members. *Ann N Y Acad Sci* 2009;**1173**:633–9.

26. Liesenfeld O. Oral infection of C57BL/6 mice with *Toxoplasma gondii*: a new model of inflammatory bowel disease? *J Infect Dis* 2002;**185**(Suppl. 1):S96–S101.

27. Blank M, Asherson RA, Cervera R, Shoenfeld Y. Antiphospholipid syndrome infectious origin. *J Clin Immunol* 2004;**24**:12–23.

28. Chen M, Aosai F, Norose K, Mun HS, Ishikura H, Hirose S, et al. *Toxoplasma gondii* infection inhibits the development of lupus-like syndrome in autoimmune (New Zealand Black x New Zealand White) F1 mice. *Int Immunol* 2004;**16**:937–46.

29. Adams EM, Hafez GR, Carnes M, Wiesner JK, Graziano FM. The development of polymyositis in a patient with toxoplasmosis: clinical and pathologic findings and review of literature. *Clin Exp Rheumatol* 1984;**2**:205–8.

30. Tomairek HA, Saeid MS, Morsy TA, Michael SA. *Toxoplasma gondii* as a cause of rheumatoid arthritis. *J Egypt Soc Parasitol* 1982;**12**:17–23.
31. Mousa MA, Soliman HE, el Shafie MS, Abdel-Baky MS, Aly MM. Toxoplasma seropositivity in patients with rheumatoid arthritis. *J Egypt Soc Parasitol* 1988;**18**:345–51.
32. Balleari E, Cutolo M, Accardo S. Adult-onset Still's disease associated to *Toxoplasma gondii* infection. *Clin Rheumatol* 1991;**10**:326–7.
33. Tozzoli R, Barzilai O, Ram M, Villalta D, Bizzaro N, Sherer Y, et al. Infections and autoimmune thyroid diseases: parallel detection of antibodies against pathogens with proteomic technology. *Autoimmun Rev* 2008;**8**:112–15.
34. Wasserman EE, Nelson K, Rose NR, Rhode C, Pillion JP, Seaberg E, et al. Infection and thyroid autoimmunity: a seroepidemiologic study of TPOaAb. *Autoimmunity* 2009;**42**:439–46.
35. Lidar M, Langevitz P, Barzilai O, Ram M, Porat-Katz BS, Bizzaro N, et al. Infectious serologies and autoantibodies in inflammatory bowel disease: insinuations at a true pathogenic role. *Ann N Y Acad Sci* 2009;**1173**:640–8.
36. Zinger H, Sherer Y, Goddard G, Berkun Y, Barzilai O, Agmon-Levin N, et al. Common infectious agents prevalence in antiphospholipid syndrome. *Lupus* 2009;**18**:1149–53.
37. Lidar M, Lipschitz N, Langevitz P, Barzilai O, Ram M, Porat-Katz BS, et al. Infectious serologies and autoantibodies in Wegener's granulomatosis and other vasculitides: novel associations disclosed using the Rad BioPlex 2200. *Ann NY Acad Sci* 2009;**1173**:649–57.
38. Sagi L, Baum S, Agmon-Levin N, Sherer Y, Katz BS, Barzilai O, et al. Autoimmune bullous diseases the spectrum of infectious agent antibodies and review of the literature. *Autoimmun Rev* 2011;**10**:527–35.
39. Wilcox MH, Powell RJ, Pugh SF, Balfour AH. Toxoplasmosis and systemic lupus erythematosus. *Ann Rheum Dis* 1990;**49**:254–7.
40. Noel I, Balfour AH, Wilcox MH. Toxoplasma infection and systemic lupus erythematosus: analysis of the serological response by immunoblotting. *J Clin Pathol* 1993;**46**:628–32.
41. Berkun Y, Zandman-Goddard G, Barzilai O, Boaz M, Sherer Y, Larida B, et al. Infectious antibodies in systemic lupus erythematosus patients. *Lupus* 2009;**18**:1129–35.
42. Fischer S, Agmon-Levin N, Shapira Y, Porat Katz BS, Graell E, Cervera R, et al. *Toxoplasma gondii*: bystander or cofactor in rheumatoid arthritis. *Immunol Res* 2013;**56** (2–3):287–92.
43. Washino T, Moroda M, Iwakura Y, Aosai F. *Toxoplasma gondii* infection inhibits Th17-mediated spontaneous development of arthritis in interleukin-1 receptor antagonist-deficient mice. *Infect Immun* 2012;**80**(4):1437–44.
44. Lo Schiavo A, Ruocco E, Brancaccio G, Caccavale S, Ruocco V, Wolf R. Bullous pemphigoid: etiology, pathogenesis, and inducing factors: facts and controversies. *Clin Dermatol* 2013;**31**(4):391–9.
45. Garweg JG, de Kozak Y, Goldenberg B, Boehnke M. Anti-retinal autoantibodies in experimental ocular and systemic toxoplasmosis. *Graefes Arch Clin Exp Ophthalmol* 2010;**248**(4):573–84.
46. Shapira Y, Agmon-Levin N, Selmi C, Petríková J, Barzilai O, Ram M, et al. Prevalence of anti-toxoplasma antibodies in patients with autoimmune diseases. *J Autoimmun* 2012;**39**(1–2):112–16.
47. Shapira Y, Agmon-Levin N, Shoenfeld Y. Defining and analyzing geoepidemiology and human autoimmunity. *J Autoimmun* 2010;**34**:J168–77.
48. Shapira Y, Agmon-Levin N, Shoenfeld Y. Geoepidemiology of autoimmune rheumatic diseases. *Nat Rev Rheumatol* 2010;**6**:468–76.

49. Shapira Y, Poratkatz BS, Gilburd B, Barzilai O, Ram M, Blank M, et al. Geographical differences in autoantibodies and anti-infectious agents antibodies among healthy adults. *Clin Rev Allergy Immunol* 2012;**42**(2):154–63.

50. Fernandes JFC, Taketomi EA, Mineo JR, Miranda DO, Alves R, Resende RO, et al. Antibody and cytokine responses to house dust mite allergens and *Toxoplasma gondii* antigens in atopic and non-atopic Brazilian subjects. *Clin Immunol* 2010;**136**:148–56.

51. Cook GC. *Toxoplasma gondii* infection: a potential danger to the unborn fetus and AIDS sufferer. *Q J Med* 1990;**74**:3–19.

52. Boyer K, McLeod R. *Toxoplasmosis 1st ed*, vol. 286. New York, N.Y.: Churchill Livingstone; 1998.

53. Luft BJ, Hafner R, Korzun AH, Leport C, Antoniskis D, Bosler EM, et al. Toxoplasmic encephalitis in patients with the acquired immunodeficiency syndrome. *N Engl J Med* 1993;**329**:995–1000.

54. Henry L, Beverley JKA. Age and sex differences in the response of lymph node postcapillary venules in mice infected with *Toxoplasma gondii*. *J Exp Pathol* 1976;**57**:274–81.

55. Kittas C, Henry L. Effect of gonadectomy and oestrogen administration on the response of lymph-node post-sapillary venules to infection with *Toxoplasma gondii*. *J Pathol* 1978;**127**:129–36.

56. Kittas C, Henry L. Effect of sex hormones on the response of mice to infection with *Toxoplasma gondii*. *B J Exp Pathol* 1980;**61**:590–600.

57. Beverley JK, Fleck DG, Kwantes W, Ludlam GB. Age-sex distribution of various diseases with particular reference to toxoplasmic lymphadenopathy. *J Hyg* 1976;**76**: 215–28.

58. Phillips AN, Antunes F, Stergious G, Ranki A, Jensen GF, Bentwich Z, et al. A sex comparison of rates of new AIDS-defining disease and death in 2554 AIDS cases. *AIDS* 1994;**8**:831–5.

59. Webster JP. Rats, cats, people and parasites: the impact of latent toxoplasmosis on behaviour. *Microb Infect* 2001;**3**:1037–45.

60. Havlicek J, Gasova Z, Smith AP, Zvara K, Flegr J. Decrease of psychomotor performance in subjects with latent 'asymptomatic' toxoplasmosis. *Parasitology* 2001; **122**:515–20.

61. Flegr J, Havlicek J, Kodym P, Maly M, Smahel Z. Increased risk of traffic accidents in subjects with latent toxoplasmosis: a retrospective case-controlstudy. *BMC Infect Dis* 2002;**2**:11.

62. Torrey EF, Yolken RH. *Toxoplasma gondii* and schizophrenia. *Emerg Infect Dis* 2003;**9**:1375–80.

63. Abramsky O, Litvin Y. Autoimmune response to dopaminereceptor as a possible mechanism in the pathogenesis of Parkinson's disease and schizophrenia. *Perspect Biol Med* 1978;**22**:104–14.

64. Chen SJ, Chao YL, Chen CY, Chang CM, Wu EC, Wu CS, et al. Prevalence of autoimmune diseases in in-patients with schizophrenia: nationwide population-based study. *Br J Psychiatry* 2012;**200**:374–80.

65. Eaton WW, Byrne M, Ewald H, Mors O, Chen CY, Agerbo E, et al. Association of schizophrenia and autoimmune diseases: linkage of Danish National Registers. *Am J Psychiatry* 2006;**163**:521–8.

66. Zandi MS, Irani SR, Lang B, Waters P, Jones PB, McKenna P, et al. Disease-relevant autoantibodies in first episode schizophrenia. *J Neurol* 2011;**258**:686–8.

67. Potasman I, Araujo FG, Remington JS. Toxoplasma antigens recognized by naturally occurring human antibodies. *J Clin Microbiol* 1986;**24**:1050–4.

68. Noel I, Balfour AH, Wilcox MH. Toxoplasma infection and systemic lupus erythematosus: analysis of the serological response by immunoblotting. *J Clin Pathol* 1993; **46**:628–32.

69. Vos GH. Population studies showing cross-reactivity of *Toxoplasma gondii* antibodies with antibodies to malignant cervical tissue antigens. *S Afr Med J* 1987;**71**:78–82.

70. Yarovinsky F, Sher A. Toll-like receptor recognition of *Toxoplasma gondii*. *Int J Parasitol* 2006;**36**:255–9.

71. Marshak-Rothstein A. Toll-like receptors in systemic autoimmune disease. *Nat Rev Immunol* 2006;**6**:823–35.

72. Munoz M, Liesenfeld O, Heimesaat MM. Immunology of *Toxoplasma gondii*. *Immunol Rev* 2011;**240**:269–85.

CHAPTER 38

Malaria and Systemic Lupus Erythematosus: Complex Interactions and Reciprocal Influences

Francesca Cainelli[*,1], **Sandro Vento**[*]
[*]Department of Internal Medicine, Faculty of Medicine, University of Botswana, Gaborone, Botswana
[1]Corresponding Author: cainellifrancesca@gmail.com

1 INTRODUCTION

Malaria, the prototype parasitic infection, is still one of the most common parasitic diseases in the world and claims almost 800,000 lives every year.[1,2] It is perhaps the most powerful agent that has influenced human populations, being responsible for a number of polymorphisms, particularly of red cells. Systemic lupus erythematosus (SLE), the prototype non–organ-specific autoimmune disease, and malaria were first linked in 1968, when Brian Greenwood[3] hypothesized that malaria protected against SLE and other autoimmune diseases in West Africa. Epidemiological data subsequently indicated that SLE and other autoimmune diseases, such as sarcoidosis and multiple sclerosis, indeed occurred less frequently in areas where exposure to malaria was high.[4–6] Experimental data supported findings in humans; *Plasmodium berghei* infection early in life was shown to prevent or delay the onset of autoimmune diseases in strains of mice, in which they develop spontaneously.[7–9]

2 MECHANISMS OF MALARIA PROTECTION FROM SLE

How would malaria protect from SLE? It is well established that immunosuppression is associated with malaria infections; children infected with malaria have more severe gastrointestinal and respiratory infections than noninfected children, and efficacy of vaccination is impaired.[10] Poor mitogenic response has been observed[11] when lymphocytes are close to nitric oxide-releasing macrophages.[12] in vitro and in vivo evidence in mouse malaria favored the notion that the poor proliferative response of lympho-cytes in the animal model is mediated through nitric oxide,[13] likely through its ability to inhibit ribonucleotide reductase.[14] This led Clark et al.[14] to pro-pose a central role of nitric oxide upregulation in protection against SLE during the establishment and maintenance of tolerance to malaria.

2.1 Tumor Necrosis Factor

Tumor necrosis factor (TNF) has attracted considerable interest.[15,16] In malaria, high plasma concentrations of TNF-α are associated with more severe disease, and the highest concentrations are found in fatal cases of cere-bral malaria.[17] A polymorphism present at position −308, identified by Wilson et al.,[18] has been associated with different levels of cytokine produc-tion, and the less common TNF2 allele (−308A) has been related to a higher TNF-α transcription rate than the TNF1 allele (−308G) after in vitro acti-vation of lymphocytes with different stimuli.[19,20] In West African patients with cerebral malaria, homozygosity for the TNF2 allele was associated with a seven-fold increased risk of severe neurological complications or death.[21] The TNF2 allele was thought to be at least partly responsible for the lower incidence of SLE in Africa resulting from endemic malaria,[15,16] even though it is unclear how the absence of this powerful stimulant of the production of TNF-α would explain the high incidence of SLE in Afro-Americans, given the increased concentrations of TNF-α found in patients with SLE. Interestingly, TNF2 is part of the extended haplotype HLA-A1-B8-DR3-DQ2,[22] which is associated with high TNF-α production[23,24] and with predisposition to several autoimmune diseases.

Notwithstanding the adverse effects of homozygosity in malaria, TNF2 seems to be maintained at a similar frequency among West African and Northern European populations, suggesting that balancing pressures (e.g., possible beneficial effects in other widespread infectious diseases) in Africa likely occur to maintain the allele.[25] It must also be noted that an allele-based comparison of 21 studies, after stratification by ethnicity, failed to confirm in African-derived or Asian-derived populations the significant association of the −308A allele with SLE susceptibility observed in the European groups.[26]

2.2 Inhibitory Receptor FcγRIIb

A more recently proposed, plausible mechanism to explain SLE protection against malaria is a defunctioning, SLE-associated polymorphism of the low-affinity immunoglobulin gamma Fc region receptor II-b (FcγRIIb) in

African and Asian populations.[27] FcγRIIb is an inhibitory Fc receptor with a critical role in immune regulation. FcγRIIb-deficient mice have increased clearance of malarial parasites and are protected from death caused by cerebral malaria,[28] and in vitro data in humans demonstrate enhanced phagocytosis of *Plasmodium falciparum*-infected erythrocytes.[27] FcγRIIb dysfunction or deficiency is linked with the development of autoimmune diseases, particularly SLE, in mice and humans.[27] The single nucleotide polymorphism (SNP) FcγRIIb^{T232} that abrogates receptor function is strongly associated with susceptibility to SLE in Caucasians and Southeast Asians, with an odds ratio of 1.7.[29] The minor allele of this SNP codes for a threonine instead of an isoleucine at position 232 in the transmembrane domain of FcγRIIb and is more common in Southeast Asians and Africans than in Caucasians. The decreased inhibitory function caused by FcγRIIb^{T232} increases B-cell and myeloid cell activation, which might predispose to SLE. Homozygosity for the minor allele was associated with protection against severe malaria in an East African population (odds ratio, 0.56);[29] the proportion of children with severe malaria who are homozygous for TT is one-half of that in controls, showing that possession of the TT genotype reduces the chances of acquiring severe malaria by ∼50%.[29] This protective effect against malaria may contribute to the higher frequency of this SNP—and therefore SLE—in Africans and Southeast Asians.[29]

With its high mortality, malaria is regarded as the strongest known force for evolutionary selection in the recent history of the human genome.[30] The most cited examples of this are the retention of the sickle cell and thalassemia traits. Interestingly, with an odds ratio of 0.56, homozygous FcγRIIb^{T232} has a protective effect against malaria similar to that of heterozygous thalassemia and could therefore explain the higher frequency of the minor allele FcγRIIb^{T232} observed in Africans and Southeast Asians.[29]

2.3 Other Mechanisms

Hemozoin, the insoluble waste product of hemoglobin digestion that accumulates over time in individuals living in malaria endemic areas, could also play a role in protection against SLE because it is taken up by macrophages and affects their function.[9,31] Malaria may protect also from sarcoidosis[5,32] and multiple sclerosis;[6] in addition to TNF-α hyperproduction,[33,34] increased synthesis of natural autoantibodies with regulatory properties[35] and interference with macrophage activity[6,9,36] have been suggested as mechanisms potentially implicated in this protective effect.

3 AUTOANTIBODIES AND MALARIA

In addition to the postulated role in preventing SLE in genetically susceptible individuals, malaria is associated with autoimmunity in other ways.
Indeed, plasmodial infection induces complications that have been linked
to autoimmune reactions, such as anemia,[37–39] nephritis,[40,41] thrombocytopenia[42] and even cerebral malaria.[43,44]

Interestingly, autoimmunity could also participate in the development of
antimalarial immunity. This possibility was initially proposed by Jayawardena and colleagues,[45] who thought that the immunoglobulin (Ig) M
response during malaria infections could be partly constituted by protective
autoantibodies directed against modified determinants exposed on the
erythrocyte membrane following plasmodium infection. A few years later,
Jarra[46] suggested that the acquisition of immunity against blood-stage parasites would be possible only with the simultaneous development of an anti-
erythrocyte autoimmune response. Research by Daniel-Ribeiro[47] has since
expanded this theory. Autoantibodies of specificities comparable to those
found in autoimmune diseases have been demonstrated during the course
of both experimental murine and natural human malaria infections. Among
these are antibodies against cardiolipin,[48] cytosol proteins,[49] single- and
double-stranded DNA (dsDNA),[50–52] erythrocytes,[38,53] lymphocytes,[54]
phospholipids,[53,55] ribonucleoproteins,[51,52,56] RNA,[57] and smooth
muscle.[56,58,59] Proposed mechanisms to explain how plasmodia induce
autoimmunity include molecular mimicry, presence of altered self-antigens,
polyclonal B-cell activation or expansion of B1a cells producing natural
anti-single-stranded DNA IgM autoantibodies.[60–62]

The specificity of autoantibodies may also be related to the degree of
immunity in malaria. Although antinuclear antibodies (ANAs) can be found
at different frequencies in both chronically exposed hyperimmune individuals and acutely infected humans and experimental animals, anti-smooth
muscle and antiactin antibodies are preferentially associated with acute
malaria.[52,61]

ANAs, anti-dsDNA antibodies and neutrophil extracellular traps (where
the nucleus of an activated neutrophil loses its lobular appearance as the
nuclear membrane dissolves, mixing chromatin with cytoplasmic granules;
the neutrophil plasma membrane then ruptures, releasing the chromatin and
adherent granule proteins)[63] with adherent parasites and erythrocytes, which
could be the source of nuclear antigens, were found in more than 80% of
Nigerian children with uncomplicated *Plasmodium falciparum* malaria.[64]

Frequencies higher than 80% also were found for IgM and IgG anticardiolipin antibodies in *P. falciparum-* and *Plasmodium vivax*-infected individuals in Senegal and Myanmar;[48] IgM was higher in the cerebral malaria group and IgG prevailed in the asymptomatic *P. falciparum* carriers.[48] An increase in antiphospholipid antibodies may be due in part to polyclonal B-cell activation resulting from lack of T-cell control of B-cell proliferation and differentiation.[65] A possible plasmodial target for antiphospholipid antibodies in malaria is glycosylphosphatidylinositol, released in large amounts by the parasite during schizogony, involved in TNF-α hyperproduction, and therefore possibly a major player in the malarial disease.[33] A role for *Plasmodium*-altered membrane phospholipid as an antigen also has been proposed because phosphatidylcholine is internalised and used by the parasite for its metabolic needs, whereas phosphatidylethanolamine and phosphatidylserine are exposed and may induce antiphospholipid antibody production.[66–68]

Autoantibodies present in sera from patients with SLE react with native plasmodial antigens possibly because of the recognition of similar structures in the parasite (as in the case of neutrophil extracellular traps generating ANAs and anti-dsDNA antibodies in both SLE and malaria),[64] or of cross-reactivity between nuclear and membrane autoantigens,[69] or between DNA and phospholipids,[70] in which plasmodia are rich.

In areas of widespread malaria transmission, individuals naturally acquire clinical immunity, initially against severe disease and then against clinical manifestations. Partial antiparasite immunity develops, and adults with few or no symptoms may have plasmodia in the blood, generally at very low densities.[71] This process of developing immunity to malaria is slow and requires years of exposure to bites from infected mosquitoes. It has been suggested that if autoimmunity plays a role in immune protection against malaria, the acquisition of clinical immunity would be delayed by the same mechanisms that control the development of autoimmune responses.[52] Hence individuals would remain susceptible to malaria infection and to its clinical manifestations until an autoimmune-based antiplasmodial immune response is established and maintained.[52]

4 AUTOIMMUNITY AND PROTECTION AGAINST MALARIA

Support for the role of autoimmunity in protecting against malaria has come from a few studies done in recent years. Of sera from 109 patients with SLE tested against autologous and plasmodial antigens, 48 (44%) reacted against the parasite.[52] In addition, 26 of 55 randomly selected sera (47%; essentially those containing anti-DNA and ANAs) inhibited plasmodium growth to some extent. Conversely, a high frequency (81%) of sera of patients with malaria exhibited reactivity against autoantigens. Antibodies against nucleus-derived antigens (ANAs, anti-dsDNA and anti-single-stranded DNA) were present in 44–58% of *P. falciparum*-infected patients and in 30–57% of *P. vivax*-infected patients. Anticardiolipin antibodies were detected in 66% of *P. falciparum*-infected patients and in 40% of *P. vivax*-infected patients.[52] Similar studies done in Africa and Southeast Asia showed even higher frequencies for antibodies with the above specificities during malaria infections.[48,64,72,73] Hence patients with SLE and other autoimmune diseases can produce antibodies that recognize plasmodial antigens in the absence of plasmodial infection, SLE sera can inhibit plasmodial growth in vitro, and the presence of anti-DNA and ANAs may be important in such antiplasmodial activity.[52] Autoimmune responses may therefore influence protective immunity against malaria.[52]

More recent findings also suggest that autoimmune responses mediated by autoantibodies may present antiplasmodial activity. A study of the pattern of reactivity to plasmodial antigens of sera from 93 patients not previously exposed to malaria but who had 14 different autoimmune diseases showed that sera from patients with 13 of the autoimmune diseases reacted against *P. falciparum* by indirect fluorescent antibody test, with frequencies varying from 33 % to 100 %.[74] In addition, sera from 37 patients were tested for reactivity against *Plasmodium yoelii* 17XNL and the asexual blood-stage forms of three different *P. falciparum* strains. The frequency of reactive sera was higher against young trophozoites than schizonts, suggesting that the antigenic determinants targeted by the tested autoimmune disease sera might be more highly expressed by trophozoites.[74] Thirteen of 18 monoclonal autoantibodies tested (72%), but none of the control monoclonal antibodies, inhibited *P. falciparum* growth in vitro—in a few cases by more than 40%.[74]

5 THE PREVALENCE GRADIENT HYPOTHESIS

This chapter cannot be exhaustive unless we also examine the "prevalence gradient hypothesis",[75] in which malaria has been so much involved. Greenwood[3] observed 47 years ago that the admissions lists of a hospital in Nigeria contained few cases of patients with autoimmune diseases. Of 98,454 admissions, only 104 were classified as autoimmune disease, including 2 with SLE and 42 with rheumatoid arthritis; these figures were considerably less than expected (4- and

6-fold, respectively) on the basis of data from European hospitals.[3] Greenwood suggested that parasitic diseases, especially malaria, somehow prevented the onset of autoimmune diseases. The apparently low prevalence of SLE in West Africa[76] contrasts sharply with the high prevalence rates reported for people of African descent living in Europe or North America,[77] and with the intermediate rates in the Caribbean. These data have given rise to the prevalence gradient hypothesis,[75] which postulates that the prevalence of SLE increases as one goes from Africa to either North America or Europe. As stated before, a possible explanation for the supposed low prevalence in Africa could be that malarial and parasitic infections alter the immune response in such a way as to protect from autoimmune diseases. It must be stressed, however, that there are no actual prevalence figures from West Africa[77] and that more recent data from sub-Saharan Africa indicate that SLE may not be as rare as had been assumed.[78–80] Moreover, a study done in South London, UK, found high prevalence rates of SLE among recent immigrants from West Africa.[81] As disease rates among recent migrants are generally similar to rates in migrants' social groups in their countries of origin,[82] the high prevalence of SLE among recent migrants from West Africa suggest that SLE is not rare in West Africa and that exposure to malaria and other parasitic infections in early life does not confer long-term protection against SLE.

6 A ROLE FOR CHLOROQUINE IN THE REDUCED PREVALENCE OF SLE IN COUNTRIES WITH HIGH MALARIA PREVALENCE?

A further possibility of the relations between malaria and SLE has been raised.[83] Because the use of hydroxychloroquine may delay the onset of SLE and slow the build-up of autoantibodies,[84] the frequent use of chloroquine to treat malaria in West Africa may delay the onset and reduce the severity of SLE in people residing in those areas.[83] Among people migrating from West Africa to Europe or the USA, the risk of malaria would end and the use of chloroquine would stop, unveiling the genetic high risk of SLE in these populations.[83] Indeed, in many African countries, self-treatment of fever with over-the-counter antimalarials is common practice,[85] and in rural areas, self-treatment rates of up to 94% have been reported.[86] In addition, despite the increasing prevalence of resistance, chloroquine remains the cheapest antimalarial drug and the one most widely used for self-treatment.[87–90]

7 CONCLUSION

The relations between malaria and SLE are complex and have attracted considerable interest in the past few decades. More studies are needed to clarify the interactions and the reciprocal influences, and such studies will have to be conducted in Africa and Asia in areas where malaria is still endemic.

REFERENCES

1. World Health Organization. *World malaria report 2010*. Geneva: WHO; 2010. [Online] Available from: http://whqlibdoc.who.int/publications/2010/9789241564106_eng.pdf [Accessed on 5 January, 2014].
2. Amina K, Giuliana G, Prato M. From control to eradication of malaria: the end of being stuck in second gear? *Asian Pac J Trop Med* 2010;**3**:412–20.
3. Greenwood BM. Autoimmune disease and parasitic infections in Nigerians. *Lancet* 1968;**ii**:380–2.
4. Zoutendyk A. Auto-antibodies in South African whites, coloured and Bantu. *S Afr Med J* 1970;**44**:469–70.
5. Butcher GA. Sarcoidosis and malaria. *Immunol Today* 1995;**16**:252–3.
6. Sotgiu S, Angius A, Embry A, Rosati G, Musumeci S. Hygiene hypothesis: innate immunity, malaria and multiple sclerosis. *Med Hypotheses* 2008;**70**:819–25.
7. Greenwood BM, Herrick EM, Voller A. Suppression of autoimmune disease in NZB and (NZB x NZW) F1 hybrid mice by infection with malaria. *Nature* 1970;**226**:266–7.
8. Hentati B, Sato MN, Payelle-Brogard B, Avrameas S, Ternynck T. Beneficial effect of polyclonal immunoglobulins from malaria-infected BALB/c mice on the lupus-like syndrome of (NZB x NZW) F1 mice. *Eur J Immunol* 1994;**24**:8–15.
9. Butcher G. Autoimmunity and malaria. *Trends Parasitol* 2008;**24**:291–2.
10. Williamson WA, Greenwood BM. Impairment of the immune response to vaccination after acute malaria. *Lancet* 1978;**i**:1328–9.
11. Taylor DW, Siddiqui WA. Effect of falciparum malaria infection on the in vitro mitogen responses of spleen and peripheral blood lymphocytes from owl monkeys. *Am J Trop Med Hyg* 1978;**27**:738–42.
12. Mills CD. Molecular basis of "suppressor" macrophages, arginine metabolism via the nitric oxide synthetase pathway. *J Immunol* 1991;**146**:2719–23.
13. Rockett KA, Awburn MM, Rockett EJ, Cowden WB, Clark IA. Possible role of nitric oxide in malarial immunosuppression. *Parasite Immunol* 1994;**16**:243–9.
14. Clark IA, Al-Yanab FM, Cowden WB, Rockett KA. Does malarial tolerance, through nitric oxide, explain the low incidence of autoimmune disease in tropical Africa. *Lancet* 1996;**348**:1492–4.
15. Adebajo A, Davis P. Rheumatic diseases in African blacks. *Semin Arthritis Rheum* 1994;**24**:139–53.
16. Wilson AG, Duff GW. Genetics of tumour necrosis factor in systemic lupus erythematosus. *Lupus* 1996;**5**:87–8.
17. Kwiatkowti D, Hill AVS, Sambou I, Twumasi P, Castracane J, Manogue KR, et al. TNF concentrations in fatal cerebral, non-fatal cerebral, and uncomplicated Plasmodium falciparum malaria. *Lancet* 1990;**336**:1201–4.
18. Wilson AG, di Giovine FS, Blakemore AIF, Duff GW. Single base polymorphism in the human Tumour Necrosis Factor alpha (TNF alpha) gene detectable by NcoI restriction of PCR product. *Hum Mol Genet* 1992;**1**:353.

19. Wilson AG, Symons JA, Mcdowell TL, Mcdevitt HO, Duff GW. Effects of a polymorphism in the human tumor necrosis factor α promoter on transcriptional activation. *Proc Natl Acad Sci USA* 1997;**94**:3195–9.

20. Kroeger KM, Steer JH, Joyce DA, Abraham LJ. Effects of stimulus and cell type on the expression of the −308 tumour necrosis factor promoter polymorphism. *Cytokine* 2000;**12**:110–19.

21. McGuire W, Hill AVS, Allsopp CEM, Greenwood BM, Kwiatkowski D. Cerebral malaria is associated with a polymorphism in the promoter region of the human TNF-a, gene. *Nature* 1994;**371**:508–11.

22. Price P, Witt C, Allcock R, Sayer D, Garlepp M, Kok CC, et al. The genetic basis for the association of the 8.1 ancestral haplotype (A1, B8, DR3) with multiple immunopathological diseases. *Immunol Rev* 1999;**167**:257–74.

23. Jacob CO, Fronek Z, Lewis GD, Koo M, Hansen JA, McDevitt HO. Heritable major histocompatibility complex class II-associated differences in production of tumor necrosis factor α: relevance to genetic predisposition to systemic lupus erythematosus. *Proc Natl Acad Sci U S A* 1990;**87**:1233–7.

24. Abraham LJ, French MAH, Dawkins RL. Polymorphic MHC ancestral haplotypes affect the activity of tumour necrosis factor-alpha. *Clin Exp Immunol* 1993;**92**:14–18.

25. Wilson AG, Duff GW. Genetic traits in common diseases. *BMJ* 1995;**310**:1482–3.

26. Lee YH, Harley JB, Nath SK. Meta-analysis of TNF-alpha promoter -308 A/G polymorphism and SLE susceptibility. *Eur J Hum Genet* 2006;**14**:364–71.

27. Clatworthy MR, Willcocks L, Urban B, Langhorne J, Williams TN, Peshu N, et al. Systemic lupus erythematosus-associated defects in the inhibitory receptor FcγRIIb reduce susceptibility to malaria. *Proc Natl Acad Sci USA* 2007;**104**:7169–74.

28. Waisberg M, Tarasenko T, Vickers BK, Scott BL, Willcocks LC, Molina-Cruz A, et al. Genetic susceptibility to systemic lupus erythematosus protects against cerebral malaria in mice. *Proc Natl Acad Sci USA* 2011;**108**:1122–7.

29. Willcocks LC, Carr EJ, Niederer HA, Rayner TF, Williams TN, Yang W, et al. A defunctioning polymorphism in FCGR2B is associated with protection against malaria but susceptibility to systemic lupus erythematosus. *Proc Natl Acad Sci USA* 2010;**107**:7881–5.

30. Kwiatkowski DP. How malaria has affected the human genome and what human genetics can teach us about malaria. *Am J Hum Genet* 2005;**77**:171–92.

31. Schwarzer E, Kuhn H, Valente E, Arese P. Malaria-parasitized erythrocytes and hemozoin non-enzymatically generate large amounts of hydroxy fatty acids that inhibit monocyte functions. *Blood* 2003;**101**:722–8.

32. McNicol MW. Sarcoidosis. In: Cruickshank JK, BeeLer DG, editors. *Ethnic factors in health and disease.* London: Wright; 1989. p. 209–15.

33. Bate CA, Taverne J, Roman E, Moreno C, Playfair JH. Tumour necrosis factor induction by malaria exoantigens depends upon phospholipid. *Immunology* 1992;**75**:129–35.

34. Souza-Passos LF. Apoptosis and SLE: Another piece in the puzzle? *Rev Bras Reumatol* 1997;**37**:327–34.

35. Dighiero G. Natural autoantibodies, tolerance, and autoimmunity. *Ann NY Acad Sci* 1997;**815**:182–92.

36. Butcher GA. Malaria and macrophage function in africans: A possible link with autoimmune disease? *Med Hypotheses* 1996;**47**:97–100.

37. Zuckerman A. Autoimmunization and other types of indirect damage to host cells as factors in certain protozoan diseases. *Exp Parasitol* 1964;**15**:138–83.

38. Lefrançois G, Bouvet E, Le Bras J, Vroklans M, Simonneau M, Vachon F. Anti-erythrocyte autoimmunisation during chronic falciparum malaria. *Lancet* 1981;**2**:661–4.

39. Banic DM, Viana-Martins FS, De Souza JM, Peixoto TD, Daniel-Ribeiro C. Polyclonal B-lymphocyte stimulation in human malaria and its association with ongoing parasitemia. *Am J Trop Med Hyg* 1991;**44**:571–7.

40. Burchard GD, Ehrhardt S, Mockenhaupt FP, Mathieu A, Agana-Nsiire P, Anemana SD, et al. Renal dysfunction in children with uncomplicated, Plasmodium falciparum malaria in Tamale, Ghana. *Ann Trop Med Parasitol* 2003;**97**:345–50.

41. Elsheikha HM, Sheashaa HA. Epidemiology, pathophysiology, management and outcome of renal dysfunction associated with plasmodia infection. *Parasitol Res* 2007;**101**:1183–90.

42. Sørensen PG, Mickley H, Schmidt KG. Malaria-induced immune thrombocytopenia. *Vox Sang* 1984;**47**:68–72.

43. Lang B, Newbold CI, Williams G, Peshu N, Marsh K, Newton CR. Antibodies to voltage-gated calcium channels in children with falciparum malaria. *J Infect Dis* 2005;**191**:117–21.

44. Bansal D, Herbert F, Lim P, Deshpande P, Bécavin C, Guiyedi V, et al. IgG autoantibody to brain beta tubulin III associated with cytokine cluster-II discriminate cerebral malaria in central India. *PLoS One* 2009;**4**:e8245.

45. Jayawardena AN, Janeway Jr. CA, Kemp JD. Experimental malaria in the CBA/N mouse. *J Immunol* 1979;**123**:2532–9.

46. Jarra W. Protective immunity to malaria and anti-erythrocyte autoimmunity. *Ciba Found Symp* 1983;**94**:137–58.

47. Daniel-Ribeiro CT. Is there a role for autoimmunity in immune protection against malaria? *Mem Inst Oswaldo Cruz* 2000;**95**:199–207.

48. Consigny PH, Cauquelin B, Agnamey P, Comby E, Brasseur P, Ballet JJ, et al. High prevalence of co-factor independent anticardiolipin antibodies in malaria exposed individuals. *Clin Exp Immunol* 2002;**127**:158–64.

49. Dugué C, Perraut R, Youinou P, Renaudineau Y. Effects of anti-endothelial cell antibodies in leprosy and malaria. *Infect Immun* 2004;**72**:301–9.

50. Daniel-Ribeiro CT, de Roquefeuil S, Druilhe P, Monjour L, Homberg JC, Gentilini M. Abnormal anti-single stranded (ss) DNA activity in sera from Plasmodium falciparum infected individuals. *Trans R Soc Trop Med Hyg* 1984;**78**:742–6.

51. Zouali M, Druilhe P, Eyquem A. IgG-subclass expression of anti-DNA and anti-ribonucleoprotein autoantibodies in human malaria. *Clin Exp Immunol* 1986;**66**:273–8.

52. Zanini GM, De MouraCarvalho LJ, Brahimi K, De Souza-Passos LF, Guimarães SJ, Da Silva ME, et al. Sera of patients with systemic lupus erythematosus react with plasmodial antigens and can inhibit the in vitro growth of Plasmodium falciparum. *Autoimmunity* 2009;**42**:545–52.

53. Vivas L, O'Dea KP, Noya O, Pabon R, Magris M, Botto C, et al. Hyperreactive malarial splenomegaly is associated with low levels of antibodies against red blood cell and Plasmodium falciparum derived glycolipids in Yanomami Amerindians from Venezuela. *Acta Trop* 2008;**105**:207–14.

54. de Souza JB, Playfair JH. Anti-lymphocyte antibodies in lethal mouse malaria. II. Induction of an autoantibody specific suppressor T cell by non-lethal P. yoelii. *Clin Exp Immunol* 1983;**54**:110–16.

55. Bate CA, Taverne J, Bootsma HJ, Mason RC, Skalko N, Gregoriadis G, et al. Antibodies against phosphatidylinositol and inositol monophosphate specifically inhibit tumour necrosis factor induction by malaria exoantigens. *Immunology* 1992;**76**:35–41.

56. Daniel-Ribeiro C, Ben Slama L, Gentilini M. Anti-nuclear and anti-smooth muscle antibodies in Caucasians, Africans and Asians with acute malaria. *J Clin Lab Immunol* 1991;**35**:109–12.

57. Kreier JP, Dilley DA. Plasmodium berghei: nucleic acid agglutinating antibodies in rats. *Exp Parasitol* 1969;**26**:175–80.

58. Quakyi IA, Voller A, Hall AP, Johnson GD, Holborow DJ, Moody AH. Immunological abnormalities in Caucasians with malaria. *Immunol Lett* 1979;**1**:153–4.

59. Poels LG, van Niekerk CC, van der Sterren-Reti V, Jerusalem C. Plasmodium berghei: T cell-dependent autoimmunity. *Exp Parasitol* 1980;**49**:97–105.
60. Abu-Shakra M, Shoenfeld Y. Parasitic infection and autoimmunity. *Autoimmunity* 1991;**9**:337–44.
61. Daniel-Ribeiro CT, Zanini G. Autoimmunity and malaria: What are they doing together? *Acta Trop* 2000;**76**:205–21.
62. Yoder BJ, Goodrum KJ. Plasmodium chabaudi chabaudi: B-1 cell expansion correlates with semiresistance in BALB/cJ mice. *Exp Parasitol* 2001;**98**:71–82.
63. Urban CF, Lourido S, Zychlinsky A. How do microbes evade neutrophil killing? *Cell Microbiol* 2006;**8**:1687–96.
64. Baker VS, Imade GE, Molta NB, Tawde P, Pam SD, Obadofin MO, et al. Cytokine-associated neutrophil extracellular traps and antinuclear antibodies in plasmodium falciparum infected children under six years of age. *Malar J* 2008;**7**:41.
65. Troye-Blomberg M, Berzins K, Perlmann P. T-cell control of immunity to the asexual blood stages of the malaria parasite. *Crit Rev Immunol* 1994;**14**:131–55.
66. Haldar K. Lipid transport in Plasmodium. *Infect Agents Dis* 1992;**1**:254–62.
67. Bevers EM, Comfurius P, Zwaal RF. Regulatory mechanisms in maintenance and modulation of transmembrane lipid asymmetry: pathophysiological implications. *Lupus* 1996;**5**:480–7.
68. Sein KK, Aikawa M. The prime role of plasma membrane cholesterol in the pathogenesis of immune evasion and clinical manifestations of falciparum malaria. *Med Hypotheses* 1998;**1**:105–10.
69. Du H, Chen M, Zhang Y, Zhao MH, Wang HY. Cross-reaction of anti-DNA autoantibodies with membrane proteins of human glomerular mesangial cells in sera from patients with lupus nephritis. *Clin Exp Immunol* 2006;**145**:21–7.
70. Eilat D, Zlotnick AY, Fischel R. Evaluation of the cross-reaction between anti-DNA and anti-cardiolipin antibodies in SLE and experimental animals. *Clin Exp Immunol* 1986;**65**:269–78.
71. Perignon JL, Druilhe P. Immune mechanisms underlying the premunition against plasmodium falciparum malaria. *Mem Inst Oswaldo Cruz* 1994;**89**(Suppl. 2):51–3.
72. Arvieux J, Renaudineau Y, Mane I, Perraut R, Krilis SA, Youinou P. Distinguishing features of anti-beta2 glycoprotein I antibodies between patients with leprosy and the antiphospholipid syndrome. *Thromb Haemost* 2002;**87**:599–605.
73. Berlin T, Zandman-Goddart G, Blank M, Matthias T, Pfeiffer S, Weiss I, et al. Autoantibodies in non autoimmune individuals during infections. *Ann NY Acad Sci* 2007;**1108**:584–93.
74. Brahimi K, Martins YC, Zanini GM, Ferreira-da-Cruz Mde F, Daniel-Ribeiro CT. Monoclonal auto-antibodies and sera of autoimmune patients react with Plasmodium falciparum and inhibit its in vitro growth. *Mem Inst Oswaldo Cruz* 2011;**106**(Suppl. 1):44–51.
75. Symmons DP. Frequency of lupus in people of African origin. *Lupus* 1995;**4**:176–8.
76. Affram RK, Neequaye AR. Systemic lupus erythematosus and other rheumatic disorders: clinical experience in Accra. *Ghana Med J* 1991;**25**:299–302.
77. Bae S-C, Fraser P, Liang MH. The epidemiology of systemic lupus erythematosus in populations of African ancestry. *Arthritis Rheum* 1998;**41**:2091–9.
78. Amoura Z, Huong Du L-T, Cacoub P, Frances C, Piette JC. Systemic lupus erythematosus in patients native to West and Central Africa. *Arthritis Rheum* 1999;**42**:1560–1.
79. Wadee S, Tikly M, Hopley M. Causes and predictors of death in South Africans with systemic lupus erythematosus. *Rheumatology (Oxford)* 2007;**46**:1487–91.
80. Adelowo OO, Oguntona SA. Pattern of systemic lupus erythematosus among Nigerians. *Clin Rheumatol* 2009;**28**:699–703.

81. Molokhia M, McKeigue PM, Cuadrado M, Hughes G. Systemic lupus erythematosus in migrants from west Africa compared with Afro-Caribbean people in the UK. *Lancet* 2001;**357**:1414–15.
82. Adelstein AM, Marmot MG, Bulusu L. Migrant studies in Britain. *Br Med Bull* 1984;**40**:315–19.
83. Westlake SL, Edwards CJ. Anti-malarials and lupus in West Africa use and lupus in Africans. *Lupus* 2009;**18**:193–5.
84. James JA, Kim-Howard XR, Bruner BF, Jonsson MK, McClain MT, Arbuckle MR, et al. Hydroxychloroquinesulfate treatment is associated with later onset of systemic lupus erythematosus. *Lupus* 2007;**16**:401–9.
85. Buabeng KO, Duwiejua M, Dodoo AN, Matowe LK, Enlund H. Self-reported use of anti-malarial drugs and health facility management of malaria in Ghana. *Malar J* 2007;**6**:85.
86. Foster S. Treatment of malaria outside the formal health services. *J Trop Med Hyg* 1995;**98**:29–34.
87. Chirdan OO, Zoakah AI, Ejembi CL. Impact of health education on home treatment and prevention of malaria in Jengre, North Central Nigeria. *Ann Afr Med* 2008;**7**:112–19.
88. Adah OS, Ngo-Ndomb T, Envuladu EA, Audu S, Banwat ME, Yusuff OT, et al. Home treatment of malaria, amongst under fives presenting with fever in PHC facilities in Jos North LGA of Plateau State. *Niger J Med* 2009;**18**:88–93.
89. Watsierah CA, Jura WG, Oyugi H, Abong'o B, Ouma C. Factors determining anti-malarial drug use in a peri-urban population from malaria holoendemic region of western Kenya. *Malar J* 2010;**9**:295.
90. Nsagha DS, Njunda AL, Kamga HL, Nsagha SM, Nguedia Assob JC, Wiysonge CS, et al. Knowledge and practices relating to malaria in a semi-urban area of Cameroon: choices and sources of antimalarials, self-treatment and resistance. *Pan Afr Med J* 2011;**9**:8.

PART 5

Autoimmune diseases and infections

CHAPTER 39

Anti-*Saccharomyces cerevisiae* Antibodies Autoimmune Diseases

Eytan Cohen, Ilan Krause
Department of Medicine F, Rabin Medical Center, Beilinson Campus, Sackler Faculty of Medicine, Tel-Aviv University, Tel-Aviv, Israel

Saccharomyces cerevisiae is the most common species of the genus *Saccharomyces*, commonly known as baker's or brewer's yeast. As such, we are commonly exposed to it in our society. In recent years, anti-*S. cerevisiae* antibodies (ASCAs), directed against the phosphopeptidomannan part of the cell wall of the yeast,[1] have been identified as an important and specific serological marker for Crohn's disease (CD).[2] At present, ASCAs, combined with perinuclear antineutrophil cytoplasmic autoantibodies (pANCAs), serve as a valuable tool for the differentiation between CD and ulcerative colitis (UC) in patients with inflammatory bowel diseases (IBDs). The pathogenic significance of ASCAs is unknown, and their exact origin, as well as the epitope against which they are directed, are unclear. They are not thought to be autoantibodies, although molecular mimicry to self-antigens remains a possibility. While ASCAs are considered rather specific for CD, several recent studies suggest that a wider panel of autoimmune and rheumatic disorders may be associated with high prevalence of ASCAs.

1 CROHN'S DISEASE

IBDs are subdivided into UC and CD.[3,4] Several lines of evidence suggest that CD and UC are different diseases. However, some patients (10–20%) cannot be easily classified as having either, and a final diagnosis of intermediate colitis is made. Making an earlier and more accurate diagnosis of IBD is important because the management of CD and UC is different, especially considering that surgery may be planned. For this reason, a search for serological tests to differentiate CD from UC has been underway for a long time. The ideal serological marker should have high sensitivity and a high

Infection and Autoimmunity
http://dx.doi.org/10.1016/B978-0-444-63269-2.00041-6

specificity. In 1988, Main et al.[5] were the first to show a high titer of anti-bodies against *S. cerevisiae* among patients with CD, but not in patients with UC, using a boiled suspension of *S. cerevisiae* as the antigenic substrate in an enzyme-linked immunosorbent assay. Since then, numerous studies have been performed to assess the sensitivity and specificity of ASCAs and pANCAs in IBDs. A meta-analysis of 60 studies comprising 3841 patients with UC and 4019 patients with CD showed that in patients with CD, the combination of a positive ASCA (IgG and IgA) and a negative pANCA test yielded a sensitivity and specificity of 55% and 93%, respectively. The best specificity (100%) was seen in positive ASCA IgA and negative pANCA. In patients with UC, however, positive pANCA and a negative ASCA test yielded a sensitivity and specificity of 51% and 94%, respectively, among the entire population and a sensitivity and specificity of 70% and 93%, respectively, in the paediatric subgroup of the population.[6] It seems, therefore, that combined measurement of both pANCAs and ASCAs may be used advantageously in the subclassification of patients with IBD with intermediate colitis.

Apart from being a diagnostic tool in established IBDs, ASCAs also have been found to be a possible predictor of future development of the disease. This was discovered through analysis of data from the Israeli Defense Force Medical Corps Serum Repository, which stores serum samples obtained systematically from 5% of all enlisted recruits and from the same population upon discharge from compulsory military service. It was found that of 32 subjects who eventually developed CD, 10 had been ASCA-positive years before, whereas among 95 controls, none had been ASCA positive before ($p < 0.001$). The mean interval between ASCA detection and IBD diagnosis was 38 months.[7]

Compared with ASCA-negative patients, ASCA-positive patients with CD have a significant higher risk for early onset of the disease, ileal involvement, complicated disease and risk for surgery.[8] During medical treatment, ASCA concentrations decrease with steroid treatment but are not influenced by mesalamine.[9] Furthermore, although the presence of ASCAs does not correlate with disease activity, titers have been found to decrease after resection of damaged gut tissue in a paediatric population.[10] These titers remained unchanged in adult population.[11]

Family studies indicate that ASCAs may be used to identify individuals at risk for CD. Lindberg et al.[12] studied 26 monozygotic twin pairs with IBD for serum antibodies against whole *S. cerevisiae* and mannan in the yeast cell wall. The twins were made up of five pairs concordant and nine pairs discordant for CD and two pairs concordant and 10 pairs discordant for UC. Twins who had developed CD displayed high antibody titers towards yeast cell wall mannan in particular and to whole *S. cerevisiae* yeast of all antibody types (IgA, IgG, and IgM). In families in which at least two members were affected with CD, ASCAs were detected in 69% of patients with CD and in 20% of healthy relatives, parents or siblings.[13] Similar rates of ASCAs in first-degree relatives of patients with CD (16–25%) have been reported in other studies.[14–16] Interestingly, the prevalence of ASCAs in relatives was not associated with the ASCA status of affected family members.[13] In addition, ASCAs were found to be significantly increased in a considerable number of unaffected relatives of families with IBD, irrespective of the characteristics of their disease (UC, CD, mixed, ASCA positive, or ASCA negative).[17]

2 BEHÇET'S DISEASE

Behçet's disease (BD) is a multi-system disorder, the clinical expression of which may be dominated by mucocutaneous, articular, neurologic, urogenital, vascular, intestinal, or pulmonary manifestations.[18] BD and CD share various clinical similarities, including mucocutaneous manifestations (recurrent oral ulcers, erythema nodosum), gastrointestinal disease favoring the terminal ileum, recurrent arthritis as well as uveitis. This increases the possibility of certain etiologic and pathogenic factors common to both diseases. Krause et al.[19] found a high rate (48.1%) of ASCAs in a group of 27 patients with BD, compared to 10% in three control groups of patients with recurrent oral ulcers, patients with systemic lupus erythematosus and healthy volunteers. No correlation was found between ASCAs and any BD-associated clinical manifestations nor the presence of human leukocyte antigen B5. Nor was any difference found in the rate of major oral ulcers or in disease severity between positive- and negative-ASCA patients with BD. These findings are supported by two other studies. Oshitani et al.[20] analyzed ASCA IgG subclasses in sera from patients with IBD, healthy controls, and seven patients with intestinal BD. IgG4 ASCAs were significantly increased in patients with IBD. In the patients with intestinal BD, the concentrations of IgG1, IgG3, and IgG4 ASCAs were increased. Similarly, Kim et al.[21] reported a high prevalence (41.7%) of ASCAs in a group of 36 patients with Behçet's colitis. In this study, four of eight healthy relatives of the patients with BD also tested positive for ASCAs. In another recent study, Monselise et al.[22] evaluated the rate and clinical correlation of ASCAs in patients with BD and their healthy relatives. Of 21 patients with BD, 8 (38.1%) were found to be ASCA positive compared to 5 of 52 healthy relatives (9.6%) and none among healthy unrelated controls ($p=0.001$). Levels of ASCAs were not correlated with clinical activity and were significantly higher in patients with BD compared to their healthy relatives ($p=0.002$).

These results suggest that BD may have a similar immunologic pathogenesis to that of CD and that the presence of ASCAs may indeed prove valuable as a preclinical marker of the disease. It also is conceivable that the presence of ASCAs do not pose an increased risk for a more severe course of BD. Further prospective studies are needed to evaluate whether ASCA titers are correlated with clinical relapses of BD.

3 CELIAC DISEASE

Celiac disease is defined as a disease of the proximal small intestine, characterized by damage to the small intestinal mucosa, and is associated with permanent intolerance to gluten.[23] Clinical symptoms and abnormal small-bowel histology resolve upon removal of gluten from the diet. Whenever suspected, the diagnosis of celiac disease is verified with an intestinal biopsy and an unequivocal clinical response to a gluten-free diet. Screening for elevated concentrations of several circulating autoantibodies is helpful in selecting suspected patients for an intestinal biopsy. These serological tests include the detection of anti-endomysium and anti-gliadin antibodies. The endomysial antigen has been identified as tissue transglutaminase. Anti-endomysium antibodies, and consequently anti-tissue transglutaminase antibodies, are considered highly specific and sensitive for celiac disease.[23] Few studies of small numbers of patients with celiac disease have addressed the relation between ASCAs and the disease. Giaffer et al.[24] first reported a group of 14 patients with celiac disease in whom high levels of IgG ASCAs, although not IgA ASCAs, were found; the antibody responses were indistinguishable from those found in CD. Since then, five more studies have been published showing a prevalence of ASCAs (IgG or IgA) between 27% and 59% in celiac patients.[25–29] Interestingly, the level of ASCAs were higher in adult patients with celiac disease compared to similar paediatric patients, suggesting the level of ASCAs may be dependent on the duration of the chronic immune inflammation.[25,27–29] Moreover, in the pediatric population, a remarkable disappearance of ASCA positivity was found after successful adherence to a gluten-free diet. This suggests a faster recovery in the juvenile population.[28,29]

4 ANKYLOSING SPONDYLITIS

Ankylosing spondylitis (AS) is an inflammatory disorder of unknown cause that primarily affects the axial skeleton. AS belongs to the spondyloarthropathies (SpAs), which have pathophysiological similarities to IBD. Subclinical bowel inflammation is present in up to 68% of patients with SpA, and 7% of these patients develop CD after 24–92 months.[30] At the same time, rheumatic manifestations are common extra-intestinal manifestations of CD, and 35% of patients with CD fulfil the criteria for SpA.[31] Hoffman et al.[32] studied the concentrations of ASCAs in 26 patients with CD, 108 patients with SpA (including 43 patients with AS), 56 patients with rheumatoid arthritis (RA), and 45 healthy controls. The concentrations of IgA ASCAs were significantly higher in SpA—and more specifically in AS—than in healthy controls and patients with RA. No correlation between the presence of subclinical bowel inflammation and concentrations of IgA ASCAs was noted. In another study, Andretta et al.[33] found that, of 70 patients with SpA, 18.6% were positive for IgA ASCAs, compared to 5.2% in 57 control subjects ($p = 0.031$). Similar to the study by Hoffman et al., the concentrations of IgA ASCAs had no relation to disease activity, clinical profile or the presence of human leukocyte antigen B27. Whether patients with ASCA-positive SpA have an increased risk of developing CD remains to be evaluated.

5 AUTOIMMUNE LIVER DISEASES

The autoimmune liver diseases, namely autoimmune hepatitis, primary biliary cirrhosis (PBC), and primary sclerosing cholangitis (PSC), are chronic inflammatory disorders of unknown etiology. These are characterized by immunological features generally including a variety of circulating and characteristic autoantibodies.[34] In light of the epidemiological association between IBDs and PSC, the prevalence of ASCAs in autoimmune liver diseases was recently studied. Reddy et al.[35] reported an ASCA prevalence of 22% in 80 patients with autoimmune hepatitis, 19% in 31 patients with PBC and 20% in 15 patients with PSC. Muratori et al.,[36] on the other hand, found higher rates of ASCAs in 17 anti-mitochondrial antibody-negative patients with PBC (44%) and in 25 patients with PSC (53%). ASCA reactivity did not correlate with biochemical parameters associated with liver disease. Furthermore, in patients with PSC, ASCA positivity was not found to predict the presence of concomitant IBD. The relatively low prevalence of ASCAs in autoimmune liver diseases (20–50%) suggests it may have lower diagnostic significance. Yet it may reflect common background susceptibility with IBDs, with a higher level of expression in CD. Given that few studies have evaluated ASCAs in autoimmune liver diseases, the actual incidence, as well its clinical significance in terms of disease progression and expression, awaits further prospective, large-scale studies.

6 SLE AND APS

Dai et al.[37] were the first to show increased concentrations of ASCAs in patients with SLE. In 40 patients with active SLE, 57.5% were shown to have high concentrations of IgG ASCAs, whereas IgA ASCA levels were not significantly higher than a control group. Another recent study by Mankai et al.,[38] involving 116 patients with SLE, demonstrated IgG ASCA, IgA ASCA and ASCA (IgG or IgA) levels of 29.3%, 12.1%, and 31.9%, respectively. All concentrations were significantly higher than in a control group. A possible explanation for the increased concentrations of ASCAs in patients with SLE may be a cross-reactivity between ASCAs and one of the anti-phospholipids found in SLE, namely anti-β2 glycoprotein I (GPI). Indeed, Krause et al.[39] found high concentrations of ASCAs in 20% of patients with APS compared to 5% in healthy controls ($p < 0.05$). The presence of ASCAs was not associated with any of the wide-spectrum APS-related clinical manifestations, and further analysis revealed the presence of cross-reactive epitopes on β2-GPI and *S. cerevisiae*. Therefore, it seems that ASCAs found in patients with SLE may be the consequence of anti β2-GPI found in some of those patients. This may further explain the finding by Mankai et al.[38] of raised concentrations of ASCAs (IgG or IgA) in 31.9% of their 116 patients with SLE; the same group demonstrated a 54.3% prevalence of anti-β2-GPI (IgG or IgA). Further studies are needed to assess the relation of ASCA to patients with SLE and those with APS.

7 OTHER AUTOIMMUNE DISEASES

Graves' disease (GD) and Hashimoto's thyroiditis are autoimmune thyroid diseases. Yazici et al.[40] and Mankai et al.[41] both found elevated concentrations of ASCAs in GD, although not in Hashimoto's thyroiditis. However, there are conflicting results between the studies as to the subtype of antibody raised in GD. While Yazici et al. found higher concentrations of IgA ASCAs (but not IgG ASCAs) compared to a control group, Mankai et al. found higher concentrations of IgG ASCAs (but not IgA ASCAs) compared to a control group. In a single study by Sakly et al.,[42] ASCA (IgA or IgG) concentrations were increased in 224 Tunisian patients with type 1 diabetes mellitus. However, although patients with celiac disease were excluded from the study, by negativity of anti-endomysium antibodies and antitissue transglutaminase antibodies, the authors themselves raise the possibility that some of their patients may have had celiac disease, which is common in Tunisia. As mentioned in the section on celiac disease, ASCAs are very common in this disease, with a prevalence ranging between 27% and 59%, according to different studies.[25-29] More evidence is needed to determine the role of ASCAs in both autoimmune thyroid diseases and type 2 diabetes mellitus.

REFERENCES

1. Sendid B, Colombel JF, Jacquinot PM, et al. Specific antibody response to oligomannosidic epitopes in Crohn's disease. *Clin Diagn Lab Immunol* 1996;**3**:219–26.
2. Quinton JF, Sendid B, Reumaux D, et al. Anti-*Saccharomyces cerevisiae* mannan antibodies combined with antineutrophil cytoplasmic autoantibodies in inflammatory bowel disease: prevalence and diagnostic role. *Gut* 1998;**42**:788–91.
3. Su C, Lichtenstein GR. Recent developments in inflammatory bowel disease. *Med Clin North Am* 2002;**86**:1497–523.
4. Banerjee S, Peppercorn MA. Inflammatory bowel disease medical therapy of specific clinical presentations. *Gastroenterol Clin North Am* 2002;**31**:185–202.
5. Main J, McKenzie H, Yeaman GR, et al. Antibody to *Saccharomyces cerevisiae* (Bakers' yeast) in Crohn's disease. *BMJ* 1988;**297**:1105–6.
6. Reese GE, Constantinides VA, Simillis C, et al. Diagnostic precision of anti-*Saccharomyces cerevisiae* antibodies and perinuclear antineutrophil cytoplasmic antibodies in inflammatory bowel disease. *Am J Gastroenterol* 2006;**101**:2410–22.
7. Israeli E, Grotto I, Gilburd B, et al. Anti-*Saccharomyces cerevisiae* and antineutrophil cytoplasmic antibodies as predictors of inflammatory bowel disease. *Gut* 2005;**54**:1232–6.
8. Zhang Z, Li C, Zhao X, et al. Anti-*Saccharomyces cerevisiae* antibodies associate with phenotypes and higher risk for surgery in Crohn's disease: a meta-analysis. *Dig Dis Sci* 2012;**57**:2944–54.
9. Teml A, Kratzer V, Schneider B, et al. Anti-*Saccharomyces cerevisiae* antibodies: a stable marker for Crohn's disease during steroid and 5-aminosalicylic acid treatment. *Am J Gastroenterol* 2003;**98**:2226–31.
10. Ruemmele FM, Targan SR, Levy G, Dubinsky M, Braun J, Seidman EG. Diagnostic accuracy of serological assays in pediatric inflammatory bowel disease. *Gastroenterology* 1998;**115**:822–9.
11. Eser A, Papay P, Primas C, et al. The impact of intestinal resection on serum levels of anti-*Saccharomyces cerevisiae* antibodies (ASCA) in patients with Crohn's disease. *Aliment Pharmacol Ther* 2012;**35**:292–9.
12. Lindberg E, Magnusson KE, Tysk C, Jarnerot G. Antibody (IgG, IgA, and IgM) to Baker's yeast (*Saccharomyces cerevisiae*), yeast mannan, gliadin, ovalbumin and betalactoglobulin in monozygotic twins with inflammatory bowel disease. *Gut* 1992;**33**:909–13.

13. Sendid B, Quinton JF, Charrier G, et al. Anti-*Saccharomyces cerevisiae* mannan antibodies in familial Crohn's disease. *Am J Gastroenterol* 1998;**93**:1306–10.

14. Seibold F, Stich O, Hufnagl R, Kamil S, Scheurlen M. Anti-*Saccharomyces cerevisiae* antibodies in inflammatory bowel disease: a family study. *Scand J Gastroenterol* 2001;**36**:196–201.

15. Vermeire S, Peeters M, Vlietinck R, et al. Anti-*Saccharomyces cerevisiae* antibodies (ASCA), phenotypes of IBD, and intestinal permeability: a study in IBD families. *Inflamm Bowel Dis* 2001;**7**:8–15.

16. Glas J, Torok HP, Vilsmaier F, Herbinger KH, Hoelscher M, Folwaczny C. Anti-*Saccharomyces cerevisiae* antibodies in patients with inflammatory bowel disease and their first-degree relatives: potential clinical value. *Digestion* 2002;**66**:173–7.

17. Annese V, Andreoli A, Andriulli A, et al. Familial expression of anti-*Saccharomyces cerevisiae* mannan antibodies in Crohn's disease and ulcerative colitis: a GISC study. *Am J Gastroenterol* 2001;**96**:2407–12.

18. Kaklamani VG, Vaiopoulos G, Kaklamanis PG. Behcet's disease. *Semin Arthritis Rheum* 1998;**27**:197–217.

19. Krause I, Monselise Y, Milo G, Weinberger A. Anti-*Saccharomyces cerevisiae* antibodies— a novel serologic marker for Behcet's disease. *Clin Exp Rheumatol* 2002;**20**:S21–4.

20. Oshitani N, Hato F, Jinno Y, et al. IgG subclasses of anti *Saccharomyces cerevisiae* antibody in inflammatory bowel disease. *Eur J Clin Invest* 2001;**31**:221–5.

21. Kim BG, Kim YS, Kim JS, Jung HC, Song IS. Diagnostic role of anti-*Saccharomyces cerevisiae* mannan antibodies combined with antineutrophil cytoplasmic antibodies in patients with inflammatory bowel disease. *Dis Colon Rectum* 2002;**45**:1062–9.

22. Monselise A, Weinberger A, Monselise Y, Fraser A, Sulkes J, Krause I. Anti-*Saccharomyces cerevisiae* antibodies in Behcet's disease—a familial study. *Clin Exp Rheumatol* 2006;**24**: S87–90.

23. Cardenas A, Kelly CP. Celiac sprue. *Semin Gastrointest Dis* 2002;**13**:232–44.

24. Giaffer MH, Clark A, Holdsworth CD. Antibodies to *Saccharomyces cerevisiae* in patients with Crohn's disease and their possible pathogenic importance. *Gut* 1992;**33**:1071–5.

25. Damoiseaux JG, Bouten B, Linders AM, et al. Diagnostic value of anti-*Saccharomyces cerevisiae* and antineutrophil cytoplasmic antibodies for inflammatory bowel disease: high prevalence in patients with celiac disease. *J Clin Immunol* 2002;**22**:281–8.

26. Candelli M, Nista EC, Carloni E, Pignataro G, Rigante D, Gasbarrini A. Anti-*Saccharomyces cerevisiae* antibodies and coeliac disease. *Scand J Gastroenterol* 2003;**38**:1191–2.

27. Granito A, Zauli D, Muratori P, et al. Anti-*Saccharomyces cerevisiae* and perinuclear anti-neutrophil cytoplasmic antibodies in coeliac disease before and after gluten-free diet. *Aliment Pharmacol Ther* 2005;**21**:881–7.

28. Mallant-Hent R, Mary B, von Blomberg E, et al. Disappearance of anti-*Saccharomyces cerevisiae* antibodies in coeliac disease during a gluten-free diet. *Eur J Gastroenterol Hepatol* 2006;**18**:75–8.

29. Toumi D, Mankai A, Belhadj R, Ghedira-Besbes L, Jeddi M, Ghedira I. Anti-*Saccharomyces cerevisiae* antibodies in coeliac disease. *Scand J Gastroenterol* 2007;**42**:821–6.

30. De Keyser F, Elewaut D, De Vos M, et al. Bowel inflammation and the spondyloarthropathies. *Rheum Dis Clin North Am* 1998;**24**:785–813.

31. de Vlam K, Mielants H, Cuvelier C, De Keyser F, Veys EM, De Vos M. Spondyloarthropathy is underestimated in inflammatory bowel disease: prevalence and HLA association. *J Rheumatol* 2000;**27**:2860–5.

32. Hoffman IE, Demetter P, Peeters M, et al. Anti-*Saccharomyces cerevisiae* IgA antibodies are raised in ankylosing spondylitis and undifferentiated spondyloarthropathy. *Ann Rheum Dis* 2003;**62**:455–9.

33. Andretta MA, Vieira TD, Nishiara R, Skare TL. Anti-*Saccharomyces cerevisiae* (ASCA) and anti-endomysial antibodies in spondyloarthritis. *Rheumatol Int* 2012;**32**:551–4.

34. Krawitt EL. Autoimmune hepatitis. *N Engl J Med* 1996;**334**:897–903.

35. Reddy KR, Colombel JF, Poulain D, Krawitt EL. Anti-*Saccharomyces cerevisiae* antibodies in autoimmune liver disease. *Am J Gastroenterol* 2001;**96**:252–3.

36. Muratori P, Muratori L, Guidi M, et al. Anti-*Saccharomyces cerevisiae* antibodies (ASCA) and autoimmune liver diseases. *Clin Exp Immunol* 2003;**132**:473–6.

37. Dai H, Li Z, Zhang Y, Lv P, Gao XM. Elevated levels of serum antibodies against *Saccharomyces cerevisiae* mannan in patients with systemic lupus erythematosus. *Lupus* 2009;**18**:1087–90.

38. Mankai A, Sakly W, Thabet Y, Achour A, Manoubi W, Ghedira I. Anti-*Saccharomyces cerevisiae* antibodies in patients with systemic lupus erythematosus. *Rheumatol Int* 2013;**33**:665–9.

39. Krause I, Blank M, Cervera R, et al. Cross-reactive epitopes on beta2-glycoprotein-I and *Saccharomyces cerevisiae* in patients with the antiphospholipid syndrome. *Ann NY Acad Sci* 2007;**1108**:481–8.

40. Yazici D, Aydin SZ, Yavuz D, et al. Anti-saccaromyces cerevisiae antibodies (ASCA) are elevated in autoimmune thyroid disease ASCA in autoimmune thyroid disease. *Endocrine* 2010;**38**:194–8.

41. Mankai A, Thabet Y, Manoubi W, Achour A, Sakly W, Ghedira I. Anti-*Saccharomyces cerevisiae* antibodies are elevated in Graves' disease but not in Hashimoto's thyroiditis. *Endocr Res* 2013;**38**:98–104.

42. Sakly W, Mankai A, Sakly N, et al. Anti-*Saccharomyces cerevisiae* antibodies are frequent in type 1 diabetes. *Endocr Pathol* 2010;**21**:108–14.

CHAPTER 40

The Infectious Origin of the Anti-Phospholipid Syndrome

M. Blank*,1, E. Israeli*, R. Cervera†
*Zabludowicz Center for Autoimmune Diseases, Sheba Medical Center, affiliated to Sackler Faculty of Medicine, Tel-Aviv University, Tel-Aviv, Israel
†Department of Autoimmune Diseases, Hospital Clínic, Barcelona, Catalonia, Spain
1Corresponding Author: rcervera@clinic.cat

1 INTRODUCTION

The anti-phospholipid syndrome (APS) is characterized by the development of thrombosis and pregnancy morbidity (mainly fetal losses) in the presence of anti-phospholipid antibodies (aPLs).[1–6] These antibodies (Abs) are currently considered to be pathogenic autoantibodies directed mainly against phospholipid-binding proteins such as β2-glycoprotein-I (β2GPI). The factors causing the production of anti-β2GPI Abs remain unidentified, but an association with infectious agents has been reported. Studies of experimental APS models proved that molecular mimicry between β2GPI-related synthetic peptides and structures within bacteria, viruses, tetanus toxoid, and cytomegalovirus (CMV) is a cause of experimental APS. The explanation of how microbial and viral infections might set off APS must take into account bystander activation, altered self-molecular changes and a second hit, in addition to molecular mimicry. Basically, all individuals seem to harbor potentially autoreactive lymphocytes and Abs, due to clonal escape, as part of the innate immunity. These cells or Abs remain innocuous unless activated by a pro-inflammatory microenvironment and/or a second hit on the proper genetic and epigenetic background. Herein, we discuss the association of aPLs in an infectious state, molecular mimicry (Figure 1) as a proposed cause for the development of APS and the contribution of databases to this topic.

2 AUTOIMMUNE DISEASES AND INFECTIONS: THE ROLE OF MOLECULAR MIMICRY

There is a general consensus that autoimmune diseases have a multifactorial etiology, depending on both genetic and environmental factors. Microbial

Infection and Autoimmunity
http://dx.doi.org/10.1016/B978-0-444-63269-2.00045-3
681

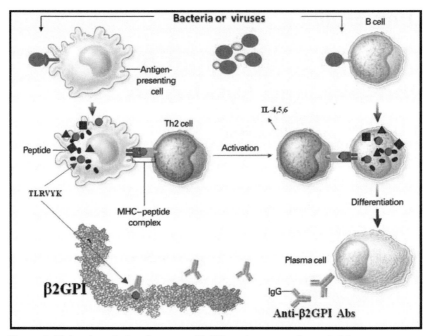

Figure 1 Molecular mimicry between β2-GPI and common bacteria/viruses.

agents or viruses can induce autoimmune diseases by a variety of mecha-nisms.[7-10] For example, proteins of certain infectious agents can act as poly-clonal activators on unique lymphocyte subsets. Viruses can preferentially infect/destroy a particular T-cell subset, leading to an imbalance in the immune response. In other instances, infectious agents can upregulate Th1 cytokines, thereby increasing selected expression of molecules such as MHC glycoproteins, as well as activation of co-stimulatory molecules. Several microbial agents have been found to encode superantigens that can selectively activate subsets of T cells. Microbes can also direct the release of cytokines and chemokines, which can act as growth, differentiation, or chemotactic factors for different Th populations and regulate the expression of MHC class I and class II molecules.

The healthy immune system is tolerant to the body's own molecules. However, among the major antigens recognized during a wide variety of bacterial, viral and parasitic diseases, many belong to conserved protein fam-ilies and share extensive sequence identity or conformational fits with host molecules, namely molecular mimicry. Antigenic similarity of either mole-cule's linear amino acid sequences or its conformational structure between antigens of infectious agents and host tissues might trigger an immune response against the shared determinant. As a result, the tolerance to auto-antigens breaks down, and the pathogen-specific immune response that is generated cross-reacts with host structures to cause tissue damage and disease. A role for molecular mimicry in the pathogenesis of autoimmune diseases has been proved in several animal models of autoimmune diseases, including rheumatic fever, allergic encephalomyelitis, experimental autoimmune uveitis and more.[10–15] Two groups of researchers found that molecular mimicry between common pathogens and β2GPI may be one of the main causes for the induction of APS.[16–18]

3 ANTI-β2GPI ANTIBODIES

3.1 β2-Glycoprotein-I

The human β2GPI molecule is a heavily glycosylated membrane-adhesion glycoprotein (326aa), present in blood plasma at a concentration of ~150-300 μg/mL.[19,20] β2GPI exhibits several properties *in vitro* that define it as an anticoagulant (e.g. the inhibition of prothrombinase activity, adenosine diphosphate-induced platelet aggregation and platelet factor IX production).[21] It has a role in the clearance of apoptotic bodies from the circulation.[22]

The β2GPI molecule was found to be immunogenic in mice and rabbits, resulting in *de novo* generation of mouse-anti-β2GPI Abs, and associated with an increased percentage of fetal resorptions (the equivalent of fetal loss in human APS), thrombocytopenia and prolonged activated partial thromboplastin time, indicating the presence of lupus anticoagulant, a presentation of experimental APS.[23–25] The importance of β2GPI as an autoantigen in experimental APS was proven by oral tolerance induced by feeding β2GPI to APS mice.[26] Anti-β2GPI Abs exert a direct pathogenic effect based on (1) the passive transfer of the Abs into naive mice induces experimental APS;[27,28] (2) in an *ex vivo* model of thrombosis, anti-β2GPI Abs affinity purified from sera of patients with APS induces thrombus formation;[29] (3) exchanging heavy and light chains between pathogenic and non-pathogenic anti-β2GPI single-chain Fv showed that the pathogenic part of the anti-β2GPI molecule is located on the CDR3 of the immunoglobulin heavy chain;[30] and (4) *in vitro* and *in vivo* studies proved that anti-β2GPI Abs activated the expression of E-selectin, intercellular adhesion molecule-1, vascular cell adhesion molecule-1, and nuclear factor-κB in monocytes and endothelial cells.[31–33]

3.2 Origin of Anti-β2GPI Antibodies in Plasma

β2GPI and cardiolipin are ubiquitous molecules. Several hypothesis for deciphering the origin of anti-phospholipid Abs were raised, such as (1) the exposure of β2GPI cryptic epitope upon binding to oxidized surfaces and negatively charged surfaces;[34,35] (2) the oxidized form of β2GPI undergoes conformational changes, presenting neoepitopes, which may induce anti-β2GPI Abs generation;[36,37] and (3) apoptotic cells present β2GPI molecules via binding to phosphatidylserine, presenting neoepitopes to the immune system and thus breaking the tolerance and inducing anti-β 2GPI Abs.[38] During the past decade, common bacteria and viruses were proved to be associated with induction of APS and evoke experimental APS.[16,17,39,40]

4 INFECTION AND ANTIPHOSPHOLIPID ANTIBODIES

4.1 Infectious Agents and the APS

Many infections may be accompanied by aPL elevations and, in some, these elevations may be accompanied by clinical manifestations of the APS. Several reviews of this important topic are deeply detailed.[39–42] Skin infections (18%), human immunodeficiency virus infection (17%), pneumonia (14%), hepatitis C virus (13%), and urinary tract infections constituted the most common infections found as "triggering" factors. In nine cases, more than one agent/organ was identified as the source of infection. Other infections less frequently associated with APS included mycoplasma (three cases), pulmonary tuberculosis (two cases), malaria (two cases), *Pneumocystis carinii* and *P. leptospirosis* in one case each. Catastrophic APS was recently reported upon.[43]

4.2 The Catastrophic APS and Infections

The catastrophic APS is an unusual and potentially fatal variant of the APS, first defined in 1992 by Asherson.[44] Since then, more than 1000 patients have been fully analyzed and documented in major publications.[44–48] "Triggering" factors, which include trauma (including both major and minor surgical trauma), anticoagulation withdrawal and a variety of carcinomas, have become increasingly apparent and were present in 51% of analyzed cases.[44–49] However, the most common, and most important, triggering factor is infection, which was identified in 24% of these patients.

Infections preceding the appearance of catastrophic APS were reported in eight patients by Rojas-Rodríguez et al.[49] The comprehensive analysis of infections and aPLs[46] has shown that 40 of these 100 cases (40%) manifested catastrophic APS, which now seems to be almost as common as the "classical" APS following a triggering infection. These infections comprised respiratory (10%), cutaneous (including infected leg ulcers) (4%), urinary tract (45%) and gastrointestinal infections (2%), general sepsis (1%) and others (3%). One patient in the latter group developed catastrophic APS following typhoid fever and has been reported in detail.[50] Another patient who developed two large vessel occlusions following typhoid fever also has recently been documented.[51] Although this patient was represented as suffering from catastrophic APS, small-vessel occlusions essential for the diagnosis of catastrophic APS were reported. One report of catastrophic APS development following malaria infection was introduced.[52] Resolution of catastrophic APS following amputation of a gangrenous limb after infection was described in two patients.[53] Molecular mimicry between a pathogen and self-antigens has been proposed as one of the major mechanisms responsible for the development of catastrophic APS following viral, bacterial or parasitic infections.

5 THE INFECTIOUS ORIGIN OF CIRCULATING ANTI-β2GPI ANTIBODIES

5.1 The Molecular Mimicry Hypothesis

We hypothesized that a molecular mimicry mechanism between a pathogen and β2GPI molecules may be the cause for APS, based on (1) a correlation between APS clinical manifestations and infectious agents in humans and (2) a strong homology between β2GPI-related peptides (target epitopes for anti-β2GPI Abs) and different common pathogens in the protein databases.

Introducing human anti-β2GPI monoclonal Abs derived from patients with APS to a hexapeptide phage display library, we previously identified several synthetic peptides as target epitopes for anti-β2GPI Abs.[32] These β2GPI-related peptides were found to be located on domain I (mimotope), domain III and domain IV. All three synthetic peptides inhibited the activation of endothelial cell *in vitro* and the induction of experimental APS in naive mice by neutralizing the pathogenic anti-β2GPI Abs. The prevalence of circulating anti-β2GPI peptide A-C Abs, directed to different domains in sera of 295 patients with APS, ranged between 18% and 47.5%.[54] Using the protein database, we found homologies between our and other peptides with common bacteria viruses, yeast and tetanus toxin.[55] To prove the involvement of molecular mimicry mechanism between the pathogen and β2GPI molecule as a cause for experimental APS, we immunized naive mice with microbial pathogens, which share structural homology with the TLRVYK hexapeptide. IgG antibodies specific to the TLRVYK peptide were affinity purified from the immunized mice on a TLRVYK column and intravenous therapy was passively infused into naive mice at day 0 of pregnancy. APS clinical parameters were evaluated in the infused mice on day 15 of pregnancy.[16] Following immunization with all the bacteria that had significant homologies, various levels of mouse anti-β2GPI Abs were observed. The highest affinity Abs for β2GPI were found in mice immunized with *Hemophilus influenzae, Neisseria gonorrhoeae* or tetanus toxoid. Mice infused with these anti-β2GPI Abs had significant thrombocytopenia, prolonged activated partial thromboplastin time and elevated percentage of fetal loss, similar to a control group of mice immunized with a pathogenic anti-β2GPI monoclonal Ab.[16] Hence, our study established a mechanism of molecular mimicry in experimental APS, demonstrating that bacteria and tetanus toxoid with a structure homologous to that of β2GPI are able to induce the generation of pathogenic anti-β2GPI Abs along with APS manifestations.[16] The concept is summarized in Figure 1. Furthermore, the β2GPI domain I-derived synthetic peptide NTLKTPRV,[32] which shares similarities with common bacterial antigens, decreased thrombogenic properties of aPLs in mice.[56] The author proposes that this peptide may have important implications in designing new modalities of prevention and/or treatment of thrombosis in APS.

Gharavi et al.[31] induced circulating anti-β2GPI Abs in naive mice by immunization with synthetic peptides conjugated to bovine serum albumin, which share some similarity with the 72-kDa human adenovirus type 2 DNA-binding protein, CMV, human CMVA, and *Bacillus subtilis*.

We believe that pathogen particles are digested and presented on macrophages, dendritic cells, or B cells. These pathogen particles are presented to T cells, which in appropriate human leukocyte antigen presentation and Th1/Th2-activated cytokine cascade expression lead to the generation of plasma cells secreting anti-β2GPI Abs, directed to the pathogen particles, which share structural homology (molecular mimicry) with the β2GPI molecule. Whether an individual develops APS depends mainly on his genetic predisposition or epigenetic scenario. The above data pave the way for the conclusion of an infection origin of APS.[16,55–57]

5.2 Association Between Various Common Pathogens and β2GPI Amino Acid Sequence

5.2.1 Helicobacter pylori Anti-β2GPI Abs and APS

Helicobacter pylori, one of the most common bacterial pathogens of humans, colonizes the gastric mucosa, where it seems to persist throughout the host's life unless the patient is treated. Colonization induces chronic gastric inflammation, which can progress to a variety of diseases ranging in severity from superficial gastritis and peptic ulcer to gastric cancer and mucosal-associated lymphoma. Strain-specific genetic diversity has been proposed to be involved in the organism's ability to cause different diseases or even to be beneficial to the infected host and participate in the lifelong chronicity of infection.[58] The disappearance of APS after *H. pylori* eradication was reported.[59]

Accumulated data show that *H. pylori* infection can affect fetal intrauterine growth, increase the risk for developing reproductive disorders or enhance platelet embolism followed by damage to arterioles.[60–62] In all these cases, the correlation to anti-β2GPI Abs or to β2GPI-related peptides should be analyzed. In one study, the screening of 50 patients with *H. pylori* infection for the presence of anti-β2GPI Abs revealed a prevalence of 33.3%.[63]

5.2.2 Streptococcus pyogenes, Anti-β2GPI Abs and APS

Rheumatic fever (RF) and subsequent rheumatic heart disease represent a relatively common connective tissue disease caused by *Streptococcus pyogenes*. Molecular mimicry, mainly between the pathogenic M protein and self structures, has been thought to be a mechanism for the development of acute RF after streptococcal pharyngitis.[14] RF and APS share a partial common clinical picture, such as involvement of the central nervous system and heart. We assumed that it may be a consequence of a cross-reactive epitope between the M-protein and the β2GPI. The β2GPI-related peptides TLRVYK and LKTPRV share homology with *S. pyogenes* M-protein (mismatch of 2). The β2GPI-related peptide TLRVYK inhibited the binding of anti-M-protein Abs from patients with RF to M-protein by 37%. Anti-β2GPI Abs could be inhibited by 23% when the M-protein binds to β2GPI.[64]

5.2.3 Borrelia burgdorferi, Anti-β2GPI Abs and APS

The spirochaete *Borrelia burgdorferi* is the cause of the neurological Lyme disease. A subset of patients (50%) with neuroborreliosis (Lyme disease) showed IgG reactivity to cardiolipin in a solid-phase ELISA.[65] Since the assay was conducted in 1987 with serum as the blocker, the reaction probably is β2GPI dependent. The β2GPI-related peptides TLRVYK and LKTPRV share homologies (mismatch 1) with *B. burgdorferi*:Q51257-a glycerol kinase, 051376 protein-glutamate methylesterase.

5.2.4 *Saccharomyces cerevisiae*, Anti-β2GPI Abs and APS

Presence of circulating anti-*Saccharomyces cerevisiae* IgA/IgG Abs (ASCAs) is one of the main markers for Crohn's disease, an idiopathic chronic inflammatory bowel disease. Oligomannose and paratuberculosis p35 and p36 antigens are epitopes of *S. cerevisiae*, defined and demonstrated in 60-70% of patients with Crohn's disease. Patients with inflammatory bowel diseases have elevated titers of circulating aCLs/anti-β2GPI Abs.[66] Episodes of thrombosis associated with Crohn's disease were described accompanied with elevated titers of anti-2GPI Abs.[66–68] ASCAs also were described in patients with another autoimmune condition – Behçet's disease (BD).[60] Some patients with BD (30–32%) have circulating anti-β2GPI Abs.[69] The association of APS with BD was suggested as a cause for the total thrombotic occlusion of the vena cava in one case.[70] So far the cross-reactivity between ASCAs and β2GPI molecules was not studied.

Using a Swiss protein database, several homologies between β2GPI-related peptides and *S. cerevisiae* were disclosed, such as TLRVYK: Q07878, the vacuolar protein sorting-associated protein VPS13, which promotes endosomal cycling of TGN membrane proteins by modulating the function of two cytosolic TGN localization signals; P53070, a mitochondrial translation optimization protein; LKTPRV:P41911, glycerol-3-phosphate dehydrogenase [NAD+] 2; P40550 and Q04182, which are adenosine triphosphate-dependent permeases PDR11 and PDR15, a multi-drug adenosine triphosphate-binding cassette transporter of the yeast plasma membrane.

5.3 Anti-β2GPI Tentative Dual Activity Associated with Infections

A wide range of specific protein–protein interactions at the cell surface and in the serum are mediated by functionally versatile 60-amino acid residue protein domains called complement control proteins (CCPs, also known as short consensus repeats), which are characterized by unique consensus sequence. Among the ligands, the β2GPI molecule contains four typical CCP modules, one atypical CPP module and key complement system proteins such as C3b and C4b anti-coagulant vitamin K-dependent protein S;

heparin; viruses such as the Epstein–Barr virus (EBV), the measles virus, enterovirus 70 and echovirus; and bacterial proteins such as M–protein of the group A *S. pyogenes* and the adhesion of *Escherichia coli*. CPP modules have been identified so far in 50 distinct mammalian proteins from plasma, the surface of many cell types, spermatozoon acrosomal matrix, retina, brain, and more.[71–73]

Using Gapped-BLAST and PSI-BLAST of a Swiss protein database, and the apoH_FASTA-file, we found a strong significant alignment ($>1e^{-11}$) between the β2GPI molecule and several infection-relevant sequences or pathogen control molecules. Herein, we present a few examples and discuss the functional relevance of anti-β2GPI Abs as natural or pathogenic autoantibodies.

5.3.1 Vaccinia Virus

Vaccinia and/or vaccinia gamma globulin are used for smallpox vaccination. Deaths were attributable to smallpox vaccination mainly by transmission of vaccinia from the smallpox vaccination, although the disease is now eradicated in most countries.[74] Domains 3 and 4 of the β2GPI molecule share a tertiary structural that is highly similar ($>1e^{-19}$) to that of the vaccinia virus and complement control protein (VCP) (Q89859). This 243-residue protein is a regulator of complement activation, and its role is to defend the virus against attack by the host complement system. β2GPI may compete with this VCP protein residue for its receptor recognition and facilitate complement activation as a response to the virus. Anti-β2GPI may act on the VCP by way of virus neutralization, thus enabling complement activation to occur.

P10998 – Complement control protein precursor (CCP) (Secretory protein 35) (Protein C3) (28 kDa protein): the vaccinia virus encodes a secretory polypeptide structurally related to CCP ($>9e^{-20}$). This polypeptide protects the virus against complement attack by inhibiting both classical and alternative pathways of complement activation. It also binds C3b and C4b. Preventing this kind of virus protection by circulating anti-β2GPI Abs causes a response to the virus.

5.3.2 Interrelation of β2GPI and Anti-β2GPI Abs in EBV

Q9DC83; O46545; Q99254-complement receptor 2 – (CR2). CR2 is the receptor for C3d, the 33-kDa fragment of the third complement component. CR2 is also the EBV receptor (EBV/C3d, CD21). CR2 binds to its two extracellular ligands, C3d and the EBV capsid glycoprotein gp350/220, through two distinct binding sites. CR2 allows C3d and EBV to induce proliferation.[75] Theoretically, different scenarios can be envisioned regarding the EBV/β2GPI/anti-β2GPI Abs interrelations: anti-β2GPI Abs may be protective Abs generated by a molecular mimicry mechanism, as described in Figure 1. These Abs may neutralize the EBV or the CR2 if they recognize a shared epitope, thus preventing infectious mononucleosis. On the other hand, they can be pathogenic, enhancing the disease if the anti-β 2GPI Abs recognize a different epitope on the EBV and on CR2. The presence of circulating anti-β2GPI Abs was described in patients with infectious mononucleosis with no correlation to disease activity.[76] However, a wide range of populations that are exposed to EBV have anti-β2GPI Abs. Patients with APS have very high titers of anti-EBV associated with anti-β2GPI with no infectious mononucleosis (unpublished data).

Q16744; Q29530-complement receptor 1 (CR1): there is controversy regarding the CR1 as an inducer or inhibitor of B-cell activation. At this stage, the question of whether β2GPI can function as a mimetic of CR1 or CR2 is speculative, as well as the role of anti-β2GPI in B-cell activation in response to a pathogen.

5.4 A Cross-Point with Innate Immunity

Toll-like receptors (TLRs) are pattern recognition receptors that trigger innate immunity, providing both immediate protective responses against pathogens and instructing the adaptive immune response.[77] Accumulating evidence has paved the way to explaining the importance of TLRs in promoting autoimmune conditions.[78–80] Different studies revealed that common molecular patterns of microorganisms such as lipopolysaccharide (LPS) are recognized by TLR4 or TLR2. β2GPI is a carrier molecule of LPS. Studies using surface plasmon resonance revealed that a synthesised peptide (LAFWKTDA) from domain V of β2GPI was able to compete for binding of β2GPI to LPS. The AFWKTDA sequence is completely conserved in all mammals. The peptide containing the LPS binding site attenuated the inhibition by β2GPI in a cellular model of LPS-induced tissue factor expression. The importance of TLRs in the procoagulative state of endothelial cells in APS was proposed a decade ago,[33] showing the role of the MyD88 transduction signaling pathway in endothelial cell activation by anti-β2GPI. Moreover, the ultimate proof of TLR4/LPS in APS came from *in vivo* studies by Pierangeli et al.,[81] who showed the pathogenic role of TLR4 in APS by studying thrombogenic aPL activity in LPS non-responsive (LPS $-/-$) mice and the association between *tlr4* gene polymorphisms and APS in patients.

6 THERAPEUTIC CONSIDERATIONS

Based on the data summarized above, there is strong evidence for an infectious etiology of APS. This raises the big issue of instituting antibiotic therapy as prevention and/or interventional therapy, especially in catastrophic APS. More information will be required in the future to solve this enigma. The disease progression depends on whether the mechanism of the disease is "hit and run", leading to bystander activation, or a continuous stimulation of the immune system, leading to a burden of proinflammatory cytokines, attenuation of the number of T regulatory and B regulatory cells, all the protecting immune network. A study in which the APS was abrogated by the eradication of *H. pylori* with antibiotic therapy[59] points to the effect of the continuous presence of the bacteria on the induction of the disease. In another study using an experimental APS model, treatment with ciprofloxacin improved the clinical picture by inducing the expression of interleukin-3 and granulocyte-macrophage colony-stimulating factor.[82] These seminal works support the addition of antibiotics to combination therapy for patients with APS.

7 CONCLUSIONS

Molecular mimicry is one of the mechanisms by which experimental APS can be initiated in association with the presence of pathogens. Shared epitopes between β2GPI-related synthetic peptides and bacteria or viruses, as well as their ability to induce experimental APS in mice, prove the existence of molecular mimicry between pathogens and autoantigens in APS. The β2GPI molecule as a carrier of LPS and LPS as a "second hit" for the pathogenic activity of the anti-β2GPI molecule both support the concept of an infectious origin of APS. Yet the mere presence of self-determinants on a virus or bacteria does not necessarily result in disease. The full-blown APS emerges only if the appropriate genetic predisposition exists.

REFERENCES

1. Harris EN, Gaharavi AE, Boey ML, Patel BM, Mackworth-Young CG, Loizou S, et al. Anticardiolipin antibodies: detection by radioimmunoassay and association with thrombosis in systemic lupus erythematosus. *Lancet* 1983;**2**:1211–14.

2. Hughes GRV, Harris EN, Gharavi AE. The anti-cardiolipin syndrome. *J Rheumatol* 1986;**13**:486–9.

3. Asherson RA, Cervera R, Piette JC, Shoenfeld Y. Milestones in the antiphospholipid syndrome. In: Asherson RA, Cervera R, Piette JC, Shoenfeld Y, editors. *The antiphospholipid syndrome II—autoimmune thrombosis.* Amsterdam: Elsevier; 2002.

4. Galli M, Comfurious P, Massen C, Hemker MH, Be-Bates PJ, van-Breda P, et al. Anticardiolipin antibodies (ACA) directed not to cardiolipin but to a plasma protein cofactor. *Lancet* 1990;**335**:1544–7.

5. Cervera R, Cervera R, Piette JC, Font J, et al. Antiphospholipid syndrome: clinical and immunologic manifestations and patterns of disease expression in a cohort of 1,000 patients. *Arthritis Rheum* 2002;**46**:1019–27.

6. Shoenfeld Y. Systemic antiphospholipid syndrome. *Lupus* 2003;**4**:97–8.

7. Oldstone MB. Molecular mimicry and immune-mediated diseases. *FASEB J* 1998;**12**:1255–65.

8. Albert LJ, Inman RD. Molecular mimicry and autoimmunity. *N Engl J Med* 1999;**341**:2068–74.

9. Regner M, Lambert PH. Autoimmunity through infection or immunization? *Nature Immunol* 2001;**2**:185–8.

10. Wucherpfennig KW. Structural basis of molecular mimicry. *J Autoimmunity* 2001;**16**:293–302.

11. Sfriso P, Ghirardello A, Botsios C, Tonon M, Zen M, Bassi N, et al. Infections and autoimmunity: the multifaceted relationship. *J Leukoc Biol* 2010;**87**:385–95.

12. Singh VK, Kalra HK, Yamaki K, Abe T, Donoso LA, Shinohara T. Molecular mimicry between a uveitopathogenic site of S-antigen and viral peptides. Induction of experimental autoimmune uveitis in Lewis rats. *J Immunol* 1990;**144**:1282–7.

13. Zhao ZS, Granucci F, Yeh L, Schaffer PA, Cantor H. Molecular mimicry by herpes simplex virus-type 1: autoimmune disease after viral infection. *Science* 1998;**279**:1344–7.

14. Guilherme L, Kalil J, Cunningham M. Molecular mimicry in the autoimmune pathogenesis of rheumatic heart disease. *Autoimmunity* 2006;**39**:31–9.

15. Levin MC, Lee SM, Kalume F, Morcos Y, Dohan Jr. FC, Hasty KA, et al. Autoimmunity due to molecular mimicry as a cause of neurological disease. *Nat Med* 2002;**8**:509–13.

16. Blank M, Krause I, Fridkin M, Keller N, Kopolovic J, Goldberg I, et al. Bacterial induction of autoantibodies to beta2-glycoprotein-I accounts for the infectious etiology of antiphospholipid syndrome. *J Clin Invest* 2002;**109**:797–804.

17. Shoenfeld Y. Etiology and pathogenetic mechanisms of the anti-phospholipid syndrome unraveled. *Trends Immunol* 2003;**24**:2–4.

18. Gharavi AE, Pierangeli SS, Espinola RG, Liu X, Colden-Stanfield M, Harris EN. Antiphospholipid antibodies induced in mice by immunization with a cytomegalovirus-derived peptide cause thrombosis and activation of endothelial cells *in vivo. Arthritis Rheum* 2002;**46**:545–52.

19. Schwarzenbacher R, Zeth K, Diederichs K, Gries A, Kostner GM, Laggner P, et al. Crystal structure of human beta2-glycoprotein I: implications for phospholipid binding and the antiphospholipid syndrome. *EMBO J* 1999;**18**:6228–39.

20. Bouma B, de Groot PG, Jean MH, van den Elsen JML, Ravelli RBG, Schouten A, et al. Adhesion mechanism of human beta$_2$-glycoprotein I to phospholipids based on its crystal structure. *EMBO J* 1999;**18**:5166–74.

21. Brighton TA, Hogg PJ, Dai YP, Murray BH, Chong BH, Chesterman CN. Beta 2 lycoprotein I in thrombosis: evidence for a role as a natural anticoagulant. *Br J Haematol* 1996;**93**:185–94.

22. Manfredi AA, Rovere P, Heltai S, Galati G, Nebbia G, Tincani A, et al. Apoptotic cell clearance in systematic lupus erythematosus II. Role of b2glycoprotein I. *Arthritis Rheum* 1998;**41**:215–23.

23. Gharavi AE, Summaritano LR, Wen J, Elkon EB. Induction of antiphospholipid antibodies by immunization with ß$_2$-glycoprotein I (apolipoprotein H). *J Clin Invest* 1992;**90**:1105–11.

24. Pierangeli SS, Harris EN. Induction of phospholipid-binding antibodies in mice and rabbits by immunization with human ß$_2$-glycoprotein I or anticardiolipin antibodies alone. *Clin Exp Immunol* 1993;**93**:269–73.

25. Blank M, Faden D, Tincani A, Kopolovic J, Goldberg I, Gilburd B, et al. Immunization with anticardiolipin cofactor (beta-2-glycoprotein I) induces experimental antiphospholipid syndrome in naive mice. *J Autoimmun* 1994;**7**:441–55.

26. Blank M, George J, Barak V, Tincani A, Koike T, Shoenfeld Y. Oral tolerance to low dose ß$_2$-glycoprotein I: immunomodulation of experimental antiphospholipid syndrome. *J Immunol* 1998;**161**:5303–12.

27. Branch DW, Dudley DJ, Mitchell MD, Creighton KA, Abott TM, Hammond E, et al. Immunoglobulin G fractions from patients with anti-phospholipid antibodies cause fetal death in BALBA/c mice: a model for autoimmune fetal loss. *Am J Obstet Gynecol* 1990;**163**:210–16.

28. Blank M, Cohen J, Toder V, Shoenfeld Y. Induction of primary anti-phospholipid syndrome in mice by passive transfer of anti-cardiolipin antibodies. *Proc Natl Acad Sci USA* 1991;**88**:3069–73.

29. Pierangeli SS, Liu X, Espinola R, Olee T, Zhu M, Harris NE, et al. Functional analyses of patient-derived IgG monoclonal anticardiolipin antibodies using in vivo thrombosis and in vivo microcirculation models. *Thromb Haemost* 2000;**84**:388–95.

30. Blank M, Waisman A, Mozes E, Koike T, Shoenfeld Y. Characteristics and pathogenic role of anti-beta2-glycoprotein I single-chain Fv domains: induction of experimental antiphospholipid syndrome. *Int Immunol* 1999;**11**:1917–26.

31. Gharavi AE, Pierangeli SS, Colden-Stanfield M, Liu XW, Espinola RG, Harris EN. GDKV-induced antiphospholipid antibodies enhance thrombosis and activate endothelial cells *in-vivo* and in-vitro. *J Immunol* 1999;**163**:2922–7.

32. Blank M, Shoenfeld Y, Cabilli S, Heldman Y, Fridkin M, Katchalski- Katzir E. Prevention of experimental antiphospholipid syndrome and endothelial cell activation by synthetic peptides. *Proc Natl Acd Sci USA* 1999;**96**:5164–8.

33. Raschi E, Testoni C, Bosisio D, Borghi MO, Koike T, Mantovani A, et al. Role of the MyD88 transduction signaling pathway in endothelial activation by antiphospholipid antibodies. *Blood* 2003;**101**:3495–500.

34. Matsuura E, Igarashi Y, Yasuda T, Triplett DA, Koike T. Anticardiolipin antibodies recognize beta 2-glycoprotein I structure altered by interacting with an oxygen modified solid phase surface. *J Exp Med* 1994;**179**:457–62.

35. de Laat B, van Berkel M, Urbanus RT, Siregar B, de Groot PG, Gebbink MF, et al. Immune responses against domain I of β(2)-glycoprotein I are driven by conformational changes: domain I of β(2)-glycoprotein I harbors a cryptic immunogenic epitope. *Arthritis Rheum* 2011;**63**:3960–8.

36. Horkko S, Miller E, Branch DW, Palinski W, Witztum JL. The epitopes for some antiphospholipid antibodies are adducts of oxidized phospholipid and beta2 glycoprotein 1 (and other proteins). *Proc Natl Acad Sci USA* 1997;**94**:10356–61.

37. Levine JS, Branch DW, Rauch J. The antiphospholipid syndrome. *N Engl J Med* 2002;**346**:752–63.

38. Rauch J, Subang R, D'Agnillo P, Koh JS, Levine JS. Apoptosis and the antiphospholipid syndrome. *J Autoimmun* 2000;**15**:231–5.

39. Asherson RA, Cervera R. Antiphospholipid antibodies and infections. *Ann Rheum Dis* 2003;**62**:388–93.

40. Cervera R, Asherson RA, Acevedo ML, Gómez-Puerta JA, Espinosa G, de la Red G, et al. Antiphospholipid syndrome triggered by Infections: a report of two cases and a review of clinical presentations in 100 patients. *Ann Rheum Dis* 2004;**63**:1312–17.

41. Zandman–Goddard G, Blank M, Shoenfeld Y. Antiphospholipid antibodies and infections—drugs. In: Asherson RA, Cervera R, Shoenfeld Y, Piette J-C, editors. *The antiphospholipid syndrome II. Autoimmune thrombosis*. Elsevier, Amsterdam; 2002. p. 343–58.

42. de Groot PG, Urbanus RT. The significance of autoantibodies against β2-glycoprotein I. *Blood* 2012;**120**:266–74.

43. Durkin ML, Marchese D, Robinson MD, Ramgopal M. Catastrophic antiphospholipid syndrome (CAPS) induced by influenza A virus subtype H1N1. *BMJ Case Rep* 2013;**2013**. pii: bcr2013200474. doi:10.1136/bcr-2013-200474. [Epub ahead of print].

44. Asherson RA. The catastrophic antiphospholipid syndrome. *J Rheumatol* 1992;**19**:508–12.

45. Cervera R, Piette JC, Font J, Khamashta MA, Shoenfeld Y, Camps MT, et al. Antiphospholipid syndrome: clinical and immunologic manifestations and patterns of disease expression in a cohort of 1,000 patients. *Arthritis Rheum* 2002;**46**:1019–27.

46. Asherson R, Cervera R, de Groot PG, Erkan D, Boffa MC, Piette JC, et al. Catastrophic antiphospholipid syndrome: international consensus statement criteria and treatment guidelines. *Lupus* 2003;**12**:530–4.

47. Cervera R, Bucciarelli S, Espinosa G, Erkan D, Shoenfeld Y, Asherson RA, et al. Catastrophic antiphospholipid syndrome (CAPS): update from the 'CAPS Registry'. *Lupus* 2010;**19**:412–18.

48. Berman H, Rodríguez-Pintó I, Cervera R, Gregory S, de Meis E, Rodrigues CE, et al. Pediatric catastrophic antiphospholipid syndrome: descriptive analysis of 45 patients from the "CAPS Registry" *Autoimmun Rev* 2014;**13**:157–62.

49. Rojas-Rodriguez J, Garcia-Carrasco M, Ramos-Casals M, Enriquez-Coronel G, Colchero C, Cervera R, et al. Catastrophic antiphospholipid syndrome: clinical description and triggering factors in 8 patients. *J Rheumatol* 2000;**27**:238–40.

50. Uhtman I, Taher A, Khalil I, Bizriu A-R, Gharavi AE. Catastrophic antiphospholipid syndrome associated with typhoid fever: comment on the article by Hayem et al. *Arthritis Rheum* 2002;**46**:850–5.

51. Uhtman IW, Gharavi AE. Viral infections and antiphospholipid antibodies. *Semin Arthritis Rheum* 2002;**31**:256–63.

52. Ehrenfeld M, Bar-Natan M, Sidi Y, Schwartz E. Antiphospholipid antibodies associated with severe malaria infection. *Lupus* 2002;**11**:S611.

53. Amital H, Levy Y, Davidson C, Lundberg I, Harju A, Kosach Y, et al. Catastrophic antiphospholipid syndrome: remission following leg amputation in 2 cases. *Semin Arthritis Rheum* 2001;**31**:127–32.

54. Shoenfeld Y, Krause I, Kvapil F, Sulkes J, Font J, von Landenberg P, et al. Euro-APS forum.Prevalence and clinical correlations of antibodies against six β2-glycoprotein-I-related peptides in the antiphospholipid syndrome. *J Clin Immunol* 2003;**23**:377–83.

55. Blank M, Shoenfeld Y. Beta-2-glycoprotein-I, infections, antiphospholipid syndrome and therapeutic considerations. *Clin Immunol* 2004;**112**:190–9.

56. Pierangeli SS, Blank M, Liu X, Espinola R, Fridkin M, Ostertag MV, et al. A peptide that shares similarity with bacterial antigens reverses thrombogenic properties of antiphospholipid antibodies in vivo. *J Autoimmun* 2004;**22**:217–25.

57. Shoenfeld Y, Blank M, Cervera R, Font J, Raschi E, Meroni PL. Infectious origin of the antiphospholipid syndrome. *Ann Rheum Dis* 2006;**65**:2–6.

58. Alm RA, Ling LSL, Moir DT, King BL, Brown ED, Doig PC, et al. Genomic-sequence comparison of two unrelated isolates of the human gastric pathogen *Helicobacter pylori*. *Nature* 1999;**397**:176–80.

59. Cicconi V, Carloni E, Franceschi F, Nocente R, Silveri NG, Manna R, et al. Disappearance of antiphospholipid antibodies syndrome after *Helicobacter pylori* eradication. *Am J Med* 2001;**111**:163–4.

60. Eslick GD, Yan P, Xia HH, Murray H, Spurrett B, Talley NJ. Foetal intrauterine growth restrictions with Helicobacter pylori infection. *Aliment Pharmacol Ther* 2002;**16**:1677–82.
61. Figura N, Piomboni P, Ponzetto A, Gambera L, Lenzi C, Vaira D, et al. Helicobacter pylori infection and infertility. *Eur J Gastroenterol Hepatol* 2002;**14**:663–9.
62. Aguejouf O, Mayo K, Monteiro L, Doutremepuich F, Doutremepuich C, Megraud F. Increase of arterial thrombosis parameters in chronic Helicobacter pylori infection in mice. *Thromb Res* 2002;**108**:245–8.
63. Sorice M, Circella A, Misasi R, Pittoni V, Garofalo T, Cirelli A, et al. Cardiolipin on the surface of apoptotic cells as a possible trigger for antiphospholipids antibodies. *Clin Exp Immunol* 2000;**122**:277–84.
64. Blank M, Krause I, Magrini L, Spina G, Kalil J, Jacobsen S, et al. Overlapping humoral autoimmunity links rheumatic fever and the antiphospholipid syndrome. *Rheumatology (Oxford)* 2006;**45**:833–41.
65. Benhamou C, Gauvain JB, Meyer O, Bardet M, Caplan F, Luthier F, et al. Anti-cardiolipin antibodies in Lyme disease. *Rev Rhum Mal Osteoartic* 1987;**54**:397–9.
66. Aichbichler BW, Petritsch W, Reicht GA, Wenzl HH, Eherer AJ, Hinterleitner TA, et al. Anti-cardiolipin antibodies in patients with inflammatory bowel disease. *Dig Dis Sci* 1999;**44**:852–6.
67. Thong BY, Chng HH, Ang CL, Ho MS. Recurrent venous thromboses, anti-cardiolipin antibodies and Crohn's disease. *QJM* 2002;**95**:253–5.
68. Koutroubakis IE, Petinaki E, Anagnostopoulou E, Kritikos H, Mouzas IA, Kouroumalis EA, et al. Anti-cardiolipin and anti-beta2-glycoprotein I antibodies in patients with inflammatory bowel disease. *Dig Dis Sci* 1998;**43**:2507–12.
69. Houman H, Lamloum M, Ben Ghorbel I, Khiari-Ben Salah I, Miled M. Vena cava thrombosis in Behcet's disease. Analysis of a series of 10 cases. *Ann Med Interne (Paris)* 1999;**150**:587–90.
70. Mukai Y, Tsutsui H, Todaka K, Mohri M, Hirai N, Arai H, et al. Total occlusion of inferior vena cava in a patient with antiphospholipid antibody syndrome associated with Behcet's disease. *Jpn Circ J* 2001;**65**:837–8.
71. Barzilai O, Sherer Y, Ram M, Izhaky D, Anaya JM, Shoenfeld Y. Epstein-Barr virus and cytomegalovirus in autoimmune diseases: are they truly notorious? A preliminary report. *Ann N Y Acad Sci* 2007;**1108**:567–77.
72. Wiles AP, Shaw G, Bright J, Perczel A, Campbell ID, Barlow PN. NMR Studies of a viral protein that mimics the regulators of complement activation. *J Mol Biol* 1997;**272**:253–5.
73. Ben-Chetrit E, Wiener-Well Y, Fadeela A, Wolf DG. Antiphospholipid antibodies during infectious mononucleosis and their long term clinical significance. *J Clin Virol* 2013;**56**:312–15.
74. Breman JG, Isao Arita I, Fenne F. Preventing the return of smallpox. *N Eng J Med* 2003;**348**:463–6.
75. Bouillie S, Barel M, Frade R. Signaling through the EBV/C3d receptor (CR2, CD21) in human B lymphocytes: activation of phosphatidylinositol 3-kinase *via* a CD19-independent pathway. *J Immunol* 1999;**162**:136–43.
76. Sorice M, Pittoni V, Griggi T, Losardo A, Leri O, Magno MS, et al. Specificity of anti-phospholipid antibodies in infectious mononucleosis: a role for anti-cofactor protein antibodies. *Clin Exp Immunol* 2000;**120**:301–6.
77. Medzhitov R, Janeway Jr. C. Innate immunity. *N Eng J Med* 2000;**343**:338–44.
78. Krieg AM. A role for toll in autoimmunity. *Nat Immunol* 2002;**3**:423–4.
79. Leadbetter EA, Rifkin IR, Marshak-Rothstein A. Toll-like receptors and activation of autoreactive B cells. *Curr Dir Autoimmun* 2003;**6**:105–22.
80. Mills KH. TLR-dependent T, cell activation in autoimmunity. *Nat Rev Immunol* 2011;**11**:807–22.

81. Pierangeli SS, Vega-Ostertag ME, Raschi E, Liu X, Romay-Penabad Z, De Micheli V, et al. Toll-like receptor and antiphospholipid mediated thrombosis: in vivo studies. *Ann Rheum Dis* 2007;**66**:1327–33.
82. Blank M, George J, Fishman P, Levy Y, Toder V, Savion S, et al. Ciprofloxacin immunomodulation of experimental antiphospholipid syndrome associated with elevation of interleukin-3 and granulocyte-macrophage colony-stimulating factor expression. *Arthritis Rheum* 1998;**41**:224–32.

CHAPTER 41

Infections and Systemic Lupus Erythematosus

Susanna Esposito[*,1], **Samantha Bosis**[*], **Margherita Semino**[*],
Donato Rigante[†]
[*]Department of Pathophysiology and Transplantation, Pediatric Highly Intensive Care Unit, Università degli Studi di Milano, Fondazione IRCCS Ca' Granda Ospedale Maggiore Policlinico, Milan, Italy
[†]Institute of Pediatrics, Università Cattolica Sacro Cuore, Rome, Italy
[1]Corresponding Author: susanna.esposito@unimi.it

1 INTRODUCTION

Systemic lupus erythematosus (SLE) is a chronic autoimmune disease that may affect any organ and presents a protean spectrum of clinical manifestations. The global incidence of SLE is 6–35 new cases per 100,000 per year, with a higher frequency among women than men (90% of patients are women of reproductive age).[1] In Northern Europe, the prevalence rates of SLE range from approximately 40 cases per 100,000 whites to more than 200 per 100,000 among blacks. In the United States, the prevalence varies between 3.2 and 250 per 100,000 in different ethnic groups.[2–12] This disease is rare in Africa but is common in African descendants around the world. Specifically, both incidence and prevalence among people of African or Asian background are approximately two to three times higher than in the white population; moreover, the disease is more common in Aboriginal Australians and some Native American groups of Canada and the United States. SLE can occur at any age, but it manifests more frequently after 5 years of age, with increased prevalence after the first decade of life.[7,13,14] Incidence and prevalence of SLE in adults are considerably higher than in children (<1 per 100,000 among children <16 years old in Europe and North America).[2]

At the molecular level, the disease is characterized by a persistent inflammatory state that is detrimental to multiple organs, including the skin, joints, vessels, kidneys, serous membranes, central nervous system, and blood. Such chronic damage is due to both immune dysregulation and hyper-production of different autoantibodies and immune complexes. Clinical manifestation is characterized by ethnicity, sex, age, and

Infection and Autoimmunity
http://dx.doi.org/10.1016/B978-0-444-63269-2.00046-5

697

socioeconomic factors.[1,15,16] Diagnosis of SLE is based on the criteria established by the American College of Rheumatology and the more recent Systemic Lupus International Collaborating Clinics classification criteria, drafted in 2012.[17,18] These criteria include the presence of dermatologic signs, arthritis and serositis variably combined with renal, neurologic, and hematologic disorders. Additional diagnostic criteria are immunologic abnormalities typical in SLE, such as anti-nuclear antibodies (80–90% of patients), double-strand DNA-directed autoantibodies (58–70% of patients), and antibodies directed to other nuclear antigens such as histones and small nuclear ribonucleoproteins (in a minor group of patients). Four or more criteria (including at least one clinical and one immunological) are necessary for the diagnosis of SLE. Criteria can be satisfied either serially or simultaneously during any interval of observation and in the absence of any another explanation in the patient's clinical picture.[17,18] The typical course of SLE is insidious, slow and progressive and presents cycles of remission and acute phases, which can be potentially and rapidly become fatal. Classical symptoms at the onset or during exacerbation of the disease are fever, fatigue, anorexia, myalgia, and weight loss, all of which are variously intertwined with specific organ-related inflammatory signs.[4,5] Because the overall outcome is highly variable, ranging from remission to death, the long-term prognosis still remains poor.

In recent years life expectancy for subjects with SLE has greatly improved, nowadays reaching a 15-year survival rate of 80%.[2,6] Pediatric SLE (starting at an age <16 years) is usually more aggressive than adult SLE and often severely involves major organs, including the kidneys and central nervous system. Moreover, SLE in childhood is associated with increased mortality risk and reduced remission rates. Major causes of death include renal disease, severe disease flares with significant organ damage and infections.[3,6]

The etiology and pathogenesis of SLE remain unknown. It is believed that SLE represents a complex multi-factorial disease arising from a combination of genetic susceptibility and hormonal and environmental factors (including infections, exposure to ultraviolet radiation, medications, drugs, and chemicals), which lead to the production and perpetuation of aberrant autoimmune responses.

Infections were recently shown to be highly associated with the onset and/or exacerbations of SLE, and their causative and/or protective role has been largely emphasized in the medical literature.[19–22] The aim of this review was to screen the medical literature of the past 15 years and investigate the role of infectious agents in the pathogenesis of SLE.

2 INFECTIONS AND AUTOIMMUNITY

Host defence against microbial agents is based on the ability of the immune system to distinguish "self" from "non-self" molecules. In patients with SLE, such ability is lost, and autoantibodies (SLE-specific and/or typical of different rheumatologic diseases) are found in the blood. The reason for the presence of these autoantibodies is still under debate; however, they are useful biomarkers for SLE diagnosis.

It has been reported that aberrations of the physiological and protective processes of the immune system may occur during viral, bacterial, parasitic, or fungal infections in genetically prone subjects.[20,21] In particular, the association between infections and autoimmunity has been a topic of discussion among researchers for a long time, and many theories have been suggested to explain the autoreactivity observed in some individuals.

Different etiopathogenetic mechanisms have been associated with the activation of autoreactive T and B cells, and it has been hypothesized that these mechanisms are mediated by diverse infectious agents. For example, molecular mimicry is one of these, and it is based on the activation of autoimmune responses by microbial peptides that possess a structure similar to human self-antigens. A variety of viruses and bacteria can produce superantigens that bind the variable domain of T-cell receptors, and a wide variety of major histocompatibility complex (MHC) class II molecules. This process activates a large number of T lymphocytes with different antigenic specificities and induces autoimmune reactions. The enhanced presentation of autoantigens by antigen-presenting cells at the site of inflammation could be followed by the priming of large numbers of T cells. This process of "epitope spreading" might contribute to the development of autoimmune responses. Another suggested mechanism, known as "bystander activation", is characterized by the increase of cytokine production, which induces the expansion of previously activated T cells within the inflammatory site. Another possibility is that lymphotropic viruses might activate lymphocytes, causing increased production of antibodies and circulating immune complexes, which might damage the host's tissues and organs. Dysregulation of the apoptotic pathway in host cells might also be a possible mechanism, either by exposing nuclear material to the immune system or causing the production of autoantibodies against nuclear structures. Finally, insufficient clearance of infectious agents and the absent or suboptimal functioning of C4 and/or C1q complement system proteins, which has been observed in patients with immunodeficiencies, might induce autoreactive T- and B-cell responses.

Recent data showed that altered expressions of particular microRNAs from infected B lymphocytes might produce autoantibodies.[22,23] Moreover, it was demonstrated that many viruses induce the expression of type 1 interferon (INF) genes (INF-1 and other INF-related cytokines); this mechanism, known as "interferon signature", was shown to exert a relevant role in many autoimmune diseases.[24,25] Other recent studies demonstrated the role of hypomethylated bacterial and viral DNA in inducing immune changes similar to those observed in patients with SLE.[26]

Specifically during childhood, the developing immune system might be vulnerable to external factors, such as infectious agents. Autoimmunity might be triggered through the cumulative effect of repeated infections, which might be clinically apparent, pauci-symptomatic, or asymptomatic.[27–29]

Clinical manifestations of SLE are closely related to the presence of specific autoantibodies, which can be induced by particular infectious agents. In particular, researchers have shown that high IgM titers against the rubella virus were associated with psychosis or depression among patients with neuropsychiatric SLE.[30] Other authors demonstrated that high titers of Epstein–Barr virus (EBV) antibodies were correlated with skin and joint manifestations of SLE.[31] More recent studies revealed that infections might induce regulatory CD4+/CD25+ T cells, which might suppress host immune responses against self- or non-self molecules. All these findings suggest that infections might play a direct role in the overall regulation of immunity, either protecting from or facilitating the onset of the autoimmune disease.[32–35]

3 VIRUSES AND PATHOGENESIS OF SLE

Copious reports in the medical literature associate viral infections and SLE.[36] EBV has long been suggested as a potential trigger of SLE. Since 1971, many efforts have attempted to find a correlation between EBV and autoimmune diseases. Studies in this direction used patients with SLE who had higher anti-EBV antibody titers compared to healthy subjects.[37,38] Some studies reported a 99% prevalence of EBV infection in young patients with SLE compared with a 70% prevalence in a control group.[39,40] Specifically, a study published in 2001 including 192 patients with SLE demonstrated that all but one had been exposed to EBV, suggesting the etiological contribution of this virus.[41] Patients with SLE compared to healthy controls also have been shown to possess elevated titers of anti-EBNA-1 and EBV-VCA IgA, as well as EBV-EA/D, EBV-EA/R IgG and IgA.[1] Moon and co-workers[42] showed that EBV load (measured by real-time polymerase chain reaction) in the sera from patients with SLE was increased 15- to 40-fold compared to control subjects. These results suggested that EBV has an active lytic cycle with high viral replication in patients with SLE.[42,43] Moreover, it has been hypothesized that EBV-infected B cells might also express virus-encoded anti-apoptotic molecules, therefore becoming resistant to apoptosis.[44] Several groups demonstrated that the increased production of INF by T cells (mediated by EBV) is another mechanism that induces autoimmunity.[19,45–47] Repeated or re-activated EBV infection, which results in increased seroprevalence of EBV IgA and IgG, may be also associated with SLE.[48] Different EBV antigens can exhibit structural, molecular or functional mimicry with SLE antigens or other critical immune-regulatory components. When infected by EBV, immunocompetent subjects show little or no EBV messenger RNA expression; in contrast, patients with SLE have abnormal expression of 4 viral mRNAs (BZLF-1, LMP-1 E 2 and EBNA-1) in their peripheral blood mononuclear cells, indicating an active replication or re-activation of the virus in these patients. Evaluating the levels of EBV mRNA in PBMCs, researchers found a 1.7-fold increase of BCRF-1, EBNA-1, and LMP-2 mRNAs in patients with SLE compared to controls. All these findings lead to the conclusion that controlling EBV infection seems to be difficult in patients with active SLE.[1]

In the past 15 years, studies of human endogenous retroviruses (HERVs) have led to the conclusion that HERVs are potential and very important contributors to several autoimmune diseases, including SLE. In this regard, several groups showed that HERVs were first integrated into the human genome 30–40 million years ago and therefore may be the possible molecular link between the human genome and environmental factors in SLE pathogenesis. According to these studies, HERV-encoded proteins should be considered self-antigens and should be tolerated by the host's immune system (although they may trigger the breakdown of immunologic tolerance).[49–51] HERVs might also affect the expression of genes regulating both the immune response and acquired tolerance.[52] In addition, autoantibodies to an endogenous retroviral element-encoded nuclear protein autoantigen, HRES-1, are detectable in a distinct subset of patients with SLE.[53]

The existence of transfusion-transmitted viruses (TTVs), which are characterized by high genetic diversity, has recently been discovered. Their prevalence is higher in patients with SLE compared to healthy subjects. Both the higher TTV prevalence and the molecular mimicry with the

HERV-encoded nuclear proteins might contribute to the generation of anti-nuclear antibodies, abnormal T- and B-cell functions and self-reactivity in patients with SLE.[40]

HTLV-1 and HIV-1 retroviruses also have been implicated in the pathogenesis of SLE.[54] Specifically, either dysregulation of the apoptotic mechanism and a shift from a T-helper type 1 (Th1) towards a T-helper type 2 (Th2) cytokine profile has been observed in patients with SLE and with HIV infection.[55] Moreover, both types of patients probably share a common mechanism mediating the subversion of apoptosis and production of autoantibodies.[50,56]

A variety of rheumatologic manifestations, mainly rheumatoid arthritis, systemic vasculitis and SLE, can be encountered in the course of parvovirus B19 infections. Parvovirus infections might be accompanied by transient subclinical autoimmunity, which also mimics or exacerbates SLE in pre-disposed individuals.[57] Similarities in both clinical and serological param-eters following parvovirus infection and SLE at the onset may lead to a less accurate diagnosis between these two conditions. Indeed, parvovirus B19 infection mimicking SLE usually fulfils fewer than 4 ACR criteria for SLE; in addition, it rarely includes hemolytic anemia or cardiac or renal abnor-malities, and it is usually associated with short-lived low titers of autoantibodies.[58]

Several studies have demonstrated a correlation between cytomegalovi-rus (CMV) infection and SLE. The presence of anti-CMV IgM or CMV-DNA has been detected in patients with initial symptoms of SLE, showing the hypothetical etiological role of the virus.[59,60] In particular, CMV infec-tions have been associated with "vascular" SLE, showing more frequent Raynaud's phenomenon and less frequent typical kidney involvement.[61]

The relationship between hepatitis C virus (HCV) and SLE has not yet been defined. Some studies demonstrated a significantly higher prevalence of HCV infection among patients with SLE compared to healthy controls,[62] but this correlation has not been confirmed.[63,64]

Among RNA viruses, C-type oncorna viruses are supposedly associated with SLE. However, although extensive studies have been conducted, the presence of C-type oncorna viruses in lymphoblastoid cell lines harboring endogenous EBV, derived from patients with active SLE, has not been yet demonstrated. In this respect, other studies showed a non-specific increase in the titer of antibodies against measles and parainfluenza type 1 in patients with SLE.[43] However, a relevant role for these agents in trigger-ing the onset of SLE has not been suggested to date.

4 THE RELATIONSHIP BETWEEN BACTERIA AND SLE

Bacterial infections might also play a role in the development of SLE. The inflammation triggered by any bacteria induces cellular damage and increases the presence of cellular debris, activating B lymphocytes or promoting the release of autoantibodies.[25,65] The presence of a bacterial infection triggers the immune system through specific products, such as bacterial lipopolysaccharides or nucleic acid-containing immune complexes. Pathogen-associated molecular patterns interact with Toll-like receptors (TLRs) and non-TLR internal receptors of antigen-presenting cells, monocytes and B and T lymphocytes. The binding of TLRs induces the release of IFN from plasmacytoid dendritic cells, leading to the production of pro-inflammatory cytokines and destabilizing innate immunity processes.[43,66,67] Recent clinical studies have placed new emphasis on the role of TLRs, specifically TLR7 and TLR9, in the promotion of autoantibody production. Pharmacologic modulation of TLR-directed pathways might offer new additional therapeutic approaches for the treatment of SLE.[68]

5 PARASITES AND DEVELOPMENT OF SLE

Parasitic infections may induce variable immunomodulatory effects. The relationship between parasitic infections and autoimmunity remains to be elucidated.[69] There is still no definite agreement about parasitic involvement in the pathogenesis of SLE, but a possible link between *Toxoplasma gondii* and rheumatoid arthritis was recently proposed.[70]

6 THE PROTECTIVE EFFECT OF INFECTIOUS AGENTS FROM AUTOIMMUNE PROCESSES

It was demonstrated that some infectious agents have a protective rather a causative role towards the development of SLE.[32] The beneficial effects of viral, parasitic, and fungal infections have been explained, deriving from a shift towards a more predominant Th2 immunological phenotype.[70] Based on this approach, infections might confer a generic protection from autoimmunity. Therefore, the recent increase in the incidence of autoimmune diseases among children in Western countries could be related to the theory of a reduced infectious pressure due to improved hygienic-sanitary conditions.[71]

Furthermore, animal models provide evidence that various autoimmune diseases are suppressed by helminthic infections.[72] Infections with *Plasmodium falciparum*, the protozoan causing the most severe form of malaria, are believed to generate a lower risk of developing SLE.[73] This hypothesis is reflected in the observation that, although people of African descent have higher rates of SLE than whites, the prevalence of SLE in Africa is low, particularly when associated with the presence of malaria.[72–74] Animal models suggest protection for SLE nephropathy through *T. gondii* infection.[32,75] *Schistosoma mansoni* and *Schistosoma japonicum* also have been related to protective effects towards autoimmune diseases.[76]

Infections could also be protective for SLE by other mechanisms, such as antigenic competition, which could induce decreased responses against self-antigens.[77,78] Bacteria and viruses could also protect against autoimmune diseases acting on TLRs; the binding between pathogens and TLRs could trigger the production of cytokines that could down-regulate autoimmune responses.[78]

Helicobacter pylori seronegativity has been related to an increased risk of development of SLE, suggesting again that this pathogen might exert a protective role.[79,80] Finally, hepatitis B virus (HBV) has been hypothesized as having a protective role because of the lower prevalence of anti-HBV antibodies in patients with SLE compared to healthy subjects. All these data confirm the immunomodulatory effects of HBV infection, probably mediated by IFN production, which might protect an infected subject from the pathogenesis of autoimmune diseases, including SLE.[81]

7 GENETIC PREDISPOSITION TO SLE AND INFECTIONS

The primary involvement of genetics in SLE was shown by the high concordance rate in monozygotic twins (approximately 25%) compared with dizygotic twins (only 2%).[82] However, genetic risk factors for SLE, including complement and mannose-binding lectin (MBL) deficiency, impaired IFN release, and STAT4 protein (a transcription factor belonging to the signal transducer and activator of transcription protein family) production,[22] are complex and still not well established. Immune deficiency might result in insufficient clearance of exogenous pathogens during infections, therefore increasing the risk of autoimmunity.[43,83,84]

In addition, different genes located in the human leucocyte antigen (HLA) locus and involved in the regulation of the immune system are associated with SLE.[22,82] Susceptibility loci on HLA-DR2 and two non-MHC immune regulatory genes (*CTLA* and *PTPN22*) were related to the risk of developing SLE.[85] In addition, the innate immune system has been suggested as having a role in the autoimmune response, as proved by recent studies of TLR7 and TLR9.[68,86] Although several studies suggested that the interaction of genetic factors with infectious agents may have a strong role in autoimmunity, this topic is still controversial, and further research is needed to better understand their dynamic interplay.

Recent studies have finally indicated that a peculiar genetic background may increase the risk of serious infections in SLE. Patients with MBL deficiency, associated with homozygous MBL variant alleles, have been reported to be at increased risk of infections. Patients with SLE who are homozygous for MBL variant alleles had a fourfold increase in the incidence of infections.[87] Furthermore, it was shown that at least one third of patients with SLE with a C1q deficiency may suffer from recurrent bacterial infections, including otitis media, meningitides, and pneumonia.[88]

8 VACCINATIONS AND SLE

There is plenty of medical literature reporting that SLE might be triggered by vaccinations. The existing data do not directly link the vaccines and the autoimmune phenomena in a causal relationship, but a temporal connection has nevertheless been described. Bacterial and viral components, or adjuvants of vaccines, have been associated with SLE onset or flare-up. One study in particular described five healthy patients who developed SLE 2–3 weeks after immunization with a combination of vaccines for typhoid, influenza, meningococcus, tetanus toxoid, measles, mumps, and rubella.[89]

Several case reports have associated the hepatitis B vaccine with SLE, but unfortunately no studies have ascertained any causal relationship. Data of the safety and efficacy of this vaccination for patients with SLE have not yet been established.[90] Associations between influenza vaccination and SLE are rare; however, the safety and efficacy of this vaccine have been clearly proven in patients with SLE.[91] Finally, Hidalgo-Tenorio and colleagues[92] demonstrated more than 10 years ago that pneumococcal vaccination is not associated with substantial changes in the evolution of SLE.[92]

9 THE RISK OF INFECTIONS IN SLE

Despite the improvement in the management of SLE in the past 15 years, infections represent a leading cause of morbidity and mortality for these patients. The common sites of infections are respiratory airways, urinary tract, soft tissue, and skin. Bacteria are the most common implicated agents, followed by viruses and fungi. Among gram-positive bacteria, *Streptococcus pneumoniae* is the most common cause of respiratory tract infections, whereas *Staphylococcus aureus* causes skin, soft-tissue, bone, and joint infections. Gram-negative bacteria such as *Escherichia coli* are most commonly involved in urinary tract infections. Also, *Klebsiella pneumoniae* and *Pseudomonas* spp. are frequent causes of infections in patients with SLE.[93,94]

Pneumococcal invasive soft-tissue infections, such as cellulitis and fascitis, are uncommon.[95] Septicemia, mainly caused by *S. aureus*, *E. coli*, and *Salmonella* spp., has been described in patients with SLE and is associated with poor long-term outcomes.[96] The incidence rate of tuberculosis (TB) is higher in patients with SLE, depending on the specific geographical area in which they live. In this regard, the prevalence of TB among patients with SLE in endemic areas is 5%.[97] Patients with SLE are also susceptible to opportunistic infections, but non-tuberculous mycobacterial infections also have been described. These infections tend to develop later in the course of the disease compared to those caused by *Mycobacterium tuberculosis*.[98]

Viral infections commonly reported in patients also are mostly related to the varicella-zoster virus, CMV, and human papillomavirus. Severe and atypical manifestations caused by CMV, mostly with respiratory or gastro-intestinal symptoms and SLE flare-like manifestations, have been described.[99] Some studies demonstrated a higher risk of hepatitis B re-activation in patients with SLE, even if this situation has been mostly reported in patients with lymphoma.[100]

Among fungal infections, those from *Candida* spp., *Pneumocystis jiroveci*, and *Cryptococcus neoformans* are frequently reported in patients with SLE. Common manifestations of *C. neoformans* are meningitis and pneumonia, whereas *P. jiroveci* and *Candida albicans* lead to severe pulmonary and genitourinary or gastrointestinal tract infections, respectively.[101]

The higher rate of infections in patients suffering from SLE can be explained by different causes. They can be primarily caused by immune system dysfunction, which involves phagocyte activity, chemotaxis and identification of exogenous pathogens. They can be caused secondarily by cytokine production and pathogen clearance, which can lead to a reduced ability to respond to infections. Finally, they can be caused by neutropenia or lymphopenia resulting from a dysfunctional macrophage-monocyte system. Hypogammaglobulinemia and impaired complement function can be also found in subjects with SLE, justifying the vulnerability to infections of these patients.[102] The risk of infection is significantly associated with disease activity, particularly with the Systemic Lupus Erythematosus Disease Activity Index, a global score index developed for the assessment of SLE activity.[103]

10 DRUGS AND INFECTIONS IN SLE

Pharmacological measures of SLE revolve around four main classes of drugs: non-steroidal anti-inflammatory drugs, antimalarials, corticosteroids, and cytotoxic or immunosuppressive agents (e.g. cyclophosphamide, azathioprine, mycophenolate mofetil, cyclosporine).

Cyclophosphamide and azathioprine are the two most commonly used cytotoxic agents; in combination with corticosteroids, these need to be used early to prevent or minimize irreversible damage to major organs. Potential side effects of corticosteroids and cytotoxic agents include infections, particularly bacterial ones. Drug types and doses are also crucial for patients with SLE because they define the magnitude of risk of becoming infected. In this regard, prolonged high-dose therapy with cyclophosphamide in leukocytopenic patients has been correlated with significant risk of infectious diseases, especially when associated with glucocorticoids.[101] Corticosteroids have been associated with susceptibility to infections because of their anti-inflammatory activity, which interferes with T-lymphocyte-mediated immunity, the monocyte and macrophage system and endothelial cells. Long duration of systemic treatments (>3 weeks) and high dosages also are associated with a greater probability of developing infections.[104]

New biological drugs such as rituximab (an anti-CD20 monoclonal antibody) have been recently introduced for the treatment of severe and refractory manifestations of SLE. Related side effects include higher risk of infections (mild and severe), mostly from *Pneumonia* or sepsis because of bacterial pathogens; however, it has been demonstrated that these tend to occur especially within the first 6 months of administration.[102,105] The efficacy and safety of belimumab (a human monoclonal antibody that inhibits B-cell activating factor, also known as B-lymphocyte stimulator) in SLE has been demonstrated in two randomized controlled studies. Data show that serious infections are reported in 8% of adult patients with SLE.[106] Antimalarial drugs, which are prescribed for cutaneous or mild articular manifestations of SLE, were shown to be protective from parasitic as well as viral, fungal, and bacterial infections in subjects with SLE.[107,108] Their use has allowed for the reduction of corticosteroid and immunosuppressive drug doses, leading to reduced risk of infectious complications. All these data suggest that it is crucial to find the lowest corticosteroid dose and the least number of immunosuppressant agents sufficient to control the clinical manifestations of SLE or prevent SLE re-activation. It is also useful to closely monitor patients and vaccinate them against preventable diseases.

11 CONCLUSION

The etiopathogenesis of SLE is still obscure and remains far from completely elucidated. Environmental and genetic factors have been implicated in the induction and progression of this disease. Among infections, EBV, parvovirus B19, retrovirus, and CMV infections in particular might play a pivotal role in the pathogenesis of SLE. The multi-faceted interactions between infections and autoimmunity reveal many possibilities for either causative or protective associations. Indeed, some infections (primarily protozoan infections) might confer protection from autoimmune processes, depending on the unique interaction between microorganisms and the host. Further studies are needed to conclude that infectious agents are indeed one of the causes of SLE and to address the potential clinical sequelae of infections in the field of autoimmunity.

ACKNOWLEDGMENTS

The authors declare no conflict of interest. This review was supported by a grant from the Italian Ministry of Health (Bando Giovani Ricercatori 2009).

REFERENCES

1. Draborg AH, Duus K, Houen G. Epstein-Barr virus and systemic lupus erythematosus. *Clin Dev Immunol* 2013;**2013**:1–10.
2. Rahman A, Isenberg DA. Systemic lupus erythematosus. *N Engl J Med* 2008;**358**:929–39.
3. Habibi S, Saleem MA, Ramanan AV. Juvenile systemic lupus erythematosus: review of clinical features and management. *Indian Pediatr* 2011;**48**:879–87.
4. O'Neill S, Cervera R. Systemic lupus erythematosus. *Best Pract Res Clin Rheumatol* 2010;**24**:841–55.
5. Hoffman IE, Lauwerys BR, De Keyser F, Huizinga TW, Isenberg D, Cebecauer L, et al. Juvenile- onset systemic lupus erythematosus: different clinical and serological pattern than adult-onset systemic lupus erythematosus. *Ann Rheum Dis* 2009;**68**:412–15.
6. Doria A, Iaccarino L, Ghirardello A, Zampieri S, Arienti S, Sarzi-Puttini P, et al. Long-term prognosis and causes of death in systemic lupus erythematosus. *Am J Med* 2006;**119**:700–6.

7. Petty RE, Laxer RM. Systemic lupus erythematosus. In: Cassidy JT, Petty RE, Laxer RM, Lindsley CB, editors. *Textbook of pediatric rheumatology*. Philadelphia, PA: Elsiever Saunders; 2005. p. 342–91.

8. Brunner HI, Gladman DD, Ibanez D, Urowitz MD, Silverman ED. Difference in disease features between childhood-onset and adult-onset systemic lupus erythematosus. *Arthritis Rheum* 2008;**58**:556–62.

9. Samanta A, Roy S, Feehally J, Symmons DP. The prevalence of systemic lupus erythematosus in whites and Indian Asian immigrants in Leicester city, UK. *Br J Rheumatol* 1992;**31**:679–82.

10. Serdula MK, Rhoads GG. Frequency of systemic lupus erythematosus in different ethnic groups in Hawaii. *Arthritis Rheum* 1979;**22**:328–33.

11. Huang JL, Yao TC, See LC. Prevalence of pediatric systemic lupus erythematosus and juvenile chronic arthritis in a Chinese population: a nation-wide prospective population-based study in Taiwan. *Clin Exp Rheumatol* 2004;**22**:776–80.

12. Kurahara DK, Grandinetti A, Fujii LL, Tokuda AA, Galario JA, Han MJ, et al. Visiting consultant clinics to study prevalence rates of juvenile rheumatoid arthritis and childhood systemic lupus erythematosus across dispersed geographic areas. *J Rheumatol* 2007;**34**:425–29.

13. Lehman TJ, McCurdy DK, Bernstein BH, King KK, Hanson V. Systemic lupus erythematosus in the first decade of life. *Pediatrics* 1989;**83**:235–39.

14. Taddio A, Rossetto E, Rosé CD, Brescia AM, Bracaglia C, Cortis E, et al. Prognostic impact of atypical presentation in pediatric systemic lupus erythematosus: results from a multicenter study. *J Pediatr* 2010;**156**:972–77.

15. Font J, Cervera R, Espinosa G, Pallarés L, Ramos-Casals M, Jiménez S, et al. Systemic lupus erythematosus (SLE) in childhood: analysis of clinical and immunological findings in 34 patients and comparison with SLE characteristics in adults. *Ann Rheum Dis* 1998;**57**:456–59.

16. Rood MJ, ten Cate R, van Suijlekom-Smit LW, den Ouden EJ, Ouwerkerk FE, Breedveld FC, et al. Childhood-onset systemic lupus erythematosus: clinical presentation and prognosis in 31 patients. *Scand J Rheumatol* 1999;**28**:222–26.

17. Tan EM, Cohen AS, Fries JF, Masi AT, McShane DJ, Rothfield NF, et al. The 1982 revised criteria for the classification of systemic lupus erythematosus. *Arthritis Rheum* 1982;**25**:1271–77.

18. Petri M, Orbai AM, Alarcòn GS, Gordon C, Merrill JT, Fortin PR, et al. Derivation and validation of the systemic lupus erythematosus. International collaborating clinics classification criteria for systemic lupus erythematosus. *Arthritis Rheum* 2012;**64**:2677–86.

19. Zandman-Goddard G, Solomon M, Rosman Z, Peeva E, Shoenfeld Y. Environment and lupus-related diseases. *Lupus* 2012;**21**:241–50.

20. Rigante D, Mazzoni MB, Esposito S. The cryptic interplay between systemic lupus erythematosus and infections. *Autoimmun Rev* 2014;**13**:96–102.

21. Barzilai O, Ram M, Shoenfeld Y. Viral infection can induce the production of autoantibodies. *Curr Opin Rheumatol* 2007;**19**:636–43.

22. Sebastiani GD, Galeazzi M. Infection-genetics relationship in systemic lupus erythematosus. *Lupus* 2009;**18**:1169–75.

23. Barzilai O, Sherer Y, Ram M, Izhaky D, Anaya JM, Shoenfeld Y. Epstein-Barr virus and cytomegalovirus in autoimmune diseases: are they truly notorious? A preliminary report. *Ann N Y Acad Sci* 2007;**1108**:567–77.

24. Koutouzov S, Mathian A, Dalloul A. Type-I interferons and systemic lupus erythematosus. *Autoimmun Rev* 2006;**5**:554–62.

25. Santana-de Anda K, Gómez-Martín D, Díaz-Zamudio M, Alcocer-Varela J. Interferon regulatory factors: beyond the antiviral response and their link to the development of autoimmune pathology. *Autoimmun Rev* 2011;**11**:98–103.

26. Sekigawa I, Kawasaki M, Ogasawara H, Kaneda K, Kaneko H, Takasaki Y, et al. DNA methylation: its contribution to systemic lupus erythematosus. *Clin Exp Med* 2006;**6**:69–106.

27. Kivity S, Agmon-Levin N, Blank M, Shoenfeld Y. Infections and autoimmunity-friends or foes? *Trends Immunol* 2009;**30**:409–14.

28. Arbuckle MR, Gross T, Scofield RH, Hinshaw LB, Chang AC, Taylor Jr FB, et al. Lupus humoral autoimmunity induced in a primate model by short peptide immunization. *J Invest Med* 1998;**46**:58–65.

29. Edwards CJ, Syddall H, Goswami R, Goswami P, Dennison EM, Cooper C. Infections in infancy and the presence of antinuclear antibodies in adult life. *Lupus* 2006;**15**:213–17.

30. Zandman-Goddard G, Berkun Y, Barzilai O, Boaz M, Ram M, Anaya JM, et al. Neuropsychiatric lupus and infectious triggers. *Lupus* 2008;**17**:380–84.

31. Zandman-Goddard G, Berkun Y, Barzilai O, Boaz M, Blank M, Ram M, et al. Exposure to Epstein-Barr virus infection is associated with mild systemic lupus erythematosus disease. *Ann N Y Acad Sci* 2009;**1173**:658–63.

32. Praprotnik S, Sodin-Semrl S, Tomsic M, Shoenfeld Y. The curiously suspicious: infectious disease may ameliorate an ongoing autoimmune destruction in systemic lupus erythematosus patients. *J Autoimmun* 2008;**30**:37–41.

33. Keynan Y, Card CM, McLaren PJ, Dawood MR, Kasper K, Fowke KR. The role of regulatory T cells in chronic and acute viral infections. *Clin Infect Dis* 2008;**46**:1046–52.

34. Bopp T, Jonuleit H, Schmitt E. Regulatory T cells. The renaissance of the suppressor T cells. *Ann Med* 2007;**39**:322–34.

35. Doria A, Sarzi-Puttini P, Shoenfeld Y. Infections, rheumatism and autoimmunity: the conflicting relationship between humans and their environment. *Autoimmun Rev* 2008;**8**:1–4.

36. Perl A. Mechanisms of viral pathogenesis in rheumatic disease. *Ann Rheum Dis* 1999;**58**:454–61.

37. Evans AS. EB-virus antibody in systemic lupus erythematosus. *Lancet* 1971;**1**:1023–24.

38. De Carvalho JF, Pereira RM, Shoenfeld Y. The mosaic of autoimmunity: the role of environmental factors. *Front Biosci* 2009;**1**:501–9.

39. James JA, Kaufman KM, Farris AD, Taylor-Albert E, Lehman TJ, Harley JB. An increased prevalence of Epstein Barr virus infection in young patients suggests a possible etiology for systemic lupus erythematosus. *J Clin Invest* 1997;**100**:3019–26.

40. Gergely Jr P, Pullmann R, Stancato C, Otvos Jr. L, Koncz A, Blazsek A, et al. Increased prevalence of transfusion transmitted virus and cross reactivity with immunodominant epitopes of the HRES-1/p28 endogenous retroviral autoantigen in patients with systemic lupus erythematosus. *Clin Immunol* 2005;**116**:124–34.

41. James JA, Neas BR, Moser KL, Hall T, Bruner GR, Sestak AL, et al. Systemic lupus erytemathosus in adults is associated with previous Epstein Barr virus exposure. *Arthritis Rheum* 2001;**44**:1122–26.

42. Moon UY, Park SJ, Oh ST, Kim WU, Park SH, Lee SH, et al. Patients with systemic lupus erythematosus have abnormally elevated Epstein-Barr virus load in blood. *Arthritis Res Ther* 2004;**6**:295–302.

43. Francis L, Perl A. Infection in systemic lupus erythematosus: friend or foe? *Int J Clin Rheumatol* 2010;**5**:59–74.

44. Zandman-Goddard G, Shoenfeld Y. Infections and SLE. *Autoimmunity* 2005;**38**:473–85.

45. Kang I, Quan T, Nolasco H, Park SH, Hong MS, Crouch J, et al. Defective control of latent Epstein-Barr virus infection in systemic lupus erythematosus. *J Immunol* 2004;**172**:1287–94.

46. Blank M, Shoenfeld Y, Perl A. Cross-talk of the environment with the host genome and the immune system through endogenous retroviruses in systemic lupus erythematosus. *Lupus* 2009;**18**:1136–43.

47. Poole BD, Scofield RH, Harley JB, James JA. Epstein-Barr virus and molecular mimicry in systemic lupus erythematosus. *Autoimmunity* 2006;**39**:63–70.
48. Parks CG, Cooper GS, Hudson LL, Dooley MA, Treadwell EL, St. Clair EW, et al. Association of Epstein-Barr virus with systemic lupus erythematosus. *Arthritis Rheum* 2005;**52**:1148–59.
49. Tugnet N, Rylance P, Roden D, Trela M, Nelson P. Human endogenous retroviruses (HERVs) and autoimmune rheumatic disease: is there a link? *Open Rheumatol J* 2013;**7**:13–21.
50. Pullmann R, Bonilla E, Phillips PE, Middleton FA, Perl A. Haplotypes of the HRES-1 endogenous retrovirus are associated with development and disease manifestations of systemic lupus erythematosus. *Arthritis Rheum* 2008;**58**:532–40.
51. Yoshiki T, Mellors RC, Strand M, August JT. The viral envelope glycoprotein of murine leukemia virus and the pathogenesis of immune complex glomerulonephritis of New Zealand mice. *J Exp Med* 1974;**140**:1011–27.
52. Perl A, Nagy G, Koncz A, Gergely P, Fernandez D, Doherty E, et al. Molecular mimicry and immunomodulation by the HRES-1 endogenous retrovirus in SLE. *Autoimmunity* 2008;**41**:287–97.
53. Perl A, Colombo E, Dai H, Agarwal R, Mark KA, Banki K, et al. Antibody reactivity to the HRES-1 endogenous retroviral element identifies a subset of patients with systemic lupus erythematosus and overlap syndromes. Correlation with antinuclear antibodies and HLA class II alleles. *Arthritis Rheum* 1995;**38**:1660–71.
54. Perl A, Fernandez D, Telarico T, Phillips PE. Endogenous retroviral pathogenesis in lupus. *Curr Opin Rheumatol* 2010;**22**:483–92.
55. Gergely P, Perl A, Poor G. Possible pathogenic nature of the recently discovered TT virus: does it play a role in autoimmune rheumatic diseases? *Autoimmun Rev* 2006;**6**:5–9.
56. Emlen W, Niebur JA, Kadera R. Accelerated in vitro apoptosis of lymphocytes from patients with systemic lupus erythematosus. *J Immunol* 1994;**152**:3685–92.
57. Pavlovic M, Kats A, Cavallo M, Shoenfeld Y. Clinical and molecular evidence for association of SLE with parvovirus B19. *Lupus* 2010;**19**:783–92.
58. Aslanidis S, Pyrpasopoulou A, Kontotasios K, Doumas S, Zamboulis C. Parvovirus B19 infection and systemic lupus erythematosus: activation of aberrant pathway? *Eur J Int Med* 2008;**19**:314–18.
59. Hayashi T, Lee S, Ogasawara H, Sekigawa I, Iida N, Tomino Y, et al. Exacerbation of systemic lupus erythematosus related to cytomegalovirus infection. *Lupus* 1998;**7**:561–64.
60. Nawata M, Seta N, Yamada M, Sekigawa I, Lida N, Hashimoto H. Possible triggering effect of cytomegalovirus infection on systemic lupus erythematosus. *Scand J Rheumatol* 2001;**30**:360–62.
61. Stratta P, Canavese C, Ciccone G, Santi S, Quaglia M, Ghisetti V, et al. Correlation between ctytomegalovirus infection and Reynaud's phenopmenon in lupus nephris. *Nephron* 1999;**82**:145–54.
62. Ramos-Casals M, Font J, García-Carrasco M, Cervera R, Jiménez S, Trejo O, et al. Hepatitis C virus infection mimicking systemic lupus erythematosus: study of hepatitis C virus infection in a series of 134 Spanish patients with systemic lupus erythematosus. *Arthritis Rheum* 2000;**43**:2801–6.
63. Karakov Y, Dilek K, Güllülü M, Yavuz M, Ersoy A, Akalyn H, et al. Prevalence of hepatitis C virus antibody in patients with systemic lupus erythematosus. *Ann Rheum Dis* 1997;**56**:570–71.
64. Mercado U, Avendaño-Reyes M, Araiza-Casillas R, Díaz-Molina R. Prevalence of antibodies against hepatitis C and B viruses in patients with systemic lupus erythematosus. *Rev Gastroenterol Mex* 2005;**70**:399–401.

65. Green NM, Marshak-Rothstein A. Toll-like receptor driven B cell activation in the induction of systemic autoimmunity. *Semin Immunol* 2011;**23**:106–12.
66. Pisetsky DS. The role of innate immunity in the induction of autoimmunity. *Autoimmun Rev* 2008;**8**:69–72.
67. Corthésy B. Role of secretory IgA in infection and maintenance of homeostasis. *Autoimmun Rev* 2013;**12**:661–65.
68. Kim WU, Sreih A, Bucala R. Toll-like receptors in systemic lupus erythematosus; prospects for therapeutic intervention. *Autoimmun Rev* 2009;**8**:204–8.
69. Munz C, Lunemann GD, Getts MT, Miller SD. Antiviral immune responses: trigger of or triggered by autoimmunity? *Nat Rev Immunol* 2009;**9**:246–58.
70. Fischer S, Agmon-Levin N, Shapira Y, Porat Katz BS, Graell E, Cervera R, et al. *Toxoplasma gondii*: bystander or cofactor in rheumatoid arthritis. *Immunol Res* 2013;**56**: 287–92.
71. Vercelli D. Mechanisms of hygiene hypothesis-molecular or otherwise. *Curr Opin Immunol* 2006;**18**:733–37.
72. Zandman-Goddard G, Shoenfeld Y. Parasitic infection and autoimmunity. *Lupus* 2009;**18**:1144–48.
73. Clatworthy MR, Willcocks L, Urban B, Langhorne J, Williams TN, Peshu N, et al. Systemic lupus erythematosus-associated defects in the inhibitory receptor FcγRIIb reduce susceptibility to malaria. *Proc Natl Acad Sci USA* 2007;**104**:7169–74.
74. Greenwood B, Corrah T. Systemic lupus erythematosus in African immigrants. *Lancet* 2001;**358**:1182.
75. Chen M, Aosai F, Norose K, Mun HS, Ishikura H, Hirose S, et al. *Toxoplasma gondii* infection inhibits the development of lupus-like syndrome in autoimmune (New Zeland black X New Zeland white) F1 mice. *Int Immunol* 2004;**16**:937–46.
76. Harnett W, Harnett MM. Molecular basis of worm-induced immunomodulation. *Parasite Immunol* 2006;**28**:535–43.
77. Liu G, Zhao Y. Toll-like receptors and immune regulation: their direct and indirect modulation on regulatory CD4+ CD25+ T cells. *Immunology* 2007;**122**:149–56.
78. Bach JF. Protective role of infections and vaccinations on autoimmune diseases. *J Autoimmun* 2001;**16**:347–53.
79. Sawalha AH, Schmid WR, Binder SR, Bacino DK, Harley JB. Association between systemic lupus erythematosus and *Helicobacter pylori* seronegativity. *J Rheumatol* 2004;**3**:1546–50.
80. Amital H, Govoni M, Maya R, Meroni PL, Ori B, Shoenfeld Y, et al. Role of infectious agents in systemic rheumatic diseases. *Clin Exp Rheumatol* 2008;**26**:S27–32.
81. Ram M, Anaya JM, Barzilai O, Izhaky D, Porat Katz BS, Blank M, et al. The putative protective role of hepatitis B virus (HBV) infection from autoimmune disorders. *Autoimmun Rev* 2008;**7**:621–25.
82. Graham RR, Ortmann W, Rodine P, Espe K, Langefeld C, Lange E, et al. Specific combinations of HLA-DR2 and DR3 class II haplotypes contribute graded risk for disease susceptibility and autoantibodies in human SLE. *Eur J Hum Genet* 2007;**15**: 823–30.
83. Schulze C, Munoz LE, Franz S, Sarter K, Chaurio RA, Gaipl US, et al. Clearance deficiency—a potential link between infections and autoimmunity. *Autoimmun Rev* 2008;**8**:5–8.
84. Van Ghelue M, Moens U, Bendiksen S, Rekvig OP. Autoimmunity to nucleosomes related to viral infection: a focus on hapten carrier complex formation. *J Autoimmun* 2003;**20**:171–82.
85. Shoenfeld Y, Gilburd B, Abu-Shakra M, Amital H, Barzilai O, Berkun Y, et al. The mosaic of autoimmunity: genetic factors involved in autoimmune diseases—2008. *Isr Med Assoc J* 2008;**10**:3–7.

86. Papadimitraki ED, Choulaki C, Koutala E, Bertsias G, Tsatsanis C, Gergianaki I, et al. Expansion of tall-like receptor 9-expressing B cells in active systemic lupus erythematosus: implication for the induction and maintenance of the autoimmune process. *Arthritis Rheum* 2006;**54**:3601–11.

87. Garred P, Voss A, Madsen HO, Junker P. Association of mannose-binding lectin gene variation with disease severity and infections in a population-based cohort of systemic lupus erythematosus patients. *Genes Immun* 2001;**2**:442–50.

88. Walport MJ, Davies KA, Botto M. C1q and systemic lupus erythematosus. *Immunobiology* 1998;**99**:265.

89. Aron-Maor A, Shoenfeld Y. Vaccination and systemic lupus erithematosus: the bidirectional dilemmas. *Lupus* 2001;**10**:237–40.

90. Dell' Era L, Esposito S, Corona F, Principi N. Vaccination of children and adolescents with rheumatic diseases. *Rheumatology (Oxford)* 2011;**50**:1358–65.

91. Del Porto F, Lagana B, Biselli R, Donatelli I, Campitelli L, Nisini R, et al. Influenza vaccine administration in patients with systemic lupus erythematosus and rheumatoid arthritis. Safety and immunogenicity. *Vaccine* 2006;**24**:3217–23.

92. Hidalgo-Tenorio C, Jiménez-Alonso J, de Dios Luna J, Tallada M, Martínez-Brocal A, Sabio JM. Urinary tract infections and lupus erythematosus. *Ann Rheum Dis* 2004;**63**:431–37.

93. Gladman DD, Husain F, Ibañez D, Urowitz MB. The nature and outcome of infection in systemic lupus erythematosus. *Lupus* 2002;**11**:234–39.

94. Hill MD, Karsh J. Invasive soft tissue infections with *Streptococcus pneumoniae* in patients with systemic lupus erythmatosus: case report and review of the literature. *Arthitis Rheum* 1997;**40**:1716–19.

95. Marcos M, Fernandez C, Soriano A, Marco F, Martinez JA, Almela M, et al. Epidemiology and clinical outcomes of bloodstream infections among lupus patients. *Lupus* 2011;**20**:965–71.

96. Erdozain JG, Ruiz-Irastorza G, Egurbide MW, Martinez Beriot Xoa A, Aguirre C. High risk of tuberculosis in systemic lupus erythematosus? *Lupus* 2006;**15**:232–35.

97. Mok MY, Wong SS, Chan TM, Fong DY, Wong WS, Lau CS. Non-tuberculous mycobacterial infection in patients with systemic lupus erythematosus. *Rheumatology* 2007;**46**:280–84.

98. Rider JR, Ollier WE, Lock RJ, Brookes ST, Pamphilon DH. Human cytomegalovirus infections and systemic lupus erythematosus. *Clin Exp Rheumatol* 1997; **15**:405–9.

99. Ramos-Casals M, Cuadrado MJ, Alba P, Sanna G, Brito-Zerón P, Bertolaccini L, et al. Acute viral infections in patients with systemic lupus erythematosus: description of 23 cases and review of the literature. *Medicine* 2008;**87**:311–18.

100. Pryor BD, Bologna SG, Kahl LE. Risk factors for serious infection during treatment with cyclophosphamide and high-dose corticosteroids for systemic lupus erythematosus. *Arthritis Rheum* 1996;**39**:1475–82.

101. Danza A, Ruiz-Irastorza G. Infection risk in systemic lupus erythematosus patients: susceptibility factors and preventive strategies. *Lupus* 2013;**22**:1286–94.

102. Bosch X, Guilabert A, Pallarés L, Cerveral R, Ramos-Casals M, Bové A, et al. Infections in systemic lupus erythematosus: a prospective and controlled study of 110 patients. *Lupus* 2006;**15**:584–89.

103. Dixon WG, Kezouh A, Bernatsky S, Suissa S. The influence of systemic glucocorticoid therapy upon the risk of non-serious infection in older patients with rheumatoid arthritis: a nested case-control study. *Ann Rheum Dis* 2010;**70**:956–60.

104. Diaz-Lagares C, Pérez-Alvarez R, Garcìa-Hernàndez FJ, Ayala-Gutiérrez MM, Callejas JL, Martínez-Berriotxoa A, et al. Rates of, and risk factors for, severe infections in patients with sistemic autoimmune diseases receiving biological agents off-label. *Arthritis Res Ther* 2011;**13**:R112.

105. Navarra SV, Guzman RM, Gallacher AE, Hall S, Levy RA, Jimenez RE, et al. Efficacy and safety of belimumab in patients with active systemic lupus erythematosus: a randomized, placebo controlled, phase 3 trial. *Lancet* 2011;**377**:721–31.
106. Sisò A, Ramos-Casals M, Bové A, Brito-Zerón P, Soria N, Muñoz S, et al. Previous antimalarial therapy in patients diagnosed with lupus nephritis: influence on outcomes and survival. *Lupus* 2008;**17**:281–88.
107. Sciascia S, Ceberio L, Garcia-Fernandez C, Roccatello D, Karim Y, Cuadrado MJ. Systemic lupus erythematosus and infections: clinical importance of conventional and upcoming biomarkers. *Autoimmun Rev* 2012;**12**:157–63.
108. Sciascia S, Bertolaccini ML, Baldovino S, Roccatello D, Khamashta MA, Sanna G. Central nervous system involvement in systemic lupus erythematosus: overview on classification criteria. *Autoimmun Rev* 2013;**12**:426–29.

CHAPTER 42

Infections and Idiopathic Inflammatory Myopathies

M. Zen, M. Gatto, E. Borella, L. Iaccarino, A. Ghirardello, A. Doria[1]
Division of Rheumatology, Department of Medicine, University of Padova, Padova, Italy
[1]Corresponding Author: adoria@unipd.it

1 IDIOPATHIC INFLAMMATORY MYOPATHIES: CLASSIFICATION, PATHOGENESIS, AND DIAGNOSIS

Idiopathic inflammatory myopathies (IIM) are a group of chronic, multifactorial, acquired, systemic diseases of unknown cause characterized by muscle inflammation and damage.[1] A variety of clinical manifestations and immunologic abnormalities may be observed in patients with IIM, including autoantibodies directed against ubiquitous cytoplasmic or nuclear antigens.[2]

The IIM are classified among connective tissue diseases (CTDs), and from a clinicopathologic perspective they fall into four major categories:[3] dermatomyositis (DM), polymyositis (PM), necrotizing immune-mediated myositis (NIMM), and inclusion body myositis (IBM). In addition, overlap syndromes, cancer-associated myositis, and other forms including rare focal and diffuse variants have been identified.

The cause of IIM is still unclear, although it has been postulated that environmental factors (including viral or bacterial infectious agents) may trigger an abnormal autoimmune response in genetically susceptible individuals. Certain human leukocyte antigen (HLA) alleles on chromosome 6, in particular HLA-DQA1*0501 and HLA-DRB1*0301, have been associated with IIM.[4,5] The presence of T and B cells in muscle biopsies together with the detection of autoantibodies in the majority of patients with IIM suggest that immune mechanisms are involved in the pathogenesis of these diseases and that T and B cells play a pathogenic role.[5]

An autoimmune response characterized by autoantibody generation in response to nuclear and cytoplasmic autoantigens can be found in about 60–80% of patients affected with IIM.[2] Some of these autoantibodies are

Infection and Autoimmunity
http://dx.doi.org/10.1016/B978-0-444-63269-2.00052-0

specific for IIM (myositis-specific antibodies, MSAs); others can be detected in other autoimmune diseases (myositis-associated antibodies, MAAs).[2] Whether these autoantibodies have a direct role in the pathogenesis of IIM or whether they are an epiphenomenon is not completely understood,[6,7] but recent studies suggest that certain MSAs can be pathogenetic by becoming endogenous type I interferon inducers by peripheral blood mononuclear cells.[8,9] MSAs are a marker of IIM. Using standard techniques (e.g. immunofluorescence on HEp-2 cells), MSAs can be found in about 40% of patients with IIM. Because of the low sensitivity, the absence of these antibodies does not certainly exclude the diagnosis of IIM, but their detection has a strong positive predictive value for disease diagnosis.

Autoantigens for MSAs identified to date include four different groups of proteins: the aminoacyl-tRNA synthetases (ARSs), the nuclear Mi-2 protein, components of the signal recognition particle (SRP), and some intracellular enzymes. Each MSA is associated with specific clinical features in addition to myositis.[10] The most common MSAs, which are found in approximately 30% of patients with myositis, target the ARSs. Antibodies against 8 of the 20 ARSs have been described to date: anti-histidyl (anti-Jo-1), anti-threonyl (anti-PL-7), anti-alanyl (anti-PL-12), anti-glycyl (anti-EJ), anti-isoleucyl (anti-OJ), anti-asparaginyl (anti-KS), anti-phenylalanyl (anti-Zo), and anti-tyrosyl (anti-Ha) tRNAs.[11,12] The most common one is the anti-Jo-1 antibody, which is detected in 20-30% of cases. Patients with anti-ARS autoantibodies are affected with the so-called anti-synthetase syndrome, which is characterised by myositis, arthritis, Raynaud's phenomenon, interstitial lung disease, and hand skin lesions (so-called mechanic's hands).

Anti-Mi-2 antibodies are considered a specific serological marker of DM and are detected in about one fifth of patients with IIM. They are associated with relatively acute onset, good response to therapy and good prognosis.[13,14] Patients with anti-SRP autoantibodies usually have a severe, acute, necrotizing myositis with severe prognosis and poor response to therapy.[15] Biopsy differentiates NIMM from the other IIM because it demonstrates marked muscle necrosis with regeneration in the absence of an inflammatory infiltrate.

Anti-CADM-140, anti-p155/140, anti-NXP-2 (p140), anti-SAE, anti-200/100, and anti-Mup44 are other newly described MSAs. Anti-155/140 is observed in malignancy-associated or juvenile DM and anti-CADM-140/MDA5 is associated with a form of clinically amyopathic DM characterized by rapidly progressive interstitial lung disease and poor prognosis.[16,17]

MAAs can be found in sera from up to 50% of patients with IIM. The most important antigenic targets of MAAs are the PM/Scl nucleolar antigen, the nuclear Ku antigen (p70/p80), small nuclear ribonucleoproteins (RNP) and cytoplasmic RNP (RoRNP).

Anti-PM/Scl autoantibodies are found in patients with PM, scleroderma or PM overlap with scleroderma;[2] anti-Ku autoantibodies are generally found in patients with myositis overlap with other CTDs;[2] anti-small nuclear RNP antibodies are found in patients with myositis and in patients with CTD overlap syndrome; antibodies directed against Ro/SSA 60 kDa, Ro/SSA 52 kDa and La/SSB proteins (components of the RoRNP complex) are almost exclusively found in patients affected with systemic lupus erythematosus and Sjögren's syndrome.

It has been demonstrated that high serum concentrations of some auto-antibodies are associated with specific clinical features (i.e. anti-synthetase syndrome),[18,19] whereas others seem to be associated with a worse outcome (i.e. non-Jo-1 ARS autoantibodies and antibodies to SRP).[13,20–22] Interestingly, a recent study comparing anti-Jo1-positive patients with and without anti-Ro52 autoantibodies found that overall outcome was poorer and survival was reduced in those with anti-Ro52 autoantibodies.[21]

Muscle biopsy is useful in IIM diagnosis and shows inflammatory infiltrates, necrotic areas, fibrosis and atrophy; regenerating fibres can also be observed.[3] In DM, the inflammatory infiltrate is more prominent in the perivascular area than in the perimysial and endomysial areas and it is mainly composed by CD4+ T cells, B cells, and macrophages. Conversely, the cellular infiltrate of PM is characterized by a predominance of CD8+ T cells and macrophages and it is localized in the endomysial area.[23,24] In NIMM, muscular biopsy shows myofibre necrosis, minimal endomysial and perivascular inflammatory infiltrate, and in some cases focal endomysial fibrosis.[25] Immunostaining of muscle biopsies shows macrophages around necrotic fibres with very few lymphocytes.[26] The lack of inflammatory cell infiltrate argues against a pathogenic role for cytotoxic T cells and suggests that an antibody-dependent complement-mediated lysis may be responsible for tissue damage, with the macrophages as the final effector cells.[27]

IIM can be clinically undefined at the beginning, leading to difficulties in early diagnosis and correct classification. IIM affect both men and women of all ages. Childhood myositis is defined when the onset occurs before the age of 18. DM occurs in both children and adults and in women more than in men; PM is more common after the second decade of life, and IBM usually occurs in men and women over the age of 50.

The clinical hallmarks of IIM are a progressive proximal muscle weakness with increased serum muscle enzymes (creatinine phosphokinase, aldolase, and lactic dehydrogenase); increased myoglobin serum concentrations; and characteristic electromyographic alterations. Other clinical features are arthralgia or arthritis, skin rash (mainly in DM) and pulmonary, gastrointestinal, cardiac, and renal abnormalities.

2 INFECTIONS AND MYOSITIS

Several studies were carried out in an attempt to identify the possible relationships between infections and autoimmune diseases. Experimental and epidemiological studies of humans suggest that a relationship does exist, and that it is biunivocal: infections can act as triggers for disease development and flare-up, whereas the disease itself, and its treatment, can predispose to infections.

2.1 Infections as a Trigger of IIM

A striking association between environmental factors and myositis has not been identified yet. However, seasonal and geographic clustering of myositis has been reported, indicating that a common environmental factor, such as a bacterial or viral infection, could trigger the onset of disease.[28] Infection with a variety of viruses can generate self-limiting myalgias and, rarely, myositis.[29] Although attempts to identify viral DNA/RNA in muscle biopsies failed to support any particular viral agent in the majority of cases of IIM, several mouse models showed that viral infection can produce muscle inflammation resembling histopathologic abnormalities found in humans.

2.1.1 Infectious Agents in Animal Models of Myositis
Animal models have been used to clarify the possible pathogenetic role of viruses in myositis. None of these models exactly replicated the complexity of human disease, but by reproducing isolated aspects of the muscle pathology found in humans they provided insight into the pathogenesis of IIM. One model of PM, based on Ross River virus infection in different knockout mice, showed that the complement system and macrophages are critical determinants of tissue inflammation.[30,31] It was shown that mononuclear cell infiltration of muscle was necessary to produce functional weakness in a mouse model of viral infection with Coxsackievirus B (CVB);[32] in the same model, the presence of muscle inflammation without weakness

following inoculation with specific mutant strains of CVB underlined the potential role of co-existing non-immune pathological mechanisms.

Other infectious models for IIM have been developed in the past 10 years, including murine myositis induced by viruses (e.g. the Chikungunya virus[33]) and protozoa, including *Trypanosoma cruzi*[34] and *Leishmania infantum*.[35] In these models, protozoal infection caused a multi-phasic disorder replicating many histopathologic features of PM, including perivascular CD4+ T-cell infiltration, endomysial CD8+ cell invasion of non-necrotic fibres, and up-regulation of major histocompatibility complex class I molecules in muscle fibres. These animal models provide clear evidence that infections can cause muscle inflammation, which can subsequently become self-sustaining and chronic.

2.1.2 Infectious Agents in IIM Induction in Humans

Many infectious agents have been proposed as initiating factors for IIM, including Epstein-Barr virus (EBV), parvoviruses, enteroviruses, and retroviruses, in particular human immunodeficiency virus (HIV) and human T-lymphotropic virus (HTLV), *Toxoplasma* and *Borrelia*.[36] Viral infection might initiate the inflammatory process in the muscle; the process then becomes self-sustaining in predisposed individuals (e.g. subjects who cannot mount the counter-inflammatory response because of genetic defects).[37,38]

A case-control study[39] showed a higher frequency of anti-Epstein-Barr nuclear antigen 1 (EBNA1) antibodies in patients with DM and PM at disease onset compared with healthy matched controls. Moreover, the EBV genome was detected more frequently in patients than in the matched healthy controls. Moreover, two case reports described the development of PM[40] and DM[41] after EBV infection.

Enteroviruses also have been isolated in the muscles of patients with myositis.[37] Among them, CVB is considered a potential casual agent in the induction of chronic muscle diseases such as PM and DM because of its tropism for muscle. CVB particles, viral RNA, and antiviral antibodies have been isolated from few patients with IIM or myocarditis.[37]

Data regarding parvovirus B19 are more controversial. Three case reports suggested an association,[42–44] but the viral DNA and viral capsid proteins were not found in muscle tissue sections in two case series,[45,46] and a case-control study did not find an increased prevalence of anti-parvovirus B19 immunoglobulin (Ig) G in the plasma of patients with juvenile DM.[47]

Many cases of PM attributed to HIV infection have been reported, but no studies have yet been able to demonstrate the virus within muscle fibres.

Thus, the direct role of HIV in PM induction remains controversial.[48] However, four cases of IBM after exposure to HIV infection[49] and four cases of DM secondary to HIV infection have been described to date.[50] With regard to DM, myositis appeared 6-18 months after HIV infection was detected, and no autoantibodies were detected in the majority of cases. No data regarding virus or viral RNA detection in biopsies were reported.

An association of PM with HTLV-1 infection also was found. An epidemiological study in Jamaica showed that the rate of anti-HTLV-1 antibodies in patients with PM was significantly higher than that in the general population.[51] In addition, in a study of three patients affected with PM anti-HTLV-1, antibodies were detected in sera of all the patients.[52] This study suggested that HTLV-1-induced PM is not due to direct viral infection in muscle fibres but to a T-cell-mediated autoimmune process that is initiated by HTLV-1 infection.[52] A study conducted in the south of Japan (where HTLV-1 is endemic) showed a higher rate of anti-HTLV-1 antibodies in patients with IBM compared with the general population.[53]

Case reports suggested a possible association between the onset of IIM and viral hepatitis, including hepatitis C[54] and B virus infection,[55] as well as an association with hepatitis B vaccination.[56,57] Some recent case reports highlighted the occurrence of benign acute myositis after influenza virus infection,[58–60] suggesting a possible role of these viruses in the induction of IIM. Elevated levels of antibodies to *Toxoplasma* also have been reported in IIM,[61] but no convincing evidence for a pathogenetic role of this infection in IIM has been provided.

2.1.3 Hypothesis of Induction of the Autoimmune Response

Several hypothesis for the potential mechanisms involved in the development of autoimmune responses following infection have been put forwards. The ability of a host to defend itself against pathogens is mediated by receptors known as pattern-recognition receptors. By triggering pattern-recognition receptors and increasing the function of antigen-presenting cells, microbes can act as adjuvants for the immune response. In this highly inflammatory environment, an autoimmune response can be triggered if autoreactive cells are present.

Some potential mechanisms have been proposed to explain the role of infectious agents in IIM induction: (1) The interaction of microbes with cellular proteins of the host may induce changes in these proteins that are then no longer recognized as "self" by the host immune system. (2) Infection makes accessible some cellular antigens that the immune system has never before encountered. (3) Microbes carry antigenic sites that "mimic" amino acid sequences in the normal host proteins (molecular mimicry). (4) Infection causes a pro-inflammatory milieu that favors the so-called bystander activation of different T- and B-cell clones. (5) Infections trigger so-called epitope spreading. (6) Induction of the production of human antibodies carrying pathogenic idiotypes (anti-idiotypic antibodies). Thus, a pathogen could initiate an immune reaction in the muscle, which then continues after the virus is eliminated, becoming self-sustaining. From this point of view, the anti-ARS antibodies could be "footprints" of previous viral infections.[62] It has been suggested that they arise following a break of tolerance due to the interaction of a virus with the synthetase during viral replication.

2.2 Infections as Comorbidity in Patients with IIM

Patients with IIM have a high risk of developing infections. This increased risk is the result of immune abnormalities characteristic of the disease as well as an effect of the use of immunosuppressive therapy for IIM.[63] Infections have been described in up to 37% of patients with IIM, and they are important causes of death, especially pulmonary infections (Table 1).[63–76] Soft-tissue and dermal infections caused by *Staphylococcus aureus* are frequent in patients with calcinosis cutis, whereas oesophageal dysfunction and ventilatory insufficiency can predispose to aspiration pneumonia.

In a recent case series of 279 patients with PM or DM, more than one-third of patients (37.3%) developed severe infections, including pyogenic (68.3%) and non-pyogenic/opportunistic infections (31.7%).[74] In this study, pyogenic infections were more commonly due to aspiration pneumonia and calcinosis cutis infection, whereas opportunistic infections were mainly due to fungi (40% of cases), especially *Candida albicans* and *Pneumocystis jiroveci*.[74]

In a cohort of 160 patients with PM or DM, infections accounted for 15% of deaths,[75] and in a series of 156 patients, 3 patients (12.5% of observed deaths) died from opportunistic infections, and other 8 patients (33.3% of observed deaths) died because of non-opportunistic infections, mainly aspiration pneumonia.[63] In another study, the main causes of death among 77 patients were cancer (47% of cases) and pulmonary complications (35% of cases).[64] When considering the global survival rate, a study of 197 patients with IIM showed 1-, 5-, and 10-year survival rates of 85%, 75%, and 67%, respectively.[73] The major causes of death were malignancies and infections.

The use of methotrexate, azathioprine, and infliximab and a higher median daily dose of corticosteroids seem to be risk factors for infections.[74] Conversely, we and other groups recently reported the safety of the use of rituximab in patients with refractory IIM.[77–79] It also has been demonstrated

Table 1 Infections and Mortality in IIM Cohorts

References	Year	Patients (n)	Length of Follow-up, Median (Range), or Mean (±SD)	Mortality rate (%)	Deaths Due to Infections (% of Total Deaths)
Marie et al.[64]	2001	77	4 (0.2-24)	22.1	28.9
Sultan et al.[65]	2002	46	20 (0.5-26)	13	33.3
Danko et al.[66]	2004	162	8.4 (0.4-26)	12.3	0
Marie et al.[63]	2005	156	NA	27.7	20.5
Airio et al.[67]	2006	248	20 (or until death)	60.1	4.1
Torres et al.[68]	2006	107	10 (or until death)	27.5	25.8
Tani et al.[69]	2006	23	4 (1-6)	8.7	49.4
Ng et al.[70]	2009	55	9 (0.3-35)	10.9	33.0
Chen et al.[71]	2010	192	3.6 (3.1)	18.8	41.5
Mustafa and Dahbour[72]	2010	30	6.5 (0.2-28)	20	100
Yamasaki et al.[73]	2011	197	4.7 (1.17-9.5)	26.9	27.8
Marie et al.[74]	2011	279	3 (1-22)	11.1	67.1
Schiopu et al.[75]	2012	160	4.6 (IQR 1.7-8.8)	16.9	14.7
Lymaie et al.[76]	2012	364	4.8 (NA)	25.3	22

NA, not available; IQR, interquartile range.

that older age, muscle weakness, dysphonia and esophageal dysfunction are more common in patients with infections compared with those without.[74] Thus, patients with IIM with severe organ involvement and active myositis, especially when treated with high doses of prednisone or immunosuppressive agents, should be carefully monitored for infections to reduce mortality and improve prognosis.

REFERENCES

1. Rider LG, Miller FW. Deciphering the clinical presentations, pathogenesis, and treatment of the idiopathic inflammatory myopathies. *JAMA* 2011;**305**:183–90.
2. Tansley S, Gunawardena H. The evolving spectrum of polymyositis and dermatomyositis–moving toward clinicoserological syndromes: a critical review. *Clin Rev Allerg Immunol* 2014; [epub ahead of print].
3. Lazarou IN, Guerne PA. Classification, diagnosis, and management of idiopathic inflammatory myopathies. *J Rheumatol* 2013;**40**(5):550–64.
4. Reed AM, Ytterberg SR. Genetic and environmental risk factors for idiopathic inflammatory myopathies. *Rheum Dis Clin North Am* 2002;**28**(4):891–916.

5. Chinoy H, Lamb JA, Ollier WE, Cooper RG. Recent advances in the immunogenetics of idiopathic inflammatory myopathy. *Arthritis Res Ther* 2011;**13**:216.
6. Betteridge ZE, Gunawardena H, McHugh NJ. Novel autoantibodies and clinical phenotypes in adult and juvenile myositis. *Arthritis Res Ther* 2011;**3**(2):209.
7. Lundberg IE, Datsmalki M. Possible pathogenic mechanisms in inflammatory myopathies. *Rheum Dis Clin N Am* 2002;**28**:799–822.
8. Gunawardena H, Betteridge ZE, McHugh NJ. Myositis-specific autoantibodies: their clinical and pathogenic significance in disease expression. *Rheumatology (Oxford)* 2009;**48**(6):607–12.
9. Eloranta ML, Barbasso Helmers S, Ulfgren AK, Ronnblom L, Alm GV, Lundberg IE. A possible mechanism for endogenous activation of the type I interferon system in myositis patients with anti-Jo1 or anti-Ro 52/anti-Ro 60 autoantibodies. *Arthritis Rheum* 2007;**56**(9):3112–24.
10. Hamaguchi Y, Kuwana M, Hoshino K, Hasegawa M, Kaji K, Matsushita T, et al. Clinical correlations with dermatomyositis-specific autoantibodies in adult Japanese patients with dermatomyositis: a multicenter cross-sectional study. *Arch Dermatol* 2011;**147**:391–8.
11. Betteridge Z, Gunawardena H, North J, Slinn J, McHugh N. Anti-synthetase syndrome: a new autoantibody to phenylalanyl transfer RNA synthetase (anti-Zo) associated with polymyositis and interstitial pneumonia. *Rheumatology (Oxford)* 2007;**46**:1005–8.
12. Hervier B, Devilliers H, Stanciu R, Meyer A, Uzunhan Y, Masseau A, et al. Hierarchical cluster and survival analyses of antisynthetase syndrome: phenotype and outcome are correlated with anti-tRNA synthetase antibody specificity. *Autoimmun Rev* 2012;**12**:210–17.
13. Suzuki S, Hayashi YK, Tsuburaya R, Kuwana M, Suzuki N, Nishino I. Myopathy associated with antibodies to signal recognition particle: disease progression and neurological outcome. *Arch Neurol* 2012;**69**(6):728–32.
14. Komura K, Fujimoto M, Matsushita T, Kaji K, Kondo M, Hirano T, et al. Prevalence and clinical characteristics of anti-Mi-2 antibodies in Japanese patients with dermatomyositis. *J Dermatol Sci* 2005;**40**:215–17.
15. Casciola-Rosen L, Mammen AL. Myositis autoantibodies. *Curr Opin Rheumatol* 2012;**24**(6):602–8.
16. Fujimoto M, Hamaguchi Y, Kaji K, Matsushita T, Ichimura Y, Kodera M, et al. Myositis-specific anti-155/140 autoantibodies target transcription intermediary factor 1 family proteins. *Arthritis Rheum* 2012;**64**:513–22.
17. Sato S, Hirakata M, Kuwana M, Suwa A, Inada S, Mimori T, et al. Autoantibodies to a 140-kd polypeptide, CADM-140, in Japanese patients with clinically amyopathic dermatomyositis. *Arthritis Rheum* 2005;**52**:1571–6.
18. Hall JC, Casciola-Rosen L, Samedy L-A, Werner J, Owoyemi K, Danoff SK, et al. Anti-MDA5-associated dermatomyositis: expanding the clinical spectrum. *Arthritis Care Res (Hoboken)* 2013;**65**(8):1307–15.
19. Labirua-Iturburu A, Selva-O'Callaghan A, Vincze M, Danko K, Vencovsky J, Fisher B, et al. Anti-PL-7 (anti-threonyl-tRNA synthetase) antisynthetase syndrome: clinical manifestations in a series of patients from a European multicenter study (EUMYONET) and review of the literature. *Medicine* 2012;**91**(4):206–11.
20. Aggarwal R, Cassidy E, Fertig N, Koontz DC, Lucas M, Ascherman DP, et al. Patients with non-Jo-1 anti-tRNA-synthetase autoantibodies have worse survival than Jo-1 positive patients. *Ann Rheum Dis* 2014;**73**(1):227–32.
21. Marie I, Hatron PY, Dominique S, Cherin P, Mouthon L, Menard JF, et al. Short-term and long-term outcome of anti-Jo1-positive patients with anti-Ro52 antibody. *Semin Arthritis Rheum* 2012;**41**(6):890–9.

22. Trallero-Araguás E, Rodrigo-Pendás JÁ, Selva-O'Callaghan A, Martínez-Gómez X, Bosch X, Labrador-Horrillo M, et al. Usefulness of anti-p155 autoantibody for diagnosing cancer-associated dermatomyositis: a systematic review and meta-analysis. *Arthritis Rheum* 2012;**64**(2):523–32.

23. Engel AG, Arahata K. Mononuclear cells in myopathies. Quantitation of functionally distinct subsets, recognition of antigen-specific cell-mediated cytotoxicity in some diseases, and implications for the pathogenesis of the different inflammatory myopathies. *Hum Pathol* 1986;**17**:704–21.

24. Greenberg SA. Proposed immunologic models of the inflammatory myopathies and potential therapeutic implications. *Neurology* 2007;**69**(21):2008–19.

25. Liang C, Needham M. Necrotizing autoimmune myopathy. *Curr Opin Rheumatol* 2011;**23**(6):612–19.

26. Sadeh M, Dabby R. Steroid-responsive myopathy: immune-mediated necrotizing myopathy or polymyositis without inflammation? *J Clin Neuromuscul Dis* 2008;**9**:341–4.

27. Dalakas MC. Review: an update on inflammatory and autoimmune myopathies. *Neuropathol Appl Neurobiol* 2011;**37**:226–42.

28. Leff RL, Burgess SH, Miller FW, Love LA, Targoff IN, Dalakas MC, et al. Distinct seasonal patterns in the onset of adult inflammatory myopathy in patients with anti Jo-1 and anti-Signal recognition particle autoantibodies. *Arthritis Rheum* 1991;**34**:1391–7.

29. Crum-Cianflone NF. Bacterial, fungal, parasitic and viral myositis. *Clin Microbiol Rev* 2008;**21**:473–94.

30. Morrison TE, Fraser RJ, Smith PN, Mahalingam S, Heise MT. Complement contributes to inflammatory tissue destruction in a mouse model of River virus-induced disease. *J Virol* 2007;**81**:5132–43.

31. Lidbury BA, Rulli NE, Suhrbier A, Smith PN, McColl SR, Cunningham AL, et al. Macrophage-derived proinflammatory factors contribute to the development of arthritis and myositis after infection with an arthrogenic alphavirus. *J Infect Dis* 2008;**197**:1585–93.

32. Sandager MM, Nugent JL, Schulz WL, Messner RP, Tam PE. Interactions between multiple genetic determinants in the 5'UTR and VP1 capsid control pathogenesis of chronic post-viral myopathy caused by coxsackievirus B1. *Virology* 2008;**372**:35–47.

33. Morrison TE, Oko L, Montgomery SA, Whitmore AC, Lotstein AR, Gunn BM, et al. A mouse model of chikungunya virus-induced musculoskeletal inflammatory disease: evidence of arthritis, tenosynovitis, myositis, and persistence. *Am J Pathol* 2011;**178**:32–40.

34. Andersson J, Englund P, Sunnemark D, Dahlstedt A, Westerblad H, Nennesmo I, et al. CBA/J mice infected with Trypanosoma cruzi: an experimental model for inflammatory myopathies. *Muscle Nerve* 2003;**27**:442–8.

35. Paciello O, Wojcik S, Gradoni L, Oliva G, Trapani F, Iovane V, et al. Syrian hamster infected with Leishmania infantum: a new experimental model for inflammatory myopathies. *Muscle Nerve* 2010;**41**:355–61.

36. Gan L, Miller FW. State of the art: what we know about infectious agents and myositis. *Cur Opinion Rheumatol* 2011;**23**:585–94.

37. Douche-Aourik F, Berlier W, Feasson L, Bourlet T, Harrath R, Omar S, et al. Detection of enterovirus in human skeletal muscle from patients with chronic inflammatory muscle disease or fibromyalgia and healthy subjects. *J Med Virol* 2003;**71**:540–7.

38. Leff RL, Love LA, Miller FW, Greenberg SJ, Klein EA, Dalakas MC, et al. Viruses in idiopathic inflammatory myopathies: absence of candidate viral genomes in muscle. *Lancet* 1992;**339**:1192–4.

39. Chen DY, Chen YM, Lan JL, Chen HH, Hsieh CW, Wey SJ, et al. Polymyositis/dermatomyositis and nasopharyngeal carcinoma: the Epstein–Barr virus connection? *J Clin Virol* 2010;**49**:290–5.

40. Tsutsumi S, Ohga S, Nomura A, Takada H, Sakai S, Ohshima K, et al. CD4-CD8- T-cell polymyositis in a patient with chronic active Epstein–Barr virus infection. *Am J Hematol* 2002;**71**:211–15.

41. Singh R, Cuchacovich R, Gomez R, Vargas A, Espinoza LR, Gedalia A. Simultaneous occurrence of diabetes mellitus and juvenile dermatomyositis: report of two cases. *Clin Pediatr (Phila)* 2003;**42**:459–62.

42. Magro CM, Iwenofu OH, Kerns MJ, Nuovo GJ, Dyrsen ME, Segal JP. Fulminant and acceleratedpresentation of dermatomyositis in two previously healthy young adult males: a potential role for endotheliotropic viral infection. *J Cutan Pathol* 2009;**36**:853–8.

43. Chandrakasan S, Singh S, Ratho RK, Kumar S, Mishra B. Anasarca as the presenting manifestation of parvovirus B19 associated juvenile dermatomyositis. *Rheumatol Int* 2009;**29**:565–7.

44. Lewkonia RM, Horne D, Dawood MR. Juvenile dermatomyositis in a child infected with human parvovirus B19. *Clin Infect Dis* 1995;**21**:430–2.

45. Chevrel G, Borsotti JP, Miossec P. Lack of evidence for a direct involvement for muscle infection by parovirus B19 in the pathogenesis of inflammatory myopathies: a follow-up study. *Rheumatology* 2003;**42**:349–52.

46. Chevrel G, Calvet A, Belin V, Miossec P. Dermatomyositis associated with the presence of parvorvirus B19 DNA in muscle. *Rheumatology* 2000;**39**:1037–9.

47. Mamyrova G, Rider LG, Haagenson L, Wong S, Brown KE. Parvovirus B19 and onset of juvenile dermatomyositis. *JAMA* 2005;**294**:2170–1.

48. Johnson RW, Williams FM, Kazi S, Dimachie MM, Reveille JD. Human immunodeficiency virus-associated polymyositis: a longitudinal study outcome. *Arthritis Rheum* 2003;**49**:172–8.

49. Dalakas MC, Rakocevic G, Shatunov A, Goldfarb L, Raju R, Salajegheh M. Inclusion body myositis with human immunodeficiency virus infection: four cases with clonal expansion of viral-specific T cells. *Ann Neurol* 2007;**61**:466–75.

50. Carroll MB, Holmes R. Dermatomyositis and HIV infection: case report and review of the literature. *Rheumatol Int* 2011;**31**:673–9.

51. Gilbert DT, Morgan O, Smikle MF, Simeon D, Barton EN. HTLV-1 associated polymyositis in Jamaica. *Acta Neurol Scand* 2001;**104**:101–4.

52. Saito M, Higuchi I, Saito A, Izumo S, Usuku K, Bangham CR, et al. Molecular analysis of T cell clonotypes in muscle-infiltrating lymphocytes from patients with human T lymphotropic virus type 1 polymyositis. *J Infect Dis* 2002;**186**:1231–41.

53. Matsuura E, Umehara F, Nose H, Higuchi I, Matsuoka E, Izumi K, et al. Inclusion body myositis associated with human T-lymphotropic virus-type I infection: eleven patients from an endemic area in Japan. *J Neuropathol Exp Neurol* 2008;**67**:41–9.

54. Yakushiji Y, Satoh J, Yukitake M, Yamaguchi K, Nakamura I, Nishino I, et al. Interferon beta-responsive inclusion body myositis in a hepatitis C virus carrier. *Neurology* 2004;**63**:587–8.

55. Nojima T, Hirakata M, Sato S, Fujii T, Suwa A, Mimori T, et al. A case of polymyositis associated with hepatitis B infection. *Clin Exp Rheumatol* 2000;**18**:86–8.

56. Ramirez-Rivera J, Vega-Cruz AM, Jaume-Anselmi F. Polymyositis: rare complication of hepatitis B vaccination: an unusual cause of toxic shock syndrome. *Bol Assoc Med PR* 2003;**95**:13–16.

57. Altman A, Szyper-Kravitz M, Shoenfeld Y. HBV vaccine and dermatomyositis: is there an association? *Rheumatol Int* 2008;**28**:609–12.

58. Heiner JD, Ball VL. A child with benign acute childhood myositis after influenza. *J Emerg Med* 2010;**39**:316–19.

59. Koliou M, Hadjiloizou S, Ourani S, Demosthenous A, Hadjidemetriou A. A case of benign acute childhood myositis associated with influenza A (H1N1) virus infection. *Clin Microbiol Infect* 2010;**16**:193–5.

60. Rubin E, De la Rubia L, Pascual A, Domínguez J, Flores C. Benign acute myositis associated with H1N1 influenza A virus infection. *Eur J Pediatr* 2010;**169**:1159–61.

61. Cuomo G, D'Abrosca V, Rizzo V, Nardiello S, La Montagna G, Gaeta GB, et al. Severe polymyositis due to *Toxoplasma gondii* in an adult immunocompetent patient: a case report and review of the literature. *Infection* 2013;**41**:859–62.

62. Messner RP. Pathogenesis of idiopathic inflammatory myopathies. In: Wortmann LR, editor. *Diseases of skeletal muscle*. Philadelphia: Lippincott Williams & Wilkins; 2000. p. 111–27.

63. Marie I, Hachulla E, Chérin P, Hellot MF, Herson S, Levesque H, et al. Opportunistic infections in polymyositis and dermatomyositis. *Arthritis Rheum* 2005;**53**:155–65.

64. Marie I, Hachulla E, Hatron PY, Hellot MF, Levesque H, Devulder B, et al. Polymyositis and dermatomyositis: short term and longterm outcome, and predictive factors. *J Rheumatol* 2001;**28**:2230–7.

65. Sultan SM, Ioannou Y, Moss K, Isenberg DA. Outcome in patients with idiopathic inflammatory myositis: morbidity and mortality. *Rheumatology (Oxford)* 2002;**41**:22–6.

66. Danko K, Ponyi A, Constantin T, Borgulya G, Szegedi G. Long-term survival of patients with idiopathic inflammatory myopathies according to clinical features: a longitudinal study of 162 cases. *Medicine (Baltimore)* 2004;**83**:35–42.

67. Airio A, Kautiainen H, Hakala M. Prognosis and mortality of polymyositis and dermatomyositis patients. *Clin Rheumatol* 2006;**25**:234–9.

68. Torres C, Belmonte R, Carmona L, Gómez-Reino FJ, Galindo M, Ramos B, et al. Survival, mortality and causes of death in inflammatory myopathies. *Autoimmunity* 2006;**39**:205–15.

69. Tani K, Tomioka R, Sato K, Furukawa C, Nakajima T, Toyota Y, et al. Comparison of clinical course of polymyositis and dermatomyositis: a follow-up study in Tokushima University Hospital. *J Med Invest* 2007;**54**:295–302.

70. Ng KP, Ramos F, Sultan SM, Isenberg DA. Concomitant diseases in a cohort of patients with idiopathic myositis during long-term follow-up. *Clin Rheumatol* 2009;**28**:947–53.

71. Chen IJ, Tsai WP, Wu YJ, Luo SF, Ho HH, Liou LB, et al. Infections in polymyositis and dermatomyositis: analysis of 192 cases. *Rheumatology (Oxford)* 2010;**49**(12):2429–37.

72. Mustafa KN, Dahbour SS. Clinical characteristics and outcomes of patients with idiopathic inflammatory myopathies from Jordan 1996-2009. *Clin Rheumatol* 2010;**29** (12):1381–5.

73. Yamasaki Y, Yamada H, Ohkubo M, Yamasaki M, Azuma K, Ogawa H, et al. Longterm survival and associated risk factors in patients with adult-onset idiopathic inflammatory myopathies and amyopathic dermatomyositis: experience in a single institute in Japan. *J Rheumatol* 2011;**38**:1636–43.

74. Marie I, Ménard JF, Hachulla E, Chérin P, Benveniste O, Tiev K, et al. Infectious complications in polymyositis and dermatomyositis: a series of 279 patients. *Semin Arthritis Rheum* 2011;**41**:48–60.

75. Schiopu E, Phillips K, MacDonald PM, Crofford LJ, Somers EC. Predictors of survival in a cohort of patients with polymyositis and dermatomyositis: effect of corticosteroids, methotrexate, and azathioprine. *Arthritis Res Ther* 2012;**14**:22.

76. Limaye V, Hakendorf P, Woodman RJ, Blumbergs P, Roberts-Thomson P. Mortality and its predominant causes in a large cohort of patients with biopsy-determined inflammatory myositis. *Intern Med J* 2012;**42**(2):191–8.

77. Nalotto L, Iaccarino L, Zen M, Gatto M, Borella E, Domenighetti M, et al. Rituximab in refractory idiopathic inflammatory myopathies and antisynthetase syndrome: personal experience and review of the literature. *Immunol Res* 2013;**56**(2–3):362–70.

78. Munoz-Beamud F, Isenberg DA. Rituximab as an effective alternative therapy in refractory idiopathic inflammatory myopathies. *Clin Exp Rheumatol* 2013;**31**(6):896–903.

79. Couderc M, Gottenberg JE, Mariette X, Hachuilla E, Sbilia J, Fain O, et al. Efficacy and safety of rituximab in the treatment of refractory inflammatory myopathies in adults: results from the AIR registry. *Rheumatology (Oxford)* 2011;**50**(12):2283–9.
80. Hashish L, Trieu EP, Sadanandan P, Targoff IN. Identification of autoantibodies to tyrosyl-tRNA synthetase in dermatomyositis with features consistent with antisynthetase syndrome. *Arthritis Rheum* 2005;**52**(Suppl. 9):s312.

CHAPTER 43

Rheumatoid Arthritis and Infections: More Than an Association?

Hussein Mahajna[1], Naim Mahroum, Howard Amital
Department of Medicine 'B', Sheba Medical Center, Tel-Hashomer, Sackler Faculty of Medicine,
Tel-Aviv University, Tel-Aviv, Israel
[1]Corresponding Author: Hmahajna@gmail.com

Rheumatoid arthritis (RA) is a systemic disease that manifests mainly as erosive polyarthritis; however, almost any organ within the human body might be involved. Untreated RA causes disabling destruction of joints, enhanced atherosclerosis and many other deleterious health consequences, which ultimately lead to accelerated morbidity rates and shorter longevity.

Despite our better understanding of the clinical spectra of RA, its etiology remains obscure. Among many other causes, infections seem to play a dominant role in the disease pathogenesis.[1] It is believed that an individual who carries a certain genetic predisposition and is exposed to certain endogenous and environmental factors (such as female hormones or smoking) and encounters a specific infection might consequently develop RA.[2–6] Several human leukocyte antigen (HLA) alleles, such as HLA-DRB1 and HLA-DRB4, have been particularly associated with RA.[7–9]

Among all environmental risk factors, smoking is believed to have the strongest link to the development of RA. Moreover, chemical constituents of smoke were found to enhance the generation of anti–citrullinated peptide antibodies. Smokers often suffer from a more severe form of the disease and respond less favorably to biological therapies.[8,10–13]

Infections are believed to contribute to the maturation of the immune system, directing it from the innate to the adaptive forms, and therefore play a seminal part in the induction of autoimmunity.[14–16] Söderlin et al.[17] systematically screened patients who presented with new-onset arthritis for preceding infections caused by *Salmonella typhimurium*, *Salmonella enteritidis*, *Yersinia enterocolitica*, *Campylobacter jejuni*, *Borrelia burgdorferi*,

Infection and Autoimmunity
http://dx.doi.org/10.1016/B978-0-444-63269-2.00065-9

Chlamydia trachomatis, Chlamydia pneumoniae and parvovirus B19 and found that the laboratory test results in 45% of the subjects indicated that a recent infection preceded their symptoms. Remission rates in cases of infection preceding arthritis were higher among subjects without antecedent arthritis. In another study, these authors found that 16% of patients with RA thought that an infection preceded their disease and 1.2% believed that a prior vaccination was related to it.[18]

A cross-sectional study compared titers of immunoglobulin G against *Mycoplasma pneumonia* in sera taken from patients with RA and from healthy patients; the presence of high anti-*Mycoplasma* immunoglobulin G was significantly associated with RA (odds ratio, 2.34; $P < 0.001$).[19] Another clue supporting this association was derived from the well-known and successful use of the RA treatment minocycline, which was also an effective antibiotic against *Mycoplasma* infections.[20]

CMV also has been mentioned in the pathogenesis of RA; CMV antibodies were recorded in patients with RA, and viral DNA has been identified in synovial tissue using DNA in situ hybridization and polymerase chain reaction. Furthermore, CMV seropositivity was shown to be associated with the expansion of $CD^{4+}CD^{28-}$ and $CD^{8+}CD^{28-}$ T cells in patients with RA.[21]

Another herpes virus that has been thought to play a significant role in the pathogenesis of RA is the Epstein-Barr virus (EBV); although there are some circumstantial data supporting this hypothesis, there is a lack of solid evidence. EBV is a ubiquitous virus that is easily recognized by antibodies but hardly ever eliminated; it is a classical infectious agent that has the capacity to trigger chronic immune complex diseases. This association is underlined by the finding of EBV viral DNA in the synovial tissue of patients with RA. In addition, EBV antigens are recognized by anti-citrullinated peptide antibodies. Impaired cytotoxic T-cell function has been detected in patients with RA infected by EBV—a finding attributed to abnormal signaling of the lymphocytic-activation molecule-associated protein.[21]

In a recent study using sera taken from 1595 patients with 23 different autoimmune diseases testing before EBV and CMV infection, a serological indication of higher rates of EBV supported the notion of a higher association between EBV and multiple autoimmune diseases, including RA.[22]

The association between *Helicobacter pylori* (HP) and RA has not been entirely determined. Most investigators have referred to a link between RA and HP by associating the effect of HP eradication on RA disease activity. However, the conclusions are controversial; some studies showed that patients benefit from HP eradication and others do not, thus suggesting that HP plays a possible defensive role through mechanisms involving oral tolerance.[23]

Data regarding the association between citrullination of connective tissue proteins such as vimentin, filaggrin, collagen and fibronectin and the pathogenesis of RA are mounting. Citrullination is a post-translational modification of arginine side chains catalyzed by peptidylarginine deiminase (PAD) enzymes, which induces a change in the protein structure, antigenicity and function. Citrullination might act as the facilitator that modifies known "self-antigens" to foreign, unrecognized proteins that are vulnerable to the immune reaction. In RA, it is thought that "stressful" environmental risk factors such as smoking and infections induce PAD synthesis and function.

Four anti-cyclic citrullinated peptides (CCPs) have been extensively characterized and reported, and they were found to convey diagnostic and prognostic features. These peptides appeared on the fibrinogen, vimentin, collagen type II and α-enolase molecules. They all are abundant in connective tissue.[24]

Proteus mirabilis is an additional bacteria that was highly suspected of being involved in the etiopathogenesis of RA. Although the hypothesis is still controversial within the rheumatological world, several studies suggest that it might have a role in the pathogenesis of RA. Studies have shown high levels of antibodies against *Proteus* peptides in patients with RA compared to healthy subjects. Furthermore, a positive correlation between antibody titers and the inflammatory parameters of erythrocyte sedimentation rate and C-reactive protein scores was observed.[25]

Gingival infection caused by *Porphyromonas gingivalis* is another that is associated with RA. It is postulated that this microbe causes a citrullination process in human proteins that leads to a cascade causing autoimmunity.[26] Periodontitis, in which *P. gingivalis* is a major pathogenic bacterium, has been linked to RA in epidemiological studies, and they share similar genomic and environmental associations. It is also the only bacterium identified that expresses endogenous citrullinated proteins and its own bacterial PAD enzyme.[24] Antibody titers to *P. gingivalis* are significantly increased in patients with RA and significantly correlated with anti-CCP antibody isotypes that are specific to RA.[27] Additional studies indicate that the major synovial targets of the RA-specific anti-CCP autoantibodies are deamidated forms of the α- and β-chains of fibrin. Other studies confirmed that bacterial PAD produced by *P. gingivalis* has the capacity of deamidating arginine in fibrin found in the periodontal lesion.[28] Citrullination of HLA binding peptides causes a 100-fold increase in peptide–major histocompatibility complex affinity and leads to the activation CD4(+)T cells in HLA DRB1 0401 transgenic mice.[28]

These PAD-engendered antigens, presented in association with major histocompatibility complex molecules by antigen-presenting cells, ultimately lead to production of the anti-CCP antibody. The anti-CCP antibodies form immune complexes with citrullinated proteins, which bind inflammatory cells via their Fc receptors and induce inflammation and joint destruction through various immune cascades, just as in RA.[28]

A recent study demonstrated a correlation between colonization of a specific intestinal bacteria, *Prevotella copri*, and the development of RA. This bacteria was identified in the intestines of 75% of patients with new-onset RA compared to 21% of normal healthy individuals. According to this study, *P. copri* could be a causative factor in developing RA. But this is not enough to conclude that colonization may be an RA-inducing factor. To confirm a causative role for this bacteria, prospective studies of healthy individuals carrying *P. copri* in their intestine compared to other healthy non-carriers should be carried out.[29,30] Similar to previous indications and associations, no prospective studies have been conducted to prove the relationship between these infections and the development of RA.

These data support previous reports indicating that infections may play a seminal role in autoimmunity in general and in the pathogenesis of RA in particular. In the coming years we believe that researchers will pursue the exact mechanisms by which this association is executed.

REFERENCES

1. Benedek TG. The history of bacteriologic concepts of rheumatic fever and rheumatoid arthritis. *Semin Arthritis Rheum* 2006;**36**(2):109–23.
2. Arnson Y, Shoenfeld Y, Amital H. Effects of tobacco smoke on immunity, inflammation and autoimmunity. *J Autoimmun* 2010;**34**(3):J258–65.
3. Perricone C, Agmon-Levin N, Shoenfeld Y. Novel pebbles in the mosaic of autoimmunity. *BMC Med* 2013;**11**:101.
4. Shoenfeld Y, Blank M, Abu-Shakra M, et al. The mosaic of autoimmunity: prediction, autoantibodies, and therapy in autoimmune diseases–2008. *Isr Med Assoc J* 2008;**10**(1):13–19.
5. Shoenfeld Y, Zandman-Goddard G, Stojanovich L, et al. The mosaic of autoimmunity: hormonal and environmental factors involved in autoimmune diseases–2008. *Isr Med Assoc J* 2008;**10**(1):8–12.
6. Shoenfeld Y, Gilburd B, Abu-Shakra M, et al. The mosaic of autoimmunity: genetic factors involved in autoimmune diseases–2008. *Isr Med Assoc J* 2008;**10**(1):3–7.

7. Bieber V, Cohen AD, Freud T, Agmon-Levin N, Gertel S, Amital H. Autoimmune smoke and fire—coexisting rheumatoid arthritis and chronic obstructive pulmonary disease: a cross-sectional analysis. *Immunol Res* 2013;**56**(2–3):261–6.

8. Goldman K, Gertel S, Amital H. Anti-citrullinated peptide antibodies is more than an accurate tool for diagnosis of rheumatoid arthritis. *Isr Med Assoc J* 2013;**15**(9):516–19.

9. van der Woude D, Rantapaa-Dahlqvist S, Ioan-Facsinay A, et al. Epitope spreading of the anti-citrullinated protein antibody response occurs before disease onset and is associated with the disease course of early arthritis. *Ann Rheum Dis* 2010;**69**(8):1554–61.

10. Canhao H, Rodrigues AM, Mourao AF, et al. Comparative effectiveness and predictors of response to tumour necrosis factor inhibitor therapies in rheumatoid arthritis. *Rheumatology (Oxford)* 2012;**51**(11):2020–6.

11. Park SJ, Shin JI. The effect of smoking on response and drug survival in rheumatoid arthritis patients treated with their first anti-TNF drug: comments on the article by Soderlin et al. *Scand J Rheumatol* 2012;**41**(5):411–12.

12. Soderlin MK, Petersson IF, Geborek P. The effect of smoking on response and drug survival in rheumatoid arthritis patients treated with their first anti-TNF drug. *Scand J Rheumatol* 2012;**41**(1):1–9.

13. Willemze A, van der Woude D, Ghidey W, et al. The interaction between HLA shared epitope alleles and smoking and its contribution to autoimmunity against several citrullinated antigens. *Arthritis Rheum* 2011;**63**(7):1823–32.

14. Bogdanos DP, Smyk DS, Invernizzi P, et al. Infectome: a platform to trace infectious triggers of autoimmunity. *Autoimmun Rev* 2013;**12**(7):726–40.

15. Meron MK, Amital H, Shepshelovich D, et al. Infectious aspects and the etiopathogenesis of rheumatoid arthritis. *Clin Rev Allergy Immunol* 2010;**38**(2–3):287–91.

16. Rigante D, Mazzoni MB, Esposito S. The cryptic interplay between systemic lupus erythematosus and infections. *Autoimmun Rev* 2014;**13**(2):96–102.

17. Soderlin MK, Kautiainen H, Puolakkainen M, et al. Infections preceding early arthritis in southern Sweden: a prospective population-based study. *J Rheumatol* 2003;**30**(3):459–64.

18. Soderlin MK, Bergsten U, Svensson B. Patient-reported events preceding the onset of rheumatoid arthritis: possible clues to aetiology. *Musculoskeletal Care* 2011;**9**(1):25–31.

19. Ramirez AS, Rosas A, Hernandez-Beriain JA, et al. Relationship between rheumatoid arthritis and Mycoplasma pneumoniae: a case-control study. *Rheumatology (Oxford)* 2005;**44**(7):912–14.

20. Langevitz P, Bank I, Zemer D, Book M, Pras M. Treatment of resistant rheumatoid arthritis with minocycline: an open study. *J Rheumatol* 1992;**19**(10):1502–4.

21. Barzilai O, Sherer Y, Ram M, Izhaky D, Anaya JM, Shoenfeld Y. Epstein-Barr virus and cytomegalovirus in autoimmune diseases: are they truly notorious? A preliminary report. *Ann N Y Acad Sci* 2007;**1108**:567–77.

22. Barzilai O, Sherer Y, Ram M, Izhaky D, Anaya JM, Shoenfeld Y. Epstein-Barr virus and cytomegalovirus in autoimmune diseases: are they truly notorious? A preliminary report. *Ann N Y Acad Sci* 2007;**1108**:567–77.

23. Amedei A, Bergman MP, Appelmelk BJ, et al. Molecular mimicry between *Helicobacter pylori* antigens and H+, K+ −adenosine triphosphatase in human gastric autoimmunity. *J Exp Med* 2003;**198**(8):1147–56.

24. Wegner N, Lundberg K, Kinloch A, et al. Autoimmunity to specific citrullinated proteins gives the first clues to the etiology of rheumatoid arthritis. *Immunol Rev* 2010;**233**(1):34–54.

25. Rashid T, Ebringer A. Rheumatoid arthritis in smokers could be linked to Proteus urinary tract infections. *Med Hypotheses* 2008;**70**(5):975–80.

26. Karlson EW, Deane K. Environmental and gene-environment interactions and risk of rheumatoid arthritis. *Rheum Dis Clin North Am* 2012;**38**(2):405–26.

27. Liao YT, He L, Meng HX, Li P, Sha YQ, Wang XY. Detection of periodontal pathogens from saliva of type 2 diabetic patients in urban area of Beijing. *Zhonghua Kou Qiang Yi Xue Za Zhi* 2013;**48**(3):144–9.

28. Liao F, Li Z, Wang Y, Shi B, Gong Z, Cheng X. Porphyromonas gingivalis may play an important role in the pathogenesis of periodontitis-associated rheumatoid arthritis. *Med Hypotheses* 2009;**72**(6):732–5.

29. Scher JU, Abramson SB. Periodontal disease, Porphyromonas gingivalis, and rheumatoid arthritis: what triggers autoimmunity and clinical disease? *Arthritis Res Ther* 2013;**15**(5):122.

30. Scher JU, Sczesnak A, Longman RS, et al. Expansion of intestinal Prevotella copri correlates with enhanced susceptibility to arthritis. *Elife* 2013;**2**:e01202.

CHAPTER 44

Infection and Systemic Sclerosis

Alexandra Balbir-Gurman[*,†,1], **Yolanda Braun-Moscovici**[*,†]

[*]B. Shine Rheumatology Unit, Rambam Health Care Campus, Haifa, Israel
[†]Bruce and Ruth Rappoport Faculty of Medicine, Technion-Israel Institute of Technology, Haifa, Israel
[1]Corresponding Author: a_balbir@rambam.health.gov.il

1 INTRODUCTION

Systemic sclerosis (SSc) is a chronic autoimmune disease (AID) characterized by microangiopathy, inflammation, autoantibody production, and fibrosis. SSc has a diverse presentation and severity related to the extent of skin and internal organ fibrosis.[1] Main SSc features include Raynaud's phenomenon (RP), digital ulcers (DUs), lung and heart involvement, renal crisis, gastric antrum vascular ectasia, telangiectasias, arthropathy, myopathy, and gastrointestinal tract (GIT) dysmotility. Abnormal immune response in SSc is attributed to a higher number of CD4+ and γ/δ-T cell receptor (TCR)+lymphocytes and a reduced number of CD8+ T lymphocytes, release of Tumor Necrosis Factor alpha (TNF-α), interleukins (IL-1, IL-6, IL-1R), Transforming Growth Factor beta (TGF-β) and Connective Tissue Growth Factor (CTGF), and chemokines that are crucial for sending leukocytes to the area of cell damage and producing autoantibodies to topoisomerase (ATA), centromere (ACA), RNA polymerase, endothelial cells (ECs), fibrillin, and others.

Some authors have connected SSc etiology to genetic predisposition related to Major Histocompatibility Complex (MHC) class II, mainly Human Leukocyte Antigen (HLA) DRB[2] and environmental factors (e.g., silica, epoxy resins, solvents). A higher incidence of antibodies to infective microorganisms in SSc patients, as well as infectious complications in SSc patients, supports the hypothesis that infection could be linked to SSc.[3,4] We review existing data on infections and SSc.

2 INFECTION AS POSSIBLE FACTOR IN SSc PATHOGENESIS

Microorganisms may induce abnormal autoimmune response in patients with SSc via several mechanisms.

Infection and Autoimmunity
http://dx.doi.org/10.1016/B978-0-444-63269-2.00073-8

735

- Adjuvant effect:

    An infective agent triggers Toll-like receptors (TLRs) leading to the activation of antigen presenting cells and lymphocytes, as well as the amplification of the immune response.
- Molecular mimicry:

    TCRs may recognize the proteins of the host and the infecting organisms in the same way.
- Microchimerism:

    Infections may trigger an interaction between γ/δ T cells and auto-reactive microchimeric T lymphocytes.
- Bystander activation:

    The presence of a virus stimulates an inflammatory cascade with proinflammatory cytokine production, progressing to bystander activation and autoreactivity with recognizing of superantigens.
- Release of self-antigens:

    Invasion by a virus leads to the apoptosis of infected cells and excessive release of self-antigens.

Several viruses have been linked to SSc pathogenesis, including human parvovirus B19 (hPVB19), human cytomegalovirus (hCMV), Epstein–Barr virus (EBV), and human herpes virus (hHHV).

2.1 Human Parvovirus B19

hPVB19 is an ssDNA nonenveloped capsid virus with three genomes: Structural Viral Protein (VP1), VP2, and Non-structural Viral Protein (NS1). When hPVB19 binds to the P antigen on erythrocytes, erythroid line cells, megakaryocytes, ECs, fetal liver cells and heart cells,[5] this binding may result in aplastic anemia, erythema infectiosum, myocarditis, myositis, rheumatoid arthritis (RA), systemic lupus erythematosus and vasculitis. hPVB19 induces changes in synovial fibroblasts phenotype similar to those seen in RA.[6] hPVB19 may induce the production of antinuclear antibodies (ANA). Patients with persistent hPVB19 infection produce anti-VP Immunoglobulin G (IgG) antibodies responsible for associated clinical features: rash caused by antibodies to keratin; arthritis caused by antibodies to collagen type II; anti-phospholipid syndrome caused by antibodies to phospholipids. Virus protein NS1 may induce cytotoxicity, excess TNF-α and IL-6, and immune complex formation.[7,8] Among nine SSc patients seropositive for hPVB19, three had positive polymerase chain reaction (PCR) in the skin, and three had it in bone marrow.[9] Researchers also demonstrated the persistence of VP1 and VP2 genotypes and viral mRNA in the skin and bone marrow of patients with SSc.[10] In addition, the hPVB19 genome was detected in the myocardium of SSc patients with myocarditis[11] and in lung tissue of patient with scleroderma lung disease (SLD).[12]

2.2 Cytomegalovirus

hCMV belongs to the B-Herpesviridae family with enveloped dsDNA. After acute episodes, latent hCMV is incorporated into mononuclear and ECs. This incorporation may be followed by apoptosis, abnormal clearance of damaged cytoplasmic and nuclear proteins, induction of abnormal immune response and activation of epitope spreading.[13] Researchers have implicated hCMV in several vasculopathies, such as atherosclerosis, allograft rejection and graft-versus-host disease.[14–16] In interferon (IFN) deficient mice, total body irradiation resulted in microangiopathy, myofibroblasts proliferation, and upregulation of TGF-β only in animals infected with CMV.[17] hCMV-related chemokine receptor US28 induced smooth muscle cell proliferation.[18] hCMV may interact with TLRs and dendritic cells with IFN-α production, B cell stimulation, and autoantibody production.[19] CMV also induced neo-intima formation in immune-compromised mice.[20] Homology between hCMV protein UL70 and topoisomerase was demonstrated.[21] hCMV releases its vasculotoxicity via late protein UL94 and ECs surface integrin Novelantigen-2 (NAG2). In addition, researchers have observed the binding of anti-UL94 and anti-NAG2 antibodies to ECs and fibroblasts inducing ECs apoptosis and fibroblasts proliferation.[22,23] High levels of anti-hCMV, anti-UL94 and anti-NAG2 antibodies were reported in SSc patients.[24–27] SSc following hCMV infection was reported as well.[27] Microchimerism may be responsible for the infiltration of skin and affected tissues by maternal cells. Thus, hCMV may cause the proliferation of microchimeric T cells.[28]

During severe hCMV infection, one SSc patient reportedly showed significant improvement, and the authors of that study suggested that hCMV "halted" the main SSc pathogenic pathways (molecular mimicry, upregulation of TGF-β1, expression of integrins)[29], as might happen with Hematopoietic stem cell transplantation (HSCT).

2.3 Epstein–Barr Virus

EBV has a unique capacity to infect and persist in B lymphocytes.[30] CD8 + T cells are responsible for the deletion of infected B cells. In SSc, the number of

CD8 + T cells falls, and the deletion of infected B lymphocytes is impaired. The pathologic vicious cycle includes circulation of autoreactive EBV-infected B cells and their targeting of specific organs followed by the tropism of CD4+ helpers, tissue and B cell damage, and release of EBV.[31,32] Recently, evidence has linked EBV to the HLA DRB1 and HLA-DQB1 regions of MHC class II.[33]

Studies have documented elevated IgM to EBV capsid antigen in patients with SSc.[34] SSc developed in a child with infectious mononucleosis.[35] Reactivity of IgG and IgM to EBV extractable antigen was high in SSc patients,[36] and in five lung biopsies from SLD patients, EBV DNA was detected.[37]

2.4 Other Viruses

Authors have also reported a connection between SSc and hepatitis C virus (HCV).[38–40] New-onset SSc was reported in an HCV patient under IFN-α therapy.[41–43] Fatal cryoglobulinemic vasculitis was reported in four SSc patients.[44] Reactivation of HHV-6 not related to immunosuppression was observed in 37 SSc patients.[45] In several cases, immunization against viruses was closely related to the onset of AID[46]: morphea developed after HBV and antitetanus immunization,[47–49] and the morphea appeared at the site of vaccination.[50]

Some viral infections may cause direct endothelial damage (hCMV), molecular mimicry (hPVB19), cytotoxicity (hPVB19, EBV) with cell breakdown, and production of superantigens (hPVB19, hCMV, EBV), B cell activation (EBV), microchimerism, and T cell response (hCMV).[51–54]

2.5 Bacterial Infections

Data on bacteria and SSc pathogenesis is conflicting. Screens for the presence of bacterial infection in 18 skin biopsies from SSc patients, for Chlamydia infections, and for "Pan Bacteria" PCR were negative.[55] Positive antibodies to *Borrelia burgdorferi* and high titers of ANA were reported in morphea patients in one study but not confirmed in another.[56,57] *Helicobacter pylori* (HP) is a gram-negative bacillus linked to peptic disease and gastric tumors.[58,59] Eradication of HP led to resolution or improvement of primary RP,[60] but it was not confirmed in SSc patients.[61] High rates of a virulent HP strain, with expression of cytotoxin-associated gene A, correlated with severe GIT involvement and tenosynovitis.[62] HP-related gastric lymphoma was cured after eradication of HP, and the course of SSc was uneventful.[63]

3 THE ROLE OF INFECTION IN THE COURSE OF SSc

Infection in the course of SSc may be serious: 24.5–52.7% of non-SSc-related deaths were attributed to infection.[64–67] Among nine SSc patients in intensive care units, three had severe infections on admission, and seven patients died (five from fatal sepsis).[68] Ischemic DUs appeared in about 30% of SSc patients, and more than 50% of DUs were infected, leading to delayed healing, necrosis, gangrene, and amputations. Ischemic skin ulcers are localized above bony prominences, and they are extremely prone to infection that may be complicated by osteomyelitis, septic arthritis, and sepsis. *Staphylococcus aureus* and *Escherichia coli* were the main pathogens in such cases, followed by *Pseudomonas aeruginosa, Enterococcus fecalis*, and *Staphylococcus epidermidis*.[69–71]

In SSc patients with esophageal hypomotility, aspiration pneumonia and sepsis were often reported in non-scleroderma-related deaths. A high rate of invasive pneumococcal disease was also reported in SSc patients,[72] and the presence of microorganisms in bronchialveolar lavage has been correlated with the deterioration of lung functions.[73] SSc patients with pneumatosis cystoides intestinales developed Klebsiela peritonitis and septic arthritis, and later fatal aspiration pneumonia.[74] Among rare infections, researchers have reported nocardia,[75] candida,[70] *Mycobacterium kansasii*,[76] actinomycosis,[77] and *Cryptococcus neoformans*[78]. The use of proton pump inhibitors in SSc increased the risk of *Clostridium difficile*.[79] Treatment with oral cyclophosphamide for SLD was complicated by pneumonia, related to neutropenia.[80] Fatal Gram-negative sepsis in a patient with SLD developed 6 months after cyclophosphamide followed by rituximab treatment,[81] and fatal opportunistic infection has been reported in an SSc patient after allogenic HSCT.[82] Multiple studies have shows that aggressive immunosuppression and autologous HSCT can be accompanied by multiple infectious events SSc patients, including fatal EBV-associated lymphoma (1), CMV-gastroenteritis (1), central line-related bacteremia (11) and hHHV reactivation (6).[83] Lung transplantation in seven SLD patients was also complicated by bacterial pneumonia (9) and hHHV (1).[84]

4 CONCLUSIONS

Given the pathogenic complexity and unknown etiology of SSc, infection, especially involving several viruses (hPVB19, hCMV, EBV), seems to be a likely cause, particularly in genetically predisposed patients. The mechanism of viral invasion and behavior in the affected host's immune cells, including autoimmune mechanisms such as the adjuvant effect, molecular mimicry, microchimerism, and autoreactivity, may support this suggestion. Is infection a consequence of abnormal host defence or does it trigger the emergence of SSc? This remains a question to be resolved. Bacterial infections have a negative impact on SSc course and prognosis. An awareness of the main infectious complications of SSc serves the clinical approach through early recognition, proper treatment, and improved outcome.

REFERENCES

1. van den Hoogen F, Khanna D, Fransen J, Johnson SR, Baron M, Tyndall A, et al. 2013 classification criteria for systemic sclerosis: an American College of Rheumatology/European League against Rheumatism collaborative initiative. *Arthritis Rheum* 2013;**65**:2737–47.
2. Azzouz DF, Rak JM, Fajardy I, Allanore Y, Tiev KP, Farge-Bancel D, et al. Comparing HLA shared epitopes in French Caucasian patients with scleroderma. *PLoS One* 2012;**7**: e36870.
3. Hamamdzic D, Kasman LM, LeRoy EC. Role of infectious agents in the pathogenesis of systemic sclerosis. *Curr Opin Rheumatol* 2002;**14**:694–8.
4. Jimenez SA, Batuman O. Immunopathogenesis of systemic sclerosis: possible role of retroviruses. *Autoimmunity* 1993;**16**:225–33.
5. Kerr JR. Pathogenesis of human parvovirus B19 in rheumatic disease. *Ann Rheum Dis* 2000;**59**:672–83.
6. Ray NB, Nieva DR, Seftor EA, Khalkhali-Ellis Z, Naides SJ. Induction of an invasive phenotype by human parvovirus B19 in normal human synovial fibroblasts. *Arthritis Rheum* 2001;**44**:1582–6.
7. Zakrzewska K, Corcioli F, Carlsen KM, Giuggioli D, Fanci R, Rinieri A, et al. Human parvovirus B19 (B19V) infection in systemic sclerosis patients. *Intervirology* 2009;**52**:279–82.
8. Lunardi C, Tinazzi E, Bason C, Dolcino M, Corrocher R, Puccetti A. Human parvovirus B19 infection and autoimmunity. *Autoimmun Rev* 2008;**8**:116–20.
9. Magro CM, Nuovo G, Ferri C, Crowson AN, Giuggioli D, Sebastiani M. Parvoviral infection of endothelial cells and stromal fibroblasts: a possible pathogenetic role in scleroderma. *J Cutan Pathol* 2004;**31**:43–50.
10. Ferri C, Zakrzewska K, Longombardo G, Giuggioli D, Storino FA, Pasero G, et al. Parvovirus B19 infection of bone marrow in systemic sclerosis patients. *Clin Exp Rheumatol* 1999;**17**:718–20.
11. Pieroni M, De Santis M, Zizzo G, Bosello S, Smaldone C, Campioni M, et al. Recognizing and treating myocarditis in recent-onset systemic sclerosis heart disease: potential utility of immunosuppressive therapy in cardiac damage progression. *Semin Arthritis Rheum* 2014;**43**:526–35.
12. Ghinoi A, Mascia MT, Giuggioli D, Magistro R, Barbolini G, Magro CM, et al. Coexistence of non-specific and usual interstitial pneumonia in a patient with severe cystic scleroderma lung involvement and parvovirus B19 infection. *Clin Exp Rheumatol* 2005;**23**:431–3.
13. Zhou YF, Yu ZX, Wanishsawad C, Shou M, Epstein SE. The immediate early gene products of human cytomegalovirus increase vascular smooth muscle cell migration,

proliferation, and expression of PDGF beta-receptor. *Biochem Biophys Res Commun* 1999;**256**:608–13.

14. Magro CM, Crowson AN, Ferri C. Cytomegalovirus-associated cutaneous vasculopathy and scleroderma sans inclusion body change. *Hum Pathol* 2007;**38**:42–9.

15. Pandey JP, LeRoy EC. Human cytomegalovirus and the vasculopathies of autoimmune diseases (especially scleroderma), allograft rejection, and coronary restenosis. *Arthritis Rheum* 1998;**41**:10–15.

16. Lunardi C, Dolcino M, Peterlana D, Bason C, Navone R, Tamassia N, et al. Endothelial cells' activation and apoptosis induced by a subset of antibodies against human cytomegalovirus: relevance to the pathogenesis of atherosclerosis. *PLoS One* 2007;**2**:e473.

17. Hamamdzic D, Harley RA, Hazen-Martin D, LeRoy EC. MCMV induces neointima in IFN-gammaR-/- mice: intimal cell apoptosis and persistent proliferation of myofibroblasts. *BMC Musculoskelet Disord* 2001;**2**:3.

18. Streblow DN, Soderberg-Naucler C, Vieira J, Smith P, Wakabayashi E, Ruchti F, et al. The human cytomegalovirus chemokine receptor US28 mediates vascular smooth muscle cell migration. *Cell* 1999;**99**:511–20.

19. York MR, Nagai T, Mangini AJ, Lemaire R, van Seventer JM, Lafyatis R. A macrophage marker, Siglec-1, is increased on circulating monocytes in patients with systemic sclerosis and induced by type I interferons and toll-like receptor agonists. *Arthritis Rheum* 2007;**56**:1010–20.

20. Presti RM, Pollock JL, Dal Canto AJ, O'Guin AK, Virgin 4th. HW. Interferon gamma regulates acute and latent murine cytomegalovirus infection and chronic disease of the great vessels. *J Exp Med* 1998;**188**:577–88.

21. Muryoi T, Kasturi KN, Kafina MJ, Cram DS, Harrison LC, Sasaki T, et al. Antitopoisomerase I monoclonal autoantibodies from scleroderma patients and tight skin mouse interact with similar epitopes. *J Exp Med* 1992;**175**:1103–9.

22. Lunardi C, Dolcino M, Peterlana D, Bason C, Navone R, Tamassia N, et al. Antibodies against human cytomegalovirus in the pathogenesis of systemic sclerosis: a gene array approach. *PLoS Med* 2006;**3**:e2.

23. Michelson S, Alcami J, Kim SJ, Danielpour D, Bachelerie F, Picard L, et al. Human cytomegalovirus infection induces transcription and secretion of transforming growth factor beta 1. *J Virol* 1994;**68**:5730–7.

24. Lunardi C, Bason C, Navone R, Millo E, Damonte G, Corrocher R, et al. Systemic sclerosis immunoglobulin G autoantibodies bind the human cytomegalovirus late protein UL94 and induce apoptosis in human endothelial cells. *Nat Med* 2000;**6**:1183–6.

25. Neihart M, Kuchen S, Distler O, Bruhlmann P, Michel BA, Gay RA, et al. Increased serum level of antibodies against human cytomegalovirus and prevalence of autoantibodies in systemic sclerosis. *Arthritis Rheum* 1999;**42**:389–92.

26. Namboodiri AM, Rocca KM, Kuwana M, Pandey JP. Antibodies to human cytomegalovirus protein UL83 in systemic sclerosis. *Clin Exp Rheumatol* 2006;**24**:176–8.

27. Pastano R, Dell'Agnola C, Bason C, Gigli F, Rabascio C, Puccetti A, et al. Antibodies against human cytomegalovirus late protein UL94 in the pathogenesis of scleroderma-like skin lesions in chronic graft-versus-host disease. *Int Immunol* 2012;**24**:583–91.

28. Artlett CM, Smith JB, Jimenez SA. Identification of fetal DNA and cells in skin lesions from women with systemic sclerosis. *N Engl J Med* 1998;**338**:1186–91.

29. Moinzadeh P, Khan K, Ong VH, Denton CP. Sustained improvement of diffuse systemic sclerosis following human cytomegalovirus infection offers insight into pathogenesis and therapy. *Rheumatology (Oxford)* 2012;**51**:2296–8.

30. Niller HH, Wolf H, Minarovits J. Regulation and dysregulation of Epstein-Barr virus latency: implications for the development of autoimmune diseases. *Autoimmunity* 2008;**41**:298–328.

31. Fattal I, Shental N, Molad Y, Gabrielli A, Pokroy-Shapira E, Oren S, et al. Epstein-Barr virus antibodies mark systemic lupus erythematosus and scleroderma patients negative for anti-DNA. *Immunology* 2014;**141**:276–85.

32. Pender MP. CD8+ T-cell deficiency, Epstein-Barr virus infection, vitamin D deficiency, and steps to autoimmunity: a unifying hypothesis. *Autoimmune Dis* 2012;**2012**:189096.

33. Rubicz R, Yolken R, Drigalenko E, Carless MA, Dyer TD, Bauman L, et al. A genome-wide integrative genomic study localizes genetic factors influencing antibodies against Epstein-Barr virus nuclear antigen 1 (EBNA-1). *PLoS Genet* 2013;**9**:e1003147.

34. Arnson Y, Amital H, Guiducci S, Matucci-Cerinic M, Valentini G, Barzilai O, et al. The role of infections in the immunopathogensis of systemic sclerosis—evidence from serological studies. *Ann NY Acad Sci* 2009;**1173**:627–32.

35. Urano J, Kohno H, Watanabe T. Unusual case of progressive systemic sclerosis with onset in early childhood and following infectious mononucleosis. *Eur J Pediatr* 1981;**136**:285–9.

36. Vaughan JH, Valbracht JR, Nguyen MD, Handley HH, Smith RS, Patrick K, et al. Epstein-Barr virus-induced autoimmune responses. I. Immunoglobulin M autoantibodies to proteins mimicking and not mimicking Epstein-Barr virus nuclear antigen-1. *J Clin Invest* 1995;**95**:1306–15.

37. Tsukamoto K, Hayakawa H, Sato A, Chida K, Nakamura H, Miura K. Involvement of Epstein-Barr virus latent membrane protein 1 in disease progression in patients with idiopathic pulmonary fibrosis. *Thorax* 2000;**55**:958–61.

38. Abu-Shakra M, Sukenik S, Buskila D. Systemic sclerosis: another rheumatic disease associated with hepatitis C virus infection. *Clin Rheumatol* 2000;**19**:378–80.

39. Yamamoto M, Yamamoto T, Tsuboi R. Discoid lupus erythematosus in a patient with scleroderma and hepatitis C infection. *Rheumatol Int* 2010;**30**:969–71.

40. Poggi G, Villani L, Sottotetti F, Tagliaferri B, Montagna B, Amatu A, et al. Treatment of chronic hepatitis C in a patient affected by systemic sclerosis. *Gastroenterol Res Pract* 2009;**2009**:475390.

41. Beretta L, Caronni M, Vanoli M, Scorza R. Systemic sclerosis after interferon-alpha therapy for myeloproliferative disorders. *Br J Dermatol* 2002;**147**:385–6.

42. Solans R, Bosch JA, Esteban I, Villardell M. Systemic sclerosis developing in association with the use of after interferon alpha therapy for chronic viral hepatitis. *Clin Exp Rheumatol* 2004;**22**:625–8.

43. Tahara H, Kojima A, Hirokawa T, Oyama T, Naganuma A, Maruta S, et al. Systemic sclerosis after interferon alphacon-1 therapy for hepatitis C. *Intern Med* 2007;**46**:473–6.

44. Giuggioli D, Manfredi A, Colaci M, Manzini CU, Antonelli A, Ferri C. Systemic sclerosis and cryoglobulinemia: our experience with overlapping syndrome of scleroderma and severe cryoglobulinemic vasculitis and review of the literature. *Autoimmun Rev* 2013;**12**:1058–63.

45. Broccolo F, Drago F, Cassina G, Fava A, Fusetti L, Matteoli B, et al. Selective reactivation of human herpesvirus 6 in patients with autoimmune connective tissue diseases. *J Med Virol* 2013;**85**:1925–34.

46. Molina V, Shoenfeld Y. Infection, vaccines and other environmental triggers of autoimmunity. *Autoimmunity* 2005;**38**:235–45.

47. Benmously Mlika R, Kenani N, Badri T, Hammami H, Hichri J, Haouet S, et al. Morphea profunda in a young infant after hepatitis B vaccination. *J Am Acad Dermatol* 2010;**63**:1111–2.

48. Schmutz JL, Posth M, Granel F, Trechot P, Barbaud A. Localized scleroderma after hepatitis B vaccination. *Presse Med* 2000;**29**:1046.

49. Drago F, Rampini P, Lugani C, Rebora A. Generalized morphoea after antitetanus vaccination. *Clin Exp Dermatol* 1998;**23**:142.

50. Torrelo A, Suárez J, Colmenero I, Azorín D, Perera A, Zambrano A. Deep morphea after vaccination in two young children. *Pediatr Dermatol* 2006;**23**:484–7.

51. Grossman C, Dovrish Z, Shoenfeld Y, Amital H. Do infections facilitate the emergence of systemic sclerosis? *Autoimmun Rev* 2011;**10**:244–7.

52. Randone SB, Guiducci S, Cerinic MM. Systemic sclerosis and infections. *Autoimmun Rev* 2008;**8**:36–40.

53. Amital H, Govoni M, Maya R, Meroni PL, Ori B, Shoenfeld Y, et al. Role of infectious agents in systemic rheumatic diseases. *Clin Exp Rheumatol* 2008;**26**:S27–32.

54. Moroncini G, Mori S, Tonnini C, Gabrielli A. Role of viral infections in the etiopathogenesis of systemic sclerosis. *Clin Exp Rheumatol* 2013;**31**:3–7.

55. Mayes MD, Whittum-Hudson JA, Oszust C, Gérard HC, Hudson AP. Lack of evidence for bacterial infections in skin in patients with systemic sclerosis. *Am J Med Sci* 2009;**337**:233–5.

56. Prinz JC, Kutasi Z, Weisenseel P, Pótó L, Battyáni Z, Ruzicka T. "Borrelia-associated early-onset morphea": a particular type of scleroderma in childhood and adolescence with high titer antinuclear antibodies? Results of a cohort analysis and presentation of three cases. *J Am Acad Dermatol* 2009;**60**:248–55.

57. Dillon WI, Saed GM, Fivenson DP. Borrelia burgdorferi DNA is undetectable by polymerase chain reaction in skin lesions of morphea, scleroderma, or lichen sclerosus et atrophicus of patients from North America. *J Am Acad Dermatol* 1995;**33**:617–20.

58. Kalabay L, Fekete B, Czirják L, Horváth L, Daha MR, Veres A, et al. Helicobacter pylori infection in connective tissue disorders is associated with high levels of antibodies to mycobacterial hsp65 but not to human hsp60. *Helicobacter* 2002;**7**:250–6.

59. Radić M, Kaliterna DM, Bonacin D, Vergles JM, Radić J, Fabijanić D, et al. Is Helicobacter pylori infection a risk factor for disease severity in systemic sclerosis? *Rheumatol Int* 2013;**33**:2943–8.

60. Gasbarrini A, Massari I, Serricchio M, Tondi P, De Luca A, Franceschi F, et al. Helicobacter pylori eradication ameliorates primary Raynaud's phenomenon. *Dig Dis Sci* 1998;**43**:1641–5.

61. Sulli A, Seriolo B, Savarino V, Cutolo M. Lack of correlation between gastric Helicobacter pylori infection and primary or secondary Raynaud's phenomenon in patients with systemic sclerosis. *J Rheumatol* 2000;**27**:1820–1.

62. Danese S, Zoli A, Cremonini F, Gasbarrini A. High prevalence of Helicobacter pylori type I virulent strains in patients with systemic sclerosis. *J Rheumatol* 2000;**27**:1568–9.

63. Arnaud L, Chryssostalis A, Terris B, Pavy S, Chaussade S, Kahan A, et al. Systemic sclerosis and gastric MALT lymphoma. *Joint Bone Spine* 2006;**73**:105–8.

64. Sampaio-Barros PD, Bortoluzzo AB, Marangoni RG, Rocha LF, Del Rio AP, Samara AM, et al. Survival, causes of death, and prognostic factors in systemic sclerosis: analysis of 947 Brazilian patients. *J Rheumatol* 2012;**39**:1971–8.

65. Foocharoen C, Siriphannon Y, Mahakkanukrauh A, Suwannaroj S, Nanagara R. Incidence rate and causes of infection in Thai systemic sclerosis patients. *Int J Rheum Dis* 2012;**15**:277–83.

66. Hashimoto A, Tejima S, Tono T, Suzuki M, Tanaka S, Matsui T, et al. Predictors of survival and causes of death in Japanese patients with systemic sclerosis. *J Rheumatol* 2011;**38**:1931–9.

67. Tyndall AJ, Bannert B, Vonk M, Airò P, Cozzi F, Carreira PE, et al. Causes and risk factors for death in systemic sclerosis: a study from the EULAR Scleroderma Trials and Research (EUSTAR) database. *Ann Rheum Dis* 2010;**69**:1809–15.

68. Shalev T, Haviv Y, Segal E, Ehrenfeld M, Pauzner R, Levy Y, et al. Outcome of patients with scleroderma admitted to intensive care unit. A report of nine cases. *Clin Exp Rheumatol* 2006;**24**:380–6.

69. Steen V, Denton CP, Pope JE, Matucci-Cerinic M. Digital ulcers: overt vascular disease in systemic sclerosis. *Rheumatology (Oxford)* 2009;**48**:19–24.

70. Alivernini S, De Santis M, Tolusso B, Mannocci A, Bosello SL, Peluso G, et al. Skin ulcers in systemic sclerosis: determinants of presence and predictive factors of healing. *J Am Acad Dermatol* 2009;**60**:426–35.

71. Giuggioli D, Manfredi A, Colaci M, Lumetti F, Ferri C. Scleroderma digital ulcers complicated by infection with fecal pathogens. *Arthritis Care Res (Hoboken)* 2012;**64**:295–7.

72. Wotton CJ, Goldacre MJ. Risk of invasive pneumococcal disease in people admitted to hospital with selected immune-mediated diseases: record linkage cohort analyses. *J Epidemiol Community Health* 2012;**66**:1177–81.

73. De Santis M, Bosello S, La Torre G, Capuano A, Tolusso B, Pagliari G, et al. Functional, radiological and biological markers of alveolitis and infections of the lower respiratory tract in patients with systemic sclerosis. *Respir Res* 2005;**6**:96.

74. Balbir-Gurman A, Brook OR, Chermesh I, Braun-Moscovici Y. Pneumatosis cystoides intestinalis in scleroderma-related conditions. *Intern Med J* 2012;**42**:323–9.

75. Auzary C, Mouthon L, Soilleux M, Cohen P, Boiron P, Guillevin L. Localized subcutaneous Nocardia farcinica abscess in a women with overlap syndrome between scleroderma and polymyositis. *Ann Med Interne (Paris)* 1999;**150**:582–4.

76. Gerster JC, Duvoisin B, Dudler J, Berner IC. Tenosynovitis of the hand caused by Mycobacterium kansasii in a patient with scleroderma. *J Rheumatol* 2004;**31**:2523–5.

77. Marie I, Lahaxe L, Levesque H, Heliot P. Pulmonary actinomycosis in a patient with diffuse systemic sclerosis treated with infliximab. *QJM* 2008;**101**:419–21.

78. Zhou HX, Ning GZ, Feng SQ, Jia HW, Liu Y, Feng HY, et al. Cryptococcosis of lumbar vertebra in a patient with rheumatoid arthritis and scleroderma: case report and literature review. *BMC Infect Dis* 2013;**13**:128.

79. Laria A, Zoli A, Gremese E, Ferraccioli GF. Proton pump inhibitors in rheumatic diseases: clinical practice, drug interactions, bone fractures and risk for infection. *Reumatismo* 2011;**63**:5–10.

80. Tashkin DP, Elashoff R, Clements PJ, Goldin J, Roth MD, Furst DE, et al. Cyclophosphamide versus placebo in scleroderma lung disease. *N Engl J Med* 2006;**354**:2655–66.

81. Braun-Moscovici Y, Butbul-Aviel Y, Guralnik L, Toledano K, Markovits D, Rozin A, et al. Rituximab: rescue therapy in life-threatening complications or refractory autoimmune diseases: a single center experience. *Rheumatol Int* 2013;**33**:1495–504.

82. Nash RA, McSweeney PA, Nelson JL, Wener M, Georges GE, Langston AA, et al. Allogeneic marrow transplantation in patients with severe systemic sclerosis: resolution of dermal fibrosis. *Arthritis Rheum* 2006;**54**:1982–6.

83. Nash RA, McSweeney PA, Crofford LJ, Abidi M, Chen CS, Godwin JD, et al. High-dose immunosuppressive therapy and autologous hematopoietic cell transplantation for severe systemic sclerosis: long-term follow-up of the US multicenter pilot study. *Blood* 2007;**110**:1388–96.

84. Shitrit D, Amital A, Peled N, Raviv Y, Medalion B, Saute M, et al. Lung transplantation in patients with scleroderma: case series, review of the literature, and criteria for transplantation. *Clin Transplant* 2009;**23**:178–83.

CHAPTER 45

Infection and Spondyloarthropathies

Michael Ehrenfeld
Rheumatic Disease Unit, Zabludowicz Center for Autoimmune Diseases, Chaim Sheba Medical Center, Tel Hashomer, Israel

1 INTRODUCTION

Spondyloarthropathies (SpAs) are a group of inflammatory rheumatic diseases characterized by axial and/or peripheral arthritis associated with enthesitis, dactylitis, and potential extra-articular manifestations involving the eyes, heart, lung, skin, gut, and genitourinary tract. This group of diseases includes the prototypical disease ankylosing spondylitis (AS), reactive arthritis (ReA) or spondyloarthritis, psoriatic arthritis (PsA) or spondyloarthritis, SpA associated with inflammatory bowel disease (IBD) (e.g. Crohn's disease or ulcerative colitis), undifferentiated SpA (uSpA), and juvenile-onset spondyloarthritis.[1-3] The two subsets of SpAs are those largely involving axial disease (AS and axial SpA) and those with predominantly peripheral manifestations (ReA, PsA, and IBD-associated SpA). The entire SpA group shares multiple clinical and radiological features, as well as common genetic predisposing factors.[3] SpAs typically involve the sacroiliac joints with sacroiliitis accompanied by a clinical presentation of inflammatory back pain, which often occurs with associated peripheral arthropathy, as well as the absence of rheumatoid factor and subcutaneous nodules. As a group, the SpAs tend toward familial aggregation and varying association with HLA-B27,[4] depending on the SPA subgroup and the population studied. However, researchers have identified a variety of other genes associated with this group of diseases. Although the strongest HLA-B27 association is with AS, its prevalence is also increased in other SpA subgroups.[4] The observed similarities in clinical manifestations and genetic predisposition suggest that these disorders share some pathogenic mechanisms. Despite the fact that the risk of developing SpA, and specifically AS, is largely genetically determined, genetic susceptibility is not sufficient, because an environmental

Infection and Autoimmunity
http://dx.doi.org/10.1016/B978-0-444-63269-2.00074-X

trigger must initiate the disease. Furthermore, the contribution that HLA–B27 makes to AS remains unknown. The overall prevalence of this group of SpAs is similar to that of rheumatoid arthritis.[5] New ASAS classification criteria for SpAs have been set in recent years and are now generally accepted and applied in clinical studies, using objective criteria, such as the presence of both HLA–B27 and specific MRI features, as well as other factors.[6–8] The new classification also gave birth to the novel entity of nonradiographic axial SpA, which is intended to describe patients not satisfying the modified New York Criteria.[9,10]

2 PATHOGENESIS OF SpAs AND ENVIRONMENTAL ASPECTS

The exact aetiology and pathogenesis of the SpAs remain unclear, but strong evidence suggests that genetics play a major role in an individual's susceptibility to this group of diseases. However, nongenetic environmental factors[11,12] seem to trigger certain responses in the genetically predisposed, leading to the release of proinflammatory cytokines such as tumor necrosis factor (TNF)–alfa. Researchers have evaluated the relative degrees to which environmental and genetic factors contribute to SpA pathogenesis, using the high degree of concordance of AS among twins.[11,13,14] Based on these studies and analyses, genetics contribute more than 90% of the overall causes of AS. Furthermore, the environmental factors contributing to the pathogenesis of SpAs are probably ubiquitous, such as enteric bacteria. Authors have long proposed infection as a triggering factor for SpAs, expressing varying degrees of certainty about this relationship for different SpA subgroups. Infection appears to be a probable trigger in ReA and a possible trigger in AS, but its role in PsA and IBD arthropathy remains unresolved.[15] HLA–B27 transgenic rats, which provide the animal model of AS, do not develop SpA when they are bred in a germ-free environment, and once transferred to a regular environment, the rats go on to develop a multisystem disease with features of SpA, including colitis, gastritis, peripheral arthritis, psoriasiform skin lesions, epididimo-orchitis, and spondylitis.[16] The HLA–B27 gene consists of multiple different alleles that encode over 100 different subtypes, many of which have yet to be studied for their disease association.[13] Although we still do not fully understand how HLA–B27 predisposes the individual to AS and related SpA, some of the known subtypes of HLA–B27 are prevalent enough that their relative strength of association with AS can be compared. HLA–B27 screening now yields a highly important marker used in the classification, diagnosis and referral of possible SpA patients to specialists.[7,17,18] HLA-B27-positive patients with AS have a significantly younger age of disease-onset, a higher prevalence of acute anterior uveitis and hip joint involvement and a higher rate of familial occurrence.[19,20] Further genetic epidemiological studies, as well as modern genomics- and proteomics-based approaches, have suggested the existence of at least six other predisposing genes for this group of diseases. Among these are HLA-B60 and HLA-DRB1 for AS, and HLA-Cw*0602, HLA-B38, and HLA-B39 for PsA. Recent genome-wide association studies have identified several novel non-MHC genetic associations with AS. AS appears to be connected to genes involved in peptide editing for loading onto class 1 MHC molecules, such as the endoplasmic reticulum aminopeptidase-1 (ERAP1 gene, formerly known as the ARTS-1 gene). AS may also be associated with genes such as IL1R2, IL-1A, ANTXR2, and gene deserts at 2p15 and 21q22.[12,21] In addition, cytokine genes, such as IL-1A and those involved in the Th17 network (IL-23R gene), have been associated with IBD and psoriasis. The association of AS with this gene has been reported to occur in multiple different populations but not in the Chinese population, and was first suggested when researchers asserted that the Th17 lymphocyte pathway may be involved in the disease. These findings imply the possibility of a therapy using an antibody that inhibits Th17 activity,[22] and, in fact, the most recent data indicate that structural damage is significantly inhibited in patients with PsA who were treated with Ustekinumab, a human (IL)-12 and IL-23 antagonist, which was recently approved by the FDA and the European Commission.[23] Similarly, a recent, small, open-label study showed that Ustekinumab was comparable to TNF-inhibitors in treating AS, with regard to the response rate and partial remission rate.[24] IL-22 was recently identified as a possible mediator of new-bone formation, as compared to other cytokines in animal models of arthritis and enthesitis.[25] Thus, IL-22 should be further studied for its potential therapeutic effects as a disease modifier in AS. The exact molecular mechanisms and pathways involved in the association between HLA-B27 and SpA remain unclear, but researchers have put forward several hypotheses in an attempt to explain the possible role of HLA-B27 in the pathogenesis of SpAs.[26] CD4+ and CD8+ B-27 reactive T cells have been both found to be related to the pathology of SpAs, and it has thus been suggested that the presentation of "arthritogenic" peptides to these CD4+ and CD8+ T cells might lead to SpA associated with certain HLA-B27 subtypes.[27,28] This hypothesis entails that a breakdown of tolerance to certain self-peptides occurs in AS as a consequence of mimicry between self-peptides, certain arthritis-causing peptides and pathogen-derived peptides.[29,30] Except for bacteria, which clearly trigger ReA (see chapter 3.1 on ReA below), this clear association has not been established in any of the other SpAs, but researchers have long known that some forms of SpAs may be triggered by enterobacterial infections, and certain subtypes share sequence homologies with these bacterial antigens, such as *Klebsiella pneumonia* nitrogenase.[31,32] Thus, the true significance of this molecular mimicry theory remains unclear, and future studies must use modern techniques to test the candidate peptides that have already been identified.[33,34] The two other active hypotheses address the possible ways in which HLA-B27 molecules mediate arthritis. The first hypothesis proposes that the condition is driven by increased endoplasmic reticulum stress triggered by misfolding of HLA-B27 heavy chains (the "free heavy chain hypothesis"). The second hypothesis points to the activation of the unfolded B27 protein response (UPR), by which these proteins may accumulate on antigen-presenting cells, activating NK cell response.[35,36] However, notably, none of these hypotheses has been well established as an explanation of the predominant pathogenic pathway in AS.

3 INTERRELATIONSHIPS BETWEEN BACTERIAL INFECTIONS AND SpAs

3.1 Reactive Arthritis

ReA is an inflammatory type of arthritis triggered by a preceding enteric or urogenital bacterial infection, often in patients bearing the HLA-B27 antigen. The usual time interval between the extra-articular infection and arthritis onset is between 2 and 4 weeks. The asymmetrical type of peripheral arthritis is typically accompanied by dactylitis and enthesitis, as well as by sacroiliitis and spondylitis in almost 50% of cases. A wide range of extra-articular features seen in ReA include cervicitis, vulvovaginitis, salpingitis, and prostatitis. Typical skin manifestations include oral ulcers, erythema nodosum, and ophthalmic involvement such as conjunctivitis and, occasionally, even cardiac involvement. In the case of ReA, the sero-negative type periphcral arthritis or SpA usually follows infections with *Yersinia enterocolitica*, *Salmonella typhimurium* and *enteritides*, *Shigella flexneri*, *Chlamydia trachomatis*, *Ureaplasma urealyticum*, and *Campylobacter jejuni*.[37] Other pathogenic organisms have been implicated in ReA, but with less frequent associations. ReA is a sterile arthritis, as opposed to infective or septic arthritis, and, as a result, the causative bacterial agent cannot be isolated from the synovial fluid. Researchers have used polymerase chain reaction (PCR) technology in an attempt to detect bacterial nucleotide sequences in the tissues or synovial fluids of patients with ReA. This type of approach has repeatedly enabled the demonstration of bacterial products in synovial tissue or fluid for all of the definite bacterial triggers of ReA, even years after the initial infection.[38,39] Thus, researchers do not yet understand the pathogenesis of ReA in detail, but they currently assume that the intracellular persistence of the pathogen causes an immune reaction resulting in arthritis. *C. trachomatis* and *Chlamydia pneumoniae* are now well accepted as causative agents in ReA.[40] Although *C. pneumonia* and *C. trachomatis* infections are very common, the incidence of arthritis associated with the these bacteria is unknown, largely because both are often asymptomatic; however, *C. pneumonia* arthritis is probably less common then arthritis triggered by *C. trachomatis*. A study has demonstrated an increased frequency of *Chlamydia*-positive synovial tissue samples, as determined by PCR, in patients with chronic uSpA.[41] Subsequent to this finding, researchers showed the efficacy of a combined antibiotic regimen in patients with uSpA and Chlamydial DNA detected by PCR in peripheral blood or in synovial fluid.[42] The role of long-term antibiotic therapy for the eradication of persistent intra-articular pathogens in chronic cases is still under investigation. Genetic susceptibility clearly plays some role in the pathophysiology of ReA. The prevalence of HLA-B27 in affected *Chlamydia*-associated ReA individuals ranges from approximately 40% to 50%,[37] but this close relationship could not be confirmed with *Campylobacter*-associated ReA[43,44] or in some population-based studies and analyses of disease outbreaks.[45] A recent study investigated the prevalence of anti-*Campylobacter* antibodies in a cohort of ReA patients, comparing them to a group of healthy blood donors.[46] The authors showed that 44–62% of the ReA cases were associated with *Campylobacter* infection. These findings indicated that *Campylobacter*-seropositivity (both IgA and IgG) was significantly higher than the seropositivity of other triggering pathogens considered (e.g. *Helicobacter pylori*, *Mycoplasma pneumoniae*, *Y. enterocolitica*, and *Borrelia afzelii*). Thus, the authors concluded that *Campylobacter* infection plays an important role in the development of ReA.

3.2 Ankylosing Spondylitis

Over the years, several studies have suggested a pathogenic role for *K. pneumoniae* in AS, demonstrating increased fecal carriage of *K. pneumoniae* during active disease.[47–49] Others were unable to confirm these findings, however.[50] Researchers proposed several hypotheses following the demonstration of this association. The molecular mimicry theory for *Klebsiella* and the HLA-B27 antigen postulated an antigenic cross-reactivity of microbial and host determinants. Although a few investigators were able to show some degree of sequence homology between HLA-B27 and the nitrogenase enzyme of *K. pneumoniae*, they had difficulty proving this relationship as a pathogenic pathway.[31,32,51,52] Other possible hypotheses regarding the infectious, pathogenic role of *Klebsiella* in AS faced similar difficulties. In keeping with the molecular mimicry theory, other studies have indicated that CD4+ and CD8+ T cells are stimulated by *Klebsiella* HSP60 in the majority of patients with AS, a response that could not be demonstrated in normal controls.[53] More recent data suggest no differences in cellular or humoural immune responses (which were previously thought to be present) with respect to *Klebsiella* in patients with AS, unaffected family members or normal controls.[50,54] Furthermore, acute infection with *K. pneumoniae* is not followed by ReA, as are infections with *Salmonella* or *Yersinia*. Thus, so far, the pathogenic role of *Klebsiella* in patients with AS remains controversial. In a large retrospective population survey of 1080 AS patients, compared to a cohort of 102 patients with prolapsed lumbar discs, infections were relatively common in the 3 months preceding the first symptoms.[54] Among the study group, 4.6% reported a gastrointestinal infection, 2.5% a urinary tract infection, and 2.6% a respiratory infection. The authors concluded that infections were potential triggers for the onset of AS, but the low rates suggest that infections are only a small part of the environmental milieu that combines with the genetic predisposition, leading to the development of this chronic inflammatory disease. Similar to the possible link between *Klebsiella* carriage in the stool and AS, another group suggested that the stool carriage of *Bacteroides* could also be implicated as a potential causative agent of AS, because the authors were able to demonstrate a significantly higher prevalence of sulphate-reducing bacteria in the group of AS patients.[55] A recent Chinese case-control study attempted to investigate the presence of anti-*C. pneumoniae* antibodies in patients with AS, in order to determine whether there was an association between the presence of these organisms and disease activity.[56] The authors studied 79 AS patients and 73 normal controls, measuring IgG, IgA, and IgM antibodies, as well as using the Bath Ankylosing Spondylitis Disease Activity Index. The authors considered the presence of *C. pneumoniae* IgM or IgA antibodies, to be proof of a recent *C. pneumoniae* infection. The authors were able to confirm that recent

C. pneumoniae infections occur frequently in AS patients, and they showed that IgM antibodies correlated with active disease. As a result, they postulated that *C. pneumoniae* infection may be a triggering factor for active AS. These intriguing associations between bacterial infection and AS obviously deserve further study in order to establish their potential pathogenc, aetiological roles in this disease.

4 PSORIATIC ARTHRITIS

Studies have suggested that a variety of genetic, immunological and environmental factors contribute to PsA pathogenesis.[57,58] Genetic evidence indicates that psoriasis and PsA probably have distinct genes that drive their pathogenesis, progression, and severity.[59] Class I antigens (HLA-B13, HLA-B57, HLA-B39, HLA-Cw6, and HLA-Cw7) have consistently shown a positive association with psoriasis and PsA in population studies, and the strongest association is with HLA-Cw6.[60,61] Various studies have also asserted that a preceding *Streptococcal* infection could be triggering psoriasis and PsA in a genetically prone subject. In one of these studies, *Streptococcus* infection could be shown in about 50% of PsA patients versus none of those with RA.[62] In support of this concept, researchers demonstrated high levels of anti-peptidoglycan antibodies in PsA patients, noting that peptidoglycan is the major component of streptococcal cell walls.[63] However, other studies could not confirm this association between a preceding infection with *Streptococcus* and PsA, however. Aside from Streptococci, few other bacteria have been suggested as a trigger of psoriasis including *Staphylococcus aureus* and *Candida albicans*. For patients with existing psoriasis, the prevalence of PsA reportedly ranges from 6% to 42%[64,65] in Caucasian populations, as opposed to the estimated population-based prevalence between 0.02% and 0.2%.[66,67] A recent case-control study investigated the association between various potential environmental exposures, including infections, and the development of PsA in such patients with psoriasis.[68] Infections requiring antibiotics were found to be significantly associated (OR 1.7, 95% CI 1.00–2.77) with the development of PsA.

5 INFLAMMATORY BOWEL DISEASE-ASSOCIATED SPONDYLOARTHROPATHY

Arthritis is the most common extraintestinal manifestation of IBD, affecting over 20% of the patients in one series of 700 patients.[69] It may present as peripheral or axial arthritis. Research investigating the prevalence of CARD15/NOD2 gene polymorphisms associated with Crohn's disease showed that these commonly occur in SpA patients with chronic gut inflammation. In contrast, the prevalence of these NOD2 variants was unaltered in SpA patients without gut inflammation or with acute gut inflammation.[70] This observation suggests that microscopic gut inflammation may be a critical factor when comparing genetic predisposition to IBD and SpA. The co-existence of AS and intestinal inflammation has been known for a long time.[71]

Between 5% and 10% of patients with AS develop clinically diagnosed IBD, and a further 70% of patients with AS can be shown by endoscopy to have subclinical asymptomatic gut inflammation.[71–74] Gastrointestinal infection with *Campylobacter*, *Salmonella*, *Shigella*, or *Yersinia* has been shown to precede inflammatory arthritis in ReA. Researchers have not established a similar sequence of events in other subgroups of SpA so far. However, a few studies have investigated the role of bacteria in the pathogenesis of IBD, suggesting several bacteria with a potential to cause these diseases. Of these candidate bacteria, the following should be noted: *Helicobacter*, *Escherichia coli*, sulphate-reducing bacteria, *Mycobacterium paratuberculosis*, *Listeria*, *Chlamydia*, *Bacteroides*, and *Enterococcus*.[75,76] The gut flora play an important role in maintaining gastrointestinal integrity and good health, but a fair amount of data supports the notion that the gut microbiome also plays an important role in IBD. Because no single bacteria was found to be clearly pathogenic for IBD, a recent theory suggests a "pathogenic community" of existing bacteria might predispose an individual with IBD when the healthy gut is disrupted in response to host genetics, leading to repeated exposures over time.[77] Notably, about one quarter of the individuals undergoing intestinal bypass surgery develop a typical arthritis-dermatitis syndrome as a consequence of antibiotic-responsive bacterial overgrowth in the residual small bowel blind loop.[78,79] Thus, further studies are needed to clarify the relationship between the host genetic factors determining IBD risk and the gut microbiome.

6 UNDIFFERENTIATED SPONDYLOARTHRITIS

uSpA is a milder or early form of SpA that likely develops into one of the defined subgroups of SpA, and it is thus used to describe manifestations of SpA in patients who do not meet criteria for any of the well-defined forms of SpA.[80] It may not be proper therefore to classify uSpA as a separate SpA subgroup because of the patient's possible future transition from uSpA to one of the SpA subgroups. Like AS, uSpA is linked to HLA-B27 and other HLA alleles, suggesting that this subgroup of SpAs is also genetically determined.[81] Over half of patients with uSpA saw their condition evolve into classical AS in a 10-year follow-up.[3,82] Few studies support a preceding infection in this subgroup of SpA as well. *C. trachomatis*, *C. pneumonia* and a few other organisms may contribute to the aetiology of uSpA. These studies were supported by PCR-based screening assays,[83,84] and they shed some light on the potential transition from uSpA to ReA.[83]

In conclusion, infections play a role in the development of SpAs. This relationship is best manifested in ReA. The interplay of these infections with genetics, and mainly the presence of HLA-B27, contributes to the development of SpA and ankylosing spondylitis.

REFERENCES

1. Gladman DD. Psoriatic arthritis. *Rheum Dis Clin North Am* 1998;**24**:829–44.
2. De Keyser F, Elewaut D, De Vos M, De Vlam K, Cuvelier C, Mielants H, et al. Bowel inflammation and spondyloarthropathies. *Rheum Dis Clin North Am* 1998;**24**:785–813.
3. Zochling J, Brandt J, Braun J. The current concept of spondyloarthropathies with special emphasis on undifferentiated spondyloarthritis. *Rheumatology* 2005;**44**:1483–91.
4. Taurog JD. The role of HLA-B27 in spondyloarthropathies. *J Rheumatol* 2010;**37**:2606–12.
5. Saraux A, Guillemin F, Guggenbuhl P, Roux CH, Fardellone P, Le Bihan E, et al. Prevalence of spondyloarthropathies in France: 2001. *Ann Rheum Dis* 2005;**64**:1431–5.
6. Rudwaleit M, Landewé R, van der Heijde D, Listing J, Brandt J, Braun J, et al. The development of Assessment of SpondyloArthritis international Society classification criteria for axial spondyloarthropathies (part I): classification of paper patients by expert opinion including uncertainty appraisal. *Ann Rheum Dis* 2009;**68**:770–6.
7. Rudwaleit M, van der Heijde D, Landewé R, Listing J, Akkoc N, Brandt J, et al. The development of Assessment of SpondyloArthritis international Society classification criteria for axial spondyloarthropathies (part II): validation and final selection. *Ann Rheum Dis* 2009;**68**:777–83.
8. Sieper J, Rudwaleit M, Kahn MA, Braun J. Concepts and epidemiology of spondyloarthritis. *Best Pract Res Clin Rheumatol* 2006;**20**:401–17.
9. Wallis D, Haroon N, Ayearst R, Carty A, Inman RD. Ankylosing spondylitis and non-radiographic axial spondyloarthritis: part of a common spectrum or distinct diseases? *J Rheumatol* 2013;**40**:2038–41.
10. Sieper J, van der Heijde D. Nonradiographic axial spondyloarthritis: new definition of an old disease? *Arthritis Rheum* 2013;**65**:543–51.
11. Pedersen OB, Svendsen AJ, Ejstrup L, Skytthe A, Harris JR, Junker P. Ankylosing spondylitis in Danish and Norwegian twins: occurrence and relative importance of genetic vs. environmental effectors in disease causation. *Scand J Rheumatol* 2008;**37**:120–6.
12. Alvarez-Navarro C, López de Castro JA. ERAP1 in ankylosing spondylitis: genetics, biology and pathogenetic role. *Curr Opin Rheumatol* 2013;**25**:419–25.
13. Kahn MA. Polymorphism of HLA-B27: 105 subtypes currently known. *Curr Rheumatol Rep* 2013;**15**:362.

14. Brown MA, Kennedy LG, MacGregor AJ, Darke C, Duncan E, Shatford JL, et al. Susceptibility to ankylosing spondylitis in twins: the role of genes, HLA, and the environment. *Arthritis Rheum* 1997;**40**:1823–8.

15. Inman RD, Stone MA. Infection and spondyloarthritis. In: Waisman M, van der Heijde D, Reveille J, editors. *Ankylosing spondylitis and spondyloarthropathies.* Philadelphia, PA: Mosby Elsevier; 2006. p. 38–52.

16. Taurog JD, Maika SD, Satumtira N, Dorris ML, McLean IL, Yanagisawa H, et al. Inflammatory disease in HLA-B27 transgenic rats. *Immunol Rev* 1999;**169**:209–23.

17. Rudwaleit M, Sieper J. Referral strategies for early diagnosis of axial spondyloarthitis. *Nat Rev Rheumatol* 2012;**8**:262–8.

18. Rudwaleit M, van der Heijde D, Landewé R, Akkoc N, Brandt J, Chou CT, et al. The Assessment SpondyloArthritis international Society classification criteria for peripheral spondyloarthritis and for spondyloarthritis in general. *Ann Rheum Dis* 2011;**70**:25–31.

19. Feldtkeller E, Kahn MA, vasn der Heijde D, van der Linden S, Braun J. Age at disease onset and diagnosis delay in HLA-B27 negative vs positive patients with ankylosing spondylitis. *Rheumatol Int* 2003;**23**:61–6.

20. Kahn MA, Kushner I, Braun WE. Comparison of clinical features in HLA-B27 positive and negative patients with ankylosing spondylitis. *Arthritis Rheum* 1977;**20**:909–12.

21. Wellcome Trust Case Control Consortium, Australo-Anglo-American Spondylitis Consortium (TASC), Burton PR et al. Association scan of 14,500 nonsynonymus SNP's in four diseases identifies autoimmunity variants. *Nast Genet* 2007;**39**:1329–37.

22. Krueger GG, Langley RG, Leonardi C, Yeilding N, Guzzo C, Wang Y, et al. A human interleukin-12/23 monoclonal antibody for the treatment of psoriasis. *N Engl J Med* 2007;**356**:580–92.

23. McInnes IB, Kavanaugh A, Gottlieb AB, Puig L, Rahman P, Ritchlin C, et al. Efficacy and safety of ustekinumab in patients with active psoriatic arthritis: 1 year results of the phase 3, multicentre, double-blind, placebo-controlled PSUMMIT 1 trial. *Lancet* 2013;**382**:780–9.

24. Poddubnyy D, Calhoff J, Listing J, Sieper J. Ustekinumab for the treatment opf patients with active ankylosing spondylitis: results of a 28-week, prospective, open-label, proof-of-concept study (TOPAS). *Arthritis Rheum* 2013;**65**:766.

25. Sherlock JP, Joyce-Shaikh B, Turner SP, Chao CC, Sathe M, Grein J, et al. IL-23 induces spondyloarthropathy by acting on ROR-gammat+CD3+CD4-CD8-entheseal resident T cells. *Nat Med* 2012;**18**:1069–76.

26. Ehrenfeld M. Geoepidemiology: the environment and spondyloarthropathies. *Autoimmun Rev* 2010;**9**:A325–9.

27. Boyle LH, Goodall JC, Opat SS, Gaston JS. The recognition of HLA-B27 by human CD4(+) T lymphocytes. *J Immunol* 2001;**167**:2619–24.

28. Roddis M, Carter RW, Sun MY, Weissensteiner T, McMichael AJ, Bowness P, et al. Fully functional HLA-B27-restricted CD4 + as well as CD8 + T cell responses in TCR transgenic mice. *J Immunol* 2004;**172**:155–61.

29. Lopez de Castro JA. HLA-B27 and the pathogenesis of spondyloarthropathies. *Immunol Lett* 2007;**108**:27–33.

30. Robinson PC, Brown MA. Genetics of ankylosing spondylitis. *Mol Immunol* 2014;**57**:2–11.

31. Tani Y, Tiwana H, Hukuda S, Nishioka J, Fielder M, Wilson C, et al. Antibodies to Klebsiella, Proteus and HLA-B27 peptides in Japanese patients with ankylosing spondylitis and rheumatoid arthritis. *J Rheumatol* 1997;**24**:109–14.

32. Ebringer A, Ahmadi K, Fielder M, Rashid T, Tiwana H, Wilson C, et al. Molecular mimicry: the geographical distribution of immune responses to *Klebsiella* in ankylosing spondylitis and its relevance to therapy. *Clin Rheumatol* 1996;**15**(Suppl.1):57–61.

33. Ben Dror L, Barnea E, Beer I, Mann M, Admon A. The HLA-B★2705 peptidome. *Arthritis Rheum* 2010;**62**:420–9.

34. Lopez de Castro JA. The HLA-B27 peptidome: building on the cornerstone. *Arthritis Rheum* 2010;**62**:316–19.
35. Chapman DC, Williams DB. ER quality control in the biogenesis of MHC class I molecules. *Semin Cell Dev Biol* 2010;**21**:512–19.
36. Smith J, Mäker-Hermann E, Colbert RA. Pathogenesis of ankylosing spondylitis: current concepts. *Best Pract Res Clin Rheumatol* 2006;**20**:571–9.
37. Carter JD, Hudson AP. Reactive arthritis: clinical aspects and medical management. *Rheum Dis Clin North Am* 2009;**35**:21–44.
38. Braun J, Tuszewski M, Eggens U, Mertz A, Schauer-Petrowskaja C, Döring E, et al. Nested polymerase chain reaction strategy simultaneously targeting DNA sequences of multiple bacterial species in inflammatory joint diseases. I. Screening of synovial fluid samples of patients with spondyloarthropathies and other arthritides. *J Rheumatol* 1997;**24**:1092–100.
39. Viitanen AM, Arstila TP, Lahesmaa R, Granfors K, Skurnik M, Toivanen P. Application of the polymerase chain reaction and immunoflourescence to the detection of bacteria in *Yersinia*-triggered reactive arthritis. *Arthritis Rheum* 1991;**34**:89–96.
40. Carter JD, Hudson AP. The evolving story of *Chlamydia*-induced reactive arthritis. *Curr Opin Rheumatol* 2010;**22**:424–30.
41. Gérad HC, Whittum-Hudson JA, Carter JD, Hudson AP. The pathogenic role of Chlamydia in spondyloarthritis. *Curr Opin Rheumatol* 2010;**22**:363–7.
42. Carter JD, Espinoza LR, Inman RD, Sneed KB, Ricca LR, Vasey FB, et al. Combination antibiotics as a treatment for chronic Chlamydia-induced reactive arthritis: a double-blind, placebo-controlled, prospective trial. *Arthritis Rheum* 2010;**62**:1298–307.
43. Hannu T, Mattila L, Rautelin H, Pelkonen P, Lahdenne P, Siitonen A. *Camylobacter*-triggered reactive arthritis: a population-based study. *Rheumatology (Oxford)* 2002;**41**:312–8.
44. Pope JE, Krizova A, Garg AX, Thiessen-Philbrook H, Ouimet JM. *Campylobacter* reactive arthritis: a systematic review. *Semin Arthritis Rheum* 2007;**37**:48–55.
45. Leirisalo-Repo M, Hannu T, Mattila L. Microbial factors in spondyloarthropathies: insights from population studies. *Curr Opin Rheumatol* 2003;**15**:408–12.
46. Zautner AE, Johann C, Strubek A, Busse C, Tareen AM, Masanta WO, et al. Seroprevalence of camylobacteriosis and relevant post-infectious sequel. *Eur J Clin Microbiol Infect Dis* 2014;**33**(6):1019–27. http://dx.doi.org/10.1007/s10096-013-2040-4, Epub.
47. Ebringer A. The relationship between *Klebsiella* infection and ankylosing spondylitis. *Baillieres Clin Rheumatol* 1989;**3**:321–38.
48. Ebringer R. Acute anterior uveitis and faecal carriage of gram-negative bacteria. *Br J Rheumatol* 1988;**27**(suppl. 2):42–5.
49. Ebringer R, Cooke D, Cawdell DR, Cowling P, Ebringer A. Ankylosing spondylitis: *Klebsiella* and HLA-B27. *Clin Rheumatol* 1977;**16**:190–6.
50. Stone MA, Payne U, Schentag C, Rahman R, Pacheco-Tena C, Inman RD. Comparative immune responses to candidate arthritogenic bacteria do not confirm a role for Klebsiella pneumoniae in the pathogenesis of familial ankylosing spondylitis. *Rheumatology (Oxford)* 2004;**43**:148–55.
51. Schwimmbeck PL, Yu DT, Oldstone MB. Autoantibodies to HLA B27 in the sera of HLA B27 patients with ankylosing spondylitis and Reiter's syndrome. Molecular mimicry with *Klebsiella pneumoniae* as potential mechanism of autoimmune disease. *J Exp Med* 1987;**166**:173–81.
52. Albert LJ, Inman RD. Molecular mimicry and autoimmunity. *N Engl J Med* 1999;**341**:2068–74.
53. Zambrano-Zaragoza F, García-Latorre E, Dominguez-López MI. CD4 and CD8 T cell response to the rHSP60 from *Klebsiella pneumoniae* in peripheral blood mononuclear cells from patients with ankylosing spondylitis. *Rev Invest Clin* 2005;**57**:555–62.
54. Zochling J, Bohl-Buhler MH, Baraliakos X, Feldtkeller E, Braun J. Infection and work stress are potential triggers of ankylosing spondylitis. *Clin Rheumatol* 2006;**25**:660–6.

55. Stebbings S, Munro K, Simon MA. Comparison of faecal microflora of patients with ankylosing spondylitis and controls using molecular methods of analysis. *Rheumatology (Oxford)* 2002;**41**:1395–401.

56. Feng XG, Xu XJ, Ye S, Lin YY, Chen P, Zhang XJ, et al. Recent *Chlamydia pneumoniae* infection is highly associated with active ankylosing spondylitis in a Chinese cohort. *Scand J Rheumatol* 2011;**40**:289–91.

57. Chimenti MS, Ballanti E, Perricone C, Cipriani P, Giacomelli R, Perricone R. Immunomodulation in psoriatic arthritis: focus on cellular and molecular pathways. *Autoimmun Rev* 2013;**12**:599–606.

58. Winchester R, Minevich G, Steshenko V, Kirby B, Kane D, Greenberg DA, et al. HLA associations reveal genetic heterogeneity in psoriatic arthritis and in the psoriasis phenotype. *Arthritis Rheum* 2012;**64**:1134–44.

59. Wittkowski KM, Leonardi C, Gottlieb A, Menter A, Krueger GG, Tebbey PW, et al. Clinical symptoms of skin, nails, and joints manifest independently in patients with concomitant psoriasis and psoriatic arthritis. *PLoS One* 2011;**6**:e20279.

60. Duffin KC, Chandran V, Gladman DD, Krueger GG, Elder JT, Rahman P. Genetics of psoriasis and psoriatic arthritis: update and future direction. *J Rheumatol* 2008;**35**:1449–53.

61. Gladman DD, Farewell VT. HLA studies in psoriatic arthritis: current situation and future needs. *J Rheumatol* 2003;**30**:4–6.

62. Wang Q, Vasey FB, Mahfood JP, Valeriano J, Kanik KS, Anderson BE, et al. V2 regions of 16S ribosomal RNAs used as molecular marker for the species identification of *Streptococci* in peripheral blood and synovial fluid from patients with psoriatic arthritis. *Arthritis Rheum* 1999;**42**:2055–9.

63. Rahman MU, Ahmed S, Schumacher HR, Zeiger AR. High levels of antipeptidoglycan antibodies in psoriatic and other seronegative arthritides. *J Rheumatol* 1990;**17**:621–5.

64. Gladman DD, Antoni C, Mease P, Clegg DO, Nash P. Psoriatic arthritis: epidemiology, clinical features, course, and outcome. *Ann Rheum Dis* 2005;**64**(Suppl. 2):14–7.

65. Ibrahim G, Waxman R, Helliwell PS. The prevalence of psoriatic arthritis in people with psoriasis. *Arthritis Rheum* 2009;**61**:1373–8.

66. Shbeeb M, Uramoto KM, Gibson LE, O'Fallon WM, Gabriel SE. The epidemiology of psoriatic arthritis in Olmsted County, Minnesota, USA, 1982–1991. *J Rheumatol* 2000;**27**:1247–50.

67. O'Neill T, Silman AJ. Psoriatic arthritis. Historical background and epidemiology. *Baillieres Clin Rheumatol* 1994;**8**:245–61.

68. Eder L, Law T, Chandran V, Shanmugarajah S, Shen H, Rosen CF, et al. Association between environmental factors and onset of psoriatic arthritis in patients with psoriasis. *Arthritis Care Res* 2011;**63**:1091–7.

69. Greenstein AJ, Janowitz HD, Sachar DB. The extra-intestinal complications of Crohn's disease and ulcerative colitis: a study of 700 patients. *Medicine* 1976;**55**:401–12.

70. Laukens D, Peeters H, Marichal D, Vander Cruyssen B, Mielants H, Elewaut D, et al. CARD15 gene polymorphisms in patients with spondyloarthropathies identify a specific phenotype previously related tyo Crohn's disease. *Ann Rheum Dis* 2005;**64**:930–5.

71. Mielants H, Veys EM, Goemaere S, Goethals K, Cuvelier C, De Vos M. Gut inflammation in the spondyloarthropathies: clinical, radiologic, biologic and genetic features in relation to the type of histology. A prospective study. *J Rheumatol* 1991;**18**:1542–51.

72. Thomas GP, Brown MA. Genetics and genomics of ankylosing spondylitis. *Immunol Rev* 2010;**233**:162–80.

73. Van Praet L, Van de Bosch FE, Jacques P, Carron P, Jans L, Colman R, et al. Microscopic gut inflammation in axial spondyloarthritis: a multiparametric predictive model. *Ann Rheum Dis* 2013;**72**:414–17.

74. Leirisalo-Repo M, Turunen U, Stenman S. High frequency of silent inflammatory bowel disease in spondyloarthropathy. *Arthritis Rheum* 1994;**37**:23–31.
75. Lidar M, Langevitz P, Shoenfeld Y. The role of infection in inflammatory bowel disease: initiation, exacerbation and protection. *Isr Med Assoc J* 2009;**11**:558–63.
76. Rhee KJ, Wu S, Wu x. Induction of persistent colitis by a human commensal, entero-toxigenic *Bacteroides fragilis* in wild-type C57BL/6 mice. *Infect Immun* 2009;**77**:1708–18.
77. Baker PI, Love DR, Ferguson LR. Role of gut microbiota in Crohn's disease. *Expert Rev Gastroenterol Hepatol* 2009;**3**:535–46.
78. Wands JR, LaMont JT, Mann E, Isselbacher KJ. Arthritis associated with intestinal-bypass procedure for morbid obesity. Complement activation and characterization of circulating cryoproteins. *N Engl J Med* 1976;**294**:121–4.
79. Drenick EJ, Ahmed AR, Greenway F, Olerud JE. Cutaneous lesions after intestinal bypass. *Ann Intern Med* 1980;**93**:557–9.
80. Cruzat V, Cuchacovich R, Espinoza LR. Undifferentiated spondyloarthritis: recent clinical and therapeutic advances. *Curr Rheumatol Rep* 2010;**12**:311–17.
81. Liao HT, Lin KC, Chen CH, Liang TH, Lin MW, Tsai CY, et al. Human leukocyte antigens in undifferentiated spondyloarthritis. *Semin Arthritis Rheum* 2007;**37**:198–201.
82. Zeidler H, Mau W, Kahn MA. Undifferentiated spondyloarthropathies. *Rheum Dis Clin NA* 1992;**18**:187–202.
83. Carter JD, Gérard HC, Espinoza LR, Ricca LR, Valerian J, Snelgrove J, et al. *Chlamydiae* as etiologic agents in chronic undifferentiated spondyloarthritis. *Arthritis Rheum* 2009;**60**:1311–16.
84. Siala M, Godoura R, Younes M, Fourati H, Cheour I, Meddeb N, et al. Detection and frequency of *Chalmydia trachomatis* DNA in synovial samples from Tunisian patients with reactive arthritis and undifferentiated oligoarthritis. *FEMS Immunol Med Microbiol* 2009;**55**:178–86.

CHAPTER 46

Infection and Behçet Disease

J. Correia[*,1], A. Campar[*], C. Ferrão[†], S. Silva[†], C. Vasconcelos[*]
[*]Clinical Immunology Unit, Centro Hospitalar do Porto, Portugal
[†]Clinical Medicine Department, Centro Hospitalar do Porto, Portugal
[1]Corresponding Author: joaoacorr@gmail.com

1 INTRODUCTION

Behçet's disease (BD) is a chronic, relapsing, multi-system disorder of unknown etiology.[1] Regarding the etiology of the disease, much research has focused on genetics, immunology and infection. The clinical manifestations are related to an inflammatory vasculitis that can affect almost any tissue[2]: mucocutaneous, ocular, neurological, vascular, gastrointestinal and cardiac. BD has a wide geographical distribution; being more prevalent in the Middle East, the Mediterranean basin and the Far East (80-370 in 100,000) and rare in North Europe and North America (0.6 in 100,000).[3]

Criteria for the classification of BD have been proposed by the International Study Group[4] (Table 1); these were reviewed in 2006 at the International Conference of BD, in Lisbon, Portugal, with the creation of the International Criteria for BD[5] (Table 2). These new criteria include vascular manifestations and propose a double scoring for genital ulcers, uveitis and retinal vasculitis.

Here we review the role of infection in pathogenesis in Behçet's syndrome and as a trigger to Behçet's exacerbations. Our aim is also to describe common and opportunistic infections in patients with BD.

2 BEHÇET'S PATHOGENESIS AND INFECTION

In recent decades there has been an enormous effort to understand the pathogenesis of BD. One interesting fact is the association between BD and Mediterranean fever gene mutations, which seem to be increased in patients with BD.[6] Although some advances have been made regarding genetic susceptibility and immunology,[7] we still know little about the role of infection in the pathogenesis of this disease.

Infection and Autoimmunity
http://dx.doi.org/10.1016/B978-0-444-63269-2.00055-6

Table 1 ISG Criteria
ISG Criteria (1990)

Recurrent oral ulceration	Minor aphthous, major aphthous or herpetiform ulcerations observed by a physician or reported by patient. Recurrent at least three times in one 12-month period

Plus any two of the following:

Recurrent genital ulceration	Recurrent genital aphthous ulceration or scarring observed by a physician or reported by patient
Eye lesions	Anterior or posterior uveitis, cells in vitreous on slit lamp examination or retinal vasculitis observed by ophthalmologist
Skin lesions	Erythema nodosum-like lesion observed by physician or patient, pseudofolliculitis, papulopustular lesions or acneiform nodules consistent with disease
Positive pathergy test	An erythematous papule, ≥ 2 mm at 48 h after a prick with a sterile #20–22 needle obliquely in avascular skin to a depth of 5 mm

Table 2 ICBD Criteria
ICBD Criteria (Lisbon 2006)

Diagnosis if ≥3 points:

Oral ulcers	1
Skin lesions	1
Vascular lesions	1
Positive pathergy test	1
Genital ulcers	2
Uveitis or retinal vasculitis	2

The most accepted theory related to infectious agents concerns the concept of molecular mimicry, in which pathogens act like autoantigens even in the absence of active infection.[8] The most studied and implicated bacterial agent is *Streptococcus sanguinis*. Several articles associating this agent with the pathogenesis of the disease have been published. In 1997, Kaneko et al. showed that streptococcal antigens induce the production of pro-inflammatory cytokines by peripheral blood mononuclear cells.[9] In fact, levels of *S. sanguinis* in oral flora are elevated in BD patients when compared with healthy controls.[10] On the other hand, sera from patients with active BD and patients with *S. sanguinis* infection both stimulate the expression of α-enolase in human endothelial cells, which in turn increases inflammation in the former by reacting with anti-α-enolase antibodies.[11] Another study compared the expression of heterogeneous nuclear ribonucleoprotein A2/B1 (a target antigen for BD) in endothelial cells. The study used sera from patients with BD and healthy controls and cultured *S. sanguinis*. The results showed that *S. sanguinis* infection and the sera from patients with BD are both inflammatory stimuli for heterogeneous nuclear ribonucleoprotein.[12] Sang Ho et al. also showed that patients with BD with a high titer of anti-streptolysin O (streptococcal antibodies tests) had a higher incidence of tonsillitis and erythema nodosum lesions.[13] However, the stimulation of T cells in patients with BD is not specific for this bacteria and is shared with other species,[14] leading to the hypothesis of a non-specific lymphocytic cell hypersensitivity.

This process may be mediated by heat shock proteins (HSP) that are synthesized by both prokaryotic and eukaryotic cells and expressed in stress conditions induced by, for example, microbial stimulus. In fact, there is 60% homology between human and bacterial HSP.[15] On the other hand, serum concentrations of human HSP and anti-HSP are elevated in patients with BD compared with healthy controls,[16] in mucocutaneous ulcers and erythema nodosum[17,18] and in ocular flares (uveitis).[19] Another study published in 2005 proved that oral bacteria from periodontal sites and saliva (namely *Prevotella intermedia*, *Fusobacterium nucleatum*, and *Capnocytophaga* spp. from subgingival plaque samples and *Streptococcus mitis* from saliva samples) produce HSP and therefore inflammation in BD.[20] Once again this process refers to molecular mimicry. Finally, in 2008, the conjunctival flora of patients with BD during an inactive period was studied,[21] and there was significant colonization by *Staphylococcus aureus*, *Moraxella* spp. and *Streptococcus* spp. compared with the control group.

Herpes simplex virus (HSV) also has been implicated in the pathogenesis of BD. Studies using polymerase chain reaction detected HSV type 1 in peripheral blood and in oral, genital, and intestinal ulcers compared with healthy controls.[22,23] Despite these results, the role of HSV in the pathology of BD remains elusive.

Several studies try to associate other microorganisms with the pathogenesis of this disease, including *Mycoplasma* spp.,[24] *Borrelia burgdorferi*,[25] *Helicobacter pylori*,[26,27] hepatitis A, B, C, E, and G[28] and human immunodeficiency virus,[29,30] but to date the evidence is weak.

3 INFECTION AS A TRIGGER TO BD EXACERBATIONS

BD has a chronic, relapsing course.[31] Little is known about its triggers, but infection is presumed to be implicated. In fact, some of the typical manifestations appear in relation to infectious conditions or with the presence of infectious agents. The most frequent reports refer to mucocutaneous involvement,[32,33] and although it was thought that cutaneous lesions such as pustules were mainly sterile, Hatemi et al.[32] demonstrated the contrary. However, it was impossible to determine whether infection was related to Behçet's pathogenesis or secondary to the disease itself. Furthermore, exacerbations of BD after tooth extraction[34,35] or gingival infection[33,36] have been described, and agents like *Staphylococcus*[33,36] or *Streptococcus* spp.[34] were implicated.

Other reports have described the association between infection and reactivation of the disease. Lellouche et al.[37] describe a case of recurrent aortic prosthetic dehiscence in which each disease exacerbation was concomitant with *Streptococcus agalactiae* infection and finally resolved after adequate antibiotic therapy plus immunosuppression. Yildirim et al.[38] reported a case of a patient with BD who developed a pulmonary artery aneurism; microbiological analysis revealed *Staphylococcus epidermidis*, which was successfully treated with vancomycin. A report about anti-*Saccharomyces cerevisiae* antibody and cumulative relapse rates of BD showed no association, although a tendency to have intestinal complications more likely to require surgical treatment was found in patients with this antibody.[39] Interestingly, the same antibody is also characteristically present in patients with Crohn's disease. Finally, a study published in 2005[40] showed that prophylactic benzathine penicillin combined with colchicine seems to be more effective than colchicine alone in controlling mucocutaneous manifestations of BD as well as preventing their relapse.

Despite the limited existing data, all these findings suggest that efforts to obtain microbiological isolates might be of interest. In addition, appropriate antibiotic therapy could play a role in dealing with some of the exacerbations of BD.

4 COMMON INFECTIONS IN BD PATIENTS

The spectrum of infections among patients with BD includes opportunistic infections resulting from immunosuppressive drugs (discussed in the next section) and common infections. *Staphylococcus* spp. is the most frequently agent isolated in mucocutaneous BD. One important paper published in 2004 proved that pustular skin lesions in BD are not sterile,[32] unlike as previously thought. The authors studied patients with BD who had active pustules during follow-up and were not receiving any kind of immunosuppression and compared them with patients with acne vulgaris. They found a significant prevalence of *S. aureus* in the unusual acne sites in patients with BD, whereas coagulase-negative staphylococci were less common. The gram-negative anerobic bacilli *Prevotella* was also more prevalent in the pustules of patients with BD. Another study in 1995 reported a patient with a gingival infection with methicillin-resistant *S. aureus* (MRSA) who improved after vancomycin administration and extraction of the carious teeth.[33] MRSA infection is described in the literature, for example, necrotizing folliculitis in a patient who had abruptly stopped taking colchicine and azathioprine and was successfully treated with cotrimoxazole plus ofloxacine.[41] A recurrent leg ulcer infected with a *Pseudomonas* agent also was described in 2013.[42] The patient was treated with antibiotics and colchicine plus corticoids.

With respect to viruses, Sun et al.[43] suggested that the Epstein–Barr virus (EBV) could be present and infect the epithelial cells of pre-ulcerative oral aphthous lesions. An oral hairy leukoplakia caused by EBV infection in a human immunodeficiency virus-negative patient with BD was published in 2005.[44]

Although surprisingly not described in the literature, localized fungal infections, such as those caused by oropharyngeal *Candida* spp., also are common. Topical anti-fungals together with antibiotics for bacterial mucosal infections should be part of the treatment.

In ocular BD, in 2000 Kiratli et al. described a pre-septal *S. aureus* abscess after cryotherapy for uveitis.[45] The patient was treated with systemic antibiotics and surgical drainage with good recovery. In 2011, another case of ocular infection was described after insertion of an intravitreal implant: cytomegalovirus endotheliitis was treated with oral valganciclovir but resulted in a poor visual outcome.[46]

Concerning vascular BD, in 2007 Erkan Yildirim et al. described a patient with BD with a pulmonary artery aneurysm probably due to *S. epidermidis*.[38] The aneurysm was successfully treated with a right upper lobectomy and antibiotic therapy with vancomycin. The relationship between vasculitis and *S. epidermidis* infection in the development of aneurysm is still unknown. Another aneurysm localized to the aortic arch, mimicking an infectious one in a patient receiving colchicine and cyclosporine, also was published.[47] Nevertheless, the presence of infection was not proven. Finally, in 2010, an aneurysm of the right iliac artery infected with *Salmonella* in a patient with BD was reported.[48]

In gastrointestinal BD, localized infections such as those caused by cytomegalovirus,[49] *Mycobacterium tuberculosis*[50] and *Clostridium difficile* have been described.[51] In 2010, a cerebral abscess was found in a patient previously diagnosed with neuro-Behçet syndrome. Unsurprisingly, the lesions were sterile.[52] Iliopoulos et al. described tuberculous meningoencephalitis in a patient with BD.[53] A hemophagocytic syndrome[54] in a patient with BD was described in 2005; it was related to EBV and solved with steroid therapy.

An interesting paper was published in 2007 describing a patient with BD who presented with multiple pulmonary abscesses that did not improve with antibiotics.[55] Culture of the bronchoalveolar lavage samples revealed no bacteria. The patient improved only after immunosuppression (corticoids plus colchicine) was started. Finally, two localized tuberculosis infections were diagnosed in patients with BD: a bacillary ganglionar disease[56] in an untreated woman who showed a good response to anti-bacillary therapy (rifampicin, isoniazid, ethambutol, and pyrazinamide) plus colchicine because of her arthritis and oral ulcers, and tuberculous thyroiditis in a woman who also showed a good response to anti-bacillary therapy.[57]

In our cohort of 147 patients with BD, we observed two serious infections by MRSA, both in leg ulcers and requiring hospital admission for intravenous antibiotic therapy with vancomycin. Another patient with ocular and mucocutaneous BD who was receiving infliximab treatment was diagnosed with lung and peritoneal tuberculosis. Two weeks after the antibacillary therapy was started, she died from acute cardiac insufficiency, fulfilling the clinical criteria for Takotsubo syndrome.

5 INFECTIOUS COMPLICATIONS OF IMMUNOSUPPRESSIVE DRUGS IN BD

Typical organ involvement in BD ranges from mucocutaneous lesions to ocular, vascular, neurological, gastrointestinal and cardiac manifestations.[31] Treatment options[58] include a wide range of drugs, from topical to systemic corticosteroids, other immunosuppressive drugs and, finally, more recent therapies such as antagonists of tumor necrosis factor (TNF)-α or anti-CD20. Selection of these drugs depends not only on the organs involved in BD but also on the severity of the disease.

Most of the drugs used have a significant immunosuppressive effect; consequently, one of the most feared adverse events is infection. Although no systematic review regarding this issue has been published, several reports[59–70] have described important opportunistic infections secondary to bacteria, fungal, protozoa and viral agents. Different infections are expected to complicate the use of various drugs, depending on the diverse mechanisms of action and consequent effects on the immune system. Corticosteroid actions[71–73] result in a qualitative defect of phagocytic function, neutropenia, lymphocytopenia, suppression of normal delayed hypersensitivity reactions and, in high doses, defective humoral immunity. A wide spectrum of microbiologic agents[63,74–76] can complicate the use of steroids, including gram-negative or –positive bacteria,[67,68] mycobacteria, fungi[69] and virus. Azathioprine use may cause lymphopenia and reduced immunoglobulin synthesis,[57,77] but when azathioprine is used alone, opportunistic infections are uncommon. Cyclophosphamide causes manly neutropenia, and frequent associated infections have been described, as in the treatment of Wegener's granulomatosis,[78] secondary to either bacterial or fungal agents. Cyclosporine A inhibits calcineurin action,[79] and consequently a defective cell-mediated immunity is expected. Methotrexate can induce bone marrow suppression; reduce neutrophil chemotaxis and immunoglobulin synthesis,[80,81] as has been described for rheumatoid arthritis; and is associated with opportunistic infections such as those caused by *Pneumocystis jirovecii* and herpes zoster. Newer agents such as infliximab[59–61] and adalimumab,[3,82] which are monoclonal antibodies with high affinity for human TNF-α, are associated with significant infections secondary to mycobacteria,[59,60,83] fungi[64] and viruses.[66] Most data refer to patients with rheumatoid arthritis who are treated with anti-TNF-α agents. These infections occur more frequently in patients with risk factors[84,85] such as some comorbidities, primary immunosuppression or immunosuppression secondary to associated conditions or risk exposure. The paucity of signs and symptoms with atypical clinical presentation of infections in this context constitutes a diagnostic challenge and requires a high level of suspicion.[86]

Finally, rituximab, a monoclonal antibody against the protein CD20, can be used in severe cases of ocular BD.[58] It results in induced peripheral B lymphocytopenia and potential decreased immunoglobulin levels with repeated treatments, but so far no significant increase of opportunistic infections has been shown.[87–89] Despite the lack of data on the long-term use of rituximab, monitoring immunoglobulin levels is advisable when maintenance therapy is being considered. Progressive multifocal leukoencephalopathy[90–93] should be included in the differential diagnosis of any new (or aggravated) neurological symptoms in patients who are heavily immunosuppressed, particularly those with neuro-Behçet syndrome, in which the distinction between a neurological manifestation of the disease and an infectious side effect of the immunosuppressive therapy can be especially difficult. Thus, recommendations in the setting of patients being treated with biological agents are as follows:[86] immunization against *Pneumococcus* and *Influenzae*; exclusion of hypogammaglobulinemia when initiating biological treatment, particularly rituximab, repeated before additional courses and in the event of an active infection; severe infections should be anticipated, immunosuppressive agents should be suspended and pre-emptive antibiotic therapy should be initiated until infection is definitively ruled out; supportive treatment with intravenous immunoglobulin might be provided on an individual basis and according to other risk factors; screening for latent tuberculosis before anti-TNF therapy, initiation of anti-TNF agents after 1 month of prophylactic treatment for latent TB and patients receiving treatment with anti-TNF agents should avoid high-risk activities associated with endemic mycosis in their geographic areas.

6 CONCLUSIONS

Infection seems to be implicated in many aspects of BD. Some evidence supports the influence of infectious agents, particularly of the streptococci group, in its pathogenesis. Sparse descriptions sustain the thesis that infection can be a trigger for exacerbations of BD. Regarding the infectious complications diagnosed in these patients, we highlight those caused by staphylococci, including MRSA. Other infections are related to immunosuppressive therapy and do not seem to differ from those found in other autoimmune diseases. Prospective long-term studies are needed to define any advantages in antibiotic prophylaxis and in the use of antibiotic-associated immunosuppression, both in controlled BD as well as in its flares.

REFERENCES

1. Alpsoy E, Akman A. Behçet's disease: an algorithmic approach to its treatment. *Arch Dermatolol Res* 2009;**301**:693–702.
2. Hatemi G, Yazici H. Infection and Behçet's disease. In: Shoenfeld Y, Rose N, editors. *Infection and autoimmunity*. 1st ed. Netherlands: Elsevier; Sept 2004. p. 629–35.
3. Cho SB, Cho S, Bang D. New insights in the clinical understanding of Behçet's disease. *Yonsei Med J* 2012;**53**(1):35–42.
4. International Study Group for Behçet's Disease. Criteria for diagnosis of Behçet's Disease. *Lancet* 1990;**335**:1078–80.
5. International Team for the Revision of the international Criteria for Behçet's Disease. Revision of the international criteria for Behçet's disease (ICBD). *Clin Exp Rheumatol* 2006;**24**:S14–15.
6. Tasliyurt T, Yigit S, Rustemoglu A, Gul U, Ates O. Common MEFV gene mutations in Turkish patients with Behçet's disease. *Gene* 2013;**530**(1):100–3. http://dx.doi.org/10.1016/j.gene.2013.08.026.
7. Chambrun M, Wechsler B, Geri G, Cacoub P, Saadoun D. New insights into the pathogenesis of Behçet's disease. *Autoimmun Rev* 2012;**11**:687–9.

8. Galeone M, Colucci R, D'Erme A, Moretti S, Lotti T. Potencial infectious etiology of Behçet's disease. *Pathol Res Int* 2012;**2012**:595380. http://dx.doi.org/10.1155/2012/595380.

9. Kaneko F, Oyama N, Nishibu A. Streptococcal Infection in the Pathogenesis of Behçet's disease and clinical effects of minocycline on the disease symptoms. *Yonsei Med J* 1997;**38** (6):444–54.

10. Kaneko F, Oyama N, Yanagihori H, Isogai E, Yokota K, Oguma K. The role of streptococcal hypersensitivity in the pathogenesis of Behçet's Disease. *Eur J Dermatol* 2008;**18** (5):489–98. http://dx.doi.org/10.1684/ejd.2008.0484.

11. Cho S, Zheng Z, Cho SB, Choi MJ, Lee KH, Bang D. Streptococcus sanguinis and the sera of patients with Behçet's disease stimulate membrane expression of α-enolase in human dermal microvascular endothelial cells. *Arch Dermatol Res* 2013;**305**(3):223–32. http://dx.doi.org/10.1007/s00403-012-1298-1.

12. Cho SB, Zheng Z, Cho S, Ahn KJ, Choi MJ, Kim DY, et al. Both the sera of patients with Behçet's disease and Streptococcus sanguis stimulate membrane expression of hnRNP A2/B1 in endothelial cells. *Scand J Rheumatol* 2013;**42**(3):241–6. http://dx.doi.org/10.3109/03009742.2012.733728.

13. Sang Ho O, Kyu-Yeop L, Lee JH. Clinical manifestations associated with high titer of anti-streptolysin O in Behçet's disease. *Clin Rheumatol* 2008;**27**:999–1003.

14. Hiroshata S, Oka H, Mizushima Y. Streptococal-related antigens stimulate production of IL- and interferon-gamma by T-cells from patients with Behçet's disease. *Cell Immunol* 1992;**140**:410–19.

15. Amoura Z, Guillaume M, Caillat Zucman S, Wechsler B, Piette JC. Pathophysiology of Behçet's disease. *Rev Med Interne* 2006;**27**:843–53.

16. Birtas-Atesoglu E, Inanc N, Yavuz S, Ergun T, Direskeneli H. Serum levels of free heat shock protein 70 and anti-HSP70 are elevated in Behçet's disease. *Clin Exp Rheumatol* 2008;**26**(4 Suppl. 50):S96–8.

17. Ergun T, Ince U, Eksioglu-Demiralp H, Gurbuz O, Direskeneli E, Gurses L, et al. HSP 60 expression in mucocutaneous lesions of Behçet's disease. *J Am Acad Dermatol* 2001;**45**:904–9.

18. Deniz E, Guc U, Buyukbabani N, Gul A. HSP60 expression in recurrent oral ulcerations of Behçet's disease. *Oral Surg Oral Med Pathol Oral Radiol Endod* 2010;**110**:196–200.

19. Sahebari M, Hashemzadeh K, Mahmoudi M, Saremi Z, Mirfeizi Z. Diagnostic yield of heat shock protein 70 (HSP-70) and anti-HSP-70 in Behçet's-induced uveitis. *Scand J Immunol* 2013;**77**(6):476–81. http://dx.doi.org/10.1111/sji.12045.

20. Miura T, Ishihara K, Kato T, Kimizuka R, Miyabe H, Ando T, et al. Detection of heat shock proteins but not superantigen by isolated oral bacteria from patients with Behçet's disease. *Oral Microbiol Immunol* 2005;**20**(3):167–71.

21. Gündüz A, Gündüz A, Cumurcu T, Seyrek A. Conjunctival flora in Behçet patients. *Can J Ophthalmol* 2008;**43**(4):476–9. http://dx.doi.org/10.3129/i08-089.

22. Lee S, Bang D, Cho YH, Lee ES, Sohn S. Polymerase chain reaction reveals herpes simplex virus DNA in saliva of patients with Behçet's disease. *Arch Dermatolol Res* 1996;**288**:179–83.

23. Sohn S, Lee ES, Bang D, Lee S. Behçet's disease-like symptoms induced by the herpes simplex virus DNA in ICR mice. *Eur J Dermatol* 1998;**8**:21–3.

24. Zouboulis CC, Turnbull JR, Mühlradt PF. Association of Mycoplasma fermentans with Adamantiades-Behçet's disease. *Adv Exp Med Biol* 2003;**528**:191–4.

25. Onen F, Tuncer D, Akar S, Birlik M, Akkoc N. Seroprevalence of Borrelia burgdorferi in patients with Behçet's disease. *Rheumatolol Int* 2003;**23**:289–93.

26. Hasni SA. Role of Helicobacter pylori infection in autoimmune diseases. *Curr Opin Rheumatol* 2012;**24**(4):429–34. http://dx.doi.org/10.1097/BOR.0b013e3283542d0b.

27. Ersoy O, Ersoy R, Yayar O, Demirci H, Tatlican S. H pylori infection in patients with Behçet's disease. *World J Gastroenterol* 2007;**13**(21):2983–5.

28. Aksu K, Kabasakal Y, Sayiner A, Keser G, Oksel F, Bilgiç A, et al. Prevalences of hepatitis A, B, C and E viruses in Behçet's disease. *Rheumatology (Oxford)* 1999;**38** (12):1279–81.

29. Zhang X, Li H, Li T, Zhang F, Han Y. Distinctive rheumatic manifestations in 98 patients with human immunodeficiency virus infection in China. *J Rheumatol* 2007;**34**(8):1760–4.

30. Mahajan VK, Sharma NL, Sharma VC, Sharma RC, Sarin S. Behçet's disease with HIV infection: response to antiretroviral therapy. *Indian J Dermatol Venereol Leprol* 2005;**71** (4):276–8.

31. Alpsoy E. Behçet's disease: treatment of mucocutaneous lesions. *Clin Exp Rheumatol* 2005;**23**:532–9.

32. Hatemi G, Bahar H, Uysal S, Mat C, Gogus F, Masatlioglu S, et al. The pustular skin lesions in Behçet's syndrome are not sterile. *Ann Rheum Dis* 2004;**63**(11):1450–2.

33. Suga Y, Tsuboi R, Kobayashi S, Ogawa H. A case of Behçet's disease aggravated by gingival infection with methicilin-resistant Staphylococcus aureus. *Br J Dermatol* 1995;**133** (2):319–21.

34. Mizushima Y, Matsuda T, Hoshi K, Ohno S. Induction of Behçet's disease symptoms after dental treatment and streptococcal antigen skin test. *J Rheumatol* 1988;**15** (6):1029–30.

35. Choi S, Choi Y, Kim J, Lee S, Park M, Kim B, et al. A case of recurrent Neuro-Behçet's disease after tooth extraction. *J Korean Med Sci* 2010;**25**(1):185–7.

36. Mora P, Kamberi E, Manzotti F, Zavota L, Orsoni JG. Staphylococcus aureus and autoimmune uveitis reactivation in childhood: a possible correlation? *Ital J Pediatr* 2009;**35** (1):34. http://dx.doi.org/10.1186/1824-7288-35-34.

37. Lellouche N, Belmatoug N, Bourgoin P, Logeart D, Acar C, Cohen-Solal A, et al. Recurrent valvular replacement due to exacerbation of Behçet's disease by Streptococcus agalactiae infection. *Eur J Intern Med* 2003;**14**(2):120–2.

38. Yıldırım E, Koçer B, Kaplan T, Sakıncı Ü. The possible role of Staphylococcus epidermidis in the development of pulmonary artery aneurysm in Behçet's disease. *Turkish J Thorac Cardiovasc Surg* 2007;**15**(3):260–2.

39. Choi CH, Kim TI, Kim BC, Shin SJ, Lee SK, Kim WH, et al. Anti-Saccharomyces cerevisiae antibody in intestinal Behçet's disease patients: relation to clinical course. *Dis Colon Rectum* 2006;**49**(12):1849–59.

40. Al-Waiz MM, Sharquie KE, A-Qaissi MH, Havani RK. Colchicine and benzathine penicillin in the treatment of Behçet disease: a case comparative study. *Dermatol Online J* 2005;**11**(3):3.

41. Trad S, Saadoun D, Barete S, Frances C, Piette JC, Wechsler B. Necrotizing folliculitis in Behçet's disease. *Rev Med Interne* 2009;**30**(3):268–70. http://dx.doi.org/10.1016/j.revmed.2008.06.007.

42. Salem B, Ichrak K, Hanène N, Safouane C, Maher B. Recurrent and superinfected leg ulcers in Behçet's disease. *Pan Afr Med J* 2013;**14**:139. http://dx.doi.org/10.11604/pamj.2013.14.139.1785.

43. Sun A, Chang JG, Chu CT, Liu BY, Yuan JH, Chiang CP. Preliminary evidence for an association of Epstein-Barr virus with pre-ulcerative oral lesions in patients with recurrent aphthous ulcers or Behçet's disease. *J Oral Pathol Med* 1998;**27**(4):168–75.

44. Schiødt M, Nørgaard T, Greenspan JS. Oral hairy leukoplakia in an HIV-negative woman with Behçet's syndrome. *Oral Surg Oral Med Oral Pathol Oral Radiol Endod* 1995;**79**(1):53–6.

45. Kiratli H, Bilgiç S, Mojab SS. Preseptal abscess formation following ocular cryotherapy for Behçet's uveitis. *Ophthalmic Surg Lasers* 2000;**31**(1):66–8.

46. Park UC, Kim SJ, Yu HG. Cytomegalovirus endotheliitis after fluocinolone acetonide (Retisert) implant in a patient with Behçet uveitis. *Ocul Immunol Inflamm* 2011;**19**(4):282–3. http://dx.doi.org/10.3109/09273948.2011.580075.

47. Kojima N, Sakano Y, Ohki S, Misawa Y. Rapidly growing aortic arch aneurysm in Behçet's disease. *Interact Cardiovasc Thorac Surg* 2011;**12**(3):502–4. http://dx.doi.org/10.1510/icvts.2010.260976.

48. Oudaïna W, Rhissassi B, Lagmouchi M, Aboulmakarim S, Bensaid Y, Zouhdi M. Complications of infected aneurysm due to Salmonella enteritidis: a case report. *Ann Biol Clin* 2010;**68**(1):104–6. http://dx.doi.org/10.1684/abc.2010.0405.

49. Mikami S, Nakase H, Ueno S, Matsuura M, Sakurai T, Chiba T. Involvement of cytomegalovirus infection in the ileal lesions of the patient with Behçet's disease. *Inflamm Bowel Dis* 2007;**13**(6):802–3.

50. Kapan M, Karabicak I, Aydogan F, Kusaslan R, Kisacik B. Intestinal perforation due to miliary tuberculosis in a patient with Behçet's disease. *Mt Sinai J Med* 2006;**73**(5):825–7.

51. Shukla A, Tolan Jr. RW. Behçet's disease presenting with pseudomembranous colitis and progression to neurological involvement: case report and review of the literature. *Clin Pediatr (Phila)* 2012;**51**(12):1197–201. http://dx.doi.org/10.1177/0009922811436339.

52. Tokgoz S, Ogmegul A, Mutluer M, Kivrak AS, Ustun ME. Cerebral abscesses in Behçet's disease: a case report. *Turk Neurosurg* 2012;**22**(1):116–18. http://dx.doi.org/10.5137/1019-5149.JTN.3297-10.2.

53. Iliopoulos A, Kedikoglou S, Laxanis S, Kourouklis S, Katsaros E. A case of tuberculous meningoencephalitis in a patient with Behçet's disease. *Clin Rheumatol* 2006;**25**(1):121–2.

54. Lee SH, Kim SD, Kim SH, Kim HR, Oh EJ, Yoon CH, et al. EBV-associated haemophagocytic syndrome in a patient with Behçet's disease. *Scand J Rheumatol* 2005;**34**(4):320–3.

55. Nakajima H, Sawaguchi H, Tsuji F, Miyamoto T, Miyara T, Tohda Y, et al. Case of Behçet's disease with frequent recurrence of multiple pulmonary abscess-like opacities. *Arerugi* 2007;**56**(10):1301–5.

56. Cho S, Lee K, Lee J, Bang D, Cho SB. Detection of tuberculous lymphadenopathy by positron emission tomography/computed tomography in a patient with Behçet's disease. *Acta Derm Venereol* 2011;**91**(4):470–1. http://dx.doi.org/10.2340/00015555-1079.

57. Chung SY, Oh KK, Chang HS. Sonographic findings of tuberculous thyroiditis in a patient with Behçet's syndrome. *J Clin Ultrasound* 2002;**30**(3):184–8.

58. Alpsoy E. New evidence-based treatment approach in Behçet's disease. *Pathol Res Int* 2012;**2012**. http://dx.doi.org/10.1155/2012/871019, Article ID 871019.

59. Skvara H, Duschek N, Karlhofer F. De novo tuberculosis during infliximab therapy in a patient with Behçet disease. *J Dtsch Dermatol Ges* 2009;**7**(7):616–19. http://dx.doi.org/10.1111/j.1610-0387.2009.07040.

60. Malkin J, Shrimpton A, Wiselka M, Barer MR, Duddridge M, Perera N. Olecranon bursitis secondary to Mycobacterium kansasii infection in a patient receiving infliximab for Behçet's disease. *J Med Microbiol* 2009;**58**:371–3. http://dx.doi.org/10.1099/jmm.0.006809-0.

61. Borhani Haghighi A, Safari A, Nazarinia MA, Habibagahi Z, Shenavandeh S. Infliximab for patients with neuro-Behçet's disease: case series and literature review. *Clin Rheumatol* 2011;**30**(7):1007–12. http://dx.doi.org/10.1007/s10067-011-1726-1.

62. Kotter I, Aepinus C, Graepler F, Gartner V, Eckstein A, Stubiger N, et al. HHV8 associated Kaposi's sarcoma during triple immunossupressive treatment with cyclosporine A, azathioprine, and prednisolone for ocular Behçet's disease and complete remission of both disorders with interferon alpha. *Ann Rheum Dis* 2001;**60**:83–6.

63. Santo M, Levy A, Levy MJ, Weinberger A, Mor R, Avidor I, et al. Pneumonectomy in pulmonary mucormycosis complicating Behçet's disease. *Postgrad Med J* 1986;**62**(728):485–6.
64. Kluger N, Poirier P, Guilpain P, Baixench MT, Cohen P, Paugam A. Cryptococcal meningitis in a patient treated with infliximab and mycophenolate mofetil for Behçet's disease. *Int J Infect Dis* 2009;**13**(5):e325. http://dx.doi.org/10.1016/j.ijid.2008.11.007.
65. Seddon ME, Thomas MG. Invasive disease due to Epidermophyton floccosum in an immunocompromised patient with Behçet's syndrome. *Clin Infect Dis* 1997;**25**(1):153–4.
66. Sari I, Birlik M, Gonen C, Akar S, Gurel D, Onen F, et al. Cytomegalovirus colitis in a patient with Behçet's disease receiving tumor necrosis factor alpha inhibitory treatment. *World J Gastroenterol* 2008;**14**(18):2912–14.
67. Auzary C, Du Boutin LTH, Wechlers B, Chollet P, Piette JC. Disseminated nocardiosis presenting as a flare of Behçet's disease. *Rheumatology* 2001;**40**:949–52.
68. Pamuk GE, Pamuk ON, Tabak F, Mert A, Ozturk R, Aktuglu Y. Systemic Nocardia infection in a patient with Behçet's disease. *Rheumatology* 2001;**40**:597–9.
69. Carbia SG, Chain M, Acuña K, Dei-Cas I, Glorio R, Malah V, et al. Disseminated cryptococcosis with cutaneous lesions complicating steroid therapy for Behçet's disease. *Int J Dermatol* 2003;**42**(10):821–3.
70. Korkmaz C, Aydinli A, Erol N, Yildirim N, Akgtün Y, Inci R, et al. Widespread nocardiosis in two patients with Behçet's disease. *Clin Exp Rheumatol* 2001;**19**(4):459–62.
71. Seror P, Pluvinage P, d'Andre FL, et al. Frequency of sepsis after local corticosteroid injection (an inquiry on 1160000 injections in rheumatological private practice in France). *Rheumatology (Oxford)* 1999;**38**:1272–4.
72. Fauci AS, Dale DC. The effect of in vivo hydrocortisone on subpopulations of human lymphocytes. *J Clin Invest* 1974;**53**:240–6.
73. Butler WT, Rossen RD. Effects of corticosteroids on immunity in man. I. Decreased serum IgG concentration caused by 3 or 5 days of high doses of methylprednisolone. *J Clin Invest* 1973;**52**:2629–40.
74. Saag KG, Koehnke R, Caldwell JR, Brasington R, Burmeister LF, Zimmerman B, et al. Low dose long-term corticosteroid therapy in rheumatoid arthritis: an analysis of serious adverse events. *Am J Med* 1994;**96**:115–23.
75. Williams AJ, Zardawi I, Walls J. Disseminated aspergillosis in high dose steroid therapy. *Lancet* 1983;**1**:1222.
76. Wollheim FA. Acute and long-term complications of corticosteroid pulse therapy. *Scand J Rheumatol* 1984;**54**:27–32.
77. Segal BH, Sneller MC. Infectious complications of immunosuppressive therapy in patients with rheumatic diseases. *Rheum Dis Clin North Am* 1997;**23**:219–37.
78. Bradley JD, Brandt KD, Katz BP. Infectious complications of cyclophosphamide treatment for vasculitis. *Arthritis Rheum* 1989;**32**:45–53.
79. Schreiber SL, Crabtree GR. The mechanism of action of cyclosporin A and FK506. *Immunol Today* 1992;**13**:136–42.
80. Van der Veen MJ, van der Heide A, Kruize AA, et al. Infection rate and use of antibiotics in patients with rheumatoid arthritis treated with methotrexate. *Ann Rheum Dis* 1994;**53**:224–8.
81. Lang B, Riegel W, Peters T, et al. Low dose methotrexate therapy for rheumatoid arthritis complicated by pancytopenia and Pneumocystis carinii pneumonia. *J Rheumatol* 1991;**18**(8):1257–9.
82. Saadoun D, Bodaghi B, Bienvenu B, Wechsler B, Sene D, Trad S, et al. Biotherapies in inflammatory ocular disorders: interferons, immunoglobulins, monoclonal antibodies. *Autoimmun Rev* 2013;**12**(7):774–83.

83. Eleftheriou D, Melo M, Marks SD, Tullus K, Sills J, Cleary G, et al. Biologic therapy in primary systemic vasculitis of the young. *Rheumatology (Oxford)* 2009;**48**:978–86.

84. Martin-Mola E, Balsa A. Infectious complications of biologic agents. *Rheum Dis Clin North Am* 2009;**35**(1):183–99.

85. Saketkoo LA, Espinoza LR. Impact of biologic agents on infectious diseases. *Infect Dis Clin North Am* 2006;**20**(4):931–61.

86. Campar A, Isenberg DA. Life-threatening complications of biological therapies. In: Khamastha M, Ramos-Casals M, editors. *Autoimmune diseases: complex and acute situations.* 1st ed; 2011. p. 375–403.

87. Cohen SB, Emery P, Greenwald MW, Dougados M, Furie RA, Genovese MC, et al. for the REFLEX Trial Group. Rituximab for rheumatoid arthritis refractory to anti-tumor necrosis factor therapy: results of a multicenter, randomized, double-blind, placebo-controlled, phase III trial evaluating primary efficacy and safety at twenty-four weeks. *Arthritis Rheum* 2006;**54**(9):2793–806.

88. Keystone E, Fleischmann R, Emery P, Furst DE, van Vollenhoven R, Bathon J, et al. Safety and efficacy of additional courses of rituximab in patients with active rheumatoid arthritis: an open-label extension analysis. *Arthritis Rheum* 2007;**56**(12):3896–908.

89. Fleischmann RM. Safety of biologic therapy in rheumatoid arthritis and other autoimmune diseases: focus on rituximab. *Semin Arthritis Rheum* 2009;**38**(4):265–80.

90. Kelesidis T, Daikos G, Boumpas D, Tsiodras S. Does rituximab increase the incidence of infectious complications? A narrative review. *Int J Infect Dis* 2011;**15**:e2–e16.

91. Carson KR, Focosi D, Major EO, Petrini M, Richey EA, West DP, et al. Monoclonal antibody-associated progressive multifocal leucoencephalopathy in patients treated with rituximab, natalizumab, and efalizumab: a Review from the Research on Adverse Drug Events and Reports (RADAR). *Lancet Oncol* 2009;**10**(8):816–24.

92. Carson K, Evens A, Richey E, Habermann T, Focosi D, Seymour J, et al. Progressive multifocal leukoencephalopathy after rituximab therapy in HIV-negative patients: a report of 57 cases from the Research on Adverse Drug Events and Reports project. *Blood* 2009;**113**(20):4834–40.

93. Salliot C, Dougados M, Gossec L. Risk of serious infections during rituximab, abatacept and anakinra treatments for rheumatoid arthritis: meta-analyses of randomised placebo-controlled trial. *Ann Rheum Dis* 2009;**68**(1):25–32.

CHAPTER 47

Vasculitides and Hepatitis C Infection

Melanie Deutsch, Dimitrios Vassilopoulos[1]

2nd Department of Medicine and Laboratory, University of Athens Medical School, Hippokration General Hospital, Athens, Greece
[1]Corresponding Author: dvassilop@med.uoa.gr

1 INTRODUCTION

Vasculitis in the setting of chronic hepatitis C virus (HCV) infection occurs in different forms. The most common form is a small-vessel vasculitis caused by the deposition of immune complexes containing cryoglobulins, that is, HCV-associated cryoglobulinemic vasculitis (CV). Involvement of medium-sized vessels is an uncommon finding in HCV-associated CV, whereas there are increasing reports of medium-sized vasculitis occurring in the setting of chronic HCV infection (polyarteritis nodosa [PAN]-like). This chapter reviews the epidemiological, pathogenetic, clinical, and laboratory findings in HCV-associated vasculitis as well as the currently available therapeutic approaches.

2 HCV-ASSOCIATED CV

2.1 Definition

HCV-associated CV is a clinical syndrome that develops in a subset of patients with HCV-associated mixed cryoglobulinemia (MC). There are currently no widely accepted diagnostic or classification criteria for HCV-associated CV or for CV in general. CV was defined by the 2012 International Chapel Hill Consensus Conference on the Nomenclature of Systemic Vasculitides as a "vasculitis with cryoglobulin immune deposits affecting small vessels (predominantly capillaries, venules, or arterioles) and associated with serum cryoglobulins. Skin, glomeruli, and peripheral nerves are often involved".[1] HCV-associated CV was subcategorized in the group of "vasculitides associated with a probable etiology".

 An international group of experts recently proposed preliminary classification criteria for CV based on various clinical and laboratory findings[2]

Infection and Autoimmunity
http://dx.doi.org/10.1016/B978-0-444-63269-2.00021-0

(Table 1). When these criteria were applied in an independent cohort of patients with HCV-associated CV, they revealed a sensitivity of 88% and specificity of 96%, whereas in patients with HCV-unrelated CV, the sensitivity and specificity were 89% and 90%, respectively.[3] Further validation of these criteria in larger cohorts of patients with various types of vasculitides are needed.

Despite these difficulties, most experts agree that a number of serologic, pathologic, and clinical findings should be present for an accurate diagnosis of HCV-associated CV:[4,5]

- Active chronic HCV infection should be documented by the presence of anti-HCV antibodies and HCV RNA in the serum using established methods.[6]
- Circulating MC (type II or III, according to the classification proposed by Brouet et al.[7]) measured by an appropriate method must be present in the serum of infected patients (cryoglobulinemia).[5] Given that cryoglobulinemia is a common laboratory finding of patients with chronic HCV infection (12–56%),[4] clinical and pathological findings strongly suggestive of vasculitic involvement should be present.

Table 1 Preliminary Classification Criteria for Cryoglobulinemic Vasculitis

---

A. Questionnaire item: at least *two* of the following:
   a)   Do you remember one or more episodes of small red spots on your skin, particularly involving the lower limbs?
   b)   Have you ever had red spots on your lower extremities, which leave a brownish color after their disappearance?
   c)   Has a doctor ever told you that you have viral hepatitis?
B. Clinical item: at least *three* of the following four (present or past)
   a)   Constitutional symptoms: fatigue, low-grade fever, fibromyalgia
   b)   Articular involvement: arthalgias, arthritis
   c)   Vascular involvement: purpura, skin ulcers, necrotizing vasculitis, hyperviscosity syndrome, Raynaud's phenomenon
   d)   Neurologic involvement: peripheral neuropathy, cranial nerve involvement, vasculitic CNS involvement
C. Laboratory item: at least *two* of the following three (present)
   a)   Reduced serum C4
   b)   Positive serum rheumatoid factor
   c)   Positive serum M component

Patients are classified as having cryoglobulinemic vasculitis (CV) if *at least two* of the three items (questionnaire, clinical, laboratory) were positive.
The patient must be positive for serum cryoglobulins in *at least two* determinations at ≥ 12 weeks.
From Ref. 2.

- Clinical findings suggestive of vasculitis, including purpura, neuropathy (distal symmetric polyneuropathy or mononeuritis multiplex [MNM]), membranoproliferative glomerulonephritis [MPGN], and skin ulcerations or digital necrosis. Clinical findings suggestive of gastrointestinal, cardiac or central nervous system (CNS) vasculitic involvement may be present, albeit rarely.
- Pathological findings of small-vessel vasculitis affecting the skin (leukocytoclastic purpura), nerves, muscles, or other involved organs are extremely helpful in making the correct diagnosis. The documentation of the presence of immune complexes in affected vessels, either by immunofluorescence or electron microscopy (kidneys), is an additional important diagnostic tool.

2.2 Epidemiology

The frequency of HCV-associated CV has not been investigated in large epidemiological studies. However, the prevalence of MC is closely related to the geographic variation of HCV infection. The worldwide prevalence of HCV infection has been estimated to be approximately 2%.[8] Although, as mentioned earlier, the prevalence of cryoglobulinemia is reported consistently in the range between 12% and 56% in HCV-infected individuals, the frequency of HCV-associated CV is significantly lower.[4,9] In a prospective study of 1614 patients with HCV infection, Cacoub et al.[10] found an overall frequency of vasculitis of 1%, whereas in patients with cryoglobulinemia the frequency was 2–3%. The disease is more common in patients with longer disease duration.[4]

Extrapolating from these data, one can assume that the prevalence of HCV-associated CV in the general population should range between 0.01% and 0.3% (based on the prevalence of HCV infection in the studied population). However, this estimate is probably an overestimation, because most studies examining the frequency of cryoglobulinemia and HCV-associated CV in patients with HCV are biased (referral and patient selection bias). Geographical variation exists: the disease is more common in Southern Europe compared to Northern Europe and the United States.[4] The mean age of patients with HCV-associated CV is approximately 40–60 years, and there seems to be a female predominance (female-to-male ratio of 3:1), with no racial predilection.[11,12]

2.3 Pathogenesis

Cryoglobulins are produced by clonally expanded B-cells in the bone marrow and liver of HCV-infected patients. The majority of these clonally expanded B-cells produce monoclonal immunoglobulin (Ig) M with rheumatoid factor (RF) activity that has a specific cross-reacting idiotype (WA). These germline-encoded WA-producing B-cells (usually V_H1-69+ B1 cells) are detected in approximately 10% of HCV-infected patients[13] and are triggered to produce IgM RF by HCV viral particles and the core protein.[14] B-cell activating factor produced by dendritic cells plays a significant role in maintaining these clonally expanded B-cells.

The produced IgM RF forms large, cold-precipitable immune complexes with IgG, viral RNA, and proteins such the core and NS3 proteins.[14,15] These immune complexes then bind to the C1q and through its specific receptor (C1qR) to endothelial cells, leading to the initiation of the inflammatory cascade that results to small-vessel vasculitis characteristic of HCV-associated CV.[4,14] The role of other cell subpopulations in the pathogenesis of HCV-associated CV has recently been explored. More specifically, regulatory T-cells (T_{Regs}) are decreased in these patients, potentially leading to the unopposed action of autoreactive effector T-cells.[16]

2.4 Clinical Characteristics

2.4.1 Skin Manifestations

Deposition of cryoglobulins (with or without associated HCV) in skin vessels leads to a localized inflammatory reaction that is expressed clinically by a number of skin manifestations, including purpura, leg ulcers and, more rarely, digital necrosis.[11,17] The hallmark of HCV-associated CV is the appearance of purpuric lesions in the lower extremities. Palpable purpura has been reported in 65–90% of cases; in most cases it represents the presenting manifestation of the disease.[11,14,17] Typically, its appearance follows an intermittent pattern, whereas the lesions tend to be nonpruritic with a predilection for the lower extremity.[4] Purpuric lesions are found more commonly in limbs with venous insufficiency, and their disappearance is followed by residual skin hyperpigmentation, which can last for prolonged periods of time.

Biopsies of purpuric lesions show leukocytoclastic vasculitis with a predominance of mononuclear cells and neutrophils.[18] Immunofluorescent studies reveal the deposition of IgM and C3 in the vessel walls in approximately 80% of cases. Attempts to detect HCV RNA in skin biopsies from patients with HCV-associated CV have given conflicting results: some studies show the presence of HCV virions in vessel walls,[18,19] whereas other studies failed to reproduce these findings.[20] The appearance of leg ulcers is another common skin manifestation of HCV-associated CV (30–40%)

Table 2 Demographic and Clinical Characteristics of Patients with Hepatitis C Virus-Associated Cryoglobulinemic Vasculitis ACV

Characteristic	
Mean age, years (range)	50 (40–60)
Female-to-male ratio	3:1
Purpura	65–90%
Arthralgia	40–80%
Leg ulcers	30–40%
Peripheral neuropathy	17–65%
Renal involvement	20–35%
Sicca syndrome	6–36%
Raynaud's phenomenon	3–40%

Data from Refs. 5, 28, 36–38.

(Table 2).[4] The ulcers typically are localized in the lower extremities (above the malleoli) in association with purpuric lesions. Other less common skin manifestations include digital necrosis, nodules, and urticarial lesions with variable histopathologic findings.[4]

2.4.2 Nerve Involvement

The predominant form of nerve involvement in HCV-associated CV is vasculitic peripheral neuropathy, detected in 17–60% of patients (Table 2)[4,14] in the form of either a symmetric distal polyneuropathy ($\sim$80%) or as MNM ($\sim$10%). Patients with distal polyneuropathy present with a painful symmetric neuropathy with predominant sensory findings (paresthesias).[21] Electromyographic studies reveal an axonal sensory neuropathic process, whereas nerve or muscle biopsies from the affected areas show inflammatory vascular lesions in the majority of cases ($\sim$83%).[21] These inflammatory lesions take the form of vasculitis of the small vessels or infiltration of the vessel wall by mononuclear cells, without necrosis.[22] A direct pathogenetic role for HCV has been postulated based on the detection of HCV RNA in epineural cells by sensitive assays (reverse-transcriptase polymerase chain reaction).[21,23,24] HCV RNA has been found in endothelial cells, infiltrating mononuclear cells, or immune complexes deposited in the arterial wall. Despite its presence, local viral replication as evidenced by the detection of its replicative (negative) strand has not been documented so far.[21] MNM is another less common neurological manifestation with prominent inflammatory vascular lesions in pathological specimens[21] and IgM deposition by immunofluorescent studies,[25] whereas HCV RNA has not been found in the affected muscles or nerves of such patients.[21]

CNS involvement is a rare, life-threatening manifestation of generalized HCV-associated CV and has a high mortality rate.[26] A number of clinical manifestations have been observed, including cerebrovascular accidents, seizures, encephalopathy, dizziness, and dementia. The mechanism by which brain lesions are produced is unclear. In a prospective study, patients with HCV-associated CV underwent clinical evaluation (neuropsychological tests) and cerebral magnetic resonance imaging studies.[27] The majority (89%) of patients had a deficiency in one or more of the 10 cognitive domains examined; the number of impaired cognitive functions was significantly higher in patients with HCV-associated CV than in patients with HCV or healthy controls. Similarly, magnetic resonance imaging analysis showed that patients with HCV-associated CV had a higher mean number of total and periventricular white matter high-intensity signals than HCV controls and healthy controls, respectively. These findings suggest specific CNS inflammatory involvement in patients with HCV-associated CV. Interpretation of these limited data is problematic because detailed analysis, including angiography and/or brain biopsy, has not been performed in each case.

2.4.3 Renal Involvement

Kidney involvement is present in 20–35% of patients with HCV-associated CV patients (Table 2).[4,14,28,29] The most common form of renal involvement is diffuse MPGN (80%).[29,30] Less common forms include focal MPGN, mesangial proliferative glomerulonephritis, membranous nephropathy, and focal segmental glomerulosclerosis.[29,30]

Renal involvement typically develops during the evolution of HCV-associated systemic MC, with only 15% of cases displaying a concomitant renal and extrarenal involvement at presentation.[31] Most patients present with asymptomatic proteinuria (subnephrotic range, ~40%), followed by nephrotic (21%) or acute nephritic syndrome (14%).[29] Difficult to control hypertension (70–80%) is a characteristic finding in these patients.[4,14,28,29] HCV-associated MPGN usually follows a fluctuating course with frequent episodes of exacerbation. Approximately 15% of patients develop end-stage renal disease and require dialysis during long-term follow-up.[32] Although data on the clinical course and prognosis of non-MPGN forms of HCV-associated renal disease are limited, no significant differences with MPGN have been observed.

Renal biopsies in patients with MPGN reveal the typical histological findings of an immune complex-mediated glomerulonephritis characterized by hypercellular glomeruli (mainly by infiltrating monocytes/macrophages), subendothelial and endocapillary deposits and IgM/IgG and C3 glomerular deposition.[29,30] In some cases, characteristic intraluminal thrombi composed of deposited immune complexes are noted.[29,30] As is the case with peripheral neuropathy in patients with HCV-associated CV, HCV RNA has been detected in kidney tissues in a number of studies, but its direct pathogenetic role has not been proven.[33–35] Searches for HCV-encoded proteins in kidney biopsies have given inconsistent results so far.[33–35] In two long-term follow-up studies, the presence of renal involvement at baseline was among the strongest predictors of poor prognosis and decreased survival.[11,12]

2.4.4 Other Clinical Manifestations

A number of other clinical manifestations have been described in patients with HCV-associated CV, including arthralgias (40–80%), arthritis (10%), sicca syndrome (6–36%), and Raynaud's phenomenon (3–40%).[5,28,36–38] Given that some of these manifestations occur also in cryoglobulin-negative patients with chronic HCV infection, their true association with HCV-associated CV is unknown.

Pulmonary,[5,11,14] heart[39] and gastrointestinal (GI)[14,40] involvement are serious but rare (<5%) manifestations of HCV-associated CV. Lung involvement takes the form of mild interstitial fibrosis, whereas cardiac involvement presents as congestive heart failure (dilated or hypertrophic cardiomyopathy) that is reversible with aggressive immunosuppressive therapy.[39] Ischemic abdominal pain is always present in patients with GI involvement, and half of them develop life-threatening complications such as intestinal bleeding and/or acute abdomen.[40]

2.5 Laboratory Findings

The hallmark of HCV-associated CV is the presence of mixed cryoglobulins in the serum. Cryoglobulins are Igs with distinct physicochemical characteristics illustrated by their tendency to precipitate at temperatures below 37 °C.[5,36] They are immune complexes composed of IgM with RF activity, either monoclonal (type II) or polyclonal (type III), directed against polyclonal IgG immunoglobulins. Intermediate forms of mixed cryoglobulins composed of oligoclonal IgM-RF also have been observed.[5,36] Special attention to blood draw and sample handling for the accurate measurement of circulating cryoglobulins has been emphasized.[5,36]

A number of studies examined the frequency of type II or III cryoglobulins in patients with chronic HCV infection.[41] The majority of patients with predominant liver disease without associated extrahepatic diseases demonstrate type III cryoglobulins.[41] In contrast, most patients with symptomatic HCV-associated CV are positive for type II cryoglobulins (58–82%).[11,12,15] Analysis of these mixed cryoglobulins revealed that they form complexes with HCV proteins (mainly from the core and NS3 regions), and they bind the C1q complement fraction.[15]

Patients with HCV-associated CV display a number of autoimmune laboratory findings (see Table 3). Among them, the detection of elevated titers of RF (68–75%) is the most prevalent.[5,36,38] Other laboratory findings include low levels of C4, indicating immune-complex formation and tissue deposition, and the presence of autoantibodies such as antinuclear, smooth muscle, actin and, more rarely, antimitochondrial or antithyroid antibodies (Table 3). It should be mentioned that patients with chronic hepatitis C without cryoglobulinemia demonstrate a similar array of autoantibodies, indicating a chronic polyclonal activation of B lymphocytes in these patients. Patients with HCV-associated CV generally display much higher titer or percentage of positive RF tests compared to HCV patients without circulating cryoglobulins.[9]

The activity and chronicity of the underlying liver disease in patients with circulating cryoglobulins or HCV-associated CV is a debatable issue. One large-scale study[42] and a meta-analysis[41] showed that advanced fibrosis/cirrhosis is present in 32–40% of patients with cryoglobulinemia compared to 12–17% of patients with HCV without cryoglobulins. The presence of severe fibrosis at the time of diagnosis of HCV-associated CV is strongly associated with poor long-term prognosis in these patients.[39] On the contrary, in a recent long-term cohort study from Italy, the cumulative probability of developing cirrhosis after 15 years of follow-up was lower in patients with CV (14%) compared to patients without

Table 3 Laboratory Findings in Hepatitis C Virus–Associated Cryoglobulinemic Vasculitis ACV
Characteristic

Rheumatoid factor	68–75%
Low C4	50–85%
Antinuclear antibodies	12–32%
Smooth muscle actin antibodies	~23%
Antimitochondrial antibodies	~10%
Antithyroid antibodies	~10%

Data from Refs, 28, 36, 38

cryoglobulins (25%), but there was no difference in their overall survival.[43] Differences in the design of these studies (cross sectional versus prospective) and possibly selection bias may explain these discrepancies.

2.5.1 Prognosis of HCV-associated CV

Two large-scale studies published the past decade[11,12] evaluated the long-term survival of patients with HCV-associated CV. The 5- and 10-year survival rates were 75% and 56–63%, respectively. Baseline factors associated with poor prognosis included kidney involvement, advanced age, male sex, and severe liver fibrosis.[11,12]

2.6 Therapy

Therapy for patients with HCV-associated CV is a challenging task for physicians.[4,14,44] The goals of therapy are clear: eradicate the responsible causative agent (HCV) and suppress the vasculitic inflammatory process. The recent advances in the antiviral treatment of chronic hepatitis C offer new therapeutic options for these patients.[45]

2.6.1 Antiviral Therapy
2.6.1.1 Interferon-α

Interferon (IFN)-α remains the most important agent in the treatment of chronic HCV infection.[6] Bonomo et al.[46] used IFN-α for the treatment of HCV-associated CV in 1987, even before the discovery of HCV.[46] Following the discovery of HCV and its clear association with MC, a number of small randomized and open trials examined the role of standard IFN-α therapy in patients with HCV-associated CV.[6] About 75% of the patients demonstrated partial or complete clinical response at the end of therapy (6–12 months), but approximately 70% of these patients relapsed after treatment was discontinued.[6] Furthermore, clinical improvement was noted predominantly in skin lesions (purpura) and less so in renal and neurological manifestations.[6] The inability of standard IFN-α monotherapy to provide a sustained clinical response is directly related to its low rate of viral clearance (~15%).

2.6.2 Combination Antiviral Therapy (Interferon-α and Ribavirin)

Multicenter, randomized clinical trials at the end of the last decade confirmed the superiority of a combination scheme consisting of standard IFN-α and ribavirin over standard IFN-α monotherapy in patients with chronic hepatitis C.[45,47] This was also the case for HCV-associated CV, although the long-term efficacy was limited by an inability to achieve viral clearance in the majority of patients.[48]

The introduction of pegylated IFNs (Peg-IFNs) has increased the efficacy of the combination scheme in patients with chronic hepatitis C. Until recently, the combination of a peg-IFN-α—according to the HCV genotype—and ribavirin for 6–12 months was the optimal therapeutic approach for treatment-naive patients with chronic hepatitis C. With this regimen, 50–80% of patients clear the virus, achieving the so-called sustained viral response, defined as undetectable HCV RNA, 6 months after the end of antiviral treatment. Combination therapy with Peg-IFN-α (-2α or -2β) and ribavirin has been explored in a number of open-label studies of patients with HCV-associated CV; they showed an overall virological and clinical response of approximately 54% and 73%, respectively.[49–54]

However, antiviral treatment should be administered in patients with an underlying vasculitis with great caution and knowledge of its potential severe side effects. In addition to the known contraindications and side effects of IFN-α and ribavirin treatment,[55] IFN-α also has the potential to exacerbate underlying skin,[56] nerve, or renal[57] lesions in patients with HCV-associated CV. Ribavirin is contraindicated in patients with moderate to severe renal dysfunction (creatinine clearance <50 mL/min), whereas reduction in the dose of Peg-IFN-α is needed in such patients.[44]

2.6.3 The Era of Triple Therapy (Direct-Acting antivirals Together with Peg-IFN and Ribavirin)

During the past 5 years, real progress has been made regarding the therapy of genotype 1 chronic hepatitis C. Several small molecules targeting crucial pathways in HCV replication have been developed.[45] Among these, telaprevir and boceprevir are the first protease inhibitors approved for the therapy of this group of patients.[45] Together with Peg-IFN-α and ribavirin (triple therapy), a significant increase in sustained viral response (~25%) was observed in all subgroups of patients who underwent treatment.[45] However, during the same time period, the adverse events of the new treatment approach also increased, making this therapy schema difficult and applicable to only a limited number of patients.

There has been only one open-label prospective study of a cohort of 23 patients with HCV-associated CV treated with triple therapy for 24 weeks.[58] All patients previously received antiviral treatment with Peg-IFN and ribavirin and were either nonresponders or relapsers. HCV RNA was undetectable at week 24 in 70% of patients, and a complete clinical response was achieved in 57% of patients. Despite a satisfactory virological response, as expected, a high rate of side effects was documented, including anemia (74%, of whom 39% required red blood cell transfusion), neutropenia (78%), thrombocytopenia (65%), bacterial infections (53%), and telaprevir-associated skin eruption (30%). This study demonstrates poor tolerance of the triple therapy in HCV-associated CV, making it an unlikely treatment option in the future. The development of IFN-α-free regimens represents a potential breakthrough in the treatment of chronic hepatitis C, which may apply also to HCV-associated CV.

2.6.4 Immunosuppressive Therapy

Immunosuppressive therapy is used in patients with severe or life-threatening disease and as adjunctive therapy in patients with mild to moderate disease activity mainly involving the skin.[4,14,47] Moreover, immunosuppressive therapy is needed in some patients who experience clinical relapse or persistence of CV despite viral eradication.[59] The goals of immunosuppressive therapy are to suppress the production of the pathogenic cryoglobulins by B cells and to down-regulate the host immune response that is responsible for the localized vascular inflammatory process.[14,47]

Most data regarding immunosuppressive agents are available for corticosteroids and cyclophosphamide. Before the discovery of HCV, patients with severe "essential" MC were frequently treated with a combination of corticosteroids, cyclophosphamide, and plasmapheresis in an uncontrolled fashion, with mixed results.[32] In a 1-year randomized, controlled study, corticosteroids used alone achieved clinical response in only 17% of patients with HCV-associated CV, whereas there was no additional clinical benefit when they were added to IFN-α compared to IFN-α alone.[60]

The administration of immunosuppressive therapy in patients with a chronic viral infection raises reasonable concerns about their short- and long-term side effects. Short-term corticosteroid use in patients with chronic hepatitis C is associated with a transient increase in HCV RNA levels, but acute deterioration of liver function during or after therapy is rare.[61] Similarly, short courses of cyclophosphamide therapy were not linked to acute liver failure in a large study of Italian patients with HCV-associated MPGN.[31] Collectively, these limited data suggest that short-term immunosuppressive therapy is not associated with acute liver toxicity in patients with HCV-associated vasculitis.

2.6.5 Apheresis

Plasma exchange or plasmapheresis is used temporally in patients with severe- or life-threatening manifestations of HCV-associated CV, including rapidly deteriorating glomerulonephritis, skin necrosis, CNS, or motor neuropathy and hyperviscosity syndrome.[62] It is usually administered in combination with corticosteroids and/or cyclophosphamide to prevent a rebound phenomenon after the discontinuation of plasmapheresis. Controlled data on its efficacy are not available, but anecdotal evidence supports its use in patients with life-threatening disease.

2.6.6 New Immunosuppressive or Immunomodulatory Agents
2.6.6.1 Rituximab

Biologic agents that specifically target those elements of the immune system that participate in the pathogenesis of HCV-associated CV are currently under investigation for the treatment of this disorder. So far, most data are available for rituximab (RTX), a B-cell-depleting agent (chimeric monoclonal antibody against CD20); more than 200 patients have been treated with this agent over the past decade (reviewed by Ferri et al.[63]). This agent is already being licenced for use in patients with B-cell non-Hodgkin's lymphomas and antineutrophil cytoplasmic antibody-associated vasculitides. RTX has been used either as monotherapy (antiviral resistant or intolerant disease) or in combination with antiviral therapy (Peg-IFN-α and ribavirin) in patients with HCV-associated CV.

2.6.7 RTX Monotherapy

In initial open studies, RTX monotherapy was used in patients with resistance to antivirals (IFN-α) and/or steroids; complete clinical response rates ranged from 36% to 73%. Relapses occurred in approximately one third of patients (36%) after a mean period of 6.7 months.[64] Two recent prospective, randomized trials assessed the efficacy of RTX monotherapy in patients who had resistance, intolerance, or contraindications to antiviral therapy.[65,66] The clinical response rate at 6 months ranged from 71% to 83%, whereas the response rate with conventional immunosuppressive therapy ranged between 3.5% and 8%, respectively. In general, therapy was well tolerated, without significant effects on liver function or HCV viral load. Moreover, RTX was found to be safe even in cirrhotic patients with HCV-associated MC.[67]

2.6.8 RTX and Antiviral Therapy (Peg-IFN-α and Ribavirin)

The combination of RTX with classical antiviral treatment (Peg-IFN-α and ribavirin) has been tested in a small number of patients with HCV-associated CV. In an earlier study of 16 patients treated with this regimen, the complete clinical response rate was 62% after 6 months of treatment.[68] In two more recent open-label controlled clinical trials, antiviral therapy (Peg-IFN-α and ribavirin) was compared to combination therapy (Peg-IFN-α and ribavirin plus rituximab) in a mixed population of patients (antiviral naive and resistant).[52,53] The overall complete clinical response rate of combination therapy ranged from 54%[53] to 73%,[52] without a statistically significant difference from the response obtained by antiviral therapy alone.

Nevertheless, combination therapy induced a clinical response earlier (in approximately 5 months, compared to 8 months with antiviral therapy alone) and was associated with better renal outcomes (81% vs. 40%) and a longer time to relapse (15 vs. 3 months).[52] The therapy was well tolerated without any significant side effects. It should be mentioned that, in one study, RTX was administered together with the antiviral therapy,[53] whereas, in the second study, RTX was administered first (every week x 4), followed by antiviral therapy.[52] However, because of the small number of patients in these studies and the heterogeneity of the study designs, the results must be interpreted with caution.

2.6.9 Interleukin-2 Treatment

The safety and efficacy of the administration of low-dose interleukin-2 in 10 patients with HCV-associated CV refractory to conventional immunosuppressives and RTX was recently investigated in a phase 1/2a study.[69] Interleukin-2 increased the number of T_{Regs} and was associated with clinical improvement in 8 of 10 patients as well as reduction of serum cryoglobulins. Furthermore, down-regulation of various inflammatory genes was noted. No important adverse events were reported. These preliminary results indicate an alternative immunomodulatory therapeutic approach in patients with HCV-associated CV that merits further investigation.

2.6.10 Treatment Algorithm for HCV-Associated CV

In the absence of well-designed randomized controlled trials evaluating the efficacy and safety of different therapeutic regimens, the therapeutic algorithm for patients with HCV-associated CV is based mainly on expert opinion. The management of HCV-associated CV should be designed on an individual basis, based on the severity of vasculitic involvement, the status of the underlying liver disease and the virological characteristics of each patient.

In treatment naive patients with mild to moderate disease activity (purpura, arthralgias/arthritis, mild sensory neuropathy, and mild protein-uria/hematuria with normal creatinine values), antiviral therapy with Peg-IFN-α and ribavirin should be offered in addition to symptomatic ther-apy. The duration of treatment and dose of these agents should be decided after consultation with a hepatologist and according to the most recent guidelines.[55,70]

In patients with severe disease (rapidly progressive glomerulonephritis; motor neuropathy; CNS, GI, or myocardial involvement; digital necrosis), combination therapy with immunosuppressives and antivirals should be tried. Currently, it seems safer to start with immunosuppressives to achieve immediate disease control, followed later by antiviral therapy. Immunosup-pressives usually include a combination of corticosteroids and cyclophospha-mide or rituximab. The choice between cyclophosphamides and rituximab should be made after balancing the risk and benefit for the individual patient and the experience of the physician providing care. In patients with life-threatening disease or hyperviscocity syndrome, plasmapheresis can also be added to immunosuppressives.

3 HCV-ASSOCIATED MEDIUM-SIZED VASCULITIS

Medium-sized vasculitis was considered an uncommon manifestation of chronic hepatitis C. Two recent large-scale epidemiological studies indi-cated an increasing frequency of HCV-associated medium-sized vasculitis, representing 20% of all HCV-related vasculitides in one study[38] and approx-imately 6% of an unselected population of patients with hepatitis C in another study.[71]

Patients with HCV-associated medium-sized vasculitis had more severe acute systemic disease manifestations resembling classic PAN[38] compared to patients with HCV-associated CV. Compared to patients with HBV-associated medium vessel vasculitis (PAN-like), they more often display skin involvement (purpura) and hypertension, whereas GI involvement is not so prevalent.[38] Biopsies of involved tissues demonstrate a necrotizing medium-sized vasculitis with mononuclear and polymorphonuclear cell infiltration (see Figure 1), and angiographic studies reveal characteristic microaneurysms

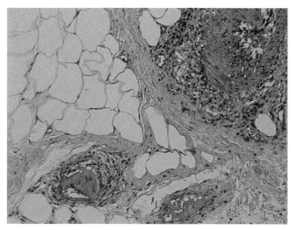

Figure 1 Biopsy from a skin lesion (hematoxylin and eosin stain) in a patient with chronic hepatitis C presenting with fever, polyarthritis, hypertension, and mononeuritis multiplex. The findings are typical of a medium-sized vasculitis (hepatitis C virus–associated, polyarteritis nodosa–like). *Courtesy of Dr. A. Pantelidaki.*

or stenoses in 64% of cases.[38] Clinical remission was induced initially by a combination of antiviral and immunosuppressive therapies in almost 80% of cases, but relapses were more common (28%) compared to HBV-associated medium vessel vasculitis (10%).

4 HCV AS A CAUSATIVE FACTOR IN OTHER AUTOIMMUNE DISEASES INCLUDING VASCULITIDES

There has been some epidemiological evidence that HCV could be involved in different autoimmune diseases. A large multinational study including 1322 patients with 18 different autoimmune diseases and 236 matched healthy controls showed a higher prevalence of anti-HCV positivity in these patients (8.7%) compared to the healthy controls (0.4%).[72] However, this study also included patients with MC and Hashimoto thyroiditis. Moreover, another study of 54 patients with granulomatosis with polyangiitis (Wegener's granulomatosis) indicated that anti-HCV antibodies were found significantly more often compared to the healthy population (30% vs. 0%).[73] These data, together with some case reports, indirectly suggest a possible link of other vasculitides with HCV. More studies are needed to substantiate these findings.

REFERENCES

1. Jennette JC, Falk RJ, Bacon PA, Basu N, Cid MC, Ferrario F, et al. 2012 revised International Chapel Hill Consensus Conference Nomenclature of Vasculitides. *Arthritis Rheum* 2013;**65**:1–11.
2. De Vitas, Soldano F, Isola M, Monti G, Gabrielli A, Tzioufas A, et al. Preliminary classification criteria for the cryoglobulinaemic vasculitis. *Ann Rheum Dis* 2011;**70**: 1183–90.
3. Quartuccio L, Isola M, Corazza L, Maset M, Monti G, Gabrielli A, et al. Performance of the preliminary classification criteria for cryoglobulinaemic vasculitis and clinical manifestations in hepatitis C virus-unrelated cryoglobulinaemic vasculitis. *Clin Exp Rheumatol* 2012;**30**:S48–52.
4. Ramos-Casals M, Stone JH, Cid MC, Bosch X. The cryoglobulinaemias. *Lancet* 2012;**379**:348–60.
5. Dammacco F, Sansonno D, Piccoli C, Tucci FA, Racanelli V. The cryoglobulins: an overview. *Eur J Clin Invest* 2001;**31**:628–38.
6. Vassilopoulos D, Calabrese LH. Hepatic C virus infection and vasculitis. Implications of antiviral and immunosuppressive therapies. *Arthritis Rheum* 2002;**46**:585–97.
7. Brouet JC, Clauvel JP, Danon F, Klein M, Seligmann M. Biologic and clinical significance of cryoglobulins. A report of 86 cases. *Am J Med* 1974;**57**:775–88.
8. El-Serag HB. Epidemiology of viral hepatitis and hepatocellular carcinoma. *Gastroenterology* 2012;**142**:1264–73.
9. Vassilopoulos D, Younossi ZM, Hadziyannis E, Boparai N, Yen-Lieberman B, Hsi E, et al. Study of host and virological factors of patients with chronic HCV infection and associated laboratory or clinical autoimmune manifestations. *Clin Exp Rheumatol* 2003;**21**:S101–11.
10. Cacoub P, Poynard T, Ghillani P, Charlotte F, Olivi M, Piette JC, et al. Extrahepatic manifestations of chronic hepatitis C. MULTIVIRC Group. Multidepartment Virus C. *Arthritis Rheum* 1999;**42**:2204–12.
11. Ferri C, Sebastiani M, Giuggioli D, Cazzato M, Longombardo G, Antonelli A, et al. Mixed cryoglobulinemia: demographic, clinical, and serologic features and survival in 231 patients. *Semin Arthritis Rheum* 2004;**33**:355–74.
12. Terrier B, Semoun O, Saadoun D, Sene D, Resche-Rigon M, Cacoub P. Prognostic factors in patients with hepatitis C virus infection and systemic vasculitis. *Arthritis Rheum* 2011;**63**:1748–57.
13. Knight GB, Gao L, Gragnani L, Elfahal MM, De Rosa FG, Gordon FD, et al. Detection of WA B cells in hepatitis C virus infection: a potential prognostic marker for cryoglobulinemic vasculitis and B cell malignancies. *Arthritis Rheum* 2010;**62**:2152–9.
14. Dammacco F, Sansonno D. Therapy for hepatitis C virus-related cryoglobulinemic vasculitis. *N Engl J Med* 2013;**369**:1035–45.
15. Minopetrou M, Hadziyannis E, Deutsch M, Tampaki M, Georgiadou A, Dimopoulou E, et al. Hepatitis C virus (HCV)-related cryoglobulinemia: cryoglobulin type and anti-HCV profile. *Clin Vaccine Immunol* 2013;**20**:698–703.
16. Boyer O, Saadoun D, Abriol J, Dodille M, Piette JC, Cacoub P, et al. CD4+CD25+ regulatory T-cell deficiency in patients with hepatitis C-mixed cryoglobulinemia vasculitis. *Blood* 2004;**103**:3428–30.
17. Terrier B, Cacoub P. Cryoglobulinemia vasculitis: an update. *Curr Opin Rheumatol* 2013;**25**:10–18.
18. Crowson AN, Nuovo G, Ferri C, Magro CM. The dermatopathologic manifestations of hepatitis C infection: a clinical, histological, and molecular assessment of 35 cases. *Hum Pathol* 2003;**34**:573–9.

19. Agnello V, Abel G. Localization of hepatitis C virus in cutaneous vasculitic lesions in patients with type II cryoglobulinemia. *Arthritis Rheum* 1997;**40**:2007–15.
20. Mangia A, Andriulli A, Zenarola P, Lomuto M, Cascavilla I, Quadri R, et al. Lack of hepatitis C virus replication intermediate RNA in diseased skin tissue of chronic hepatitis C patients. *J Med Virol* 1999;**59**:277–80.
21. Authier FJ, Bassez G, Payan C, Guillevin L, Pawlotsky JM, Degos JD, et al. Detection of genomic viral RNA in nerve and muscle of patients with HCV neuropathy. *Neurology* 2003;**60**:808–12.
22. Lidove O, Cacoub P, Maisonobe T, Servan J, Thibault V, Piette JC, et al. Hepatitis C virus infection with peripheral neuropathy is not always associated with cryoglobulinaemia. *Ann Rheum Dis* 2001;**60**:290–2.
23. Bonetti B, Scardoni M, Monaco S, Rizzuto N, Scarpa A. Hepatitis C virus infection of peripheral nerves in type II cryoglobulinaemia. *Virchows Arch* 1999;**434**:533–5.
24. De Martino L, Sampaolo S, Tucci C, Ambrosone L, Budillon A, Migliaresi S, et al. Viral RNA in nerve tissues of patients with hepatitis C infection and peripheral neuropathy. *Muscle Nerve* 2003;**27**:102–4.
25. David WS, Peine C, Schlesinger P, Smith SA. Nonsystemic vasculitic mononeuropathy multiplex, cryoglobulinemia, and hepatitis C. *Muscle Nerve* 1996;**19**:1596–602.
26. Retamozo S, Diaz-Lagares C, Bosch X, Bove A, Brito-Zeron P, Gomez ME, et al. Life-threatening cryoglobulinemic patients with hepatitis C: clinical description and outcome of 279 patients. *Medicine (Baltimore)* 2013; (e-pub ahead of print).
27. Casato M, Saadoun D, Marchetti A, Limal N, Picq C, Pantano P, et al. Central nervous system involvement in hepatitis C virus cryoglobulinemia vasculitis: a multicenter case-control study using magnetic resonance imaging and neuropsychological tests. *J Rheumatol* 2005;**32**:484–8.
28. Trejo O, Ramos-Casals M, Garcia-Carrasco M, Yague J, Jimenez S, de la Red G, et al. Cryoglobulinemia: study of etiologic factors and clinical and immunologic features in 443 patients from a single center. *Medicine (Baltimore)* 2001;**80**:252–62.
29. Roccatello D, Fornasieri A, Giachino O, Rossi D, Beltrame A, Banfi G, et al. Multicenter study on hepatitis C virus-related cryoglobulinemic glomerulonephritis. *Am J Kidney Dis* 2007;**49**:69–82.
30. Beddhu S, Bastacky S, Johnson JP. The clinical and morphologic spectrum of renal cryoglobulinemia. *Medicine (Baltimore)* 2002;**81**:398–409.
31. D'Amico G. Renal involvement in hepatitis C infection: cryoglobulinemic glomerulonephritis. *Kidney Int* 1998;**54**:650–71.
32. Tarantino A, Campise M, Banfi G, Confalonieri R, Bucci A, Montoli A, et al. Long-term predictors of survival in essential mixed cryoglobulinemic glomerulonephritis. *Kidney Int* 1995;**47**:618–23.
33. Sabry AA, Sobh MA, Irving WL, Grabowska A, Wagner BE, Fox S, et al. A comprehensive study of the association between hepatitis C virus and glomerulopathy. *Nephrol Dial Transplant* 2002;**17**:239–45.
34. Rodriguez-Inigo E, Casqueiro M, Bartolome J, Barat A, Caramelo C, Ortiz A, et al. Hepatitis C virus RNA in kidney biopsies from infected patients with renal diseases. *J Viral Hepat* 2000;**7**:23–9.
35. Sansonno D, Gesualdo L, Manno C, Schena FP, Dammacco F. Hepatitis C virus-related proteins in kidney tissue from hepatitis C virus-infected patients with cryoglobulinemic membranoproliferative glomerulonephritis. *Hepatology* 1997;**25**:1237–44.
36. Ferri C, Zignego AL, Pileri SA. Cryoglobulins. *J Clin Pathol* 2002;**55**:4–13.
37. Agnello V. The etiology and pathophysiology of mixed cryoglobulinemia secondary to hepatitis C virus infection. *Springer Semin Immunopathol* 1997;**19**:111–29.

38. Saadoun D, Terrier B, Semoun O, Sene D, Maisonobe T, Musset L, et al. Hepatitis C virus-associated polyarteritis nodosa. *Arthritis Care Res (Hoboken)* 2011;**63**:427–35.
39. Terrier B, Karras A, Cluzel P, Collet JP, Sene D, Saadoun D, et al. Presentation and prognosis of cardiac involvement in hepatitis C virus-related vasculitis. *Am J Cardiol* 2013;**111**:265–72.
40. Terrier B, Saadoun D, Sene D, Scerra S, Musset L, Cacoub P. Presentation and outcome of gastrointestinal involvement in hepatitis C virus-related systemic vasculitis: a case-control study from a single-centre cohort of 163 patients. *Gut* 2010;**59**:1709–15.
41. Kayali Z, Buckwold VE, Zimmerman B, Schmidt WN. Hepatitis C, cryoglobulinemia, and cirrhosis: a meta-analysis. *Hepatology* 2002;**36**:978–85.
42. Saadoun D, Asselah T, Resche-Rigon M, Charlotte F, Bedossa P, Valla D, et al. Cryoglobulinemia is associated with steatosis and fibrosis in chronic hepatitis C. *Hepatology* 2006;**43**:1337–45.
43. Lauletta G, Russi S, Conteduca V, Sansonno L, Dammacco F, Sansonno D. Impact of cryoglobulinemic syndrome on the outcome of chronic hepatitis C virus infection: a 15-Year Prospective Study. *Medicine (Baltimore)* 2013; (e-pub ahead of print).
44. Vassilopoulos D, Calabrese LH. Viral hepatitis: review of arthritic complications and therapy for arthritis in the presence of active HBV/HCV. *Curr Rheumatol Rep* 2013;**15**:319.
45. Ghany MG, Liang TJ. Current and future therapies for hepatitis C virus infection. *N Engl J Med* 2013;**369**:679–80.
46. Bonomo L, Casato M, Afeltra A, Caccavo D. Treatment of idiopathic mixed cryoglobulinemia with alpha interferon. *Am J Med* 1987;**83**:726–30.
47. Cacoub P, Terrier B, Saadoun D. Hepatitis C virus-induced vasculitis: therapeutic options. *Ann Rheum Dis* 2014;**73**:24–30.
48. Cacoub P, Lidove O, Maisonobe T, Duhaut P, Thibault V, Ghillani P, et al. Interferon-alpha and ribavirin treatment in patients with hepatitis C virus-related systemic vasculitis. *Arthritis Rheum* 2002;**46**:3317–26.
49. Saadoun D, Resche-Rigon M, Thibault V, Piette JC, Cacoub P. Antiviral therapy for hepatitis C virus-associated mixed cryoglobulinemia vasculitis: a long-term followup study. *Arthritis Rheum* 2006;**54**:3696–706.
50. Mazzaro C, Zorat F, Caizzi M, Donada C, Di Gennaro G, Maso LD, et al. Treatment with peg-interferon alfa-2b and ribavirin of hepatitis C virus-associated mixed cryoglobulinemia: a pilot study. *J Hepatol* 2005;**42**:632–8.
51. Joshi S, Kuczynski M, Heathcote EJ. Symptomatic and virological response to antiviral therapy in hepatitis C associated with extrahepatic complications of cryoglobulimia. *Dig Dis Sci* 2007;**52**:2410–17.
52. Saadoun D, Resche RM, Sene D, Terrier B, Karras A, Perard L, et al. Rituximab plus Peg-interferon-alpha/ribavirin compared with Peg-interferon-alpha/ribavirin in hepatitis C-related mixed cryoglobulinemia. *Blood* 2010;**116**:326–34.
53. Dammacco F, Tucci FA, Lauletta G, Gatti P, De R. V. Conteduca V, et al. Pegylated interferon-alpha, ribavirin, and rituximab combined therapy of hepatitis C virus-related mixed cryoglobulinemia: a long-term study. *Blood* 2010;**116**:343–53.
54. Mazzaro C, Monti G, Saccardo F, Zignego AL, Ferri C, De VS, et al. Efficacy and safety of peginterferon alfa-2b plus ribavirin for HCV-positive mixed cryoglobulinemia: a multicentre open-label study. *Clin Exp Rheumatol* 2011;**29**:933–41.
55. Ghany MG, Strader DB, Thomas DL, Seeff LB. Diagnosis, management, and treatment of hepatitis C: an update. *Hepatology* 2009;**49**:1335–74.
56. Cid MC, Hernandez-Rodriguez J, Robert J, del Rio A, Casademont J, Coll-Vinent B, et al. Interferon-alpha may exacerbate cryoblobulinemia-related ischemic manifestations: an adverse effect potentially related to its antiangiogenic activity. *Arthritis Rheum* 1999;**42**:1051–5.

57. Ohta S, Yokoyama H, Wada T, Sakai N, Shimizu M, Kato T, et al. Exacerbation of glomerulonephritis in subjects with chronic hepatitis C virus infection after interferon therapy. *Am J Kidney Dis* 1999;**33**:1040–8.

58. Saadoun D, Resche RM, Thibault V, Longuet M, Pol S, Blanc F, et al. Peg-IFNalpha/ribavirin/protease inhibitor combination in hepatitis C virus associated mixed cryoglobulinemia vasculitis: results at week 24. *Ann Rheum Dis* 2014;**73**:831–7.

59. Levine JW, Gota C, Fessler BJ, Calabrese LH, Cooper SM. Persistent cryoglobulinemic vasculitis following successful treatment of hepatitis C virus. *J Rheumatol* 2005;**32**: 1164–7.

60. Dammacco F, Sansonno D, Han JH, Shyamala V, Cornacchiulo V, Iacobelli AR, et al. Natural interferon-alpha versus its combination with 6-methyl-prednisolone in the therapy of type II mixed cryoglobulinemia: a long-term, randomized, controlled study. *Blood* 1994;**84**:3336–43.

61. Vassilopoulos D, Calabrese LH. Management of rheumatic disease with comorbid HBV or HCV infection. *Nat Rev Rheumatol* 2012;**8**:348–57.

62. Rockx MA, Clark WF. Plasma exchange for treating cryoglobulinemia: a descriptive analysis. *Transfus Apher Sci* 2010;**42**:247–51.

63. Ferri C, Cacoub P, Mazzaro C, Roccatello D, Scaini P, Sebastiani M, et al. Treatment with rituximab in patients with mixed cryoglobulinemia syndrome: results of multicenter cohort study and review of the literature. *Autoimmun Rev* 2011;**11**: 48–55.

64. Cacoub P, Delluc A, Saadoun D, Landau DA, Sene D. Anti-CD20 monoclonal antibody (rituximab) treatment for cryoglobulinemic vasculitis: where do we stand? *Ann Rheum Dis* 2008;**67**:283–7.

65. De Vitas, Quartuccio L, Isola M, Mazzaro C, Scaini P, Lenzi M, et al. A randomized controlled trial of rituximab for the treatment of severe cryoglobulinemic vasculitis. *Arthritis Rheum* 2012;**64**:843–53.

66. Sneller MC, Hu Z, Langford CA. A randomized controlled trial of rituximab following failure of antiviral therapy for hepatitis C virus-associated cryoglobulinemic vasculitis. *Arthritis Rheum* 2012;**64**:835–42.

67. Petrarca A, Rigacci L, Caini P, Colagrande S, Romagnoli P, Vizzutti F, et al. Safety and efficacy of rituximab in patients with hepatitis C virus-related mixed cryoglobulinemia and severe liver disease. *Blood* 2010;**116**:335–42.

68. Saadoun D, Resche-Rigon M, Sene D, Perard L, Karras A, Cacoub P. Rituximab combined with Peg-interferon-ribavirin in refractory hepatitis C virus-associated cryoglobulinaemia vasculitis. *Ann Rheum Dis* 2008;**67**:1431–6.

69. Saadoun D, Rosenzwajg M, Joly F, Six A, Carrat F, Thibault V, et al. Regulatory T-cell responses to low-dose interleukin-2 in HCV-induced vasculitis. *N Engl J Med* 2011;**365**:2067–77.

70. European Association for the Study of the Liver. EASL Clinical Practice Guidelines: management of hepatitis C virus infection. *J Hepatol* 2011;**55**:245–64.

71. Ramos-Casals M, Munoz S, Medina F, Jara LJ, Rosas J, Calvo-Alen J, et al. Systemic autoimmune diseases in patients with hepatitis C virus infection: characterization of 1020 cases (The HISPAMEC Registry). *J Rheumatol* 2009;**36**:1442–8.

72. Agmon-Levin N, Ram M, Barzilai O, Porat-Katz BS, Parikman R, Selmi C, et al. Prevalence of hepatitis C serum antibody in autoimmune diseases. *J Autoimmun* 2009;**32**:261–6.

73. Lidar M, Lipschitz N, Langevitz P, Barzilai O, Ram M, Porat-Katz BS, et al. Infectious serologies and autoantibodies in Wegener's granulomatosis and other vasculitides: novel associations disclosed using the Rad BioPlex 2200. *Ann N Y Acad Sci* 2009;**1173**: 649–57.

CHAPTER 48

The Role of Infection in Inflammatory Bowel Disease: Initiation, Exacerbation and Protection

Neta Brender-Gotlieb[*], **Merav Lidar**[†,1]
[*]Department of Internal Medicine F, Sheba Medical Center, Tel Hashomer, Israel
[†]Rheumatology Unit, Sheba Medical Center, Tel Hashomer, Israel and Sackler Faculty of Medicine, Tel Aviv University, Tel Aviv, Israel
[1]Corresponding Author: merav.lidar@gmail.com

Inflammatory bowel disease (IBD) is a chronic, relapsing, multi-factorial disease affecting the digestive tract. It is comprised of two major disorders: ulcerative colitis (UC) and Crohn's disease (CD). Both have distinct pathologic and clinical characteristics yet their pathogenesis remains poorly understood.

First-degree relatives of patients with IBD are approximately 3–20 times more likely to develop the disease than the general population.[1] Environmental factors (i.e. geography, cigarette smoking, sanitation, and hygiene), ethnic origin, genetic susceptibility, infectious microbes, and a dysregulated immune system all have been implicated in causing mucosal inflammation in IBD.[2] UC and CD occur with equal frequency. Both diseases are more common among Jews, and the incidence is lower among black and Hispanic populations compared to whites. Disease onset is usually in the second or third decade of life, with a second late peak documented in UC.[3] Extraintestinal manifestations are relatively common in IBD and affect joints, skin, eyes, bile ducts, and various other organs. Inflammatory arthropathies and nephrolithiasis are more common in CD, whereas primary sclerosing cholangitis is more common in UC.[4]

The pathological and clinical characteristics of each disease have a unique pattern of distribution. UC is characterized by inflammation limited to the mucosal layer of the colon. It almost invariably involves the rectum and may

Infection and Autoimmunity
http://dx.doi.org/10.1016/B978-0-444-63269-2.00057-X

extend proximally in a continuous fashion. The histological features of UC include crypt abscesses as well as Paneth cell metaplasia. Patients with UC usually present with colicky abdominal pain and diarrhea, which may be associated with blood and/or mucus. Long-term complications of UC include strictures, dysplasia, and colorectal cancer. Transmural inflammation of the gastrointestinal (GI) tract is the hallmark of CD. This may involve the entire GI tract from the mouth to the perianal area in a skip-like pattern of distribution along the GI tract, yet the small bowel is the most commonly involved area. The histological features of CD are characterized by transmural inflammation and granulomas. These patients may present with various clinical symptoms including fatigue, prolonged diarrhea with or without gross bleeding, abdominal pain, weight loss, and fever. Long-term complications of CD include fistulas and strictures as well as phlegmon or abscess formation.[5]

1 HUMAN INTESTINAL MICROBIOTA

The human "microbiota" is an ecosystem comprising bacteria, fungi, bacteriophages, and viruses that synergistically acts as an "organ" within the host. The human GI tract contains as many as 10^{14} bacteria comprising 500 different species.[6] Colonization of the GI tract begins during birth, as the newborn is exposed to maternal and environmental microbes. However, the infant microbiota is marked by heterogeneity and instability until approximately 2–4 years of age, from which point on it resembles the adult system. The most abundant bacterial phyla found in the healthy human large intestine are gram-negative bacteroides and gram-positive firmicutes.[7]

The microbiota plays a number of key roles in the maintenance of host health, including aiding in the digestion of otherwise indigestible dietary compounds (e.g. degradation of non-digestible polysaccharides) and synthesis of vitamins and other beneficial metabolites.[8] In addition to the role of the intestinal microbiota in the digestion and absorption of nutrients, it plays an important part in immune system regulation, providing enhanced resistance against colonization by pathogenic microorganisms. The microbiota of the GI tract is critical in determining the host's susceptibility to GI infections. It has a major role in protecting the intestine against colonization by exogenous pathogens and potentially harmful indigenous microorganisms via several mechanisms, among which are direct competition for limited nutrients, maintenance of an appropriate intestinal pH and modulation of the host immune responses.[9,10]

2 IMMUNITY AND GUT MICROBIOTA

The intestinal mucosa serves as the primary barrier between the immune system and the external environment by producing a mucus layer and secreting antimicrobial proteins.[11] The innate immune system senses bacteria within the gut through Toll-like receptors (TLRs) and nucleotide-binding domain and leucine-rich repeat-containing receptors (NLRs) on macrophages and dendritic cells (DCs). Activated innate immune cells, such as mucosal DCs, constantly sample luminal microbial antigens and present them to adaptive immune cells in Peyer's patches.

In healthy hosts the pro-inflammatory pathways associated with TLR and NLR are suppressed by inhibitory molecules of both human and bacterial origin, such as cyclooxygenase-2 inhibitors; LPS; nuclear factor-κB (NF-κB) inhibitor; interferon-α/β; interleukin-10 (IL-10); TGF-β and eicosanoids. Repetitive TLR stimulation due to commensal bacterial exposure induces the down-regulation of the NF-κB pathway, with increased production of antimicrobial peptides (e.g. defensins). Similarly, chronic stimulation of NOD-2 has been demonstrated to lead to the down-regulation of pro-inflammatory cytokines (TNF-α, IL-8, IL-1β).[7]

Therefore, the host's mechanism of tolerance to the resident microbiota offers simultaneous protection from both unwanted inflammatory responses and pathogen invasion. Under normal conditions, stimulation of the mucosal immune system by gut microbiota results in a state of "low-grade physiological inflammation".[6] However, overgrowth of aggressive commensal microbes increases the number of antigens that induce pathogenic immune responses and increases mucosal permeability.

3 INTESTINAL MICROBIOTA IN IBD AND DYSBIOSIS

In IBD, the homeostatic mechanisms that allow the host organism and the commensal microbiota to co-exist are disrupted. An imbalance in the proportions of "protective" and "harmful" bacteria has been termed "dysbiosis" and is thought to be central to IBD pathogenesis. Dysregulation of host–microbe interactions can lead to inadequate or hyper-inflammatory reactions. Host genetics can contribute to dysbiosis. Mutations in specific genes lead to abnormal immune regulation and affects microbial composition.[12]

While numerous organisms have been studied as potential inciters of IBD, it is improbable that IBD results from a traditional infection. Rather, the notion that infectious agents facilitate a change from the status quo that is sufficient to allow the development of IBD is more plausible.[13] The role of infectious agents and commensal bacteria in the initiation and exacerbation of IBD on the one hand, and in protection from disease on the other, is reviewed in the following sections.

3.1 Pathogens Implicated in the Causation or Exacerbation of IBD

Infectious complications, which may arise from the disease process itself, its complications and/or the use of immunosuppressive medications, are a significant cause of morbidity and mortality in IBD. Also, intercurrent infections in these patients often present in an atypical manner, and their treatment may interfere with effective therapy in cases of active disease.[14] Whereas superinfection with intestinal pathogens may cause disease flare-ups, opportunistic pathogens are increasingly recognized due to the immunosuppressive therapy in IBD. Corticosteroids, azathioprine/6-mercaptopurine and TNF inhibitors all are associated with an increased risk for developing opportunistic infections, especially when used in combination. TNF inhibitors in particular have been linked to the re-activation of TB, which in immunosupressed individuals has a tendency to develop in an extra-pulmonary location.[15] Secondary bacterial invasion of mucosal ulcers may lead to local septic complications, including abscesses and fistulae formation, as well as to severe systemic complications such as sepsis, hepatic abscesses and endocarditis.[15] The most common organisms recovered from intra-abdominal abscesses complicating CD are *Escherichia coli*, *Bacteroides fragilis*, *Enterococcus* species and *Streptococcus viridans*.

3.2 Bacteria

3.2.1 Mycobacterium paratuberculosis

Mycobacterium avium subspecies *paratuberculosis* (*MAP*) is an extremely slow-growing, acid-fast, mycobactin-dependent, multi-species pathogen that has been associated with small-bowel inflammation in cattle (referred to as Johne's disease).[16] The histopathological similarities between CD and mycobacterial infection—notably epithelial granulomata as well as macroscopic lesions of segmental fibrosis and stenosis—have led investigators to incriminate this agent in the pathogenesis of IBD.[17] Initially, *MAP* DNA was found to be over-represented in peripheral blood of patients with CD compared to controls. When peripheral blood mononuclear cell proliferation in response to *MAP* from patients with IBD and controls without

IBD was examined using flow cytometry, increased proliferation of T cells and altered cytokine response in the patients with IBD was found. While interpreting these findings it was suggested that prior exposure to *MAP* could be involved in the pathogenesis of IBD.[18] The relative numbers of CD4+ T cells in biopsies taken from patients with CD were recently analyzed to address whether clonal expansion of T cells had occurred. The frequency of mycobacteria-reactive T cells in patients with CD ranged from 0.17% to 1.63%, whereas the responses to *E. coli* were lower, despite the higher number of *E. coli* present in the gut. Specifically, patients with CD had significantly more T-cell clones reactive against *MAP* compared to *E. coli* in comparison to no or very low numbers of *MAP*-reactive clones in patients with UC. It was demonstrated in various studies that expansion of mycobacteria reactive T cells likely occurred *in vivo* and that a high frequency of CD4+ T cells were present in intestinal biopsies from patients with CD. The high numbers of mycobacteria-reactive T cells in patients with CD suggest that an adaptive immune response to mycobacteria occurred and that these bacteria contributed to the inflammation.[19,20] In addition, it was postulated that the efficacy of both methotrexate and 6-mercaptopurine in inhibiting *MAP* growth *in vitro* explains their beneficial clinical effect in patients with IBD.[21] Finally, a systematic review and meta-analysis performed in 2007 assessed the evidence for an association between *MAP* and CD. Twenty-eight case-control studies were analyzed, comparing *MAP* in patients with CD to individuals free of IBD or patients with UC. The study showed that the association of *MAP* with CD seems to be specific but concluded that its role in the etiology of CD remains to be defined.[22]

3.2.2 E. coli

E. coli is the predominant facultative, anerobic, gram-negative bacterial species of the normal intestinal flora, where it plays an important role in maintaining normal intestinal homeostasis. Both commensal and entero-pathogenic strains of *E. coli* can inhabit the human intestinal tract. Commensal *E. coli* strains rarely cause disease, except in immunocompromised hosts or when the normal GI barriers are breached. Studies have recognized that antibody titers against *E. coli* are higher in patients with CD than in controls, and their presence is associated with a more severe disease course. On the basis of the pathogenic traits exhibited by CD-associated *E. coli*, a new pathogenic group of *E. coli* was designated as AIEC (Adherent-Invasive *E. coli*).[23] This is a true invasive pathogen, able to invade intestinal epithelial cells via a macropinocytosis-like process as well as to survive and replicate intracellularly after lysis of the endocytic vacuole.[24] Within macrophages, AIEC strains replicate and induce the release of high amounts of TNF-α, leading to granuloma formation.[25] Indeed, *E. coli* antigens and DNA were detected in 80% of CD granulomas,[26] as well as in 20–30% of ileal specimens from patients with CD compared to negligible amounts in patients with UC or controls. Taken together, these data may conclude that AIEC has a true pathogenic role in CD, more specifically in cases with ileal involvement.[24]

3.2.3 Listeria monocytogenes

Listeria monocytogenes is a gram-positive, facultative, intracellular organism that causes listeriosis in animals and humans characterized by fever, diarrhea, and other GI symptoms. The organisms are widely distributed in the environment and have been isolated from soil, vegetables, animal meat, dairy products, and water as well as from asymptomatic human and animal carriers. The GI tract is the major entry point of *L. monocytogenes* infection, in which the organism may induce aphthoid ulceration or granulomatous reactions.

Immunohistochemical studies have detected *L. monocytogenes* antigens to a much greater extent in patients with CD than in patients with UC or controls. *Listeria* antigens have been found in macrophages and giant cells distributed underneath ulcers, along fissures, around abscesses, within the lamina propria, in granulomas and in the germinal centres of mesenteric lymph nodes.[27] In addition, because *L. monocytogenes* was found at the site of colonic perforation in a patient with fulminant UC, it has been suggested that it is associated with the potential to cause and exacerbate IBD.[28]

However, the fact that *L. monocytogenes* DNA was equally detected in the intestine of patients with IBD and in controls without IBD, severely undermined causality and suggested that the apparent association between *L. monocytogenes* and IBD reflects the widespread presence of this organism in the environment.[28,29]

3.2.4 Chlamydia

Chlamydia pneumoniae, a gram-negative, obligate, intracellular bacterium, has been associated with several autoimmune diseases such as sarcoidosis and multiple sclerosis.[30] Given the predilection of *C. pneumoniae* to colonize human endothelial and epithelial tissue, it was postulated to play a pathogenic role in IBD. However, several studies failed to show an overabundance of chlamydial species in patients with IBD. *C. pneumoniae*

DNA was detected by PCR in a moderate yet similar frequency in intestinal biopsies of patients with CD and UC as well as of controls without IBD. *Chlamydia trachomatis*-specific DNA was rarely detected in the intestinal biopsies of patients with IBD and controls without IBD.[31]

3.2.5 Clostridium difficile

Clostridium difficile, an anerobic, gram-positive, spore-forming bacilli, is the most common cause of nosocomial infectious diarrhea in developed countries. Clinical colitis develops because of an overgrowth of the toxin B-expressing pathogen among commensal bacteria. Factors that increase patients' susceptibility to *C. difficile* infection (CDI) include antibiotic exposure, advanced age, hospitalization and immunosuppression.[32] The incidence and severity of CDI among patients with IBD is notable, especially in patients with UC with colonic involvement, among whom rates of surgery required because of complications of CDI are around 20%.[33] The increased incidence of CDI in patients with IBD is attributed to the susceptibility of previously damaged and chronically inflamed colonic mucosa to CDI. Also, steroid use, a staple in IBD therapy, increases the risk of CDI threefold. Awareness of the possibility of CDI in a patient with IBD is crucial because it may mimic a disease relapse, exacerbate the severity of colitis or exist as asymptomatic carriage. Because of the severity of CDI in these patients, prompt diagnosis and treatment of infection are paramount in exacerbations of IBD.[34]

3.2.6 Gastroenteritis Predisposing to IBD

Non-typhoid *Salmonella* and thermophilic *Campylobacter* have been implicated in the causation of IBD. Two large cohort studies evaluated the association of infectious gastroenteritis and IBD. The first study included 43,000 patients; the estimated incidence of IBD after an episode of gastroenteritis was 68.4 per 100,000 person-years vs. 29.7 per 100,000 person-years in the control cohort.[35] The second cohort, comprising 13,000 patients with *Salmonella/Campylobacter* gastroenteritis, similarly reported a twofold increased incidence of IBD following gastroenteritis. First-time diagnosis of IBD was reported in 107 cases who had an episode of *Salmonella* or *Campylobacter* gastroenteritis (1.2%) vs. 73 cases of IBD in unexposed individuals (0.5%). However, a history of exposure to *Salmonella/Campylobacter* did not account for the severity of IBD that ensued.[36]

3.3 Viruses

The role of viruses in the etiopathology of IBD has not been extensively studied. While enteric viruses (rotavirus, norovirus, human astrovirus, and adenovirus) are not frequently observed in patients with IBD and are not considered a trigger for active disease,[37] there is evidence to suggest that infection with cytomegalovirus (CMV), herpes simplex virus 1, human herpes virus 6, and Epstein Barr virus (EBV) may contribute to disease exacerbation.[38]

3.3.1 CMV

Cytomegalovirus (CMV) is a member of the herpesvirus family, and previous infection is evident in 40–100% of adults. Clinically significant GI CMV disease usually occurs in immunocompromised hosts.[39] Patients with IBD are at higher risk for CMV infection because of immunosuppressive medications, poor nutrition, impaired absorption of nutrients and dysfunction of the immune system.[40] A prospective study evaluating CMV infection in patients with IBD showed that female patients with pancolonic disease and active inflammation on histology who had been prescribed azathioprine in addition to corticosteroids were more likely to have evidence of CMV infection. In addition, CMV infection was associated with a higher relapse rate, more need for surgical intervention and a higher mortality rate.[41] CMV infection in patients with refractory or complicated IBD must be ruled out before aggressive immunosuppressive therapy for presumed-resistant disease is initiated.

3.3.2 Epstein–Barr Virus

EBV, a member of the herpesvirus family, is one of the most prolific human viruses, with a seroprevalence of > 90% in the adult population. Although it is not more common in patients with IBD then in healthy controls, there is evidence to suggest that EBV infection has a role in the etiopathology of IBD.[42] EBV-infected B lymphocytes are abundant in intestinal mucosal samples from patients with IBD, more so in patients who are not responsive to medical therapy, suggesting an association with increased disease activity in IBD. In addition, higher EBV replication rates are noted in patients with IBD compared to controls without IBD, regardless of their immunosuppressive state.[43] Patients with IBD taking immunosuppressive medications are at a particular risk for EBV-associated fatal and non-fatal lymphoproliferative disorders because treatment both alters the otherwise stable EBV viral load and increases the likelihood of viral reactivation.[43]

3.3.3 Mumps and Measles

The contribution of infection by measles and mumps viruses, both of which belong to the paramyxoviruses family, to IBD is controversial. Measles and mumps infections in early childhood may result in granulomatous vasculitis and hence were considered to be inciters of IBD, especially CD. A similar phenomenon also has been recognized following administration of the live attenuated MMR vaccine.[44] However, despite the histological similarity, available evidence does not support an association between vaccines containing measles and risk of IBD, nor between measles infection and IBD.[45] When linked to the fact that the mumps virus genome is not detected in intestinal specimens of patients with IBD, it may be concluded that persistent paramyxovirus infection in UC or CD is unlikely.[46]

4 INFECTIOUS AGENTS CONFERRING PROTECTION FROM IBD

Among the various chemical and biological treatment options for IBD, the use of probiotics is quite popular. The general idea is to "rebalance" the host's normal commensal flora by introducing beneficial microorganisms other than bacteria. These organisms elicit defined immune responses in the host that antagonize or inhibit the mechanisms of the immunopathology observed in IBD.

4.1 Helminths

The incidence of IBD has steadily increased in the developed world. It has been suggested that lack of exposure to helmintic infections, as a result of improved living standards and medical conditions, may have contributed to this increased incidence of IBD.

Helminths induce Th2 and Treg cells that suppress Th1 effector cells. Considering that IBD is mainly a Th1-mediated disease, it may be ameliorated by the Th2-to-Th1 shift induced by helminthic infections. This theory has led investigators to examine whether intentional colonization with intestinal helminths might be beneficial in reducing inflammation in patients with IBD.[47,48] Optimally, the helminth colonizes the intestine without invading the host, causing symptoms or creating illness. Indeed, the ova of the porcine whipworm *Trichuris suis* are capable of colonizing a human host for several weeks without causing a disease. Several studies of both animals and humans showed a reduction in the severity of colitis following the oral administration of *T. suis* ova. An immunomodulatory vaccine containing *T. suis* has been formulated, yet at this point data are not sufficient to recommend the use of helminths as part of the routine treatment of IBD.[49]

4.2 *Helicobacter pylori*

H. pylori is a gram-negative, micro-aerophilic, spiral-shaped bacterium found in the human gastric mucosa. More than 50% of the world's population harbor *H. pylori* in their upper GI tract. Infection is more prevalent in developing countries, whereas incidence is decreasing in Western countries. Although carriers are generally asymptomatic, *H. pylori* has been recognized as a major cause of gastritis and is associated with duodenal ulcer disease, gastric ulcer disease, gastric lymphoma and gastric cancer in humans.[50] Previous studies showed an inverse relationship between *H. pylori* seropositivity and IBD. Also, patients with IBD have an increased prevalence of *H. pylori*-negative gastritis. Several explanations for this observation have been given, including an inverse socioeconomic distribution between carrying *H. pylori* and IBD, the countereffect of *H. pylori* on the immune system and the inhibition of GI infections by yet-unknown bacteria that are directly linked to the development of IBD.[51] The inverse association between *H. pylori* infection and IBD was noted both *in vivo* and *in vitro*. *H. pylori* DNA was shown to suppress the release of pro-inflammatory cytokines by DCs and attenuate the severity of colitis in a mouse model of IBD. In addition, the luminal delivery of *H. pylori* genomic DNA ameliorated the severity of chronic experimental colitis.[52] Further research aimed at identifying particular strains of *H. pylori* that are likely to provide more benefit than harm is ongoing. In the meantime, *H. pylori* DNA should be regarded as a potential future treatment for IBD.

5 SUMMARY

The recognition of the important role of "dysbiosis", an imbalance between "protective" and "harmful" commensal microbiota in a host, has provided new insight into the pathogenesis of IBD. Dysregulation of host–microbe interactions leads to hyper-inflammatory reactions, resulting in the typical pathologic changes and clinical syndrome of IBD. Alterations in intestinal microbiota through genetics and environment (diet, infections, or antibiotics) ultimately lead to defective host immune responses.

In addition, infection with a pathogenic organism serves as an environmental trigger, which initiates an inflammatory response in genetically susceptible individuals. Luminal inflammation, together with loss of normal immunologic tolerance, propagate the pathogenic processes underlying the initiation of IBD. Although many pathogens have been implicated in the causation of IBD, a single pathogen has not been found to be responsible for the disease. Future research should effectively characterize the bacterial and fungal constituents of the human microbiome in healthy and IBD subsets, resulting in highly effective, nontoxic, selective intervention to treat and prevent exacerbations and recurrence of these relapsing conditions.

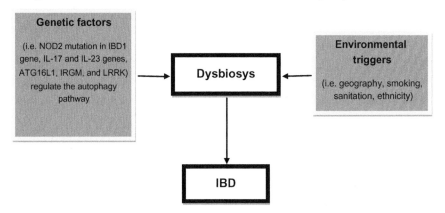

REFERENCES

1. Fielding JF. The relative risk of inflammatory bowel disease among parents and siblings of Crohn's disease patients. *J Clin Gastroenterol* 1986;**8**(6):655–7.
2. Baumgart DC, Carding SR. Inflammatory bowel disease: cause and immunobiology. *Lancet* 2007;**369**(9573):1627–40, Review.
3. Ponder A, Long MD. A clinical review of recent findings in the epidemiology of inflammatory bowel disease. *Clin Epidemiol* 2013;**5**:237–47.
4. Larsen S, Bendtzen K, Nielsen OH. Extraintestinal manifestations of inflammatory bowel disease: epidemiology, diagnosis, and management. *Ann Med* 2010;**42**(2):97–114.
5. Satsangi J, Silverberg MS, Vermeire S, Colombel JF. The Montreal classification of inflammatory bowel disease: controversies, consensus, and implications. *Gut* 2006;**55**(6):749–53.
6. Scaldaferri F, Gerardi V, Lopetuso LR, Del Zompo F, Mangiola F, Boškoski I, et al. Gut microbial flora, prebiotics, and probiotics in IBD: their current usage and utility. *Biomed Res Int* 2013;**2013**:435268.
7. Fava F, Danese S. Intestinal microbiota in inflammatory bowel disease: friend of foe? *World J Gastroenterol* 2011;**17**(5):557–66.
8. Cani PD, Delzenne NM. The role of the gut microbiota in energy metabolism and metabolic disease. *Curr Pharm Des* 2009;**15**(13):1546–58, Review.
9. Kamada N, Seo SU, Chen GY, Núñez G. Role of the gut microbiota in immunity and inflammatory disease. *Nat Rev Immunol* 2013;**13**(5):321–35.

10. Strober W. Impact of the gut microbiome on mucosal inflammation. *Trends Immunol* 2013;**34**(9):423–30.

11. Shim JO. Gut microbiota in inflammatory bowel disease. *Pediatr Gastroenterol Hepatol Nutr* 2013;**16**(1):17–21.

12. Hansen R, Thomson JM, El-Omar EM, Hold GL. The role of infection in the aetiology of inflammatory bowel disease. *J Gastroenterol* 2010;**45**(3):266–76.

13. Chassaing B, Darfeuille-Michaud A. The commensal microbiota and enteropathogens in the pathogenesis of inflammatory bowel diseases. *Gastroenterology* 2011;**140**(6): 1720–8.

14. Epple HJ. Therapy- and non-therapy-dependent infectious complications in inflammatory bowel disease. *Dig Dis* 2009;**27**(4):555–9.

15. Sartor RB. Microbial influences in inflammatory bowel diseases. *Gastroenterology* 2008;**134**(2):577–94.

16. Li L, Bannantine JP, Zhang Q, Amonsin A, May BJ, Alt D, et al. The complete genome sequence of Mycobacterium avium subspecies paratuberculosis. *Proc Natl Acad Sci USA* 2005;**102**(35):12344–9.

17. Lidar M, Langevitz P, Shoenfeld Y. The role of infection in inflammatory bowel disease: initiation, exacerbation and protection. *Isr Med Assoc J* 2009;**11**(9):558–63, Review.

18. Sibartie S, Scully P, Keohane J, O'Neill S, O'Mahony J, O'Hanlon D, et al. Mycobacterium avium subsp. Paratuberculosis (MAP) as a modifying factor in Crohn's disease. *Inflamm Bowel Dis* 2010;**16**(2):296–304.

19. Olsen I, Lundin KE, Sollid LM. Increased frequency of intestinal CD4(+) T cells reactive with mycobacteria in patients with Crohn's disease. *Scand J Gastroenterol* 2013; **48**(11):1278–85.

20. Bentley RW, Keenan JI, Gearry RB, Kennedy MA, Barclay ML, Roberts RL. Incidence of Mycobacterium avium subspecies paratuberculosis in a population-based cohort of patients with Crohn's disease and control subjects. *Am J Gastroenterol* 2008;**103**(5):1168–72.

21. Greenstein RJ, Su L, Haroutunian V, Shahidi A, Brown ST. On the action of methotrexate and 6-mercaptopurine on M. avium subspecies paratuberculosis. *PLoS One* 2007;**2**(1):e161.

22. Feller M, Huwiler K, Stephan R, Altpeter E, Shang A, Furrer H, et al. Mycobacterium avium subspecies paratuberculosis and Crohn's disease: a systematic review and meta-analysis. *Lancet Infect Dis* 2007;**7**(9):607–13.

23. Darfeuille-Michaud A, Colombel JF. Pathogenic Escherichia coli in inflammatory bowel diseases Proceedings of the 1st International Meeting on E. coli and IBD, June 2007, Lille, France. *J Crohns Colitis* 2008;**2**(3):255–62.

24. Darfeuille-Michaud A, Boudeau J, Bulois P, Neut C, Glasser AL, Barnich N, et al. High prevalence of adherent-invasive *Escherichia coli* associated with ileal mucosa in Crohn's disease. *Gastroenterology* 2004;**127**(2):412–21.

25. Glasser AL, Boudeau J, Barnich N, Perruchot MH, Colombel JF, Darfeuille-Michaud A. Adherent invasive *Escherichia coli* strains from patients with Crohn's disease survive and replicate within macrophages without inducing host cell death. *Infect Immun* 2001; **69**(9):5529–37.

26. Ryan P, Kelly RG, Lee G, Collins JK, O'Sullivan GC, O'Connell J, et al. Bacterial DNA within granulomas of patients with Crohn's disease—detection by laser capture microdissection and PCR. *Am J Gastroenterol* 2004;**99**(8):1539–43.

27. Chen W, Li D, Paulus B, Wilson I, Chadwick VS. Detection of Listeria monocytogenes by polymerase chain reaction in intestinal mucosal biopsies from patients with inflammatory bowel disease and controls. *J Gastroenterol Hepatol* 2000;**15**(10):1145–50.

28. Chiba M, Fukushima T, Koganei K, et al. Listeria monocytogenes in the colon in a case of fulminant ulcerative colitis. *Scand J Gastroenterol* 1998;**33**:778–82.

29. Chen W, Li D, Paulus B, Wilson I, Chadwick VS. Detection of Listeria monocytogenes by polymerase chain reaction in intestinal mucosal biopsies from patients with inflammatory bowel disease and controls. *J Gastroenterol Hepatol* 2000;**15**(10):1145–50.

30. Libbey JE, Cusick MF, Fujinami RS. Role of pathogens in multiple sclerosis. *Int Rev Immunol* 2013;**33**(4):266–83.

31. Müller S, Arni S, Varga L, Balsiger B, Hersberger M, Maly F, et al. Serological and DNA-based evaluation of Chlamydia pneumoniae infection in inflammatory bowel disease. *Eur J Gastroenterol Hepatol* 2006;**18**(8):889–94.

32. Shakir FA, Ali T, Bigham AC, Ballard JD, Miner Jr. PB, Philpott JR. Determination of serum antibodies to Clostridium difficile toxin B in patients with inflammatory bowel disease. *Gastroenterol Hepatol (NY)* 2012;**8**(5):313–7.

33. Rodemann JF, Dubberke ER, Reske KA, Seo da H, Stone CD. Incidence of Clostridium difficile infection in inflammatory bowel disease. *Clin Gastroenterol Hepatol* 2007; **5**(3):339–44.

34. Issa M, Vijayapal A, Graham MB, Beaulieu DB, Otterson MF, Lundeen S, et al. Impact of Clostridium difficile on inflammatory bowel disease. *Clin Gastroenterol Hepatol* 2007; **5**(3):345–51.

35. García Rodríguez LA, Ruigómez A, Panés J. Acute gastroenteritis is followed by an increased risk of inflammatory bowel disease. *Gastroenterology* 2006;**130**(6):1588–94.

36. Gradel KO, Nielsen HL, Schønheyder HC, Ejlertsen T, Kristensen B, Nielsen H. Increased short- and long-term risk of inflammatory bowel disease after salmonella or campylobacter gastroenteritis. *Gastroenterology* 2009;**137**(2):495–501.

37. Masclee GM, Penders J, Pierik M, Wolffs P, Jonkers D. Enteropathogenic viruses: triggers for exacerbation in IBD? A prospective cohort study using real-time quantitative polymerase chain reaction. *Inflamm Bowel Dis* 2013;**19**(1):124–31.

38. Magin WS, Van Kruiningen HJ, Colombel JF. Immunohistochemical search for viral and bacterial antigens in Crohn's disease. *J Crohns Colitis* 2013;**7**(2):161–6.

39. Kishore J, Ghoshal U, Ghoshal UC, Krishnani N, Kumar S, Singh M, et al. Infection with cytomegalovirus in patients with inflammatory bowel disease: prevalence, clinical significance and outcome. *J Med Microbiol* 2004;**53**(Pt. 11):1155–60.

40. Yi F, Zhao J, Luckheeram RV, Lei Y, Wang C, Huang S, et al. The prevalence and risk factors of cytomegalovirus infection in inflammatory bowel disease in Wuhan. *Central China Virol J* 2013;**10**:43.

41. Maher MM, Nassar MI. Acute cytomegalovirus infection is a risk factor in refractory and complicated inflammatory bowel disease. *Dig Dis Sci* 2009;**54**(11):2456–62.

42. Linton MS, Kroeker K, Fedorak D, Dieleman L, Fedorak RN. Prevalence of Epstein-Barr Virus in a population of patients with inflammatory bowel disease: a prospective cohort study. *Aliment Pharmacol Ther* 2013;**38**(10):1248–54.

43. Sankaran-Walters S, Ransibrahmanakul K, Grishina I, Hung J, Martinez E, Prindiville T, et al. Epstein-Barr virus replication linked to B cell proliferation in inflamed areas of colonic mucosa of patients with inflammatory bowel disease. *J Clin Virol* 2011;**50**(1):31–6.

44. Lewin J, Dhillon AP, Sim R, Mazure G, Pounder RE, Wakefield AJ. Persistent measles virus infection of the intestine: confirmation by immunogold electron microscopy. *Gut* 1995;**36**(4):564–9.

45. Daszak P, Purcell M, Lewin J, Dhillon AP, Pounder RE, Wakefield AJ. Detection and comparative analysis of persistent measles virus infection in Crohn's disease by immunogold electron microscopy. *J Clin Pathol* 1997;**50**(4):299–304.

46. Iizuka M, Saito H, Yukawa M, Itou H, Shirasaka T, Chiba M, et al. No evidence of persistent mumps virus infection in inflammatory bowel disease. *Gut* 2001;**48**(5):637–41.

47. Hunter MM, McKay DM. Review article: helminths as therapeutic agents for inflammatory bowel disease. *Aliment Pharmacol Ther* 2004;**19**(2):167–77.

48. Ruyssers NE, De Winter BY, De Man JG, Loukas A, Herman AG, Pelckmans PA, et al. Worms and the treatment of inflammatory bowel disease: are molecules the answer? *Clin Dev Immunol* 2008;**2008**:567314.

49. Summers RW, Elliott DE, Qadir K, Urban Jr JF, Thompson R, Weinstock JV. Trichuris suis seems to be safe and possibly effective in the treatment of inflammatory bowel disease. *Am J Gastroenterol* 2003;**98**(9):2034–41.

50. Brown LM. Helicobacter pylori: epidemiology and routes of transmission. *Epidemiol Rev* 2000;**22**(2):283–97.

51. Sonnenberg A, Genta RM. Low prevalence of *Helicobacter pylori* infection among patients with inflammatory bowel disease. *Aliment Pharmacol Ther* 2012;**35**(4):469–76.

52. Owyang SY, Luther J, Owyang CC, Zhang M, Kao JY. Helicobacter pylori DNA's anti-inflammatory effect on experimental colitis. *Gut Microbes* 2012;**3**(2):168–71.

CHAPTER 49

Post-Infectious Arthritis and Reactive Arthritis

Alvaro Ferreira[*,†,1], **Marta Monteiro**[*,†], **Pedro Vita**[*,†], **António Marinho**[*,†], **Carlos Vasconcelos**[*,†]

[*]Unidade de Imunologia Clínica, Centro Hospitalar do Porto, Portugal
[†]UMIB/ICBAS, Universidade do Porto, Portugal
[1]Corresponding Author: alvaro.s.ferreira@gmail.com

1 INTRODUCTION

In recent years, researchers have shown growing interest in the association between genetic susceptibility to environmental factors and the pathogenesis of autoimmune diseases. The existence of environmental *triggers*, such as bacteria, seems to induce complex mechanisms of interaction with host immunogenic factors, leading to an inflammatory response.[1–3] Reactive arthritis (ReA) is one of the diseases for which this role is better demonstrated, with agents of urinary infection (*Chlamydia trachomatis, Mycoplasma, Ureaplasma urealyticum*) or gastrointestinal infection (*Campylobacter, Salmonella, Shigella, Yersinia*) playing active roles in the pathogenesis of the disease.[1,2,4] The mechanism appears to be molecular mimicry, in which the host immune response is directed against the organism itself due to "antigenic cross-reactivity" between the host and microbial determinants. These determinants define not only the innate immune response, but also the adaptive one, leading to the long-term clinical course of ReA.[2]

ReA is thus defined as a systemic inflammatory disorder characterized by aseptic arthritis, which is triggered by an infection at a distant site, occurring in a genetically susceptible person.[5] ReA is considered a member of spondyloarthritis group, sharing clinical, radiographic, and laboratory features with the other subgroups of the disease.[3] Human leukocyte antigen (HLA)-B27 has been described in 30–80% of patients with ReA having a higher probability of presenting chronic or axial manifestations.[6,7] The risk of developing ReA is about five times higher in patients with HLA-B27.[5] The classic presentation of ReA is characterized by an asymmetric arthritis,

Infection and Autoimmunity
http://dx.doi.org/10.1016/B978-0-444-63269-2.00050-7

usually in the lower limbs, associated with urethritis, conjunctivitis, and articular or extra-articular manifestations such as enthesitis, dactylitis, or inflammatory back pain.[8,9] The minimal interval between the preceding symptoms and arthritis is thought to be between 1–7 days and 4 weeks, and 15–30% of the patients evolve to chronicity.[2]

The terms ReA and Reiter's syndrome have been used to describe the same condition. However, the latter refers more specifically to the triad of urethritis, conjunctivitis, and arthritis secondary to infectious dysentery (classical definition) or to an episode of peripheral arthritis exceeding 1 month in duration and occurring in association with urethritis or cervicitis (American College of Rheumatology definition).[5] Most patients, after all, do not have this classic triad.[9] Some authors reviewed the use of the term Reiter's syndrome, concluding that it was less commonly mentioned in the literature, and they recommended replacing it with the term[6,10] introduced by Ahvonen in 1969: ReA.[2]

Many authors assert that the term ReA should be applied only to genitourinary and gastrointestinal infections caused by the agents listed above, and other aseptic forms of arthritis following an infection should be termed *post-infectious arthritis*, including arthritis following infections caused by some viruses, bacteria, and parasites such as *Clostridium difficile*, *Cryptosporidium*, *Giardia*, *Strongyloides*, *Brucella*, *Leptospira*, *Mycobacteria*, *Neisseria*, *Staphylococcus*, and *Streptococcus*.[2,8] The barrier between ReA and post-infectious arthritis is further blurred by the demonstration of not cultivable viable bacteria and/or antigenic material in the ReA patient's joints (*Salmonella* and *Yersinia lipopolysaccharide*) and of DNA, RNA, and even metabolic activity of Chlamydia.[11] At the risk of creating more confusion, certain forms of ReA could represent authentic chronic infectious arthritis caused by slow-growing organisms that may be undetectable using standard microbiological methods. Moreover, ReA differs from other post-infectious arthritis due to its independent natural history.[5] Unfortunately, no validated criteria for the conditions exist, and the diagnosis is essentially clinical.[12] For clarity, all of the discussed forms of arthritis should be called ReA, which, according to the trigger, occurs with or without the presence of HLA-B27. In this chapter, we discuss several aspects of ReA.

2 EPIDEMIOLOGY

The estimated incidence and prevalence of ReA depends on the definition of the condition and the research methods used to identify it.[13] Furthermore, the mild forms of the disease often go undiagnosed, and the prevalence of the disease depends on the incidence of gastrointestinal and genitourinary infections in the specific population studied.[14] Nevertheless, the annual incidence based on population studies is 0.6–27/100,000,[12,15] and in Europe, it is 30/100,000.[5] The prevalence is thought to be 30–40/100,000.[15] The disease occurs worldwide, affecting young adults in the age group of 20–40 years and appearing more often in men than it does in women (3:1).[2,14,15]

3 MECHANISMS INVOLVED – HLA-B27-ASSOCIATED AND HLA-B27-NONASSOCIATED REA

Although HLA-B27 is much more frequent in patients who develop classic ReA than it is in the general population (up to 90%), HLA-B27 frequency varies widely according to the microbial agent involved and can be as low as 27% for *Salmonella* outbreaks.[16,17] Several bacteria genera have been described as causing ReA via an HLA-B27-nonassociated mechanism, including *Borrelia*, *Brucella*, *Hemophilus*, *Hafnia*, *Leptospira*, *Mycobacterium*, *Neisseria*, *Staphylococcus*, *Streptococcus*, *Ureaplasma*, and *Vibrio*.[18–31]

Neisseria gonorrhoea infections provide a paradigm for post-infectious arthritis because they can cause classic Reiter's syndrome, ReA (incomplete Reiter's)[32] and septic arthritis.[33] Gonorrhoea is a common bacterial infection transmitted almost exclusively by sexual contact. It is most prevalent in adolescent and young adults (15–24 years) living in high-density urban areas.[34]

Also, viral, fungal, and parasitic infections are known to induce ReA without the presence of HLA-B27.[20,35–39] One important aspect of HLA-B27-nonassociated ReA is that the involved bacteria are known causes of septic arthritis, and, in some cases, differential diagnosis between reactive and bacterial arthritis may be virtually impossible.[23,40,41] However, HLA-B27 most certainly represents a risk factor for arthritis severity.[42]

3.1 Induction of ReA

Human ReA greatly resembles antigen-induced arthritis in animal models, in which an animal is first systemically immunized and then challenged with the same antigen (protein or nonviable bacteria) intra-articularly.[43,44] Therefore, the patient must have a preceding infection and become naturally immunized against the etiological agent, but during this process or a second exposure to the same agent, microbial antigens reach the synovial tissue. The following CD4+ cell mediated reaction is clinically manifested as an acute arthritis.[45–50] Studies also describe cases after vaccination with killed *Salmonella*,[51] recombinant hepatitis B viral protein[52], or tetanus.[53] This reaction may become chronic if there is a continuous supply of the antigen, probably derived from hidden reservoirs or nonarticular chronic infection sites. Some of this arthritis following vaccination could represent cases of Autoimmune/inflammatory Syndrome Induced by Adjuvants (ASIA) which is also called Shoenfeld syndrome.[54] For *Yersinia*-related ReA, the reservoir seems to be the enteric submucosal tissue.[55] In a series of cases, tonsil microabscesses were the cause of a chronic ReA induced by tonsillitis that was cured by resection of the microabscesses.[56] In some cases, forborne infections, such as travellers' diarrhea, may be the trigger, and subclinical infection may also be the source of episodic or continuous exposure to an antigen.[57,58]

3.2 HLA-B27-Associated Pathogenesis

HLA-B27 is a major histocompatibility complex class I molecule that encompasses 25 glycoproteins (HLA-B*2701 to HLA-B*2725), and it is encoded on chromosome 6p. HLA-B27 is ubiquitous among cell types and is highly expressed on antigen-presenting cells. After translation and tertiary folding, HLA-B27 heavy chains form heterotrimeric complexes with β2-microglobulin and intracellular peptides derived from self-proteins, viruses, and bacteria.[59]

Despite the intensive research, the exact role of HLA-B27 in the pathogenesis of these diseases is still unclear. Molecular mimicry between HLA-B27 and bacterial molecules has been found in *Yersinia*,[60] *Shigella*,[61] and *Salmonella*.[62] This mimicry could induce tolerance and lack of clearance of these organisms. Also, studies have described the formation of unusual forms of HLA-B27 (homodimers and heterodimers) that can be recognized by T CD4+ cells[63–66] typically associated with HLA class II. β2-Microglobulin seems to inhibit the formation of usual forms, however.[67]

The dominant paradigm (arthritogenic peptide hypothesis) states that self-peptides displayed by folded HLA-B27 become the target of autoreactive CD8+ T cells because they resemble microbial peptides, which does not occur with other HLA molecules. These T cells then cause cytotoxicity resulting in chronic inflammation. This hypothesis identifies the unique peptide-binding specificity of HLA-B27 as the problem.[59]

Interestingly, HLA-B27 positively effects two of the most threatening human viral infections: in HIV infection, HLA-B27-positive patients have low viral loads, and their CD4+ T cell counts decline slowly, as does the progression of AIDS; in acute infection with the hepatitis C virus (HCV), HLA-B27 is associated with a very high rate of spontaneous viral clearance.[68]

4 IMMUNE RESPONSE TO BACTERIA

In ReA, the Th1 cytokine response (interferon (IFN)-γ, IL-2, and IL-12) is impaired, and the Th2 response (IL-4 and IL-10) predominates and contributes to bacterial persistence in the joints.[69,70] The cause of this Th1–Th2 imbalance is unknown, although there is some evidence that tumor necrosis factor (TNF)-α genotypes, which seem to be associated with low IFN-γ and TNF-α production, are present at a higher percentage in ReA patients.[71,72] Because IFN-γ and TNF-α play a crucial role in the elimination of bacteria, insufficient production of these cytokines contributes to bacterial persistence. Furthermore, lower TNF-α levels have been associated with longer disease duration.[69] These findings suggest that a defective innate immunity allows the bacterial antigens to reach the synovia, where they then initiate the T cell responses.[72]

5 IMMUNE RESPONSE TO VIRAL INFECTIONS

Viral infections are one of the environmental factors capable of triggering immunoreactivity, and they have been implicated in the etiology of various rheumatic and autoimmune diseases, when infecting individuals who have a genetic or epigenetic susceptibility to chronic immune activation conditions.[73] Viral infections related arthritis depend on other host factors, such as age, gender, history, and infectious immune response.[74] On the other hand, viral infections often trigger acute joint inflammation by different mechanisms, only causing self-limited arthritis. For example, studies have implicated parvovirus B19 and Chikungunya virus (CHIKV) in both acute and chronic arthritis, sometimes with criteria for diagnosis of rheumatoid arthritis.[74,75]

The pathogenesis of arthritis associated with viral infections is not completely understood. It is known that they could trigger autoimmunity and inflammatory joint phenomenon by different pathogenic mechanisms (Table 1) including molecular mimicry (immunologic epitope shared between the host and the microbe), bystander activation (activation of antigen–presenting cells that can stimulate preprimed autoreactive T cells) and viral persistence (constant presence of viral antigens driving the immune response).[76]

Another mechanism by which viruses may trigger autoimmune phenomena is plasmacytoid dendritic cell activation, especially through the production of high levels of type I IFN that, in turn, lead to aberrant immune

Table 1 Pathogenic Mechanisms of Virus Related Arthritis

Virus	HBV	HCV	HIV	Parvovirus	Alphaviruses	HTLV-I	Rubella
Genome	DNA	RNA	Retrovirus	Single-stranded DNA	Single-stranded RNA	Retrovirus	Single-stranded RNA
Arthritogenic mechanisms	Immune complex deposition in synovia	Cryoglobulins formation Immune complexes deposition Direct tissue injury	Direct action of the virus	Immune complexes formation Activity of VP1u Inadequate humoral immune response Persistence in synoviocytes Cytotoxicity Up-regulation of inflammatory cytokines Autoantibodies production	Cytokines production Activation of MMPs Induces apoptosis in synovial tissue	Production of protein "Tax-1" in host cells Secretion of pro-inflammatory cytokines	Persistently infects synoviocytes and condrocytes Promotes inadequate humoral immune response Immune complexes formation

HBV, hepatitis B virus; HCV, hepatitis C virus; HTLV-I, human T-cell lymphotropic virus type I; MMPs, matrix metalloproteinases.

responses and the development of autoimmune disease. Plasmocitoid dendritic cells promote sensing of viral nucleic acids by intracellular expression of Toll-Like Receptor 7 (TLR7) and TLR9, and probably senses self nucleic acids through its interaction with antimicrobial peptides, like LL37.[77]

Parvovirus B19 is a single strand DNA virus of the Togavirus family, with a genome encoding two capsomer proteins, VP1 and VP2, and a nonstructural protein (NS1). VP1 contains an N-terminal region termed the VP1-unique region (VP1u), which differentiates it from VP2.[78] The suggested mechanisms relating Parvovirus B19 to chronic arthritis include deposition of immune complexes mostly secondary to humoral responses against VP1u, viral persistence, cytotoxicity, upregulation of inflammatory cytokines by NS1, the phospholipase A2-like activity of VP1u, production of autoantibodies such as rheumatoid factor (RF), antinuclear antibodies, anti-DNA, action against extractable nuclear antigens, Anti-Neutrophil Cytoplasmic Antibodies (ANCAs), antiphospholipids, and virus-related alteration of cellular immune or host reactions.[79-81] Acute polyarthritis related to Parvovirus B19 infection is thought to be due to the deposition of immune complexes, because the joint symptoms coincide with the disappearance of viremia and the appearance and specific IgG.[79] This also seems to be the mechanism by which articular inflammation is triggered in other acute viral infections, such as hepatitis and rubella.[82] The production of antiviral antibodies in synovia is another possible mechanism of rubella-related arthritis.[83]

The deposition of immune complexes also appears to be implicated in persistent arthritis. This is suggested by reports of reduced joint complaints following the administration of intravenous immunoglobulin, coinciding with the decrease in B19-positive cells in the bone marrow.[84,85] Evidence also shows that the persistence of organisms in synovial macrophages is important in the pathogenesis of viral arthritis.[86] Several alphaviruses, single-strand RNA viruses transmitted by mosquitoes, have arthritogenic capacities, including CHIKV, Sindbis virus (SINV), Ross River virus (RRV), Mayaro virus (MAYV), O'nyong-nyong virus (ONNV), and Barmah Forest virus (BFV).

SINV can replicate in human macrophages, and it stimulates the production of various cytokines, which leads to the expression of two matrix metalloproteinases (MMPs), a known mechanism in the development of arthritis. Studies have also demonstrated the involvement of the inhibitor of macrophage migration factor in the production of other inflammatory cytokines and MMPs in macrophages infected with SINV. This may explain the development of arthritis after viral infections, including CHIKV, which is considered the prototype of the diseases caused by this large group of alphaviruses.[87]

Furthermore, CHIKV has a marked cytotoxic effect, and it can induce apoptosis in vitro and in synovial tissue, as deduced by the presence of numerous lysed cells positive for polyadenosine diphosphate-ribose polymerase, whereas a high expression of MMP2 may contribute to chronic tissue injury.[86]

Hepatitis B virus (HBV)-associated polyarthritis occurs during the early phases of acute hepatitis B, when there is significant viremia. More rarely, an arthritis accompanying HBV-associated polyarteritis nodosa (PAN) may occur. In both cases, immune complexes are deposited in the synovia. Tests may also detect immune complexes containing HBsAg or HBeAg, their respective antibodies (anti-HBs and anti-HBe) and complement components.[81]

Arthritis related to HCV can be associated with cryoglobulinemia or directly connected to HCV infection,[88,89] but the most common cause of arthritis in patients infected with HCV is probably the coexistence of other inflammatory diseases such as systemic lupus, rheumatoid arthritis, and Sjogren's syndrome.[81] HCV is capable of modifying B lymphocytes through CD81 receptors, inducing polyclonal activation leading to the production of cryoglobulins, RF, and other autoantibodies.[90] The production of cryoglobulins is closely related to HCV, and cryoprecipitate contains a significant number of RNA viruses.[91] The mechanism by which HCV induces arthritis is not fully understood, but it may be due to the direct tissue injury caused by the virus, the autoimmune response that it induces or the deposition of immune complexes or cryoglobulins.[92] Another possible pathogenic mechanism could be related to the ability of the lymphocytes from cryoglobulin producers to concentrate large quantities of HCV particles on their surfaces.[93]

HIV infection is associated with various rheumatic manifestations, including ReA, and it is directly linked to infection with different pathophysiological mechanisms and clinical features. HIV-related arthritis seems mediated by the direct action of the virus, as demonstrated by the finding of tubuloreticular inclusions in synovia. In patients with "rheumatoid HIV", the p24 antigen was detected in the synovial tissue and CD4 and CD8 lymphocytes.[94] With the introduction of Highly Active Anti-Retroviral Treatment (HAART), the incidence of HIV-associated arthritis has decreased.[95,96]

In arthritis associated with the retrovirus human T-cell lymphotropic virus type I (HTLV-1), there is proliferation of synovial cells with T cells infiltration. The analysis of the synovial tissue of HTLV-1-positive patients not only confirms that lymphocytes and synoviocytes are infected by HTLV-1, but they also overexpress Tax1 transactivator protein, which induces the proliferation and secretion of proinflammatory cytokines such as TNF.[97]

6 CLINICAL MANIFESTATIONS

ReA affects people in the second to fourth decades of life, and it occurs up to 4 weeks following genitourinary (male-to-female ratio, 9:1) or enteric (male-to-female ratio, 1:1) infections.[18,98] It is a systemic disease, and serious visceral involvement is possible. Studies have not yet identified a direct correlation between extra-articular features and the associated infection, however.

ReA combines four syndromes: (i) a peripheral arthritis syndrome (an asymmetric acute or subacute oligoarthritis of the lower limbs); (ii) an enthesopathic syndrome[99]; (iii) a pelvic and axial syndrome (spinal involvement with sacroiliitis); and (iv) an extramusculoskeletal syndrome. The most frequent presentation is a nondestructive acute oligoarthritis of large lower limb joints (an average of four joints are affected). Approximately 15–30% of patients develop chronic or recurrent arthritis, sacroiliitis, or spondylitis, and most of these patients are positive for HLA-B27.[100]

Other clinical findings include diffuse swelling of an entire finger or toe, known as dactylitis[101]; enthesitis with associated heel pain, Achilles tendonitis, or pain at the insertion of the patella tendon into the tibial tubercle; inflammatory low back pain secondary to sacroiliitis or spondylitis; conjunctivitis; urethritis; prostatitis; hemorrhagic cystitis; mucopurulent cervicitis with or without easily induced cervical bleeding[98]; keratoderma blennorrhagica or pustulosis palmoplantaris; circinate balanitis; erythematous and superficial painless oral ulcers; and hyperkeratotic nail and skin lesions similar to pustular psoriasis. Proteinuria, microhematuria, or aseptic pyuria is seen in about 50% of patients with sexually acquired ReA. Studies have also reported severe systemic necrotizing vasculitis,[102] thrombophlebitis, purpura, livedo reticularis, and amyloidosis[103] as rare complications in chronic disease.[104]

Septic gonococcal arthritis without skin lesions can be confounded with a form of ReA, representing a true diagnostic challenge. The correct diagnosis of these entities may bring up several problems: strains causing gastrointestinal disease do not usually present with symptoms of urethral discharge,[33] fever is not always a rule, blood cultures are often either not collected or yield negative results, and the pauciarticular[33] form can be easily mistaken as undifferentiated spondyloarthritis or ReA.

The final diagnosis requires a high index of suspicion, and the health professional should take articular fluid for Gram stain and culture, even when the patient presents with chronic pauciarticular arthritis. *N. gonorrhoea* is isolated from synovial cultures in only 50% of the cases, however.[105] Appropriate samples, such as urethral, pharyngeal and blood cultures, can be useful adjuncts to a final diagnosis. A timely diagnosis depends on considering the possibility of *N. gonorrhoea* infection and taking a careful sexual history, and the culturing of *N. gonorrhoea* is of tremendous importance not only for a definite diagnosis but also for the determination of drug susceptibility.[106]

The most frequent presentation of virus-associated arthritis is acute symmetric polyarthritis (Table 2). HCV-associated arthritis is more often chronic in its polyarticular form, however, leading to a difficult differential diagnosis with Rheumatoid Arthritis (RA). Only 20% of cases have intermittent mono- or oligoarticular involvement of medium and large joints, and this form is rarely chronic.[107] Patients with HCV-associated mixed cryoglobulinemia usually show intermittent polyarthralgias involving the hands and knees, and less than 10% develop frank nonerosive arthritis.[89,90]

HIV-associated arthritis is usually oligoarticular and predominantly involves the lower extremities, most commonly the knees and ankles, and less frequently the wrists, metatarsophalangeal joints, elbows, and metacarpophalangeal and interphalangeal joints of the fingers. This condition tends to be self-limiting, lasting less than 6 weeks. A small number of patients have been reported as having a longer course with joint destruction, however.[108,109]

In Rubella infection symmetric or migratory arthralgias are more common than synovitis. Joint symptoms appear in about 30% of patients, with women more often affected, and articular symptoms develop within a week of the characteristic rash onset. Metacarpophalangeal and proximal interphalangeal joints are frequently affected, as are the knees, wrists, ankles, and elbows. Morning stiffness is also prominent. Periarthritis, tenosynovitis, and carpal tunnel syndrome may occur.[109,110] Similar symptoms may appear a few weeks after vaccination with live rubella vaccine. Joint manifestations usually resolve over a few days to 2 weeks, but they may persist for months to years.[110,111]

In the viremic phase, parvovirus B19 infection is frequently asymptomatic, but it can be accompanied by flulike symptoms, including transient fevers, malaise, myalgia, and headaches, and it is associated with the absence of reticulocytosis. This phase lasts for 5–6 days. The rash and joint symptoms appear within 4–6 days during the beginning of the antibody response phase. The joint involvement is far less common in children than in adults, with females being the most frequently affected group.[112] Arthralgias and arthritis can occur, beginning in a few joints but rapidly spreading, often in a rheumatoid-like distribution.[113,114]

Inflammatory polyarthritis has long been associated with alphavirus infections. The geographic area of CHIKV infection has enlarged in the last

Table 2 Clinical Characteristics of Virus Related Arthritis

Virus	HBV	HCV HCV-Associated Arthritis	HCV-Associated Mixed Cryo-Globulinemia	HIV	Parvovirus	Alphaviruses	HTLV-I	Rubella
Epidemiology								
Population at risk	– IVDUs – Persons with multiple sexual partners – Health workers	– IVDUs – Transfusion before 1992 – Persons with multiple sexual partners – Health workers		– IVDUs – Persons with multiple sexual partners – Health workers	Workers at schools or day care facilities	Travellers or inhabitants of endemic areas (Africa, South, and Southeast Asia)	– Perinatal – Sexual transmission in endemic areas (Caribbean, Japan)	Workers at schools or day care facilities
Clinical findings								
Type of joint manifestations	Polyarthritis	Polyarthritis (80%), mono/oligo-arthritis (20%)	Polyarthralgias	Assimetric oligo/polyarthritis	Polyarthritis	Polyarthritis	Polyarthritis	Polyarthralgias
Duration of arthritis	2–3 weeks	Chronic	Chronic	Less than 6 weeks Rarely chronic	2–3 weeks	Weeks to months	Chronic	Days to 2 weeks

Continued

Table 2 Clinical Characteristics of Virus Related Arthritis—cont'd

Virus	HBV	HCV		HIV	Parvovirus	Alphaviruses	HTLV-I	Rubella
		HCV-Associated Arthritis	HCV-Associated Mixed Cryo-Globulinemia					
Characteristic extra-articular manifestations	– Generalized skin rash – Fever – Myalgias		– Purpura – Peripheral neuropathy – Glomerulonephritis – Skin ulcers		– Flu-like symptoms 1 week prior to arthritis – Skin rash	– Fever – Skin rash – Myalgias – Headache – Nausea	– Vasculitis – Sjögren-like syndrome	– Low grade fever – Morbiliform skin rash – Lymphadenopathy – Lombar radiculoneuropathy
Complementary findings								
Diagnosis of associated viral infection	HBsAg (+) Anti-HBc IgM (+) ↑↑ALT/AST	Anti-HCV (+) (EIA) and HCV RNA (+) (PCR)		Anti-HIV (+) (ELISA) and HIV RNA (+) (PCR)	IgM B19 Ab (+)	Specific IgM Abs (+) and viral RNA (+) (PCR)	Anti-HTLV-I (+) (ELISA) and Western blot or HTLV-I DNA (+) PCR	Specific IgM abs (+)
RF	25% +	40–70% +	>90% +		Rarely +	Low titer + (chronic)	+	Negative
X-ray erosions	No	No	No	Rarely	No	Rarely	Yes	No

Ab, antibody; ALT, alanine aminotransferase; anti–TNF, anti–tumor necrosis factor; AST, aspartate aminotransferase; EIA, enzyme immunoassay; ELISA, enzyme-linked immunosorbent assay; HBV, hepatitis B virus; HCV, hepatitis C virus; HTLV-I, human T-cell lymphotropic virus type I; IFN-α, interferon-alpha; IVDU, intravenous injection drug user; PCR, polymerase chain reaction; RF, rheumatoid factor.
Adapted with permission from Ref. [81] (BioMed Central).

decade, with epidemic outbreaks involving many islands of the Indian Ocean and several countries in Asia and Africa.[115,116] Studies have also reported an increasing number of cases visitors returning to Europe and the United States from these regions.[117,118] In 2007, in the Ravenna region of Italy, 200 cases of CHIKV fever were identified.[119] In September 2010, autochthonous transmission of CHIKV was reported in southeastern France.[120] Virtually all CHIKV-infected patients have joint symptoms. During the acute phase, which lasts less than 2 weeks, the clinical features include fever; transient maculopapular rash, typically involving the trunk and extremities and more rarely the palms, soles, and face; conjunctivitis; myalgias and symmetric polyarthralgias; and/or polyarthritis involving the wrists, hands, ankles, and toes. Large joints (the knees and elbows) and the axis joints may be inflamed in addition to the peripheral ones.[121,122] The persistence of rheumatic manifestations is the most important clinical feature of the chronic stage of CHIKV infection. Symptoms and signs of severe polyarthritis appear in 80–90% of patients within the first 3 months. More than 60% of patients with CHIKV fever have joint stiffness and/or pains more than a year after the initial infections. Symmetrical arthritis has been described, but it can be asymmetrical and even present as oligo- or mono-arthritis.[123,124] Tenosynovitis or enthesopathy have also been described. Deformity, limitations in joint mobility, and bone erosions may also develop.[123]

ONNV fever is very similar to CHIKV fever.[125] RRV polyarthritis is often migratory, asymmetric, and incapacitating.[126] MAYV arthritis usually involves the wrists, ankles, and toes, and less commonly the elbows and knees, and it can be incapacitating and persist for months.[127] Arthritis is less common and less prominent in BFV infection than it is in other alphavirus infections.[128] Nonerosive chronic arthropathy is common after SINV infection, and 30% of patients can have joint complaints for 2 years and in some cases for 5–6 years.[129]

HTLV-1 is an established cause of inflammatory arthropathy with a presentation not much different from Rheumatoid Arthritis. Typically, it occurs as a symmetric inflammatory arthritis usually in elderly women from an endemic area, such as Caribbean countries and the southern part of Japan. It is also present in Africa, South America, Asia, and other tropical or subtropical areas. Often, HTLV-1-associated arthritis has an oligoarticular presentation affecting primarily the knees, shoulders, and wrists. RF is frequently detected, and X-rays of the affected joints only reveal erosive changes mildly different from those present in RA.[130]

Arthritis in patients with HBV is usually sudden in onset and often severe, with symmetric and simultaneous involvement of several joints, but it may also be migratory or additive. The joints of the hand and knee are most often affected, but the wrists, ankles, elbows, shoulders, and other large joints may be involved as well. Fusiform swelling occurs in the small joints of the hand as in rheumatoid arthritis. The HBV-associated arthritis appears during the preicteric phase of acute hepatitis B infection and may precede jaundice by days to weeks. It usually subsides soon after its onset, but it may persist for several weeks.[131,132] Patients with chronic active hepatitis or chronic HBV viremia may have recurrent polyarthralgia or polyarthritis.[132] Arthritis also may occur in the context of HBV-associated PAN, but only in a small proportion of patients. The most frequent manifestations, affecting nearly half of the patients, are arthralgias and myalgias.[133]

7 TREATMENT OPTIONS

In theory, ReA would be one of the best disorders to use for evaluating the efficacy of anti-infectious treatment. Although several small studies have investigated the efficacy of prolonged antibiotic monotherapy treatment, no study was able to show a clinical benefit.[134–137] Thus, a short conventional course may eradicate the triggering infection and may prevent the development of ReA, but this approach seems to have no benefit in established arthritis.[134] However, combined doxycycline and rifampin for 6–9 months seemed to be effective in treating chronic inflammatory arthritis possibly secondary to persistent *Chlamydia*.[138,139] Non-Steroid Anti-Inflammatory Drugs (NSAIDs), steroids, Disease Modifying Anti-Rheumatic Drugs (DMARDs), and anti-TNFα therapies are the mainstream approaches for ReA remission induction, and they are used in protocols similar to those employed for other forms of spondyloarthritis.

The drug treatment of viral arthritis primarily addresses symptoms, often employing NSAIDs, analgesics and, in some cases, low-dose corticosteroids for conditions such as arthritis associated with HTLV-1,[97,140] hepatitis C,[127,141] and rubella.[142] In some situations the treatment of the underlying disease is also effective in controlling the joint symptoms, as happens with hepatitis C and HIV infection. The other infections have no specific treatment.

Hydroxychloroquine and, less often, methotrexate (MTX) and penicillamine have been used to treat arthritis associated with HCV infection.[143] Studies have reported the safe and effective use of MTX for HCV-positive patients with stable liver function and close monitoring.[143,144]

Hydroxychloroquine[145,146] and sulfasalazine[147] have also shown efficacy and safety in the treatment of seronegative arthritis in HIV patients.

In addition, some authors have proposed DMARDs for the treatment of arthritis associated with HTLV-1[97] and CHIKV.[75] TNF inhibitors have been used safely in patients with hepatitis C,[144] and a small study indicated that etanercept was effective and safe for patients with hepatitis C when used with antiviral therapy.[121] TNF inhibitors were also successfully used in HIV patients with spondyloarthritis and rheumatoid arthritis,[148,149] but no studies have addressed its use in HIV-associated arthritis. The use of TNF inhibitors should be limited to patients with CD4 counts higher than $200/mm^3$ and viral loads less than 60,000 copies/mm^3.[150] Prompt treatment with third-generation cephalosporin can be curative, prevent joint damage[151] and may confirm the diagnosis in culture-negative gonococcal arthritis.[106]

8 CONCLUSIONS

Many authors only apply the term ReA to genitourinary and gastrointestinal infections caused by specific agents, using the term post-infectious arthritis for other aseptic forms of arthritis following an infection. ReA can be regarded as a form of post-infectious arthritis with clinical features, treatment and prognosis similar to those for other types of spondyloarthritis. Studies have yet to determine the role of antibiotic therapy in preventing the triggering of arthritis or the development of chronic sequels in patients with ReA, as has been proven for other post-infectious arthritis. However, if the patient has classic ReA triggered by *C. trachomatis*, antibiotics will likely eradicate the primary infection. Despite clinical differences, most authors use the term ReA for both entities. Infections can also be a source of acute self-limiting arthritis or chronic arthritis. Both of these conditions have different mechanisms and, sometimes, different specific treatments. In ReA, recurrent arthritis, enthesitis and inflammatory low back pain occur as late manifestations in many patients, requiring treatment with NSAIDs or DMARDS, as is done for patients with other types of spondyloarthritis. Finally, the lack of uniformly accepted diagnostic criteria for these two entities is a major problem in the comparison of studies.

REFERENCES

1. Astrauskiene D, Bernotiene E. New insights into bacterial persistence in reactive arthritis. *Clin Exp Rheumatol* 2007;**25**:470–9.
2. Girschick HJ, Guilherme L, Inman RD, Latsch K, Rilhe M, Sherer Y, et al. Bacterial triggers and autoimmune rheumatic diseases. *Clin Exp Rheumatol* 2008;**26**(Jan-Feb):S12–17.

3. Carter JD. Bacterial agents in spondyloarthritis: a destiny from diversity? *Best Pract Res Clin Rheumatol* 2010;**24**(5):701–14.
4. Butrimiene I, Ranceva J, Griskevicius A. Potential triggering infections of reactive arthritis. *Scand J Rheumatol* 2006;**35**(6):459–62.
5. Hamdulay SS, Glynne SJ, Keat A. When is arthritis reactive? *Postgrad Med J* 2006;**82**:446–53.
6. Keynan Y, Rimar D. Reactive arthritis—the appropriate name. *Isr Med Assoc J* 2008;**10**(4):256–8.
7. Kaarela K, Jäntti JK, Kotaniemi KM. Similarity between chronic reactive arthritis and ankylosing spondylitis. A 32-35-year follow-up study. *Clin Exp Rheumatol* 2009;**27**(2):325–8.
8. Townes JM. Reactive arthritis after enteric infections in the United States: the problem of definition. *Clin Infect Dis* 2010;**50**(2):247–54.
9. Carter JD, Hudson AP. Reactive arthritis: clinical aspects and medical management. *Rheum Dis Clin North Am* 2009;**35**(1):21–44.
10. Lu DW, Katz KA. Declining use of the eponym "Reiter's syndrome" in the medical literature, 1998-2003. *J Am Acad Dermatol* 2005;**53**(4):720–3.
11. Hannu T, Inman R, Granfors K, Leirisalo-Repo M. Reactive arthritis or post-infectious arthritis? *Best Pract Res Clin Rheumatol* 2006;**20**(3):419–33.
12. Hannu T. Reactive arthritis. *Best Pract Res Clin Rheumatol* 2011;**25**(3):347–57.
13. Rohekar S, Pope J. Epidemiologic approaches to infection and immunity: the case of reactive arthritis. *Curr Opin Rheumatol* 2009;**21**(4):386–90.
14. Zochling J, Smith EU. Seronegative spondyloarthritis. *Best Pract Res Clin Rheumatol* 2010;**24**(6):747–56.
15. Hanova P, Pavelka K, Holcatova I, Pikhart H. Incidence and prevalence of psoriatic arthritis, ankylosing spondylitis, and reactive arthritis in the first descriptive population-based study in the Czech Republic. *Scand J Rheumatol* 2010;**39**(4):310–17.
16. Tertti R, Granfors K, Lehtonen OP, Mertsola J, Mäkelä AL, Välimäki I, et al. An outbreak of Yersinia pseudotuberculosis infection. *J Infect Dis* 1984;**149**:245–50.
17. Mattila L, Leirisalo-Repo M, Koskimies S, Granfors K, Siitonen A. Reactive arthritis following an outbreak of Salmonella infection in Finland. *Br J Rheumatol* 1994;**33**:1136–41.
18. Keat A. Reiter's syndrome and reactive arthritis in perspective. *N Engl J Med* 1983;**309**(26):1606–15.
19. Ford MJ, Hurst NP, Nuki G. Reactive arthritis—infectious agents and genetic susceptibility in the pathogenesis of sero-negative arthritis. *Scott Med J* 1983;**28**:34–41.
20. Toivanen A, Toivanen P. Epidemiologic aspects, clinical features, and management of ankylosing spondylitis and reactive arthritis. *Curr Opin Rheumatol* 1994;**6**:354–9.
21. Alarcon GS, Bocanegra TS, Gotuzzo E, Hinostroza S, Carrillo C, Vasey FB, et al. Reactive arthritis associated with brucellosis: HLA studies. *J Rheumatol* 1981;**8**:621–5.
22. Winter RJD, Richardson A, Lehner MJ, Hoffbrand BI. Lung abscess and reactive arthritis: rare complications of leptospirosis. *BMJ* 1984;**288**:448–9.
23. Rush PJ, Shore A, Inman R, Gold R, Jadavji T, Laski B. Arthritis associated with Haemophilus influenzae meningitis: septic or reactive? *J Pediatr* 1986;**109**:412–15.
24. Maricic MJ, Alepa FP. Reactive arthritis after Mycobacterium avium-intracellulare infection: Poncet's disease revisited. *Am J Med* 1990;**88**:549–50.
25. Newmark JJ, Hobbs WN, Wilson BE. Reactive arthritis associated with Hafnia alvei enteritis. *Arthritis Rheum* 1994;**37**:960.
26. Deighton C. Beta-haemolytic streptococci and reactive arthritis in adults. *Ann Rheum Dis* 1993;**52**:475–82.
27. Tamura N, Kobayashi S, Hashimoto H, Hirose S-I. Reactive arthritis induced by Vibrio parahaemolyticus. *J Rheumatol* 1993;**20**:1062–3.

28. Horowitz S, Horowitz J, Taylor-Robinson D, Sukenik S, Apte RN, Bar-David J, et al. Ureaplasma urealyticum in Reiter's syndrome. *J Rheumatol* 1994;**21**:877–82.

29. Mader R, Zu'Bi A, Schonfeld S. Recurrent sterile arthritis following primary septic meningococcal arthritis. *Clin Exp Rheumatol* 1994;**12**:531–3.

30. Gutiérrez-Ureña S, Molina J, Molina JF, García CO, Cuéllar ML, Espinoza LR. Post-streptococcal reactive arthritis, clinical course, and outcome in 6 adult patients. *J Rheumatol* 1995;**22**:1710–13.

31. Siam ARM, Hammoudeh M. Staphylococcus aureus triggered reactive arthritis. *Ann Rheum Dis* 1995;**54**:131–3.

32. Rosenthal L, Olhagen B, Ek S. Aseptic arthritis after gonorrhoea. *Ann Rheum Dis* 1980;**39**(2):141–6.

33. Le Berre JP, Samy J, Garrabé E, Imbert I, Magnin J, Lechevalier D. Arthritis without urethritis: remember gonococcus. *Rev Med Interne* 2007;**28**(3):183–5.

34. Handsfield H, Spaling P. Neisseria gonorrhoea. In: Mandell GL, Bernett JE, Dolin R, editors. *Principles and practice of infectious diseases.* Philadelphia: Elsevier Churchill Livingstone; 2005. p. 2514–27.

35. Burnstein SL, Liakos S. Parasitic rheumatism presenting as rheumatoid arthritis. *J Rheumatol* 1983;**10**:514–15.

36. Woo P, Panayi GS. Reactive arthritis due to infestation with Giardia lamblia. *J Rheumatol* 1984;**11**:719.

37. Kamel M, Safwat E, Eltayeb S. Bilharzial arthropathy. Immunological findings. *Scand J Rheumatol* 1989;**18**:315–19.

38. Lee MG, Rawlins SC, Didier M, DeCeulaer K. Infective arthritis due to Blastocystis hominis. *Ann Rheum Dis* 1990;**49**:192–3.

39. Cron RQ, Sherry DD. Reiter's syndrome associated with cryptosporidial gastroenteritis. *J Rheumatol* 1995;**22**:1962–3.

40. Kortekangas P, Aro HT, Tuominen J, Toivanen A. Synovial fluid leukocytosis in bacterial arthritis vs. reactive arthritis and rheumatoid arthritis in the adult knee. *Scand J Rheumatol* 1992;**21**:283–8.

41. Toivanen P, Toivanen A. Bacterial or reactive arthritis? *Rheumatol Europe* 1995;**24** (Suppl. 2):253–5.

42. Linssen A, Feltkamp TEW. B27 positive diseases versus B27 negative diseases. *Ann Rheum Dis* 1988;**47**:431–9.

43. Greenvald RA, Diamond HS, Cooke TDV. Antigen-induced arthritis, polyarthritis, and tenosynovitis. In: Greenvald RA, Diamond HS, editors. *Handbook of animal models for the rheumatic diseases,* vol. I. Boca Raton, FL: CRC Press; 1988. p. 53–81.

44. Henderson B, Edwards JCW, Pettipher ER, Pettipher ER, Blake S. Antigen-induced arthritis. In: Henderson B, Edwards JCW, Pettipher ER, editors. *Mechanisms and models in rheumatoid arthritis.* London: Academic Press; 1995. p. 457–70.

45. Burmester GR, Daser A, Kamradt T, Krause A, Mitchison NA, Sieper J, et al. Immunology of reactive arthritides. *Annu Rev Immunol* 1995;**13**:229–50.

46. Gaston JS, Life PF, Granfors K, Merilahti-Palo R, Bailey L, Consalvey S, et al. Synovial T lymphocyte recognition of organisms that trigger reactive arthritis. *Clin Exp Immunol* 1989;**76**:348–53.

47. Sieper J, Kingsley G, Palacios-Boix A, Pitzalis C, Treharne J, Hughes R, et al. Synovial T lymphocyte-specific immune response to Chlamydia trachomatis in Reiter's disease. *Arthritis Rheum* 1991;**34**:588–98.

48. Hassell AB, Pilling D, Reynolds D, Life PF, Bacon PA, Gaston JSH. MHC restriction of synovial fluid lymphocyte responses to the triggering organism in reactive arthritis. Absence of a class I-restricted response. *Clin Exp Immunol* 1992;**88**:442–7.

49. Sieper J, Braun J, Wu P, Kingsley G. T cells are responsible for the enhanced synovial cellular immune response to triggering antigen in reactive arthritis. *Clin Exp Immunol* 1993;**91**:96–102; Hermann E. T cells in reactive arthritis. *APMIS* 1993;**101**:177–86.

50. Lahesmaa R, Shanafelt M-C, Steinman L, Peltz G. Immunopathogenesis of human inflammatory arthritis: lessons from Lyme and reactive arthritis. *J Infect Dis* 1994;**170**:978–85.

51. Calin A, Goulding N, Brewerton D. Reactive arthropathy following Salmonella vaccination [Letter]. *Arthritis Rheum* 1987;**30**:1197.

52. Hassan W, Oldham R. Reiter's syndrome and reactive arthritis in health care workers after vaccination. *BMJ* 1994;**309**:94.

53. Sahin N, Salli A, Enginar AU, Ugurlu H. Reactive arthritis following tetanus vaccination: a case report. *Mod Rheumatol* 2009;**19**(2):209–11.

54. Zafri Y, Agmon-Levin N, Paz Z, Shilton T, Shoenfeld Y. Autoimmunity following hepatitis B vaccine as part of the spectrum of 'autoimmune (auto-inflammatory) syndrome induced by adjuvants' (ASIA): analysis of 93 cases. *Lupus* 2012;**21**:146–52.

55. de Koning J, Heesemann J, Hoogkamp-Korstanje JAA, Festen JJM, Houtman PM, van Oijen PLM. Yersinia in intestinal biopsy specimens from patients with seronegative spondyloarthropathy: correlation with specific serum IgA antibodies. *J Infect Dis* 1989;**159**:109–12.

56. Kobayashi S, Ichikawa G. Reactive arthritis induced by tonsillitis: a type of 'focal infection'. *Adv Otorhinolaryngol* 2011;**72**:79–82.

57. Batz MB, Henke E, Kowalcyk B. Long-term consequences of foodborne infections. *Infect Dis Clin North Am* 2013;**27**(3):599–616.

58. Connor BA, Riddle MS. Post-infectious sequelae of travelers' diarrhea. *J Travel Med* 2013;**20**(5):303–12.

59. Zambrano-Zaragoza JF, Agraz-Cibrian JM, González-Reyes C, Durán-Avelar Mde J, Vibanco-Pérez N. Ankylosing spondylitis: from cells to genes. *Int J Inflam* 2013;**2013**, Article ID 501653,16 p.

60. Taccetti G, Trapani S, Ermini M, Falcini F. Reactive arthritis triggered by Yersinia enterocolitica: a review of 18 pediatric cases. *Clin Exp Rheumatol* 1994;**12**(6):681–4.

61. Lahesmaa R, Skurnik M, Vaara M, Leirisalo-Repo M, Nissilä M, Granfors K, et al. Molecular mimicry between HLA B27 and Yersinia, Salmonella, Shigella and Klebsiella within the same region of HLA alpha 1-helix. *Clin Exp Immunol* 1991;**86**(3):399–404.

62. Singh AK, Aggarwal A, Chaurasia S, Misra R. Identification of immunogenic HLA-B★27:05 binding peptides of Salmonella outer membrane protein in patients with reactive arthritis and undifferentiated spondyloarthropathy. *J Rheumatol* 2013;**40**(2):173–85.

63. Bird LA, Peh CA, Kollnberger S, Elliott T, McMichael AJ, Bowness P. Lymphoblastoid cells express HLA-B27 homodimers both intracellularly and at the cell surface following endosomal recycling. *Eur J Immunol* 2003;**33**(3):748–59.

64. Allen RL, O'Callaghan CA, McMichael AJ, Bowness P. Cutting edge: HLA-B27 can form a novel beta 2-microglobulin-free heavy chain homodimer structure. *J Immunol* 1999;**162**(9):5045–8.

65. Allen RL, Raine T, Haude A, Trowsdale J, Wilson MJ. Leukocyte receptor complex-encoded immunomodulatory receptors show differing specificity for alternative HLA-B27 structures. *J Immunol* 2001;**167**(10):5543–7.

66. Malik P, Klimovitsky P, Deng LW, Boyson JE, Strominger JL. Uniquely conformed peptide-containing beta 2-microglobulin-free heavy chains of HLA-B2705 on the cell surface. *J Immunol* 2002;**169**(8):4379–87.

67. Bowness P. HLA B27 in health and disease: a double-edged sword? *Rheumatology (Oxford)* 2002;**41**(8):857–68.

68. Neumann-Haefelin C. Protective role of HLA-B27 in HIV and hepatitis C virus infection. *Dtsch Med Wochenschr* 2011;**136**(7):320–4.

69. Braun J, Yin Z, Spiller I, Siegert S, Rudwaleit M, Liu L, et al. Low secretion of tumor necrosis factor alpha, but no other Th1 or Th2 cytokines, by peripheral blood

mononuclear cells correlates with chronicity in reactive arthritis. *Arthritis Rheum* 1999;**42**(10):2039–44.

70. Yin Z, Braun J, Neure L, Wu P, Liu L, Eggens U, et al. Crucial role of interleukin-10/interleukin-12 balance in the regulation of the type 2 T helper cytokine response in reactive arthritis. *Arthritis Rheum* 1997;**40**(10):1788–97.

71. Sieper J, Braun J, Kingsley GH. Report on the fourth international workshop on reactive arthritis. *Arthritis Rheum* 2000;**43**(4):720–34.

72. Wuorela M, Granfors K. Infectious agents as triggers of reactive arthritis. *Am J Med Sci* 1998;**316**(4):264–70.

73. Kerr JR. Pathogenesis of parvovirus B19 infection: host gene variability, and possible means and effects of virus persistence. *J Vet Med B Infect Dis Vet Public Health* 2005;**52**:335–9.

74. Colmegna I, Alberts-Grill N. Parvovirus B19: its role in chronic arthritis. *Rheum Dis Clin North Am* 2009;**35**:95–110.

75. Ali Ou Alla S, Combe B. Arthritis after infection with Chikungunya virus. *Best Pract Res Clin Rheumatol* 2011;**25**:337–46.

76. Fujinami RS, von Herrath MG, Christen U, Lindsay Whitton J. Molecular mimicry, bystander activation, or viral persistence: infections and autoimmune disease. *Clin Microbiol Rev* 2006;**19**:80–94.

77. Santana-de Anda K, Gomez-Martin D, Soto-Solis R. Plasmacytoid dendritic cells: key players in viral infections and autoimmune diseases. *Semin Arthritis Rheum* 2013;**43**:131–6.

78. Zuffi E, Manaresi E, Gallinella G, Gentilomi GA, Venturoli S, Zerbini M, et al. Identification of an immunodominant peptide in the parvovirus B19 VP1 unique region able to elicit a long-lasting immune response in humans. *Viral Immunol* 2001;**14**:151–8.

79. Kerr JR. Pathogenesis of human parvovirus B19 in rheumatic disease. *Ann Rheum Dis* 2000;**59**:672–83.

80. Tsay GJ, Zouali M. Unscrambling the role of human parvovirus B19 signaling in systemic autoimmunity. *Biochem Pharmacol* 2006;**72**:1453–9.

81. Vassilopoulos D, Calabrese LH. Virally associated arthritis 2008: clinical, epidemiologic, and pathophysiologic considerations. *Arthritis Res Ther* 2008;**10**:215–23.

82. Vergani D, Morgan-Capner P, Davies ET, Anderson AW, Tee DEH, Pattison JR. Joint symptoms, immune complexes and rubella. *Lancet* 1980;**1**:321–2.

83. Mims CA, Stokes A, Grahame R. Synthesis of antibodies, including antiviral antibodies, in the knee joints of patients with arthritis. *Ann Rheum Dis* 1985;**44**:734.

84. Murai C, Munakata Y, Takahashi Y, Ishii T, Shibata S, Muryoi T, et al. Rheumatoid arthritis after human parvovirus B19 infection. *Ann Rheum Dis* 1999;**58**:130–2.

85. Ogawa E, Otaguro S, Murata M, Kainuma M, Sawayama Y, Furusyo N, et al. Intravenous immunoglobulin therapy for severe arthritis associated with human parvovirus B19 infection. *J Infect Chemother* 2008;**14**:377.

86. Jaffar-Bandjee MC, Das T, Hoarau JJ. Chikungunya virus takes centre stage in virally induced arthritis: possible cellular and molecular mechanisms to pathogenesis. *Microbes Infect* 2009;**11**:1206–18.

87. Assunção-Miranda I, Bozza MT, Da Poian AT. Pro-inflammatory response resulting from Sindbis virus infection of human macrophages: implications for the pathogenesis of viral arthritis. *J Med Virol* 2010;**82**:164–74.

88. Sanzone AM, Bégué RE. Hepatitis C and arthritis: an update. *Infect Dis Clin North Am* 2006;**20**(4):877–89, vii.

89. Vassilopoulos D, Calabrese LH. Rheumatic manifestations of hepatitis C infection. *Curr Rheumatol Rep* 2003;**5**:200–4.

90. Antonelli A, Ferri C, Galeazzi M, Giannitti C, Manno D, Mieli-Vergani G, et al. HCV infection: pathogenesis, clinical manifestations and therapy. *Clin Exp Rheumatol* 2008;**26**:S39–47.

91. Agnello V, Chung RT, Kaplan LM. A role of hepatitis C virus infection in type II cryoglobulinemia. *N Engl J Med* 1992;**327**:1490–5.

92. Buskila D. Infections and rheumatic diseases hepatitis C–associated rheumatic disorders. *Rheum Dis Clin North Am* 2009;**35**:111–23.

93. Sansonno D, Lauletta G, Montrone M, Tucci FA, Nisi L, Dammacco F. Virological analysis and phenotypic characterization of peripheral blood lymphocytes of hepatitis C virus-infected patients with and without mixed cryoglobulinemia. *Clin Exp Immunol* 2006;**143**:288–96.

94. Espinoza LR, Aguilar JL, Espinoza CG, Berman A, Gutierrez F, Vasey FB, et al. HIV-associated arthropathy: HIV antigen demonstration in the synovial membrane. *J Rheumatol* 1990;**17**:1195–201.

95. Reveille JD, Williams FM. Infection and musculoskeletal conditions: rheumatologic complications of HIV infection. *Best Pract Res Clin Rheumatol* 2006;**20**(6):1159–79.

96. Walker UA, Tyndall A, Daikeler T. Rheumatic conditions in human immunodeficiency virus infection. *Rheumatology (Oxford)* 2008;**47**(7):952–9.

97. Kitajima I, Yamamoto K, Sato K, Nakajima Y, Nakajima T, Maruyama I, et al. Detection of human T cell lymphotropic virus type I proviral DNA and its gene expression in synovial cells in chronic inflammatory arthropathy. *J Clin Invest* 1991;**88**:1315–22.

98. Barth WF, Segal K. Reactive arthritis (Reiter's syndrome). *Am Fam Physician* 1999;**60**(2):499–503, 507.

99. McGonagle D, Gibbon W, Emery P. Classification of inflammatory arthritis by enthesitis. *Lancet* 1998;**352**(9134):1137–40.

100. Khan MA. Update on spondyloarthropathies. *Ann Intern Med* 2002;**136**(12):896–907.

101. Klippel JH, Dieppe PA, editors. *Practical rheumatology*. St Louis, MO: Mosby Inc.; 1995

102. Boehni U, Christen B, Greminger P, Michel BA. Systemic vasculitis associated with seronegative spondylarthropathy (Reiter's syndrome). *Clin Rheumatol* 1997;**16**(6):610–13.

103. Duarte M, Alzaga X, Sellas A, Arderiu A, Lience E. Amyloidosis in reactive arthritis. *Clin Exp Rheumatol* 1997;**15**(5):584–5.

104. Wollenhaupt J, Zeidler H. Undifferentiated arthritis and reactive arthritis. *Curr Opin Rheumatol* 1998;**10**(4):306–13.

105. O'Brien JP, Goldenberg DL, Rice PA. Disseminated gonococcal infection: a prospective analysis of 49 patients and a review of pathophysiology and immune mechanisms. *Medicine (Baltimore)* 1983;**62**:395–406.

106. Bardin T. Gonococcal arthritis. *Best Pract Res Clin Rheumatol* 2003;**17**(2):201–8.

107. Olivieri I, Palazzi C, Padula A. Hepatitis C virus infection and arthritis. *Rheum Dis Clin North Am* 2003;**29**:111–22.

108. Berman A, Cahn P, Perez H, Spindler A, Lucero E, Paz S, et al. Human immunodeficiency virus infection associated arthritis: clinical characteristics. *J Rheumatol* 1999;**26**:1158–62.

109. Mody GM, Parke FA, Reveille JD. Articular manifestations of human immunodeficiency virus infection. *Best Pract Res Clin Rheumatol* 2003;**17**:265–87.

110. Smith CA, Petty RE, Tingle AJ. Rubella virus and arthritis. *Rheum Dis Clin North Am* 1987;**13**:265–74.

111. Tingle AJ, Allen M, Petty RE, Kettyls GD, Chantler JK. Rubella-associated arthritis. I. Comparative study of joint manifestations associated with natural rubella infection and RA 27/3 rubella immunization. *Ann Rheum Dis* 1986;**45**:110.

112. Howson CP, Katz M, Johnston Jr RB, Fineberg HV. Chronic arthritis after rubella vaccination. *Clin Infect Dis* 1992;**15**:307.

113. Ager A, Chin TDY, Poland JD. Epidemic erythema infectiosum. *N Engl J Med* 1966;**275**:1326–31.

114. White DG, Woolf AD, Mortimer PP, Cohen BJ, Blake DR, Bacon PA. Human parvovirus arthropathy. *Lancet* 1985;**i**:419–21.
115. Woolf AD, Campion GV, Chiswick A, Wise S, Cohen BJ, Klouda PT, et al. Clinical manifestations of human parvovirus B19 in adults. *Arch Intern Med* 1989;**149**:1153–6.
116. Renault P, Solet JL, Sissoko D, Balleydier E, Larrieu S, Filleul L, et al. A major epidemic of Chikungunya virus infection on Réunion Island, France 2005–2006. *Am J Trop Med Hyg* 2007;**77**:727–31.
117. Lahariya C, Pradhan SK. Emergence of Chikungunya virus in Indian subcontinent after 32 years: a review. *J Vector Borne Dis* 2006;**43**:151–60.
118. Queyriaux B, Armengaud A, Jeannin C, Couturier E, Peloux-Petiot F. Chikungunya in Europe. *Lancet* 2008;**371**:723–4.
119. Simon F, Javelle E, Oliver M, Lepare-Goffart I, Marimoutou C. Chikungunya virus infection. *Curr Infect Dis* 2011;**13**:218–28.
120. Rezza G, Nicoletti L, Angelini R, Romi R, Finarelli AC, Panning M, et al. Infection with Chikungunya virus in Italy: an outbreak in a temperate region. *Lancet* 2007;**370**:1840–6.
121. Grandadam M, Caro V, Plumet S, Thiberge JM, Souares Y, Falilloux AB, et al. Chikungunya virus, southeastern France. *Emerg Infect Dis* 2011;**17**:910–13.
122. Brighton SW, Prozesky OW, de la Harpe AL. Chikungunya virus infection. A retrospective study of 107 cases. *S Afr Med J* 1983;**63**:313–15.
123. Manimunda SP, Vijayachari P, Uppoor R. Clinical progression of chikungunya fever during acute and chronic arthritic stages and the changes in joint morphology as revealed by imaging. *Trans R Soc Trop Med Hyg* 2010;**104**:392–9.
124. Borgherini G, Poubeau P, Jossaume A, Gouix A, Cotte L, Michault A, et al. Persistent arthralgia associated with Chikungunya virus: a study of 88 adult patients on Reunion Island. *Clin Infect Dis* 2008;**47**:469–75.
125. Kiwanuka N, Sanders EJ, Rwaguma EB, Kawamata J, Ssengooba FP, Najjemba R, et al. O'nyong-nyong fever in south-central Uganda, 1996–1997: clinical features and validation of a clinical case definition for surveillance purposes. *Clin Infect Dis* 1999;**29**:1243.
126. Fraser JRE. Epidemic polyarthritis and Ross River virus disease. *Clin Rheum Dis* 1986;**12**:369.
127. Pinheiro FP, Freitas RB, Travassos da Rosa JF, Gabbay YB, Mello WA, LeDuc JW. An outbreak of Mayaro virus disease in Belterra, Brazil. I. Clinical and virological findings. *Am J Trop Med Hyg* 1981;**30**:674.
128. Flexman JP, Smith DW, Mackenzie JS, Fraser JR, Bass SP, Hueston L, et al. A comparison of the diseases caused by Ross River virus and Barmah Forest virus. *Med J Aust* 1998;**169**:159.
129. Laine M, Luukkainen R, Jalava J, Ilonen J, Kuusistö P, Toivanen A. Prolonged arthritis associated with Sindbis-related (Pogosta) virus infection. *Rheumatology (Oxford)* 2002;**41**:829.
130. Masuko-Hongo K, Kato T, Nishioka K. Virus-associated arthritis. *Best Pract Res Clin Rheumatol* 2003;**17**:309–18.
131. Inman RD. Rheumatic manifestations of hepatitis B virus infection. *Semin Arthritis Rheum* 1982;**11**:406–20.
132. Csepregi A, Rojkovich B, Nemesánszky E, Poór G, Héjjas M, Horányi M. Chronic seropositive polyarthritis associated with hepatitis B virus–induced chronic liver disease: a sequel of virus persistence. *Arthritis Rheum* 2000;**43**:232.
133. Guillevin L, Mahr A, Callard P, Godmer P, Pagnoux C, Leray E, et al. Hepatitis B virus-associated polyarteritis nodosa: clinical characteristics, outcome, and impact of treatment in 115 patients. *Medicine (Baltimore)* 2005;**84**:313–22.
134. Hannu T, Mattila L, Siitonen A, Leirisalo-Repo M. Reactive arthritis following an outbreak of Salmonella typhimurium phage type 193 infection. *Ann Rheum Dis* 2002;**61** (3):264–6.

135. Sieper J, Fendler C, Laitko S, Sörensen H, Gripenberg-Lerche C, Hiepe F, et al. No benefit of long-term ciprofloxacin treatment in patients with reactive arthritis and undifferentiated oligoarthritis: a three-month, multicenter, double-blind, randomized, placebo-controlled study. *Arthritis Rheum* 1999;**42**(7):1386–96.
136. Hoogkamp-Korstanje JA, Moesker H, Bruyn GA. Ciprofloxacin v placebo for treatment of Yersinia enterocolitica triggered reactive arthritis. *Ann Rheum Dis* 2000;**59**(11):914.
137. Wakefield D, McCluskey P, Verma M, Aziz K, Gatus B, Carr G. Ciprofloxacin treatment does not influence course or relapse rate of reactive arthritis and anterior uveitis. *Arthritis Rheum* 1999;**42**(9):1894–7.
138. Carter JD, Valeriano J, Vasey FB. Doxycycline versus doxycycline and rifampin in undifferentiated spondyloarthropathy with special reference to Chlamydia-induced arthritis. A prospective, randomized 9-month comparison. *J Rheumatol* 2004;**31**(10):1973–80.
139. Carter JD, Espinoza LR, Inman RD, Sneed KB, Ricca LR, Vasey FB, et al. Combination antibiotics as a treatment for chronic Chlamydia-induced reactive arthritis: a double-blind, placebo-controlled, prospective trial. *Arthritis Rheum* 2010;**62**(5):1298–307. http://dx.doi.org/10.1002/art.27394.
140. Yin W, Hasunuma T, Kobata T, Sumida T, Nishioka K. Synovial hyperplasia in HTLV-1 associated arthropathy is induced by tumor necrosis factor-alpha produced by HTLV-1 infected CD68+ cells. *J Rheumatol* 2000;**27**:874–81.
141. Palazzi C, D'Angelo S, Olivieri I. Hepatitis C virus-related arthritis. *Autoimmun Rev* 2008;**8**:48–51.
142. Mitchell LA, Tingle AJ, Shukin R, Sangeorzan JA, McCune J, Braun DK. Chronic rubella vaccine-associated arthropathy. *Arch Intern Med* 1993;**153**:2268.
143. Nissen MJ, Fontanges E, Allam Y, Zoulim F, Trépo C, Miossec P. Rheumatological manifestations of hepatitis C: incidence in a rheumatology and non-rheumatology setting and the effect of methotrexate and interferon. *Rheumatology* 2005;**44**:1016–20.
144. Vassilopoulos D, Calabrese LH. Risks of immunosuppressive therapies including biologic agents in patients with rheumatic diseases and co-existing chronic viral infections. *Curr Opin Rheumatol* 2007;**19**:619–25.
145. Ornstein MH, Sperber K. The anti-inflammatory and antiviral effects of hydroxychloroquine in two patients with acquired immunodeficiency syndrome and active inflammatory arthritis. *Arthritis Rheum* 1996;**39**:157–61.
146. Chiang G, Sassaroli M, Louie M, Chen H, Stecher VJ, Sperber K. Inhibition of HIV-1 replication by hydroxychloroquine: mechanism of action and comparison with zidovudine. *Clin Ther* 1996;**18**:1080–92.
147. Adebajo AO, Mijiyawa M. The role of sulfasalazine in African patients with HIV-associated seronegative arthritis. *Clin Exp Rheumatol* 1998;**16**:629.
148. Ferri C, Ferraccioli G, Ferrari D, Galeazzi M, Lapadula G, Montecucco C, et al. Safety of anti-tumor necrosis factor-alpha therapy in patients with rheumatoid arthritis and chronic hepatitis C virus infection. *J Rheumatol* 2008;**35**:1944–9.
149. Cepeda EJ, Williams FM, Ishimori ML, Weisman MH, Reveille JD. The use of anti-tumor necrosis factor therapy in HIV-positive individuals with rheumatic disease. *Ann Rheum Dis* 2008;**67**:710–12.
150. Filippi J, Roger PM, Schneider SM, Durant J, Breittmayer JP, Benzaken S, et al. Infliximab and human immunodeficiency virus infection: viral load reduction and CD4 + T-cell loss related to apoptosis. *Arch Intern Med* 2006;**166**:1783–4.
151. Smith JW, Chalupa P, Shabaz Hasan M. Infectious arthritis: clinical features, laboratory findings and treatment. *Clin Microbiol Infect* 2006;**12**(4):309–14, Review.

CHAPTER 50

Nonnutritional Environmental Factors Associated with Celiac Disease: The Infectome

Aaron Lerner[*,1], **Shimon Reif**[†]

[*]Pediatric Gastroenterology and Nutrition Unit, Carmel Medical Center, B. Rappaport School of Medicine, Technion-Israel Institute of Technology, Haifa, Israel
[†]Pediatric Department, Hadassah Medical Center, Hebrew University of Jerusalem, Jerusalem, Israel
[1]Corresponding Author: lerner_aaron@clalit.org.il

1 INTRODUCTION

1.1 Celiac Disease: Epidemiology

Celiac disease (CD) is a life-long autoimmune condition[1] largely affecting the small intestine of genetically susceptible individuals. Gluten, which is the storage protein of wheat, and its alcohol-soluble gliadins often induce the disease, together with structurally related molecules found in barley and rye. Nevertheless, additional environmental factors such as infections might play a role in CD induction.[2] Tissue transglutaminase (tTG) is the autoantigen against which the abnormal immune response is directed,[3] and two main autoantibodies, antiendomysium and anti-tTG, are the most useful serological markers when screening for the disease.[3,4] Recently, two additional autoantibodies, antideaminated gliadin peptide and antineoepitope tTG, were also found to be reliable for CD screening.[5] The HLA-DQ2 and HLA-DQ8 molecules are the most important predisposing genetic factors. Recently, substantial evidence was discovered regarding the pathogenesis of CD. Researchers have also unravelled the chain of events operating in the disease, providing hope for future therapeutic strategies.[6] Furthermore, the epidemiology, prevalence and clinical presentation of CD are changing constantly, and, over time, new clinical presentations have been reported, widening clinical variability of CD.[7]

As shown in the literature, the classic clinical presentation of CD in the intestine exists only in a minority of patients, and the extraintestinal presentation is becoming more common. Studies often describe skin, endocrine,

Infection and Autoimmunity
http://dx.doi.org/10.1016/B978-0-444-63269-2.00051-9

hepatic, skeletal, hematological, gynecological, infertility, dental, and behavioral abnormalities associated with CD.[8–10] Family practitioners, hematologists, gastroenterologists and now gynecologists and neurologists are increasingly diagnosing CD during the whole lifespan. In fact, about 20% of newly diagnosed cases occur in patients who are older than 60 years of age. Several of the growing domains are the extraintestinal presentations of CD affecting the bone, presenting as osteopenia or osteoporosis, and hypercoagulability.[11–13]

1.2 Celiac Disease: Pathophysiology

Researchers are constantly unravelling the pathogenesis of CD. In this section, we present a stepwise description of the chain of events operating in CD, but we only highlight steps during which pathogens may play a role. After ingestion, the body digests gluten into multiple segments. CD induction is closely related to one of the produced segments, a 33-amino-acid peptide, corresponding to amino acid 57-89, that is resistant to luminal digestion by gastric, pancreatic and intestinal brush border proteases, yet reactive to tTG. The repertoire of gluten peptides is wider, however, and it includes some native and non-tTG-deaminated gluten peptides capable of T cell immune stimulation.[2] Interestingly, those immune peptides are polypeptides rich with proline (15%) and glutamine (35%), which form the basis for two major steps in the celiac inflammatory cascade: 1) They confer resistance to enzymatic breakdown, because the human intestine lacks prolyl endopeptidase, which can readily cleave proline-rich immunostimulatory gluten peptides. (In contrast, part of the endogenous microbiota contains this enzyme.) 2) The glutamine-rich gluten peptides are an ideal substrate for tTG deamination. The deamination is crucial for the stability and avidity of the presented peptide in the HLA-DQ groove and the recognition of T cell epitopes. Thus, upon exposure to gluten peptides, the intestinal epithelium undergoes immediate cytoskeletal rearrangement, and functional barrier integrity is lost. Interestingly, pathogens are also known for their ability to increase intestinal permeability. So, a paracellular leak and an inappropriate immune response to gluten develops. In parallel, the local innate immune system activates, with IL-15 being a key factor. Gluten 31-49 peptide induces epithelial cell damage and intraepithelial lymphocyte recruitment, and IL-15 is produced, resulting in further epithelial injury, expansion of intraepithelial lymphocytes, cytotoxic IFNγ secretion and enhancement of the dendritic cells' capacity to present antigens.

The subepithelial compartment is rich in tTG. Due to its increased avidity to the glutamine-rich gluten peptides, deamination occurs, facilitating the high-affinity binding of the resultant negatively charged glutamic acid residues, which are in key positions on gliadin peptide T-cell epitopes, to HLA-DQ2/8 molecules. The presentation of antigen to CD4 T lymphocytes in the lamina propria then results in Th1 cell-type activation and subsequent release of IFNγ, proinflammatory cytokines (IFNγ, IL-2, TNFα, TGFβ, IL-6), as well as macrophage activation.[14] The activated humeral immunity is the origin of numerous specific and associated autoantibodies.[15]

Some of the pathogenic steps are well described in the literature,. As a result, the enzyme-resistant gluten peptides, the increased intestinal permeability and the activation of the Th1 branch of the immune system can be targeted for potential future therapeutic modality, using probiotics, the pathogen's products or protozoa.[6] Thus, unravelling disease pathogenesis has fostered research and development in several bacterial manipulations, protozoa inoculation or using bacterial products modalities to treat the disorder.

1.3 The Infectome is one Aspect of the Exposome

The exposome represents all exogenous and endogenous environmental exposures that begin at preconception and carry on throughout the entire lifespan.[16] Multiple genetic, epigenetic, nutrogenetic, or pathogen-related risk factors can induce or maintain an inflammatory state and expose the body to various stimuli that provoke further autoaggression. Their exposure and association to a phenotype may help researchers identify an inducer that leads to the breakdown of tolerance, eventually resulting in an autoimmune attack.

Recently, the concept of the infectome was introduced as a means of studying all infectious factors that contribute to the development of autoimmune diseases.[16] The infectome forms the infectious part of the exposome that leads to the loss of adaptive mechanisms in the body.

Multiple clinical and experimental models of autoimmune diseases clearly demonstrate that infectious agents disrupt immunological tolerance to self-antigens and induce autoimmune disease.[17] Examples include *Streptococcus pyogenes* and rheumatic fever, *Helicobacter pylori* and autoimmune gastritis, *Trypanosome cruzi* and Chagas cardiomyopathy and *Mycoplasma* and rheumatoid arthritis. Several classical autoimmune conditions, such as systemic lupus erythematosus (SLE), multiple sclerosis, primary biliary cirrhosis and others, were also found to be related to infections.[16] Likewise, CD has a long history with the infectome.[2,18,19]

Most recently, Fumagalli and colleagues showed that signatures of environmental genetic adaptation pinpoint pathogens as the main selective pressure through human evolution. Researchers also identified the diversity of the local environment as the predominant driver of local adaptation in some autoimmune diseases, including CD.[19] The past distinction between genetic and environmental influences in autoimmunity evolvement is somewhat artificial, given that some susceptibility alleles for autoimmune diseases may be selected by pathogens.

2 INFECTION ASSOCIATED WITH CD INDUCTION

Infections may play a role in several aspects of CD.[20] Table 1 summarizes those associations.

Most of the pathogens associated with the presence or induction of CD are controversial, and researchers have not yet shown a clear causal association. Table 2 summarizes those infectious agents, with references supporting or denying the association.

An exception to the infectome–CD association is the use of hookworm as a therapeutic strategy in treating CD. It is hypothesised that the parasite induces TH2 and IL-10 cross regulation of the TH1/TH17 inflammatory response, thus supressing mucosal inflammation in CD.[49] The surveys of past

Table 1 Associations Between Infections and Celiac disease

Associations Infectome\CD	Reference
Early infection and increased incidence of CD	21
Presentation as diarrhea or malabsorption	2
Antimicrobial serology incidence is increased in CD	22,23
Parallelism between pathogens and gluten peptides	24
Positive association between antibiotic use and subsequent CD	25
Diversity and composition of microbiota in CD	26–28
Increased intestinal permeability in infections and CD	2,6,29
Tissue transglutaminase antibodies positivity in confirmed viral infections	30
Interferon drives intestinal immunopathology in viral infecttions and CD	31
Seasonal variability in infections and CD	32
Specific infectious agent related to CD	See Table 2

Table 2 Pathogens Associated with Celiac Disease: Pros and Cons

Name of Pathogens	Positive References	Negative References
Saccharomyces cerevisiae, pseudomonas, bacteroides caccae	22	
Yeast (anti-glycans)	23	
Bacteroides species	27,28	
Enterovirus, EBV, CMV, HCV	30,18,33	34–36
Rotavirus	37,38	
Adenovirus	2,18	35,36
Campylobacter jejuni	39–41	
Pneumococcus	42	
Toxoplasma gondii	43	
Tuberculosis	44	
Hepatitis B virus	45	46
Helicobacter pylori		47,48

infections and CD are also controversial, however. One study associated neonatal infections with the risk of developing CD,[50] but this observation was not replicated in another study.[51] Another study asserted that repeated infectious episodes early in life increase the risk for later CD,[21] but no such association was found in the most recent study on this relationship.[52] Because lower economical status is related to increased infectious load, one can predict higher autoimmune conditions in this population. Yet, several studies suggest, that an inferior hygiene environment exerts a protective effect on CD.[53,54]

Authors have offered several explanations for the influence of pathogens on CD occurrence or induction: molecular mimicry, increased mucosal permeability, bystander activation or proinflammatory cytokine release. Most recently, a study suggested that the environmental factor retinoic acid might act as an adjuvant that promotes rather than prevents inflammatory cellular and humeral responses to fed antigen in the presence of IL-15.[55] Taken together, these findings reveal an unexpected role for retinoic acid and IL-15 in the abrogation of tolerance to dietary antigens, as is the situation in CD. The correct pathogenic pathway through which pathogens induce autoimmunity is far from being elucidated.

3 ROTAVIRUS AND CELIAC DISEASES

In 2006, Stene and colleagues provided the first indication that a high frequency of rotavirus infections may increase the risk of CD autoimmunity in genetically predisposed children.[37] In Iranian adults with positive celiac serology, the prevalence of active rotavirus was not significantly higher, however.[56] Using a random peptide library approach, an Italian team identified a peptide (celiac peptide) recognized by serum immunoglobulins of patients with CD.[57] This peptide shares homology with the rotavirus's major neutralizing protein, VP7, and with the CD autoantigen tTG. Surprisingly, antibodies directed against the celiac peptide, purified from the sera of patients with active disease, recognized VP7. Following their original observations, the same group also demonstrated that, in active CD, a subset of anti-tTG IgA antibodies recognize the viral protein VP7, suggesting a possible involvement of rotavirus infection in CD evolvement.[38] Moreso, rotavirus can induce the same mucosal injury that gluten induces in CD, and, as mentioned above, the rotavirus–CD relationship is supported by an epidemiology study.[37]

Encouraged by their previous findings, Dolcino and colleagues observed that the antibodies directed against VP7 predict the onset of CD and induce typical features of CD in the intestinal epithelial cell-line T84.[38] Trying to explore the pathogenic pathways involved using gene-array analysis, the same group showed that those antibodies modulate genes that are involved in apoptosis, inflammation and epithelial barrier integrity, all typical features of CD. Taking together, the new data produced by Dolcino and colleagues further support the involvement of rotavirus infection in CD pathogenesis, suggesting a predictive role for the antirotavirus VP7 antibodies.

An additional aspect of the interrelationship between rotavirus and CD relates to the effects of the former on human cellular immunity and gene expression. Comparing the patterns of gene expression in peripheral blood mononuclear cells from both healthy children and children affected by rotavirus diarrhea, the authors found that the group with rotavirus diarrhea had increased expression of genes involved in B cell differentiation, maturation, activation and survival, as well as a reduction in the proportion of CD4+ and CD8+ T cells in the periphery, suggesting that rotavirus alters B and T behavior and homeostasis.[58] Most recently, Pozo-Rubio and colleagues went a step further by documenting the influences of the rotavirus vaccine on the balance between T and B lymphocytes. They found that the B cell percentage was higher in vaccinated infants.[28] Given the worldwide introduction of the rotavirus vaccine during infancy, rotavirus infection's epidemiology is going to change dramatically, and future research must address the relationship between the rotavirus vaccine and CD.

REFERENCES

1. Lerner A, Blank M, Shoenfeld Y. Celiac disease and autoimmunity. *Isr J Med Sci* 1996;**32**:33–6.
2. Reif S, Lerner A. Celiac disease and infection. In: Shoenfeld Y, Rose N, editors. *Infections and Autoimmunity*. Amsterdam: Elsevier B.V.; 2004. p. 689–92.
3. Reif S, Lerner A. Tissue transglutaminase–the key player in celiac disease: a review. *Autoimm Rev* 2004;**3**:40–5.
4. Shamir R, Eliakim R, Lahat N, Sobel E, Lerner A. ELISA assay of anti endomysial antibodies in the diagnosis of celiac disease: comparison with immunofluorescence assay of anti endomysial antibodies and tissue transglutaminase antibodies. *Isr Med Assoc J* 2002;**4**:594–6.
5. Rozenberg O, Lerner A, Pacht A, Grinberg M, Reginashvili D, Henig C, et al. A novel algorithm for childhood celiac disease serological diagnosis based upon intestinal biopsies. *Crit Rev Allerg Immunol* 2010;**42**:331–41.
6. Lerner A. New Therapeutic Strategies for Celiac Disease. *Autoimmun Rev* 2010;**9**:144–7.
7. Lerner A. Factors affecting the clinical presentation and time diagnosis of celiac disease: the Jerusalem and the West Bank-Gaza experience (editorial). *Isr J Med Sci* 1994;**30**:294–5.
8. Branski D, Ashkenazy A, Frier S, Lerner A, et al. Extra intestinal manifestation and associated disorders of celiac disease. In: Branski D, Rozen P, Kaganoff MF, editors. *Gluten-Sensitive Enteropathy From Gastrointest Res*. Basel: Karger; 1992. p. 164–75.
9. Zelnik N, Pacht A, Obeid R, Lerner A. Range of neurological disorders in patients with celiac disease. *Pediatrics* 2004;**113**:1672–6.
10. Lerner A, Makhoul B. Neurological manifestations of celiac disease in children and adults. *Europ Neurolog J* 2012;**4**:15–20.
11. Hartman C, Hino B, Lerner A, Eshach-Adiv O, Berkovitz D, Shaoul R, et al. Bone quantitative ultrasound and bone mineral density in children with celiac disease. *J Pediatr Gastroenterol Nutr* 2004;**39**:504–10.
12. Lerner A, Shapira Y, Agmon-Levin N, Pacht A, Ben-Ami Shor D, López Hoyos M, et al. The clinical significance of 25OH-vitamin D status in celiac disease. *Crit Rev Allerg Immunol* 2012;**42**:322–30.
13. Lerner A, Agmon-Levin N, Shapira Y, Gilburd B, Reuter S, Lavi L, et al. The thrombophylic network of autoantibodies in celiac disease. *BMJ Medicine* 2013;**11**:89–95.
14. Lahat N, Shapiro S, Karban A, Gerstein R, Kinarty A, Lerner A. Cytokine profile in celiac disease. *Scand J Immunol* 1999;**49**:441–6.
15. Shaoul R, Lerner A. Associated authoantibodies in celiac disease. *Autoimmun Rev* 2007;**6**:559–65.
16. Bogdanos DP, Smyk DS, Invernizzi P, Rigopoulou RI, Blank M, Sakkas L, et al. Tracing environmental markers of autoimmunity: introducing the infectome. *Immunol Res* 2013;**56**:220–40.
17. Kivity S, Agmon-levin N, Blank M, Shoenfeld Y. Infections and autoimmunity-friends or foes? *Trends Immunol* 2009;**30**:409–14.
18. Plot L, Amital H. Infectious associations of celiac disease. *Autoimmun Rev* 2009;**8**:316–9.
19. Fumagalli M, Sironi M, Pozzoli U, Ferrer-Admetla A, Pattini L, Nielsen R. Signatures of environmental genetic adaptation pinpoint pathogens as the main selective pressure through human evolution. *PLoS Genet* 2011;**7**:e1002355.
20. Lerner A. Non nutritional environmental factors associated with celiac disease: infections and vaccinations. In: Shoenfeld Y, Agmon-levin N, editors. *vaccine and autoimmunity*. Wiley pub; 2013.
21. Myleus A, Hernell O, Gothefors L, Hammarström ML, Persson LA, Stenlund H, et al. Early infections are associated with increased risk for celiac disease: an incident case-referent study. *BMC Pediatr* 2012;**12**:194–201.

22. Ashorn S, Valineva T, Kaukinen K, Ashorn M, Braun J, Raukola H, et al. Serological responses to microbial antigens in celiac disease patients during a gluten-free diet. *J Clin Immunol* 2009;**29**:190–5.
23. Papp M, Foldi I, Altorjay I, Palyu E, Udvardy M, Tumpek J, et al. Anti-microbial antibodies in celiac disease: trick or treat. *World J Gastroenterol* 2009;**15**:3891–900.
24. Bethune MT, Khosla C. Parallels between pathogens and gluten peptides in celiac sprue. *PLoS Pathog* 2008;**4**:e34.
25. Marild K, Ye W, Lebwohl B, Green PH, Blaser MJ, Card T, et al. Antibiotic exposure and the development of coeliac disease: a nationwide case-control study. *BMC Gastroenterol* 2013;**13**:109–17.
26. Wacklin P, Kaukinen K, Tuovinen E, Collin P, Lindfors K, Partanen J, et al. The duodenal microbiota composition of adult celiac disease patients is associated with the clinical manifestation of the disease. *Inflamm Bowel Dis* 2013;**19**:934–41.
27. Sanchez E, De Palma G, Capilla A, Nova E, Pozo T, Castillejo G, et al. Influence of environmental and genetic factors linked to celiac disease risk on infant gut colonization by Bacteroides species. *Appl Environ Microbiol* 2011;**77**:5316–23.
28. Pozo-Rubio T, de Palma G, Mujico Jorge R, Olivares M, Marcos A, Acuna MD, et al. Influence of early environmental factors on lymphocyte subsets and gut microbiota in infants at risk of celiac disease; The PROFICEL study. *Nutr Hosp* 2013;**28**:464–73.
29. Heyman M, Abed J, Lebreton C, Cerf-Bensussan N. Intestinal permeability in coeliac disease: insight into mechanisms and relevance to pathogenesis. *Gut* 2012;**61**:1355–64.
30. Sarmiento L, Galvan Jose A, Cabrera-Rode E, Aira L, Correa C, Sariego S, et al. Type 1 diabetes associated and tissue transglutaminase autoantibodies in pateints without type 1 diabetes and celiac disease with confirmed viral infections. *J Med Virol* 2012;**84**:1049–53.
31. Montelone G, Pender SL, Wathen NC, MacDonald TT. Interferon alfa drive T cell mediated immunopathology in the intestine. *Eur J Immunol* 2001;**31**:2247–55.
32. Tanpowpong P, Obuch JC, Jiang H, McCarty CE, Katz AJ, Leffler DA, et al. Multicenter study on season of birth and celiac disease: evidence for a new theoretical model of pathogenesis. *J Pediatr* 2013;**162**:501–4.
33. Marconcini Maira L, Fayad L, Shiozawa M, Beatriz C, Schiavon Ld Lucca, Narciso-Schiavon JL. Autoantibody profile in individuals with chronic hepatitis C. *Revista da Sociedade Brasilrira de, Medicina* 2013;**46**:147–53.
34. Gravina Antonietta G, Federico A, Masarone M, Cuomo A, Tuccillo C, Loguercio C, et al. Coeliac disease and C virus-related chronic hepatitis: a non association. *BMC Res Notes* 2012;**5**:533–7.
35. Carlsson AK, Lindberg BA, Bredberg AC, Hyoty H, Ivarsson SA. Enterovirus infection during pregnancy is not a risk factor for celiac disease in the offspring. *J Pediatr Gastroenterol Nutr* 2002;**35**:649–52.
36. Lawler M, Humpheries PO, Farrelly C. Adenovirus 12 E1A gene detection by polymerase chain reaction in both normal and celiac duodenum. *Gut* 1994;**35**:1226–32.
37. Stene LC, Honeyman MC, Hoffenberg EJ, Haas JE, Sokol RJ, Emery L, et al. Rotavirus infection frequency and risk of celiac disease autoimmunity in early childhood:alongitudinal study. *Amer J Gastroenterol* 2006;**101**:2333–40.
38. Dolcino M, Zanoni G, Bason C, Tinazzi E, Boccola E, Valletta E, et al. A subset of anti-rotavirus antibodies directed against the viral protein VP7 predicts the onset of celiac disease and induces typical features of the disease in the intestinal epithelial cell line T84. *Immunol Res* 2013;**56**:465–76.
39. Sabayan B, Foroughinia F, Imanieh MH. Can Canpylobacter jejuni play a role in development of celiac disease? A hypothesis. *World J Gastroenterol* 2007;**13**:4784–5.
40. Riddle MS, Murray JA, Cash BD, Pimentel M, Porter CK. Pathogen-specific risk of celiac disease following bacterial causes of foodborne illness: a retrospective cohort study. *Dig Dis Sci* 2013;**58**:3242–5.

41. Verdu EF, Mauro M, Bourgeois J, Armstrong D. Clinical onset of celiac disease after an episode of Campylobacter jejuni enteritis. *Can J Gastroenterol* 2007;**21**:453–5.

42. Ludvigsson JF, Olen O, Bell M, Ekbom A, Montgomery SM. Coeliac disease and risk of sepsis. *Gut* 2008;**57**:1074–80.

43. Mohammad Rostami-Nejad, Kamran Rostami, Cheraghipour K, Nazemalhosseini Mojarad E, Volta U, Al Dulaimi D, et al. Celiac disease increases the risk of Toxoplasma gondii infection in a large cohot of pregnant women. *Amer J Gastroenterol* 2011;**106**:548–9.

44. Ludvigsson JF, Sanders DS, Maeurer M, Jonsson J, Grunewald J, Wahlström J. Risk of tuberculosis in a large sample of patients with celiac disease—a nationwide cohort study. *Aliment Pharmacol Ther* 2011;**33**:689–96.

45. Iglesias S, vazquer Rodrigues S, Ulla Rocha JL, Baltar Arias R, Díaz Saá W, Barrio Antoranz J, et al. Onset of celiac disease after acute hepatitis B infection. *Gastroenterol Hepatol* 2010;**33**:17–20.

46. Ouakaa-Kchaou A, Gargouri D, Kharrat J, Ghorbel A. Relationship between hepatitis B virus infection and celiac disease. *Hepat Mon* 2010;**10**:313–14.

47. Aydogdu S, Cakir M, Yuksekkaya HA, Tumgor G, Baran M, Arikan C, et al. Helicobacter pylori infection in children with celiac disease. *Scand J Gastroenterol* 2008;**43**:1088–93.

48. Rostami-Nejad M, Rostami K, Yamaoka Y, Mashayekhi R, Molaei M, Dabiri H, et al. Clinical and histological presentation of helicobacter pylori and gluten related gastroenteropathy. *Arch Iran Med* 2011;**14**:115–18.

49. McSorly HJ, Gaze S, Daveson J, Jones D, Anderson RP, Clouston A, et al. Suppression of inflammatory immune responses in celiac disease by experimental hookworm infection. *PLoS One* 2011;**6**:e24092.

50. Sandberg-bennich S, Dahlquist G. kallen B. Coeliac disease is associated with intrauterine growth and neonatal infections. *Acta Paediatr* 2002;**91**:30–3.

51. Marild K, Stephansson O, Montgomery S, Murray JA, Ludvigsson JF. Pregnancy outcome and risk of celiac disease in offspring; a nationwide case-control study. *Gastroenterology* 2011;**142**:39–45 e33.

52. Welander A, Tjernberg AR, Montgomery SM, Ludvigsson J, Ludvigsson JF. Infectious disease and risk of later celiac disease in childhood. *Pediatrics* 2010;**125**:e530–6.

53. Kondrashova A, Mustalahti K, Kaukinen K, Viskari H, Volodicheva V, Haapala AM, et al. Lower economic status and inferior environment may protect against celiac disease. *Ann Med* 2008;**40**:223–31.

54. Plot L, Amital H, Barzilai O, Ram M, Bizzaro N, Shoenfeld Y. Infections may have a protective role in the etiopathogenesis of celiac disease. *Ann NY Acad Sci* 2009;**1173**:670–4.

55. DePaolo RW, Abadie V, Tang F, Fehlner-Peach H, Hall JA, Wang W, et al. Co-adjuvant effects of retinoic acid and IL-15 induce inflammatory innunity to dietary antigens. *Nature* 2011;**471**(7337):220–4.

56. Rostami-Nejad M, Rostami K, Sanaei M, Mohebbi SR, Al-Dulaimi D, Nazemalhosseini-Mojarad E, et al. Rotavirus and celiac autoimmunity among adults with nonspecific gastrointestinal symptoms. *Saudi Med J* 2010;**31**:891–4.

57. Zanoni G, Navone R, Lunardi C, Tridente G, Bason C, Sivori S, et al. In celiac disease, a subset of autoantibodies against transglutaminase binds toll-like receptor 4 and induces activation of monocytes. *PLoS Med* 2006;**3**:e358.

58. Wang Y, Dennehy PH, Keyserling HI, Tang K, Gentsch JR, Glass RI, et al. Rotavirus infection alters peripheral T-cell homeostasis in children with acute diarrhea. *J Virol* 2007;**81**:3904–12.

CHAPTER 51

Infection and Autoimmune Liver Diseases

Daniel S. Smyk[*], Eirini I. Rigopoulou[†], Pietro Invernizzi[‡], Dimitrios P. Bogdanos[*,†,1]

[*]Division of Transplantation Immunology and Mucosal Biology, King's College London School of Medicine at King's College Hospital, London, UK
[†]Department of Rheumatology, School of Health Sciences, University of Thessaly, Larissa, Greece
[‡]Liver Unit and Center for Autoimmune Liver Diseases, Humanitas Clinical and Research Center, Rozanno, Milan, Italy
[1]Corresponding Author: dimitrios.bogdanos@kcl.ac.uk

1 PRIMARY BILIARY CIRRHOSIS

Primary biliary cirrhosis (PBC) is an autoimmune liver disease (AiLD) affecting the small and medium-sized intrahepatic bile ducts.[1-4] Periportal inflammation progresses to fibrosis then cirrhosis and eventual liver failure. The hallmark of PBC is the presence of antimitochondrial antibodies (AMA), which are directed against the E2 subunit of pyruvate dehydrogenase (PDC-E2).[5-7] In a minority of cases, AMA may also be directed against the branched-chain 2-oxoacid dehydrogenase complex (BCOADC) and/or the 2-oxoglutarate dehydrogenase complex (OGDC), and the E1α and E1β subunits of PDC have also been identified as subdominant autoantigenic targets.[5-7] These diseases are also characterized by PBC-specific responses against nuclear-body antigens, including sp100 and promyelocytic leukemia protein (PML), as well as gp210 and Nup62 nuclear-envelope antigens.

Numerous environmental, genetic and epigenetic factors have been implicated in the development of PBC (Figure 1), including infectious triggers[8] (Table 1). Some of those are distinct from the ones closely linked with the pathogenesis of autoimmune hepatitis (AIH) (Tables 2 and 3). This chapter discusses the numerous infectious triggers investigated in relation to PBC. These primarily include bacteria, but we also consider the role of viruses in the disease.

1.1 Escherichia coli

Due to the high incidence of recurrent urinary tract infections (rUTI) in PBC patients, *Escherichia coli* (*E. coli*), which is the most common cause of

Infection and Autoimmunity
http://dx.doi.org/10.1016/B978-0-444-63269-2.00075-1

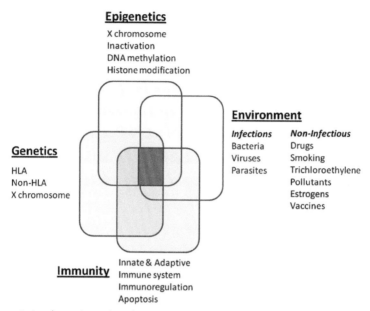

Epigenetics
X chromosome
Inactivation
DNA methylation
Histone modification

Environment

Infections   *Non-Infectious*
Bacteria   Drugs
Viruses   Smoking
Parasites   Trichloroethylene
                  Pollutants
                  Estrogens
                  Vaccines

Genetics
HLA
Non-HLA
X chromosome

Immunity   Innate & Adaptive
                Immune system
                Immunoregulation
                Apoptosis

Figure 1 A close interplay between genetic, epigenetic, environmental and immunological factors is closely associated with the development of primary biliary cirrhosis. The degree of participation of these factors varies between studies. For some of those factors (e.g., epigenetic), the data are limited.

rUTI, has likely been implicated in the pathogenesis of PBC more often than any other organism.[9,10] In recent years, several large epidemiological studies have noted a higher incidence of rUTI among PBC patients,[11,12] and new epidemiological data have demonstrated that episodes of rUTI precede the diagnosis of PBC.[13,14]

Researchers have suggested molecular mimicry and immunological cross reactivity involving *E. coli* and human PDC-E2 homologues as a possible mechanism, because several highly conserved sequences are shared between the microbial and the human antigens surrounding the core epitopic regions (Figure 2).[15,16] *E. coli* and human PDC-E2 cross-reactive antibodies do exist.[17] Additionally, motifs shared by human PDC-E2 and *E. coli* are targets of PBC-specific responses at the CD4 and CD8 T cell level,[18] which has also been suggested by experimental studies.[19,20] Immunological cross-reactive antibodies and cellular responses have also been found against the major human PDC-E2 autoepitopic region and several other *E. coli* sequences irrelevant to *E. coli* PDC-E2.[9,21,22] Among the 16 T cell clones specific for *E. coli* OGDC-E2, 13 responded to human OADC-E2 autoepitopes

Table 1 Major Features of Studies Investigating Pathogenic Links Between Bacterial Agents and Primary Biliary Cirrhosis (PBC). The Type of Study Varies and Includes Clinical Observations, Epidemiological Data and Virological or Immunological Analyses. The Table Also Presents Data on Experimental Models of the Disease. The Strength of Support Differs Between Studies (Reviewed in 8,62)

Infectious Agent	Nature of the Study	Major Findings (in Support or Against a Link)
Escherichia coli	Bioinformatics Clinical observation Epidemiological Immunological Experimental animal model	*E. coli* shares amino-acid similarity/motifs with the human autoepitope (in support), but this homology is not remarkable (against). Bacteriuria is more frequent in PBC than in controls (in support). Bacteriuria is equally prevalent in PBC patients and controls (in support). Bacteriuria is not present in the majority of the affected individuals (against). History of urinary tract infection is more frequently reported in patients than in controls (in support). History of infection precedes disease (in support). Women with rUTI have disease-specific AMA and PBC-related ANA (in support). There is evidence of B and T cell cross-reactive immunity (in support). The frequency of the anti–*E. coli* antibody to human PDC–E2 mimics is 100-fold lower compared to that against the human autoepitope (against). Infection induces AMA and causes PBC-like disease in experimental models (in support). There is a lack of evidence in support of the induction of PBC-like disease involving human mitochondrial autoantigen–mimics originated from *E. coli* (against).

Continued

Table 1 Major Features of Studies Investigating Pathogenic Links Between Bacterial Agents and Primary Biliary Cirrhosis (PBC). The Type of Study Varies and Includes Clinical Observations, Epidemiological Data and Virological or Immunological Analyses. The Table Also Presents Data on Experimental Models of the Disease. The Strength of Support Differs Between Studies (Reviewed in 8,62)—cont'd

Infectious Agent	Nature of the Study	Major Findings (in Support or Against a Link)
Novosphingobium aromaticivorans	Bioinformatics Immunological Microbiological Experimental animal model	The amino acid homology between this bacterium and the human autoepitope is the best so far reported (in support). Anti-microbial cross-reactive antibodies are often present in patients and relatives (in support). Patients with PBC often have positive fecal cultures (in support). Infection induces AMA and causes PBC-like disease (in support). The disease is transferable (in support).
Lactobacillus delbrueckii	Bioinformatics Immunological	Identities shared by microbial/self are many, and the homology is the best so far described between human PDC-E2 and a microbial mimic not related to OADC antigens (in support). There is evidence of cross-reactive antibodies (in support). A woman develops PBC after lactobacilli vaccination. Antibodies are also found in controls (in support). No evidence of T cell cross-reactivity or experimental animal model data supports an involvement (against).
Mycobacterium gordonae	Microbiological Immunological Bioinformatics Immunological	Microbiological evidence of the mycobacterium is not specific for PBC (against). The presence of cross-reactive antibodies has been obtained by independent investigators (in support). Researchers have confirmed amino acid homology between mycobacterial hsp65 and human PDC-E2 (in support). Antimycobacterial antibodies are specific for *M. gordonae* (against).
H. pylori	Immunological	

Agent	Type	Evidence
Betaretroviruses	Immunological	There is a lack of cross-reactive B and T cell responses (against).
	Virological	Anti-*Helicobacter* antibodies are similarly present in patients and controls (against). Prevalence is higher in patients than in controls in another study (in support).
	Virological	Antiviral antibodies are present in PBC patients (in support).
	Virological	MMTV has been cloned from PBC patients (in support). There is a lack of molecular evidence (against). The virus is less prevalent in PBC livers than in other liver diseases (against).
	Experimental animal model	Retroviral sequences have been identified in a murine model of PBC (in support).
	Clinical	There is inconclusive data regarding the efficacy of antiviral treatment (against). Date supporting a link are not reproducible (against).
Chlamydia pneumoniae	Immunological	There is an increased prevalence of antibodies in PBC patients compared to controls (in support), but data are not reproducible (against).
Toxoplasma gondii	Immunological	There is an increased prevalence of antibodies in patients compared to controls (in support), but results have been obtained in a single study (against).
Epstein–Barr virus	Virological	Increased EBV DNA levels have been found in patients compared to controls (in support).
	Immunological	The prevalence of EBV early antigen-specific antibodies is higher in PBC patients (in support). There is a lack of cross reactivity (against).
Pseudomonas aeruginosa	Immunological	There is evidence of T cell cross reactivity (in support).
Human cytomegalovirus	Immunological	There is a lack of cross-reactive antibodies (against).
Haemophilus influenzae	Immunological	There is a lack of cross-reactive antibodies (against).

Table 2 Infectious and Noninfectious Risk Factors for Autoimmune Hepatitis (AIH). Although No Epidemiological Studies have been Preformed, Several Small Studies have Identified Several Risk Factors Associated with AIH Development. This Table Summarizes some of the Risk Factors that have a Stronger Evidence Base

Risk Factor	Examples
Infectious agents	Hepatitis C virus, Hepatitis A virus, Epstein–Barr virus, Herpes simplex virus-1
Genetics (AIH type 1)	Female sex; HLA-DRB1*0301, DRB1*0401, DRB1*0405 (Japanese), DRB1*0404 (Chinese), DRB1*1301 (South American)
Genetics (AIH type 2)	Female sex; HLA-DRB1*03, DRB1*06, DRB1*07, DRB1*15, DQB1*0201
Non-HLA genes	CTLA4, TNFA*2, TNFRSF6, CD45, Fok (vitamin D receptor) polymorphisms
Ethnicity	Increased rates and more advanced presentation among people of African descent or South American patients; decreased rates among Caucasians and Japanese
Xenobiotics	Multiple medications and environmental toxins implicated; trichloroethylene has a stronger link than most
Other	Increased age correlated with more advanced presentation; associated with more complications in pregnancy and post-partum disease flares

Table 3 Major Risk Factors Identified in Primary Biliary Cirrhosis (PBC) and Autoimmune Hepatitis (AIH).[62] PBC is an Autoimmune Liver Disease for which Particular Risk Factors have been Consistently Identified in Large Epidemiological Studies. Although Large Epidemiological Studies are Lacking for AIH, Several Risk Factors have been Identified. This Table Compares some of the Risk Factors Identified in PBC in Relation to AIH

Factor	PBC	AIH
Viruses	Weak Associations: betaretroviruses, EBV	Strong association: HCV, weak Associations: HSV-1, EBV
Microbial	Strong Associations: *E. coli* (recurrent urinary tract infections) *N. aromaticivorans*	No associations
Female sex	Very strong associations	Strong associations
HLA associations	Weak associations	Very strong associations
Genomewide association studies	Multiple genes identified	Not performed
Smoking	Found to be an association	Unknown
Estrogenic immunomodulation	Association with estrogen deficiency; oral contraceptives appear to be protective	Disease flares postpartum
Family history	Higher rates of PBC and autoimmune disease among first-degree relatives of PBC patients	Not as strong as in PBC

Species	Protein	aa position																Similarity (%)	Identities	Double Reactivity
Cytomegalovirus	Capsid assembly protein UL47	V120$_{663-677}$	V	T	P	N	V	D	L	L	A	E	L	M	A	R	S	10/15 (67%)	5	2/55 (3.6%)
H. influenzae	tRNA (uracil-5-)-methyltranferase	TRMA$_{205-219}$	Q	N	S	E	G	D	L	L	E	L	Y	C	G	N	G	8/15 (53%)	6	3/55 (5.4%)
P. aeruginosa	Diaminopimelate decarboxylase	DCDA$_{335-349}$	A	L	A	E	G	D	L	L	A	V	R	S	A	G	A	9/15 (60%)	7	2/55 (3.6%)
H. pylori	Urease beta subunit	UREB$_{22-36}$	R	L	G	D	T	D	L	I	A	E	V	E	H	D	Y	13/15 (86.6%)	7	1/55 (1.8%)
Human	PDC-E2	PDC-E2$_{212-226}$	K	L	S	E	G	D	L	L	A	E	I	E	T	D	K			
E.coli	ATP-dependent clp X	CLPX$_{280-294}$	K	A	S	E	G	E	L	L	A	Q	V	E	P	E	D	14/15 (93%)	8	3/55 (5.4%)
E.coli	ATP-dependent helicase hrpA	HRPA$_{153-167}$	L	M	T	D	G	I	L	L	A	E	I	Q	Q	D	R	12/15 (80%)	7	15/55 (27.3%)
E.coli	Periplasmic maltose-binding protein	MALE$_{95-109}$	G	Y	A	Q	S	G	L	L	A	E	I	T	P	D	K	11/15 (73%)	7	16/55 (29.1%)
E.coli	Fatty acid oxidation complex alpha	FADP$_{605-619}$	D	A	V	E	D	L	L	A	E	V	S	Q	P	K		9/15 (60%)	6	11/55 (20%)
E.coli	(P)ppGpp synthetase II	SPOT$_{517-531}$	L	A	T	L	D	D	L	L	A	E	I	G	L	G	N	9/15 (60%)	6	10/55 (18.2%)
E.coli	Nitrate reductase 2	NARW$_{61-85}$	G	Q	A	M	V	D	L	L	A	E	Y	E	K	V	G	8/15 (53%)	6	6/55 (10.9%)

Figure 2 Amino acid sequence similarities between the major PBC-specific mitochondrial autoepitope and infectious mimics. The figure shows the amino acid sequence alignment between the E2 subunit of the human pyruvate dehydrogenase complex (PDC-E2)212–226 and its microbial mimics from *E. coli* or other pathogens. Amino acids are provided in standard single-letter code. Identities are in bold, and conservative substitutions are in italics. The last column indicates double reactivity to self and microbial peptides expressed in absolute numbers and percentages (%) in 55 patients with primary biliary cirrhosis.[21]

from PDC-E2, OGDC-E2 and BCOADC-E2[23]. Interestingly, of the several human PDC-E2-mimicking *E. coli* homologues identified so far, very few have been recognized as immunological targets in sera or peripheral blood mononuclear cells from patients with PBC. This finding indirectly points toward the immunobiological significance of those few mimics that are targeted by B and T cells.

Despite this indication, several studies have also provided evidence against the role of *E. coli* in the development of PBC, including data supporting a 100-fold lower antibody cross recognition of the *E. coli* PDC-E2 mimic compared to the human homologue, as well as those against *E. coli* BCOADC and OGDC in serum samples from patients with PBC. Also, there appears to be lack of reactivity against short, linear epitopic regions of human PDC-E2 and the corresponding sequences in *E. coli* PDC-E2 (reviewed in 8), a finding that supports the notion that molecular mimicry at the B cell level most likely involves larger peptidyl sequences instead of short peptides. This lack of reactivity may be due to structural differences, because a 3D model of the predicted structure of human and *E. coli* PDC-E2 has shown significant differences between the two, which may account for a possible lack of cross reactivity targeting short, linearized epitopes.[9] In fact, a series of studies have convincingly demonstrated that antibody responses against PDC-E2 are mainly conformational in nature. Nevertheless, the strength of the data supporting cross-reactive T cell responses further indicates that *E. coli* could be a potential trigger of PBC in susceptible individuals.

Recent evidence in support of a pathogenic link between *E. coli* and PBC comes from work conducted on *E. coli*-infected NOD.B6 *Idd10/Idd18* mice. This work shows that the infected mice develop antimitochondrial antibodies and more importantly autoimmune cholangitis resembling the human disease.[24] It remains to be seen whether the human PDC-E2 homologues originated from *E. coli* are pivotal for the induction of the pathological features seen in this experimental model, however.

1.2 Novosphingobium aromaticivorans

Novosphingobium aromaticivorans is another bacterium that has been investigated in relation to the pathogenesis of PBC, both in regard to prevalence and molecular-level presentation. The first report incriminating *N. aromaticivorans* as a potential pathogen responsible for PBC induction found that two proteins from *N. aromaticivorans* were homologous with human PDC-E2 and other OADC antigens, and that 100% of PBC patients who had AMA against PDC-E2 reacted against two of its bacterial domains.[25] Authors have also noted that reactivity against *N. aromaticivorans* was 10 times stronger than that of *E. coli*.[26] Among the AMA-negative patients with PBC, 12% showed reactivity against *N. aromaticivorans*. Several studies have also found the prevalence of *N. aromaticivorans* to be higher in PBC patients. A study of Icelandic PBC patients and their first-degree relatives found that 25% of both patient and relative groups had *N. aromaticivorans* in fecal samples and that individuals with antibodies against *N. aromaticivorans* also had PBC.[27] Selmi et al.[25] found that a quarter of PBC patients had detectable *N. aromaticivorans*, although this proportion was not significantly different from those of healthy controls and individuals living in the same households as PBC patients. That study also noted the ability of *N. aromaticivorans* to metabolize xenobiotics and estrogens, which is of interest because other studies have demonstrated the protective effects of estrogen against the development of PBC.[25]

Work on an animal model has demonstrated that the inoculation of mice with *N. aromaticivorans* induced the production of antibodies against PDC-E2, in addition to PBC-like liver histopathology.[28] Disease induction is achieved only in the presence of NKT cells responding to *N. aromaticivorans* cell wall alpha-glycuronosylceramides that are presented by CD1d molecules. This set of experiments underlines the importance of NKT induction by microbial species in the development of PBC.[28] The transfer of T cells from inoculated mice to noninfected mice appeared to reproduce the disease, although early treatment with antibiotics appeared to prevent autoantibody production and liver pathology.[28]

Of interest, *N. aromaticivorans*-infected mice appear to develop less severe disease than do *E. coli*-infected mice. Also, the titers of AMA are higher in the latter mice than in the former. Such data further underline the fact that the degree of pathogenic significance varies among infectious agents. Whether infection with a particular agent induces a specific disease course, such as slow versus rapid progression, remains undefined.

1.3 Lactobacillus delbrueckii

The current evidence suggesting *Lactobacillus delbrueckii* as a potential trigger of PBC comes from both immunological studies of cross reactivity between bacterial antigens and the major PDC-E2 epitope and from a case study of PBC following *L. delbrueckii* immunization. A study of PBC patients has shown that IgG antibody reactivity to the beta-galactosidase of *L. delbrueckii* subsp. *bulgaricus* (anti-$BGAL_{266-280}$) mimics the human PDC-E2 autoepitope.[29] IgG3 antibodies directed to $BGAL_{266-280}$ were almost exclusively present in the PBC patient cohort, being totally absent in the control cohorts. This study confirmed cross-reactive antibodies against the beta-galactosidase mimic and the major autoepitope of PDC-E2 ($PDC-E2_{212-226}$).[29] The evidence of several mimics from various infectious agents has led to the formulation of the hypothesis of a multiple-hit mechanism of molecular mimicry operating in PBC (Figure 3). In relation to *Lactobacillus*, the remaining

Step 1: A microbe and an infectious agent share antigenic mimicry

E. coli

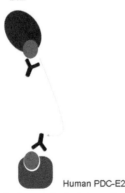

Human PDC-E2

Figure 3 A simplified overview of the multiple-hit molecular mimicry mechanism. The prerequisite for the initiation of cross-reactive responses is the identification of antigenic mimics involving a microbial epitopic region and a self-epitope (Step 1). The figure
Continued

Step 2: Several microbial epitopes share antigenic mimicry with an autoepitope
A multiple hit mechanism

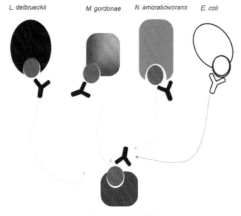

Human PDC-E2

Step 3: Other self-mimicking epitopes within the same microbe may exist

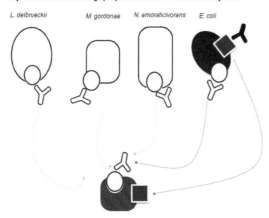

Human PDC-E2

Figure 3—cont'd   illustrates two mimics, one from *E. coli* and another from the human pyruvate dehydrogenase complex, which are the major target autoantigens in primary biliary cirrhosis. The antigenic mimicry initiates cross-reactive responses. In other words, urinary tract infection induces antibodies against a specific epitope from an *E. coli* antigen that mimics an autoepitopic region of PDC-E2. Such a homology leads to the initiation of antibodies cross-reacting with the microbial and self-epitopes. An alternative scenario (Step 2) postulates that various infectious agents share amino acid homologies with the same autoepitope. That scenario implies a multiple-hit mechanism of molecular mimicry. Another hypothesis suggests that one microbial antigen may contain more than one epitopic region shared with the respective autoepitopic sequences within an autoantigen (Step 3). Such mimicries have been identified and reported by studies investigating the role of molecular mimicry in autoimmune diseases such as primary biliary cirrhosis and autoimmune hepatitis.[8]

evidence consists of a case report in which a 39-year-old female developed PBC (with AMA positivity) following vaccination with *L. delbrueckii* for recurrent vaginitis.[30] Characterization of the AMA demonstrated a predominance of IgG3, which targeted PDC-E2$_{212-226}$, with reactivity to the *L. delbrueckii* subsp. *bulgaricus* self-mimicking BGAL$_{266-280}$ sequence.[30] Further evidence linking or refuting the role of *L. delbrueckii* in PBC are currently needed, because no experimental studies based on infected mice with this agent have been reported.

1.4 Mycobacteria

The histological feature of granulomas in PBC biopsy material has lead to speculation that typical and atypical mycobacteria, which are commonly associated with granulomatous lesions, may be involved in PBC pathogenesis.[3] Although AMA has been detected in patients with pulmonary tuberculosis and leprosy,[31,32] mycobacterial DNA has not been detected in liver samples from PBC patients.[33] Studies in Spain have demonstrated a high prevalence of antibodies against *Mycobacterium gordonae*, specifically against its 65 kDa-heat shock protein (hsp65).[34,35] Further studies have shown amino acid similarities between hsp65 and the major mitochondrial auto-epitope of PDC-E2.[36] However, subsequent studies in the UK could not find a link between mycobacteria and PBC.[36] The current evidence does not suggest a role for mycobacteria in the pathogenesis of PBC.[37]

1.5 Chlamydia pneumoniae

Few studies have proposed a pathogenic role for *Chlamydia pneumoniae* in the loss of immunological tolerance that leads to the development of PBC.[38,39] Those studies are based on the more frequent serological detection of antichlamydial antibodies in PBC patients than in pathological and healthy controls. Some authors have suggested that antichlamydial reactivity seen in patients with PBC is not biologically meaningful, and it is likely an epiphenomenon due to cross recognition of chlamydial OADC with human OADC antigens.[40] Also, *C. pneumoniae* DNA has not been detected in liver tissue from PBC patients.[38,39] Currently, the evidence suggesting a role for *C. pneumoniae* in the development of PBC is insufficient, and the limited existing data further underlines the weakness of the potential link.

1.6 *Helicobacter* species

Evidence suggesting a role for *Helicobacter* species (*H. pylori* and *H. hepaticus*) has come from the observation of the high prevalence of anti-*Helicobacter* antibodies in the serum and bile of PBC patients, as well as from animal models of PBC-like pathology following *Helicobacter* infection.[41–43] More recent studies have challenged data suggesting that anti-*H. pylori* antibodies are similarly present in patients with PBC and age-matched controls (51% vs. 46%),[44] showing that antibodies against *H. pylori* are more frequently present in patients with PBC than in controls (54% vs. 31%).[45]

Some authors have proposed molecular mimicry as a mechanism associating the microbe and the disease at the immunological level, because the *H. pylori* urease beta subunit sequence shares amino acid similarity with the human PDC-E2$_{212-226}$ autoepitope (Figure 2).[46] However, no reactivity to the *H. pylori* urease beta mimic has been observed at the B or the CD4 T cell levels, ruling out the possibility that *H. pylori* is involved in the loss of immunological tolerance seen in PBC.[47]

The data is also limited in regard to investigations on the 16S rRNA gene in livers from patients with PBC, suggesting *Propionibacterium acne* as an agent that could be involved in the formation of disease-specific granulomas in PBC. Antibodies against *Toxoplasma gondii* are present in 71% patients with PBC compared to 40% in healthy controls.[45] Interestingly, the reported difference in the seroprevalence of anti-*T. gondii* antibodies has not been noted in the past, because this parasite was never linked with the pathogenesis of PBC. Several other bacterial agents have been considered likely infectious triggers of PBC, but the data are limited and not replicable among studies.

1.7 Viral infections

One study has suggested that infection with a virus resembling mouse mammary tumor virus (MMTV) might be a pathogenic cause of PBC.[48] However, external groups have not reproduced these results, and currently, no universally accepted evidence suggests a viral etiology to PBC.[49,50] The betaretrovirus-PBC connection has been based on the results of an early study demonstrating the existence of antiretroviral antibodies in patients with PBC. This study provided data showing viral particles in biliary epithelial cells isolated from patients with PBC. The same investigators have cloned a human betaretroviral sequence highly homologous to MMTV. Also, retroviral sequences were isolated from experimental autoimmune cholangitis resembling the human disease.[51] Increased expression of MMTV gag and env was found in the liver tissue of the affected mice.[51] Among the experimental animals tested, only the NOD.c3c4 mice demonstrated aberrant expression of PDC-E2-like proteins in the bile ducts. Other strains expressed such protein in the splenic tissue but not in the liver.[51] In the same study, a significant correlation between the induction of PBC-specific AMA and anti-MMTV antibodies was noted in the sera of NOD and NOD. c3c4 mice with production.[51] Based on these results, the Canadian group has hypothesized that this betaretrovirus can infect biliary epithelial cells, leading to an increase of PDC-E2 expression on the cell surface. The virus may then incorporate PDC-E2 or exits along with PDC-E2 in exosomes.[52] The antigen presentation of PDC-E2 and viral proteins induces immune responses to the major mitochondrial autoantigen and the viral proteins expressed on the biliary epithelium.[52] Other studies have not replicated these data, however, raising concerns as to whether the reported link between the virus and the disease really exists.[49,50] Although MMTV is present in liver specimens obtained from PBC patients, this virus also occurs in livers from patients with various liver diseases, and, therefore, it lacks disease-specificity. In fact, one study has reported that the virus occurred more frequently in normal livers than it did in the livers of patients with PBC.[53] Thus, the treatment of PBC patients with a combination of antiviral agents should be questioned, especially because such treatments are not efficacious and evidence indicates resistance to treatment with biochemical rebound.[54]

2 AUTOIMMUNE HEPATITIS

Autoimmune hepatitis (AIH) is an AiLD characterized by the immune-mediated destruction of the hepatocytes. The disease is associated with elevated transaminases, the presence of disease-related autoantibodies, raised IgG, and histological evidence of interface hepatitis.[55] Autoantibody profiling is useful in dividing AIH into types 1 or 2.[55–57] ANAs and smooth muscle antibodies (SMAs) are characteristic of type 1 AIH, with anti-liver-kidney microsomal antigen type 1 (anti-LKM1) and anti-liver cytosol type 1 (anti-LC1) antibodies being found in type 2.[56,57] Several pathogens have been implicated in the development of AIH, most of which are viruses (Figure 4).[58] This section discusses the potential roles of the hepatitis C virus (HCV), the Epstein–Barr virus (EBV), and the herpes simplex virus 1 (HSV1) in relation to AIH.

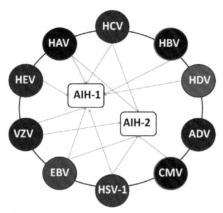

Figure 4 Viruses associated with autoimmune hepatitis 1 (AIH-1) and AIH-2. Some viral triggers are associated with either AIH-1 or AIH-2, and others are associated with both forms of AIH.[62] HAV, hepatitis A virus; HBV, hepatitis B virus; HCV, hepatitis C virus; HDV, hepatitis D virus; HEV, hepatitis E virus; ADV, adenovirus; CMV, cytomegalovirus; HSV-1, herpes simplex virus 1; EBV, Epstein–Barr virus; VZV, varicella zoster virus.

2.1 Hepatitis C virus

For many years, studies have explored the potential role of the hepatitis C virus (HCV) in the development of AIH, due to the presence of AIH-specific autoantibodies in patients chronically infected with HCV. Approximately 40% of patients with HCV infection are seropositive for ANA, SMA, and, to a lesser extent, anti-LKM1 antibodies (less than 10%). In addition, anti-HCV antibodies have been detected in patients with AIH but with no evidence of on-going HCV infection.

These observations have led to speculation regarding molecular mimicry between HCV components and AIH-specific autoantigens. Data obtained by independent studies demonstrated cross-reactive responses between HCV and cytochrome P450 2D6, the sole autoantigen of anti-LKM1 antibodies. Molecular mimicry and immunological cross reactivity operate at the B and T (CD4) cell levels,[59] and they are preferably seen in HCV–infected patients bearing an HLA-B51 genetic background.[60] Research has described amino acid similarities between AIH-related smooth muscle and nuclear autoantigens, and several of those are cross-recognized by anti-HCV antibodies targeting self-mimicking viral epitopes. Such cross reactivities may explain the presence of AIH-specific ANA and SMA during viral infection.[60] The current evidence linking HCV with AIH is not as strong as that described for the connection between other viruses and autoimmune diseases. Nevertheless, HCV infection has been associated with various autoimmune phenomena seen in patients with AIH.[61] As a final note, the high prevalence of HCV infection is disproportionate to the low prevalence of AIH, which further negates a link between the two conditions.

2.2 Hepatitis A and B

Several case reports describe the development of AIH following hepatitis A virus (HAV) infection.[62] When histopathologically assessed, liver specimens from individuals with acute HAV infection have features indistinguishable from those seen in AIH. Seropositivity for AIH-related autoantibodies such as ANA, SMA and anti-asialoglycoprotein receptor (anti-ASGPR) antibodies have been noted in patients infected with HAV and hepatitis B virus (HBV).[62] As such, it may be the case that HAV/HBV infection may trigger a humoral immune response to liver antigens, leading to the subsequent induction of the liver disease. One study prospectively followed relatives of AIH patients with regular serum sampling for AIH markers, and it found that, in three of these cases, the relative developed AIH type 1 (with anti-ASGPR positivity) following infection with HAV.[63] Two of these three individuals also had suppressor-inducer T cell defects.[63] In addition, a study in Brazil has shown that the protracted form of HAV is closely associated with the possession of HLA DRB1*1301, an allele that also confers susceptibility to pediatric AIH-1 characterized by anti-F-actin-specific SMA.[64] Currently, there is insufficient molecular, immunological and epidemiological data to link HAV or HBV with AIH. Despite the reported link, the body of data is relatively small, and the connection between HAV or HBV and AIH is arguably weaker than that related to HCV.

2.3 Epstein–Barr virus

A study has reported the development of AIH in first-degree relatives of AIH patients following infection with Epstein–Barr virus (EBV).[65] Similar case reports of AIH following EBV infection have also been reported in the literature.[62] Much like the hepadnaviridae, acute EBV infection of the liver may histologically resemble AIH.[62] To date, no large studies have investigated the role of EBV in the development of AIH, including studies of molecular mimicry and cross reactivity.[60]

2.4 Herpes simplex virus 1

One study has noted that the immunodominant regions of CYP2D6 share homologous regions with herpes simplex virus 1 (HSV-1) and HCV, and this observation has led to speculation that AIH type 2 cases may be related to HSV-1.[60] The ICP4 protein of HSV-1 shares antigenic determinants with the HCV RNA polymerase. Thus, mimicking sequences are targeted by cross-reactive responses supporting a multi-hit mechanism of molecular mimicry through which HSV, HCV and probably EBV contribute to the development of anti-LKM1 antibodies in patients with AIH-2.[60] Despite this assertion, the prevalence of anti-HSV-1 antibodies in AIH patients is similar to that in healthy controls.

REFERENCES

1. Hohenester S, Oude-Elferink RP, Beuers U. Primary biliary cirrhosis. *Semin Immunopathol* 2009;**31**(3):283–307 [Review].
2. Invernizzi P, Selmi C, Gershwin ME. Update on primary biliary cirrhosis. *Dig Liver Dis* 2010;**42**(6):401–8 [Research Support, N.I.H., Extramural Review].
3. Kaplan MM, Gershwin ME. Primary biliary cirrhosis. *N Engl J Med* 2005;**353** (12):1261–73[Review].
4. Poupon R. Primary biliary cirrhosis: a 2010 update. *J Hepatol* 2010;**52**(5):745–58 [Review].
5. Bogdanos DP, Komorowski L. Disease-specific autoantibodies in primary biliary cirrhosis. *Clin Chim Acta* 2011;**412**(7–8):502–12[Review].
6. Bogdanos DP, Invernizzi P, Mackay IR, Vergani D. Autoimmune liver serology: current diagnostic and clinical challenges. *World J Gastroenterol* 2008;**14**(21):3374–87 [Review].
7. Bogdanos DP, Baum H, Vergani D. Antimitochondrial and other autoantibodies. *Clin Liver Dis* 2003;**7**(4):759–77[Review] vi.
8. Smyk DS, Rigopoulou EI, Bogdanos DP. Potential roles for infectious agents in the pathophysiology of primary biliary cirrhosis: what's new? *Curr Infect Dis Rep* 2013;**15** (1):14–24.
9. Bogdanos DP, Baum H, Vergani D, Burroughs AK. The role of E. coli infection in the pathogenesis of primary biliary cirrhosis. *Dis Markers* 2010;**29**(6):301–11[Review].
10. Burroughs AK, Rosenstein IJ, Epstein O, Hamilton-Miller JM, Brumfitt W, Sherlock S. Bacteriuria and primary biliary cirrhosis. *Gut* 1984;**25**(2):133–7[Research Support, Non-U.S. Gov't].
11. Gershwin ME, Selmi C, Worman HJ, Gold EB, Watnik M, Utts J, et al. Risk factors and comorbidities in primary biliary cirrhosis: a controlled interview-based study of 1032 patients. *Hepatology* 2005;**42**(5):1194–202[Research Support, N.I.H., Extramural Research Support, U.S. Gov't, P.H.S.].
12. Parikh-Patel A, Gold EB, Worman H, Krivy KE, Gershwin ME. Risk factors for primary biliary cirrhosis in a cohort of patients from the united states. *Hepatology* 2001;**33** (1):16–21[Research Support, U.S. Gov't, P.H.S.].
13. Varyani FK, West J, Card TR. Primary biliary cirrhosis does not increase the risk of UTIs following diagnosis compared to other chronic liver diseases? *Liver Int* 2013;**33**(3):384–8 [Comparative Study Research Support, Non-U.S. Gov't].
14. Varyani FK, West J, Card TR. An increased risk of urinary tract infection precedes development of primary biliary cirrhosis. *BMC Gastroenterol* 2011;**11**:95[Research Support, Non-U.S. Gov't].
15. Bogdanos DP, Choudhuri K, Vergani D. Molecular mimicry and autoimmune liver disease: virtuous intentions, malign consequences. *Liver* 2001;**21**(4):225–32[Review].

16. Burroughs AK, Butler P, Sternberg MJ, Baum H. Molecular mimicry in liver disease. *Nature* 1992;**358**(6385):377–8[Comparative Study Letter].

17. Butler P, Valle F, Hamilton-Miller JM, Brumfitt W, Baum H, Burroughs AK. M2 mitochondrial antibodies and urinary rough mutant bacteria in patients with primary biliary cirrhosis and in patients with recurrent bacteriuria. *J Hepatol* 1993;**17**(3):408–14.

18. Van de Water J, Ishibashi H, Coppel RL, Gershwin ME. Molecular mimicry and primary biliary cirrhosis: premises not promises. *Hepatology* 2001;**33**(4):771–5[Review].

19. Shimoda S, Nakamura M, Shigematsu H, Tanimoto H, Gushima T, Gershwin ME, et al. Mimicry peptides of human PDC-E2 163-176 peptide, the immunodominant T-cell epitope of primary biliary cirrhosis. *Hepatology* 2000;**31**(6):1212–16[Research Support, Non-U.S. Gov't Research Support, U.S. Gov't, P.H.S.].

20. Shimoda S, Van de Water J, Ansari A, Nakamura M, Ishibashi H, Coppel RL, et al. Identification and precursor frequency analysis of a common T cell epitope motif in mitochondrial autoantigens in primary biliary cirrhosis. *J Clin Invest* 1998;**102**(10):1831–40 [Research Support, U.S. Gov't, P.H.S.].

21. Bogdanos DP, Baum H, Grasso A, Okamoto M, Butler P, Ma Y, et al. Microbial mimics are major targets of crossreactivity with human pyruvate dehydrogenase in primary biliary cirrhosis. *J Hepatol* 2004;**40**(1):31–9[Research Support, Non-U.S. Gov't].

22. Bogdanos DP, Baum H, Butler P, Rigopoulou EI, Davies ET, Ma Y, et al. Association between the primary biliary cirrhosis specific anti-sp100 antibodies and recurrent urinary tract infection. *Dig Liver Dis* 2003;**35**(11):801–5[Research Support, Non-U.S. Gov't].

23. Tanimoto H, Shimoda S, Nakamura M, Ishibashi H, Kawano A, Kamihira T, et al. Promiscuous T cells selected by Escherichia coli: OGDC-E2 in primary biliary cirrhosis. *J Autoimmun* 2003;**20**(3):255–63[In Vitro Research Support, U.S. Gov't, P.H.S.].

24. Wang JJ, Yang GX, Lu L, Tsuneyama K, Kronenberg M, Véla JL, Lopez-Hoyos M, He XS, Ridgway WM, Leung PS, Gershwin ME. Escherichia coli infection induces autoimmune cholangitis and anti-mitochondrial antibodies in non-obese diabetic (NOD).B6 (Idd10/IDD18) mice. *Clin Exp Immunol* 2014;**175**(2):192–201. http://dx.doi.org/10.1111/cei.12224.

25. Selmi C, Balkwill DL, Invernizzi P, Ansari AA, Coppel RL, Podda M, et al. Patients with primary biliary cirrhosis react against a ubiquitous xenobiotic-metabolizing bacterium. *Hepatology* 2003;**38**(5):1250–7[Research Support, U.S. Gov't, P.H.S.].

26. Padgett KA, Selmi C, Kenny TP, Leung PS, Balkwill DL, Ansari AA, et al. Phylogenetic and immunological definition of four lipoylated proteins from Novosphingobium aromaticivorans, implications for primary biliary cirrhosis. *J Autoimmun* 2005;**24**(3):209–19.

27. Olafsson S, Gudjonsson H, Selmi C, Amano K, Invernizzi P, Podda M, et al. Antimitochondrial antibodies and reactivity to N. aromaticivorans proteins in Icelandic patients with primary biliary cirrhosis and their relatives. *Am J Gastroenterol* 2004;**99**(11):2143–6.

28. Mattner J, Savage PB, Leung P, Oertelt SS, Wang V, Trivedi O, et al. Liver autoimmunity triggered by microbial activation of natural killer T cells. *Cell Host Microbe* 2008;**3**(5):304–15[Research Support, N.I.H., Extramural Research Support, Non-U.S. Gov't].

29. Bogdanos DP, Baum H, Okamoto M, Montalto P, Sharma UC, Rigopoulou EI, et al. Primary biliary cirrhosis is characterized by IgG3 antibodies cross-reactive with the major mitochondrial autoepitope and its Lactobacillus mimic. *Hepatology* 2005;**42**(2):458–65 [Research Support, Non-U.S. Gov't].

30. Bogdanos D, Pusl T, Rust C, Vergani D, Beuers U. Primary biliary cirrhosis following Lactobacillus vaccination for recurrent vaginitis. *J Hepatol* 2008;**49**(3):466–73[Case Reports].

31. Gilburd B, Ziporen L, Zharhary D, Blank M, Zurgil N, Scheinberg MA, et al. Antimitochondrial (pyruvate dehydrogenase) antibodies in leprosy. *J Clin Immunol* 1994;**14**(1):14–19[Research Support, Non-U.S. Gov't].

32. Klein R, Wiebel M, Engelhart S, Berg PA. Sera from patients with tuberculosis recognize the M2a-epitope (E2-subunit of pyruvate dehydrogenase) specific for primary biliary cirrhosis. *Clin Exp Immunol* 1993;**92**(2):308–16[Research Support, Non-U.S. Gov't].

33. O'Donohue J, McFarlane B, Bomford A, Yates M, Williams R. Antibodies to atypical mycobacteria in primary biliary cirrhosis. *J Hepatol* 1994;**21**(5):887–9.

34. Vilagut L, Pares A, Vinas O, Vila J, Jimenez de Anta MT, Rodes J. Antibodies to mycobacterial 65-kD heat shock protein cross-react with the main mitochondrial antigens in patients with primary biliary cirrhosis. *Eur J Clin Invest* 1997;**27**(8):667–72[Research Support, Non-U.S. Gov't].

35. Vilagut L, Vila J, Vinas O, Pares A, Gines A, Jimenez de Anta MT, et al. Cross-reactivity of anti-Mycobacterium gordonae antibodies with the major mitochondrial autoantigens in primary biliary cirrhosis. *J Hepatol* 1994;**21**(4):673–7[Comparative Study Research Support, Non-U.S. Gov't].

36. Bogdanos DP, Pares A, Baum H, Caballeria L, Rigopoulou EI, Ma Y, et al. Disease-specific cross-reactivity between mimicking peptides of heat shock protein of Mycobacterium gordonae and dominant epitope of E2 subunit of pyruvate dehydrogenase is common in Spanish but not British patients with primary biliary cirrhosis. *J Autoimmun* 2004;**22**(4):353–62[Comparative Study Research Support, Non-U.S. Gov't].

37. Smyk DS, Bogdanos DP, Pares A, Liaskos C, Billinis C, Burroughs AK, et al. Tuberculosis is not a risk factor for primary biliary cirrhosis: a review of the literature. *Tuberc Res Treat* 2012;**2012**:218183.

38. Abdulkarim AS, Petrovic LM, Kim WR, Angulo P, Lloyd RV, Lindor KD. Primary biliary cirrhosis: an infectious disease caused by Chlamydia pneumoniae? *J Hepatol* 2004;**40**(3):380–4.

39. Leung PS, Park O, Matsumura S, Ansari AA, Coppel RL, Gershwin ME. Is there a relation between Chlamydia infection and primary biliary cirrhosis? *Clin Dev Immunol* 2003;**10**(2–4):227–33[Research Support, U.S. Gov't, P.H.S.].

40. Taylor-Robinson D, Sharif AW, Dhanjal NS, Taylor-Robinson SD. Chlamydia pneumoniae infection is an unlikely cause of primary biliary cirrhosis. *J Hepatol* 2005;**42**(5):779–80[Comment Letter].

41. Nilsson HO, Castedal M, Olsson R, Wadstrom T. Detection of Helicobacter in the liver of patients with chronic cholestatic liver diseases. *J Physiol Pharmacol* 1999;**50**(5):875–82 [Comparative Study Research Support, Non-U.S. Gov't].

42. Nilsson HO, Taneera J, Castedal M, Glatz E, Olsson R, Wadstrom T. Identification of Helicobacter pylori and other Helicobacter species by PCR, hybridization, and partial DNA sequencing in human liver samples from patients with primary sclerosing cholangitis or primary biliary cirrhosis. *J Clin Microbiol* 2000;**38**(3):1072–6 [Research Support, Non-US Gov't].

43. Nilsson I, Lindgren S, Eriksson S, Wadstrom T. Serum antibodies to Helicobacter hepaticus and Helicobacter pylori in patients with chronic liver disease. *Gut* 2000;**46**(3):410–14[Research Support, Non-U.S. Gov't].

44. Durazzo M, Rosina F, Premoli A, Morello E, Fagoonee S, Innarella R, et al. Lack of association between seroprevalence of Helicobacter pylori infection and primary biliary cirrhosis. *World J Gastroenterol* 2004;**10**(21):3179–81.

45. Shapira Y, Agmon-Levin N, Renaudineau Y, Porat-Katz BS, Barzilai O, Ram M, et al. Serum markers of infections in patients with primary biliary cirrhosis: evidence of infection burden. *Exp Mol Pathol* 2012;**93**(3):386–90.

46. Bogdanos DP, Pares A, Rodes J, Vergani D. Primary biliary cirrhosis specific antinuclear antibodies in patients from Spain. *Am J Gastroenterol* 2004;**99**(4):763–4 [Comment Letter] author reply 5.

47. Boomkens SY, de Rave S, Pot RG, Egberink HF, Penning LC, Rothuizen J, et al. The role of Helicobacter spp. in the pathogenesis of primary biliary cirrhosis and primary sclerosing cholangitis. *FEMS Immunol Med Microbiol* 2005;**44**(2):221–5[Comparative Study].

48. Mason A, Xu L, Shen Z, Fodera B, Joplin R, Neuberger J, et al. Patients with primary biliary cirrhosis make anti-viral and anti-mitochondrial antibodies to mouse mammary tumor virus. *Gastroenterology* 2004;**127**(6):1863–4[Comment Letter] author reply 4-5.
49. Selmi C. The evidence does not support a viral etiology for primary biliary cirrhosis. *J Hepatol* 2011;**54**(6):1315–16.
50. Selmi C, Ross SR, Ansari AA, Invernizzi P, Podda M, Coppel RL, et al. Lack of immunological or molecular evidence for a role of mouse mammary tumor retrovirus in primary biliary cirrhosis. *Gastroenterology* 2004;**127**(2):493–501.
51. Zhang G, Chen M, Graham D, Subsin B, McDougall C, Gilady S, et al. Mouse mammary tumor virus in anti-mitochondrial antibody producing mouse models. *J Hepatol* 2011;**55**(4):876–84[Research Support, Non-U.S. Gov't].
52. Wasilenko ST, Mason GE, Mason AL. Primary biliary cirrhosis, bacteria and molecular mimicry: what's the molecule and where's the mimic? *Liver Int* 2009;**29**(6):779–82 [Comment Editorial].
53. Johal H, Scott GM, Jones R, Camaris C, Riordan S, Rawlinson WD. Mouse mammary tumour virus-like virus (MMTV-LV) is present within the liver in a wide range of hepatic disorders and unrelated to nuclear p53 expression or hepatocarcinogenesis. *J Hepatol* 2009;**50**(3):548–54.
54. Mason AL, Lindor KD, Bacon BR, Vincent C, Neuberger JM, Wasilenko ST. Clinical Trial: Randomized controlled trial of zidovudine and lamivudine for patients with primary biliary cirrhosis stabilized on ursodiol. *Aliment Pharmacol Ther* 2008;**28**:886–94.
55. Floreani A, Liberal R, Vergani D, Mieli-Vergani G. Autoimmune hepatitis: contrasts and comparisons in children and adults—a comprehensive review. *J Autoimmun* 2013;**46**:7–16.
56. Bogdanos DP, Mieli-Vergani G, Vergani D. Autoantibodies and their antigens in autoimmune hepatitis. *Semin Liver Dis* 2009;**29**(3):241–53[Review].
57. Liberal R, Mieli-Vergani G, Vergani D. Clinical significance of autoantibodies in autoimmune hepatitis. *J Autoimmun* 2013;**46**:17–24.
58. Vento S, Cainelli F. Is there a role for viruses in triggering autoimmune hepatitis? *Autoimmun Rev* 2004;**3**(1):61–9.
59. Kammer AR, van der Burg SH, Grabscheid B, Hunziker IP, Kwappenberg KM, Reichen J, et al. Molecular mimicry of human cytochrome P450 by hepatitis C virus at the level of cytotoxic T cell recognition. *J Exp Med* 1999;**190**(2):169–76[Comparative Study Research Support, Non-U.S. Gov't].
60. Bogdanos DP, Lenzi M, Okamoto M, Rigopoulou EI, Muratori P, Ma Y, et al. Multiple viral/self immunological cross-reactivity in liver kidney microsomal antibody positive hepatitis C virus infected patients is associated with the possession of HLA B51. *Int J Immunopathol Pharmacol* 2004;**17**(1):83–92.
61. Ferrari SM, Fallahi P, Mancusi C, Colaci M, Manfredi A, Ferri C, et al. HCV-related autoimmune disorders in HCV chronic infection. *Clin Ter* 2013;**164**(4):e305–12.
62. Smyk DS, Bogdanos DP, Rigopoulou EI. Risk factors for autoimmune hepatitis: from genes and pregnancy to vaccinations and pollutants. *Immuno Gastroenterol* 2013;**2**:29–37.
63. Vento S, Garofano T, Di Perri G, Dolci L, Concia E, Bassetti D. Identification of hepatitis A virus as a trigger for autoimmune chronic hepatitis type 1 in susceptible individuals. *Lancet* 1991;**337**(8751):1183–7.
64. Fainboim L, Canero Velasco MC, Marcos CY, Ciocca M, Roy A, Theiler G, et al. Protracted, but not acute, hepatitis A virus infection is strongly associated with HLA-DRB*1301, a marker for pediatric autoimmune hepatitis. *Hepatology* 2001;**33**(6):1512–17.
65. Vento S, Guella L, Mirandola F, Cainelli F, Di Perri G, Solbiati M, et al. Epstein–Barr virus as a trigger for autoimmune hepatitis in susceptible individuals. *Lancet* 1995;**346** (8975):608–9[Case Reports].

CHAPTER 52

Acute and Chronic Infections: Their Role in Immune Thrombocytopenia

Zahava Vadasz[1], Elias Toubi
Division of Allergy and Clinical Immunology, Bnai-Zion Medical Center, Faculty of Medicine, Technion, Haifa, Israel
[1]Corresponding Author: Zahava.vadas@b-zion.org.il

1 INTRODUCTION

Immune thrombocytopenic purpura (ITP) is defined as one of the classical autoimmune disorders, mainly characterized by thrombocytopenia (platelet count $<100 \times 10^3$ mL), platelet destruction by the spleen and morphologic abnormalities of megakaryocytes, including their altered maturation. ITP was proven to be the result of specific antiplatelet autoantibodies, a diagnosis strengthened by the autoimmune origin of this disease.[1,2] When ITP occurs as the only clinical symptom, lacking any evidence of systemic disease(s), it is classified as primary ITP; this is the diagnosis in 80% of all cases. Secondary ITP is only considered when infectious, malignant or other autoimmune diseases are responsible for the underlying condition.[3] Furthermore, it is well accepted to classify ITP into the following three phases: (1) the new-onset phase, which lasts 3 months from diagnosis; (2) persistent ITP, which lasts between 3 and 12 months from diagnosis; and (3) chronic ITP, which lasts more than 12 months from diagnosis.[4] Cellular immunity, namely CD4 effector T cells, is considered to be the main conductor in the development of ITP. Early studies showed that when platelets isolated from patients with ITP were incubated with autologous lymphocytes, increased interleukin (IL)-2 production occurred. These responsive lymphocytes were proved to be CD4 T cells and were demonstrated to specifically react against modified glycoprotein (GP) IIb/IIIa on activated platelets.[5] Aiming to better understand this process, GPIIb/GPIIIa-reactive T-cell lines generated from

Infection and Autoimmunity
http://dx.doi.org/10.1016/B978-0-444-63269-2.00056-8

patients with ITP were cultured with autologous freshly isolated splenic macrophages, B cells or dendritic cells. Macrophages induced the proliferation of GPIIb/IIIa-reactive T-cell lines without being exposed to exogenous antigens; however, both B cells and dendritic cells required glycoprotein peptides to stimulate T cells. Cultured macrophages that captured opsonized platelets promoted anti-GPIIb/IIIa antibody production in mixed cultures of autologous GPIIb/IIIa-reactive T-cell lines and B cells.[6] In the thymus, T cells lose either CD4 or CD8 antigens and thus are released as either CD4+ effector or CD8+ cytotoxic T lymphocytes. Some self-reactive T cells survive thymic depletion and persist in peripheral blood, becoming autoreactive and mediating autoimmunity. Normally, autoreactive T cells are controlled by many peripheral self-tolerance mechanisms, such as altered costimulatory molecules or failure of T regulatory cell (Treg) function. When self-tolerance fails, CD4+ T effector cells react with specific antigens presented by major histocompatibility complex class II molecules in association with the proper expression of costimulatory molecules. When T cells of patients with ITP were stimulated by platelet antigens, the production of both Th1- and Th2-related cytokines was increased. Th1 cells produce IL-2, IFNs and tumor necrosis factor, whereas Th2 cells produce IL-4, IL-13, and IL-10, all of which play a role in directing cell-mediated immune responses and in reacting to different pathogens involved in the pathogenesis of ITP. The role of Th17 (recently known to play a role in the process of autoimmunity) in the pathogenesis of chronic ITP also was evaluated. Higher levels of IL-17A and Th17-related cytokines, and obviously IL-17-producing CD4-T cells, were observed in patients with ITP.[7–9] In addition, CD4+ effector T cells are intensively recruited into the bone marrow and lymph nodes of patients with ITP. In this respect, T-cell surface expression of chemokine receptors such as CXCRI and CXCR4 was significantly increased in patients with ITP compared to healthy individuals. Also, the number of CD3 T cells in bone marrow but not in peripheral blood, together with increased Fas expression in these cells, was documented, thus emphasizing the importance of cellular immunity in ITP.[10]

As mentioned above, T-cell-mediated immune response is central in the pathogenesis of ITP, but the role of humoral immunity, mainly autoimmunity, seems to be no less important. Using antigen-specific assays such as immunoprecipitation, immunoblotting and antigen capture techniques, specific autoantibodies against multiple glycoproteins on activated platelets were found to have a crucial pathogenic role in the development of ITP. Of these autoantibodies, anti-GPIIb/GPIIIa and/or GPIb/GPIX were identified most often.[11] The positive finding of these autoantibodies is considered a diagnostic hallmark of ITP, with a sensitivity of 49–60% and a specificity of 78–93%; however, negative results do not rule out this diagnosis.[12] The most likely explanation for not finding these autoantibodies is that other mechanisms are involved in the pathophysiology of ITP, such as T-cell-dependent activation and the destruction of platelets following the exposure to many cross-reactive pathogens. The persistent destruction of platelets by macrophages induces the continuous processing and presentation of the above membrane glycoproteins by antigen-presenting cells, which is a crucial step for the generation of pathogenic antiplatelet antibodies.

One of the contributing factors in the development of the above-described autoimmunity, which leads to the development of ITP, is the imbalance between the over-activity of effector CD4+ T cells and the altered function of Tregs.[13] In patients with ITP, naturally occurring CD4+CD25+ Tregs were usually both functionally impaired and reduced in number. Aiming to further establish this finding, Tregs were evaluated using flow cytometry analyses in 44 patients with acute ITP. In this study, the number of Tregs was significantly lower in patients with severe ITP and in those positive for anti-GPIIb/GPIIIa antibodies. Of special interest is the fact that the number of those cells increased in patients when they were considered to be in full remission, especially in those after splenectomy.[14] In another study, the frequency of circulating CD4+CD25+Foxp3+ Tregs was comparable both in patients with ITP and in healthy individuals. However, stored Tregs from patients with chronic ITP ($n = 13$) demonstrated a twofold reduction of in $vitro$ immunosuppressive activity when compared to healthy controls ($n = 10$; $p < 0.05$). This impaired suppression was specific to Tregs, as shown by cross-mixing experiments with T cells from controls, suggesting that functional defects in Tregs are involved in the pathogenesis of ITP.[15] In spite of their pivotal role in maintaining peripheral immune tolerance, a very small and clinically ineffective number of natural Tregs are found in peripheral blood. In this respect, Zhang et al. demonstrated that platelet GP-specific induced Tregs could be generated de $novo$ from nonregulatory CD4+CD25-CD45RA+ cells in patients with ITP and induced both antigen-specific and linked suppression. They also showed that Toll-like receptor pathway is the dominant one related to the GP-specific tolerance.[16]

Although it is accepted that most ITP cases are considered to be primary, infection-induced (both acute and chronic) ITP is still common and should therefore be always considered when differential diagnosis of ITP is discussed. Many well-identified pathogens were shown to cross-react with self-antigens and induce the activation of effector T cells and/or induce numerical and functional alterations of Tregs, increasing the development of specific autoimmunity in ITP.

In this review we focus on the role of different pathogens known to be involved in the development of both acute and chronic ITP. We also discuss the various mechanisms by which these pathogens could possibly lead to the development of ITP and how to treat ITP in such patients.

2 ACUTE INFECTIONS AND ITP

2.1 Pathogenesis

Acute ITP is considered to be ITP that endures for 6 months or less. Most patients with acute ITP are children. Affected children are young (peak age, approximately 5 years) and previously healthy, and they typically present with the sudden onset of petechiae or purpura a few days or weeks after an infectious illness. In a subset of affected children, a specific virus can be identified, such as varicella zoster virus, rubella, the Epstein–Barr virus, influenza, or cytomegalovirus, indicating an etiological role for preceding viral infection in these children with ITP. Boys and girls are equally affected, and the illness resolves within 6 months in more than 70% of children, irrespective of whether they receive therapy.[17]

Of the many mechanisms contributing to infectious-induced acute ITP, we should point out platelet destruction, which has been attributed to the over-expression of viral antigens; the binding of immune complexes; the generation of anti-viral antibodies cross-reactive with platelet antigens (molecular mimicry); and the formation of autoantibodies through "epitope spread". Infectious-induced thrombocytopenia also was attributed to infected megakaryocytes or defects in platelet surfaces and accelerated clearance.[3] The basis for molecular mimicry lies in the fact that host proteins may have antigenic determinants similar to those exhibited by microbial pathogens or viral agents. Consequently, in the course of infection, an immune response mounted against the invading pathogen produces antibodies that have the ability to cross-react with host tissue, namely platelets. "Epitope spread" denotes the process by which the immune system acquires recognition of new self-determinants. These determinants are usually presented at sub-optimal concentrations and therefore escape detection by the central tolerance screening system in the thymus and are not eliminated. These self-determinants might share cross-reactivity with cryptic epitopes present on invading microbial pathogens or viral agents. Therefore, when cryptic epitopes are exposed in an immune response, T-cell activation sets up an inflammatory cascade that can lead to platelet destruction. Platelet auto-antigens from either the platelets or infectious agents are processed by antigen-presenting cells within the spleen in the context of major histocompatibility complex class II molecules on T helper cells. Co-signaling pathways are established, such as the activation of T helper cells and the activation and differentiation of autoreactive B cells.[3]

3 ITP-CYTOMEGALOVIRUS

Cytomegalovirus (CMV) commonly causes severe congenital thrombocytopenia and delayed platelet recovery after bone marrow transplantation. CMV can infect megakaryocytes, progenitor cells and supporting stroma. Acute ITP can occur in both immunocompetent and immunosuppressed people. The literature is full of conflicting case and series presentations regarding the beneficial effects of anti-viral therapy and platelet recovery. In one of these studies, 3 of 28 children and 3 of 80 adults with typical ITP were shown to have CMV in their urine, but there was no correlation between urinary viral clearance and the resolution of thrombocytopenia; in another study, platelet counts improved in four refractory patients after treatment for CMV.[3,18,19] Although thrombocytopenia is recognized as a complication of acute CMV infection, the underlying mechanism is unclear. These fall into two categories: (1) the production of antiplatelet antibodies (e.g. CMV-related thrombocytopenia) and direct cytotoxic effects to bone marrow progenitor cells (e.g. megakaryocytes) and (2) stromal marrow cells that result in decreased platelet production (e.g. CMV-induced thrombocytopenia). Treatment choices include the use of anti-viral therapies, but in some cases immunomodulatory agents also are considered.[20–22]

4 ITP-VARICELLA ZOSTER VIRUS

Approximately 2–5% of otherwise healthy children hospitalized with primary varicella zoster virus (VZV) develop severe thrombocytopenia. Within 5 days of the exanthem, patients present with the abrupt onset of bleeding, prominently at extracutaneous sites. Here, ITP could also be the result of VZV infecting megakaryocytes, leading to the inhibition of platelet production or resulting in the release of platelets expressing viral markers. In cases of hemorrhagic varicella, megakaryocytes undergo degeneration of nuclei and vacuolization, adsorption of viral antigens onto platelets, or desialylation of platelet GPs.[23] Thrombocytopenia can be a harbinger of viral dissemination, which can eventually result in purpura fulminans. Exposure to corticosteroids within the preceding 3 months may increase this risk. Spontaneous resolution in non-fulminant cases generally occurs within 2 weeks. The utility of anti-viral therapy in hastening resolution of thrombocytopenia is unproven.

Less often, thrombocytopenia develops days to several weeks after the resolution of infection and is characterized by reduced platelet survival with a normal-appearing bone marrow (ITP-VZV).[3,24] Antibodies to known platelet GPs and uncharacterized platelet antigens that do not cross-react with VZV have been demonstrated.[25] Complement-fixing anti-viral antibodies that cross-react with approximately 50-kDa and approximately 100-kDa antigens on normal platelets disappear as the infection resolves. ITP-VZV typically resolves spontaneously within 1–3 weeks, but occasionally the course is protracted and requires ITP therapy.[26,27]

5 ITP AND H1N1 INFECTION

Several reports suggested the evolvement of acute ITP following influenza vaccination; however, only a few proved this association to be evidence based. Whereas typical thrombocytopenia and purpureal rash develop 2–3 weeks after vaccination, influenza-associated thrombocytopenia generally develops during the onset of illness. The pathogenic mechanism by which influenza-associated ITP evolves is not fully understood. Some suggest the existence of shortened platelet survival time and enhanced clearance of platelets in the circulation. Previous studies showed that leukopenia and thrombocytopenia often are associated with severe novel 2009 H1N1 influenza infection. The treatment that was suggested in the literature of these cases included anti-viral therapy and intravenous high-dose methylprednisolone or intravenous immunoglobulin (IVIG) therapy given immediately after the diagnosis. In these cases, platelet counts returned to normal after few days.[28]

6 ITP AND HEPATITIS A INFECTION

Acute hepatitis A infection is generally a self-limited disease in childhood. Hepatitis A virus (HAV) infection can be subclinical, anicteric, or icteric. Younger children more frequently have asymptomatic infection or mild nonspecific symptoms with hepatitis A. Transient hematologic disturbances due to myelosuppression in the course of HAV infection are also well known. Autoimmune manifestations, such as immune thrombocytopenic purpura, aplastic anemia, and hemophagocytic syndrome, were rarely described in acute hepatitis A. ITP occurring during the course of acute hepatitis A may be related to the presence of transient anti-cardiolipin and anti-phospholipid antibodies, antiplatelet antibodies or circulating immune complexes. Only a few case reports concerning ITP during the acute phase of HAV were published. In these reports, thrombocytopenia occurred in association with anti-cardiolipin antibody positivity or chole-static hepatitis A. The authors suggested that thrombocytopenia may be the result of viral-associated immune-mediated peripheral destruction. In some of these reports, the ITP was the only manifestation of acute hepatitis A, and other manifestations, such as jaundice, vomiting, or abdominal pain, were absent. Further studies are required to explain the cause of thrombocytopenia-associated hepatitis A. Acute hepatitis A should be considered in the differential diagnosis of ITP in children.[29,30]

7 ITP AFTER VACCINATION

The issue of acute ITP following childhood vaccination has received a clinical and health attention during the last decade. Therefore, a large multi-site study of 1.8 million children was conducted to examine the risk of ITP after all childhood vaccines.[31] In this study, no evidence of an increased risk of ITP for any of the common childhood vaccines other than the measles, mumps and rubella (MMR) vaccine in younger children was found. In this survey, the diagnosis of ITP was infrequent in the 1- to 3-year-old age group. It was demonstrated that serious sequelae after vaccine-associated ITP were rare: only one child among 1.8 million vaccinated children was described as having an event that required the emergency transfusion of platelets. New data pointing to an association of ITP with hepatitis A, Tdap, and VAR vaccines in older children. In the 12- to 18-month-old age group, no increased risk of ITP after VAR, Hep A, DTaP, IPV, Hib, or PCV vaccination was found. In this age group, there is an elevated risk for ITP after the MMRV; the measles, mumps, and rubella components in the MMRV are essentially identical to MMR itself. Although several elevated risks for acute ITP were found to be of statistical significance in older children (such as in the human papillomavirus, the trivalent inactivated influenza and meningococcal conjugate vaccines), the estimated rates among older children are less stable because there are fewer cases of ITP to use in statistical analyses. The findings related to hepatitis A, Tdap, and VAR should be considered as hypothesis-generating rather than as conclusive evidence that these vaccines are associated with ITP because of the rarity of ITP in these age groups. Regarding possible biologic mechanisms, it is unclear why these vaccines would trigger acute ITP in older age groups but not in younger children. Thus, although it is important to consider the elevated risk of ITP after Hep A, VAR, and Tdap in older children to be real, these results must be interpreted with caution. The vast majority of the ITP cases in this survey were acute and mild. In addition, not all these cases developed serious permanent complications. These clinical findings are consistent with previous studies of vaccine-associated ITP in this regard. ITP after vaccination may have a similar clinical course as ITP from other causes. Other reports regarding the risk of ITP in association with vaccines other than MMR support the rarity of this phenomenon. This information on ITP after vaccines other than MMR has come from the Vaccine Adverse Event Reporting System (VAERS). There have been three reports of ITP after whole-cell DTP vaccine[31] and one after the DT vaccine have been published in the VAERS, but no case reports of ITP after hepatitis A, VAR, or Tdap were published. In another study from Canada based on an active surveillance system for vaccine adverse events, 28 cases of ITP after the DTP or DTaP vaccine were reported, compared with 77 reported after the MMR vaccine and only 10 reports after VAR; there were no reports after Hep A vaccination because children do not routinely receive this in Canada.[32] In a recently published report from the VAERS, there were 478 reports of ITP after the MMR vaccine alone or in combination with other vaccines, 47 cases reported after the VAR vaccine, 32 after the hepatitis A vaccine and only 8 after the Tdap vaccine.[33] Studies of the genetics of ITP, including ITP-associated vaccines, are ongoing, but it is assumed that there likely is a genetic predisposition, as in other immune-mediated diseases.[34] It is important to note that the sample size in these surveys was large enough to confirm that ITP is a rare complication following vaccination.

8 ITP AFTER THE MMR VACCINE

As stated above, acute ITP after vaccination is considered to be rare. However, in many cohorts, acute ITP was reported after MMR vaccination and therefore disserves further attention. The estimated incidence of ITP after MMR vaccination is 1 in 40,000 doses, which is five- to sixfold higher than acute ITP in childhood. In this case, ITP is defined as thrombocytopenia developing within 42 days of exposure. Most cases occur after initial vaccination during the second year of life and were demonstrated to be predominant in males. Thrombocytopenia can be severe ($<50,000/mm^3$) but is responsive to IVIG or corticosteroids.[35,36] Most affected children (>80%) recover within 2 months, typically within 2–3 weeks, and less than 10% evolve into chronic ITP. This course simulates the pattern of acute childhood ITP.[36,37] The precise pathophysiology is unknown, although antibodies to GPIIb/IIIa determinants were identified in a few patients, similar to primary ITP.[38] It is recommended that those patients in remission or with stable ITP receive all recommended immunizations because the incidence of ITP after MMR vaccination is 10- to 20-fold lower than after natural infection. Delays in vaccination are appropriate during the resolution of acute ITP or immunosuppressive treatment.[3]

9 CHRONIC INFECTIONS AND ITP

When ITP evolves a few weeks after acute infections, it is mostly transient and, as mentioned earlier, it resolves spontaneously within a few months. Contrary to this condition, chronic infections are typically associated with long-lasting ITP, thus leading to the persistence of chronic ITP. In this section we focus on some of the chronic infections known to contribute to the development of chronic ITP.

9.1 Hepatitis C Virus and Chronic ITP

Hepatitis C virus (HCV) is one of the persisting viruses with the ability to evade the immune response and to evolve into a chronic state in the majority of infected individuals. In addition to being the most common viral infection causing liver disease, HCV is considered to be the most immunogenic virus reported to persist in association with high autoimmunity, namely the increased incidence of autoantibodies such as anti-nuclear and anti-cardiolipin antibodies and rheumatoid factor.[39] This is why thrombocytopenia was reported to be present in patients infected with chronic HCV even when clinical symptoms are still absent. When the evidence for HCV infection in 250 adult patients with ITP (fulfilling the diagnostic criteria of the American Society of Hematology) was assessed, it was found to be positive in 30% of these patients.[40] The prevalence of ITP among patients with HCV also was evaluated and was suggested to be greater than would be expected in general by chance. In one study the incidence rate of ITP among HCV-infected individuals was compared to that of matched HCV-uninfected individuals. It was indicated that HCV infection is indeed associated with an elevated risk of developing ITP (hazard ratio, 1.8; 95% confidence interval, 1.4–2.3) among both untreated and treated patients.[41] In another study, and to further support the above finding, the platelet count in HCV-positive patients was found to be lower than in HCV-negative patients (26 ± 9 vs. $49 \pm 30 \times 10^9$/L, respectively; $p < 0.02$).[42]

9.1.1 Pathophysiology

Many pathogenic mechanisms are reported to be involved in the development of ITP related to HCV infection. Of these, the most relevant is the finding of high-affinity binding of HCV to platelet membranes and the subsequent binding of anti-HCV antibodies to platelets, theoretically leading to increased phagocytosis of platelets. Of special relevance is the improvement of thrombocytopenia following successful IFN therapy in HCV-infected patients.[43] Another mechanism worth mentioning is the possible sequestration of platelets in the enlarged spleen due to portal hypertension. In addition, reduced hepatic production of thrombopoietin and bone marrow suppression due to HCV infection also were reported.[44,45] Aiming to evaluate humoral immune mechanisms and their role in the development of thrombocytopenia in chronic HCV infection, anti-platelet antibodies were assessed in 50 patients with HCV infection (30 with thrombocytopenia and 20 with normal platelet count). The frequency of platelet-associated immunoglobulin (PAIg) in thrombocytopenic HCV-positive patients, as measured by flow cytometry, was 86.7%, 83.3%, 46.7%, and 33.3% for total PAIg, PAIgG, PAIgM, and PAIgA, respectively. Platelet-specific antibodies were found in 26 of 30 patients (86.7%), suggesting that these autoantibodies represent a common mechanism for inducing thrombocytopenia in patients with chronic HCV infection.[46]

9.1.2 The Treatment of HCV-Related ITP

Following the initiation of steroids, a significant increase in thrombocyte count was noticed in patients in whom chronic ITP was related to HCV infection. However, steroids caused an elevation of hepatic transaminases, HCV viral load and elevated serum bilirubin concentrations. IVIGs were documented to be effective in increasing platelet counts in both HCV-seropositive and HCV-seronegative patients. Finally, IFN-α was proved to be efficient in decreasing HCV RNA in correlation with a significant increase of thrombocytes in HCV-positive adult patients with ITP.[47,48] Eltrombopag is a small-molecule nonpeptide oral platelet growth factor that acts as an agonist to the thrombopoietin receptor. Thus, it was logical to assess the benefit of this drug in HCV-associated ITP. After 4 weeks of therapy, the thrombocyte count increased to $\geq 100 \times 109/L$ in 75%, 79%, and 95% of patients treated with 30, 50, and 75 mg of eltrombopag, respectively, compared with no response in placebo patients ($p < 0.001$). Also, significantly more patients in the eltrombopag treatment groups completed 12 weeks of anti-viral therapy compared with those treated with placebo, and those treated with eltrombopag had a greater increase in platelet counts at the end of the anti-viral treatment phase.[49,50] Because of this, patients in whom thrombocytopenia persists should be screened for HCV infection and should be treated for this infection first, and only thereafter should classical treatments for ITP be added.

9.2 *Helicobacter Pylori* and ITP

Helicobacter Pylori, a gram-negative bacterium, was previously reported as a causative pathogen of chronic gastritis and peptic ulcer, as well as one of the contributing factors in the development of gastric adenocarcinoma. The incidence of *H. pylori* infection was reported to involve half of the world's population, becoming one of the most attractive pathogens considered in association with many immune-mediated diseases, such as chronic urticaria, autoimmunity and ITP. Since the first report by Gasbarrini et al.[51] more than a decade ago, several other authors have tried to assess a possible correlation between *H. pylori* infection and the development of ITP. In some of these studies the prevalence of infection in adult patients with ITP was different from that reported in the general healthy population; however, many others could not confirm this finding.[52] Of special interest was the attempt to evaluate the possibility that bacterium eradication was followed by an increase in platelet count, but other authors did not confirm such positive results. In an attempt to clarify this issue, 17 different studies including 788 patients with ITP were considered to be suitable for meta-analysis and the evaluation of whether *H. pylori* is indeed responsible for the development of ITP and whether its eradication could possibly change the course of ITP.[53] Looking into these studies, it seems that an increase in platelet count in patients with ITP receiving eradication treatment was noticed, particularly when compared with untreated patients. Here, the success of eradicating *H. pylori* was highly beneficial in improving ITP.

9.2.1 *Pathophysiology of* H. pylori *and Its Relation to ITP*

As in many infections, molecular mimicry between epitopes of any pathogen and self-antigens are proposed as one of the important mechanisms in autoimmunity. Here, the expression of the CagA antigen on *H. pylori* is suggested to play a pathogenic role in evoking autoimmune responses. Support for the hypothesis of CagA + strains playing a pathophysiological role in ITP comes from an Italian study showing that the prevalence of the *H. pylori cagA* gene was significantly higher in patients with ITP than in healthy individuals.[54] In this respect, Takahashi et al. were able to show that platelet-associated IgG from 12 of 18 patients with ITP recognized the antigenic *H. pylori* cagA protein and that these cross-reactive antibody levels decreased following *H. pylori* eradication.[55] Another study reported data from eight patients with ITP and pointed to the occurrence of molecular mimicry mechanisms between the cagA antigen and a similar platelet peptide of 55 kDa, as well as the disappearance of anti-cagA antibodies in all these patients following efficient eradication of *H. pylori*. These results support the notion that cross-reacting autoantibodies against cagA could partially contribute to the pathogenesis of ITP.[56] Further support for molecular mimicry in ITP comes from another study where antibodies against *H. pylori* urease B cross-reacted with human platelet GPIIIa and were able to inhibit platelet aggregation.[57] A role for lipopolysaccharide (LPS) bacteria also has been suggested by a study were the existence of anti-platelet antibodies to LPS are able to enhance Fc-dependent platelet phagocytosis. Here again, *H. pylori* eradication was associated with decreased phagocytic capacity and the modulation of the inhibitory Fcγ receptor IIB in peripheral blood monocytes. These studies may explain why thrombocytopenia becomes severe in some patients who suffer from infectious diseases and how their thrombocytopenia improves when they successfully cure these infections.[58] A shift towards a Th1 immune response is noticed both during *H. pylori* infection and in the process of active ITP. Therefore, one can assume that *H. pylori* infection is a driving factor that facilitates the persistence of chronic ITP.[59]

9.2.2 Treatment

The issue of whether *H. pylori* eradication is indeed beneficial in improving ITP was assessed in a prospective study in which 37 patients with ITP were treated with triple therapy irrespective of the presence or absence of *H. pylori*. Therapeutic response of a platelet count $>100 \times 10^9$/L at 24 weeks was documented in 16 of 26 responding *H. pylori*-positive patients (62%); however, therapeutic response was not noticed in any of the *H. pylori*-negative patients. In addition, anti-GPIIb/IIIa antibody-producing B cells were significantly decreased at 12 and 24 weeks in *H. pylori*-positive responders ($p < 0.0001$), but much less so in non-responders ($p = 0.02$) and not at all in *H. pylori*-negative patients.[60] In another study, platelet count was evaluated in a group of 25 *H. pylori*-positive patients with chronic ITP who were randomized to receive or not receive treatment for *H. pylori* infection. Complete response was defined by an increase in platelet count of $>150 \times 10^9$/L; a partial response occurred when platelet count was increased $>50 \times 10^9$/L 6 months after eradication therapy. A significant increase in platelet counts was observed in 46.2% of those in whom *H. pylori* was successfully eradicated (4 presenting a complete response and 2 presenting only a partial response) but was 0% in those in whom eradication failed ($p < 0.01$).[61]

10 HUMAN IMMUNODEFICIENCY VIRUS (HIV) AND ITP

Thrombocytopenia is commonly observed among HIV-infected individuals and many studies report an occurrence in 5–30% of these patients.[62] ITP may appear at any stage during HIV infection, but in most patients thrombocytopenia was noticed during advanced stages of HIV infection. Thrombocytopenia also was found to be more severe among patients with HIV who were injection drug users, particularly when compared with homosexual patients with HIV. This observation was explained by the finding of a higher incidence of co-infection with HCV in the group of drug users with HIV.[63,64]

In a retrospective study, medical records of 55 HIV-positive patients in association with thrombocytopenia were analyzed. In more than half of these patients, thrombocytopenia was associated with opportunistic diseases such as tuberculosis, CMV and CNS toxoplasmosis. One could notice a predominance of homosexual patients with HIV and only a few with a history of intravenous drug use.[65] HIV-associated thrombocytopenia is rarely severe (platelet counts are mostly $>50 \times 109$/L), and therefore bleeding is rare. Severe thrombocytopenia in patients with advanced HIV infection is frequently observed when other cytopenias are present, namely when pancytopenia is caused by hypocellular bone marrow.[66]

10.1 Pathophysiology

The mechanisms by which ITP evolves in HIV-infected patients is complex. Various mechanisms, either alone or in combination, can lead to this: (1) increased platelet sequestration by the spleen, thus shortening their life span and (2) altered production of platelets, unrelated to the extent of thrombopoietin production. Different mechanisms were shown to be dependent on the stage of HIV infection. In early HIV infection, thrombocytopenia was noticed to be the result of peripheral platelet destruction, whereas in advanced stages (decreased CD4 T-cell count) thrombocytopenia was predominantly the result of decreased platelet production and failed hematopoiesis.[67] One of the leading causes of insufficient platelet production is the direct inhibition of megakaryocytes because of their infection by HIV. HIV infects megakaryocytes via the binding of both CD4 and co-receptors. Once internalized, HIV causes microscopic intracellular abnormalities such as blebbing of surface membrane and vacuolization of the megakaryocyte cytoplasm. Platelet destruction evolves because of the production of cross-reacting antiplatelet antibodies and the development of immune complexes. Some of these antibodies are directed against the integrin subunit GPIIIa, which was found in circulating immune complexes and can cross-react with the epitope region of HIV. These cross-reacting antibodies are potent in inducing complement-independent platelet fragmentation following the generation of reactive oxygen species.[68,69] Underlying opportunistic infections (viral, mycobacterial, and others), Kaposi's sarcoma, and anti-viral therapies also are responsible for the development of thrombocytopenia during HIV infection.

10.2 Treatment

Because the severity of ITP is related with the degree of HIV viral load and the extent of CD4+ T-cell depletion, it is obvious to consider anti-viral therapy as a first-line therapy for ITP in these patients. Anti-viral monotherapy was shown to be somehow efficacious in improving platelet counts in HIV-induced thrombocytopenia; however, combined anti-viral therapies later seemed to have a larger beneficial effect. The increased experience with highly active anti-retroviral therapy (HAART) supported the association of this combined therapy with a better improvement of ITP in HIV-infected patients. A recent study assessing 55 HIV-positive patients with thrombocytopenia evaluated the beneficial effect of HAART. While being treated with other drugs such as steroids and IVIG, HAART was started with the goal of improving thrombocytopenia in 20% of patients. The study concluded that HAART was followed by a significant increase in thrombocytes after 3 months of therapy, suggesting that this therapy was a beneficial one in treating ITP secondary to HIV infection.[70,71]

11 CONCLUSIONS

Infections (both viral and bacterial) are frequent causes of ITP, the pathogenesis of which remains complex and, in some cases, unknown. Of the many mechanisms to be considered in these cases is platelet destruction, the development of anti-platelet autoantibodies and the generation of anti-viral antibodies, cross-reactions with platelet antigens (molecular mimicry) and others. The issue of to what extent anti-viral/bacterial therapy could be efficient in improving platelet counts remains the subject of many studies. Further studies of large cohorts with infectious disease are required to better establish all of these issues.

REFERENCES

1. Cines DB, Blanchette VS. Immune thrombocytopenic purpura. *N Engl J Med* 2002; **346**:995–1008.
2. McMillan R. The pathogenesis of chronic immune thrombocytopenic purpura. *Semin Hematol* 2007;**44**:S3–S11.
3. Cines DB, Bussel JB, Liebman HA, Luning Park ET. The ITP syndrome: pathogenic and clinical diversity. *Blood* 2009;**113**:6511–21.
4. Rodeghiero F, Stasi R, Gemsheimer T, et al. Standardization of terminology, definitions and outcome criteria in immune thrombocytopenic purpura of adults and children: report from an international working group. *Blood* 2009;**113**:2386–93.
5. Kuwana M, Ikeda Y. The role of autoreactive T-cells in the pathogenesis of idiopathic thrombocytopenic purpura. *Int J Hematol* 2005;**81**:106–12.
6. Kuwana M, Okazaki Y, Ikeda Y. Splenic macrophages maintain the anti-platelet autoimmune response via uptake of opsonized platelets with immune thrombocytopenic purpura. *J Thromb Haemost* 2009;**7**:322–9.
7. Zhang F, Chu X, Wang L, Zhu Y, Li L, Ma D, et al. Cell-mediated lysis of autologous platelets in chronic idiopathic thrombocytopenic purpura. *Eur J Haematol* 2006; **76**:427–31.
8. Rocha AM, Souza C, Rocha GA, et al. The levels of IL-17A and of the cytokines involved in TH17 cell commitment are increased in patients with chronic immune thrombocytopenia. *Haematologica* 2011;**96**:1560–4.
9. Hemdan NY, Birkenmeier G, Wichmann G, Abu El-Saad AM, Krieger T, Conrad K, et al. Interleukin-17-producing T helper cells in autoimmunity. *Autoimmun Rev* 2010;**9**:785–92.
10. Olsson B, Ridell B, Carlsson L, Jacobsson S, Wadenvik H. Recruitment of T cells into bone marrow of ITP patients possibly due to elevated expression of VLA-4 and CX3CR1. *Blood* 2008;**112**:1078–84.
11. Provan D, Stasi R, Newland AC, et al. International consensus report on the investigation and management of primary immune thrombocytopenia. *Blood* 2010;**115**:168–86.
12. McMilan R, Wang L, Tani P. Prospective evaluation of the immunobead assay for the diagnosis of adult chronic immune thrombocytopenic purpura. *J Thromb Haemost* 2003;**1**:485–91.
13. Miyara M, Gorochov G, Ehrenstein M, Musset L, Sakaguchi S, Amoura Z. Human FoxP3+ regulatory T cells in systemic autoimmune diseases. *Autoimm Rev* 2011; **10**:744–55.

14. Sakakura M, Wada H, Tawara I, et al. Reduced CD4+CD25+ T cells in patients with idiopathic thrombocytopenic purpura. *Thromb Res* 2007;**120**:187–93.
15. Yu J, Heck S, Patel V, et al. Defective circulating CD25 regulatory T cells in patients with chronic immune thrombocytopenic purpura. *Blood* 2008;**112**:1325–8.
16. Zhang XL, Peng J, Sun JZ, et al. De novo induction of platelet-specific CD4(+)CD25 (+) regulatory T cells from CD4(+)CD25(-) cells in patients with idiopathic thrombocytopenic purpura. *Blood* 2009;**113**:2568–77.
17. George JN, Woolf SH, Raskob GE, et al. Idiopathic thrombocytopenic purpura: a practice guideline developed by explicit methods for the American Society of Hematology. *Blood* 1996;**88**:3–40.
18. Wright JG. Severe thrombocytopenia secondary to asymptomatic cytomegalovirus infection in an immunocompetent host. *J Clin Pathol* 1992;**45**:1037–8.
19. Psaila B, Bussel JB. Refractory immune thrombocytopenic purpura: current strategies for investigation and management. *Br J Haematol* 2008;**143**:16–26.
20. Sugioka T, Kubota Y, Wakayama K, Kimura S. Severe steroid-resistant thrombocytopenia secondary to cytomegalovirus infection in an immunocompetent adult. *Intern Med* 2012;**51**:1747–50.
21. Yaari S, Koslowsky B, Wolf D, Chajek-Shaul T, Hershcovici T. CMV-related thrombocytopenia treated with foscarnet: a case series and review of the literature. *Platelets* 2010;**21**:490–5.
22. Papagianni A, Economou M, Tsoutsou E, Athanassiou-Metaxa M. CMV-related immune thrombocytopenic purpura or CMV-induced thrombocytopenia? *Br J Haematol* 2010; **149**:454–5.
23. Rand ML, Wright JF. Virus-associated idiopathic thrombocytopenic purpura. *Transfus Sci* 1998;**19**:253–9.
24. Feusner JH, Slichter SJ, Harker LA. Mechanisms of thrombocytopenia in varicella. *Am J Hematol* 1979;**7**:255–64.
25. Mayer JL, Beardsley DS. Varicella-associated thrombocytopenia: autoantibodies against platelet surface glycoprotein V. *Pediatr Res* 1996;**40**:615–9.
26. Yeager AM, Zinkham WH. Varicella-associated thrombocytopenia: clues to the etiology of childhood idiopathic thrombocytopenic purpura. *Johns Hopkins Med J* 1980;**146**:270–4.
27. Welch RH. Thrombcytopenic purpura and chickenpox. *Arch Dis Child* 1956;**31**:38–41.
28. Lee CY, Wu MC, Chen PY, Chou TY, Chan YJ. Acute immune thrombocytopenic purpura in an adolescent with 2009 novel H1N1 influenza A virus infection. *J Chinese Med Assoc* 2011;**74**:425–7.
29. Tanir G, Aydem C, Tuygun N, Kaya Z, Yarali. Immune thrombocytopenic purpura as sole manifestation in a case of acute hepatitis A. *Turk J Gastroenterol* 2005;**16**(4):217–19.
30. Ertem D, Acar Y, Pehlivanoglu E. Autoimmune complications associated with hepatitis A virus infection in children. *Ped Infect Dis J* 2001;**20**:809–11.
31. O'Leary ST, Glanz JM, McClure DL, et al. The risk of immune thrombocytopenic purpura after vaccination in children and adolescents. *Pediatrics* 2012;**129**:248–54.
32. Sauvé LJ, Scheifele D. Do childhood vaccines cause thrombocytopenia? *Paediatr Child Health (Oxford)* 2009;**14**(1):31–2.
33. Woo EJ, Wise RP, Menschik D, et al. Thrombocytopenia after vaccination: case reports to the US Vaccine Adverse Event Reporting System, 1990-2008. *Vaccine* 2011; **29**(6):1319–23.
34. Bergmann AK, Grace RF, Neufeld EJ. Genetic studies in pediatric ITP: outlook, feasibility, and requirements. *Ann Hematol* 2010;**89**(Suppl. 1):S95–S103.
35. France EK, Glanz J, Xu S, et al. Risk of immune thrombocytopenic purpura after measles-mumps-rubella immunization in children. *Pediatrics* 2008;**121**:e687–92.

36. Black C, Kaye JA. MMR vaccine and idiopathic thrombocytopaenic purpura. *Br J Clin Pharmacol* 2003;**55**:107–11.

37. Jadavji T, Scheifele D, Halperin S. Thrombocytopenia after immunization of Canadian children, 1992 to 2001. *Pediatr Infect Dis J* 2003;**22**:119–22.

38. Schattner A. Consequence or coincidence? The occurrence, pathogenesis and significance of autoimmune manifestations after viral vaccines. *Vaccine* 2005;**23**:3876–86.

39. Toubi E, Kessel A, Goldstein L, Slobodin G, Sabo E, Shmuel Z, et al. Enhanced peripheral T-cell apoptosis in chronic hepatitis C virus infection: association with liver disease severity. *J Hepatol* 2001;**35**:774–80.

40. Rajan SK, Espina BM, Liebman HA. Hepatitis C virus-related thrombocytopenia: clinical and laboratory characteristics compared with chronic immune thrombocytopenic purpura. *Br J Haematol* 2005;**129**:818–24.

41. Chiao EY, Engels EA, Kramer JR, et al. Risk of immune thrombocytopenic purpura and autoimmune hemolytic anemia among 12908 US veterans with hepatitis C virus infection. *Arch Intern Med* 2009;**169**:357–63.

42. Sakuraya M, Murakami H, Uchiumi H, et al. Steroid refractory chronic idiopathic thrombocytopenic purpura associated with hepatitis C virus infection. *Eur J Haematol* 2002;**68**:49–53.

43. Hamaia S, Li C, Allain JP. The dynamics of hepatitis C virus binding to platelets, and 2 mononuclear cell lines. *Blood* 2001;**98**:2293–300.

44. Peck-Radosavljevic M. Thrombocytopenia in liver disease. *Can J Gastroenterol* 2000;**14**:60D–6D.

45. Iga D, Tomimatsu M, Endo H, et al. Improvement of thrombocytopenia with disappearance of HCV RNA in patients treated by interferon-alpha therapy: possible etiology of HCV-associated immune thrombocytopenia. *Eur J Haematol* 2005;**75**:417–23.

46. Aref S, Sleem T, El Menshawy N, et al. Antiplatelet antibodies contribute to thrombocytopenia associated with chronic hepatitis C virus infection. *Hematology* 2009;**14**:277–81.

47. Ramos-Casals M, Garcia-Carrasco M, Lopez-Medrano F, et al. Severe autoimmune cytopenias in treatment-naïve hepatitis C virus infection: clinical description of 35 cases. *Medicine (Baltimore)* 2003;**82**:87–96.

48. Rajan S, Liebman HA. Treatment of hepatitis C related thrombocytopenia with interferon alpha. *Am J Hematol* 2001;**68**:202–9.

49. McHutchison JG, Dusheiko G, Shiffman ML, et al. Eltrombopag for thrombocytopenia in patients with cirrhosis associated with hepatitis C. *N Eng J Med* 2007;**357**:2227–36.

50. Saleh MN, Bussel JB, Cheng G, Meyer O, Bailey CK, Aming M, et al. Safety and efficacy of Eltrombopag for treatment of chronic immune thrombocytopenia: results of the long-term, open-labeled EXTEND study. *Blood* 2013;**121**:537–45.

51. Gasbarrini A, Franceschi F, Tartaglioni R, et al. Regression of autoimmune thrombocytopenia after eradication of Helicobacter pylori. *Lancet* 1998;**352**:878.

52. Fujimura K. Helicobacter pylori infection and idiopathic thrombocytopenic purpura. *Int J Haematol* 2005;**81**:113–18.

53. Franchini M, Cruciani M, Mengoli C, Pizzolo G, Veneri D. Effect of Helicobacter pylori eradication on platelet count in idiopathic thrombocytopenic purpura: a systematic review and meta-analysis. *J Antimicrob Chemother* 2007;**60**:237–46.

54. Emilia Luppi M, Zucchini P, et al. Helicobacter pylori infection and chronic immune thrombocytopenic purpura: long-term results of bacterium eradication and association with bacterium virulence profiles. *Blood* 2007;**110**:3833–41.

55. Takahashi T, Yujiri T, Shinohara K, et al. Molecular mimicry by Helicobacter pylori CagA protein may be involved in the pathogenesis of H. pylori associated chronic idiopathic thrombocytopenic purpura. *Br J Haematol* 2004;**124**:91–6.

56. Franceschi F, Christodoulides N, Kroll MH, et al. Helicobacter pylori and idiopathic thrombocytopenic purpura. *Ann Intern Med* 2004;**140**:766–7.
57. Bai Y, Wang Z, Bai X, et al. Cross-reaction of antibody against Helicobacter pylori urease B with platelet glycoprotein IIIa and its significance in the pathogenesis of immune thrombocytopenic purpura. *Int J Hematol* 2009;**89**:142–9.
58. Semple JW, Aslam R, Kim M, et al. Platelet-bound lipopolysaccharide enhances Fc receptor-mediated phagocytosis of IgG-opsonized platelets. *Blood* 2007;**109**:4803–5.
59. Guo C, Chu X, Shi Y, et al. Correlation of Th1-dominant cytokine profiles by high-dose dexamethasone in patients with chronic idiopathic thrombocytopenic purpura. *J Clin Immunol* 2007;**27**:557–62.
60. Asahi A, Kuwana M, Suzuki H, et al. Effects of Helicobacter pylori eradication regimen on antiplatelet autoantibody response in infected and uninfected patients with idiopathic thrombocytopenic purpura. *Haematologica* 2006;**91**:1436–7.
61. Suzuki T, Matsushima M, Masui A, et al. Effect of Helicobacter pylori eradication in patients with chronic idiopathic thrombocytopenic purpura randomized controlled trial. *Am J Gastroenterol* 2005;**100**:1265–70.
62. Carbonara S, Fiorentino G, Serio G, et al. Response of severe HIV associated thrombocytopenia to highly active antiretroviral therapy including protease inhibitors. *J Infect* 2001;**42**:251–6.
63. Sloand EM, Klein HG, Banks SM, et al. Epidemiology of thrombocytopenia in HIV infection. *Eur J Haematol* 1992;**48**:168–72.
64. Burbano X, Miguez MJ, Lecusay R, et al. Thrombocytopenia in HIV-infected drug users in the HAART era. *Platelets* 2001;**12**:456–61.
65. Marks KM, Clarke RM, Bussel JB, Talal AH, Glesby MJ. Risk factors for thrombocytopenia in HIV-infected persons in the era of potent antiretroviral therapy. *J Acquir Immune Defic Syndr* 2009;**52**:595–9.
66. Mientjes GH, van Ameijden EJ, Mulder JW, et al. Prevalence of thrombocytopenia in HIV-infected and non-HIV infected drug users and homosexual men. *Br J Haematol* 1992;**82**:615–19.
67. Cole JL, Marzec UM, Gunthel CJ, et al. Ineffective platelet production in thrombocytopenic human immunodeficiency virus-infected patients. *Blood* 1998;**91**:3239–46.
68. Najean Y, Rain JD. The mechanism of thrombocytopenia in patients with HIV infection. *J Lab Clin Med* 1994;**123**:415–20.
69. Nardi MA, Liu LX, Karpatkin S. GPIIIa- (49-66) is a major pathophysiologically relevant antigenic determinant for anti-platelet GPIIIa of HIV-1 related immunologic thrombocytopenia. *Proc Natl Acad Sci USA* 1997;**94**:7589–94.
70. Scaradavou A, Woo B, Woloski BM, et al. Intravenous anti-D treatment of immune thrombocytopenic purpura: experience in 272 patients. *Blood* 1997;**89**:2689–700.
71. Scaradavou A. HIV-related thrombocytopenia. *Blood Rev* 2002;**16**:73–6.

CHAPTER 53

Viral Infections and Type 1 Diabetes

Alessandro Antonelli[1], Silvia Martina Ferrari, Andrea Di Domenicantonio, Ele Ferrannini, Poupak Fallahi
Department of Clinical and Experimental Medicine, University of Pisa, Pisa, Italy
[1]Corresponding Author: alessandro.antonelli@med.unipi.it

1 INTRODUCTION

Diabetes mellitus type 1 (also known as type 1 diabetes, or T1D; formerly insulin-dependent diabetes) is a form of diabetes mellitus that results from autoimmune destruction of insulin-producing β-cells in the pancreas.[1] The subsequent lack of insulin leads to increased blood glucose. The classical symptoms are polyuria, polydipsia, polyphagia, and weight loss. Incidence varies from about 35 per 100,000 in Scandinavia to 1 per 100,000 in Japan and China.[2] Untreated, T1D is ultimately fatal, but the disease can be controlled with supplemental insulin. Insulin is most commonly administered by injection at periodic intervals several times per day, though other options, such as insulin pumps, exist. Transplantation of both the entire pancreas and pancreatic islet cells is a possible cure in some cases. T1D can be distinguished from type 2 by autoantibody testing, glutamic acid decarboxylase autoantibodies (GADA), islet cell autoantibodies, insulinoma-associated (IA-2) autoantibodies, and zinc transporter autoantibodies (ZnT8) are present in individuals with type 1 diabetes, but not type 2.[1]Other autoantibodies also have been associated with T1D.[3,4] The C-peptide assay, which measures endogenous insulin production, can also be used to determine disease.[1]

T1D is induced by one or more of the following: genetic susceptibility, a diabetogenic trigger and/or exposure to a driving antigen.[5] T1D is a polygenic disease, meaning many different genes contribute to its onset. The strongest gene, *IDDM1*, is located in the major histocompatibility complex (MHC) class II region on chromosome 6. Certain variants of this gene increase the risk for T1D. Such variants include *DRB1 0401, DRB1 0402, DRB1 0405, DQA 0301, DQB1 0302*, and *DQB1 0201*, which are common in North Americans of European ancestry and in Europeans. Some variants also seem to be

Infection and Autoimmunity
http://dx.doi.org/10.1016/B978-0-444-63269-2.00047-7

protective.[5,6] Among identical twins, when one twin has T1D, the other twin has it only 30–50% of the time. Despite having exactly the same genome, one twin had the disease, while the other did not; which suggests environmental factors, in addition to genetic factors, can influence disease prevalence.[6]

Other indications of environmental influence include the presence of a 10-fold difference in occurrence among Caucasians living in different areas of Europe and a tendency of people who migrate to acquire the incidence of the disease in the destination country.[5] It has been proposed that T1D is a virus-triggered autoimmune response in which the immune system attacks virus-infected cells along with the β-cells in the pancreas. The Coxsackie virus family or rubella is implicated, although the evidence is inconclusive.[7,8] However, not everyone infected by the suspected virus develops T1D. For this reason, the presence of a genetic vulnerability has been suggested, and there is indeed an observed inherited tendency to develop T1D.[9] Here, we review the literature about the possible association of T1D and viruses in humans.

2 EPIDEMIOLOGY

In recent decades there has been a rapid rise in the incidence of T1D, especially among children younger than the age of 5.[10] In Europe, from 1989 to 2003 the average annual increase was 3.9%—too fast to be accounted for by genetics alone.[11] A putative role for viral infections in the development of T1D comes from epidemiological studies that have shown a significant geographical variation in incidence, a seasonal pattern to disease presentation[10,12,13] and an increased incidence of diabetes after enterovirus epidemics.[14] Furthermore, an intrafamilial spread of enterovirus infections at the clinical onset of T1D was observed.[15]

Several other viruses have been proposed to contribute to T1D in epidemiological studies: (1) increased rates of T1D following epidemics of mumps were observed[16]; (2) the incidence of childhood diabetes was associated with both mumps and rubella infection[17]; and (3) the relationship between rubella and T1D is predominantly based on follow-up studies of congenital rubella syndrome, which suggest that in utero infection may lead to T1D.[18] Hepatitis C virus (HCV) has been associated with the appearance of T1D and type 2 diabetes (T2D).

3 ENTEROVIRUS–COXSACKIE VIRUS B

Enteroviruses are ubiquitous; they are transmitted via the fecal-oral route and replicate primarily in the gut. Systemic infection may lead to dissemination to other target organs. The methodology used to detect enterovirus infection critically influenced the results of research.

A systematic review of evidence from published controlled studies of the relationship between Coxsackie B virus serology and incident or prevalent T1D[19] do not provide convincing evidence for or against an association between Coxsackie B virus infection and T1D. The problem with using antibodies as a marker is the possible involvement of several viral serotypes.

On the other hand, a meta-analysis of studies using molecular methods of enterovirus detection by Yeung et al.[20] found a significant association between enterovirus infection and T1D-related autoimmunity and clinical T1D. The majority of published studies have used reverse-transcriptase polymerase chain reaction to detect enterovirus RNA in blood samples.

Oikarinen et al.[21] reported more frequent enterovirus detection in the mucosa of the small intestine in patients with T1D. However, Mercalli et al.[22] found no evidence of enteroviruses in the small-intestine biopsy samples from 25 patients at different stages of T1D.[22] Two studies also reported detection of enteroviruses in islets and in β-cells.[23,24] Taken together, these studies suggest that enteroviruses are more frequently detected in patients with T1D; however, enteroviruses may well infect patients with T1D after disease onset. Available longitudinal studies investigating the potential link between enterovirus infections and islet autoimmunity or T1D (studies from Finland [DIPP, DiMe, and TRIGR studies], the United States [DAISY study], Norway [MIDIA study], Germany [BABYDIAB and Baby-diet studies], and Australia [VIGR study]) were reviewed by Yeung et al.[20] and Stene and Rewers,[25] who found inconsistent results regarding temporal association.

An association between CVB and high circulating levels of interferon (IFN)-α (which is considered a strong marker of viral infection) in patients with T1D was found in 50% patients who were positive for IFN-α at various stages of T1D but not in healthy individuals.[26] Furthermore, persistent infection of human pancreatic islets by the Coxsackievirus was associated with IFN-α synthesis in β-cells.[27]

Yoon et al. first demonstrated the presence of a virus in the pancreas of a child with diabetic ketoacidosis.[28] Subsequent inoculation of mouse, monkey, and human cell cultures with homogenates of the pancreas led to the identification of a diabetogenic variant of CVB4.[28]

The more recent analysis using *in situ* hybridization of pancreas from 65 patients with T1D compared to controls demonstrated the presence of enteroviral RNA in islet cells and in some duct cells but not in exocrine tissue.[29] The same authors also found that typical enterovirus receptors were expressed in primary human islets exclusively in β-cells.[29] The presence of CVB4 was also found in the pancreatic islets of three of six T1D organ donors analyzed.[23] In a study of a large cohort of pancreas of 72 patients with recent onset T1D, the presence of VP-I enteroviral protein in islets was found in 44 of 72 samples compared with only 3 of 50 neonatal and pediatric controls. VP-I staining was restricted to insulin-positive cells.[24]

The mechanism by which CVB4 induces diabetes is not fully understood. In a study of enterovirus strains isolated from T1D patients at clinical presentation of T1D revealed β-cell tropism and clearly affected the function of the β-cell. In addition, the infection caused a clear increase in the number of dead cells.[30] In another study the expression of pro-inflammatory cytokine genes (interleukin [IL]-1α, IL-1β, and tumor necrosis factor [TNF]-α) that also mediate cytokine-induced β-cell dysfunction correlated with the lytic potential of a virus. Temporally increasing levels of gene expression of double-stranded RNA recognition receptors, antiviral molecules, cytokines and chemokines were detected for all studied virus strains. Lytic CVB5 infection also down-regulated genes involved in glycolysis and insulin secretion.[31]

Global gene expression profiling of isolated human islets exposed to CVB5 infection and to pro-inflammatory cytokines to simulate an insulitis situation revealed a wide pattern of altered genes. Several pro-inflammatory cytokines (e.g. IL-1, IL-15 receptor agonist) and chemokines (e.g. CXCL10) have been shown to be up-regulated by the genes encoding for the MHC class I and class II. Prolonged exposure to these conditions resulted in β-cell destruction.[32]

The inflammatory condition due to viral infection may also lead to bystander activation of autoreactive T cells as a consequence of enhanced autoantigen presentation by B cells through MHC class I. It is interesting that both lytic and non-lytic CVB4 strains are able to up-regulate CXCL10 secretion from human islets during infections, contributing to islet inflammation in T1D.[33]

Molecular mimicry also has been proposed as an inductive or accelerating mechanism of T1D. Molecular mimicry between p2C of Coxsackie B-like enteroviruses and GAD65 has been observed, albeit limited to the HLA DR3–positive subpopulation of T1D patients.[34]

Furthermore, the results obtained with human paired sera, collected during enterovirus infection, indicated that enterovirus infection in humans may also occasionally induce a humoral response that cross-reacts with β-cell autoantigen tyrosine phosphatase (IA-2/IAR).[35]

Although HLA genes admittedly are involved in T1D susceptibility, recent genome-wide association studies identified more than 20 loci associated with T1D.[36] Interestingly, some of the loci are associated with antiviral activities. An association between T1D and single-nucleotide polymorphisms in the IFN-induced helicase 1 (*IFIH1*) gene that encodes melanoma differentiation-associated protein 5 (MDA5), a cytoplasmic sensor of viruses, especially CVB, has been found.[37] Upon viral infection, MDA5 stimulates the production of type 1 IFNs, which are mediators of the innate antiviral immune response and are able to play a role in the activation of the adaptive immune response. This viral sensor is expressed at low levels in human pancreatic islets. Rare variants of *IFIH1* through lost or reduced expression of the protein are protective against T1D.[38,39] Elevated *IFIH1* levels in response to enteroviruses may have an increased capacity to stimulate dendritic cells and elevate production of pro-inflammatory cytokines, which may promote the development of T1D. A current hypothesis is that a weaker immune response to enterovirus (associated with the minor alleles) should be mirrored by increased replication of enterovirus. However, to date, no clear association between *IFIH1* polymorphisms and enterovirus detection in the gut or in the blood has been found.[40,41]

A theory that has attracted some attention entails that viral infections may interfere with T-cell selection in the thymus. CVB4 was found to infect the thymus of experimentally infected mice and to profoundly affect T-cell maturation.[42] *In vitro* studies indicate that CVB4 has the ability to infect human thymocytes.[43] It is uncertain, however, whether these experimental data bear any relevance to the natural course of T1D.

4 RUBELLA VIRUS AND T1D

Rubella is a single-stranded RNA-enveloped virus and member of the Togavirus family. Several reports have shown an increased prevalence of T1D in patients with congenital rubella.[44,45]

Among patients with congenital rubella syndrome, the frequencies of the HLA antigens DR2 and DR3 are decreased in nondiabetic subjects, whereas they are increased in rubella-positive patients who also developed T1D, suggesting that T1D develops only in subjects that have genetic susceptibility to developing T1D. Controversial results about the percentage of subjects with antibodies against islet cells among patients with congenital rubella syndrome compared with noninfected subjects have been reported.[45,46]

Infection of neonatal hamsters with rubella indeed induces diabetes, providing experimental evidence for a causal relationship between rubella infection and the development of T1D.[47] Results from *in vitro* and *in vivo* studies indicate that rubella is able to infect human pancreatic β-cells[47,48] and reduce insulin secretion.[48] Molecular mimicry could be implicated in the diabetogenic effect of rubella virus. In fact, T cells of patients with congenital rubella and T1D were found to be cross-reactive with rubella virus peptides and GAD protein determinants.[49]

5 MUMPS VIRUS AND T1D

The mumps virus is an enveloped single-stranded virus belonging to the paramyxovirus family. Mumps virus was one of the first viruses implicated in the development of human T1D: (1) a high frequency of children with mumps appeared to have islet cell antibodies and occasionally developed overt diabetes,[50] and (2) mumps outbreaks were associated with an increase in the incidence of T1D 2–4 years later.[16] The mechanism through which mumps might be involved in the development of T1D is not clear. *In vitro* studies have shown that (1) human β-cells could be infected with the mumps virus; [51] (2) mumps infection of a human insulinoma cell line induced the release of IL-1 and IL-6;[52] and (3) pancreatic β-cells infected with mumps virus had increased expression of only HLA class I molecules.[53] On the basis of these results, it has been hypothesized that the release of cytokines and the increased expression of HLA molecules by infected β-cells may lead to an immune response against the β-cells or may exacerbate pre-existing autoimmune processes against β-cells.

Several studies have explored the effect of mumps vaccinations on either increasing or decreasing the incidence of T1D. One study suggested that the elimination of natural mumps by mumps–measles–rubella vaccination may have decreased the risk for T1D in Finland; a possible causal relationship was substantiated by the observed concomitant decrease in the levels of mumps antibodies in diabetic children.[54] Low levels of mumps antibodies induced by mumps–measles–rubella vaccinations in T1D children suggested decreased responsiveness rather than a different number of past infections in these patients.[55] However, the results of other studies concluded that there is no association with childhood mumps vaccinations and the development of islet autoimmunity[56] or T1D.[57]

6 HCV AND T1D

An association between HCV infection and the development of T1D has been hypothesized because some studies found markers of pancreatic auto-immunity in a small proportion of patients with chronic HCV hepatitis.[58–61] In particular, among Egyptian children with T1D a relatively high preva-lence of HCV antibody seropositivity was found.[59] Chen et al.[62] described a case of a 66-year-old man who developed acute HCV infection after trans-fusion. One year later, the patient presented with diabetic ketoacidosis, and tests for C-peptide confirmed that he had T1D. Testing of pre- and post-operative serum specimens demonstrated that the patient developed positive tests for islet cells and GADA 4 weeks after transfusion, concurrent with the development of acute HCV infection. The simultaneous development of HCV infection and diabetes-related autoantibodies suggested a relationship between HCV and T1D.[62] Masuda et al.[63] described a 22-year-old woman who had diabetic ketoacidosis. Her serum aspartate aminotransferase and alanine aminotransferase concentrations were 158 and 1220 IU/L, respec-tively, and GADA level was 12.4 IU/mL. Upon viral examinations, HCV antibody was negative, whereas HCV-RNA was positive. Based on these findings, she was diagnosed as having autoimmune diabetes and acute hepatitis C. These findings suggested that the progression of autoimmune diabetes might have been accelerated because of the infection with HCV.[63]

Several mechanisms have been proposed to be involved in such a pro-gression. A direct destruction of β-cells by viral infection could be a good explanation. This hypothesis was recently supported by Masini et al.,[64] who showed a direct cytopathic effect of HCV at the islet cell level.

Furthermore, HCV infection could initiate an immune reaction against β-cells. Some authors suggested the involvement of a process of molecular mimicry as a trigger of HCV-related autoimmunity.[65] Indeed, GAD65 shares similar amino acids in common with antigenic regions on the HCV polyprotein.[66] Of interest, the HCV/self-homologous autoantigenic regions also are mimicked by other microbial agents. Such mimics may give rise to β-cell autoimmunity through a "multiple-hit" mechanism of molecular mimicry.[65,67] Cross-reactive immunity does not exclude the possibility of the involvement of additional factors such as pro-inflammatory cytokines.[66] Another possibility regards the induction of antibody reactivity against GAD and the development of full-blown diabetes mediated by IL-18 and other pro-inflammatory cytokines. In particular, IL-18 is presumed to play a pathogenetic role in T1D; it especially seems to be involved in the acceleration of the development of overt disease.[63,68,69] IL-18 can induce both a T helper (Th) 1 and Th2 response, depending on its surrounding cytokine circumstances,[70] and it has been shown to play a pathogenic role in several diseases,[70] including acute hepatic injury.[71] Other pro-inflammatory cytokines, such as TNF-α and IL-1β, that are elevated in patients with acute hepatitis[72] can also induce autoimmune diabetes.[73,74]

Chronic HCV infection has been associated with a high prevalence of T2D.[75–78] The type of diabetes manifested by patients with chronic HCV infection is not the classical T2D. The labelling of HCV-positive patients as having T2D is purely conventional; the lines separating T1D from latent autoimmune diabetes and from T2D are fading away as new pathogenetic information is obtained.[79] Three studies[76,77,80] previously reported that HCV-positive patients with T2D were leaner than T2D controls and showed significantly lower low-density lipoprotein cholesterol and lower systolic and diastolic blood pressure. An immune-mediated mechanism for HCV-related mixed cryoglobulinemia-associated diabetes has been postulated,[76] and a similar pathogenesis might be involved in diabetes in HCV-positive patients. This hypothesis is strengthened by the finding that autoimmune phenomena in T2D patients are more common than previously thought.[3,4,81] On the above-mentioned bases, it has been hypothesized that HCV infection of β-cells[64] may act by up-regulating *CXCL10* gene expression and secretion (as previously shown in human hepatocytes), recruiting Th1 lymphocytes that secrete IFN-γ and TNF-α and that induce *CXCL10* secretion by β-cells, thus perpetuating the immune cascade, which may lead to the appearance of β-cell dysfunction in genetically predisposed subjects. This hypothesis has recently been confirmed by a study that demonstrates higher serum concentrations of *CXCL10* in HCV-positive patients with T2D compared to those without.[82,83] Furthermore, it was recently shown that increased serum *CXCL10* and normal chemokine (C-C motif) ligand 2 concentrations signal a predominant Th1-driven autoimmune process, which shifts towards Th2 immunity after 2 years from diagnosis in children with newly diagnosed T1D.[84]

7 CONCLUSION

Genetic predisposition seems to be a major component in the development of T1D; however, environmental factors also play an important role in the expression of the disease. Among them, viruses seem to be implicated in the pathogenesis of T1D in humans. A putative role for viral infections in the development of T1D comes from epidemiological studies that have shown a significant geographical variation in incidence, a seasonal pattern to disease presentation and an increased incidence of diabetes after enterovirus epidemics. A strong body of evidence suggests an important role for CVB in the development of T1D. However, several other viruses, such as mumps, congenital rubella infection, and HCV, have been proposed to contribute to T1D in humans.

Viruses may directly infect and destroy pancreatic β-cells or may trigger or contribute to β-cell-specific autoimmunity with or without β-cell infection. Unequivocal evidence that viruses can cause diabetes comes from animal models. However, there is no direct evidence that viruses can cause diabetes in humans. It is difficult to study the role of viruses in the development of T1D in humans. Large prospective cohort studies in prediabetic or genetically susceptible individuals as well as patients with newly diagnosed T1D are needed to understand the viral etiology of T1D in humans.

REFERENCES

1. Daneman D. Type 1 diabetes. *Lancet* 2006;**367**:847–58.
2. Kasper DL, Braunwald E, Hauser S, Longo D, Jameson JL, Fauci AS. *Harrison's principles of internal medicine*. 16th ed. New York: McGraw-Hill; 2005.
3. Antonelli A, Baj G, Marchetti P, Fallahi P, Surico N, Pupilli C, et al. Human anti-CD38 autoantibodies raise intracellular calcium and stimulate insulin release in human pancreatic islets. *Diabetes* 2001;**50**:985–91.
4. Antonelli A, Tuomi T, Nannipieri M, Fallahi P, Nesti C, Okamoto H, et al. Autoimmunity to CD38 and GAD in type I and type II diabetes: CD38 and HLA genotypes and clinical phenotypes. *Diabetologia* 2002;**45**:1298–306.
5. Bluestone JA, Herold K, Eisenbarth G. Genetics, pathogenesis and clinical interventions in type 1 diabetes. *Nature* 2010;**464**:1293–300.
6. Bartsocas CS, Gerasimidi-Vazeou A. Genetics of type 1 diabetes mellitus. *Pediatr Endocrinol Rev* 2006;**3**:508–13.
7. Fairweather D, Rose NR. Type 1 diabetes: virus infection or autoimmune disease? *Nat Immunol* 2002;**3**:338–40.
8. Toniolo A, Onodera T, Yoon JW, Notkins AL. Induction of diabetes by cumulative environmental insults from viruses and chemicals. *Nature* 1980;**288**:383–5.
9. Donner H, Rau H, Walfish PG, Braun J, Siegmund T, Finke R, et al. CTLA4 alanine-17 confers genetic susceptibility to Graves' disease and to type 1 Diabetes mellitus. *J Clin Endocrinol Metab* 2007;**82**:143–6.
10. Diamond Project Group. Incidence and trends of childhood type 1 diabetes worldwide 1990-1999. *Diabet Med* 2006;**23**:857–66.
11. Patterson C, Dahlquist G, Gyürüs E, Green A, Soltész G, EURODIAB Study Group. Incidence trends for childhood type 1 diabetes in Europe during 1989-2003 and predicted new cases 2005-20: a multicentre prospective registration study. *Lancet* 2009;**373**:2027–33.

12. Green A, Patterson CC, EURODIAB TIGER Study Group, Europe and Diabetes. Trends in the incidence of childhood-onset diabetes in Europe 1989-1998. *Diabetologia* 2001;**44**:B3–8.
13. Kimpimaki T, Kupila A, Hamalainen AM, Kukko M, Kulmala P, Savola K, et al. The first signs of B-cell autoimmunity appear in infancy in genetically susceptible children from the general population: the Finnish Type 1 Diabetes Prediction and Prevention Study. *J Clin Endocrinol Metab* 2001;**86**:4782–8.
14. Wagenknecht LE, Roseman JM, Herman WH. Increased incidence of insulin-dependent diabetes mellitus following an epidemic of coxsackievirus B5. *Am J Epidemiol* 1991;**133**:1024–31.
15. Salvatoni A, Baj A, Bianchi G, Federico G, Colombo M, Toniolo A. Intrafamilial spread of enterovirus infections at the clinical onset of type 1 diabetes. *Pediatr Diabetes* 2013;**14**:407–16.
16. Hyoty H, Leinikki P, Reunanen A, Ilonen J, Surcel HM, Rilva A, et al. Mumps infections in the etiology of type 1 (insulin-dependent) diabetes. *Diabetes Res* 1988;**9**:111–16.
17. Ramondetti F, Sacco S, Comelli M, Bruno G, Falorni A, Iannilli A, et al. Type 1 diabetes and measles, mumps and rubella childhood infections within the Italian Insulin-dependent Diabetes Registry. *Diabet Med* 2012;**29**:761–6.
18. Burgess MA, Forrest JM. Congenital rubella and diabetes mellitus. *Diabetologia* 2009;**52**:369–70.
19. Green J, Casabonne D, Newton R. Coxsackie B virus serology and type 1 diabetes mellitus: a systematic review of published case–control studies. *Diabet Med* 2004;**21**:507–14.
20. Yeung WC, Rawlinson WD, Craig ME. Enterovirus infection and type 1 diabetes mellitus: systematic review and meta-analysis of observational molecular studies. *BMJ* 2011;**342**:d35.
21. Oikarinen M, Tauriainen S, Honkanen T, Oikarinen S, Vuori K, Kaukinen K, et al. Detection of enteroviruses in the intestine of type 1 diabetic patients. *Clin Exp Immunol* 2008;**151**:71–5.
22. Mercalli A, Lampasona V, Klingel K, Albarello L, Lombardoni C, Ekström J, et al. No evidence of enteroviruses in the intestine of patients with type 1 diabetes. *Diabetologia* 2012;**55**:2479–88.
23. Dotta F, Censini S, van Halteren AG, Marselli L, Masini M, Dionisi S, et al. Coxsackie B4 virus infection of cells and natural killer cell insulitis in recent-onset type 1 diabetic patients. *Proc Natl Acad Sci USA* 2007;**104**:5115–20.
24. Richardson SJ, Willcox A, Bone AJ, Foulis AK, Morgan NG. The prevalence of enteroviral capsid protein vp1 immunostaining in pancreatic islets in human type 1 diabetes. *Diabetologia* 2009;**52**:1143–51.
25. Stene LC, Rewers M. Immunology in the clinic review series; focus on type 1 diabetes and viruses: the enterovirus link to type 1 diabetes: critical review of human studies. *Clin Exp Immunol* 2012;**168**:12–23.
26. Chehadeh W, Weill J, Vantyghem MC, Alm G, Lefèbvre J, Wattré P, et al. Increased level of interferon-alpha in blood of patients with insulin-dependent diabetes mellitus: relationship with coxsackievirus B infection. *J Infect Dis* 2000;**181**:1929–39.
27. Chehadeh W, Kerr-Conte J, Pattou F, Alm G, Lefèbvre J, Wattré P, et al. Persistent infection of human pancreatic islets by coxsackievirus B is associated with alpha interferon synthesis in beta cells. *J Virol* 2000;**74**:10153–64.
28. Yoon JW, Austin M, Onodera T, Notkins AL. Isolation of a virus from the pancreas of a child with diabetic ketoacidosis. *N Engl J Med* 1979;**300**:1173–9.
29. Ylipaasto P, Klingel K, Lindberg AM, Otonkoski T, Kandolf R, Hovi T, et al. Enterovirus infection in human pancreatic islet cells, islet tropism in vivo and receptor involvement in cultured islet beta cells. *Diabetologia* 2004;**47**:225–39.

30. Elshebani A, Olsson A, Westman J, Tuvemo T, Korsgren O, Frisk G. Effects on isolated human pancreatic islet cells after infection with strains of enterovirus isolated at clinical presentation of type 1 diabetes. *Virus Res* 2007;**124**:193–203.
31. Ylipaasto P, Smura T, Gopalacharyulu P, Paananen A, Seppänen-Laakso T, Kaijalainen S, et al. Enterovirus-induced gene expression profile is critical for human pancreatic islet destruction. *Diabetologia* 2012;**55**:3273–83.
32. Ylipaasto P, Kutlu B, Rasilainen S, Rasschaert J, Salmela K, Teerijoki H, et al. Global profiling of coxsackievirus- and cytokine-induced gene expression in human pancreatic islets. *Diabetologia* 2005;**48**:1510–22.
33. Berg AK, Tuvemo T, Frisk G. Enterovirus markers and serum CXCL10 in children with type 1 diabetes. *J Med Virol* 2010;**82**:1594–9.
34. Vreugdenhil GR, Geluk A, Ottenhoff TH, Melchers WJ, Roep BO, Galama JM. Molecular mimicry in diabetes mellitus: the homologous domain in coxsackie B virus protein 2C and islet autoantigen GAD65 is highly conserved in the coxsackie B-like enteroviruses and binds to the diabetes associated HLA-DR3 molecule. *Diabetologia* 1998;**41**:40–6.
35. Härkönen T, Lankinen H, Davydova B, Hovi T, Roivainen M. Enterovirus infection can induce immune responses that cross-react with beta-cell autoantigen tyrosine phosphatase IA-2/IAR. *J Med Virol* 2002;**66**:340–50.
36. Concannon P, Rich SS, Nepom GT. Genetics of type 1A diabetes. *N Engl J Med* 2009;**360**:1646–54.
37. Hühn MH, McCartney SA, Lind K, Svedin E, Colonna M, Flodström-Tullberg M. Melanoma differentiation-associated protein-5 (MDA-5) limits early viral replication but is not essential for the induction of type 1 interferons after Coxsackievirus infection. *Virology* 2010;**401**:42–8.
38. Nejentsev S, Walker N, Riches D, Egholm M, Todd JA. Rare variants of IFIH1, a gene implicated in antiviral responses, protect against type 1 diabetes. *Science* 2009;**324**:387–9.
39. Liu S, Wang H, Jin Y, Podolsky R, Reddy MV, Pedersen J, et al. IFIH1 polymorphisms are significantly associated with type 1 diabetes and IFIH1 gene expression in peripheral blood mono- nuclear cells. *Hum Mol Genet* 2009;**18**:358–65.
40. Witsø E, Tapia G, Cinek O, Pociot FM, Stene LC, Rønningen KS. Polymorphisms in the innate immune IFIH1 gene, frequency of enterovirus in monthly fecal samples during infancy, and islet autoimmunity. *PLoS One* 2011;**6**:e27781.
41. Cinek O, Tapia G, Witsø E, Kramna L, Holkova K, Rasmussen T, et al. Enterovirus RNA in peripheral blood may be associated with the variants of rs1990760, a common type 1 diabetes associated polymorphism in IFIH1. *PLoS One* 2012;**7**:e48409.
42. Chatterjee NK, Hou J, Dockstader P, Charbonneau T. Coxsackievirus B4 infection alters thymic, splenic, and peripheral lymphocyte repertoire preceding onset of hyperglycemia in mice. *J Med Virol* 1992;**38**:124–31.
43. Brilot F, Geenen V, Hober D, Stoddart CA. Coxsackievirus B4 infection of human fetal thymus cells. *J Virol* 2004;**78**:9854–61.
44. Menser MA, Forrest JM, Bransby RD. Rubella infection and diabetes-mellitus. *Lancet* 1978;**1**:57–60.
45. Ginsberg-Fellner F, Witt ME, Yagihashi S, Dobersen MJ, Taub F, Fedun B, et al. Congenital rubella syndrome as a model for type 1 (insulin-dependent) diabetes mellitus: increased prevalence of islet cell-surface antibodies. *Diabetologia* 1984;**27**:87–9.
46. Viskari H, Paronen J, Keskinen P, Simell S, Zawilinska B, Zgorniak-Nowosielska I, et al. Humoral beta-cell autoimmunity is rare in patients with the congenital rubella syndrome. *Clin Exp Immunol* 2003;**133**:378–83.
47. Rayfield EJ, Kelly KJ, Yoon JW. Rubella virus-induced diabetes in the hamster. *Diabetes* 1986;**35**:1278–81.

48. Numazaki K, Goldman H, Wong I, Wainberg MA. Infection of cultured human fetal pancreatic islet cells by rubella virus. *Am J Clin Pathol* 1989;**91**:446–51.
49. Ou D, Mitchell LA, Metzger DL, Gillam S, Tingle AJ. Cross-reactive rubella virus and glutamic acid decarboxylase (65 and 67) protein determinants recognised by T cells of patients with type I diabetes mellitus. *Diabetologia* 2000;**43**:750–62.
50. Helmke K, Otten A, Willems W. Islet cell antibodies in children with mumps infection. *Lancet* 1980;**2**:211–12.
51. Prince G, Jenson AB, Billups L, Notkins AL. Infection of human pancreatic beta cell cultures with mumps virus. *Nature* 1978;**27**:158–61.
52. Cavallo MG, Baroni MG, Toto A, Gearing AJ, Forsey T, Andreani D, et al. Viral infection induces cytokine release by beta islet cells. *Immunology* 1992;**75**:664–8.
53. Parkkonen P, Hyöty H, Koskinen L, Leinikki P. Mumps virus infects beta cells in human fetal islet cell cultures upregulating the expression of HLA class I molecules. *Diabetologia* 1992;**35**:63–9.
54. Hyöty H, Hiltunen M, Reunanen A, Leinikki P, Vesikari T, Lounamaa R, et al. Decline of mumps antibodies in type 1 (insulin-dependent) diabetic children and a plateau in the rising incidence of type 1 diabetes after introduction of the mumps–measles–rubella vaccine in Finland. Childhood Diabetes in Finland Study Group. *Diabetologia* 1993;**36**:1303–8.
55. Hiltunen M, Hyöty H, Leinikki P, Akerblom HK, Tuomilehto J, Vesikari T. Low mumps antibody levels induced by mumps-measles-rubella vaccinations in type 1 diabetic children. *Diabet Med* 1994;**11**:942–6.
56. Hummel M, Füchtenbusch M, Schenker M, Ziegler AG. No major association of breast-feeding, vaccinations, and childhood viral diseases with early islet autoimmunity in the German BABYDIAB Study. *Diabetes Care* 2000;**24**:969–74.
57. DeStefano F, Mullooly JP, Okoro CA, Chen RT, Marcy SM, Ward JI, et al. Childhood vaccinations, vaccination timing, and risk of type 1 diabetes mellitus. *Pediatrics* 2001;**108**: E112.
58. Ando H, Nagay Y, Yokoyama M, Takamura T, Kobayashi K. Antibodies to GAD in diabetic patients with chronic hepatitis C. *Diabet Med* 1998;**15**:797–8.
59. Hieronimus S, Fredenrich A, Tran A, Benzaken S, Fénichel P. Antobodies to GAD in chronic hepatitis C patients. *Diabetes Care* 1997;**20**:1044.
60. Mason AL, Lau JYN, Hoang N, Qian K, Alexander GJ, Xu L, et al. Association of diabetes mellitus and chronic hepatitis C virus infection. *Hepatology* 1999;**29**:328–33.
61. Piquer S, Hernadez C, Enriquez J, Ross A, Esteban JI, Genescà J, et al. Islet cell and thyroid antibody in patients with hepatitis C virus infection: effect of treatment with interferon. *J Lab Clin Med* 2001;**137**:38–42.
62. Chen LK, Chou YC, Tsai ST, Hwang SJ, Lee SD. Hepatitis C virus infection-related Type 1 diabetes mellitus. *Diabet Med* 2005;**22**:340–3.
63. Masuda H, Atsumi T, Fujisaku A, Shimizu C, Yoshioka N, Koike T. Acute onset of type 1 diabetes accompanied by acute hepatitis C: the potential role of proinflammatory cytokine in the pathogenesis of autoimmune diabetes. *Diabetes Res Clin Pract* 2007;**75**:357–61.
64. Masini M, Campani D, Boggi U, Menicagli M, Funel N, Pollera M, et al. Hepatitis C virus infection and human pancreatic beta-cell dysfunction. *Diabetes Care* 2005;**28**:940–1.
65. Bogdanos DP, Choudhuri K, Vergani D. Molecular mimicry and autoimmune liver disease: virtuous intentions, malign consequences. *Liver* 2001;**21**:225–32.
66. Bogdanos DP, Rigopoulou EI. Viral/self-mimicry and immunological cross-reactivity as a trigger of hepatic C virus associated autoimmune diabetes. *Diabetes Res Clin Pract* 2007;**77**:155–6.

67. Bogdanos DP, Lenzi M, Okamoto M, Rigopoulou EI, Muratori P, Ma Y, et al. Multiple viral/self immunological cross-reactivity in liver kidney microsomal antibody positive hepatitis C virus infected patients is associated with the possession of HLA B51. *Int J Immunopathol Pharmacol* 2004;**17**:83–92.

68. Hanifi-Moghaddam P, Schloot NC, Kappler S, Seissler J, Kolb H. An association of autoantibody status and serum cytokine levels in type 1 diabetes. *Diabetes* 2003;**52**:1137–42.

69. Oikawa Y, Shimada A, Kasuga A, Morimoto J, Osaki T, Tahara H, et al. Systemic administration of IL-18 promotes diabetes development in young nonobese diabetic mice. *J Immunol* 2003;**171**:5865–75.

70. Nakanishi K, Yoshimoto T, Tsutsui H, Okamura H. Interleukin IL-18 is a unique cytokine that stimulates both Th1 and Th2 responses depending on its cytokine milieu. *Cytokine Growth Factor Rev* 2001;**12**:53–72.

71. Yumoto E, Higashi T, Nouso K, Nakatsukasa H, Fujiwara K, Hanafusa T, et al. Serum gamma-interferon-inducing factor (IL-18) and IL-10 levels in patients with acute hepatitis and fulminant hepatic failure. *J Gastroenterol Hepatol* 2002;**17**:285–94.

72. Torre D, Zeroli C, Giola M, Ferrario G, Fiori GP, Bonetta G, et al. Serum levels of interleukin-1 alpha, interleukin-1 beta, interleukin-6, and tumor necrosis factor in patients with acute viral hepatitis. *Clin Infect Dis* 1994;**18**:194–8.

73. Eizirik DL, Mandrup-Poulsen T. A choice of death-the signal-transduction of immune-mediated beta-cell apoptosis. *Diabetologia* 2001;**44**:2115–33.

74. Thomas HE, Irawaty W, Darwiche R, Brodnicki TC, Santamaria P, Allison J, et al. IL-1 receptor deficiency slows progression to diabetes in the NOD mouse. *Diabetes* 2004;**53**:113–21.

75. Noto H, Raskin P. Hepatitis C infection and diabetes. *J Diabetes Complications* 2006;**20**:113–20.

76. Antonelli A, Ferri C, Fallahi P, Sebastiani M, Nesti C, Barani L, et al. Type 2 diabetes in hepatitis C-related mixed cryoglobulinaemia patients. *Rheumatology (Oxford)* 2004;**43**:238–40.

77. Antonelli A, Ferri C, Fallahi P, Pampana A, Ferrari SM, Goglia F, et al. Hepatitis C Virus Infection: Evidence for an association with type 2 diabetes. *Diabetes Care* 2005;**28**:2548–50.

78. Mehta SH, Brancati FL, Strathdee SA, Pankow JS, Netski D, Coresh J, et al. Hepatitis C virus infection and incident type 2 diabetes. *Hepatology* 2003;**38**:50–6.

79. Gale EA. Latent autoimmune diabetes in adults: a guide for the perplexed. *Diabetologia* 2005;**48**:2195–9.

80. Skowronski M, Zozulińska D, Juszczyk J, Wierusz-Wysocka B. Hepatitis C virus infection: evidence for an association with type 2 diabetes. *Diabetes Care* 2006;**29**:750.

81. Pupilli C, Giannini S, Marchetti P, Lupi R, Antonelli A, Malavasi F, et al. Autoantibodies to CD38 (ADP-ribosyl cyclase/cyclic ADP-ribose hydrolase) in Caucasian patients with diabetes: effects on insulin release from human islets. *Diabetes* 1999;**48**:2309–15.

82. Antonelli A, Ferri C, Ferrari SM, Colaci M, Fallahi P. Immunopathogenesis of HCV-related endocrine manifestations in chronic hepatitis and mixed cryoglobulinemia. *Autoimmun Rev* 2008;**8**:18–23.

83. Antonelli A, Ferri C, Ferrari SM, Colaci M, Sansonno D, Fallahi P. Endocrine manifestations of hepatitis C virus infection. *Nat Clin Pract Endocrinol Metab* 2009;**5**:26–34.

84. Antonelli A, Fallahi P, Ferrari SM, Pupilli C, d'Annunzio G, Lorini R, et al. Serum Th1 (CXCL10) and Th2 (CCL2) chemokine levels in children with newly diagnosed type 1 diabetes: a longitudinal study. *Diabet Med* 2008;**25**:1349–53.

CHAPTER 54

Infection and Autoimmune Thyroid Diseases

Sara Salehi Hammerstad[*,†], Ronald Villanueva[*], Yaron Tomer[*,1]
[*]Division of Endocrinology, Diabetes, and Bone Disease, Department of Medicine, Mount Sinai School of Medicine, New York, New York, USA
[†]Division of Pediatric Endocrinology and Diabetes, Oslo University Hospital, Oslo, Norway
[1]Corresponding Author: Yaron.Tomer@mssm.edu

1 INTRODUCTION

Autoimmune thyroid diseases (AITDs) include a number of conditions that have in common cellular and humoral immune responses targeted at the thyroid gland. AITDs mainly include Graves' disease (GD) and Hashimoto's thyroiditis (HT), both of which involve infiltration of the thyroid by T and B cells that react with thyroid antigens, producing thyroid autoantibodies, with the resultant clinical manifestations of hyperthyroidism in GD and hypothyroidism in HT (reviewed in Refs. 1,2). While the etiology of the immune response to the thyroid remains unknown, the current paradigm is that AITDs are complex diseases in which susceptibility genes and environmental triggers act in concert to initiate the autoimmune response to the thyroid. In this review we focus on the contribution of one environmental factor—infection—to the pathogenesis of AITDs. We examine the pertinent data relating to the role of infectious organisms in the development of AITDs, with an emphasis on the mechanisms by which infection may trigger AITDs.

2 GD AND INFECTION

GD is an autoimmune disease characterized by hyperthyroidism and diffuse goiter with or without associated ophthalmopathy and dermopathy.[1] GD is organ specific and is associated with the production of thyrotropin receptor

Infection and Autoimmunity
http://dx.doi.org/10.1016/B978-0-444-63269-2.00048-9

(TSHR-Ab). These autoantibodies stimulate the TSH receptor to increase iodide uptake and cyclic-AMP production, thereby inducing the production and secretion of excess thyroid hormones.[3]

2.1 Epidemiological Data

Evidence for genetic factors implicated in the development of AITDs is now widely accepted. However, it is also recognized that the development of AITDs may be triggered by environmental factors, including infectious agents. Cox et al.[4] found seasonality in the diagnosis of GD, but the data failed to reach statistical significance. In another study, Phillips et al.[5] found that the incidence of thyrotoxic patients who had TSH receptor and anti-microsomal antibodies varied markedly between towns in England, but this study remains to be confirmed. Moreover, significantly increased prevalence of non-secretors (individuals with an inability to secrete the water-soluble glycoprotein form of the ABO blood group antigens into saliva) was reported in patients with GD.[6–8] Since non-secretors are known to have increased susceptibility to infection,[7] these findings lend further support to the notion that an infective agent may play a part in the pathogenesis of GD. Indeed, Valtonen and co-workers found serological evidence for a recent bacterial or viral infection in 36% of patients with newly diagnosed GD and in only 10% of controls.[9] An increased frequency of antibodies to the influenza B virus also was found in patients with thyrotoxicosis.[10]

A homology has been reported to exist between some amino acid sequences of thyroid autoantigens and a number of gram-positive and gram-negative bacteria.[11] Moreover, 5 of 12 GD IgG preparations displaced radio-labelled bovine TSH from the bacterial binding proteins.[12] These findings imply that anti-TSH receptor antibodies could be produced by cross-reaction between bacterial proteins and the TSH receptor.

2.2 *Yersinia* Infection and GD

Primarily known to cause outbreaks of food poisoning, *Yersinia enterocolitica* (YE) also has been associated with various autoimmune phenomena.[13] The relationship between YE infection and AITDs has been reported by many groups since early 1970s, albeit with conflicting results. Studies of patients with YE infections demonstrated that the sera of these patients contained autoantibodies to thyroid epithelium,[14,15] although these may be of the "natural" autoantibody variety.[16] Conversely, a large proportion of patients with GD were reported to have antibodies to *Yersinia*,[17] and many different *Yersinia* antigens cross-react with thyroid antigens,[18] although with uncertain affinity. Wenzel et al. found antibodies to plasmid-encoded release proteins of YE in 72% of patients with GD, in 81% of patients with recurrent disease, as well as in 35% of unmatched controls.[19] Arscott et al. examined the serological reactivity of sera from patients with GD to *Yersinia* release proteins 2–5, as well as the ability of these *Yersinia* release proteins to stimulate T-lymphocyte proliferation in patients with GD, but they could not confirm the findings of Wenzel et al. However, two patients with GD demonstrated significant proliferative responses to the release proteins in their peripheral blood mononuclear cells (PBMCs) and proliferation of intrathyroidal lymphocytes, suggesting that the relationship of this pathogen with GD may be due to T-cell cross-recognition and not serological cross-reactivity.[20] Another study showed a high incidence of *Yersinia* agglutinating antibodies measured in blood samples from 65 patients with GD compared to patients with HT, patients with multi-nodular goiter and controls.[21] Furthermore, a higher prevalence of antibodies to *Yersinia* is reported in a twin with GD compared to their healthy twin.[22] By contrast, an earlier study from Canada showed no differences in the mean levels of *Yersinia* antibodies to serotypes 3 and 9 between patients with GD, nontoxic goiter and autoimmune rheumatic disease and normal controls.[23]

A large study of 803 female relatives of patients with AITD and 100 healthy controls from the Netherlands showed that IgG and IgA antibodies to the outer membrane of *Yersinia* were higher in relatives of patients with AITD compared to controls. However, among euthyroid relatives, no difference in the prevalence of TPO antibodies was found between those who were *Yersinia* antibody positive or negative.[24] Results from the recent follow-up of the same cohort could not find any relationship between *Yersinia* seroactivity and the development of GD.[25]

Weiss et al. demonstrated a saturable binding site for TSH on YE,[26] and the binding of radio-labelled TSH to *Yersinia* was shown to be inhibited by GD immunoglobulins;[27] however, none of these observations show that infection with *Yersinia* leads directly or indirectly to the development of AITDs. However, it is possible that the hypothesized cross-reaction between *Yersinia* antibodies and thyroid antigens is secondary to a recurrent epitope or a reflection of a related but unknown infection.[28] In addition, a 200-bp fragment of *Yersinia* complementary DNA was successfully amplified using TSH receptor oligonucleotide primers, and a radio-labelled TSHR probe gave several discrete bands of hybridization with digested YE DNA, albeit under low stringency conditions.[29]

In addition, T-cell-mediated immunity towards YE has been reported in patients with GD.[30] However, similar data have been demonstrated in rheumatoid arthritis.[31] Further evidence supporting the role of *Yersinia* infection in thyroid autoimmunity comes from a study of rats that demonstrated the induction of lymphocytic thyroiditis after immunization with the YE purified outer membrane protein.[32]

The possibility of *Yersinia*-specific immune responses being merely reflective of the "natural" immune response deserves serious consideration in view of the low-affinity interactions and the lack of predictability in the published studies. Moreover, most patients with *Yersinia* infection do not develop GD.[33] Hence, it is possible that while *Yersinia* antigens, which are homologous to the TSH receptor can induce the production of anti-TSH receptor antibodies, this immune response is transitory and does not precipitate GD.

2.3 Enterovirus and GD

It has been hypothesized that certain HLA subtypes interacting with infectious triggers, including enteroviruses, can contribute to the development of GD. Kraemer et al. found that the frequency of HLA-B15, -B21 and -DR3 was increased in patients with GD compared with healthy individuals and that an association between the HLA-DR3 antigen and lymphocytotoxic antibodies was observed (i.e. IgGs from patients with GD were cytotoxic to HLA-DR3+ normal B cells). Absorption with the Coxsackie B virus completely inhibited the lymphocytotoxic reactions against HLA-DR3+ B cells, suggesting a role for Coxsackie-reactive HLA-DR3 antibodies as a contributing factor to the development of GD.[34] However, in a recent Norwegian cohort, no significant association was reported between HLA genotype and the occurrence of human enterovirus gut infection in 190 healthy infants.[35] Nested PCRs performed on blood samples from 21 patients with newly diagnosed GD were investigated in an attempt to amplify the enterovirus genome, but no RNA from Coxsackie or related viruses were detected.[36] Thyroid tissue from 46 patients with GD and 24 control subjects were recently directly examined for visualization of enteroviral RNA and the virus protein VP1. The results showed that the rate of simultaneous detection of the enteroviral genome and VP1 in thyroid tissue was significantly higher in patients with GD compared to controls ($p < 0.05$).[37] However, further studies are needed to show the causality.

2.4 Endogenous and Exogenous Retroviruses and GD

Retroviruses have been implicated in the induction of GD, but data supporting this view remain unsubstantiated. Bottazzo's group reported the existence of retroviral sequences in the thyroid and PBMCs of patients with GD.[38] Using antibodies against foamy virus (FV) gag protein, Wick et al. detected a signal on immunofluorescence in thyroid tissue sections from 7 patients with GD.[39] Lagaye at al. detected the presence of FV DNA in 19 of 29 French patients with GD using PCR.[40] Using Southern blot and PCR, subsequent analysis of DNA from four of these patients confirmed the presence of FV DNA, but the same study did not detect any FV DNA in samples from another cohort of 41 German patients with GD.[41] Another study of 28 patients with GD found no FV DNA using immunofluorescence, RIPA and Western blot.[42] The last two negative studies leave the possibility of artifactual contamination of the French samples. Analyses by ELISA and Western blot also found no FV antibodies in 45 African patients with GD.[43] Yanagawa et al. detected the gag region sequence of the human spumaretrovirus from DNA extracted from PBMCs and thyroid tissue in both Caucasian and African Americans patients with GD and in controls.[44] Moreover, FV gag, env, and LTR sequences were detected by nested PCR in 13 of 24 Korean patients with GD (peripheral blood lymphocytes), and in 7 patients all three regions were amplified. However, 9 of 23 normal controls also were positive for at least one locus under the same conditions.[45] Thus, there is presently no evidence for FV as a causative factor for GD.

DNA extracted from thyroid glands of 5 patients with GD was hybridized with a probe containing the gag region of HIV-I. The results showed positive bands in the thyroid DNA of each of the patients; these apparently were absent in control samples.[38] However, these results were not confirmed by Humphrey et al.[46] or Tominaga et al.[47] An increased risk for thyroid pathology in HIV-infected patients is reported in some studies.[48] However, it should be remembered that most studies include mainly patients receiving highly active anti-retroviral therapy.

High reverse transcriptase activity, a marker for retroviral infection, was demonstrated in thyroid tissue extracts from patients with GD compared to thyroids from patients with thyroid adenomas or carcinomas.[49] An uncharacterized retroviral-like factor (p15E) also has been detected in the serum of patients with GD but is absent in controls, suggesting the involvement of endogenous retroviruses.[50] Tas and co-workers suggested that the origin of the p15E-related factors may be an exogenous infection with an as yet unknown retrovirus possessing determinants with structural homology with an endogenous retrovirus.[51] Jaspan et al. reported that 87.5% (35 of 40) of patients with GD had a positive reaction against a prototypic strain of a human intracisternal A-type retroviral particle type 1 (HIAP-1), compared with only 2% of healthy controls, 10% of patients with multi-nodular goiter, and 15% of patients with type 1 DM.[52] A study of 35 members of 3 kindreds with a high prevalence of GD reported a possible interaction between HIAP-1 and HLA susceptibility haplotypes. When HLA susceptibility genes and HIAP-1 were co-detected (in a total of 15 members from the 3 kindreds), the incidence of GD was 100%, 67%, and 80%, in each kindred, respectively. The association between the occurrence of both anti-HIAP-1 antibody positivity and HLA susceptibility and the presence of GD was highly significant $(p < 0.001)$.[53] Another group further investigated these findings on the background of experiments on H9 cells co-cultured with homogenates of salivary glands from patients with Sjögren's syndrome.[54] Fierbracci et al. co-cultured the H9 T-cell line with thyroid homogenate and viable thyrocytes prepared from the thyroids of patients with GD, but after 24 weeks, no HIAP-1 particles were detected by electron microscopy.[55] Yokoi et al. found a high incidence of HTLV-II proviral DNA fragments in the DNA of peripheral blood leukocytes from patients with AITD: this occurred in 51.5% of patients with HT and 11.8% of patients with GD compared to only 1.9% of diseased controls, and 1.0% of healthy controls. However, no antibodies to HTLV-II were detected.[56] Another study did not implicate the involvement of HTLV-1 in the development of GD.[57]

To help explain a possible relationship between retroviruses and thyroid autoimmunity, a homology between the HIV-I Nef protein and the human TSH has been suggested.[58] There was 66% homology demonstrated within a 166-bp region encoding a unique portion of the hTSHR, with a segment in which 7 of 10 consecutive amino acids were identical. However, when sera from 10 patients with GD and 10 controls were tested for reactivity against an 18-amino acid peptide containing this segment of homology, there was no significant difference in the degree of interaction.[48]

Nevertheless, this does not exclude a conformational B-cell epitope or the presence of a T-cell epitope.

3 AUTOIMMUNE (HASHIMOTO'S) THYROIDITIS AND INFECTION

Autoimmune thyroiditis is characterized by infiltration of the thyroid by lymphocytes, gradual destruction of the gland associated with cytotoxic T-cells, and production of various secondary polyclonal thyroid autoantibodies, notably anti-TPO and anti-Tg.[2] The etiology of Hashimoto's disease is still unknown; however, genetic and environmental factors have been implicated in its pathogenesis.[2]

3.1 Evidence for the Involvement of Infection in the Etiology of Autoimmune Thyroiditis

Serological evidence for a recent bacterial or viral infection was demonstrated in patients with HT,[9] and lymphoid thyroiditis was described after immunization with group A streptococcal vaccine.[59] In addition, it was reported that autoimmune thyroiditis may be associated with a significantly increased frequency of antibodies that react to HIV-1 Western blot proteins in patterns not diagnostic for HIV.[60] Viral-like particles have been detected in thyroids of humans with AITDs; however, since these viral-like particles also were demonstrated in normal thyroids and in other tissues, their significance is unclear at present.[61]

Wenzel et al. reported that antibodies against *Yersinia* release proteins raised in rabbits showed specific bands on Western blots with thyroid epithelial cell homogenates, and one band could be blocked by purified TPO.[62] Further evidence suggesting that infection is involved in the etiology of HT comes from studies of T-cell function in the disease. It was reported that the lymphocytes in thyroids affected by HT have a restricted antigenic response, suggesting their triggering by a specific antigenic stimulus, perhaps an infection.[63]

3.2 Viral Hepatitis and HT

The association of hepatitis C with HT has been widely studied. There also have been a few reports of hepatitis B as possibly being associated with HT. Because of the increasing prevalence of viral hepatitis, especially hepatitis C, the use of interferon (IFN) has become widespread. It is thus important to study patients with viral hepatitis before receiving IFN, since IFN is a known immunomodulator that can trigger AITD.

Both hepatitis B and HT occur frequently in Down's syndrome. May and Kawanishi found a threefold increase in the frequency of HT in patients with Down's syndrome who were carriers of the HbsAg compared to patients with Down's syndrome who are negative for the HbsAg. They postulated that this might be explained by cytokine/cellular immune abnormalities due to extra-genetic material in chromosome 21.[64] However, hepatitis B alone has not been found to be associated with an increased incidence of thyroid autoimmunity.[65,66]

There have been numerous studies reporting varying concentrations of abnormal thyroid antibodies (TAbs) in patients with hepatitis C. Several studies found no significant correlation between the presence of hepatitis C before IFN treatment and the presence of TAbs.[67-71] Other studies showed a significant association between hepatitis C and HT and/or TAb positivity. Abnormal concentrations of TAbs in up to 42% of patients with hepatitis C have been reported.[72-78,65] Some studies showed that these IFN-naive patients with hepatitis C and associated HT tended to be older and female.[66,72,75,79] There also have been reports of a high prevalence of anti-HCV antibodies in patients with HT, suggesting this could be induced by HCV infection,[80,81] but this was not confirmed by other investigators.[76,82] Hepatitis C RNA also was present in thyroid tissue from hepatitis C-positive patients,[83] and a recent study showed that Hepatitis C virus can infect human cells *in vitro*.[84] Furthermore, Akeno et al. demonstrated that CD81 expressed on thyrocytes can bind hepatitis virus C envelope proteins E1 and E2, inducing cytokine production.[85]

While the epidemiological data are inconclusive, we still believe that hepatitis C may trigger thyroiditis, maybe via bystander activation mechanisms. The latest studies focus on the induction of autoimmune thyroiditis by treatment in these patients;[86] hence, further investigation of IFN-naive hepatitis C is required.

3.3 Retroviruses and HT

Retroviruses also have been purported to be involved in the development of HT. A high incidence of HTLV-II proviral DNA fragments was found in peripheral blood lymphocytes from patients with AITD. Although no antibodies for HTLV-II could be detected, and thus HTLV-II infection could not be confirmed, HTLV-II proviral DNA fragments were demonstrated in 51.5% of patients with HT compared to 1.9% of diseased controls and 1% of healthy controls.[56] The same authors found HTLV-I protein and messenger RNA in thyroid follicular cells in one of two patients with HT, although no virus particles were found on electron microscopy.[87] This same group measured TAbs in blood donors. Donors with both HTLV-I antibodies and TAbs tended to be more prevalent compared to donors without the HTLV-I antibody. However, the frequency of TAbs was significantly higher only in young male donors with HTLV-I Ab than those without HTLV-I Ab ($p < 0.05$). Also, detection of HTLV-II proviral DNA was significantly higher ($p < 0.001$) in donors with TAb than in those without, regardless of HTLV-I infection. The authors suggested that HTLV-I infection and the presence of HTLV-II proviral DNA may be independently related to the development of AITD.[88] Akamine et al. found a high prevalence of TAbs in patients with adult T-cell leukemia and HTLV-I carriers compared to healthy controls. Furthermore, for those subjects positive for TAbs, 40% of HTLV-I carriers, 19% of patients with adult T-cell leukemia, and 7.5% of controls had hypothyroidism ($p < 0.005$).[89] The observed prevalence of HTLV-I seropositivity also was shown to be significantly higher in patients with HT compared to controls.[57] Matsuda et al. observed a significantly higher HTLV-1 viral load in peripheral blood from patients with HT compared to asymptomatic HTLV-I carriers.[90] These epidemiological studies demonstrate that HTLV-I seropositivity seems to be a risk factor for thyroid autoimmunity in Japan. A study of *CTLA-4* gene polymorphisms and HTLV-I infection in Japanese patients showed that there was a significantly higher frequency of the exon 1 G allele of *CTLA-4* in patients with HT with HTLV-I Ab compared to those without HTLV-I Ab. However, HTLV-I Ab were not associated with *CTLA-4* polymorphisms in either patients with HT or controls, suggesting that if HTLV-1 is indeed a factor in the development of HT, it is a purely an environmental one.[91]

3.4 *Yersinia* and HT

YE has been suspected of being involved in the development of HT. An early study reported finding *Yersinia* antibodies in all seven patients with HT compared to a low prevalence (<8%) in controls.[17] The most prevalent serotype, with the highest titers, was serotype 3. Chatzipanagiotou and co-workers reported a 14-fold prevalence of class-specific antibodies to *Yersinia* plasmid-encoded outer proteins in patients with HT compared to healthy blood donors and those with non-postinfectious rheumatic disorders.[92]

A Japanese study found that antibodies to serotype 5, but not serotype 3, were significantly higher in HT ($p < 0.001$ vs. controls) and that a significantly increased incidence of antibodies to serotypes 6 and 9 was seen only in patients with HT.[93] This was not confirmed by a Canadian study, which found no significant difference in the serological reactivity to serotypes 3 and 9 of *Yersinia* in patients with AITD versus controls.[23] A more recent prospective study, including 790 euthyroid women who were relatives of patients with AITD, found no causal relationship between *Yersinia* infection and the development of autoimmune thyroiditis in a 5-year follow-up.[25] Furthermore, looking at twin pairs discordant for TAbs, Hansen et al. showed that YE antibodies did not confer an increase risk of thyroid autoimmunity.[94]

3.5 Helicobacter pylori

Helicobacter pylori is another infectious agent purported to be involved in the development of HT. De Luis and co-workers determined that the prevalence of *H. pylori* infection was markedly increased in patients with HT (85.7%) compared with the controls with nontoxic multi-nodular goiter (40%), and patients with Addison's disease (45.4%). Furthermore, a positive linear regression was found between levels of anti-TPO antibodies and anti-*H. pylori* IgG in patients with HT ($n = 21$; $r = 0.79$; $p < 0.01$), and anti-*H. pylori* IgG levels were higher in patients with HT than controls.[95] Figura et al. found that the prevalence of CagA-positive *H. pylori* was significantly higher in patients with AITD (56%) compared to controls (24.2%) ($p < 0.01$).[96] Furthermore, the prevalence of seropositivity was reported higher in 90 children with AITD compared to 70 age- and sex-matched controls ($p < 0.05$), and a similar tendency was observed in a group of patients with Turner syndrome.[97] Another study showed a different distribution of *H. pylori* antibodies: 39% IgA positive and 13% CagA positive in patients with AITD vs. 7% and 20%, respectively, in controls.[98] Tomasi et al. included 302 patients who underwent gastroscopy for dyspeptic symptoms. No association was reported between serpositivity for *H. pylori* and positive TAbs.[99]

3.6 Enterovirus and HT

Enteroviral infection has been reported to be associated with a number of autoimmune diseases; however, a clear relationship with autoimmune thyroiditis is still unclear. Desailloud et al. detected enterovirus RNA by PCR in 25% of thyroid tissue from an unselected group of patients who underwent thyroidectomy.[100] However, no relationship was observed between enterovirus RNA and autoimmune thyroiditis. The frequency of detection of enteroviral RNA by *in situ* hybridization and capsid protein VP1 by immunohistochemistry in thyroid tissue from 46 patients with newly diagnosed HT showed no significant difference with 24 controls.[101] The authors also reported pronounced tissue destruction, lymphocyte infiltration and increased expression of MxA1 (a surrogate marker for the *in situ* production of IFN) and concluded that the disease had started much earlier and the triggering factors might have been cleared.

4 MECHANISMS OF INDUCTION OF AUTOIMMUNITY BY INFECTIOUS AGENTS

The central feature of the immune system is specificity. The specificity of the immune response is maintained by complex mechanisms, which include the unique structures of secreted and non-secreted antigen receptors on lymphocytes and the elaborate interactions that occur between cells involved in the immune response. Together they form an interconnecting regulatory network that controls immune reactions. Infectious agents may induce autoimmunity by influencing any of the stages of the immune response, namely, the encounter with an antigen, the recognition of an antigen as non-self, the activation of the various effector arms of the immune system and the regulation of the immune response.

4.1 Viral-Induced Changes in Self-Antigen Expression

Viral infection may theoretically (1) alter self-antigens, (2) lead to the virus becoming a persistent endogenous antigen, or (3) cause the revelation of previously non-exposed, or rarely exposed, antigens. Alterations in normal body components can develop during infections as a result of the release of bacterial or viral products, expression of viral antigens on host cells, or tissue injury caused by the accompanying inflammatory reaction.[102] For example, it has been shown that Coxsackie virus B4 infection produces diabetes in mice by inducing increased expression of a 64,000-M islet autoantigen in infected mice.[103] This autoantigen is believed to be the primary target protein in the anti-beta cell autoimmune reaction that characterizes the insulitis of type 1 diabetes mellitus.[104] Further evidence that viral-induced modification of self-antigens may cause autoimmune disease comes from a study by Whittingham et al. in which a patient developed Sjögren's syndrome after protracted infectious mononucleosis.[105] The authors were able to show that the autoimmune reaction developed as a consequence of the association of viral RNA with the La nucleoprotein, resulting in a break in immunologic tolerance and induction of anti-SSB antibodies, leading to autoimmune sialoadenitis. The mechanism of altered self-antigens has not been reported to operate in thyroid autoimmunity. However, one observation of interest is the finding of GD and Graves' ophthalmopathy in patients who received external radiation over the thyroid region. The radiation may have altered thyroid antigens or their expression, thereby inducing an autoimmune reaction.[106] However, it cannot be ruled out that the development of GD in these patients was a consequence of immune dysregulation induced by irradiation of the thymic region.

Persistent expression of viral antigens on host cells is another mechanism by which an infecting organism, mainly viruses, may alter self constituents and induce autoimmunity. This phenomenon has been shown to occur in infections with endogenous retroviruses. Adams et al.[107] reported that if endogenous retroviral expression does not develop neonatally and is delayed until adulthood, then an autoimmune reaction ensues. As discussed earlier, endogenous retroviral protein expression has been reported in autoimmune thyroid disease[34,44,55] and in Sjögren's syndrome,[108–110] and it has been shown that when transgenic mice expressing LCMV antigens in pancreatic beta cells are challenged with LCMV they produce lymphocytic infiltrates in their beta cells and develop signs of IDDM.[111,112]

In addition, antigens not normally exposed to the immune circuit may become significant antigens for the first time. This may be important in viral-induced murine encephalitis and cardiac myositis and in the formation of sperm antibodies after vasectomy.[113,114]

4.2 Molecular Mimicry

Molecular mimicry is defined as structural similarity between antigens coded by different genes. Molecular mimicry has long been implicated as a mechanism by which microbes can induce autoimmunity.[115] The best known example is rheumatic fever, in which antigenic cross-reactivity between cardiac tissue and streptococcal polysaccharides is believed to induce an autoimmune reaction targeted at the heart valves.[116,117] Antigenic similarity between infectious agents and host cell proteins is common, and in one analysis of 600 monoclonal antibodies raised against a large variety of viruses, it was found that 4% of the monoclonal antibodies cross-reacted with host determinants expressed in uninfected tissues.[118] The clinical importance of molecular mimicry between mycobacteria and self-antigen was highlighted by the observation that patients treated with BCG immunotherapy developed arthritis.[119] Furthermore, anti–DNA antibodies were shown to have amino acid sequence homology with anti-*Klebsiella pneumonia* Waldenström monoclonal antibody, and when normal PBMCs were stimulated with *Klebsiella* antigens, they secreted a common anti-DNA (16/6) idiotype.[120] The 16/6 idiotype also has been found in the serum of patients with the parasitic infections filariasis and schistosomiasis.[121]

Mice infected with reovirus type 1 developed an autoimmune polyendocrinopathy and generated a panel of autoantibodies directed against normal pancreas, pituitary, and gastric mucosa, suggesting an antigenic similarity between a reoviral antigen and an endocrine tissue antigen.[122,123] Serreze and colleagues[124] reported that antibodies directed against the p73 antigen, an endogenous retroviral gene product, are cross-reactive with anti–insulin antibodies. The authors suggested that anti-p73 autoantibodies are involved in inducing beta cell destruction in NOD mice. Likewise, Talal et al. demonstrated that 22 of 61 patients with SLE produced antibodies to the p24 gag protein of HIV-1.[125] Moreover, Sm (a ribonucleoprotein involved in the generation of mRNA) was shown to partially inhibit the antibody binding of the p24 gag protein, suggesting immunologic cross-reactivity between the p24 gag protein and the Sm autoantigen.[115]

Homology between microbial and host tissue antigens does not necessarily mean that an autoimmune response will emerge upon infection with that microbe. To prove that a sequence homology leads to autoimmunity, it is necessary to show that challenging the host with the microbial antigen leads to an autoimmune response unrelated to direct infection of the target tissues. An example of such an experiment was provided by Fujinami and Oldstone. They used myelin basic protein, which has been shown to have significant homology with several viral proteins including hepatitis B virus polymerase.[126] When the authors injected a hepatitis B virus polymerase derived peptide into rabbits, the animals developed lesions in the central nervous system similar to the autoimmune disease induced by injection of myelin basic protein.[126]

As discussed earlier, molecular mimicry was reported between YE and the TSH.[15,17] Moreover, a saturable binding site for TSH was demonstrated on YE.[26] Wolf and co-workers demonstrated that IgG of individuals convalescing from *Yersinia* infections produced concentration-dependent inhibition of TSH binding to thyroid membranes,[33] perhaps as a consequence of cross-reactivity between antigenic determinants on YE and the TSH receptor. Hargreaves et al. recently provided a mechanistic framework for molecular mimicry in GD in which early precursor B cells are expanded by YE porins to undergo somatic hypermutation to acquire a cross-reactive pathogenic response to TSHR.[127]

Another finding suggesting a possible role for molecular mimicry in AITD was that 42% of sera from patients with lepromatous leprosy contained anti-thyroglobulin antibodies compared to 3% of sera from the controls.[128] Molecular mimicry also has been suggested between retroviral sequences and the TSH receptor;[48] however, these findings remain to be confirmed.

4.3 Alterations in the Idiotypic Network

As first envisioned by Jerne,[129] auto-anti-idiotypic antibodies are generated in the course of the normal immune response to a foreign invading pathogen and serve to regulate the normal immune response. Anti-idiotypic antibodies produced during the primary immune response carry the internal image of the epitopes on the pathogen, which bind to its receptor in the host. Consequently, the development of receptor-binding anti-idiotypes can be harmful to the host and initiate autoimmunity.[130] Williams and co-workers were able to produce a monoclonal antibody (called 9BG5) in BALB/c mice that could strongly bind to reovirus type 3 and neutralize its infectivity. Moreover, an anti-idiotype monoclonal antibody that was found to bind to 9BG5 and inhibit its interaction with HA3 was produced. The same authors then demonstrated that the anti-idiotype bore the internal image of the receptor-binding epitope on reovirus type 3; this anti-idiotype could induce changes in cells upon binding to their HA3 receptors, similar to those induced by the virus itself.[131] Therefore, the damage caused by certain viruses does not involve their direct effect on target cells but rather an immunologic attack by anti-idiotypic antibodies on viral receptors. There are now reports supporting the notion that anti-idiotypes bearing internal images of viral antigens participate in the induction of several autoimmune diseases (reviewed in Ref. 130). Myasthenia gravis developed in five individuals a few weeks after rabies virus vaccination. The rabies virus has been shown to bind to acetyl-choline receptor;[132] therefore, it is possible that the antiviral response induced anti-idiotypic antibodies that also acted as anti-receptor antibodies and bound to the acetyl-choline receptor, thus inducing an autoimmune disease.

Alterations in the idiotypic network have been implicated in the pathogenesis of GD based on the findings that the immunization of animals with

TSH led to the development of anti-idiotypic antibodies that recognized and activated the TSH receptor.[133] Moreover, we were able to induce experimental autoimmune thyroiditis in mice (a model of human autoimmune thyroiditis) by immunizing them with anti-thyroglobulin antibodies, which induced an anti-idiotypic reaction.[134]

4.4 Immune Complex Formation

Antigens produced by an infectious organism can form immune complexes with antibodies generated against them, thus leading to the development of autoimmunity. The best known example of this phenomenon is immune thrombocytopenia that follows viral infection. The virus triggers the production of antibodies that can form immune complexes with the viral antigens. The immune complexes then attach to platelets, which are damaged as innocent bystanders.[102]

Immune complex formation also has been implicated in the pathogenesis of certain parasitic diseases (for a review see Ref. 135). In patients with malaria the development of nephrotic syndrome has been associated with the deposition of immune complexes in the renal glomeruli.[135] Similarly, immune complex deposition has been implicated in the pathogenesis of glomerulonephritis associated with schistosomiasis, and circulating immune complexes also were found in patients with leishmaniasis.[135] Immune complexes have been well documented in AITDs,[136–139] and there are reports of glomerulonephritis and immune complex deposition with thyroglobulin antigen recognized within the complexes.[140] However, whether these immune complexes are induced by infection remains to be shown.

4.5 Heat Shock Proteins and Thyroid Autoimmunity

Cells in different organisms respond to elevated temperatures by synthesizing new proteins called heat shock proteins (HSPs). HSP synthesis can also be induced by other stressful stimuli, including exposure to oxidative radicals, alcohol or heavy metals, anoxia and infection.[141] Since HSPs are highly conserved among different species and are widespread in bacterial cells, it is believed that they carry vital cellular functions during stress and in resting conditions (reviewed in Ref. 142); therefore, HSPs are produced in small quantities under normal conditions. By interacting with other intracellular proteins and altering their folding and unfolding, HSPs serve four vital cellular functions: (1) HSPs assist in the assembly of polypeptides into their final tertiary structures,[143] (2) HSPs assist in the intracellular transport of other proteins by maintaining them in a conformation suitable for transport into cellular organelles (e.g. mitochondria),[144] (3) HSPs can bind and temporarily inactivate other proteins such as the steroid receptor,[145] and (4) HSPs participate in protein degradation.[142]

HSPs have been shown to be strongly immunogenic, and in view of their high degree of conservation between different species and their presence in many infectious agents, they may be involved in the induction of autoimmune diseases. During the course of a bacterial infection, an antibody and T-cell response to the microbe's HSPs is induced. These antibodies and T cells may then cross-react with self-HSPs containing conserved epitopes. Moreover, the stress of the infection itself and the inflammation accompanying it may generate increased synthesis of self-HSPs, thereby enhancing the autoimmune response.[146] Production of self-HSPs can also be induced by a concomitant viral infection. Increased levels of anti-HSP antibodies have been reported in SLE[147] and rheumatoid arthritis.[148]

Recent studies have suggested a role for HSPs in the pathogenesis of type 1 diabetes mellitus. Cohen and co-workers demonstrated that a pancreatic beta cell target antigen in OD mice is a molecule that is cross-reactive with HSP65 of *Mycobacterium tuberculosis*. The authors showed that the onset of beta cell destruction was associated with spontaneous development of anti-HSP65 T lymphocytes and antibodies.[149] Only a few studies have examined the possible association of HSPs with AITDs, although this is an active area of investigation. Ratanachaiyavong et al. reported an association between GD and a specific RFLP of the HSP70 gene.[150] In addition, HSP72 was demonstrated in thyroid specimens from patients with GD and HT but not in controls.[151] Heufelder et al.[152] reported increased surface expression of a 72-kDa HSP in retro-ocular and pretibial fibroblasts from patients with GD with severe ophthalmopathy and pretibial myxedema but not in fibroblasts from unaffected sites from the same patients and controls. Moreover, the same group suggested that in patients with GD, IgG enhanced HSP72 expression in cultured retroorbital fibroblasts in a dose-dependent manner.[153] In contrast, Sztankay et al. demonstrated that culture thyroid endothelial cells from patients with GD express the same amount of HSP72 than thyroid cells from controls. IFN-γ increased the expression of HSP72 under basal culture conditions and after heat shock treatment.[154] The authors concluded that environmental and local factors may facilitate the induction of HSP72. Furthermore, enhanced staining for HSP60 was demonstrated in oncocytes (eosinophilic cells with an increased number of mitochondria) in thyroid and adrenal autoimmune diseases as well as in unrelated conditions where oncocytes were identified.[155]

These studies imply that AITD is associated with an autoimmune response to certain HSPs. However, it is possible that self-HSP production is not the primary event triggering autoimmunity, but a secondary response to the tissue damage induced by the autoimmune process itself. Their role in etiology, however, requires clarification.

4.6 Induction of MHC Antigens on Non-Immune Cells

Infection can lead to an autoimmune reaction associated with the expression of MHC antigens on non-immune cells. As proposed by Bottazzo et al.,[156] a local viral infection may cause the production of IFN-γ or other cytokines in the target organ, which in turn induce HLA class II molecule expression for the first time in non-immune cells (e.g. epithelial cells); this can lead to presentation of autoantigens and activation of autoreactive T cells. Indeed, expression of HLA-DR antigens by thyroid epithelial cells has been demonstrated in thyroids from patients with AITD but was absent in normal tissues.[157] The mechanisms leading to this unusual expression of MHC class II molecules in thyroid cells have been investigated (for a review see Ref. 158 Rat and human thyroid cells can be induced to express MHC class II antigens by recombinant IFN-γ, TNF α and TSH itself.[159] Neufeld et al. demonstrated that cultured rat thyroid cells (derived from a rat thyroid cell line) infected with reovirus types 1 and 3 were induced to express MHC class II antigens in a dose-dependent manner.[160] Furthermore, a viral thyroiditis caused by infecting either the thyroid or the immune cells was demonstrated in an avian model, as discussed earlier.[161] Thyroid follicular epithelial cells bearing MHC class II determinants were shown to be able to present pre-processed viral peptide antigens to cloned human T cells,[162] but unfortunately the thyroid cells used contained other potential antigen-presenting cells. Further evidence, however, came from studies in which thyroid-reactive T-cell clones were specifically reactive to cloned autologous thyroid cells in the total absence of antigen-presenting cells.[163] Moreover, Kawakami et al. showed that *in vivo* induction of MHC class II molecules on thyrocytes by IFN-γ can induce autoimmune thyroiditis in mice.[164]

Viruses can also induce the expression of MHC class II molecules independent of cytokine secretion. Massa et al. showed that a neurotropic murine hepatitis virus can directly induce the expression of La antigen on astrocytes in tissue culture and not through release of cytokines.[165]

Retroviruses also have been shown to enhance MHC class I molecule expression.[166] However, there are reports showing reduced expression of MHC molecules by cells infected *in vitro* with some viruses.[167–169] It has been reported that cytomegalovirus infection of primary cultures of thyroid cells resulted in the induction of HLA-DR expression on thyroid follicular cells.[170] These findings support the view that infection may induce MHC class II molecule expression on thyroid cells and that these cells may act as antigen-presenting cells and may be involved in the induction of AITDs.

4.7 Microbiome and Autoimmunity

Increasing attention has recently been given to the human microbiome and its role in the etiopathogenesis of autoimmunity in diseases such as arthritis, psoriasis and Crohn's disease (mechanisms are reviewed in Ref. 171). The gut, as a physical barrier, and its microbial flora is a primary site of interaction between microorganisms and the immune system. The co-existence of gut inflammation and thyroid autoimmunity has been reported. Cindoruk and co-workers reported that 20 of 50 patients with HT had histologic findings consistent with lymphocytic colitis, compared to 1 of 22 control subjects.[172] Impaired intestinal morphology and function also is reported in autoimmune thyroiditis.[173] However, at this time, little information is available regarding gut microbial composition in patients with AITD.

4.8 Epigenetic Interactions in AITD

The way in which environmental triggers interact with susceptibility genes to cause disease is still not clear. It recently became apparent that environmental agents can interact with susceptibility genes through epigenetic modulation. While the exact definition of epigenetics is somewhat controversial, we define epigenetic effects as effects on gene expression and regulation that are not coded in the DNA sequence and are mitotically stable, that is, long lasting. Epigenetic effects include regulation of gene expression by DNA methylation, histone modifications, and micro-RNA interactions.[174,175] In several autoimmune diseases such as rheumatoid arthritis,[176] epigenetic changes have been shown to be important in the pathogenesis of the disease. Similarly, epigenetic alterations are likely to be critical to the role of infection in triggering AITDs.[177] Indeed, recent data from our laboratory suggest that IFN-α (which is a key cytokine secreted during viral infections) can epigenetically modify the promoter of the thyroglobulin gene by interacting with a susceptibility gene variant.[178] Therefore, it is plausible that viral infectious agents can trigger AITD by epigenetically modifying the expression or function of key genes in the thyroid.

5 CONCLUSION

The paradigm that infection may trigger autoimmunity is old, however, most data supporting this paradigm is indirect. The literature examined in this review points to the possibility of the involvement of bacterial and viral agents in the pathogenesis of GD and HT. Various mechanisms have been proposed to explain the induction of autoimmunity by infection, but it seems that two possibilities may be important to thyroid autoimmunity, namely molecular mimicry and the induction of MHC class II antigens. However, the association between AITD and infections may be merely coincidental and not etiological. To address this question, more studies using direct approaches (e.g. isolation of the infecting organisms from thyroids of patients with AITD and induction of AITD in experimental animals by viruses) are needed. However, it should be remembered that there is a latent period between exposure to infectious agents and clinically apparent autoimmune disease, making it difficult to identify triggering infectious agents.

ACKNOWLEDGMENTS

This work was supported in part by National Institutes of Health Grants DK61659, DK067555, and DK073681; The Department of Veterans Affairs, Veterans Health Administration; and The Unger Vetlesen Fund.

REFERENCES

1. Davies TF. Graves' diseases: pathogenesis. In: Braverman LE, Utiger RD, editors. *Werner and Ingbar's the thyroid: a fundamental and clinical text.* Philadelphia: Lippincott Williams & Wilkens; 2000. p. 518–30.
2. Weetman AP. Autoimmune thyroiditis: predisposition and pathogenesis. *Clin Endocrinol (Oxf)* 1992;**36**:307–23.
3. McDougall IR. Graves' disease. Current concepts. *Med Clin North Am* 1991;**75**:79–95.
4. Cox SP, Phillips DI, Osmond C. Does infection initiate Graves disease? A population based 10 year study. *Autoimmunity* 1989;**4**:43–9.
5. Phillips DI, Barker DJ, Rees SB, Didcote S, Morgan D. The geographical distribution of thyrotoxicosis in England according to the presence or absence of TSH-receptor antibodies. *Clin Endocrinol (Oxf)* 1985;**23**:283–7.

6. Collier A, Patrick AW, Toft AD, Blackwell CC, James V, Weir DM. Increased prevalence of non-secretors in patients with Graves' disease: evidence for an infective aetiology? *Br Med J (Clin Res Ed)* 1988;**296**:1162.

7. Toft AD, Blackwell CC, Saadi AT, Wu P, Lymberi P, Soudjidelli M, et al. Secretor status and infection in patients with Graves' disease. *Autoimmunity* 1990;**7**:279–89.

8. Blackwell CC, Collier A, Patrick AW, James V, Weir DM, Toft AD. Secretor state in autoimmune thyroid disease. *J Endocrinol* 1988;**117**(Suppl. 1):282.

9. Valtonen VV, Ruutu P, Varis K, Ranki M, Malkamaki M, Makela PH. Serological evidence for the role of bacterial infections in the pathogenesis of thyroid diseases. *Acta Med Scand* 1986;**219**:105–11.

10. Joasoo A, Robertson P, Murray IP. Letter: viral antibodies in thyrotoxicosis. *Lancet* 1975;**2**:125.

11. Benvenga S, Santarpia L, Trimarchi F, Guarneri F. Human thyroid autoantigens and proteins of Yersinia and Borrelia share amino acid sequence homology that includes binding motifs to HLA-DR molecules and T-cell receptor. *Thyroid* 2006;**16**:225–36.

12. Byfield PGH, Copping S, David SC, Barclay FE, Borriello SP. Interactions of TSH and Graves' IgG with bacterial binding proteins. *J Endocrinol* 1988;**117**(Suppl. 1):283.

13. Laitinen O, Leirisalo M, Skylv G. Relation between HLA-B27 and clinical features in patients with yersinia arthritis. *Arthritis Rheum* 1977;**20**:1121–4.

14. Lidman K, Eriksson U, Norberg R, Fagraeus A. Indirect immunofluorescence staining of human thyroid by antibodies occurring in *Yersinia enterocolitica* infections. *Clin Exp Immunol* 1976;**23**:429–35.

15. Gripenberg M, Miettinen A, Kurki P, Linder E. Humoral immune stimulation and anti-epithelial antibodies in Yersinia infection. *Arthritis Rheum* 1978;**21**:904–8.

16. Tomer Y, Shoenfeld Y. The significance of natural autoantibodies. *Immunol Invest* 1988;**17**:389–424.

17. Shenkman L, Bottone EJ. Antibodies to Yersinia enterocolitica in thyroid disease. *Ann Intern Med* 1976;**85**:735–9.

18. Ingbar SH, Weiss M, Cushing GW, Kasper DL. A possible role for bacterial antigens in the pathogenesis of autoimmune thyroid disease. In: Pinchera A, Ingbar SH, McKenzie JM, Fenzi GF, editors. *Thyroid autoimmunity*. New York: Plenum Press; 1987. p. 35–44.

19. Wenzel BE, Heesemann J, Wenzel KW, Scriba PC. Antibodies to plasmid-encoded proteins of enteropathogenic Yersinia in patients with autoimmune thyroid disease. *Lancet* 1988;**1**:56.

20. Arscott P, Rosen ED, Koenig RJ, Kaplan MM, Ellis T, Thompson N, et al. Immunoreactivity to Yersinia enterocolitica antigens in patients with autoimmune thyroid disease. *J Clin Endocrinol Metab* 1992;**75**:295–300.

21. Corapcioglu D, Tonyukuk V, Kiyan M, Yilmaz AE, Emral R, Kamel N, et al. Relationship between thyroid autoimmunity and Yersinia enterocolitica antibodies. *Thyroid* 2002;**12**:613–17.

22. Brix TH, Hansen PS, Hegedus L, Wenzel BE. Too early to dismiss Yersinia enterocolitica infection in the aetiology of Graves' disease: evidence from a twin case-control study. *Clin Endocrinol (Oxf)* 2008;**69**:491–6.

23. Resetkova E, Notenboom R, Arreaza G, Mukuta T, Yoshikawa N, Volpe R. Seroreactivity to bacterial antigens is not a unique phenomenon in patients with autoimmune thyroid diseases in Canada. *Thyroid* 1994;**4**:269–74.

24. Strieder TG, Wenzel BE, Prummel MF, Tijssen JG, Wiersinga WM. Increased prevalence of antibodies to enteropathogenic Yersinia enterocolitica virulence proteins in relatives of patients with autoimmune thyroid disease. *Clin Exp Immunol* 2003;**132**:278–82.

25. Effraimidis G, Tijssen JG, Strieder TG, Wiersinga WM. No causal relationship between Yersinia enterocolitica infection and autoimmune thyroid disease: evidence from a prospective study. *Clin Exp Immunol* 2011;**165**:38–43.

26. Weiss M, Ingbar SH, Winblad S, Kasper DL. Demonstration of a saturable binding site for thyrotropin in Yersinia enterocolitica. *Science* 1983;**219**:1331–3.
27. Heyma P, Harrison LC, Robins-Browne R. Thyrotrophin (TSH) binding sites on Yersinia enterocolitica recognized by immunoglobulins from humans with Graves' disease. *Clin Exp Immunol* 1986;**64**:249–54.
28. Thyroid disease and antibodies to Yersinia. *Lancet* 1977;**1**:734-5.
29. Burman KD, Lukes YGGP. Molecular homology between the human TSH receptor and Yersinia enterocolitica (abstract). *Thyroid* 1991;**1**(Suppl. 1):S62.
30. Bech K, Clemmensen O, Larsen JH, Bendixen G. Thyroid disease and Yersinia. *Lancet* 1977;**1**:1060–1.
31. Toivanen A, Granfors K, Lahesmaa-Rantala R, Leino R, Stahlberg T, Vuento R. Pathogenesis of Yersinia-triggered reactive arthritis: immunological, microbiological and clinical aspects. *Immunol Rev* 1985;**86**:47–70.
32. Ebner S, Alex S. KTAMHJWB. Immunization with Yersinia enterocolitica purifies outer membrane protein induces lymphocytic thyroiditis in the BB/WOR rat (abstract). *Thyroid* 1991;**1**(Suppl):S28.
33. Wolf MW, Misaki T, Bech K, Tvede M, Silva JE, Ingbar SH. Immunoglobulins of patients recovering from Yersinia enterocolitica infections exhibit Graves' disease-like activity in human thyroid membranes. *Thyroid* 1991;**1**:315–20.
34. Kraemer MH, Donadi EA, Tambascia MA, Magna LA, Prigenzi LS. Relationship between HLA antigens and infectious agents in contributing towards the development of Graves' disease. *Immunol Invest* 1998;**27**:17–29.
35. Witso E, Cinek O, Tapia G, Rasmussen T, Stene LC, Ronningen KS. HLA-DRB1-DQA1-DQB1 genotype and frequency of enterovirus in longitudinal monthly fecal samples from healthy infants. *Viral Immunol* 2012;**25**:187–92.
36. Pichler R, Maschek W, Hatzl-Griesenhofer M, Huber H, Luger C, Binder L, et al. Enterovirus infection—a possible trigger for Graves' disease? *Wien Klin Wochenschr* 2001;**113**:204–7.
37. Hammerstad SS, Tauriainen S, Hyoty H, Paulsen T, Norheim I, Dahl-Jorgensen K. Detection of enterovirus in the thyroid tissue of patients with Graves' disease. *J Med Virol* 2013;**85**:512–18.
38. Ciampolillo A, Marini V, Mirakian R, Buscema M, Schulz T, Pujol-Borrell R, et al. Retrovirus-like sequences in Graves' disease: implications for human autoimmunity. *Lancet* 1989;**1**:1096–100.
39. Wick G, Grubeck-Loebenstein B, Trieb K, Kalischnig G, Aguzzi A. Human foamy virus antigens in thyroid tissue of Graves' disease patients. *Int Arch Allergy Immunol* 1992;**99**:153–6.
40. Lagaye S, Vexiau P, Morozov V, Guenebaut-Claudet V, Tobaly-Tapiero J, Canivet M, et al. Human spumaretrovirus-related sequences in the DNA of leukocytes from patients with Graves' disease. *Proc Natl Acad Sci USA* 1992;**89**:10070–4.
41. Schweizer M, Turek R, Reinhardt M, Neumann-Haefelin D. Absence of foamy virus DNA in Graves' disease. *AIDS Res Hum Retroviruses* 1994;**10**:601–5.
42. Heneine W, Musey VC, Sinha SD, Landay A, Northrup G, Khabbaz R, et al. Absence of evidence for human spumaretrovirus sequences in patients with Graves' disease. *J Acquir Immune Defic Syndr Hum Retrovirol* 1995;**9**:99–101.
43. Mahnke C, Kashaiya P, Rossler J, Bannert H, Levin A, Blattner WA, et al. Human spumavirus antibodies in sera from African patients. *Arch Virol* 1992;**123**:243–53.
44. Yanagawa T, Ito K, Kaplan EL, Ishikawa N, DeGroot LJ. Absence of association between human spumaretrovirus and Graves' disease. *Thyroid* 1995;**5**:379–82.
45. Lee H, Kim S, Kang M, Kim W, Cho B. Prevalence of human foamy virus-related sequences in the Korean population. *J Biomed Sci* 1998;**5**:267–73.
46. Humphrey M, Mosca J, Baker Jr. JR, Drabick JJ, Carr FE, Burke DS, et al. Absence of retroviral sequences in Graves' disease. *Lancet* 1991;**337**:17–18.

47. Tominaga T, Katamine S, Namba H, Yokoyama N, Nakamura S, Morita S, et al. Lack of evidence for the presence of human immunodeficiency virus type 1-related sequences in patients with Graves' disease. *Thyroid* 1991;**1**:307–14.

48. Burch HB, Nagy EV, Lukes YG, Cai WY, Wartofsky L, Burman KD. Nucleotide and amino acid homology between the human thyrotropin receptor and the HIV-1 Nef protein: identification and functional analysis. *Biochem Biophys Res Commun* 1991;**181**:498–505.

49. Nagasaka A, Nakai A, Oda N, Kotake M, Iwase K, Yoshida S. Reverse transcriptase is elevated in the thyroid tissue from Graves' disease patients. *Clin Endocrinol (Oxf)* 2000;**53**:155–9.

50. Tas M, de Haan-Meulman M, Kabel PJ, Drexhage HA. Defects in monocyte polarization and dendritic cell clustering in patients with Graves' disease. A putative role for a non-specific immunoregulatory factor related to retroviral p15E. *Clin Endocrinol (Oxf)* 1991;**34**:441–8.

51. Tas M, de Haan-Meulman M, Drexhage HA. An immunosuppressive factor shring homology with the p15E protein leukomogenic retroviruses is present in the serum of patients with Grave's disease. In: Scherbaum WA, Bogner U, Weinheimer B, Botazzo GF, editors. *Autoimmune thyroiditis. Approaches towards its etiological differentiation*. Berlin: Springer-Verlag; 1991. p. 197–202.

52. Jaspan JB, Luo H, Ahmed B, Tenenbaum S, Voss T, Sander DM, et al. Evidence for a retroviral trigger in Graves' disease. *Autoimmunity* 1995;**20**:135–42.

53. Jaspan JB, Sullivan K, Garry RF, Lopez M, Wolfe M, Clejan S, et al. The interaction of a type A retroviral particle and class II human leukocyte antigen susceptibility genes in the pathogenesis of Graves' disease. *J Clin Endocrinol Metab* 1996;**81**:2271–9.

54. Deas JE, Thompson JJ, Fermin CD, Liu LL, Martin D, Garry RF, et al. Viral induction, transmission and apoptosis among cells infected by a human intracisternal A-type retrovirus. *Virus Res* 1999;**61**:19–27.

55. Fierabracci A, Upton CP, Hajibagheri N, Bottazzo GF. Lack of detection of retroviral particles (HIAP-1) in the H9 T cell line co-cultured with thyrocytes of Graves' disease. *J Autoimmun* 2001;**16**:457–62.

56. Yokoi K, Kawai H, Akaike M, Mine H, Saito S. Presence of human T-lymphotropic virus type II-related genes in DNA of peripheral leukocytes from patients with autoimmune thyroid diseases. *J Med Virol* 1995;**45**:392–8.

57. Mizokami T, Okamura K, Ikenoue H, Sato K, Kuroda T, Maeda Y, et al. A high prevalence of human T-lymphotropic virus type I carriers in patients with antithyroid antibodies. *Thyroid* 1994;**4**:415–9.

58. Burch HB, Nagy E, Cai WY, Wartofsky L, Carr FE. Investigation of functional homology between the HIV-1 nef protein and the human thyrotropin receptor (hTSH-R) (abstract). *Thyroid* 1991;**1**(Suppl. 1):S-65.

59. Tonooka N, Leslie GA, Greer MA, Olson JC. Lymphoid thyroiditis following immunization with group A streptococcal vaccine. *Am J Pathol* 1978;**92**:681–90.

60. Drabick JJ, Horning VL, Lennox JL, Coyne PE, Oster CN, Knight RD, et al. A retrospective analysis of diseases associated with indeterminate HIV western blot patterns. *Mil Med* 1991;**156**:93–6.

61. Volpe R. Pathogenesis of autoimmune thyroid disease. In: Ingbar SH, Braverman LE, editors. *The thyroid: a fundamental and clinical text*. Philadelphia: JB Lippincott Co.; 1986.

62. Wenzel BE, Gutekunst R, Heesemann J. Hashimoto's thyroiditis and enterpathogenic *Yersinia enterocolitica*. In: Scherbaum WA, Weinheimer B, Bogner U, Botazzo GF, editors. *Autoimmune thyroiditis. Approaches towards its etiological differentiation*. Berlin: Springer-Verlag; 1991. p. 205–10.

63. Katzin WE, Fishleder AJ, Tubbs RR. Investigation of the clonality of lymphocytes in Hashimoto's thyroiditis using immunoglobulin and T-cell receptor gene probes. *Clin Immunol Immunopathol* 1989;**51**:264–74.

64. May P, Kawanishi H. Chronic hepatitis B infection and autoimmune thyroiditis in Down syndrome. *J Clin Gastroenterol* 1996;**23**:181–4.

65. Antonelli A, Ferri C, Pampana A, Fallahi P, Nesti C, Pasquini M, et al. Thyroid disorders in chronic hepatitis C. *Am J Med* 2004;**117**:10–13.

66. Huang MJ, Tsai SL, Huang BY, Sheen IS, Yeh CT, Liaw YF. Prevalence and significance of thyroid autoantibodies in patients with chronic hepatitis C virus infection: a prospective controlled study. *Clin Endocrinol (Oxf)* 1999;**50**:503–9.

67. Loviselli A, Oppo A, Velluzzi F, Atzeni F, Mastinu GL, Farci P, et al. Independent expression of serological markers of thyroid autoimmunity and hepatitis virus C infection in the general population: results of a community-based study in north-western Sardinia. *J Endocrinol Invest* 1999;**22**:660–5.

68. Metcalfe RA, Ball G, Kudesia G, Weetman AP. Failure to find an association between hepatitis C virus and thyroid autoimmunity. *Thyroid* 1997;**7**:421–4.

69. Boadas J, Rodriguez-Espinosa J, Enriquez J, Miralles F, Martinez-Cerezo FJ, Gonzalez P, et al. Prevalence of thyroid autoantibodies is not increased in blood donors with hepatitis C virus infection. *J Hepatol* 1995;**22**:611–15.

70. Blot E, Kerleau JM, Levesque H, Heron F, Menard JF, Buffet-Janvresse C, et al. Does hepatitis c virus-related autoimmune thyroiditis exist? Reflections on a controlled study of 58 consecutive subjects. *Rev Med Interne* 1999;**20**:220–5.

71. Nduwayo L, Bacq Y, Valat C, Goudeau A, Lecomte P. Thyroid function and autoimmunity in 215 patients seropositive for the hepatitis C virus. *Ann Endocrinol (Paris)* 1998;**59**:9–13.

72. Ganne-Carrie N, Medini A, Coderc E, Seror O, Christidis C, Grimbert S, et al. Latent autoimmune thyroiditis in untreated patients with HCV chronic hepatitis: a case-control study. *J Autoimmun* 2000;**14**:189–93.

73. Tran A, Quaranta JF, Benzaken S, Thiers V, Chau HT, Hastier P, et al. High prevalence of thyroid autoantibodies in a prospective series of patients with chronic hepatitis C before interferon therapy. *Hepatology* 1993;**18**:253–7.

74. Pateron D, Hartmann DJ, Duclos-Vallee JC, Jouanolle H, Beaugrand M. Latent autoimmune thyroid disease in patients with chronic HCV hepatitis. *J Hepatol* 1992;**16**:244–5.

75. Fernandez-Soto L, Gonzalez A, Escobar-Jimenez F, Vazquez R, Ocete E, Olea N, et al. Increased risk of autoimmune thyroid disease in hepatitis C vs hepatitis B before, during, and after discontinuing interferon therapy. *Arch Intern Med* 1998;**158**:1445–8.

76. Preziati D, La RL, Covini G, Marcelli R, Rescalli S, Persani L, et al. Autoimmunity and thyroid function in patients with chronic active hepatitis treated with recombinant interferon alpha-2a. *Eur J Endocrinol* 1995;**132**:587–93.

77. Deutsch M, Dourakis S, Manesis EK, Gioustozi A, Hess G, Horsch A, et al. Thyroid abnormalities in chronic viral hepatitis and their relationship to interferon alfa therapy. *Hepatology* 1997;**26**:206–10.

78. Custro N, Montalto G, Scafidi V, Soresi M, Gallo S, Tripi S, et al. Prospective study on thyroid autoimmunity and dysfunction related to chronic hepatitis C and interferon therapy. *J Endocrinol Invest* 1997;**20**:374–80.

79. Marazuela M, Garcia-Buey L, Gonzalez-Fernandez B, Garcia-Monzon C, Arranz A, Borque MJ, et al. Thyroid autoimmune disorders in patients with chronic hepatitis C before and during interferon-alpha therapy. *Clin Endocrinol (Oxf)* 1996;**44**:635–42.

80. Duclos-Vallee JC, Johanet C, Trinchet JC, Deny P, Laurent MF, Duron F, et al. High prevalence of serum antibodies to hepatitis C virus in patients with Hashimoto's thyroiditis. *BMJ* 1994;**309**:846–7.

81. Tran A, Quaranta JF, Beusnel C, Thiers V, De SM, Francois E, et al. Hepatitis C virus and Hashimoto's thyroiditis. *Eur J Med* 1992;**1**:116–18.

82. Wong S, Mehta AE, Faiman C, Berard L, Ibbott T, Minuk GY. Absence of serologic evidence for hepatitis C virus infection in patients with Hashimoto's thyroiditis. *Hepatogastroenterology* 1996;**43**:420–1.

83. Bartolome J, Rodriguez-Inigo E, Quadros P, Vidal S, Pascual-Miguelanez I, Rodriguez-Montes JA, et al. Detection of hepatitis C virus in thyroid tissue from patients with chronic HCV infection. *J Med Virol* 2008;**80**:1588–94.

84. Blackard JT, Kong L, Huber AK, Tomer Y. Hepatitis C virus infection of a thyroid cell line: implications for pathogenesis of hepatitis C virus and thyroiditis. *Thyroid* 2013;**23**:863–70.

85. Akeno N, Blackard JT, Tomer Y. HCV E2 protein binds directly to thyroid cells and induces IL-8 production: a new mechanism for HCV induced thyroid autoimmunity. *J Autoimmun* 2008;**31**:339–44.

86. Mammen JS, Ghazarian SR, Rosen A, Ladenson PW. Patterns of interferon-alpha-induced thyroid dysfunction vary with ethnicity, sex, smoking status, and pretreatment thyrotropin in an international cohort of patients treated for hepatitis C. *Thyroid* 2013;**23**:1151–8.

87. Kawai H, Mitsui T, Yokoi K, Akaike M, Hirose K, Hizawa K, et al. Evidence of HTLV-I in thyroid tissue in an HTLV-I carrier with Hashimoto's thyroiditis. *J Mol Med (Berl)* 1996;**74**:275–8.

88. Mine H, Kawai H, Yokoi K, Akaike M, Saito S. High frequencies of human T-lymphotropic virus type I (HTLV-I) infection and presence of HTLV-II proviral DNA in blood donors with anti-thyroid antibodies. *J Mol Med (Berl)* 1996;**74**:471–7.

89. Akamine H, Takasu N, Komiya I, Ishikawa K, Shinjyo T, Nakachi K, et al. Association of HTLV-I with autoimmune thyroiditis in patients with adult T-cell leukaemia (ATL) and in HTLV-I carriers. *Clin Endocrinol (Oxf)* 1996;**45**:461–6.

90. Matsuda T, Tomita M, Uchihara JN, Okudaira T, Ohshiro K, Tomoyose T, et al. Human T cell leukemia virus type I-infected patients with Hashimoto's thyroiditis and Graves' disease. *J Clin Endocrinol Metab* 2005;**90**:5704–10.

91. Tomoyose T, Komiya I, Takara M, Yabiku K, Kinjo Y, Shimajiri Y, et al. Cytotoxic T-lymphocyte antigen-4 gene polymorphisms and human T-cell lymphotrophic virus-1 infection: their associations with Hashimoto's thyroiditis in Japanese patients. *Thyroid* 2002;**12**:673–7.

92. Chatzipanagiotou S, Legakis JN, Boufidou F, Petroyianni V, Nicolaou C. Prevalence of Yersinia plasmid-encoded outer protein (Yop) class-specific antibodies in patients with Hashimoto's thyroiditis. *Clin Microbiol Infect* 2001;**7**:138–43.

93. Asari S, Amino N, Horikawa M, Miyai K. Incidences of antibodies to Yersinia enterocolitica: high incidence of serotype O5 in autoimmune thyroid diseases in Japan. *Endocrinol Jpn* 1989;**36**:381–6.

94. Hansen PS, Wenzel BE, Brix TH, Hegedus L. Yersinia enterocolitica infection does not confer an increased risk of thyroid antibodies: evidence from a Danish twin study. *Clin Exp Immunol* 2006;**146**:32–8.

95. de Luis DA, Varela C, de La CH, Canton R, de Argila CM, San Roman AL, et al. *Helicobacter pylori* infection is markedly increased in patients with autoimmune atrophic thyroiditis. *J Clin Gastroenterol* 1998;**26**:259–63.

96. Figura N, Di CG, Lore F, Guarino E, Gragnoli A, Cataldo D, et al. The infection by *Helicobacter pylori* strains expressing CagA is highly prevalent in women with autoimmune thyroid disorders. *J Physiol Pharmacol* 1999;**50**:817–26.

97. Larizza D, Calcaterra V, Martinetti M, Negrini R, De SA, Cisternino M, et al. *Helicobacter pylori* infection and autoimmune thyroid disease in young patients: the disadvantage of carrying the human leukocyte antigen-DRB1*0301 allele. *J Clin Endocrinol Metab* 2006;**91**:176–9.

98. Sterzl I, Hrda P, Potuznikova B, Matucha P, Hana V, Zamrazil V. Autoimmune thyroiditis and *Helicobacter pylori*—is there a connection? *Neuro Endocrinol Lett* 2006;**27** (Suppl. 1):41–5.

99. Tomasi PA, Dore MP, Fanciulli G, Sanciu F, Realdi G, Delitala G. Is there anything to the reported association between *Helicobacter pylori* infection and autoimmune thyroiditis? *Dig Dis Sci* 2005;**50**:385–8.
100. Desailloud R, Goffard A, Page C, Kairis B, Fronval S, Chatelain D, et al. Detection of enterovirus RNA in postoperative thyroid tissue specimens. *Clin Endocrinol (Oxf)* 2009;**70**:331–4.
101. Hammerstad SS, Jahnsen FL, Tauriainen S, Hyoty H, Paulsen T, Norheim I, et al. Inflammation and increased myxovirus resistance protein a expression in thyroid tissue in the early stages of Hashimoto's thyroiditis. *Thyroid* 2013;**23**:334–41.
102. Shoenfeld Y, Cohen IR. Infection and autoimmunity. In: Sela M, editor. *The Antigens.* New York: Academic Press; 1987. p. 307–25.
103. Gerling I, Chatterjee NK, Nejman C. Coxsackievirus B4-induced development of antibodies to 64,000-Mr islet autoantigen and hyperglycemia in mice. *Autoimmunity* 1991;**10**:49–56.
104. Baekkeskov S, Landin M, Kristensen JK, Srikanta S, Bruining GJ, Mandrup-Poulsen T, et al. Antibodies to a 64,000 Mr human islet cell antigen precede the clinical onset of insulin-dependent diabetes. *J Clin Invest* 1987;**79**:926–34.
105. Whittingham S, McNeilage J, Mackay IR. Primary Sjogren's syndrome after infectious mononucleosis. *Ann Intern Med* 1985;**102**:490–3.
106. Wasnich RD, Grumet FC, Payne RO, Kriss JP. Graves' ophthalmopathy following external neck irradiation for nonthyroidal neoplastic disease. *J Clin Endocrinol Metab* 1973;**37**:703–13.
107. Adams TE, Alpert S, Hanahan D. Non-tolerance and autoantibodies to a transgenic self antigen expressed in pancreatic beta cells. *Nature* 1987;**325**:223–8.
108. Garry RF, Fermin CD, Hart DJ, Alexander SS, Donehower LA, Luo-Zhang H. Detection of a human intracisternal A-type retroviral particle antigenically related to HIV. *Science* 1990;**250**:1127–9.
109. Flescher E, Talal N. Do viruses contribute to the development of Sjogren's syndrome? *Am J Med* 1991;**90**:283–5.
110. Talal N, Dauphinee MJ, Dang H, Alexander SS, Hart DJ, Garry RF. Detection of serum antibodies to retroviral proteins in patients with primary Sjogren's syndrome (autoimmune exocrinopathy). *Arthritis Rheum* 1990;**33**:774–81.
111. Ohashi PS, Oehen S, Buerki K, Pircher H, Ohashi CT, Odermatt B, et al. Ablation of "tolerance" and induction of diabetes by virus infection in viral antigen transgenic mice. *Cell* 1991;**65**:305–17.
112. Oldstone MB, Nerenberg M, Southern P, Price J, Lewicki H. Virus infection triggers insulin-dependent diabetes mellitus in a transgenic model: role of anti-self (virus) immune response. *Cell* 1991;**65**:319–31.
113. Alexander NJ, Anderson DJ. Vasectomy: consequences of autoimmunity to sperm antigens. *Fertil Steril* 1979;**32**:253–60.
114. Rival C, Wheeler K, Jeffrey S, Qiao H, Luu B, Tewalt EF, et al. Regulatory T cells and vasectomy. *J Reprod Immunol* 2013;**100**(1):66–75.
115. Oldstone MB. Molecular mimicry and autoimmune disease. *Cell* 1987;**50**:819–20.
116. Williams Jr. RC. Molecular mimicry and rheumatic fever. *Clin Rheum Dis* 1985;**11**:573–90.
117. Delunardo F, Scalzi V, Capozzi A, Camerini S, Misasi R, Pierdominici M, et al. Streptococcal-vimentin cross-reactive antibodies induce microvascular cardiac endothelial proinflammatory phenotype in rheumatic heart disease. *Clin Exp Immunol* 2013;**173**:419–29.
118. Srinivasappa J, Saegusa J, Prabhakar BS, Gentry MK, Buchmeier MJ, Wiktor TJ, et al. Molecular mimicry: frequency of reactivity of monoclonal antiviral antibodies with normal tissues. *J Virol* 1986;**57**:397–401.

119. Hughes RA, Allard SA, Maini RN. Arthritis associated with adjuvant mycobacterial treatment for carcinoma of the bladder. *Ann Rheum Dis* 1989;**48**:432–4.
120. el-Roiey A, Gross WL, Luedemann J, Isenberg DA, Shoenfeld Y. Preferential secretion of a common anti-DNA idiotype (16/6 Id) and anti-polynucleotide antibodies by normal mononuclear cells following stimulation with Klebsiella pneumoniae. *Immunol Lett* 1986;**12**:313–9.
121. Thomas MA, Frampton G, Isenberg DA, Shoenfeld Y, Akinsola A, Ramzy M, et al. A common anti-DNA antibody idiotype and anti-phospholipid antibodies in sera from patients with schistosomiasis and filariasis with and without nephritis. *J Autoimmun* 1989;**2**:803–11.
122. Haspel MV, Onodera T, Prabhakar BS, McClintock PR, Essani K, Ray UR, et al. Multiple organ-reactive monoclonal autoantibodies. *Nature* 1983;**304**:73–6.
123. Haspel MV, Onodera T, Prabhakar BS, Horita M, Suzuki H, Notkins AL. Virus-induced autoimmunity: monoclonal antibodies that react with endocrine tissues. *Science* 1983;**220**:304–6.
124. Serreze DV, Leiter EH, Kuff EL, Jardieu P, Ishizaka K. Molecular mimicry between insulin and retroviral antigen p73. Development of cross-reactive autoantibodies in sera of NOD and C57BL/KsJ db/db mice. *Diabetes* 1988;**37**:351–8.
125. Talal N, Garry RF, Schur PH, Alexander S, Dauphinee MJ, Livas IH, et al. A conserved idiotype and antibodies to retroviral proteins in systemic lupus erythematosus. *J Clin Invest* 1990;**85**:1866–71.
126. Fujinami RS, Oldstone MB. Amino acid homology between the encephalitogenic site of myelin basic protein and virus: mechanism for autoimmunity. *Science* 1985;**230**:1043–5.
127. Hargreaves CE, Grasso M, Hampe CS, Stenkova A, Atkinson S, Joshua GW, et al. Yersinia enterocolitica provides the link between thyroid-stimulating antibodies and their germline counterparts in Graves' disease. *J Immunol* 2013;**190**:5373–81.
128. Bonomo L, Dammacco F, Pinto L, Barbieri G. Thyroglobulin antibodies in leprosy. *Lancet* 1963;**2**:807–9.
129. Jerne NK. Towards a network theory of the immune system. *Ann Immunol (Paris)* 1974;**125C**:373–89.
130. Tomer Y, Shoenfeld Y. Idiotypes, anti-idiotypic antibodies and autoimmunity. In: Khamashta MA, Font J, Hughes GRV, editors. *Autoimmune conncetive tissue diseases.* Barcelona: Ediciones Doyma; 1993. p. 27–37.
131. Williams WV, Guy HR, Cohen JA, Weiner DB, Greene MI. Structure and regulation of internal image idiotypes. *Chem Immunol* 1990;**48**:185–208.
132. Lentz TL, Burrage TG, Smith AL, Crick J, Tignor GH. Is the acetylcholine receptor a rabies virus receptor? *Science* 1982;**215**:182–4.
133. Islam MN, Pepper BM, Briones-Urbina R, Farid NR. Biological activity of anti-thyrotropin anti-idiotypic antibody. *Eur J Immunol* 1983;**13**:57–63.
134. Tomer Y, Gilburd B, Sack J, Davies TF, Meshorer A, Burek CL, et al. Induction of thyroid autoantibodies in naive mice by idiotypic manipulation. *Clin Immunol Immunopathol* 1996;**78**:180–7.
135. Abu-Shakra M, Shoenfeld Y. Parasitic infection and autoimmunity. *Autoimmunity* 1991;**9**:337–44.
136. Brohee D, Delespesse G, Debisschop MJ, Bonnyns M. Circulating immune complexes in various thyroid diseases. *Clin Exp Immunol* 1979;**36**:379–83.
137. Kalderon AE, Bogaars HA. Immune complex deposits in Graves' disease and Hashimoto's thyroiditis. *Am J Med* 1977;**63**:729–34.
138. Mariotti S, DeGroot LJ, Scarborough D, Medof ME. Study of circulating immune complexes in thyroid diseases: comparison of Raji cell radioimmunoassay and specific thyroglobulin-antithyroglobulin radioassay. *J Clin Endocrinol Metab* 1979;**49**:679–86.

139. Nielsen CH, Hegedus L, Leslie RG. Autoantibodies in autoimmune thyroid disease promote immune complex formation with self antigens and increase B cell and CD4+ T cell proliferation in response to self antigens. *Eur J Immunol* 2004;**34**:263–72.

140. Jordan SC, Buckingham B, Sakai R, Olson D. Studies of immune-complex glomerulonephritis mediated by human thyroglobulin. *N Engl J Med* 1981;**304**:1212–15.

141. Lindquist S. The heat-shock response. *Annu Rev Biochem* 1986;**55**:1151–91.

142. Latchman DS. Heat shock proteins and human disease. *J R Coll Physicians Lond* 1991;**25**:295–9.

143. Hemmingsen SM, Woolford C, van der Vies SM, Tilly K, Dennis DT, Georgopoulos CP, et al. Homologous plant and bacterial proteins chaperone oligomeric protein assembly. *Nature* 1988;**333**:330–4.

144. Chirico WJ, Waters MG, Blobel G. 70K heat shock related proteins stimulate protein translocation into microsomes. *Nature* 1988;**332**:805–10.

145. Sanchez ER, Toft DO, Schlesinger MJ, Pratt WB. Evidence that the 90-kDa phosphoprotein associated with the untransformed L-cell glucocorticoid receptor is a murine heat shock protein. *J Biol Chem* 1985;**260**:12398–401.

146. Lamb JR, Young DB. T cell recognition of stress proteins. A link between infectious and autoimmune disease. *Mol Biol Med* 1990;**7**:311–21.

147. Minota S, Koyasu S, Yahara I, Winfield J. Autoantibodies to the heat-shock protein hsp90 in systemic lupus erythematosus. *J Clin Invest* 1988;**81**:106–9.

148. Tsoulfa G, Rook GA, Van-Embden JD, Young DB, Mehlert A, Isenberg DA, et al. Raised serum IgG and IgA antibodies to mycobacterial antigens in rheumatoid arthritis. *Ann Rheum Dis* 1989;**48**:118–23.

149. Elias D, Markovits D, Reshef T, van der Zee R, Cohen IR. Induction and therapy of autoimmune diabetes in the non-obese diabetic (NOD/Lt) mouse by a 65-kDa heat shock protein. *Proc Natl Acad Sci USA* 1990;**87**:1576–80.

150. Ratanachaiyavong S, Demaine AG, Campbell RD, McGregor AM. Heat shock protein 70 (HSP70) and complement C4 genotypes in patients with hyperthyroid Graves' disease. *Clin Exp Immunol* 1991;**84**:48–52.

151. Bahn RS, Heufelder AEGCGJ. Immunohistochemical detection and localization of a 72 kDa heat shock protein (HSP) in Graves' and Hashimoto's thyroid glands. *Thyroid* 1991;**1**(Suppl. 1):62.

152. Heufelder AE, Wenzel BE, Gorman CA, Bahn RS. Detection, cellular localization, and modulation of heat shock proteins in cultured fibroblasts from patients with extrathyroidal manifestations of Graves' disease. *J Clin Endocrinol Metab* 1991;**73**:739–45.

153. Heufelder AE, Wenzel BE, Bahn RS. Graves' immunoglobulins (GD-IgG) induce and bind to stress-induced proteins in retroocular fibroblasts form patients with Graves' ophthalmopathy (GO). *Thyroid* 1991;**1**(Suppl. 1):21.

154. Sztankay A, Trieb K, Lucciarini P, Steiner E, Grubeck-Loebenstein B. Interferon gamma and iodide increase the inducibility of the 72 kD heat shock protein in cultured human thyroid epithelial cells. *J Autoimmun* 1994;**7**:219–30.

155. Mallard K, Jones DB, Richmond J, McGill M, Foulis AK. Expression of the human heat shock protein 60 in thyroid, pancreatic, hepatic and adrenal autoimmunity. *J Autoimmun* 1996;**9**:89–96.

156. Bottazzo GF, Pujol-Borrell R, Hanafusa T, Feldmann M. Role of aberrant HLA-DR expression and antigen presentation in induction of endocrine autoimmunity. *Lancet* 1983;**2**:1115–19.

157. Hanafusa T, Pujol-Borrell R, Chiovato L, Russell RC, DONIACH D, Bottazzo GF. Aberrant expression of HLA-DR antigen on thyrocytes in Graves' disease: relevance for autoimmunity. *Lancet* 1983;**2**:1111–15.

158. Davies TF, Piccinini LA. Intrathyroidal MHC class II antigen expression and thyroid autoimmunity. *Endocrinol Metab Clin North Am* 1987;**16**:247–68.

159. Platzer M, Neufeld DS, Piccinini LA, Davies TF. Induction of rat thyroid cell MHC class II antigen by thyrotropin and gamma-interferon. *Endocrinology* 1987;**121**: 2087–92.
160. Neufeld DS, Platzer M, Davies TF. Reovirus induction of MHC class II antigen in rat thyroid cells. *Endocrinology* 1989;**124**:543–5.
161. Carter JK, Smith RE. Rapid induction of hypothyroidism by an avian leukosis virus. *Infect Immun* 1983;**40**:795–805.
162. Londei M, Lamb JR, Bottazzo GF, Feldmann M. Epithelial cells expressing aberrant MHC class II determinants can present antigen to cloned human T cells. *Nature* 1984;**312**:639–41.
163. Davies TF. Cocultures of human thyroid monolayer cells and autologous T cells: impact of HLA class II antigen expression. *J Clin Endocrinol Metab* 1985;**61**:418–22.
164. Kawakami Y, Kuzuya N, Watanabe T, Uchiyama Y, Yamashita K. Induction of experimental thyroiditis in mice by recombinant interferon gamma administration. *Acta Endocrinol (Copenh)* 1990;**122**:41–8.
165. Massa PT, Dorries R, Ter MV. Viral particles induce Ia antigen expression on astrocytes. *Nature* 1986;**320**:543–6.
166. Wilson LD, Flyer DC, Faller DV. Murine retroviruses control class I major histocompatibility antigen gene expression via a trans effect at the transcriptional level. *Mol Cell Biol* 1987;**7**:2406–15.
167. Maudsley DJ, Morris AG. Regulation of IFN-gamma-induced host cell MHC antigen expression by Kirsten MSV and MLV I. Effects on class I antigen expression. *Immunology* 1989;**67**:21–5.
168. Maudsley DJ, Morris AG. Regulation of IFN-gamma-induced host cell MHC antigen expression by Kirsten MSV and MLV II. Effects on class II antigen expression. *Immunology* 1989;**67**:26–31.
169. Eager KB, Williams J, Breiding D, Pan S, Knowles B, Appella E, et al. Expression of histocompatibility antigens H-2K, -D, and -L is reduced in adenovirus-12-transformed mouse cells and is restored by interferon gamma. *Proc Natl Acad Sci USA* 1985;**82**:5525–9.
170. Khoury EL, Pereira L, Greenspan FS. Induction of HLA-DR expression on thyroid follicular cells by cytomegalovirus infection in vitro. Evidence for a dual mechanism of induction. *Am J Pathol* 1991;**138**:1209–23.
171. Costello ME, Elewaut D, Kenna TJ, Brown MA. Microbes, the gut and ankylosing spondylitis. *Arthritis Res Ther* 2013;**15**:214.
172. Cindoruk M, Tuncer C, Dursun A, Yetkin I, Karakan T, Cakir N, et al. Increased colonic intraepithelial lymphocytes in patients with Hashimoto's thyroiditis. *J Clin Gastroenterol* 2002;**34**:237–9.
173. Sasso FC, Carbonara O, Torella R, Mezzogiorno A, Esposito V, Demagistris L, et al. Ultrastructural changes in enterocytes in subjects with Hashimoto's thyroiditis. *Gut* 2004;**53**:1878–80.
174. Jungel A, Ospelt C, Gay S. What can we learn from epigenetics in the year 2009? *Curr Opin Rheumatol* 2010;**22**:284–92.
175. Barski A, Cuddapah S, Cui K, Roh TY, Schones DE, Wang Z, et al. High-resolution profiling of histone methylations in the human genome. *Cell* 2007;**129**:823–37.
176. Karouzakis E, Gay RE, Gay S, Neidhart M. Epigenetic control in rheumatoid arthritis synovial fibroblasts. *Nat Rev Rheumatol* 2009;**5**:266–72.
177. Eschler DC, Hasham A, Tomer Y. Cutting edge: the etiology of autoimmune thyroid diseases. *Clin Rev Allergy Immunol* 2011;**41**:190–7.
178. Stefan M, Jacobson EM, Huber AK, Greenberg DA, Li CW, Skrabanek L, et al. Novel variant of thyroglobulin promoter triggers thyroid autoimmunity through an epigenetic interferon alpha-modulated mechanism. *J Biol Chem* 2011;**286**:31168–79.

CHAPTER 55

Pemphigus and Infection

Ayelet Ollech[*], **Emillia Hodak**[*,†], **Daniel Mimouni**[*,†,1]
[*]Department of Dermatology, Rabin Medical Center, Petach Tikva, Israel
[†]Sackler Faculty of Medicine, Tel Aviv University, Tel Aviv, Israel
[1]Corresponding Author: mimouni@post.tau.ac.il

1 INTRODUCTION

Autoimmune diseases are assumed to be initiated or triggered by a complex interaction of environmental factors in a genetically susceptible individual. Pemphigus is a group of autoimmune organ-specific mucocutaneous blistering disorders with an established immunological basis. The first study to shed light on the autoimmune mechanism of pemphigus was conducted in 1964 by Beutner and Jordon.[1] Using direct and indirect immunofluorescence, the authors detected IgG depositions in intercellular spaces of the epidermis of patients with pemphigus as well as circulating serum autoantibodies directed against the keratinocyte cell surface. Further studies showed that these autoantibodies are pathogenic and can induce the formation of intraepithelial blisters,[2,3] the clinical hallmark of pemphigus. Almost two decades later, Anhalt and colleagues[4] observed the formation of blisters and erosions in neonatal mice following the passive transfer of IgG from patients with pemphigus. The pemphigus antigens were defined as desmoglein 3 and desmoglein 1, two transmembrane glycoprotein compounds of the desmosome.

2 CLINICAL VARIANTS OF PEMPHIGUS

The major clinical variants of pemphigus are pemphigus vulgaris, pemphigus foliaceus, and paraneoplastic pemphigus. All are characterized histologically by cell-to-cell detachment of epidermal and mucosal epithelial cells (acantholysis) due to IgG autoantibodies directed against the desmosomal adhesion molecules of the affected epithelium. Recent studies described IgA pemphigus, a form of pemphigus involving IgA rather than IgG autoantibodies against the desmosomal adhesion molecules. These autoantibodies can be visualized using the direct IF technique.

Infection and Autoimmunity
http://dx.doi.org/10.1016/B978-0-444-63269-2.00049-0

919

Pemphigus vulgaris is the most common form of pemphigus in North America and Europe. Like many other autoimmune diseases, the pathophysiology is well defined but the etiology is unknown, and the suspected trigger of the autoimmune response is an interaction of exogenous factors in genetically susceptible individuals. Human leukocyte antigen (HLA) DR4, DR14, DQ1, and DQ3 alleles have been implicated in the genetic susceptibility to pemphigus. Studies report a high prevalence of pemphigus vulgaris in Jews of Eastern European origin, with a predominance of DRB1*0402 (HLA-DR4) and DQB1*0503. The target antigens in pemphigus vulgaris are desmogleins 1 and 3. Potential exogenous factors that may trigger the autoimmune process include infections, drugs, physical trauma, ultraviolet rays, ionizing radiation, neoplasms, contact allergens, nutritional factors, and emotional stress.[5]

The lesions of pemphigus vulgaris typically occur first in the oropharyngeal mucosa and subsequently in the skin. Other mucosa, such as the genitalia and conjunctiva, may be involved as well. The primary skin lesions consist of flaccid bullae that break to form a large painful erosion that usually fails to heal in the absence of specific intervention. The skin lesions may occur in all parts of the body, although the scalp, face, and trunk are the most common sites affected.

Pemphigus vegetans is a rare subgroup of pemphigus vulgaris representing a reactive pattern to the autoimmune insult of pemphigus vulgaris or a response of long-lasting lesions that are resistant to therapy. Pemphigus vegetans is characterized by flaccid blisters that become erosions and then form fungoid vegetations or papillomatous proliferations, especially in intertriginous areas and on the scalp or face.

Pemphigus foliaceus is divided into two clinical groups: Brazilian pemphigus (endemic pemphigus, fogo selvagem) and pemphigus erythematosus (Senear–Usher syndrome). The etiology of Brazilian pemphigus is unknown, but epidemiological data suggest that it is triggered by an environmental factor found in certain regions of Brazil. Pemphigus erythematosus has features of both pemphigus foliaceus and systemic lupus erythematosus. Pemphigus foliaceus is associated with HLA-DR14 and DQ1 alleles. The target antigen is desmoglein 1. The clinical presentation is distinct from that of pemphigus vulgaris: mucosal involvement is extremely unusual and mainly "seborrheic" areas, such as the scalp, face, and upper trunk, are involved. In addition, blisters are not always present because of the superficial level of epidermal separation. Pemphigus foliaceus has the least morbidity of all forms of pemphigus.

Herpetiform pemphigus is a variant mainly of pemphigus foliaceus and less commonly of pemphigus vulgaris. The target antigen is desmoglein 1 in the majority of cases and desmoglein 3 in the remainder. Herpetiform pemphigus clinically presents as erythematous urticarial plaques and tense vesicles in a herpetiform arrangement. Histological findings include eosinophilic spongiosis and subcorneal pustules, with minimal or no apparent acantholysis. Sometimes patients have features of pemphigus foliaceus or vulgaris or the disease evolves into these forms. Herpetiform pemphigus may have a more chronic course than pemphigus vulgaris.[6]

Paraneoplastic pemphigus was first described in 1990.[7] It is nearly always associated with an underlying neoplasm. Two-thirds of patients have a pre-existing malignancy, usually non-Hodgkin's lymphoma, chronic lymphocytic lymphoma, or Castleman's disease; in the remainder, the disease serves as a marker for an occult malignancy. Anti-desmoplakin 1 and 2, envoplakin, periplakin and the recently discovered alpha-2 macroglobulin-like 1 protein, known previously as the 170-kDa protein, are the autoantibodies that are characteristically present in patients with paraneoplastic pemphigus.[8] Autoantibodies against desmogleins 1 and 3 as well as plectin are occasionally identified.[9] The typical clinical picture consists of a polymorphous eruption on the skin (pemphigus-like blisters, bullous pempigoid-like blisters, erythema multiforme-like or lichenoid eruption) along with intractable stomatitis.

Two forms of drug-related pemphigus exist: drug-induced pemphigus and pemphigus-like drug eruption.

Drug-induced pemphigus has the pathomechanism of a true autoimmune disease: Unlike more common drug eruptions, it persists even after withdrawal of the causal drug. The clinical features are mostly those of pemphigus vulgaris. The main drugs involved are thiols and derivatives such as d-penicillamine, captopril, and penicillin.[10] The drugs' sulfhydryl groups are incorporated into the keratinocyte molecular structure, causing antigenic conformational changes, the formation of anti-desmoglein 1 and 3 antibodies, and acantholysis. They may also cause an immune imbalance, amplifying the acantholysis. Other suspect drugs are phenols, such as cephalosporin and aspirin, which induce the release of interleukin (IL)-α and tumor necrosis factor-α from keratinocytes, which are known to be involved in acantholysis in pemphigus vulgaris, in addition to angiotensin-converting enzyme inhibitors, non-steroidal anti-inflammatory drugs, and biologic immunomodulators.[5]

Drug-induced pemphigus is distinguished from the less frequent pemphigus-like drug eruption, which eventually resolves after withdrawal of the causal drug, even in the absence of treatment. This type is character-ized clinically mostly by features of pemphigus foliaceous and histologically by irregular acantholysis. The acantholysis directly interferes with the adhe-sive function of the desmogleins without the production of antibodies.

IgA pemphigus is a variant of pemphigus that involves IgA rather than IgG autoantibodies against desmogleins 1 and 3, desmocollin 1, and other undefined antigens. No etiological agent has been identified, and the exact pathogenic role of IgA antibodies in the disease is still unclear. Two subsets of IgA pemphigus have been described: subcorneal pustular dermatosis and intra-epidermal neutrophilic type. Clinically, patients present with a vesicu-lopustular eruption that tends to coalesce to form an annular or circinate pat-tern on the skin, mainly in skin folds and on the trunk and rarely in mucous membranes.[11]

3 CLINICAL EVIDENCE OF AN INFECTIOUS AGENT

3.1 Viruses and Pemphigus

Only rarely has pemphigus been described in association with infectious agents, although many early studies sought to isolate a virus from pemphigus lesions or to find clear serological evidence of a recent viral infection. Given the numerous methodological limitations, the casual association between pemphigus and viral infection is yet unclear. Individual reports documented the onset or relapse of pemphigus following or coincident with infection by varicella zoster virus (VZV),[12] Epstein–Barr virus (EBV),[13,14] human immu-nodeficiency virus,[15,16] or cytomegalovirus (CMV).[17] Most of the cases involved herpes simplex virus (HSV) infection. Krain[18] was the first to describe a severe precedent HSV infection in 2 of 59 patients with pemphi-gus vulgaris. In 1996, Ruocco and colleagues,[19] in a review of the literature, found 13 cases of virus-associated pemphigus: CMV in 1, EBV in 1, VZV in 2, and HSV in 10 (one case was related to both VZV and HSV). Seven cases were proven by viral culture and five by serology.

To demonstrate the presence of viruses in patients with pemphigus, early investigators inoculated animals with fluid from blisters or samples of skin, blood, or urine from affected patients.[20–24] This was followed by tissue cul-ture experiments,[25–27] with inconsistent results, and more recently by other serologic studies, such as complement fixation, which yielded disappointing findings.[28] In 1999, Tufano et al.,[29] using polymerase chain reaction (PCR), identified the DNA sequence of HSV (types 1 and 2) in 50% of peripheral blood mononuclear cells and 71% of skin biopsies derived from 20 patients with pemphigus; results in the control cases were all negative. Given that HSV DNA in skin lesions has been reported in true virus-induced diseases, the authors concluded that HSV may trigger pemphigus. However, their failure to detect HSV in all pemphigus cases might suggest that viral infection is only an occasional trigger.

A possible association of pemphigus with human herpes virus type 8 (HHV-8) was demonstrated in 1997 by Memar and colleagues[30] using PCR, Southern blot hybridization, and automated sequencing of the PCR products. The study included 12 patients, 6 with pemphigus vulgaris and 6 with pemphigus foliaceus, and 12 controls, 2 with Kaposi's sarcoma and 10 healthy individuals. Interestingly, lesional skin from 4 patients with pemphigus vulgaris, all 6 patients with pemphigus foliaceus, and both controls with Kaposi's sarcoma tested positive for HHV-8 DNA. The HHV-8 DNA sequences differed among all 6 specimens from the pemphigus foliaceus subgroup, whereas 3 of the 4 specimens from the pemphigus vulgaris subgroup were identical. HHV-8 DNA was absent from all normal human skin samples analyzed. The researchers concluded that it is possible that HHV-8 has a tropism for pemphigus lesions. In a later study, Wang et al.[31] identified HHV-8 DNA sequences in 30.8% of peripheral blood mononuclear cells and 36.1% of skin lesions from patients with pemphigus, in addition to a higher IgG titer to HHV-8 in 34.5%.

3.2 Bacteria and Pemphigus

The role of bacteria or other microorganisms in pemphigus is speculative and, so far, solid data are lacking. A recent study by Amagai et al.[32] demonstrated that *Staphylococcus aureus* toxin is involved in the mechanism of cell–cell detachment in staphylococcal scalded skin syndrome (SSSS), a transient, generalized and superficial exfoliative disease. Specifically, the researchers noted that the exfoliative toxin produced by the bacterium binds and cleaves desmoglein 1, the target antigen in pemphigus foliaceus. However, there is no evidence that such a mechanism initiates the acantholysis in pemphigus and, to the best of our knowledge, pemphigus foliaceus has never been associated with *S. aureus* infection.

3.3 Vaccination and Pemphigus

There are two reports of patients in whom new-onset oral pemphigus vulgaris developed within 1 month[33] or 7–10 days (on two occasions)[34] after influenza vaccination. In addition, Cozzani et al.[35] described the appearance of pemphigus, probably foliaceus, 7 days after intramuscular vaccination against tetanus and diphtheria in a 7-year-old girl. In this specific case, the authors recognized that while the relationship might be causal, there was a possibility that the vaccine vehicle, which contained a thiol group, was the culprit. Korang et al.[36] reported an extremely unusual case of exacerbation of pemphigus foliaceus after tetanus vaccination; this exacerbation was accompanied by the production of autoantibodies directed against paraneoplastic pemphigus antigens. In other reports, pemphigus occurred following a first anthrax vaccination (adsorbed),[37] typhoid booster,[38] antirabies vaccination (10-day delay),[39] and hepatitis B vaccinations (3-month delay).[40]

4 POSSIBLE PATHOGENESIS

Several mechanisms that might explain the potential association of infection with pemphigus have been suggested. First, viral infections may stimulate the immune system, leading to the up-regulation and activation of the cellular and humoral response. In individuals with a genetic predisposition to pemphigus, such immune system stimulation may lead to the production and secretion of interferons (IFNs) and ILs. Specifically, IFN-γ is known to induce the expression of HLA class II antigens on keratinocyte cell membranes, thereby immunologically activating the structural site of pemphigus. In this context, chronic viral infection may cause an overproduction of IL-4 and IL-10, which are responsible for shifting from a T helper 1 to a T helper 2 immune response, further enhancing antibody production.[41] ILs can also directly cause acantholysis, as shown in reports of pemphigus associated with INF and IL-2 therapy.[42]

Second, viruses can alter the structure of cell proteins both in infected cells and in nearby cells that are not actually penetrated.[43] In pemphigus, these new antigens may interact and form complexes with the histocompatibility system to produce immunogenic antigens, inducing structural changes in the proteins of the keratinocyte host cell membrane.

Third, infection of a keratinocyte by a virus may destroy the intracellular proteins that are important for self-tolerance, thereby exposing antigens to the immune system. It also is possible that viruses cross-react with proteins of the keratinocyte cell membrane through molecular mimicry, exposing immunologically protected autoantigens such as desmoglein 1 and 3 and leading to the production of autoantibodies and an autoimmune response.[5,44]

In addition, viruses might induce the production of anti-idiotype antibodies against monoclonal antibodies generated against a specific virus.

For example, one group found that anti-idiotype antibodies to monoclonal antibodies generated against Coxsackie B4 virus antigen also react with surface antigens of other cells.[25]

Finally, viruses may interact directly with lymphocytes and alter the normal immune mechanism. The alteration can occur at several levels: infection of T lymphocytes, leading to lymphocyte activation and the production of autoreactive B lymphocytes; infection of suppressor T lymphocytes, leading to their destruction and preventing their defensive action against autoimmune process; and infection of B lymphocytes, leading to cell activation and the production of autoimmune antibodies.

5 THERAPEUTIC ASPECTS

No therapeutic implications of a possible role for viruses in pemphigus have been reported in the literature. The administration of anti-herpetic medications such as acyclovir was prompted in some cases by emerging evidence of a possible role for HSV in initiating the autoimmune process in pemphigus. However, it apparently had no effect on the natural course of the disease. Because erosive stomatitis is the first clinical presentation in 50% of pemphigus cases, many patients are treated with antiviral agents arising from misdiagnosis, with no response.

In infected patients with preexisting pemphigus, it is unclear whether the infection serves as a trigger of an exacerbation of the disease or occurs as a consequence of the immunosuppressive treatment the patient is receiving. In a few case reports of concurrent pemphigus and HSV infection, alleviation of the oral lesions was noted with anti-herpetic therapy.[19,45] However, a report of three patients with HSV-1 infection concurrent with a clinical flare-up of pemphigus showed no correlation with increased anti-desmoglein-specific IgG. The authors concluded that the HSV disease was a secondary infection, perhaps one facilitated by the immunosuppressive therapy.[46]

6 SUMMARY

An etiopathogenic role for infectious agents in pemphigus cannot be ruled out. Solid evidence from prospective studies using novel techniques of viral and bacterial detection at the initial phase of the disease is needed.

REFERENCES

1. Beutner EH, Jordon RE. Demonstration of skin antibodies in sera of pemphigus vulgaris patients by indirect immunofluorescent staining. *Proc Soc Exp Biol Med* 1964; **117**:505–10.
2. Schiltz JR, Michel B. Production of epidermal acantholysis in normal human skin in vitro by the IgG fraction from pemphigus serum. *J Invest Dermatol* 1976;**67**:254–60.
3. Farb RM, Dykes R, Lazarus GS. Anti-epidermal-cell-surface pemphigus antibody detaches viable epidermal cells from culture plates by activation of proteinase. *Proc Natl Acad Sci USA* 1978;**75**:459–63.
4. Anhalt GJ, Labib RS, Voorhees JJ, Beals TF, Diaz LA. Induction of pemphigus in neonatal mice by passive transfer of IgG from patients with the disease. *N Engl J Med* 1982;**306**:1189–96.
5. Lo Schiavio A, Brancaccio G, Ruocco E, Caccavale S, Ruocco V, Wolf R. Bullous pemphigus. Etiology, pathogenesis, and inducing or triggering factors: facts and controversies. *Clin Dermatol* 2013;**31**:391–9.
6. Joly P, Litrowski N. Pemphigus group (vulgaris, vegetans, foliaceus, herpetiformis, brasiliensis). *Clin Dermatol* 2011;**29**(4):432–6.
7. Anhalt GJ, Kim SC, Stanley JR, Korman NJ, Jabs DA, Kory M, et al. Paraneoplastic pemphigus. An autoimmune mucocutaneous disease associated with neoplasia. *N Engl J Med* 1990;**323**:1729–35.
8. Schepens I, Jaunin F, Begre N, Laderach U, Marcus K, Hashimoto T, et al. The protease inhibitor alpha-2-macroglobulin-like-1 is the p170 antigen recognized by paraneoplastic pemphigusautoantibodies in human. *PLoS One* 2010;**5**:e12250.
9. Mimouni D, Anhalt GJ, Lazarova Z, Aho S, Kazerounian S, Kouba DJ, et al. Paraneoplastic pemphigus in children and adolescents. *Br J Dermatol* 2002;**147**:725–32.
10. Heymann D, Chodick G, Kramer E, Green M, Shalev V. Pemphigus variant associated with penicillin use. *Arch Dermatol* 2007;**143**:704–7.
11. Tsuruta D, Ishii N, Harmada T, Ohyama B, Fukuda S, Koga H, et al. IgA pemphigus. *Clin Dermatol* 2011;**29**:437–42.
12. Goon AT, Tay YK, Tan SH. Pemphigus vulgaris following varicella infection. *Clin Exp Dermatol* 2001;**26**:661–3.
13. Markitziu A, Pisanty S. Pemphigus vulgaris after infection by Epstein-Barr virus. *Int J Dermatol* 1993;**32**:917–18.
14. Barzilai O, Sherer Y, Ram M, Izhaky D, Anaya JM, Shoenfeld Y. Epstein-Barr virus and cytomegalovirus in autoimmune diseases: are they truly notorious? A preliminary report. *Ann NY Acad Sci* 2007;**1108**:567–77.
15. Splaver A, Silos S, Lowell B, Valenzuela R, Kirsner RS. Case report: pemphigus vulgaris in a patient infected with HIV. *AIDS Patient Care STDS* 2000;**14**:295–6.
16. Hodgson TA, Fidler SJ, Speight PM, Weber JN, Porter SR. Oral pemphigus vulgaris associated with HIV infection. *J Am Acad Dermatol* 2003;**49**:313–15.
17. Ruocco V, Rossi A, Satriano RA, Sacerdoti G, Astarita C, Pisani M. Pemphigus foliaceus in a haemophilic child: cytomegalovirus induction? *Acta Derm Venereol* 1982;**62**:534–7.
18. Krain LS. Pemphigus. Epidemiologic and survival characteristics of 59 patients, 1955-1973. *Arch Dermatol* 1974;**110**:862–5.
19. Ruocco V, Wolf R, Ruocco E, Baroni A. Viruses in pemphigus: a casual or causal relationship? *Int J Dermatol* 1996;**35**:782–4.
20. Grace AW, Suskind FH. An agent, transmissible to mice, obtained during a study of pemphigus vulgaris. *Proc Soc Exp Biol Med* 1937;**37**:324–6.

21. Grace AW, Suskind FH. An investigation of the etiology of pemphigus vulgaris: the isolation of transmissible agent from a fourth case of the disease. *J Invest Dermatol* 1939;**2**:1–13.
22. Grace AW. The etiologic agent of pemphigus vulgaris. *Bull NY Acad Med* 1946; **22**:480–1.
23. Dostrovsky A, Gurevitch I, Ungar H. On the question of the aetiology of pemphigus vulgaris and dermatitis herpetiformis (Duhring's disease): a clinical experimental study. *Br J Dermatol* 1938;**50**:412–35.
24. Werth J. Beitrage zur virusatiologie des pemphigus vulgaris. *Archiv Dermatol Syphilis* 1938;**176**:382–90.
25. Ahmed AR, Rosen GB. Viruses in pemphigus. *Int J Dermatol* 1989;**28**:209–17.
26. Siegl G, Hahn EE. A paramyxovirus-like virus isolated from pemphigus-disease in man. *Arch Gesamte Virusforsch* 1969;**28**:41–50.
27. Angulo JJ. Attempts to isolate a virus from pemphigus foliaceus cases. *Arch Dermatol Syphilol* 1954;**69**:472–4.
28. Dahl MV, Katz SI, Scott RM, et al. Viral studies in pemphigus. *J Invest Dermatol* 1974;**62**:96–9.
29. Tufano MA, Baroni A, Buommino E, Ruocco E, Lombardi ML, Ruocco V. Detection of herpesvirus DNA in peripheral blood mononuclear cells and skin lesions of patients with pemphigus by polymerase chain reaction. *Br J Dermatol* 1999;**141**:1033–9.
30. Memar OM, Rady PL, Goldblum RM, Yen A, Tyring SK. Human herpesvirus 8 DNA sequences in blistering skin from patients with pemphigus. *Arch Dermatol* 1997;**133**:1247–51.
31. Wang GQ, Xu H, Wang YK, Gao XH, Zhao Y, He C, et al. Higher prevalence of human herpesvirus 8 DNA sequence and specific IgG antibodies in patients with pemphigus in China. *J Am Acad Dermatol* 2005;**52**:460–7.
32. Amagai M, Matsuyoshi N, Wang ZH, Andl C, Stanley JR. Toxin in bullous impetigo and staphylococcal scalded-skin syndrome targets desmoglein 1. *Nat Med* 2000;**6**:1275–7.
33. Mignogna MD, Muzio LL. Pemphigus induction by influenza vaccination. *Int J Dermatol* 2000;**39**:800.
34. De Simone C, Caldarola G, D'agostino M, Zampetti A, Amerio P, Feliciani C. Exacerbation of pemphigus after influenza vaccination. *Clin Exp Dermatol* 2008;**33**: 718–20.
35. Cozzani E, Cacciapuoti M, Parodi A, Rebora A. Pemphigus following tetanus and diphtheria vaccination. *Br J Dermatol* 2002;**147**:188–9.
36. Korang K, Ghohestani R, Krieg T, Uitto J, Hunzelmann N. Exacerbation of pemphigus foliaceus after tetanus vaccination accompanied by synthesis of auto-antibodies against paraneoplastic pemphigus antigens. *Acta Derm Venereol* 2002;**82**:482–3.
37. Muellenhoff M, Cukrowski T, Morgan M, Dorton D. Oral pemphigus vulgaris after anthrax vaccine administration: association or coincidence? *J Am Acad Dermatol* 2004;**50**:136–9.
38. Bellaney GJ, Rycroft RJ. Pemphigus vulgaris following a hyperimmune response to typhoid booster. *Clin Exp Dermatol* 1996;**21**:434–6.
39. Yalcin B, Alli N. Pemphigus vulgaris following antirabies vaccination. *J Dermatol* 2007;**34**:734–5.
40. Berkun Y, Mimouni D, Shoenfeld Y. Pemphigus following hepatitis B vaccination—coincidence or causality? *Autoimmunity* 2005;**38**(2):117–19.
41. Vercelli D, Jabara HH, Lauener RP, Geha RS. IL-4 inhibits the synthesis of IFN-gamma and induces the synthesis of IgE in human mixed lymphocyte cultures. *J Immunol* 1990;**144**:570–3.

42. Ramseur WL, Richards F, Duggan DB. A case of fatal pemphigus vulgaris in association with beta interferon and interleukin-2 therapy. *Cancer* 1989;**63**:2005–7.
43. Johnson RT. The possible viral etiology of multiple sclerosis. *Adv Neurol* 1975;**13**:1–46.
44. Isacson P. Myxoviruses and autoimmunity. *Prog Allergy* 1967;**10**:256–92.
45. Hale EK, Bystrin AG. Atypical herpes simplex can mimic a flare of disease activity in patients with pemphigus vulgaris. *J Eur Acad Dermatol Venereol* 1999;**13**:221–3.
46. Caldarola G, Kneisel A, Hertl M, Feliciani C. Herpes simplex virus infection in pemphigus vulgaris: clinical and immunological considerations. *Eur J Dermatol* 2008;**18**:440–3.

CHAPTER 56

Infections and Autoimmune Renal Diseases

Vasiliki Kalliopi Bournia[*], **Maria G. Tektonidou**[†,1]

[*]First Department of Propeudeutic and Internal Medicine, Laikon General Hospital, Athens, Greece
[†]First Department of Internal Medicine, Medical School, University of Athens, Laikon General Hospital, Athens, Greece
[1]Corresponding Author: mtektonidou@gmail.com

1 INTRODUCTION

Autoimmune diseases are a broad range of related conditions characterized by a disruption in self-tolerance, causing the body's own immune system to mount an inflammatory reaction against self-tissues. Autoimmune diseases can be either systemic or organ specific. Kidneys are among the organs most frequently affected by systemic autoimmune disorders. Immune mechanisms are also important in some forms of primary glomerulonephritis, such as IgA nephritis, membranous nephropathy, and membranoproliferative glomerulonephritis, characterized by the presence of autoantibodies directed either to glomeruli, podocytes or components of the immune system.[1] Despite the increased prevalence of autoimmune diseases, collectively affecting 14.7 to 23.5 million people in the United States,[2] knowledge regarding the pathogenesis of these conditions is still limited. Several studies have provided evidence for the role of genetic predisposition in the development of autoimmunity. However, it is believed that exposure to offending environmental agents is also required.[3,4] Environmental agents are categorized into chemical, physical and biologic agents, the latter including mostly infections.[5] Different viruses, bacteria or parasites have been implicated in the pathogenesis of autoimmune conditions that commonly affect the kidneys through mechanisms of molecular mimicry. Other possible mechanisms include interaction with pattern recognition receptors such as Toll-like receptors (TLRs), superantigens, revelation of sequestered autoantigens through tissue damage or the interaction of microbial factors with self-proteins and the formation of neoantigens.[4,6] In this review we describe the available evidence for the role of infections in the pathogenesis of

Infection and Autoimmunity
http://dx.doi.org/10.1016/B978-0-444-63269-2.00066-0

autoimmune renal diseases such as IgA nephropathy, membranous nephropathy, anti-glomerular basement membrane (GBM) disease (Goodpasture's disease), anti-neutrophil cytoplasmic autoantibody (ANCA)-associated vasculitides, Henoch-Schönlein purpura, cryoglobulinemia, and lupus nephritis.

2 IGA NEPHROPATHY

IgA nephropathy, the most common primary glomerulonephritis, is typically expressed as macroscopic hematuria coinciding with or directly following a mucosal infection, usually of the upper respiratory tract. It is characterized by an increase of circulating, poorly galactosylated IgA1 O-glycoforms and deposition of IgA1 immune complexes in the mesangium, followed by mesangial cell activation and proliferation, segmental glomerulosclerosis and tubulointerstitial scarring[7] (Figure 1).

There are two subclasses of human IgA, designated IgA1 and IgA2, which differ structurally in the presence of an 18-amino acid sequence located in the hinge region of IgA1. This region bears up to nine potential O-glycosylation sites (serine or threonine residues), six of which (at most) can simultaneously carry O-glucans. An antigen (*Helicobacter pylori*) encountered at the mucosal surface generates IgA1 with significantly lower galactosylation compared to the IgA1 generated following antigen exposure within the systemic compartment (tetanus toxoid).[8] However, mucosal IgA1 plasma cell numbers are reduced and mucosal IgA1 secretion is impaired in IgA nephropathy,[9] whereas B cells from bone marrow seem

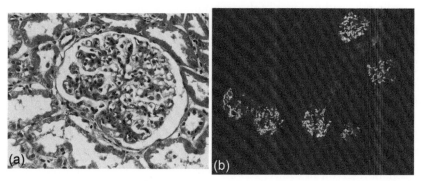

Figure 1 Immunoglobulin A nephropathy. (a) IgA nephropathy with mesangial proliferative glomerulonephritis (hematoxylin and eosin stain; magnification ×400). (b) Immunofluorescence shows diffuse global mesangial staining for IgA (fluorescein isothiocyanate anti-human IgA, magnification ×40).

to be the main source of aberrantly glycosylated IgA1 in these patients.[10] Poorly galactosylated IgA1 molecules can self-aggregate, bind to glucan-specific IgG or bind to antigens, thus forming immune complexes. It has been suggested that glucan-specific antibodies are in fact directed against glycoproteins on the microbial cell surface but recognize poorly galactosylated IgA1 O-glycoforms as a result of molecular mimicry. This hypothesis offers an explanation for the relationship between mucosal infections and exacerbations of IgA nephropathy.[7] Immune complexes containing poorly galactosylated IgA1 escape hepatic clearance and preferentially accumulate in the kidneys, where they bind with high affinity to mesangial cells, resulting in their proliferation and pro-inflammatory and pro-fibrotic transformation.[11] Moreover, polymeric, aggregated or poorly galactosylated IgA can activate the alternative complement pathway, resulting in cell injury, inflammation and further aggravation of renal disease.[12]

Reduced mucosal response to viral or bacterial antigens further contributes to the pathogenesis of IgA nephropathy. Defective antigen clearance and prolonged antigenic challenge for B cells could eventually trigger the production of nephritogenic IgA.[13] RNA from group B Coxsackie enteroviruses,[14] DNA and antigens from human cytomegalovirus,[15] *Staphylococcus aureus* cell envelope antigens[16] and *Hemophilus parainfluenzae* antigens[17] all have been detected in renal biopsies from patients with IgA nephropathy. In addition, experimental IgA nephropathy has been induced in mouse models through oral or intraperitoneal immunization with *H. parainfluenzae*[18] or through intranasal administration of the Sendai virus.[19] Interestingly, experimental models of antigen-induced IgA nephropathy have been reproduced in mice exhibiting impaired oral tolerance, such as Th2-prone BALB/c mice[20] and in transgenic animals carrying a dysregulation of lymphotoxin-like inducible protein. TLR4 expression is up-regulated in circulating monocytes of patients with IgA nephropathy, especially in those with proteinuria and heavy microscopic hematuria.[21] Furthermore, ligation of B-cell TLR4 by bacterial lipopolysaccharides induces methylation of the *Cosmc* gene, the molecular chaperone of C1GalT1, leading to reduced galactosylation of IgA1.[22]

One further point of interest regarding the contribution of infections in the pathogenesis of IgA nephropathy is the potential role of tonsillectomy as a means of treatment. The rationale for tonsillectomy is to remove an important reservoir of pathogens multiplying in tonsil crypts, B lymphocytes and macrophages of lymphoid tonsil follicles, as well as to reduce the gut-associated lymphoid tissue mass, which is an important source of aberrantly glycosylated IgA1.[23] In a retrospective study of 118 patients with IgA nephropathy, renal survival rates were significantly better in the group with tonsillectomy compared to the group without tonsillectomy at 240 months' follow-up (89.6% vs. 63.7%; $P = 0.0329$, log-rank test).[19] Nevertheless, well-designed randomized, placebo-controlled trials testing the therapeutic effect of tonsillectomy in IgA nephropathy are lacking.

3 MEMBRANOUS NEPHROPATHY

Membranous nephropathy is an autoimmune disease usually associated with a nephrotic syndrome, which is characterized by sub-epithelial deposition of immune complexes, leading to thickening of glomerular capillary walls. In approximately 75% of cases no underlying etiology is found, and the condition is considered idiopathic. The most common causes of secondary membranous nephropathy include infections, especially with hepatitis B virus (HBV), drugs, systemic lupus erythematosus (SLE), and neoplasms. The natural course of the disease is variable; some patients show spontaneous, complete or partial remission and others progress to end-stage renal disease.[24] The exact pathogenesis of membranous nephropathy remains obscure. Nearly 70% of patients with idiopathic membranous nephropathy have circulating antibodies against the M-type phospholipase A2 receptor, a 185-kDa glycoprotein that is normally located on the surface of human podocytes. These autoantibodies are mainly IgG4, which is the predominant immunoglobulin subclass in glomerular deposits.[25]

Membranous nephropathy is the most common renal manifestation in patients with HBV infection. As far as pathogenesis is concerned, it is believed that formation and deposition of immune complexes, predominantly in the sub-epithelial region of the glomerulus, in a genetically predisposed patient with chronic HBV infection can activate complement and lead to glomerular injury.[26] Different HBV antigens and HBV DNA and RNA have been detected in renal tissue from patients with HBV-related membranous nephropathy.[27] However, a pivotal role has been attributed to HBeAg, since it is thought that it is able to traverse the GBM and form sub-epithelial immune complex deposits because of its low molecular weight.[28] Clearance of HBeAg has been related to remission of proteinuria.

4 ANTI-GBM DISEASE (GOODPASTURE'S DISEASE)

Anti-GBM disease is an organ-specific autoimmune disorder characterized by circulating and deposited autoantibodies targeted against the non-collagenous carboxy-terminal (NC1) domain of the α3 chain of type IV collagen. This rare condition (one new case per million population per year) typically presents as a renal-pulmonary syndrome with rapidly progressive glomerulonephritis and pulmonary hemorrhage.[29] Onset of symptoms is commonly preceded by a flu-like illness.[30] Renal biopsy reveals severe crescentic glomerulonephritis and linear deposition of IgG antibodies along the GBM, frequently accompanied by complement (C3) deposits[31] (Figure 2). Circulating anti-GBM antibodies are usually detected by ELISA or Western blotting. A number of animal models have shown that passive transfer of serum or kidney eluate IgG from patients with Goodpasture's disease resulted in the development of rapidly progressive glomerulonephritis.[32,33] The pathogenic role of anti-GBM antibodies is further supported by the correlation of their levels with disease activity.[34]

Patients with Goodpasture's disease also present circulating antibodies specific for the α5NC1 domain of type IV collagen, the major epitope of which was recently mapped to a region called EA–α5.[35] Type IV collagen consists of a family of six α-chains (α1 to α6). The α3, α4, and α5 chains assemble in a triple helical protomer. Two such protomers associate through C-terminal NC1 domains to form a hexamer that in its cross-linked formation is stabilized by novel sulfilimine bonds. Cross-linked α345NC1 hexamers harbor cryptic epitopes that do not bind antibodies unless the hexamer is dissociated. It is hypothesized that factors such as post-translational modifications, oxidation damage, or proteolytic cleavage can alter the quaternary structure of the hexamer, unmask hidden epitopes, induce autoantibody

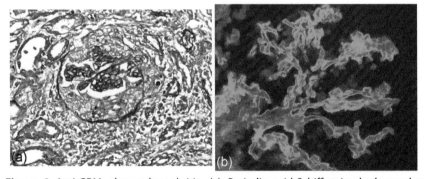

Figure 2 Anti-GBM glomerulonephritis. (a) Periodic acid-Schiff-stained glomerulus showing a large circumferential cellular crescent and segmental disruption of Bowman's capsule in a patient with anti-GBM glomerulonephritis (magnification ×200). (b) Linear immunofluorescence for IgG along the glomerular capillary walls in anti-GBM glomerulonephritis (fluorescein isothiocyanate anti-IgG, magnification ×400).

production and enable binding of antibodies to antigens.[29,31] Furthermore, environmental triggers such as exposure to organic solvents, cigarette smoking or viral infections can inhibit the enzyme responsible for the formation of sulfilimine bonds, rendering α345NC1 hexamers more susceptible to conformational transitions.[29,31]

Although anti-GBM disease is considered the prototype for autoantibody-mediated autoimmunity, recent studies have indicated an increasingly important role for T-cell-mediated mechanisms in the pathogenesis of this condition. Arends et al. showed that a single nephritogenic T-cell epitope (pCol$_{28-40}$) of the NC1 domain of the α3 chain of type IV collagen can induce glomerulonephritis in a rat model.[36] The authors examined seven microbial peptides identified by their sequence homology to the critical residue motif of pCol$_{28-40}$ (xxtTxNPsxx) and recognized three such peptides that could induce modest to severe glomerulonephritis as well as anti-GBM antibodies in immunized rats. The most nephritogenic of these peptides derived from *Clostridium botulinum* could also induce pulmonary hemorrhage. This study was the first to provide experimental evidence linking molecular mimicry to the pathogenesis of anti-GBM disease.[36]

5 ANCA-ASSOCIATED VASCULITIDES

The term *ANCA-associated vasculitis* refers to a group of systemic autoimmune diseases characterized by necrotizing inflammation of small vessels. The ANCA-associated vasculitides comprise granulomatosis with polyangiitis (formerly known as Wegener's granulomatosis), microscopic polyangiitis and its renal-limited form, and Churg-Strauss syndrome.[37] All three diseases can involve the kidney, causing glomerulonephritis with a paucity of immune deposits. ANCAs are directed against components of neutrophil granules and monocyte lysosomes, predominantly proteinase-3 (PR-3) in Wegener's granulomatosis and myeloperoxidase in the case of microscopic polyangiitis and Churg-Strauss syndrome.[31] Recent evidence suggests a potential pathogenetic role for ANCAs. In patients with Wegener's granulomatosis, an increasing ANCA titer has been associated with clinical relapses[38] that could be prevented by early reconstitution of treatment.[39]

Several lines of evidence implicate infections as triggering factors in the pathogenesis of ANCA-associated vasculitis. Chronic nasal carriage of *S. aureus* was reported in 63% of patients with Wegener's granulomatosis and was related to an increased risk of relapsing disease (relative risk, 7.16),[40] whereas co-treatment with trimoxazole effectively reduced the incidence of relapses (relative risk, 0.4).[41] It has been postulated that chronic *S. aureus* infection of the upper airways could induce low-grade inflammation, creating the pro-inflammatory cytokine milieu required for the priming of neutrophils.[31,37] A second hypothesis states that *S. aureus*-derived superantigens could activate B and/or T cells. In a retrospective cohort study by Popa et al., 82% of patients with Wegener's granulomatosis were nasal carriers of *S. aureus*, and 73% of them carried at least one superantigen-positive strain. The presence of *S. aureus* strains expressing the toxic shock toxin-1 superantigen conferred a 13.3 relative risk for relapsing disease.[42] Furthermore, Tadema et al. showed that CpG motifs that are highly prevalent in bacterial DNA can trigger production of ANCAs by autoreactive B lymphocytes *in vitro*.[43] Antibodies against complementary PR-3 peptides were recently identified in patients with Wegener's granulomatosis. Complementary PR-3 is generated from the anti-sense DNA strand encoding for PR-3 and was found to have strong homology with peptides from *S. aureus, Entameba histolytica* and Ross river virus. It is therefore believed that these pathogens could induce the production of antibodies to complementary PR-3 by mechanisms of molecular mimicry, which in turn could generate anti-idiotypic antibodies with affinity to PR-3.[44] In addition, Kain et al. showed that almost all patients with focal necrotizing glomerulonephritis have autoantibodies to the extracellular domain of human lysosomal membrane protein-2 (LAMP-2).[45] LAMP-2 is a heavily glycosylated membrane protein that mediates cell adhesion, cellular homeostasis, and antigen presentation. When detected by indirect IF, antibodies to human LAMP-2 produce a cytoplasmic ANCA pattern. In patients with focal necrotizing glomerulonephritis, these antibodies recognize an epitope (designated P41-49) with 100% homology to FimH, an adhesive protein of gram-negative bacteria such as *Escherichia coli* and *Klebsiella pneumoniae*. It is believed that immune response to FimH during infection with fimbriated gram-negative pathogens can induce anti-LAMP-2 antibodies through molecular mimicry.[45]

Finally, circumstantial evidence indicates that in addition to bacterial infections, other pathogens such as viruses and protozoa could also contribute to the pathogenesis of ANCA-associated vasculitides. More specifically, a higher level of autoantibodies against hepatitis C virus (HCV), *Toxoplasma gondii, H. pylori*, cytomegalovirus and Epstein-Barr virus have been described in patients with Wegener's granulomatosis.[46] Although parvovirus B19 also has been proposed as one of the most prominent contributors to the initiation of the vasculitic process,[47] other studies have refuted this connection.[48]

6 HENOCH-SCHÖNLEIN PURPURA

Henoch-Schönlein purpura is an acute small-vessel leukocytoclastic vasculitis predominantly affecting the pediatric population; it is associated with IgA1 deposition in vessel walls and renal mesangium. It is characterized by cutaneous purpura on the buttocks and the lower extremities, arthritis, abdominal pain, gastrointestinal bleeding and, in approximately 40% of cases, nephritis.[49] Cases of Henoch-Schönlein purpura show a seasonal distribution, with lowest incidence during the summer months,[50] and are usually preceded by an upper respiratory tract infection.[51]

The disease has been associated with a wide variety of infectious agents, such as *Bartonella henselae*,[52] parvovirus B19,[53] *S. aureus*,[54] *H. pylori*,[55] *Mycoplasma pneumoniae*,[56] Coxsackievirus,[57] and HBV.[58] However, the strongest association has been reported with group A beta-hemolytic *Streptococcus*, found in 20–50% of patients.[6] In one study, 30% of children with nephritis due to Henoch-Schönlein purpura had mesangial deposition of nephritis-associated plasmin receptor, a group A streptococcal antigen with possible implications in the pathogenesis of the disease.[59] Likewise, another study reported deposits of IgA-binding streptococcal M-protein in the mesangium and skin vessels of these patients.[60] Interestingly, a temporal association between hospitalizations for group A beta-hemolytic *Streptococcus*, *S. aureus* or parainfluenza virus and hospitalizations for Henoch-Schönlein purpura has been found.[61] The role of infections in the development of Henoch-Schönlein purpura is further stressed by the fact that some patients improve following tonsillectomy.[62] Potential development of Henoch-Schönlein purpura as a response to vaccine antigens has also been suggested, yet this linkage has been considered coincidental since the number of reported cases is small.[51]

7 CRYOGLOBULINEMIAS

Cryoglobulinemia is associated with multiple conditions including autoimmune disorders, malignancies, and infections, which are characterized by the presence of immunoglobulins that precipitate *in vitro* at temperatures less than 37°C and produce organ damage (cryoglobulins).[63] Type I cryoglobulins are simple monoclonal immunoglobulins, usually of the IgM or, less frequently, of the IgG or IgA class, or consisting of light chains. Type I cryoglobulins are related to lymphoproliferative disorders. Types II and III cryoglobulins are encountered in mixed cryoglobulinemias and consist of a monoclonal (in type II) or polyclonal (in type III) immunoglobulin, usually of the IgM and, rarely, of the IgG or IgA class. These display rheumatoid factor activity and bind the Fc portion of polyclonal IgG. Mixed cryoglobulinemias represent 80% of all cases and are commonly associated with connective tissue diseases, lymphoproliferative disorders, and chronic infections.

In a large cohort of patients, cryoglobulinemia was associated with infections in 75% of cases; 73% of these cases were positive for HCV, 19% for human immunodeficiency virus, and 3% for HBV.[64] The clinical syndrome related to cryoglobulinemic vasculitis is characterized mainly by cutaneous, renal, articular, and peripheral nervous system involvement. Renal manifestations develop in 20–30% of patients with mixed cryoglobulinemia,[65] including new-onset hypertension, proteinuria with microscopic hematuria and renal insufficiency, most commonly in the context of a type I membranoproliferative glomerulonephritis with sub-endothelial deposits.[66] The pivotal role of HCV in the pathogenesis of cryoglobulinemic vasculitis is supported by studies demonstrating the presence of HCV core and E2 proteins in skin and renal biopsies of patients.[67] A central event in the etiopathogenesis of HCV-related mixed cryoglobulinemia is a clonal autoreactive B-lymphocyte expansion resulting from the chronic immune stimulation by a persisting HCV infection. Finally, a strong indication for the pathogenetic role of HCV infection in the development of cryoglobulinemic vasculitis and membranoproliferative glomerulonephritis is provided by the clinical observation that treatment of the infection with interferon-α frequently leads to improvement of proteinuria and renal function. In contrast, cessation of therapy often leads to recurrence of the disease.[68]

8 LUPUS NEPHRITIS

Lupus nephritis is one of the most frequent and potentially devastating manifestations of SLE and is related to chronic kidney disease and inflammation. The exact cause is unknown, but sex, genetic predisposition, infections, and environmental factors may play a role in the pathogenesis of lupus nephritis. Infections are known to trigger SLE flares. Nucleic acids released from netting or apoptotic neutrophils activate innate and adaptive immunity via viral nucleic acid- TLRs.[69] A possible mechanism is that pathogens bind to TLRs, thus activating immune cell subsets and inducing the release of cytokines, chemokines and type I interferons that also contribute to autoimmune tissue injury in SLE.[69,70] For example, in the kidneys of patients with SLE, activation of TLR7 and TLR9 expressed on dendritic cells infiltrating macrophages and B cells promotes release of pro-inflammatory cytokines such as IL-6 or CCL2, which in turn enhance glomerular or tubulointerstitial inflammation. Similarly, ligation of TLR2 and TLR4 by bacterial wall components strongly activates glomerular endothelial cells and podocytes.[70]

9 CONCLUSIONS

The role of infections in the pathogenesis of autoimmune renal diseases is supported by both clinical and experimental data. In many cases, such as IgA nephropathy, Henoch-Schönlein purpura, Goodpasture's disease and lupus nephritis, symptoms develop or are exacerbated following infections. In the case of IgA nephropathy and Henoch-Schönlein purpura, experimental evidence suggests that impaired mucosal response to microbial antigens could trigger synthesis of poorly galactosylated nephritogenic IgA1. In membranous nephropathy, a potential infectious agent could reveal cryptic epitopes of the phospholipase A2 receptor 1 peptide, enhancing its antigenicity. Likewise, in Goodpasture's disease microbial pathogens possibly induce autoantibody formation by facilitating conformational transition of α345NC1 hexamers, whereas in ANCA-associated vasculitides, nasal carriage of *S. aureus* strains has been related to clinical relapses through activation of the immune system by superantigens or mechanisms of molecular mimicry. In cryoglobulinemia, a prominent association with chronic HCV infection has been described; this leads to clonal autoreactive B-cell expansion, synthesis of mixed type cryoglobulins, and deposition of immune complexes in the glomerulus. TLR receptor and complement activation also have been implicated in the complex pathogenetic process of all these diseases.

REFERENCES

1. Segelmark M, Hellmark T. Autoimmune kidney diseases. *Autoimmun Rev* 2010;**9**(5): A366–71.
2. *Progress in Autoimmune Diseases Research. Report to Congress, National Institutes of Health, The Autoimmune Diseases Coordinating Committee.* March 2005.
3. Wahren-Herlenius M, Dörner T. Immunopathogenic mechanisms of systemic autoimmune disease. *Lancet* 2013;**382**(9894):819–31.
4. Pollard KM, Kono DH. Requirements for innate immune pathways in environmentally induced autoimmunity. *BMC Med* 2013;**11**:100.
5. Miller FW, Alfredsson L, Costenbader KH, Kamen DL, Nelson LM, Norris JM, et al. Epidemiology of environmental exposures and human autoimmune diseases: findings from a National Institute of Environmental Health Sciences Expert Panel Workshop. *J Autoimmun* 2012;**39**(4):259–71.

6. Yang YH, Chuang YH, Wang LC, Huang HY, Gershwin ME, Chiang BL. The immunobiology of Henoch-Schönlein purpura. *Autoimmun Rev* 2008;**7**(3):179–84.

7. Barratt J, Feehally J. Primary IgA nephropathy: new insights into pathogenesis. *Semin Nephrol* 2011;**31**(4):349–60.

8. Smith A, Molyneux K, Feehally J, Barratt J. O-glycosylation of serum IgA1 antibodies against mucosal and systemic antigens in IgA nephropathy. *J Am Soc Nephrol* 2006;**17** (12):3520–8.

9. Roodnat J, de Fijter J, van Kooten C, Daha M, van Es L. Decreased IgA1 response after primary oral immunization with live typhoid vaccine in primary IgA nephropathy. *Nephrol Dial Transplant* 1999;**14**(2):353–9.

10. Buck K, Smith A, Molyneux K, El-Barbary H, Feehally J, Barratt J. B-cell O-galactosyltransferase activity, and expression of O-glycosylation genes in bone marrow in IgA nephropathy. *Kidney Int* 2008;**73**(10):1128–36.

11. Novak J, Vu H, Novak L, Julian B, Mestecky J, Tomana M. Interactions of human mesangial cells with IgA and IgA-containing immune complexes. *Kidney Int* 2002;**62** (2):465–75.

12. Wyatt R, Julian B. Activation of complement in IgA nephropathy. *Am J Kidney Dis* 1988;**12**(5):437–42.

13. Coppo R, Amore A, Peruzzi L, Vergano L, Camilla R. Innate immunity and IgA nephropathy. *J Nephrol* 2010;**23**(6):626–32.

14. Takahashi A, Kawasaki Y, Yoshida K, Mochizuki K, Isome M, Honzumi K, et al. Detection of enteroviruses in renal biopsies from patients with immunoglobulin A nephropathy. *Pediatr Nephrol* 2005;**20**(11):1578–82.

15. Müller G, Müller C, Engler-Blum G, Kühn W, Risler T, Bohle A, et al. Human cytomegalovirus in immunoglobulin A nephropathy: detection by polymerase chain reaction. *Nephron* 1992;**62**(4):389–93.

16. Kai H, Shimizu Y, Hagiwara M, Yoh K, Hirayama K, Yamagata K, et al. Post-MRSA infection glomerulonephritis with marked Staphylococcus aureus cell envelope antigen deposition in glomeruli. *J Nephrol* 2006;**19**(2):215–19.

17. Yamamoto C, Suzuki S, Kimura H, Yoshida H, Gejyo F. Experimental nephropathy induced by Haemophilus parainfluenzae antigens. *Nephron* 2002;**90**(3):320–7.

18. Amore A, Coppo R, Nedrud J, Sigmund N, Lamm M, Emancipator S. The role of nasal tolerance in a model of IgA nephropathy induced in mice by Sendai virus. *Clin Immunol* 2004;**113**(1):101–8.

19. Xie Y, Nishi S, Ueno M, Imai N, Sakatsume M, Narita I, et al. The efficacy of tonsillectomy on long-term renal survival in patients with IgA nephropathy. *Kidney Int* 2003;**63**(5):1861–7.

20. Sharmin S, Shimizu Y, Hagiwara M, Hirayama K, Koyama A. Staphylococcus aureus antigens induce IgA-type glomerulonephritis in Balb/c mice. *J Nephrol* 2004;**17** (4):504–11.

21. Coppo R, Camilla R, Amore A, Peruzzi L, Daprà V, Loiacono E, et al. Toll-like receptor 4 expression is increased in circulating mononuclear cells of patients with immunoglobulin A nephropathy. *Clin Exp Immunol* 2010;**159**(1):73–81.

22. Qin W, Zhong X, Fan J, Zhang Y, Liu X, Ma X. External suppression causes the low expression of the Cosmc gene in IgA nephropathy. *Nephrol Dial Transplant* 2008;**23** (5):1608–14.

23. Coppo R. Can a dysregulated mucosal immune system in IgA nephropathy be controlled by tonsillectomy? *Nephrol Dial Transplant* 2010;**25**(8):2395–7.

24. Ponticelli C, Glassock R. Glomerular diseases: membranous nephropathy-a modern view. *Clin J Am Soc Nephrol* 2014;**9**(3):609–16.

25. Beck L, Bonegio R, Lambeau G, Beck D, Powell D, Cummins T, et al. M-type phospholipase A2 receptor as target antigen in idiopathic membranous nephropathy. *N Engl J Med* 2009;**361**(1):11–21.
26. Chan TM. Hepatitis B, and renal disease. *Curr Hepat Rep* 2010;**9**(2):99–105.
27. Lai KN, Ho RT, Tam JS, Lai FM. Detection of hepatitis B virus DNA and RNA in kidneys of HBV related glomerulonephritis. *Kidney Int* 1996;**50**(6):1965–77.
28. Lai KN, Lai FM, Tam JS. Comparison of polyclonal and monoclonal antibodies in determination of glomerular deposits of hepatitis B virus antigens in hepatitis B virus-associated glomerulonephritides. *Am J Clin Pathol* 1989;**92**(2):159–65.
29. Pedchenko V, Vanacore R, Hudson B. Goodpasture's disease: molecular architecture of the autoantigen provides clues to etiology and pathogenesis. *Curr Opin Nephrol Hypertens* 2011;**20**(3):290–6.
30. Wilson C, Dixon F. Anti-glomerular basement membrane antibody-induced glomerulonephritis. *Kidney Int* 1973;**3**(2):74–89.
31. Kambham N. Crescentic Glomerulonephritis: an update on Pauci-immune and Anti-GBM diseases. *Adv Anat Pathol* 2012;**19**(2):111–24.
32. Lerner R, Glassock R, Dixon F. The role of anti-glomerular basement membrane antibody in the pathogenesis of human glomerulonephritis. *J Exp Med* 1967;**126**(6):989–1004.
33. Germuth F, Choi I, Taylor J, Rodriguez E. Antibasement membrane disease. I. The glomerular lesions of Goodpasture's disease and experimental disease in sheep. *Johns Hopkins Med J* 1972;**131**(5):367–84.
34. Yang R, Hellmark T, Zhao J, Cui Z, Segelmark M, Zhao M-H, et al. Levels of epitope-specific autoantibodies correlate with renal damage in anti-GBM disease. *Nephrol Dial Transplant* 2009;**24**(6):1838–44.
35. Pedchenko V, Bondar O, Fogo A, Vanacore R, Voziyan P, Kitching A, et al. Molecular architecture of the Goodpasture autoantigen in anti-GBM nephritis. *N Engl J Med* 2010;**363**(4):343–54.
36. Arends J, Wu J, Borillo J, Troung L, Zhou C, Vigneswaran N, et al. T cell epitope mimicry in antiglomerular basement membrane disease. *J Immunol* 2006;**176**(2):1252–8.
37. Kallenberg C. Pathogenesis of ANCA-associated vasculitis, an update. *Clin Rev Allergy Immunol* 2011;**41**(2):224–31.
38. Boomsma M, Stegeman C, van der Leij M, Oost W, Hermans J, Kallenberg C, et al. Prediction of relapses in Wegener's granulomatosis by measurement of antineutrophil cytoplasmic antibody levels: a prospective study. *Arthritis Rheum* 2000;**43**(9):2025–33.
39. Tervaert J, Huitema M, Hené R, Sluiter W, The T, van der Hem G, et al. Prevention of relapses in Wegener's granulomatosis by treatment based on antineutrophil cytoplasmic antibody titre. *Lancet* 1990;**336**(8717):709–11.
40. Stegeman C, Tervaert J, Sluiter W, Manson W, de Jong P, Kallenberg C. Association of chronic nasal carriage of Staphylococcus aureus and higher relapse rates in Wegener granulomatosis. *Ann Intern Med* 1994;**120**(1):12–17.
41. Stegeman C, Tervaert J, de Jong P, Kallenberg C. Trimethoprim-sulfamethoxazole (co-trimoxazole) for the prevention of relapses of Wegener's granulomatosis. Dutch Co-Trimoxazole Wegener Study Group. *N Engl J Med* 1996;**335**(1):16–20.
42. Popa E, Stegeman C, Abdulahad W, van der Meer B, Arends J, Manson W, et al. Staphylococcal toxic-shock-syndrome-toxin-1 as a risk factor for disease relapse in Wegener's granulomatosis. *Rheumatology (Oxford)* 2007;**46**(6):1029–33.
43. Tadema H, Abdulahad W, Lepse N, Stegeman C, Kallenberg C, Heeringa P. Bacterial DNA motifs trigger ANCA production in ANCA-associated vasculitis in remission. *Rheumatology (Oxford)* 2011;**50**(4):689–96.

44. Pendergraft W, Preston G, Shah R, Tropsha A, Carter C, Jennette J, et al. Autoimmunity is triggered by cPR-3(105-201), a protein complementary to human autoantigen proteinase-3. *Nat Med* 2004;**10**(1):72–9.

45. Kain R, Exner M, Brandes R, Ziebermayr R, Cunningham D, Alderson C, et al. Molecular mimicry in pauci-immune focal necrotizing glomerulonephritis. *Nat Med* 2008;**14**(10):1088–96.

46. Lidar M, Lipschitz N, Langevitz P, Barzilai O, Ram M, Porat-Katz B-S, et al. Infectious serologies and autoantibodies in Wegener's granulomatosis and other vasculitides. *Ann N Y Acad Sci* 2009;**1173**(1):649–57.

47. Shimohata H, Higuchi T, Ogawa Y, Fujita S, Nagai M, Imaizumi M, et al. Human parvovirus B19-induced acute glomerulonephritis: a case report. *Ren Fail* 2013;**35**(1):159–62.

48. Eden A, Mahr A, Servant A, Radjef N, Amard S, Mouthon L, et al. Lack of association between B19 or V9 erythrovirus infection and ANCA-positive vasculitides: a case-control study. *Rheumatology (Oxford)* 2003;**42**(5):660–4.

49. Saulsbury F. Henoch-Schönlein purpura. *Curr Opin Rheumatol* 2010;**22**(5):598–602.

50. Atkinson S, Barker D. Seasonal distribution of Henoch-Schönlein purpura. *Br J Prev Soc Med* 1976;**30**(1):22–5.

51. Piram M, Mahr A. Epidemiology of immunoglobulin A vasculitis (Henoch-Schönlein): current state of knowledge. *Curr Opin Rheumatol* 2013;**25**(2):171–8.

52. Robinson J, Spady D, Prasad E, McColl D, Artsob H. Bartonella seropositivity in children with Henoch-Schonlein purpura. *BMC Infect Dis* 2005;**5**:21.

53. Cioc A, Sedmak D, Nuovo G, Dawood M, Smart G, Magro C. Parvovirus B19 associated adult Henoch Schönlein purpura. *J Cutan Pathol* 2002;**29**(10):602–7.

54. Eftychiou C, Samarkos M, Golfinopoulou S, Skoutelis A, Psarra A. Henoch-Schonlein purpura associated with methicillin-resistant *Staphylococcus aureus* infection. *Am J Med* 2006;**119**(1):85–6.

55. Xiong L-J, Tong Y, Wang Z-L, Mao M. Is Helicobacter pylori infection associated with Henoch-Schonlein purpura in Chinese children? a meta-analysis. *World J Pediatr* 2012;**8**(4):301–8.

56. Kaneko K, Fujinaga S, Ohtomo Y, Nagaoka R, Obinata K, Yamashiro Y. Mycoplasma pneumoniae-associated Henoch-Schönlein purpura nephritis. *Pediatr Nephrol* 1999;**13**(9):1000–1.

57. Costa M, Lisboa M, Romeu J, Caldeira J, De Queiroz V. Henoch-Schonlein purpura associated with coxsackie-virus B1 infection. *Clin Rheumatol* 1995;**14**(4):488–90.

58. Shin J, Lee J. Hepatitis B virus infection and Henoch-Schönlein purpura. *J Dermatol* 2007;**34**(2):156.

59. Masuda M, Nakanishi K, Yoshizawa N, Iijima K, Yoshikawa N. Group A streptococcal antigen in the glomeruli of children with Henoch-Schönlein nephritis. *Am J Kidney Dis* 2003;**41**(2):366–70.

60. Schmitt R, Carlsson F, Mörgelin M, Tati R, Lindahl G, Karpman D. Tissue deposits of IgA-binding streptococcal M proteins in IgA nephropathy and Henoch-Schonlein purpura. *Am J Pathol* 2010;**176**(2):608–18.

61. Weiss P, Klink A, Luan X, Feudtner C. Temporal association of Streptococcus, Staphylococcus, and parainfluenza pediatric hospitalizations and hospitalized cases of Henoch-Schönlein purpura. *J Rheumatol* 2010;**37**(12):2587–94.

62. Iwazu Y, Akimoto T, Muto S, Kusano E. Clinical remission of Henoch-Schönlein purpura nephritis after a monotherapeutic tonsillectomy. *Clin Exp Nephrol* 2011;**15**(1):132–5.

63. Ramos-Casals M, Stone JH, Cid MC, Bosch X. The cryoglobulinaemias. *Lancet* 2012;**379**(9813):348–60.

64. Trejo O, Ramos-Casals M, García-Carrasco M, Yagüe J, Jiménez S, de la Red G, et al. Cryoglobulinemia: study of etiologic factors and clinical and immunologic features in 443 patients from a single center. *Medicine* 2001;**80**(4):252–62.
65. Cordonnier D, Renversez J, Vialtel P, Dechelette E. The kidney in mixed cryoglobulinemias. *Springer Semin Immunopathol* 1987;**9**(4):395–415.
57. Terrier B, Cacoub P. Renal involvement in HCV-related vasculitis. *Clin Res Hepatol Gastroenterol* 2013;**37**(4):334–9.
67. Sansonno D, Gesualdo L, Manno C, Schena F, Dammacco F. Hepatitis C virus-related proteins in kidney tissue from hepatitis C virus-infected patients with cryoglobulinemic membranoproliferative glomerulonephritis. *Hepatology* 1997;**25**(5):1237–44.
68. Miller S, Howell D. Glomerular diseases associated with hepatitis C virus infection. *Saudi J Kidney Dis Transpl* 2000;**11**(2):145–60.
69. Allam R, Anders H-J. The role of innate immunity in autoimmune tissue injury. *Curr Opin Rheumatol* 2008;**20**(5):538–44.
70. Lech M, Anders HJ. The pathogenesis of lupus nephritis. *J Am Soc Nephrol* 2013;**24**(9):1357–66.

CHAPTER 57

Infections Associated with Retinal Autoimmunity

Barbara Detrick[*,1], **John J. Hooks**[†], **Robert Nussenblatt**[†]
[*]Department of Pathology, School of Medicine, The Johns Hopkins University, Baltimore, Maryland, USA
[†]Laboratory of Immunology, National Eye Institute, National Institutes of Health, Bethesda, Maryland, USA
[1]Corresponding Author: bdetrick@jhmi.edu

1 INFECTIONS AND AUTOIMMUNITY IN THE RETINA

Autoimmune reactivity and autoimmune disease in the eye is a rapidly expanding area of research and therapy.[1–5] Numerous studies of other body sites revealed clear links between infections and autoimmunity and autoimmune disease.[6,7] However, only a limited number of studies in which retinal disorders were evaluated to study this relationship have been reported. This chapter begins with a brief overview of infection and autoimmunity in the eye, focusing on some of the unique features of the ocular microenvironment. This is followed by specific examples of infections and autoimmunity in the retina. We highlight two human diseases triggered by *Onchocerca volvulus* or *Toxoplasma gondii* and discuss an experimental model of retinal degenerative disease, referred to as experimental coronavirus retinopathy (ECOR). This degeneration is triggered by the murine coronavirus, the mouse hepatitis virus (MHV), and is characterized by genetic predisposition and autoimmune reactivity. Finally, we explore mechanisms by which different infectious agents trigger autoimmune reactivity.

2 THE EYE: INFECTION AND AUTOIMMUNITY

The visual axis is a precious sense. The eye is an organ with known immunologic processes that are driven by both infectious and non–infectious factors. The eye is unique in that it lacks lymphatics and still enjoys an intimate relationship with the immune system. An inflammatory process nor where in the eye is called uveitis, but this term does not reflect the origin of the inflammatory process nor where in the eye it is located. While there are many descriptions of inflammatory processes in the eye, there are three major presentations

Infection and Autoimmunity
http://dx.doi.org/10.1016/B978-0-444-63269-2.00059-3

of these conditions. If the inflammatory condition is centered in the front of the eye, the process is termed an anterior uveitis. If upon examination the dominant part of the inflammation is centered in the vitreous of the eye, it is termed an intermediate uveitis. Finally, if inflammation occurs in the back of the eye and is centered in the retina or the choroid, it is termed a posterior uveitis. Clearly, inflammatory conditions may involve several parts of the eye, and if all anatomic components of the eye are involved, it is termed a panuveitis.

Eye specialists have the distinct advantage of being able to visualize directly the parts of the eye that can be involved in an inflammatory process. In addition to simple visualization, many additional tools can be readily applied. Electrophysiologic testing is easily and frequently performed. This is an excellent way to evaluate the retina's ability to react to a light stimulus. Fluorescein angiography, which uses a dye injected into a vein in the arm, allows photographs of the retina to be printed. This approach helps to visualize the vascular system and the integrity of the retina. The severity of the inflammatory response can be graded by direct visualization of the ocular inflammatory response. Most inflammatory processes that we recognize have associated cellular responses. We also know that antibody-mediated pathology, as seen in such entities as cancer-associated retinopathy, can occur but seem to do so in the distinct minority of cases.

The eye is a complex organ from the point of view of the immune system. It is known that an antigen placed into the anterior chamber of the eye induces a deviated immune response, with a marked decrease in cell-mediated responses, but intact cytotoxic and B-cell responses are maintained (1). In addition, the retina is a complicated structure; several layers are needed to turn a light stimulus into a chemical signal that is ultimately sent to the brain. A number of uveitogenic antigens have been identified and characterized at the photoreceptor level and the single layer just below it, that is, the retinal pigment epithelium (RPE) (2). Two antigens in particular, the retinal S-antigen and the inter-photoreceptor binding protein (IRBP), have been used to develop a model of autoimmune ocular disease, called experimental autoimmune uveoretinitis (3). This model has many qualities of the disease observed in humans, and it has enhanced our understanding of the underlying mechanisms that lead to disease. One major difference between this model and human disease is, of course, that it is not spontaneous. It is not clear what triggers the human disease. This chapter explores one such trigger—ocular infection. Several entities, some based on animal models, others seen in the clinic, are discussed to elucidate the possible role between infection and autoimmunity.

3 EXPERIMENTAL CORONAVIRUS RETINOPATHY

ECOR is an animal model system that we generated in the 1990s to demonstrate that a virus can trigger a progressive retinal degenerative disease.[8] Studies during the past 20 years have identified that this degenerative eye disease is composed of three basic components: a virus component, a genetic component, and a immunologic component.[9,10] In our system, we selected a naturally occurring neurotrophic strain (JHM) of MHV that infects and persists within the retina. The virus causes an acute infection marked by virus replication in distinct retinal cells, and the production of both neutralizing antibody and cytokines. This disease also has a genetic component. Different strains of mice, such as BABL/c and CD-1, were extensively studied after coronavirus infection. During the early phase of the disease (days 1–8) the virus infects and replicates within the retina of both BALB/c and CD-1 mouse strains.[11] However, only the BALB/c mice experience a late phase of the disease (days 10–140) that is marked by a retinal degeneration. CD-1 mice do not undergo the retinal degenerative phase; rather, the retina returns to a normal architecture within 20 days.

Finally, this disease is characterized by the presence of autoantibodies, specifically anti-retinal and anti-RPE antibodies. The presence of these antibodies is observed only in the BALB/c mice susceptible to retinal degeneration. These autoantibodies are absent in the CD-1 mice resistant to retinal degeneration. In summary, ECOR is a virus-triggered retinal degenerative disease that is influenced by both genetics and immune response. In the following sections we discuss in detail the virologic, pathologic, immunologic, genetic, and autoimmune factors involved in this model system.

3.1 Virologic Component of ECOR

Coronaviruses are large, enveloped, positive-strand RNA viruses that cause significant diseases in a number of animal species and humans. In animals, coronaviruses are responsible for important diseases among livestock, poultry, and laboratory rodents. Until recently, man was known to be infected with two strains of coronavirus. Either of these strains is responsible for approximately 50% of the incidence of the common cold. A new human coronavirus was discovered as the causative agent for severe acute respiratory syndrome (SARS).[12] One of the closest relatives to the human SARS-coronavirus is the murine coronavirus MHV. The JHM strain of MHV is the most thoroughly studied neurotrophic coronavirus. It causes both acute and chronic central nervous system (CNS) effects in mice and rats. Acute encephalomyelitis and chronic CNS disease have been observed in mice, whereas an autoimmune disease known as subacute demyelinating encephalomyelitis has been described in rats.

Initial studies of the ECOR system showed that inoculation of this JHM strain into the vitreous or anterior chamber of BALB/c mice resulted in retinal tissue damage.[9,10] Infectious virus could be detected within the retina between 1 and 6 days post-inoculation (PI), reaching a peak level of $10^{4.5}$ plaque-forming units/mL at day 3.[13] Virus antigen also was identified within the retina between days 2 and 6 PI.[10] On day 2, virus antigen was first detected within the RPE cells and the ciliary body epithelial cells, and this virus replication intensified at days 3 and 4. Between days 3 and 6, virus antigen also was detected in Müller-like cells that span the multiple layers of the neural retina. Virus antigen was occasionally observed within the ganglion cells. After day 7, infectious virus and viral antigen could not be detected anywhere within the retina. However, in situ hybridization studies identified that the viral RNA persisted within the retina until 60 days PI.[14] Antivirus neutralizing antibodies were first noted at day 7 PI[13] and coincided with the disappearance of infectious virus and viral antigen.

3.2 Retinal Pathology in ECOR

After inoculation with the JHM virus, two distinct patterns of retinal pathology were noted in the BALB/c mice.[10] The early phase of the disease was characterized by retinal vasculitis and perivasculitis. The late phase of the disease was marked by retinal degenerative changes. The retinal layers revealed disorganization with large areas of outer and inner segment loss. In addition, the RPE cells were morphologically abnormal, with focal RPE cell swelling or proliferation or with focal RPE cell atrophy. Analysis of retinal cell function also revealed dramatic changes.[15,16] There was a significant decrease in or complete loss of electroretinogram patterns and the disappearance of an important transport protein in the retina, IRBP.

3.3 Host Response in ECOR

The host immune response to this virus infection was evaluated by tracking the cellular infiltrate and identifying the cytokine profile within the retina.[17] Macrophages were the most prominent infiltrating cells, followed by T cells (CD4 and CD8). During the course of the disease, cytokine profiles were studied by assessing retina tissue and sera.[17] On day 4, cytokine retinal gene expression and serum protein expression revealed the presence of

IL-6, interferon (IFN-γ), and tumor necrosis factor (TNF-α) in retinas infected with the virus. The presence of IFN-γ also was associated with an up-regulation of MHC class I and II molecules on a variety of retinal cells. In contrast, MHC class I and II molecules were not identified within the normal or mock-injected retinas. It was noted that the first cell to express these MHC molecules was the RPE cell. This cell is also the first cell to express new viral antigens during infection in vivo and is persistently infected in vitro.[18] It is critically important to point out that this RPE cell has been shown to process and present retinal and non-retinal antigens to sensitized T cells, and it is up-regulated to express MHC class II molecules during retinal autoimmune and degenerative processes.[19,20]

3.4 Innate Immunity is a Key Factor

We next examined very early cytokine and chemokine profiles as a measure of the intensity of immune reactivity in mice infected with coronavirus. These studies identified a distinct difference in the early innate immune response between the susceptible and resistant mouse strains.[21] These differences are noted in the production of IFN-γ and the two chemokines triggered by IFN-γ: CXCL9 and CXCL10. For example, on day 2 and 3 PI, the BALB/c mice have high levels of IFN-γ, CXCL9 and CXCL10 in their sera. At the same time, significantly lower levels of these molecules are detected in the sera from CD-1 mice. Moreover, real-time PCR analysis of retinas confirmed that CXCL9 and CXCL10 gene expression is significantly greater in the BALB/c mice retinas compared with CD-1 mice retinas. CXCL9 and CXCL10 interact with CXCR3, which is present on activated T cells and natural killer (NK) cells, and they direct the migration of these cells to specific targets, such as the retina.[22] These studies underscore an important concept: that innate immunity directs and sets the stage for adaptive immunity. In this model system, we describe how the robust immune response in the BALB/c mouse could trigger an autoimmune component.

3.5 Genetic Factors in ECOR

The genetic constitution of the host can be a critical factor in determining the outcome of a virus infection.[11] We therefore evaluated the possible role of host genetics in ECOR. We inoculated selected strains of mice (BABL/c, C57B1, A/J, and CD-1) and examined the retinal disease. When C57B1 and A/J mice were evaluated, we observed a disease pattern similar to that

Table 1 Retinal Inflammation and Retinal Degeneration in Mice Inoculated with Coronavirus (JHM Strain)

Retinal Disease	Days	BALB/c Mice		CD-1 Mice	
		Positive/ Tested (n)	%	Positive/ Tested (n)	%
Inflammation (vasculitis)	0	0/30	0	0/20	0
	1–7	26/26	100	20/20	100
	10–45	0/30	0	0/20	0
Degeneration	0	0/30	0	0/20	0
	1–7	0/26	0	0/20	0
	10–45	30/30	100	0/20	0

observed in the BALB/c mice. However, retinal tissue damage induced by the JHM virus in the CD-1 mice was very different (Table 1). Only the early phase of the disease, consisting of retinal vasculitis, was observed. These CD-1 mice did not develop retinal degenerative disease. In fact, by day 20 PI, the retina had a normal appearance. These studies underscore the role of genetics in ECOR and showed that the genetics of the host profoundly affects the nature of retinal tissue damage.

Since the CD-1 mice did not exhibit the late retinal degenerative phase of the disease, we studied a variety of parameters and compared these findings with the data obtained from BALB/c mice. For example, during the acute phase of the disease, viral load in the retina, production of anti-virus antibody, breakdown of the blood–retina barrier, lymphoid trafficking and MHC class I and II staining were similar in both mouse strains. Only in the late phase of the disease did the two mouse strains show significant differences: one group (BALB/c mice) displayed a retinal degeneration with blood–retina barrier breakdown, and the other (CD-1 mice) showed a normal retinal architecture.

3.6 Autoimmune Component of ECOR

In ECOR, the late phase of the disease was associated with the lack of direct evidence for viral replication within the retina. This observation suggested that the continued degenerative process may be associated with alterations directly induced by virus replication during the first few days after infection or it may be associated with additional factors. Inasmuch as viruses are known to trigger autoimmune phenomena and some human retinopathies may be associated with autoantibody formation, we studied the possible production

Table 2 Anti-Retinal Antibody Production and Retinal Degeneration in Coronavirus-Inoculated Mice

Mouse	Treatment	Autoantibody in Retinal Tissue Positive/Tested (n)	Retinal Degeneration Positive/Tested (n)
BALB/c	Untreated	0/20	0/20
	Mock injection	0/15	0/15
	JHM virus	22/22	22/22
CD-1	Untreated	0/15	0/15
	Mock injection	0/15	0/15
	JHM virus	0/20	0/20

of anti-retinal autoantibodies.[23] We found that the degenerative process in the BALB/c mice was associated with the presence of anti-retinal autoantibodies (Table 2). These autoantibodies were not found in sera from normal or mock-injected mice. Furthermore, the CD-1 mice that developed an immune response in the acute disease did not develop autoantibodies.

The presence of antibodies to retinal tissue was evaluated by immuno-peroxidase staining of frozen sections of normal rat eyes. Two patterns of staining were observed in the BALB/c mice: reactivity in the neural retina and reactivity in the RPE. The anti-retinal autoantibodies first appeared as IgM class antibodies. This was later replaced by IgG class autoantibodies. The anti-RPE cell autoantibodies were predominantly of the IgG class. Therefore, those mice that failed to develop anti-retinal autoantibodies also failed to develop retinal degeneration (Table 2). These findings suggest a role for autoimmunity in the pathogenesis of ECOR.

Our latest approach towards better understand this disease process was the development of an autoantigen discovery programme. Using a mouse RPE cDNA library, we identified two retinal autoantigens, α-fodrin and villin 2, in ECOR. α-Fodrin is found in the cytoplasm of cell bodies in inner nuclear layer (INL) and retinal ganglion cell (RGC) and on the apical surface of the RPE. Villin-2 is found in both RPE cells and Müller cells. A truncated form of α-fodrin was expressed and purified. This purified α-fodrin reacted only with sera from virus-infected BALB/c mice. Moreover, CD4 T cells from virus-infected BALB/c mice specifically responded to α-fodrin peptide. These data suggest that both antibodies to α-fodrin and CD4 T cells specifically sensitized to α-fodrin may contribute to the retinal degeneration seen in the ECOR susceptible mice. It is of interest to note that autoantibodies to α-fodrin have been observed in three human diseases: glaucoma, Alzheimer's disease, and Sjögren's syndrome.

4 TOXOPLASMOSIS (*T. GONDII*)

Toxoplasmosis is a disorder that has a worldwide distribution. It is caused by the obligate intracellular parasite *T. gondii*. Over 500 million people are believed to have the disease. The organism was first described in the brain of gondii, a North African rodent, by Nicolle and Manceaux[24] in 1908 and in a rabbit by Splendore.[25] The first connection between this organism and human disease was made by Janku,[26] who described the presence of the organism in a child who died of disseminated toxoplasmosis. While suspected for a long period, it was not until the early 1950s that the parasite was shown to cause ocular disease. Helenor Campbell Wilder, working at the Armed Forces Institute of Pathology in Washington, DC, identified the organism in eyes that were believed to have other types of inflammatory processes, particularly tuberculosis.[27] It is interesting to note that a similar observation has been made more recently in Nepal, where many cases of ocular tuberculosis have been re-diagnosed as toxoplasmosis of the eye.

The cat (and perhaps related species) seems to be the definitive host of *T. gondii*. The sexual cycle is one of schizogony and gametogony, leading to the development of toxoplasma oocysts, which are 10–12 μm in size and are found uniquely in the intestinal mucosa of cats. Two forms of organisms can be found in man: cysts and tachyzoites. The tachyzoites (the proliferative intracellular form) are believed to be the cause of most tissue damage in humans, although often it is very difficult to demonstrate the presence of this stage of the organism. The bradyzoites (the latent form of the organism found in cysts) are found in host cells. Hundreds of bradyzoites (with very slow metabolic rates) have a propensity towards neural tissue, such as the eye and brain, but also are found in skeletal muscle and heart. It is assumed that attacks occur with rupture of the cysts, leading to a release of bradyzoites and then the conversion of the brayzoites to tachyzoites. The mechanisms that lead to cyst rupture are still unknown.

4.1 Clinical Features

While the hallmark of the disease is distinct, changes in the posterior portion and the front of the eye also are noted. Anterior uveitis can be seen in many patients with this disorder. This is an interesting finding, since the organism is not seen in the anterior segment of the eye, except possibly in immunocompromised individuals. In addition, there is a loss of pigment in the iris that can be observed, and this is associated with changes in the back of the eye.[28] This finding, termed Fuchs heterochromia, is thought to be an autoimmune phenomenon.

The classic finding in ocular toxoplasmosis is that of a retinal lesion, which is destructive. It is typically an oval lesion infecting all the layers of the retina and frequently many layers of the choroid. It is the result of an immune response believed to have occurred against the *Toxoplasma* organism. While there may be only one lesion, often there are multiple lesions surrounding an old, large scar; these are called satellite lesions. In addition to the lesion itself, evidence of retinal vascular leakage is seen during the active stage of the disease. It has been hypothesized that this vasculitis is caused by an immune complex-related phenomenon.

While stigmata of the disease may be present in both eyes, recurrences of the disorder typically occur only in one eye. In addition, while reactivation of the disease is believed to be due to the breakage of cysts and the presence of tachyzoites, it is rare to see this stage of the organism in the retina. Patients who are immunocompromised, such as those with acquired immunodeficiency virus, often have bilateral disease and multiple lesions, suggesting a different mechanism in these patients compared to immunocompetent patients.

4.2 Evidence for Autoimmunity

A longitudinal study of patients with ocular toxoplasmosis by Abrahams and Gregerson[28] evaluated serum antibody responses to three retinal antigens. They tested the retinal S-antigen, a "P" antigen (thought to contain rhodopsin) and a new antigen designated p59ag. They reported that all the patients initially tested showed antibody responses to all three antigens. The anti-S-antigen responses tended to decrease with clinical improvement, whereas the anti-P antibodies remained high even after resolution of the acute attack. A more recent report by Whittle and colleagues[29] looked at a larger number of patients with toxoplasmic retinochoroiditis. Using indirect immunofluorescence, they reported that 34 of 36 sera samples showed antibodies directed against the photoreceptor later of the retina. However, 6 of 16 controls showed a similar staining pattern ($p < 0.001$). Interestingly, using an enzyme immunoassay (EIA) to measure the presence of anti-S-antigen antibodies, the researchers observed that 27 of 36 sera samples from patients with toxoplasmosis retinochoroiditis were positive, but so were those from 10 of 16 normal individuals ($p > 0.05$). The antibodies seen in the two assays did not seem to run in parallel.

Our group and others have had the chance to evaluate cell-mediated responses of lymphocytes from patients with ocular toxoplasmosis. In an early study in which we examined proliferative responses from patients with various uveitic conditions, we reported that a small number of lymphocytes from patients with ocular toxoplasmosis did respond to the uveitogenic retinal S-antigen.[30] In a later study, we evaluated the proliferative cell-mediated responses in 40 patients with ocular toxoplasmosis. In addition to the retinal S-antigen, we also evaluated the response to crude *Toxoplasma* antigen and to purified antigens from the parasite.[31] We also used EIA to look for anti-S-antigen antibodies and investigated HLA phenotyping to determine whether a specific HLA type was associated with S-antigen responsiveness. Of the 40 patient's lymphocytes tested, 16 (40%) had proliferative responses with a stimulation index above 2.5 (Figure 1). There seemed to be no correlation with this responsiveness and any HLA phenotype. In addition, we were unable to demonstrate anti-S-antigen antibodies using EIA. The patients with ocular toxoplasmosis could be divided by their lymphocytes responsiveness to the various toxoplasma antigens tested. However, no correlation was seen in S-antigen responsiveness and the stimulation index to toxoplasmosis antigens.

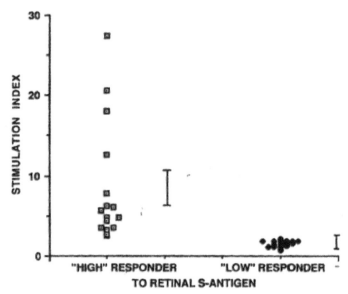

Figure 1 Proliferative responses of peripheral lymphocytes from 40 patients with ocular toxoplasmosis to the retinal S-antigen. Sixteen of these had stimulation indices above 2.5 and were designated as "high responders". This responsiveness was not correlated to either a specific HLA phenotype nor the vigor of the cell-mediated response to *Toxoplasma* antigens. *Reprinted with permission.*

A study by Vallochi et al.[32] in Brazil introduced an interesting interpretation of autoimmune reactivity in *Toxoplasma* infections. Three different retinal antigens were used to stimulate peripheral blood leukocytes (PBLs) from normal individuals, patients with mild ocular disease and patients with severe ocular disease. They found that patients with mild disease responded to one or more retinal antigens with a significantly higher frequency than patients without disease or with severe disease. Based on these findings, they suggested that the presence of cellular immune response towards retinal autoantigens is not protective against the development of ocular lesions induced by *T. gondii*, but it may protect against the development of severe disease. Autoimmune responses may protect the neural retina against the damage caused by infection with *T. gondii*. This protective effect may occur by providing the local cells with cytokines and growth factors that protect retinal cells and limit *T. gondii* replication.

5 ONCHOCERCIASIS

Infection with the nematode parasite *O. volvulus* can result in severe eye disease, often referred to as river blindness. It is estimated that approximately 18 million people in tropical Africa, the Arabian peninsula and Latin America are infected with the organism, and of these, approximately 1–2 million are blind or have severe visual impairment. Humans are infected with the helminth larvae by the bite of a black fly from the *Simulium* genus; approximately 1 year after infection, the adult female worms produce microfilariae. In fact, the adult worm can live for up to 15 years, producing 900–1900 microfilariae per day. It is the microfilariae that are able to move through subcutaneous and ocular tissues. When these microfilaria die, they incite an immune response that is associated with clinical symptoms.

5.1 Clinical Features

Onchocerciasis is one of the leading causes of blindness in the developing world. Ocular disease occurring in the anterior segment of the eye consists of corneal opacification and sclerosing keratitis, whereas ocular disease occurring in the posterior pole is characterized by retinal degeneration.[33] Clinical disease activity in the anterior segment is associated with microfilarial load, and it is generally believed that ocular pathology is a result of host-directed inflammatory responses to the nematode. In contrast, pathology associated with the retina and optic nerve has not been directly linked to microfilarial load.

5.2 Evidence for Autoimmunity

Posterior ocular onchocerciasis is characterized by atrophy of the RPE, and as lesions advance, subretinal fibrosis occurs.[34] A number of studies indicate that this retinal disease process may involve autoimmune responses. In 1987, Chan and associates[35] identified that a majority of patients with onchocerciasis had anti-retinal antibodies in their sera and vitreous. Using an immunofluorescent assay of human retina tissue, they observed reactivity in the inner retina and photoreceptor layers. During the 1990s, researchers performed a number of studies to elucidate the nature of autoimmune reactivity.[36–39] They identified a recombinant antigen in *O. volvulus* that showed immunologic cross-reactivity with a component of the RPE.[36,37] Using Western blot analysis, an antibody to a 22,000-molecular weight antigen (OV39) of *O. volvulus* recognized a 44,000-molecular weight component of the RPE cell. Subsequent studies showed that hr44 antigen is present in the optic nerve, epithelial layers of iris, ciliary body, and RPE. Although OV39 and the hr44 proteins are not homologous, they did show limited amino acid sequence identity.[40] Immunization of Lewis rats with either OV39 from *O. volvulus* of hr44 from human retinal tissue induced ocular pathology.[39] Retinal disease in the rat was characterized by extensive breakdown of the posterior blood–ocular barrier, iridocyclitis and retinitis and the activation of retinal microglia. These studies indicate that molecular mimicry between *O. volvulus* and human RPE protein may contribute to the retinopathy found in patients with onchocerciasis.

Saint André and colleagues[41] recently proposed that the predominant inflammatory response seen in the cornea of *Onchocerca*-infected animals is really directed against the endosymbiont of *Onchocerca*, *Wolbachia*. Parasite antigens and *Wolbachia* endotoxin or endotoxin-like molecules are released into the ocular microenvironment and bind to Toll-like receptor (TLR4) on stromal fibroblasts. TLR4 activation stimulates the production of neutrophil chemokines and pro-inflammatory cytokines, leading to enhanced inflammation.[42]

6 RETINOPATHIES THAT MAY HAVE INFECTIOUS/ AUTOIMMUNE ETIOLOGIES (WHITE-DOT SYNDROMES)

A large group of clinical entities have been grouped under the title "white dot syndromes". As the name infers, they are all characterized by whitish lesions of varying sizes that are found scattered throughout the fundus. Some patients have a significant associated inflammatory reaction, whereas others do not. The natural history of some may lead to significant visual handicap, whereas others may not. Some of these disorders seem to progress, yet others fade away. These disorders include such entities as acute multifocal placoid posterior pigment epitheliopathy (AMPPE), serpiginous choroiditis, the multifocal evanescent white dot syndrome, and multifocal choroiditis. The underlying cause of these diseases is unknown. Many of these disorders seem to be preceded by a viral illness, and AMPPE, was hypothesized to be due to Epstein–Barr virus infection;[43] however, this concept is no longer thought to be the case.[44] A few patients have been treated with anti-viral medications, with unclear responses. The most common therapy for all of these conditions is immunosuppression, and therapy is directed against what is believed to be an autoimmune, or least non-infectious, process in the back of the eye.

7 SUMMARY

We have reviewed the evidence implicating three distinct classes of infectious agents in the development of an autoimmune process within the retina. These data also indicate that distinct pathogenic mechanisms are involved in the induction of autoimmunity triggered by these three organisms. In *T. gondii* infections, the persistence and chronic reactivation of the organism is probably responsible for the introduction and presentation of sequestered retinal epitopes to the immune system. In *O. volvulus* infections, molecular mimicry between the organism and human RPE protein may contribute to the retinal pathology. In ECOR, similar processes are induced in coronavirus-infected mice displaying either susceptibility or resistance to retinal degeneration. However, recent evidence indicates that differences in time of induction, duration, and intensity of innate immune reactivity may contribute to autoimmune reactivity in BALB/c mice.

ACKNOWLEDGMENT

This research was supported in part by the intramural research program of the National Institutes of Health, National Eye Institute.

REFERENCES

1. Stein-Streilein J, Streilein JW. Anterior chamber associated immune deviation (ACAID): regulation, biological relevance, and implications for therapy. *Int Rev Immunol* 2002;**21**(2–3):123–52.
2. Nussenblatt RB, Whitcup S. *Fundamentals. Uveitis. Fundamentals and clinical practice.* Philadelphia, PA: W.B. Saunders; 2004, pp. 1–46.
3. Caspi RR. Understanding autoimmune uveitis through animal models. The Friedenwald Lecture. *Invest Ophthalmol Vis Sci* 2011;**52**:1872–9.

4. Forooghian F, MacDonald IM, Heckenlively JR, Heon E, Gordon LK, Hooks JJ, et al. The need for standardization of antiretinal antibody detection and measurement. *Am J Ophthalmol* 2008;**146**(4):489–95.
5. Hooks JJ, Tso MOM, Detrick B. Retinopathies associated with antiretinal antibodies. *Clin Diagn Lab Immunol* 2001;**8**(5):853–8.
6. Fujinami RS, Oldstone MB. Amino acid homology between the encephalitogenic site of myelin basic protein and virus: mechanism for autoimmunity. *Science* 1985;**230**(4729):1043–5.
7. Rose NR. The role of infection in the pathogenesis of autoimmune disease. *Semin Immunol* 1998;**10**(1):5–13.
8. Detrick B, Hooks JJ. Immune regulation in the retina. *Immunol Res* 2010;**47**(1–3):153–61.
9. Robbins SG, Detrick B, Hooks JJ. Ocular tropisms of murine coronavirus (strain JHM) after inoculation by various routes. *Invest Ophthalmol Vis Sci* 1991;**32**(6):1883–93.
10. Robbins SG, Hamel CP, Detrick B, Hooks JJ. Murine coronavirus induces an acute and long-lasting disease of the retina. *Lab Invest* 1990;**62**(4):417–26.
11. Wang Y, Burnier M, Detrick B, Hooks JJ. Genetic predisposition to coronavirus-induced retinal disease. *Invest Ophthalmol Vis Sci* 1996;**37**(1):250–4.
12. Holmes KV. SARS-associated coronavirus. *N Engl J Med* 2003;**348**(20):1948–51.
13. Wang Y, Detrick B, Yu ZX, Zhang J, Chesky L, Hooks JJ. The role of apoptosis within the retina of coronavirus-infected mice. *Invest Ophthalmol Vis Sci* 2000;**41**(10):3011–18.
14. Komurasaki Y, Nagineni CN, Wang Y, Hooks JJ. Virus RNA persists within the retina in coronavirus-induced retinopathy. *Virology* 1996;**222**(2):446–50.
15. Robbins SG, Wiggert B, Kutty G, Chader GJ, Detrick B, Hooks JJ. Redistribution and reduction of interphotoreceptor retinoid-binding protein during ocular coronavirus infection. *Invest Ophthalmol Vis Sci* 1992;**33**(1):60–7.
16. Vinores SA, Wang Y, Vinores MA, Derevjanik NL, Shi A, Klein DA, et al. Blood–retinal barrier breakdown in experimental coronavirus retinopathy: association with viral antigen, inflammation, and VEGF in sensitive and resistant strains. *J Neuroimmunol* 2001;**119**(2):175–82.
17. Hooks JJ, Wang Y, Detrick B. The critical role of IFN-gamma in experimental coronavirus retinopathy. *Invest Ophthalmol Vis Sci* 2003;**44**(8):3402–8.
18. Wang Y, Detrick B, Hooks JJ. Coronavirus (JHM) replication within the retina: analysis of cell tropism in mouse retinal cultures. *Virology* 1993;**193**(1):124–37.
19. Detrick B, Rodrigues M, Chan CC, Tso MO, Hooks JJ. Expression of HLA-DR antigen on retinal pigment epithelial cells in retinitis pigmentosa. *Am J Ophthalmol* 1986;**101**(5):584–90.
20. Percopo CM, Hooks JJ, Shinohara T, Caspi R, Detrick B. Cytokine-mediated activation of a neuronal retinal resident cell provokes antigen presentation. *J Immunol* 1990;**145**(12):4101–7.
21. Detrick B, Lee MT, Chin MS, Hooper LC, Chan C-C, Hooks JJ. Experimental coronavirus retinopathy (ECOR): retinal degeneration susceptible mice have an augmented interferon and chemokine (CXCL9, CXCL10) response early after virus infection. *J Neuroimmunol* 2008;**193**(1–2):28–37.
22. Hooks JJ, Nagineni CN, Hooper LC, Hayashi K, Detrick B. IFN-beta provides immuno-protection in the retina by inhibiting ICAM-1 and CXCL9 in retinal pigment epithelial cells. *J Immunol* 2008;**180**(6):3789–96.
23. Hooks JJ, Percopo C, Wang Y, Detrick B. Retina and retinal pigment epithelial cell autoantibodies are produced during murine coronavirus retinopathy. *J Immunol* 1993;**151**(6):3381–9.
24. Nicolle C, Manceaux L. Sur Une infection a corps de Leishman (ou organismes voisins) due Gondii. *C R Biol* 1908;**147**:763–6.

25. Splendore A. Un nuovo protozoa parassita dei conigli: incontrato nell lesioni anatomiche d'une malattia che ricorda in molti punti kala-azar dell'uomo. *Rev Soc Sci* 1908;**3**:109–12.

26. Janku J. Pathogenesis and pathologic anatomy of coloboma of macula lutea in eye of normal dimensions, and in microphthalmic eye, with parasites in the retina. *Cas Lek Cesk* 1923;**62**:1021–7.

27. Holland GN, Lewis KG, O'Connor GR. Ocular toxoplasmosis: a 50th anniversary tribute to the contributions of Helenor Campbell Wilder Foerster. *Arch Ophthalmol* 2002;**120**(8):1081–4.

28. Abrahams IW, Gregerson DS. Longitudinal study of serum antibody responses to retinal antigens in acute ocular toxoplasmosis. *Am J Ophthalmol* 1982;**93**:224–31.

29. Whittle RM, Wallace GR, Whiston RA, Dumonde DC, Stanford MR. Human anti-retinal antibodies in toxoplasma retinochoroiditis. *Br J Ophthalmol* 1998;**82**(9):1017–21.

30. Nussenblatt RB, Gery I, Ballintine EJ, Wacker WB. Cellular immune responsiveness of uveitis patients to retinal S-antigen. *Am J Ophthalmol* 1980;**89**(2):173–9.

31. Nussenblatt RB, Mittal KK, Fuhrman S, Sharma SD, Palestine AG. Lymphocyte proliferative responses of patients with ocular toxoplasmosis to parasite and retinal antigens. *Am J Ophthalmol* 1989;**107**(6):632–41.

32. Vallochi AL, da Silva Rios L, Nakamura MV, Silveira C, Muccioli C, Martins MC, et al. The involvement of autoimmunity against retinal antigens in determining disease severity in toxoplasmosis. *J Autoimmun* 2005;**24**(1):25–32.

33. Hall LR, Pearlman E. Pathogenesis of onchocercal keratitis (river blindness). *Clin Microbiol Rev* 1999;**12**(3):445–53.

34. Abiose A. Onchocercal eye disease and the impact of Mectizan treatment. *Ann Trop Med Parasitol* 1998;**92**(Suppl. 1):S11–22.

35. Chan CC, Ottesen EA, Awadzi K, Badu R, Nussenblatt RB. Immunopathology of ocular onchocerciasis. I. Inflammatory cells infiltrating the anterior segment. *Clin Exp Immunol* 1989;**77**(3):367–72.

36. Braun G, McKechnie NM, Connor V. Immunological crossreactivity between a cloned antigen of *Onchocerca volvulus* and a component of the retinal pigment epithelium. *J Exp Med* 1991;**174**(1):169–77.

37. McKechnie NM, Braun G, Kläger S, Connor V, Kasp E, Wallace G, et al. Cross-reactive antigens in the pathogenesis of onchocerciasis. *Ann Trop Med Parasitol* 1993;**87**(6):649–52.

38. McKechnie NM, Braun G, Connor V, Kläger S, Taylor DW, Alexander RA, et al. Immunologic cross-reactivity in the pathogenesis of ocular onchocerciasis. *Invest Ophthalmol Vis Sci* 1993;**34**(10):2888–902.

39. McKechnie NM, Gürr W, Braun G. Immunization with the cross-reactive antigens Ov39 from *Onchocerca volvulus* and hr44 from human retinal tissue induces ocular pathology and activates retinal microglia. *J Infect Dis* 1997;**176**(5):1334–43.

40. Braun G, McKechnie NM, Gürr W. Molecular and immunological characterization of hr44, a human ocular component immunologically cross-reactive with antigen Ov39 of *Onchocerca volvulus*. *J Exp Med* 1995;**182**(4):1121–31.

41. Saint André A, Blackwell NM, Hall LR, Hoerauf A, Brattig NW, Volkmann L, et al. The role of endosymbiotic Wolbachia bacteria in the pathogenesis of river blindness. *Science* 2002;**295**(5561):1892–5.

42. Hise AG, Gillette-Ferguson I, Pearlman E. Immunopathogenesis of *Onchocerca volvulus* keratitis (river blindness): a novel role for TLR4 and endosymbiotic Wolbachia bacteria. *J Endotoxin Res* 2003;**9**(6):390–4.

43. Tiedeman JS. Epstein-Barr viral antibodies in multifocal choroiditis and panuveitis. *Am J Ophthalmol* 1987;**103**(5):659–63.

44. Spaide RF, Sugin S, Yannuzzi LA, DeRosa JT. Epstein–Barr virus antibodies in multifocal choroiditis and panuveitis. *Am J Ophthalmol* 1991;**112**(4):410–13.

CHAPTER 58

Oral Infections and Autoimmune Diseases

Sok-Ja Janket[*,1], **Eleni Kanasi**[*], **Alison E. Baird**[†]
[*]Department of General Dentistry, Boston University, Henry M. Goldman School of Dental Medicine, Boston, Massachusetts, USA
[†]Division of Cerebrovascular Disease and Stroke, Department of Neurology, State University of New York, Downstate Medical Center, Brooklyn, NY, USA
[1]Corresponding Author: skjanket@bu.edu

1 INTRODUCTION

Autoimmunity is defined as the presence of autoreactive T or B lymphocytes in the periphery that escaped the immunological surveillance system; it may be physiological.[1] However, because of several checkpoints, as well as central and peripheral regulatory controls that destroy autoreactive cells, not all autoimmunity results in the genesis of autoimmune diseases (AIDs).[2]

What, then, are the key determinants for transforming autoimmunity into AID? The prevailing consensus of the autoimmune community seems to be that environmental factors may play an important triggering role in genetically susceptible individuals.[3] These potential triggering factors are (1) infections (bacterial, parasitic, or viral); (2) chemicals/xenobiotics; (3) adjuvants; (4) physical elements (ultraviolet radiation, electromagnetic field); and (5) hormones (estrogen, menopause, and pregnancy).

Under the condition of normal immunity, the innate immune system defends the host from invading pathogens through Toll-like receptors (TLRs). TLRs rapidly triage the molecules into "self", "non-self" or "pathogens" using pattern recognition receptors and take appropriate actions.[1,3] Altered TLR responses are hypothesized to trigger AID.[4,5] TLRs activate T helper-17 cells, which play crucial roles in the pathogenesis of AIDs. Thus, it is highly likely that recurrent infections, which could activate TLRs and Th17 cells, may contribute to the pathogenesis of AIDs. The putative role of oral infections in the pathogenesis of AID is presented in Figure 1. In addition, we critically review published evidence suggesting oral infection as a trigger for various AID.

Infection and Autoimmunity
http://dx.doi.org/10.1016/B978-0-444-63269-2.00063-5

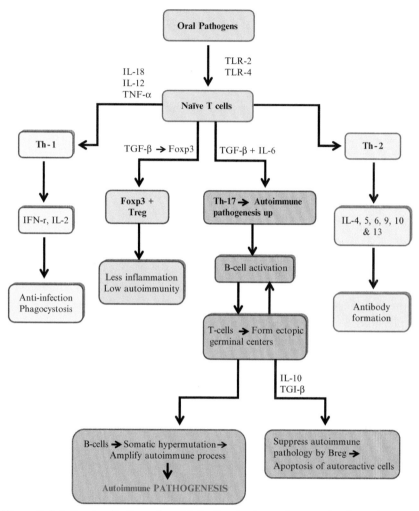

Figure 1 Putative implication of oral infection in the pathogenesis of autoimmune disease. IFN = interferon, IL = interleukin, RANKL = receptor activator of nuclear factor-κB ligand, TGF = transforming growth factor, Th = T helper cell, Treg = T regulatory cell, TNF = tumor necrosis factor.

2 ORAL INFECTIONS AND ATHEROSCLEROSIS

The role of inflammation in atheroma formation and rupture is well recognized.[6,7] Some researchers consider atherosclerosis to be an AID,[8–14] and recent experimental evidence seems to support this view. For example, local delivery of IL-2 decreased atherosclerosis by up-regulating regulatory T-cell action[15] and down-regulating Th1 cell responses in murine models.[16] In addition, atherosclerosis is quite similar to autoimmune anti-phospholipid syndrome (APS) in that both pathologies are associated with increased levels of antibodies to oxidized LDL (oxLDL), phospholipids, and heat shock proteins.[17] Furthermore, many patients with systemic lupus erythematous (SLE) die from cardiovascular complications. However, it should be noted that anti-phospholipid antibodies are expressed in many areas of human biology: diabetes, chronic kidney disease, periodontitis (PD) and ageing.[17] To make matters more complicated, periodontopathogens are known to cross-react with heat shock proteins (Choi J 2011)[17a] and oxLDL.[18]

Atherosclerosis commences when low-density lipoprotein molecules are deposited in the arterial wall and become oxidized by reactive oxygen species (or enzymes) and initiate a cascade of inflammatory reactions, expressing cytokines such as tumor necrosis factor (TNF)-α, IL-1, and IL-6, as well as matrix metalloproteinases and oxygen-activated radicals. Several studies reported abundant T-cell proliferation[19,20] and the expression of vascular adhesion molecules in atherosclerosis.[21,22] Interestingly, these immune responses could be either pro- or anti-inflammatory.[20] Similar pro- and anti-inflammatory actions of C-reactive protein were observed in a relationship between oral infections and cardiovascular mortality.[23] Therefore, the mere presence or significant correlation of molecules does not establish causality. Potential causality can only be determined by a longitudinal assessment of the relationship while controlling for all established confounding factors, since most human chronic diseases are multifactorial.

Several longitudinal studies reported positive associations of PD with atherosclerotic disease, suggesting a potential causal role for oral infection in the pathogenesis of atherosclerosis.[24–26] However, two large studies reported a null association in this same relationship.[27,28] A subsequent meta-analysis elucidated that the null results of the two large-scale epidemiologic studies were due to bias originating from imprecise PD assessment using questionnaires.[29] Since then, the relationship of oral infections to coronary artery disease has been assessed in many studies using various predictors: composite oral infection score,[30,31] salivary lysozyme[32,33] and salivary immunoglobulin A.[34] Nevertheless, confounding adjustment and determining potential causality have been especially problematic because both oral infections and atherosclerosis share common risk factors such as smoking and diabetes.

What are the key criteria necessary to establish a causal assumption? Sir Bradford Hill formulated criteria to establish potential causality in 1965, which are still used today.[35] These six criteria should be satisfied if the relationship between two factors is causal:

1. Strength: A strong association probably suggests causality. (But this does not always hold true. It could be due to unadjusted confounding.)
2. Consistency: Multiple, independent, *original* studies should report the same or similar results. (This does not always hold true either because several studies can report the same flawed results.) The aforementioned epidemiologic studies with null results were consistent, but consistently wrong. Because both studies used the same flawed diagnostic method (i.e. using a questionnaire to diagnose PD), both generated flawed results.
3. Specificity: If the exposure is specific to the outcome, causality is probable. However, in reality, the specificity in many multifactorial diseases cannot always be established.
4. Temporality: The predictor *must* occur before the outcome. This always holds true if the relationship is causal. Thus, a cross-sectional study cannot satisfy this criterion.
5. Biological gradient: This means that the higher the level of a risk factor, the higher is the disease rate. This does not always hold true, either. Some risk factors may have a threshold effect.
6. Biological plausibility: This also does not always hold true. For example, it has been shown that high glucose concentrations were associated with high rates of cardiovascular disease. Therefore, it is plausible that lowering glucose will result in lower rates of cardiovascular disease. However, this plausibility was not supported by the results of the ACCORD trial.[36]

Most criteria may or may not be satisfied even in a true causal relationship. However, the temporal relationship *must* be satisfied at all times if the relationship is causal. Several recent, reasonably well-conducted longitudinal studies with adequate adjustment of confounding linked oral infections to atherosclerosis.[23,37] Some used salivary lysozyme as a proxy for oral infection,[38] whereas others used the number of teeth as an indicator for oral infections.[23,37] In addition, several intervention studies also supported the thesis that eliminating oral infections reduced serum concentrations of atherosclerosis markers,[39,40] but another study did not.[41] The latter study was a secondary prevention trial where reversing the vascular changes that had already occurred might have been nearly impossible. In conclusion, although the status of atherosclerosis as an AID is still debatable, there is adequate longitudinal evidence that oral infections could be a trigger for atherosclerosis.

3 PD AND AIDS

3.1 Molecular Biology of PD

The most common oral infection is PD, a highly prevalent chronic infectious disease affecting 31% of the US adult population.[42] The etiology of PD is not completely understood, but it is generally accepted that oral bacteria interact with the host's immune system to cause inflammation and tissue breakdown. PD can be thought of as a state of dysregulated immunoprotection via differentially regulated cytokines or transcription factors, such as the receptor activator of NFκB ligand (RANKL), IL-1, IL-6, transforming growth factor-β and IL-17.[43] If early periodontitis is untreated, healthy periodontium (Figure 2) will deteriorate resulting in connective tissue damages, erosion of supporting bones and eventual tooth loss (Figure 3). PD could have further implications in general health because it has been linked to a number of systemic diseases and AIDs such as bacterial endocarditis,[44] adverse birth outcomes,[45] cardiovascular disease,[23] diabetes mellitus,[46–48] Crohn's disease and ulcerative colitis.[49]

The most important group of periodontal pathogens is termed the "red complex" and was identified by Socransky and colleagues. The red complex is usually found in the deeper sections of the periodontal pocket, the space between the tooth and gingival tissue created by tissue dissolution.[50] It includes *Porphyromonas gingivalis*, *Prevotella intermedia*, *Tannerella forsythia*, and *Aggregatibacter actinomycetemcomitans*. Periodontal pathogens activate the innate immune system, which recognizes the pathogen pattern via TLRs and recruits fibroblasts, osteoblasts, dendritic cells and epithelial cells.[51]

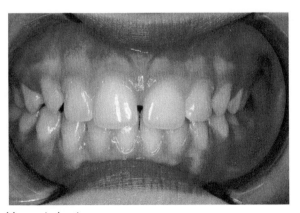

Figure 2 Healthy periodontium.

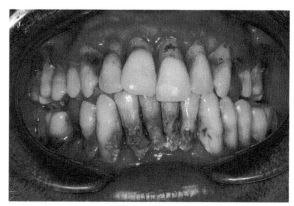

Figure 3 Unhealthy periodontium.

Some TLRs recognize gram-positive bacterial lipoteichoic acid, whereas others recognize gram-negative bacterial lipopolysaccharides, suggesting specificity in their actions.[51]

P. gingivalis and A. actinomycetemcomitans are capable of invading epithelial cells using β-1 integrins; they replicate in the connective tissue while expressing TNF-α, IL-1, IL-6, IL-8, macrophage inflammatory proteins (MIP-1-α) and stromal cell-derived factor 1.[52] In addition, multiple transcription factors become activated and induce cytokines to recruit leukocytes. These pathogens also express many toxins, including leukotoxins that down-regulate neutrophil chemotaxis.[53] This orchestration of cytokine activity leads to the activation of adaptive immunity via Th-1, Th-2, Th-17 and regulatory T cells (Tregs) in an attempt to reach homeostasis in immune responses.[54]

One major cytokine responsible for bone loss in the periodontium is RANKL.[55] RANKL is expressed mainly by osteoblasts, but it also is found in T and B lymphocytes and fibroblasts.[55] In PD, RANKL production is significantly increased by bacterial components such as the cytolethal distending toxin produced by A. actinomycetemcomitans and by P. gingivalis LPSs.[56] However, it should be noted that RANKL is expressed in any immune challenge, including exposure to oxLDLs or titanium particles.[57,58] This impressive array of cytokines and transcription factors, such as IL-17, TNF-α, RANKL, TLR2, and TLR4, is associated with PD as well as with confounding factors such as genetic polymorphisms, smoking and diabetes.[59]

Among the periodontal pathogens, P. gingivalis is the only known microorganism that expresses peptidylarginine deiminase (PAD)[60] and can citrullinate human fibrinogen, which is considered the autoantigen for rheumatoid arthritis (RA).[61] In patients with RA, antibodies to citrullinated proteins (CPAbs), such as filaggrin, keratin, vimentin, and fibrinogen, as well as antibodies to cyclic citrullinated peptides (CCPs), are found. It should be noted that CPAbs also are expressed in individuals who smoke or who have genetic traits related to human leukocyte antigen (HLA) DRB1 alleles.[62,63]

The majority of studies linking PD and AID were conducted in patients with RA who had PD, and it was difficult to determine whether any molecular changes observed were caused by PD or RA. However, a recent study reported that patients with PD without RA had elevated PAD and CPAbs, although some of the study subjects had other confounding factors, such as smoking and inflammatory vascular diseases.[64] More detailed discussions follow in the section "Oral Infections and RA".

4 IS PD A TRIGGER FACTOR FOR AID?

PD has many features resembling AID: the expression of cytokines commonly expressed in autoimmunity, as well as production of citrullinated proteins. In addition, the polymorphism of the Fcγ family of genes that controls AIDs, such as RA and SLE, was associated with PD.[65,66] Thus, confounding by shared genetics is quite possible.

Numerous studies reported that PD involved the expression of the key molecules associated with AID. For example, the lipopolysaccharide of *P. gingivalis* regulates the expression of IL-17 and IL-23,[67,68] and Th1, Th2, and Th17 disequilibrium shown in AIDs is also present in PD.[69] Also, a Th17/Treg imbalance was observed in PD.[70] Tregs, key players in AID, also were expressed in PD.[71] Furthermore, forkhead box P3 (Foxp3), RANKL, and transforming growth factor-β were overexpressed in chronic PD, suggesting the expression of molecules related to the Th2 pathway.[72,73] These studies strongly suggest that PD expresses many molecules expressed in AID and may be an AID itself. However, unequivocal evidence that PD is a trigger factor for the pathogenesis of AID is still lacking. We further review the evidence to answer the question of whether PD is a causal factor for individual AIDs because each AID has a slightly different pathogenic mechanism. The potential causal relationship between PD and AID is very complex because all the cytokines produced in PD also are expressed in settings of smoking,[74–76] obesity,[77,78] hyperlipidemia,[79] low vitamin D concentrations[80,81] and genetic linkage to Fcγ gene receptor polymorphisms.[66,82] Therefore, it is extremely important to understand the concept of confounding in clinical research so that unbiased conclusions are drawn.

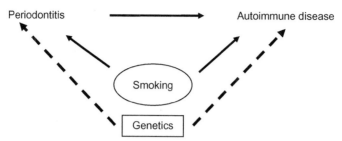

Figure 4 Confounding by smoking or genetics in periodontitis and autoimmune diseases relationship.

Let us review the relationship of smoking as a confounder in the *P. gingivalis* and AID relationship. The same formulae can be applied for obesity, dyslipidemia, low vitamin D concentrations and genetic factors.[83–85]

In a situation like that presented in Figure 4, where three factors form a triangle, we can say that smoking or genetics can be a confounding factor.[86] Without controlling for smoking or genetics, the relationship of PD and AID may be biased. One can replace smoking with other potential confounders such as low vitamin D or low estrogen concentrations. Estrogen depletion is reported to produce TNF-α and RANKL;[87] it also causes bone erosion.[88,89] Thus, T cells, B-cell activation, and the expression of RANKL are not unique to PD.

To investigate this subject, Shaddox and colleagues conducted a study in which they provided periodontal treatment and administered systemic antibiotics. Significantly reduced inflammatory cytokines induced by *P. gingivalis* LPSs, such as IFN-γ, IL-10, IL-12, IL-1β, IL-6, and TNF-α ($p < 0.05$) were observed. However, similar reductions have been observed with *Escherichia coli* LPS stimulation. Moreover, the reduction of inflammation rebounded after 3–6 months, suggesting PD is a phenotype of a genetic or confounding factor.[90] Further evidence that PD may be a manifestation of systemic pathology has emerged in a recent study in which spontaneous PD and type 2 diabetes mellitus (T2DM) were induced by feeding a high-fat diet to CD14 knockout, ovariectomized female mice. CD14 is relevant to the mechanism of recognizing LPSs via TLR4. It also was observed that this relationship was ameliorated by estrogen. This study implied that a high-fat diet increased the prevalence of periodontal pathogens and that PD might be a manifestation of a systemic condition such as T2DM or low estrogen concentrations.[91] Similar to this result, a previously published study showed that serum lipids concentrations affected periodontal status.[92] Therefore, as stated in the previous section, the lipid levels have to be controlled to establish an unbiased causal association between PD and AIDs.

Another example of systemic pathology precipitating PD in an experimental arthritis murine model was published.[93] Interestingly, PD induced by experimental arthritis expressed transcription factors RORγ and Foxp3, suggesting a potential linkage to AID. However, we are not certain whether these factors originated from PD or arthritis. One recent study reported that the RA autoantibody repertoire was higher in the PD group after controlling for smoking.[94] This study represents a slight improvement over many previous reports that did not control for any confounding factors. However, this was still a cross-sectional study, and many other factors, such as adiposity, lipid profile, and genetics, were not controlled.

IL-6 plays a crucial role in the expression of Th17 from naive T cells (Figure 1): Naive T cells may develop into Tregs or Th17, depending on the presence of IL-6. Thus IL-6 can induce cells that suppress or promote autoimmunity. IL-6 is expressed in a study of experimental PD,[95] as well as in an *ex vivo* study in which IFN-γ, IL-6, and IL-4 were identified in biopsied tissues extracted from healthy patients and patients with chronic PD but were higher in the PD group.[96] However, IL-6 is a non-specific inflammatory marker that is expressed in liver disease, cardiovascular disease, diabetes, hyperlipidemia and non-pathologic inflammatory conditions such as orthodontic tooth movement.[97] Therefore, meticulous adjustments of confounding are required.

Smoking is a strong contributor to PD and PD-related tooth loss[98] and is also a risk factor for atherosclerosis[99,100] and AIDs.[101,102] Osteoporosis is another confounding factor to be considered when evaluating the relation of PD to AIDs. The case definition of PD is based on alveolar bone, on which osteoporosis has strong influence.[103] Furthermore, osteoporosis is strongly associated with estrogen and vitamin D concentrations, both of which are important factors that may be associated with atherosclerosis[104] or AIDs.[105,106] Low vitamin D concentrations were associated with increased inflammatory responses,[107] and vitamin D deficiency was associated with elevated IL-17 and TNF-α, both of which are important cytokines in autoimmune responses[80,108,109] and with PD.[81,110] Thus, future studies should control for these parallel factors to assess the unbiased effect of PD on AIDs. Alternatively, using oral infection markers such as salivary IgA or lysozyme, which are not dependent on bone levels, will bypass this confounding.

5 ORAL INFECTIONS AND RA

RA affects 0.5-1% of the world population and is one of the most studied AIDs in relation to oral infection. Much of the work has focused on PD because RA and PD produce similar pro-inflammatory cytokines—TNF-α, IL-6, IL-1β—and share the same genetic loci via HLA DRβ1.[111] PD is twice as prevalent, and the clinical presentation of PD is more severe, in patients with RA.[112] In addition, treatment of PD mitigated RA symptoms in some studies.[113,114] Although these studies were too small to balance all confounding factors, their results indicate a potential causal link. However, behavioral factors such as smoking and genetic influence may still confound this relationship.[115]

Furthermore, new research has highlighted the potential causal link by elucidating the antibodies against citrullinated proteins that are present well before overt RA. CCPs are now used as a diagnostic marker for RA.[61] Citrullination is considered physiological[116] because this process generates ammonia, allowing the microorganism to survive in acidic environments,[117] and provides energy during anerobic growth.[118] However, in some pathologic conditions, protein citrullination may cause immune tolerance to fail, provoking RA in susceptible individuals.[119] Some researchers postulated that *P. gingivalis* might contribute to the pathogenesis of RA.[63,111] However, several confounding factors shared by these two prevalent diseases require careful assessment. After periodontal treatment, patients with PD who smoke had levels of anti-CCP similar to those in non-smoking patients with PD, suggesting that PD and smoking both express comparable amounts of CCPs and thus may equally contribute to the development of AID. The CCP levels increased incrementally in non-smoking non-PD, non-smoking PD, to smoking PD groups. It seems that PD may express CCP to a lesser degree compared to smoking but they may be synergized in patients with PD who smoke. However, 6 months after periodontal treatment, anti-CCP antibodies decreased only in non-smokers ($p < 0.05$). We interpret these results as showing that smoking is a persistent producer of CCP and that periodontal treatment may not eliminate the entire source of molecules that may trigger AID if the person is a smoker.[120]

Immunological mapping has identified a B-cell dominant epitope citrullinated enolase peptide-1 (CEP-1), which showed 82% sequence matching with *P. gingivalis* and 100% homology with α-enolase at nine amino acids, including arginine-15.[121] Thus, molecular mimicry with gingivalis enolase and human CEP-1 might be a distinct possibility in the pathogenesis of RA.

In a recent study involving a transgenic murine model, severe RA developed after injection with *P. gingivalis* enolase.[122] Yet, we have to keep in mind that murine and human models have different major histocompatibility complexes and that autoimmune response may also be different.[123] Furthermore, diabetes[124] and obesity[125] are associated with elevations in the same cytokines that PD expresses. Smoking also significantly contributes to the development of anti-CCP antibodies.[115] At this point, it seems that PD and RA are highly correlated and perhaps causally associated via molecular mimicry, but we are not yet confident enough to say that PD is a trigger for RA pathogenesis. A large prospective cohort study of asymptomatic humans is warranted; by following the cohort for 6-10 years, RA development in the participants with *P. gingivalis* enolase and others without this molecule can be examined while carefully controlling for all established confounding factors.

6 ORAL INFECTIONS AND SLE

SLE predominantly affects females of childbearing age, with a prevalence of 4-20 per 10,000. Low IL-2 is pivotal in the pathogenesis of SLE, with the resultant failure to suppress apoptosis of autoreactive T cells and increase in the expression of IL-17.[126] These hypo-performing T cells not only contribute to the pathogenesis of SLE but also cause frequent infections. Thus, increased IL-17 expression in PD[68,127] could be the result of SLE, rather than the cause. It should be noted that even cell senescence[128] and many inflammatory/ infectious diseases express IL-17.[129,130] Thus, the mere presence of a molecule cannot establish a causal association. Future longitudinal studies with careful adjustment for confounder are needed.

Although debate on the role of B cells in the pathogenesis of AID continues, defects in B-cell response and defects in B-cell tolerance may play a role in the pathogenesis of SLE.[131,132] Some patients with SLE possess antibodies to phospholipids and β2-glycoprotein I (GPI),[133] and some patients present anti-cardiolipin (aCL) autoantibodies secondary to the APS.[134] Nevertheless, the causal role of these molecules in SLE is yet to be elucidated.

7 ORAL INFECTIONS AND MULTIPLE SCLEROSIS

Multiple sclerosis (MS) is the second most prevalent AID after RA, with a prevalence of 69.1 per 100,000 person-years worldwide.[135] Although the etiopathology of MS is not clearly defined, abnormal reactions to factors such as infections, latitude, vitamin D deficiency and smoking have been implicated them as triggers.[136] Like many AIDs, the infectome or collective past infections may play a role in the pathogenesis of MS.[137] However, few studies have been conducted among patients with MS in relation to oral infections. A recent population-based study assessed the PD and MS relationship, controlling for all potential confounding factors, and reported a significant association. This study was retrospective and longitudinal and satisfied the temporal requirement for causal association.[138]

8 ORAL INFECTIONS AND APS AND OTHER CLOTTING DISORDERS

APS is an AID affecting multiple organs. APS presents venous and arterial thromboses in the setting of serological positivities to anti-phospholipid antibodies, including aCL and anti-β2-GPI antibodies. aCL levels fluctuate, and therefore it is difficult to use them as a diagnostic test; anti-β2-GPI antibodies may prove more dependable in diagnosing APS (Greco, 2000).[138a] APS can be primary or secondary to other AIDs such as SLE. The exact mechanism of pathogenesis is not known, but it is presumed that anti-phospholipid antibodies react with phospholipids of the plasma membrane and inhibit protein C, which has an anti-coagulatory function by degrading activated factor V. Consequently, coagulopathy occurs.

Elevated aCL levels have been observed in patients with PD relative to periodontally healthy individuals.[139] However, smoking, obesity[140] and metabolic syndrome[141] were not controlled for, which could have confounded this observation. It seems that many atherosclerosis risk factors also increase the level of β2-GPI. Meanwhile, it is possible that periodontal pathogens can induce aCL antibodies by molecular mimicry; these periodontal pathogens possess homology to the antigen epitope of aCL and or β2-GPI.[142,143] Nevertheless, the aforementioned confounding factors, including diabetes, metabolic syndrome or family history,[141,143,144] should be controlled for to arrive at an unbiased conclusion.

9 ORAL INFECTIONS AND SJÖGREN'S SYNDROME

Sjögren's syndrome (SS) is an autoimmune epithelitis of the salivary and lacrimal glands. Mainly CD4+ T cells infiltrate ductal tissue of these exocrine glands and cause glandular dysfunction, leading to xerostomia and xerophthalmia. Although the pathogenesis is not fully understood, salivary gland epithelitis may play a role in the initiation and perpetuation of local auto-immune responses.[145] Almost 50% of patients with SS develop extra-glandular diseases affecting epithelial lymphocytic invasion of the lung, liver, or kidney.[146] In a recent study, morphological changes in the labial gland biopsies of patients with xerostomia were associated with dyslipidemia.[147] Scardina and colleagues conducted a study of non-smoking, non-dyslipidemic, and non-diabetic patients with SS, comparing their gingival microcirculation to that of healthy controls. The patients with SS showed reduced calibre of capillaries and increased tortuosity of capillary loops, suggesting a potential association of oral mucosa and SS. Although important confounding factors such as smoking, dyslipidemia and diabetes were controlled for by restricting the cohort to one group, this was a cross-sectional study, and inverse causality is quite possible.[148]

10 ORAL INFECTIONS AND CROHN'S DISEASE/ INFLAMMATORY BOWEL DISEASE

A study found that patients with Crohn's disease or inflammatory bowel disease and chronic PD harbored significantly higher levels of *Prevotella melaninogenica*, *Staphylococcus aureus*, *Streptococcus anginosus*, *Streptococcus mutans*, and *Treponema denticola* ($P < 0.001$) compared with controls with chronic PD only.[149] However, this was a cross-sectional study where the temporal requirement of the causality establishment could not be satisfied, and no potential confounding factors, such as smoking or diabetes, were controlled for.

Although this chapter focused the role of infection in the pathogenesis of AIDs, we are qualified to comment on the implication of dental amalgam in the pathogenesis of autoimmune thyroiditis. In a small study, anti-thyroid peroxidase and anti-thyroglobulin decreased in patients with hypersensitivity to inorganic mercury after dental amalgam removal.[150] Meanwhile, no association was reported between blood and urine concentrations of mercury, which were measured by atomic absorption spectrophotometry, and diagnosis of AID.[151] Moreover, in a randomized trial investigating whether amalgam restorations (via mercury toxicity) cause developmental harm to children, the authors concluded that there was "no evidence that exposure to mercury from dental amalgam was associated with any adverse neuropsychological effects over the five-year period after placement of amalgam restorations."[152,153]

Considering the multifactorial nature of AIDs, we concur with the opinion that "[t]he goal of inducing self-tolerance to prevent autoimmune (thyroid) disease will require accurate prediction together with an antigen-specific, not blanket, therapeutic approach."[154] Future longitudinal studies with more specific objectives in at-risk populations are indicated.

11 CONCLUSIONS AND FUTURE DIRECTIONS

Notwithstanding the controversies surrounding the extent of autoimmune involvement in the pathogenesis of atherosclerosis, we conclude that there is ample longitudinal evidence to suggest that oral infection may be a causal factor for atherosclerosis. There is credible evidence for a potential causal association between RA and oral infections via molecular mimicry, although longitudinal assessment of this relationship is lacking. There is small but significant longitudinal evidence linking oral infections and MS, suggesting that oral infection may be a trigger factor. However, confirmatory data to corroborate this is needed. For the other AIDs, only rudimentary evidence is available, suggesting some association. Much more intense investigation in a longitudinal format with meticulous confounding adjustment is definitely needed to establish the causal contribution of oral infections to autoimmune pathogenesis. Some of the confounding factors that must be controlled are smoking, dyslipidemia, diabetes and genetics.

ACKNOWLEDGMENT

The authors acknowledge Homan Javaheri for his assistance with creating Figure 1.

REFERENCES

1. Salinas GF, Braza F, Brouard S, Tak PP, Baeten D. The role of B lymphocytes in the progression from autoimmunity to autoimmune disease. *Clin Immunol* 2013;**146**(1):34–45.
2. Wardemann H, Yurasov S, Schaefer A, Young JW, Meffre E, Nussenzweig MC. Predominant autoantibody production by early human B cell precursors. *Science* 2003;**301**(5638):1374–7.
3. Selmi C, Leung PS, Sherr DH, et al. Mechanisms of environmental influence on human autoimmunity: a National Institute of Environmental Health Sciences expert panel workshop. *J Autoimmun* 2012;**39**(4):272–84.
4. Lee TP, Tang SJ, Wu MF, Song YC, Yu CL, Sun KH. Transgenic overexpression of anti-double-stranded DNA autoantibody and activation of Toll-like receptor 4 in mice induce severe systemic lupus erythematosus syndromes. *J Autoimmun* 2010;**35**(4):358–67.
5. Mills KH. TLR-dependent T, cell activation in autoimmunity. *Nat Rev Immunol* 2011;**11**(12):807–22.

6. Libby P, Ridker P, Maseri A. Inflammation and atherosclerosis. *Circulation* 2002;**105**:1135–43.

7. Ridker PM, Buring JE, Shih J, Matias M, Hennekens CH. Prospective study of C-reactive protein and the risk of future cardiovascular events among apparently healthy women. *Circulation* 1998;**98**(8):731–3.

8. Shoenfeld Y, Sherer Y, Harats D. Artherosclerosis as an infectious, inflammatory and autoimmune disease. *Trends Immunol* 2001;**22**(6):293–5.

9. Bjorkbacka H, Fredrikson GN, Nilsson J. Emerging biomarkers and intervention targets for immune-modulation of atherosclerosis—a review of the experimental evidence. *Atherosclerosis* 2013;**227**(1):9–17.

10. Bartoloni E, Shoenfeld Y, Gerli R. Inflammatory and autoimmune mechanisms in the induction of atherosclerotic damage in systemic rheumatic diseases: two faces of the same coin. *Arthritis Care Res (Hoboken)* 2011;**63**(2):178–83.

11. Lakota K, Zigon P, Mrak-Poljsak K, Rozman B, Shoenfeld Y, Sodin-Semrl S. Antibodies against acute phase proteins and their functions in the pathogenesis of disease: a collective profile of 25 different antibodies. *Autoimmun Rev* 2011;**10**(12):779–89.

12. Matsuura E, Lopez LR, Shoenfeld Y, Ames PR. β2-glycoprotein I and oxidative inflammation in early atherogenesis: a progression from innate to adaptive immunity? *Autoimmun Rev* 2012;**12**(2):241–9.

13. Nussinovitch U, Shoenfeld Y. Anti-troponin autoantibodies and the cardiovascular system. *Heart* 2010;**96**(19):1518–24.

14. Nussinovitch U, Shoenfeld Y. The diagnostic and clinical significance of anti-muscarinic receptor autoantibodies. *Clin Rev Allergy Immunol* 2012;**42**(3):298–308.

15. Dietrich T, Hucko T, Schneemann C, et al. Local delivery of IL-2 reduces atherosclerosis via expansion of regulatory T cells. *Atherosclerosis* 2011;**220**(2):329–36.

16. Laurat E, Poirier B, Tupin E, et al. In vivo downregulation of T helper cell 1 immune responses reduces atherogenesis in apolipoprotein E-knockout mice. *Circulation* 2001;**104**(2):197–202.

17. Broder A, Chan JJ, Putterman C. Dendritic cells: an important link between antiphospholipid antibodies, endothelial dysfunction, and atherosclerosis in autoimmune and non-autoimmune diseases. *Clin Immunol* 2013;**146**(3):197–206.

17a. Choi J, Lee SY, Kim K, Choi BK. Identification of immunoreactive epitopes of the Porphyromonas gingivalis heat shock protein in periodontitis and atherosclerosis. *J Periodontal Res* Apr 2011;**46**(2):240–5.

18. Offenbacher S, Madianos PN, Champagne CM, et al. Periodontitis-atherosclerosis syndrome: an expanded model of pathogenesis. *J Periodontal Res* 1999;**34**(7):346–52.

19. Jonasson L, Holm J, Skalli O, Bondjers G, Hansson GK. Regional accumulations of T cells, macrophages, and smooth muscle cells in the human atherosclerotic plaque. *Arteriosclerosis* 1986;**6**(2):131–8.

20. Hansson GK, Libby P. The immune response in atherosclerosis: a double-edged sword. *Nat Rev Immunol* 2006;**6**(7):508–19.

21. Dong ZM, Chapman SM, Brown AA, Frenette PS, Hynes RO, Wagner DD. The combined role of P- and E-selectins in atherosclerosis. *J Clin Invest* 1998;**102**(1):145–52.

22. Li H, Cybulsky MI, Gimbrone Jr. MA, Libby P. Inducible expression of vascular cell adhesion molecule-1 by vascular smooth muscle cells in vitro and within rabbit atheroma. *Am J Pathol* 1993;**143**(6):1551–9.

23. Janket SJ, Baird AE, Jones JA, et al. Number of teeth, C-reactive protein, and fibrinogen and cardiovascular mortality: a 15-year follow-up study in a Finnish cohort. *J Clin Periodontol* 2014;**41**(2):131–40.

24. Beck J, Garcia R, Heiss G, Vokonas PS, Offenbacher S. Periodontal disease and cardiovascular disease. *J Periodontol* 1996;**67**:1123–37.

25. DeStefano F, Anda RF, Kahn HS, Williamson DF, Russell CM. Dental disease and risk of coronary heart disease and mortality. *BMJ* 1993;**306**(6879):688–91.

26. Wu T, Trevisan M, Genco RJ, Dorn JP, Falkner KL, Sempos CT. Periodontal disease and risk of cerebrovascular disease: the first national health and nutrition examination survey and its follow-up study. *Arch Intern Med* 2000;**160**(18):2749–55.

27. Howell T, Ridker P, Ajani U. Periodontal disease and risks of subsequent cardiovascular disease in U.S. male physicians. *J Am Coll Cardiol* 2001;**37**:445.

28. Joshipura KJ, Rimm EB, Douglass CW, Trichopoulos D, Ascherio A, Willett WC. Poor oral health and coronary heart disease. *J Dent Res* 1996;**75**(9):1631–6.

29. Janket S-J, Baird AE, Chuang S-K, Jones JA. Meta-analysis of periodontal disease and risk of coronary heart disease and stroke. *Oral Surg Oral Med Oral Pathol Oral Radiol Endod* 2003;**95**(5):559–69.

30. Mattila KJ, Valtonen VV, Nieminen M, Huttunen JK. Dental infection and the risk of new coronary events: prospective study of patients with documented coronary artery disease. *Clin Infect Dis* 1995;**20**(3):588–92.

31. Janket SJ, Qvarnstrom M, Meurman JH, Baird AE, Nuutinen P, Jones JA. Asymptotic dental score and prevalent coronary heart disease. *Circulation* 2004;**109**(9):1095–100.

32. Janket SJ, Meurman JH, Nuutinen P, et al. Salivary lysozyme and prevalent coronary heart disease: possible effects of oral health on endothelial dysfunction. *Arterioscler Thromb Vasc Biol* 2006;**26**(2):433–4.

33. Qvarnstrom M, Janket S, Jones JA, et al. Salivary lysozyme and prevalent hypertension. *J Dent Res* 2008;**87**(5):480–4.

34. Janket S, Meurman JH, Baird AE, et al. Salivary immunoglobulins and prevalent coronary artery disease. *J Dent Res* 2010;**89**(4):389–94.

35. Hennekens CH, Buring JE. *Epidemiology in medicine*. Hagerstown, MD. 21740: Lippincott Williams & Wilkins; 1987.

36. Action to Control Cardiovascular Risk in Diabetes Study G, Gerstein HC, Miller ME, et al. Effects of intensive glucose lowering in type 2 diabetes. *N Engl J Med* 2008;**358** (24):2545–59.

37. Schwahn C, Polzer I, Haring R, et al. Missing, unreplaced teeth and risk of all-cause and cardiovascular mortality. *Int J Cardiol* 2013;**167**:1430–7.

38. Jethwani K, Janket S-J, Jones JA, Baird AE, Meurman JH, Van Dyke TE. Salivary lysozyme as a predictor of cardiovascular mortality. *Arterioscler Thromb Vasc Biol* 2010;**30**(11): e183–321.

39. D'Aiuto F, Nibali L, Parkar M, Suvan J, Tonetti MS. Short-term effects of intensive periodontal therapy on serum inflammatory markers and cholesterol. *J Dent Res* 2005;**84**(3):269–73.

40. Tonetti MS, D'Aiuto F, Nibali L, et al. Treatment of periodontitis and endothelial function. *N Engl J Med* 2007;**356**(9):911–20.

41. Offenbacher S, Beck JD, Moss K, et al. Results from the Periodontitis and Vascular Events (PAVE) Study: a pilot multicentered, randomized, controlled trial to study effects of periodontal therapy in a secondary prevention model of cardiovascular disease. *J Periodontol* 2009;**80**(2):190–201.

42. Eke PI, Page RC, Wei L, Thornton-Evans G, Genco RJ. Update of the case definitions for population-based surveillance of periodontitis. *J Periodontol* 2012;**83** (12):1449–54.

43. Belibasakis GN, Meier A, Guggenheim B, Bostanci N. The RANKL-OPG system is differentially regulated by supragingival and subgingival biofilm supernatants. *Cytokine* 2011;**55**(1):98–103.

44. Chen SJ, Liu CJ, Chao TF, et al. Dental scaling and risk reduction in infective endocarditis: a nationwide population-based case-control study. *Can J Cardiol* 2013;**29** (4):429–33.

45. Heimonen A, Janket SJ, Kaaja R, Ackerson LK, Muthukrishnan P, Meurman JH. Oral inflammatory burden and preterm birth. *J Periodontol* 2009;**80**(6):884–91.

46. Genco RJ, Grossi SG, Ho A, Nishimura F, Murayama Y. A proposed model linking inflammation to obesity, diabetes, and periodontal infections. *J Periodontol* 2005;**76**(11 Suppl.):2075–84.
47. Taylor GW, Burt BA, Becker MP, Genco RJ, Shlossman M. Glycemic control and alveolar bone loss progression in type 2 diabetes. *Ann Periodontol* 1998;**3**(1):30–9.
48. Taylor GW, Loesche WJ, Terpenning MS. Impact of oral diseases on systemic health in the elderly: Diabetes mellitus and aspiration pneumonia. *J Public Health Dent Fal* 2000;**60**(4):313–20.
49. Brito F, de Barros FC, Zaltman C, et al. Prevalence of periodontitis and DMFT index in patients with Crohn's disease and ulcerative colitis. *J Clin Periodontol* 2008;**35**(6):555–60.
50. Socransky SS, Haffajee AD. Dental biofilms: difficult therapeutic targets. *Periodontol 2000* 2002;**28**:12–55.
51. Hans M, Hans VM. Toll-like receptors and their dual role in periodontitis: a review. *J Oral Sci* 2011;**53**(3):263–71.
52. Belibasakis GN, Bostanci N. The RANKL-OPG system in clinical periodontology. *J Clin Periodontol* 2012;**39**(3):239–48.
53. Kantarci A, Oyaizu K, Van Dyke TE. Neutrophil-mediated tissue injury in periodontal disease pathogenesis: findings from localized aggressive periodontitis. *J Periodontol* 2003;**74**(1):66–75.
54. Weaver CT, Hatton RD. Interplay between the TH17 and TReg cell lineages: a (co-)evolutionary perspective. *Nat Rev Immunol* 2009;**9**(12):883–9.
55. Miossec P, Korn T, Kuchroo VK. Interleukin-17 and type 17 helper T cells. *N Engl J Med* 2009;**361**(9):888–98.
56. Belibasakis GN, Brage M, Lagergard T, Johansson A. Cytolethal distending toxin upregulates RANKL expression in Jurkat T-cells. *APMIS* 2008;**116**(6):499–506.
57. Maziere C, Salle V, Gomila C, Maziere JC. Oxidized low density lipoprotein increases RANKL level in human vascular cells. Involvement of oxidative stress. *Biochem Biophys Res Commun* 2013;**440**(2):295–9.
58. Qian Y, Zhang XL, Zeng BF, Jiang Y, Shen H, Wang Q. Substance P enhanced titanium particles-induced RANKL expression in fibroblasts from periprosthetic membrane. *Connect Tissue Res* 2013;**54**(6):361–6.
59. D'Aiuto F, Parkar M, Brett PM, Ready D, Tonetti MS. Gene polymorphisms in proinflammatory cytokines are associated with systemic inflammation in patients with severe periodontal infections. *Cytokine* 2004;**28**(1):29–34.
60. McGraw WT, Potempa J, Farley D, Travis J. Purification, characterization, and sequence analysis of a potential virulence factor from Porphyromonas gingivalis, peptidylarginine deiminase. *Infect Immun* 1999;**67**(7):3248–56.
61. Wegner N, Wait R, Sroka A, et al. Peptidylarginine deiminase from Porphyromonas gingivalis citrullinates human fibrinogen and alpha-enolase: implications for autoimmunity in rheumatoid arthritis. *Arthritis Rheum* 2010;**62**(9):2662–72.
62. El-Gabalawy H. The preclinical stages of RA: lessons from human studies and animal models. *Best Pract Res Clin Rheumatol* 2009;**23**(1):49–58.
63. Routsias JG, Goules JD, Goules A, Charalampakis G, Pikazis D. Autopathogenic correlation of periodontitis and rheumatoid arthritis. *Rheumatology (Oxford)* 2011;**50**(7):1189–93.
64. Harvey GP, Fitzsimmons TR, Dhamarpatni AA, Marchant C, Haynes DR, Bartold PM. Expression of peptidylarginine deiminase-2 and -4, citrullinated proteins and anti-citrullinated protein antibodies in human gingiva. *J Periodontal Res* 2013;**48**(2):252–61.
65. Kobayashi T, Ito S, Yasuda K, et al. The combined genotypes of stimulatory and inhibitory Fc gamma receptors associated with systemic lupus erythematosus and periodontitis in Japanese adults. *J Periodontol* 2007;**78**(3):467–74.
66. Chai L, Song YQ, Leung WK. Genetic polymorphism studies in periodontitis and Fcgamma receptors. *J Periodontal Res* 2011;**47**(3):273–85.

67. Park YD, Kim YS, Jung YM, et al. Porphyromonas gingivalis lipopolysaccharide regulates interleukin (IL)-17 and IL-23 expression via SIRT1 modulation in human periodontal ligament cells. *Cytokine* 2012;**60**(1):284–93.

68. Moutsopoulos NM, Kling HM, Angelov N, et al. Porphyromonas gingivalis promotes Th17 inducing pathways in chronic periodontitis. *J Autoimmun* 2012;**39**(4):294–303.

69. Mu L, Sun B, Kong Q, et al. Disequilibrium of T helper type 1, 2 and 17 cells and regulatory T cells during the development of experimental autoimmune myasthenia gravis. *Immunology* 2009;**128**(1 Suppl.):e826–36.

70. Wang L, Wang J, Jin Y, Gao H, Lin X. Oral administration of all-trans retinoic acid suppresses experimental periodontitis by modulating the Th17/Treg imbalance. *J Periodontol* 2014;**85**:740–50.

71. Nakajima T, Ueki-Maruyama K, Oda T, et al. Regulatory T-cells infiltrate periodontal disease tissues. *J Dent Res* 2005;**84**(7):639–43.

72. Dutzan N, Gamonal J, Silva A, Sanz M, Vernal R. Over-expression of forkhead box P3 and its association with receptor activator of nuclear factor-kappa B ligand, interleukin (IL) -17, IL-10 and transforming growth factor-beta during the progression of chronic periodontitis. *J Clin Periodontol* 2009;**36**(5):396–403.

73. Matarese G, Isola G, Anastasi GP, et al. Immunohistochemical analysis of TGF-beta1 and VEGF in gingival and periodontal tissues: a role of these biomarkers in the pathogenesis of scleroderma and periodontal disease. *Int J Mol Med* 2012;**30**(3):502–8.

74. Churg A, Wang RD, Tai H, Wang X, Xie C, Wright JL. Tumor necrosis factor-alpha drives 70% of cigarette smoke-induced emphysema in the mouse. *Am J Respir Crit Care Med* 2004;**170**(5):492–8.

75. Kuschner WG, D'Alessandro A, Wong H, Blanc PD. Dose-dependent cigarette smoking-related inflammatory responses in healthy adults. *Eur Respir J* 1996;**9**(10):1989–94.

76. Semlali A, Witoled C, Alanazi M, Rouabhia M. Whole cigarette smoke increased the expression of TLRs, HBDs, and proinflammory cytokines by human gingival epithelial cells through different signaling pathways. *PLoS One* 2012;**7**(12):e52614.

77. Timper K, Grisouard J, Sauter NS, et al. Glucose-dependent insulinotropic polypeptide induces cytokine expression, lipolysis, and insulin resistance in human adipocytes. *Am J Physiol Endocrinol Metab* 2013;**304**(1):E1–E13.

78. Zhou YJ, Zhou H, Li Y, Song YL. NOD1 activation induces innate immune responses and insulin resistance in human adipocytes. *Diabetes Metab* 2012;**38**(6):538–43.

79. Larsson PT, Hallerstam S, Rosfors S, Wallen NH. Circulating markers of inflammation are related to carotid artery atherosclerosis. *Int Angiol* 2005;**24**(1):43–51.

80. Karim Y, Turner C, Dalton N, et al. The relationship between pro-resorptive inflammatory cytokines and the effect of high dose vitamin D supplementation on their circulating concentrations. *Int Immunopharmacol* 2013;**17**(3):693–7.

81. Tang X, Pan Y, Zhao Y. Vitamin D inhibits the expression of interleukin-8 in human periodontal ligament cells stimulated with Porphyromonas gingivalis. *Arch Oral Biol* 2013;**58**(4):397–407.

82. Schulz S, Schlitt A, Lutze A, et al. The importance of genetic variants in TNFalpha for periodontal disease in a cohort of coronary patients. *J Clin Periodontol* 2012;**39**(8):699–706.

83. Cha S, Choi CB, Han TU, Kang CP, Kang C, Bae SC. Association of anti-cyclic citrullinated peptide antibody levels with PADI4 haplotypes in early rheumatoid arthritis and with shared epitope alleles in very late rheumatoid arthritis. *Arthritis Rheum* 2007;**56**(5):1454–63.

84. Jagannathan R, Lavu V, Rao SR. Comparison of the proportion of non classical (CD14 + CD16 +) monocytes/macrophages in peripheral blood and gingiva of healthy individuals and chronic periodontitis patients. *J Periodontol* 2014;**85**(6):852–8.

85. Suzuki T, Ikari K, Yano K, et al. PADI4 and HLA-DRB1 are genetic risks for radiographic progression in RA patients, independent of ACPA status: results from the IORRA cohort study. *PLoS One* 2013;**8**(4):e61045.
86. Merchant AT, Pitiphat W. Directed acyclic graphs (DAGs): an aid to assess confounding in dental research. *Community Dent Oral Epidemiol* 2002;**30**(6):399–404.
87. Faienza MF, Ventura A, Marzano F, Cavallo L. Postmenopausal osteoporosis: the role of immune system cells. *Clin Dev Immunol* 2013;**2013**:575936.
88. Eghbali-Fatourechi G, Khosla S, Sanyal A, Boyle WJ, Lacey DL, Riggs BL. Role of RANK ligand in mediating increased bone resorption in early postmenopausal women. *J Clin Invest* 2003;**111**(8):1221–30.
89. Onal M, Xiong J, Chen X, et al. Receptor activator of nuclear factor kappaB ligand (RANKL) protein expression by B lymphocytes contributes to ovariectomy-induced bone loss. *J Biol Chem* 2012;**287**(35):29851–60.
90. Shaddox LM, Goncalves PF, Vovk A, et al. LPS-induced inflammatory response after therapy of aggressive periodontitis. *J Dent Res* 2013;**92**(8):702–8.
91. Blasco-Baque V, Serino M, Vergnes JN, et al. High-fat diet induces periodontitis in mice through lipopolysaccharides (LPS) receptor signaling: protective action of estrogens. *PLoS One* 2013;**7**(11):e48220.
92. Haro A, Saxlin T, Suominen AL, et al. Serum lipids modify periodontal infection—C-reactive protein association. *J Clin Periodontol* 2012;**39**(9):817–23.
93. Queiroz-Junior CM, Madeira MF, Coelho FM, et al. Experimental arthritis triggers periodontal disease in mice: involvement of TNF-alpha and the oral Microbiota. *J Immunol* 2011;**187**(7):3821–30.
94. de Pablo P, Dietrich T, Chapple IL, et al. The autoantibody repertoire in periodontitis: a role in the induction of autoimmunity to citrullinated proteins in rheumatoid arthritis? *Ann Rheum Dis* 2014;**73**:580–6.
95. Hosokawa Y, Shindo S, Hosokawa I, Ozaki K, Matsuo T. IL-6 trans-signaling enhances CCL20 production from IL-1beta-stimulated human periodontal ligament cells. *Inflammation* 2014;**37**:381–6.
96. Navarrete M, Garcia J, Dutzan N, Henriquez L, Puente J, Carvajal P. Interferon-γ. *J Periodontol* 2014;**85**:751–60.
97. Yang JH, Li ZC, Kong WD, et al. Effect of orthodontic force on inflammatory periodontal tissue remodeling and expression of IL-6 and IL-8 in rats. *Asian Pac J Trop Med* 2013;**6**(10):757–61.
98. Mai X, Wactawski-Wende J, Hovey KM, et al. Associations between smoking and tooth loss according to the reason for tooth loss: the Buffalo OsteoPerio Study. *J Am Dent Assoc* 2013;**144**(3):252–65.
99. Weinberger I, Rotenberg Z, Fuchs J, Sagy A, Friedmann J, Agmon J. Myocardial infarction in young adults under 30 years: risk factors and clinical course. *Clin Cardiol* 1987;**10**(1):9–15.
100. Winniford MD, Wheelan KR, Kremers MS, et al. Smoking-induced coronary vasoconstriction in patients with atherosclerotic coronary artery disease: evidence for adrenergically mediated alterations in coronary artery tone. *Circulation* 1986;**73**(4):662–7.
101. Arnson Y, Shoenfeld Y, Amital H. Effects of tobacco smoke on immunity, inflammation and autoimmunity. *J Autoimmun* 2010;**34**(3):J258–65.
102. Gerli R, Sherer Y, Vaudo G, et al. Early atherosclerosis in rheumatoid arthritis: effects of smoking on thickness of the carotid artery intima media. *Ann NY Acad Sci* 2005;**1051**:281–90.
103. Passos JS, Vianna MI, Gomes-Filho IS, et al. Osteoporosis/osteopenia as an independent factor associated with periodontitis in postmenopausal women: a case-control study. *Osteoporos Int* 2013;**24**(4):1275–83.

104. Grodstein F, Stampfer MJ, Colditz GA, et al. Postmenopausal hormone therapy and mortality. *N Eng J Med* 1997;**336**(25):1769–75.
105. Agmon-Levin N, Theodor E, Segal RM, Shoenfeld Y. Vitamin d in systemic and organ-specific autoimmune diseases. *Clin Rev Allergy Immunol* 2013;**45**(2):256–66.
106. Shoenfeld Y, Tincani A, Gershwin ME. Sex gender and autoimmunity. *J Autoimmun* 2012;**38**(2–3):J71–3.
107. Grant WB. Vitamin D, periodontal disease, tooth loss, and cancer risk. *Lancet Oncol* 2008;**9**(7):612–13.
108. Milovanovic M, Pesic G, Nikolic V, et al. Vitamin D deficiency is associated with increased IL-17 and TNFalpha levels in patients with chronic heart failure. *Arq Bras Cardiol* 2012;**98**(3):259–65.
109. Ranganathan P, Khalatbari S, Yalavarthi S, Marder W, Brook R, Kaplan MJ. Vitamin d deficiency, interleukin 17, and vascular function in rheumatoid arthritis. *J Rheumatol* 2013;**40**(9):1529–34.
110. Alshouibi EN, Kaye EK, Cabral HJ, Leone CW, Garcia RI. Vitamin D and periodontal health in older men. *J Dent Res* 2013;**92**(8):689–93.
111. Ogrendik M. Does periodontopathic bacterial infection contribute to the etiopathogenesis of the autoimmune disease rheumatoid arthritis? *Discov Med* 2012;**13**(72):349–55.
112. de Pablo P, Chapple IL, Buckley CD, Dietrich T. Periodontitis in systemic rheumatic diseases. *Nat Rev Rheumatol* 2009;**5**(4):218–24.
113. Al-Katma MK, Bissada NF, Bordeaux JM, Sue J, Askari AD. Control of periodontal infection reduces the severity of active rheumatoid arthritis. *J Clin Rheumatol* 2007;**13**(3):134–7.
114. Ortiz P, Bissada NF, Palomo L, et al. Periodontal therapy reduces the severity of active rheumatoid arthritis in patients treated with or without tumor necrosis factor inhibitors. *J Periodontol* 2009;**80**(4):535–40.
115. Lee HS, Irigoyen P, Kern M, et al. Interaction between smoking, the shared epitope, and anti-cyclic citrullinated peptide: a mixed picture in three large North American rheumatoid arthritis cohorts. *Arthritis Rheum* 2007;**56**(6):1745–53.
116. Gyorgy B, Toth E, Tarcsa E, Falus A, Buzas EI. Citrullination: a posttranslational modification in health and disease. *Int J Biochem Cell Biol* 2006;**38**(10):1662–77.
117. Casiano-Colon A, Marquis RE. Role of the arginine deiminase system in protecting oral bacteria and an enzymatic basis for acid tolerance. *Appl Environ Microbiol* 1988;**54**(6):1318–24.
118. Surken M, Keller C, Rohker C, Ehlers S, Bange FC. Anaerobic arginine metabolism of Mycobacterium tuberculosis is mediated by arginine deiminase (arcA), but is not essential for chronic persistence in an aerogenic mouse model of infection. *Int J Med Microbiol* 2008;**298**(7–8):657–61.
119. Klareskog L, Ronnelid J, Lundberg K, Padyukov L, Alfredsson L. Immunity to citrullinated proteins in rheumatoid arthritis. *Annu Rev Immunol* 2008;**26**:651–75.
120. Lappin DF, Apatzidou D, Quirke AM, et al. Influence of periodontal disease, Porphyromonas gingivalis and cigarette smoking on systemic anti-citrullinated peptide antibody titres. *J Clin Periodontol* 2013;**40**(10):907–15.
121. Lundberg K, Kinloch A, Fisher BA, et al. Antibodies to citrullinated alpha-enolase peptide 1 are specific for rheumatoid arthritis and cross-react with bacterial enolase. *Arthritis Rheum* 2008;**58**(10):3009–19.
122. Kinloch AJ, Alzabin S, Brintnell W, et al. Immunization with Porphyromonas gingivalis enolase induces autoimmunity to mammalian alpha-enolase and arthritis in DR4-IE-transgenic mice. *Arthritis Rheum* 2011;**63**(12):3818–23.
123. Lundberg K, Venables PJ. Epitope spreading in animal models: array of hope in rheumatoid arthritis and multiple sclerosis. *Arthritis Res Ther* 2008;**10**(6):122.

124. Khosravi R, Ka K, Huang T, et al. Tumor necrosis factor- alpha and interleukin-6: potential interorgan inflammatory mediators contributing to destructive periodontal disease in obesity or metabolic syndrome. *Mediators Inflamm* 2013;**2013**:728987.
125. Huang CJ, Acevedo EO, Mari DC, Randazzo C, Shibata Y. Glucocorticoid inhibition of leptin- and lipopolysaccharide-induced interlukin-6 production in obesity. *Brain Behav Immun* 2013;**13**:00503–5.
126. Crispin JC, Kyttaris VC, Terhorst C, Tsokos GC. T cells as therapeutic targets in SLE. *Nat Rev Rheumatol* 2010;**6**(6):317–25.
127. Schenkein HA, Koertge TE, Brooks CN, Sabatini R, Purkall DE, Tew JG. IL-17 in sera from patients with aggressive periodontitis. *J Dent Res* 2010;**89**(9):943–7.
128. Lim MA, Lee J, Park JS, et al. Increased Th17 differentiation in aged mice is significantly associated with high IL-1beta level and low IL-2 expression. *Brain Behav Immun* 2014;**35**:163–8.
129. Fuchs A, Colonna M. Innate lymphoid cells in homeostasis, infection, chronic inflammation and tumors of the gastrointestinal tract. *Curr Opin Gastroenterol* 2013;**29**(6):581–7.
130. Tsai HC, Velichko S, Hung LY, Wu R. IL-17A and Th17 cells in lung inflammation: an update on the role of Th17 cell differentiation and IL-17R signaling in host defense against infection. *Clin Dev Immunol* 2013;**2013**:267971.
131. Yurasov S, Wardemann H, Hammersen J, et al. Defective B cell tolerance checkpoints in systemic lupus erythematosus. *J Exp Med* 2005;**201**(5):703–11.
132. Zhang Z, Kyttaris VC, Tsokos GC. The role of IL-23/IL-17 axis in lupus nephritis. *J Immunol* 2009;**183**(5):3160–9.
133. Tsokos GC. Systemic lupus erythematosus. *N Engl J Med* 2011;**365**(22):2110–21.
134. Tripodi A, de Groot PG, Pengo V. Antiphospholipid syndrome: laboratory detection, mechanisms of action and treatment. *J Intern Med* 2011;**270**(2):110–22.
135. Elemek E, Almas K. Multiple sclerosis and oral health: an update. *NY State Dent J* 2013;**79**(3):16–21.
136. Ascherio A, Munger KL. Environmental risk factors for multiple sclerosis. Part I: the role of infection. *Ann Neurol Apr* 2007;**61**(4):288–99.
137. Bogdanos DP, Smyk DS, Invernizzi P, et al. Infectome: a platform to trace infectious triggers of autoimmunity. *Autoimmun Rev* 2013;**12**(7):726–40.
138. Sheu JJ, Lin HC. Association between multiple sclerosis and chronic periodontitis: a population-based pilot study. *Eur J Neurol* 2013;**20**(7):1053–9.
138a. Greco TP, Amos MD, Conti-Kelly AM, Naranjo JD, Ijdo JW. Testing for the antiphospholipid syndrome: importance of IgA anti-β2-glycoprotein I. *Lupus* 2000;**9**(1): 33–41.
139. Schenkein HA, Berry CR, Burmeister JA, et al. Anti-cardiolipin antibodies in sera from patients with periodontitis. *J Dent Res* 2003;**82**(11):919–22.
140. Kraml PJ, Syrovatka P, Potockova J, Andel M. The oxidized low-density lipoprotein/beta2-glycoprotein I complex is associated with abdominal obesity in healthy middle-aged men. *Ann Nutr Metab* 2013;**62**(1):7–13.
141. Borges RB, Bodanese LC, Muhlen CA, et al. Anti-beta2-glycoprotein I autoantibodies and metabolic syndrome. *Arq Bras Cardiol* 2011;**96**(4):272–6.
142. Chaston R, Sabatini R, Koertge TE, Brooks CN, Schenkein HA. Serum anticardiolipin concentrations in chronic periodontitis patients following scaling and root planing. *J Periodontol* 2014;**85**(5):683–7.
143. Chen YW, Nagasawa T, Wara-Aswapati N, et al. Association between periodontitis and anti-cardiolipin antibodies in Buerger disease. *J Clin Periodontol* 2009;**36**(10):830–5.
144. Mishra MN, Rohatgi S. Antiphospholipid antibodies in young Indian patients with stroke. *J Postgrad Med* 2009;**55**(3):161–4.

145. Tzioufas AG, Kapsogeorgou EK, Moutsopoulos HM. Pathogenesis of Sjogren's syndrome: what we know and what we should learn. *J Autoimmun* 2012;**39**(1–2):4–8.
146. Mavragani CP, Moutsopoulos HM. The geoepidemiology of Sjogren's syndrome. *Autoimmun Rev* 2010;**9**(5):A305–10.
147. Lukach L, Maly A, Zini A, Aframian D. Morphometrical study of minor salivary gland in xerostomic patients with altered lipid metabolism. *Oral Dis* 2014;**20**(7):714–19.
148. Scardina GA, Ruggieri A, Messina P. Periodontal disease and sjogren syndrome: a possible correlation? *Angiology* 2010;**61**(3):289–93.
149. Brito F, Zaltman C, Carvalho AT, et al. Subgingival microflora in inflammatory bowel disease patients with untreated periodontitis. *Eur J Gastroenterol Hepatol* 2013;**25**(2):239–45.
150. Sterzl I, Prochazkova J, Hrda P, Matucha P, Bartova J, Stejskal V. Removal of dental amalgam decreases anti-TPO and anti-Tg autoantibodies in patients with autoimmune thyroiditis. *Neuro Endocrinol Lett* 2006;**27**(Suppl. 1):25–30.
151. Eyeson J, House I, Yang YH, Warnakulasuriya KA. Relationship between mercury levels in blood and urine and complaints of chronic mercury toxicity from amalgam restorations. *Br Dent J* 2010;**208**(4):E7, discussion 162-163.
152. Bellinger DC, Trachtenberg F, Daniel D, Zhang A, Tavares MA, McKinlay S. A dose-effect analysis of children's exposure to dental amalgam and neuropsychological function: the New England Children's Amalgam Trial. *J Am Dent Assoc* 2007;**138**(9):1210–16.
153. Maserejian NN, Hauser R, Tavares M, Trachtenberg FL, Shrader P, McKinlay S. Dental composites and amalgam and physical development in children. *J Dent Res* 2012;**91**(11):1019–25.
154. McLachlan SM, Rapoport B. Breaking tolerance to thyroid antigens: changing concepts in thyroid autoimmunity. *Endocr Rev* 2014;**35**(1):59–105.

CHAPTER 59

Infections as a Cause of Guillain–Barré Syndrome

Eitan Israeli[*], **Nancy Agmon-Levin**[*], **Miri Blank**[*], **Joab Chapman**[‡],
Yehuda Shoenfeld[*,†,1]
[*]Center for Autoimmune Diseases, Sheba Medical Center, Tel-Hashomer, Israel
[†]Sackler Faculty of Medicine, Incumbent of the Laura Schwarz-Kip Chair for Research of Autoimmune
Diseases, Tel-Aviv University, Tel-Aviv, Israel
[‡]Department of Neurology and Sagol Center for Neurosciences, Sheba Medical Center, Tel-Hashomer, Israel
[1]Corresponding Author: shoenfel@post.tau.ac.il

1 INTRODUCTION

Guillain–Barré syndrome (GBS) is a rare autoimmune disorder, the incidence of which is estimated to be 0.6 to 4 per 100,000 persons per year worldwide. In around one-third of cases, GBS occurs a few days or weeks after the patient has symptoms of a respiratory or gastrointestinal microbial infection. The disorder is sub-acute, developing over the course of hours or days and up to 3–4 weeks. Reflexes are usually lost. Although ascending paralysis is the most common form of spread in GBS, other variants also exist, including Miller Fisher syndrome. GBS is a classical autoimmune disease, as all four major Witebsky–Rose criteria for an autoimmune disease are fulfilled. Viral and bacterial infections often are associated with GBS. Some parts of this chapter were published in a review,[1] and it is an update of the chapter by van Sorge et al. (2004)[2] published in the previous edition of this textbook.

2 DEFINITION OF GBS

GBS is a disorder in which the immune system attacks gangliosides on the peripheral nervous system. The first symptoms of this disorder include varying degrees of weakness or tingling sensations in the legs. In many instances, the weakness and abnormal sensations spread to the arms and upper body.[3]

☆ Competing interests: Y. Shoenfeld declares an association with the following organization: the US National Vaccine Injury Compensation Program. The other authors declare no competing interests.

Infection and Autoimmunity
http://dx.doi.org/10.1016/B978-0-444-63269-2.00053-2
981

These symptoms can increase in intensity until the muscles fail completely and the patient is almost totally paralyzed or there is severe dysfunction of the autonomic nervous system. In these cases, the disease is life threatening and is considered a medical emergency. Most patients, however, recover from even the most severe cases of GBS, although some continue to have some degree of weakness. GBS is rare: incidence worldwide is estimated to be 0.6 to 4 in 100,000 persons per year (Vucic, Kiernan et al.). In around one-third of cases, GBS occurs a few days or weeks after the patient has had symptoms of a respiratory or gastrointestinal microbial infection. Surgery or vaccinations occasionally trigger the syndrome. The disorder can develop over the course of hours or days, or it may take up to 3–4 weeks, and reflexes are usually lost. Because of the slowing of signals traveling along the nerve, a nerve conduction velocity test can aid in the diagnosis. The cerebrospinal fluid contains more protein than usual but a normal cell count, so a spinal tap is important for diagnosis.

3 INFECTIONS AND GBS

About a third of all cases of GBS are preceded by *Campylobacter jejuni* infection.[4] This bacterium expresses a lipooligosaccharide (LOS) molecule that mimics various gangliosides present in high concentrations in peripheral nerves. Numerous viruses also collect gangliosides as they incorporate plasma membrane from the host cell. As a result, viral infections (e.g. influenza, parainfluenza, polio, herpes) often are associated with GBS, and both bacterial and viral vaccines have been linked with the induction of the condition.[5] Numerous epidemiological studies and anecdotal cases have established an association between infections and GBS (Table 1). Kinnunen et al. (1998)[11] performed a retrospective analysis of the incidence of GBS in Finland in 1981–1986. Monthly rates showed an increased incidence of GBS from baseline (8.2 per million) in March 1985, following by a few weeks the onset of the nationwide oral poliovirus vaccine campaign and partly overlapping it. In-depth analysis of the time series suggested, however, that a change in the occurrence of GBS had already taken place before the oral poliovirus vaccine campaign. Widespread circulation of wild-type 3 poliovirus among the population immediately preceded the oral poliovirus vaccine campaign and the peak occurrence of GBS. These results demonstrate a temporal association between poliovirus infections, caused by either wild virus or live attenuated vaccine, and an episode of increased occurrence of GBS. In a review about GBS as an autoimmune disease, Shoenfeld et al.[9]

Table 1 Infectious Agents Associated with GBS

Infectious Agent	Year	Incidence (per 10⁶)	Time After Infection	References
Chikungunya virus	2009	Up 22% from baseline (3.3)	2–3 weeks	6
Influenza	1990–2005	7.3 16.6 Relative incidence	90 days 30 days	7
Coxsackieviruses; Chlamydia; CMV; M. pneumoniae; C. jejuni	Prospective	?	6 weeks	8
Echo/Coxsackie; varicela; mumps; rubella; influenza; HIV; Borrelia; M. pneumoniae; C. jejuni	1990	?	Weeks	9
C. jejuni	2003	9.5 OR	?	10
Polio (circulating type 3)	1981–1986	Increase from (8.2) baseline	Weeks	11
Hepatitis E	2009	One case	Weeks	12

cite numerous bacterial and viral infections associated with the disease. Among the viruses, echo, Coxsackie, varicella, mumps, rubella, influenza, and human immunodeficiency virus are documented as infections preceding episodes of GBS. Bacterial infections preceding GBS included *Borrelia*, *Mycoplasma pneumoniae*, and *C. jejuni*. A strong association between *C. jejuni* infection and GBS, with an odds ratio of 9.5, also was demonstrated in another study, confirming a causal association.[10] Microbiological studies carried out using 84 patients resulted in a probable diagnosis of infectious diseases etiology in 46 (55%). Coxsackieviruses (15%), *Chlamydia pneumoniae* (8%), cytomegalovirus (7%), and *M. pneumoniae* (7%) were the most frequently involved agents. Serological evidence of a *C. jejuni* infection was found in six patients (7%). The authors concluded that the etiology of antecedent diseases is distributed over a wide spectrum of pediatric infectious diseases. Most of the children who had been vaccinated showed concomitant infectious diseases, thus obscuring the causative role for GBS.[8] Another strong association between GBS and influenza infections was documented by Stowe et al. (2009).[7] The authors used the self-controlled case series method to investigate the relation of GBS with influenza vaccine and influenza-like illness using cases recorded in the General Practice Research Database from 1990 to 2005 in the United Kingdom. The relative incidence of GBS within 90 days of vaccination was 0.76 (95% confidence interval, 0.41–1.40). By contrast, the relative incidence of GBS within 90 days of an influenza-like illness was 7.35 (95% confidence interval, 4.36–12.38), with the greatest relative incidence (16.64) within 30 days (95% confidence interval, 9.37–29.54). The relative incidence was similar (0.89; 95% confidence interval, 0.42–1.89) when the analysis was restricted to a subset of validated cases. The authors found no evidence of an increased risk of GBS after seasonal influenza vaccine.

The finding of a greatly increased risk after influenza-like illness is consistent with anecdotal reports of a preceding respiratory illness in GBS and has important implications for the risk/benefit assessment that would be carried out should pandemic vaccines be deployed in the future. Two reports (2009) document an association of GBS and relatively rare viral infections: Lebrun et al. (2009)[6] reported two cases of GBS after Chikungunya virus infection on Réunion Island, which correlated with epidemiological data conferring the association between the two. Chikungunya virus is an RNA alphavirus (group A arbovirus) in the family *Togaviridae*. *Aedes aegypti* and *Aedes albopictus* are the known mosquitoes vectors. Anti-Chikungunya IgM was found in serum and CSF, although genomic products in serum and CSF were negative, which was not surprising given the brief period (4–5 days) of viremia. These findings strongly supported a disseminated acute Chikungunya infection and support the conclusion that the Chikungunya virus was probably responsible for the GBS. In 2006, the Chikungunya virus was found on Réunion Island; seroprevalence on the island was estimated to be 38.2% among 785,000 inhabitants (95% confidence interval, 35.9–40.6%). Epidemiologic data also support a causal relationship between Chikungunya infection and GBS: The incidence rate of GBS increased 22% in 2006 (26 in 787,000 persons) over the rate in 2005 (21 in 775,000 [2.7 in 10,000] persons) and then declined to a rate closer to baseline in 2007 (23 in 800,000 [2.87 in 100,000] persons). Loly et al. (2009)[12] report a case of GBS in a patient sporadically contaminated in a Western country. This is the third report of GBS in a patient with hepatitis E and the first occurring in a patient sporadically contaminated in a Western country. The authors believe it is the first description of the presence of antiganglioside GM2 antibodies in GBS associated with a hepatotropic virus, suggesting possible molecular mimicry involving gangliosides.

In all the above-mentioned reports, the time between the infection and the onset of GBS was a few weeks, ranging from 2–3 weeks to 3 months. This time period is in agreement with a temporal association between an environmental trigger and the onset of an autoimmune disease. Adding the high odds ratio of association calculated for some of these infections (9.5 for *C. jejuni*) and augmentation of the relative incidence following infection (7.3–16.6 for influenza), the conclusion that these and other bacterial and viral infections are strong environmental agents involved with the onset of GBS is quite obvious.

4 POSSIBLE MECHANISMS THAT CAN TRIGGER GBS

Most infectious agents, such as viruses, bacteria and parasites, can induce autoimmunity via a number of mechanisms. Molecular mimicry is one mechanism by which infectious agents may trigger an immune response against autoantigens. GBS, the prototype of post-infectious autoimmune diseases, ranks as the most frequent cause of acute flaccid paralysis, and *C. jejuni* is the most frequent antecedent pathogen. Epidemiological studies, which established the relationship between GBS and antecedent *C. jejuni* infection, showed that one-fourth to one-third of patients with GBS develop the syndrome after being infected. GBS was considered a demyelinating disease of the peripheral nerves, but the existence of primary "axonal GBS" has been confirmed and is now widely recognized. Ganglioside GM1 is an autoantigen for IgG antibodies in patients with axonal GBS subsequent to *C. jejuni* enteritis. *C. jejuni* strains isolated from such patients have a LOS with a GM1-like structure. To verify that molecular mimicry between an environmental agent and the peripheral nerves causes GBS, Yuki et al. (2004)[13] sensitized animals with *C. jejuni* LOS and produced a model of human GBS, generated anti-GM1 monoclonal antibody (mAb) by immunizing with the LOS, and determined the distribution of GM1 in human spinal nerve roots. As further proof that an autoimmune reaction causes neuromuscular disease, the authors also showed that anti-GM1 mAb blocked muscle action potentials in a muscle–spinal cord co-culture.

C. jejuni infection also often precedes acute motor axonal neuropathy (AMAN), a variant of GBS. Anti-GM1, anti-GM1b, anti-GD1a, and anti-GalNAc-GD1a IgG antibodies are associated with AMAN. Carbohydrate mimicry (Galbeta1-3GalNAcbeta1-4[NeuAcalpha2-3]Galbeta1-) was seen between the LOS of *C. jejuni* isolated from a patient with AMAN and human GM1 ganglioside. Sensitization with the LOS of *C. jejuni* induces AMAN in rabbits, as does sensitization with the GM1 ganglioside. Paralyzed rabbits have pathological changes in their peripheral nerves that are identical to changes seen in human GBS. *C. jejuni* infection may induce anti-ganglioside antibodies by molecular mimicry, eliciting AMAN. This verifies the causative mechanism of molecular mimicry in an autoimmune disease. To express ganglioside mimics, *C. jejuni* requires specific gene combinations that function in sialic acid biosynthesis or transfer. The knockout mutants of these landmark genes of GBS show reduced reactivity with the sera of patients with GBS and fail to induce an anti-ganglioside antibody response in mice. These genes are crucial for the induction of neuropathogenic cross-reactive antibodies.[14] Koga et al. (2006)[15] performed a comprehensive analysis of bacterial risk factors for the development of GBS after *C. jejuni* enteritis. *C. jejuni* strains carrying a sialyltransferase gene (cst-II), which is essential for the biosynthesis of ganglioside-like LOSs. Strains of *C. jejuni* from patients with GBS more frequently had LOS biosynthesis locus class A (72 of 106; 68%) than did strains from patients with enteritis (17 of 103; 17%). Class A strains predominantly were serotype HS:19 and had the *cstII* (Thr51) genotype; the latter is responsible for biosynthesis of GM1-like and GD1a-like LOSs. Both anti-GM1 and anti-GD1a monoclonal antibodies regularly bind to class A LOSs, whereas no antibody or either antibody binds to other LOS locus classes. Mass spectrometric analysis showed that a class A strain carried GD1a-like LOS as well as GM1-like LOS. Logistic regression analysis showed that serotype HS:19 and the class A locus were predictive of the development of GBS. The high frequency of the class A locus in GBS-associated strains, which was recently reported in Europe, provided the first GBS-related *C. jejuni* characteristic that is common to strains from Asia and Europe. The class A locus and serotype HS:19 seem to be linked to the *cstII* polymorphism, resulting in the promotion of both GM1-like and GD1a-like structure synthesis on LOS and, consequently, an increase in the risk of producing anti-ganglioside autoantibodies and developing GBS.

The sialyltransferase gene polymorphism may also direct the clinical features of GBS. The *C. jejuni* sialyltransferase (Cst-II) consists of 291 amino acids, and the 51st determines its enzymatic activity. Strains with cst-II

(Thr51) expressed GM1-like and GD1a-like LOS, whereas strains with cst-II (Asn51) expressed GT1a-like and GD1c-like LOS. Patients infected with the cst-II (Thr51) strains had anti-GM1 or anti-GD1a IgG antibodies and showed limb weakness. Patients infected with the cst-II (Asn51) strains had anti-GQ1b IgG antibodies and showed ophthalmoplegia and ataxia. The *cst-II* gene is responsible for the development of GBS and Fisher syndromes, and the polymorphism (Thr/Asn51) determines which syndrome develops after *C. jejuni* enteritis.[16]

5 CONCLUDING REMARKS

Judging by the evidence presented here, the etiology of GBS can be multifactorial, as in other autoimmune diseases. It involves genetic and environmental factors, may be triggered by infections or vaccinations and predisposition can be predicted by analyzing some of these factors. In a series of three enlightening reviews, Shoenfeld et al. depict the "mosaic of autoimmunity." The authors present the multi-factorial character of autoimmune diseases, including GBS, concentrate on genetic, hormonal and environmental factors and focus on the prediction and therapy of these disorders.[17–19] GBS is unique in the aspect that it can be triggered both by infection (*C. jejuni*) or vaccination (influenza, polio), and in this respect it can serve as a model for the linkage between exposure to environmental agents and autoimmune diseases. GBS is still a classical example of an autoimmune disease triggered by either infection or vaccination.

REFERENCES

1. Israeli E, Agmon-Levin N, et al. Guillain–Barré syndrome—a classical autoimmune disease triggered by infection or vaccination. *Clin Rev Allergy Immunol* 2012;**42**(2):121–30.
2. Van Sorge NM, Van der Berg LH, Jansen MD, Van der Winkel JGJ, Van der Pol WL. Infection and Guillain–Barré syndrome. In: Shoenfeld Y, Rose NR, editors. *Infection and autoimmunity*. Amsterdam-Boston-Heidelberg-London-New York: Elsevier; 2004. p. 591–612.
3. Vucic S, Kiernan MC, et al. Guillain–Barré syndrome: an update. *J Clin Neurosci* 2009;**16**(6):733–41.
4. Gruenewald R, Ropper AH, et al. Serologic evidence of Campylobacter jejuni/coli enteritis in patients with Guillain–Barré syndrome. *Arch Neurol* 1991;**48**(10):1080–2.
5. Melnick SC, Flewett TH. Role of infection in the Guillain–Barré syndrome. *J Neurol Neurosurg Psychiatry* 1964;**27**:395–407.
6. Lebrun G, Chadda K, et al. Guillain–Barré syndrome after chikungunya infection. *Emerg Infect Dis* 2009;**15**(3):495–6.

7. Stowe J, Andrews N, et al. Investigation of the temporal association of Guillain–Barré syndrome with influenza vaccine and influenzalike illness using the United Kingdom General Practice Research Database. *Am J Epidemiol* 2009;**169**(3):382–8.

8. Schessl J, Luther B, et al. Infections and vaccinations preceding childhood Guillain–Barré syndrome: a prospective study. *Eur J Pediatr* 2006;**165**(9):605–12.

9. ·Shoenfeld Y, George J, et al. Guillain–Barré as an autoimmune disease. *Int Arch Allergy Immunol* 1996;**109**(4):318–26.

10. Liu GF, Wu ZL, et al. A case-control study on children with Guillain–Barré syndrome in North China. *Biomed Environ Sci* 2003;**16**(2):105–11.

11. Kinnunen E, Junttila O, et al. Nationwide oral poliovirus vaccination campaign and the incidence of Guillain–Barré syndrome. *Am J Epidemiol* 1998;**147**(1):69–73.

12. Loly JP, Rikir E, et al. Guillain–Barré syndrome following hepatitis E. *World J Gastroenterol* 2009;**15**(13):1645–7.

13. Yuki N, Susuki K, et al. Carbohydrate mimicry between human ganglioside GM1 and Campylobacter jejuni lipooligosaccharide causes Guillain–Barré syndrome. *Proc Natl Acad Sci USA* 2004;**101**(31):11404–9.

14. Komagamine T, Yuki N. Ganglioside mimicry as a cause of Guillain–Barré syndrome. *CNS Neurol Disord Drug Targets* 2006;**5**(4):391–400.

15. Koga M, Gilbert M, et al. Comprehensive analysis of bacterial risk factors for the development of Guillain–Barré syndrome after Campylobacter jejuni enteritis. *J Infect Dis* 2006;**193**(4):547–55.

16. Yuki N. Campylobacter sialyltransferase gene polymorphism directs clinical features of Guillain–Barré syndrome. *J Neurochem* 2007;**103**(Suppl. 1):150–8.

17. Shoenfeld Y, Blank M, et al. The mosaic of autoimmunity: prediction, autoantibodies, and therapy in autoimmune diseases—2008. *Isr Med Assoc J* 2008;**10**(1):13–19.

18. Shoenfeld Y, Gilburd B, et al. The mosaic of autoimmunity: genetic factors involved in autoimmune diseases—2008. *Isr Med Assoc J* 2008;**10**(1):3–7.

19. Shoenfeld Y, Zandman-Goddard G, et al. The mosaic of autoimmunity: hormonal and environmental factors involved in autoimmune diseases—2008. *Isr Med Assoc J* 2008;**10**(1):8–12.

CHAPTER 60

Acute Disseminated Encephalomyelitis

Ravindra Kumar Garg[1]

Department of Neurology, King George Medical University, Lucknow, Uttar Pradesh, India
[1]Corresponding Author: garg50@yahoo.com

1 INTRODUCTION

Acute disseminated encephalomyelitis (ADEM) is a frequently encountered acute demyelinating disorder of the central nervous system (CNS). ADEM has been reported across the world; in resource-constrained countries it is a common pediatric emergency. ADEM is usually triggered by a preceding viral infection or immunization. ADEM predominantly involves the white matter of the brain, brain stem, optic nerves, and less frequently the spinal cord and usually has a monophasic course. Magnetic resonance imaging (MRI) often reveals demyelination that involves the white matter of the cerebral cortex and spinal cord. Relapses of ADEM are infrequent but pose a great diagnostic challenge in its differentiation from multiple sclerosis.[1,2] The International Pediatric Multiple Sclerosis Study Group recently proposed a consensus definition to distinguish multiphasic ADEM from multiple sclerosis[3,4] (Table 1). Some cases of ADEM or clinically isolated syndrome convert to chronic demyelinating disorders such as multiple sclerosis and neuromyelitis optica.

2 EPIDEMIOLOGY

ADEM predominantly affects children and young adults; however, it can occur at any age. It is more common in the winter and spring seasons.[5] Absoud and co-workers conducted a population-based study ($n = 4095$) to determine the incidence of pediatric acquired demyelinating disorders. This study used International Pediatric MS Study Group 2007 definitions and McDonald 2010 mass spectrometry imaging criteria. Acute acquired

Infection and Autoimmunity
http://dx.doi.org/10.1016/B978-0-444-63269-2.00062-3

Table 1 Revised Definitions (2012 Revision of 2007 Consensus Definitions)

Term	Definition
Acute disseminated encephalomyelitis (ADEM)	A multifocal and polysymptomatic acute demyelinating syndrome that has encephalopathy (that cannot be explained by fever) as an essential feature; neuroimaging shows focal or multifocal lesions predominantly involving white matter
Multiphasic ADEM	A new clinical event or the re-emergence of a prior clinical event meeting the criteria for ADEM but involving new anatomic areas of the CNS at least 3 months or more after the onset of the initial ADEM
Neuromyelitis optica	An acute demyelinating syndrome with optic neuritis, myelitis, and at least two of three supportive criteria: MRI evidence of a contiguous spinal cord involvement of ≥ 3 segments, neuromyelitis optica, and IgG seropositivity; brain MRI does not meeting diagnostic criteria for MS
Clinically isolated syndrome	An acute demyelinating syndrome with CNS involvement (monofocal or multifocal) but without encephalopathy, such as isolated involvement of optic nerve, cerebellum, or brain stem
Multiple sclerosis	Multiple episodes of CNS demyelination separated in time and space; diagnosis is based on the McDonald criteria

Table created based on information in Krupp et al., reference 4.

demyelinating syndromes were identified in 125 patients. The incidence of first acquired demyelinating syndrome was 9.83 per million children per year. Of these patients, 66.4% were classified as having clinically isolated syndrome, 32.0% as having ADEM, and 1.6% as having neuromyelitis optica.[6] In one study, among people younger than 20 years of age living in California, the incidence of ADEM was estimated to be 0.4 per 100,000 per year.[7] In poor and resource-constrained countries, ADEM is common because of a high incidence of many viral and bacterial infections such as measles. The Semple vaccine, an obsolete anti-rabies vaccine, is still being extensively used in poor countries; however, the exact incidence of ADEM in these countries is not known.[8,9]

3 ETIOLOGY

The occurrence of ADEM is often preceded by a vast variety of viral or bacterial infections; however, the most frequent preceding event is a non-specific upper respiratory tract infection. In several patients it is not possible to identify the responsible infectious agent.[5] Organisms that have been identified in ADEM include mumps virus, enterovirus, Epstein–Barr virus, human herpes virus-6, herpes simplex, Japanese B encephalitis virus, adenovirus, dengue virus, hepatitis C virus, *Mycoplasma pneumoniae*, *Chlamydia pneumoniae*, rotavirus, human papilloma virus, *Listeria monocytogenes*, leptospirosis, *Streptococcus pyogenes*, *Borrelia burgdorferi*, and *Rickettsia rickettsii*. The risk of ADEM is greatest following measles and rubella infection. The H1N1 influenza virus is a common viral agent responsible for ADEM.[1,2,10] Filaria and malaria can occasionally trigger ADEM in endemic regions.[11,12] Allogeneic bone marrow transplantation and stem cell transplantation are new emerging causes of ADEM.[13] Vaccinations such as rabies, measles, polio, pertussis, rubella, Japanese B encephalitis, H1N1 influenza, human papilloma virus, typhoid, hepatitis B, and tetanus antitoxin have been found to be associated with ADEM.[1,2,10]

4 PATHOGENESIS

A genetic susceptibility is likely in patients with ADEM. In a study from Korea, association with major histocompatibility complex class II alleles HLA-DRB1★1501, as well as HLA-DRB5★0101 have been demonstrated. In Russia, ADEM was found to be associated with DRB1★01 and DRB1★017(03). In Brazil, the genetic susceptibility for ADEM was significantly associated with the HLA-DQB1★0602, DRB1★1501 and DRB1★1503 alleles.[14–16]

The exact immunopathogenesis is still not known. Theiler's murine encephalomyelitis virus, which produces encephalomyelitis in mice, may serve as a model for encephalomyelitis after infection. Pathologically, Theiler's virus-induced demyelinating disease closely resembles ADEM.[17,18] The molecular mimicry theory and the inflammatory cascade theory are the two most accepted hypotheses to explain the pathogenesis of ADEM. The molecular mimicry theory is based on the assumption that some myelin antigens may share a structural similarity with antigenic determinants present on the pathogen responsible for ADEM. The antibodies produced against the infecting microorganism are thought to cross-react with myelin antigens, producing an immune response against neuronal tissue.[19–21] Alternatively, according to the inflammatory cascade theory, a CNS infection with a neurotropic virus results in the release of myelin-based autoantigens into the systemic circulation through a disrupted blood–brain barrier. The immune system reacts against these autoantigens in the peripheral blood circulation and triggers a cascade of inflammatory reaction. Autoreactive T-cell clones are generated during this process. These T cells cross the blood–brain barrier and invade the brain parenchyma, subsequently damaging the brain tissue.[22,23]

Studies of the pathogenesis of ADEM have demonstrated the effect of autoantibodies on several myelin-associated proteins. In one study, high serum immunoglobulin G titers to myelin oligodendrocyte glycoprotein were detected in 40% of children with clinical isolated syndrome and ADEM.[24] Myelin oligodendrocyte glycoprotein is a myelin antigen present at the outer surface of the myelin sheath that may trigger immune responses.[25] Profiles of serum autoantibodies against myelin antigens have been useful in distinguishing multiple sclerosis from ADEM. ADEM is characterized by the demonstration of IgG autoantibodies against myelin basic protein, proteolipid protein, myelin-associated oligodendrocyte basic glycoprotein and α-B-crystallin. Multiple sclerosis is characterized by IgM autoantibodies against myelin basic protein, proteolipid protein, myelin-associated oligodendrocyte basic glycoprotein and oligodendrocyte-specific protein.[26] The persistence or disappearance of antibodies to myelin oligodendrocyte glycoprotein may have a prognostic value. In one study, myelin oligodendrocyte glycoprotein antibodies rapidly declined in all 16 monophasic patients with ADEM and in one patient with clinically isolated syndrome. In contrast, in six of eight patients diagnosed with multiple sclerosis, the antibodies persisted, with fluctuations showing a second increase during an observation period up to 5 years.[27]

Several cytokines, including tumor necrosis factor-α, interleukin-2 and interferon-γ, are thought to be important in the immunopathogenesis of ADEM.[28] Cytokines lead to the activation of macrophages, and type 1 and type 2 helper T cells are up-regulated in CSF. Matrix metalloproteinase-9 and tissue inhibitor of matrix metalloproteinase-1 also have been shown to play some role. Matrix metalloproteinase-9 expression is associated with disruption of the blood–brain barrier.[29]

5 PATHOLOGY

The pathological hallmark of ADEM is perivenular inflammatory changes along with sleeves of perivenous demyelination. In contrast, confluent sheets of demyelination (with macrophage infiltration and reactive astrocytes) are the hallmark of multiple sclerosis. Demyelination in ADEM is limited to the region of inflammation, whereas in multiple sclerosis demyelination is extensive and plaque-like. The inflammatory lesions of ADEM consist of T lymphocytes, lipid-laden macrophages and, less frequently, neutrophil, esinophil, or plasma cell infiltrates. Axons are relatively preserved. In the advanced stages of disease, the demyelinating lesions show astrocytic proliferation with gliosis. Characteristically, in ADEM all the demyelinating lesions are of same age and predominantly affect white matter. The peripheral nervous system is more frequently involved in vaccine-associated ADEM.[30,31]

6 CLINICAL MANIFESTATIONS

Clinical manifestations of ADEM are usually poly-symptomatic and multi-focal. Full-blown clinical syndrome is often preceded by non-specific prodromal symptoms. The prodromal manifestations include fever, malaise, headache, nausea, or vomiting. Encephalopathy, the main characteristic feature of ADEM, evolves within 7 days after prodromal symptoms occur. Encephalopathy manifests as behavioral changes, including confusion, irritability and restlessness. Severe cases of encephalopathy may result in obtundation, stupor, decerebrate posturing, and coma. In addition, patients may have focal neurologic deficits such as vision impairment, hemiparesis, paraparesis, ataxia, bladder dysfunction, sensory loss, and a variety of movement disorders. Optic neuritis, resulting in vision loss, is characteristically bilateral. Ataxia is particularly common in children. There may be increased intracranial pressure with tentorial herniation in severely affected patients, resulting in death. Infrequently, the peripheral nervous system may also be involved.[32,33]

In one study, patients with perivenous demyelination (the hallmark of ADEM) were compared with a cohort of patients with confluent demyelination (the hallmark of multiple sclerosis). The patients with perivenous demyelination presented with encephalopathy, altered consciousness, headache, meningismus, CSF pleocytosis or multifocal enhancing lesions seen on MRI. Almost all the patients with perivenous demyelination had a monophasic course. In the group with confluent demyelination, 76 of 91 patients fulfilled multiple sclerosis criteria at the last follow-up (2.9 years; range, 0.1–18.8 years).[31]

7 DIAGNOSTIC WORKUP

Peripheral blood counts are usually normal, but peripheral leukocytosis can be observed. The CSF can be normal in a large number of patients. In severe and fulminant cases, the CSF may have mild lymphocytosis. Cells may be predominantly polymorphonuclear in the acute stage. CSF protein is usually elevated, but levels are only slightly >100 mg/dL. Oligoclonal IgG bands can be present in up to 25% of cases in the early stage but may disappear later.

MRI is the most efficient imaging tool for the evaluation of ADEM. MRI is able to demonstrate white matter lesions in virtually in all patients with ADEM. It also helps characterize the nature, location, activity, and size of the lesions. Demyelinating lesions are most frequently visualized on T2-weighted and fluid-attenuated inversion recovery sequences. T1-weighted sequences rarely demonstrate hypointense white matter lesions. Demyelinating lesions appear on MRI as large (>1–2 cm), multiple, asymmetric, patchy and poorly demarcated imaging abnormalities[4] (Figure 1). Lesions are typically located in the centrum semiovale at the junction of cortical grey and white matter, the cerebellum, the brainstem, and the spinal cord. Lesions occasionally affect grey matter structures such as the basal ganglia and thalamus. Among grey matter structures, the putamen is the most frequently involved.[34] In ADEM, there is no specific predilection for periventricular white matter. In addition, lesions involving the corpus callosum are rarely seen. Lesions appear hypointense on T1-weighted sequences and have increased signal intensity on T2-weighted and fluid-attenuated inversion recovery sequences. The spinal lesions of ADEM are often large and

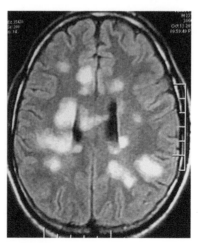

Figure 1 MRI axial fluid-attenuated inversion recovery image of brain showing multiple small, hyperintense lesions in deep white matter.

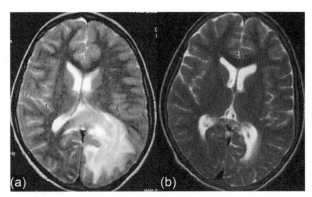

Figure 2 MRI axial fluid-attenuated inversion recovery image of brain shows a tumefactive demyelinating lesion (a). MRI shows the disappearance of lesions 3 months after methylprednisolone therapy (b).

swollen. The spinal cord lesions in multiple sclerosis are typically smaller, more discrete and involve cervical spinal segments.[35,36] In the spinal cord, demyelinating lesions dominantly affect thoracic spinal segments. Demyelinating lesions in ADEM may show a varied pattern of enhancement (patchy and fluffy, single or multiple ring-shaped, open ring, nodular, gyral, and diffuse) after contrast administration. In the presence of a large cerebral lesion with a mass effect (a tumefactive demyelinating lesion), it may be essential to biopsy the lesion to exclude an infective or a malignant disease (Figure 2). Quantitative MRI techniques such as diffusion-weighted imaging and proton magnetic resonance spectroscopy can be used to characterize and determine the stage of the lesions. ADEM lesions show restricted diffusion in the acute stage and free diffusion and a decrease in N-acetyl aspartate/choline ratios in the subacute stage.[37]

8 DIFFERENTIAL DIAGNOSIS

There is no single test that can confirm the diagnosis of ADEM. The diagnosis is based on a constellation of clinical and radiologic features. Accurate diagnosis also requires efficient exclusion of diseases that resemble ADEM. Therefore, a comprehensive workup, with the objective of excluding possibilities that mimic ADEM, should be performed. A variety of CNS infections, autoimmune disorders of the brain, and several metabolic disorders may pose a diagnostic challenge because of the similarity of clinical manifestations. Other acute demyelinating disorders such as multiple sclerosis, neuromyelitis optica, and idiopathic transverse myelitis may resemble ADEM; it is crucial to differentiate them because treatment and prognosis vary to a large extent. A variety of CNS infections presenting as acute encephalopathy need to considered in the differential diagnosis. These conditions include bacterial meningitis, viral encephalitis, and autoimmune encephalitis. The differential diagnosis should also include vasculitic syndromes such as primary CNS vasculitis, Sjögren's syndrome, systemic lupus erythematosus, and Behçet's disease. ADEM was misdiagnosed in a patient who actually had glioblastoma multiforme.[38] Lesions of the posterior reversible encephalopathy syndrome, eclampsia and hypertensive encephalopathy look similar to those of ADEM on MRI and need to be differentiated. Post-malaria neurological syndrome may present with impaired consciousness, headache, myoclonus, cerebellar ataxia, and focal neurological deficits and can clinically resemble ADEM.[39] Hemophago-cytic lymphohistiocytosis (genetic defects in the cytotoxicity of CD8 T lym-phocytes and natural killer cells) may present with encephalitic syndrome, which resembles ADEM.[40]

9 MANAGEMENT

Available treatment is largely empirical because current treatment is based on experience gained from case reports and some small series. Data from ran-domized controlled studies are not available. Immunomodulatory agents, including methylprednisolone, intravenous immunoglobulin, or plasma-pheresis, are used. There are no studies comparing the efficacy of these dif-ferent immunomodulatory therapies.

It is well accepted among experts that methylprednisolone is effective in rapidly resolving the symptoms as well as lesions of ADEM seen on MRI. Methylprednisolone is administered intravenously (20–30 mg/kg/day; max-imum 1 g/day) for 3–5 days. After methylprednisolone therapy, tapering doses of oral corticosteroids are usually given for 4–6 weeks. In patients who respond poorly to methylprednisolone, intravenous immunoglobulin G (at a dosage of 2 g/kg divided over 2–5 days) need to be considered. In ful-minant cases, plasmapheresis is an effective alternative in early stages.[41] A decompressive hemicraniectomy may be lifesaving in some seriously ill patients who have markedly increased intracranial pressure.[42] Patients with recurrent and multiphasic ADEM may require repeated administration of methylprednisolone.

10 PROGNOSIS

Most patients with ADEM recover completely following methylpredniso-lone therapy. In one series, 89% (75 of 84) of patients either completely recovered or had minor disability. None of the patients died. In this series, 11% of patients had residual deficits. The most frequently observed residual disabilities were focal motor deficits, vision loss, mental handicap and sei-zures.[43] Functional recovery is usually more rapid in children than in adults. In adults, duration of hospitalization is longer and intensive care unit admis-sion is more frequently required.[44] One study including 12 children with severe manifestations of ADEM with a mean follow-up of 6.2 years (range, 2–13.6 years) revealed that 7 children had deficits in the categories of alert-ness, memory, school performance, visual-spatial skills, and/or impulse con-trol. Children were evaluated for neuropsychological outcome using a parental questionnaire.[45]

A proportion of patients with ADEM have recurrent demyelinating epi-sodes. These relapses are called recurrent ADEM and multiphasic ADEM. In a series of 88 patients (mean duration of follow-up, 6.6 years), 90% had monophasic course and a 10% had biphasic pattern.[43] In another series, among 90 pediatric patients with ADEM, 11 had multiphasic ADEM. A multiphasic course was associated with older age, severe and prolonged focal neurologic symptoms and a distinct demyelination on MRI.[15]

11 CONVERSION TO MULTIPLE SCLEROSIS

The exact relationship of ADEM with multiple sclerosis is still not known, and it needs to be established.[35,36,46] A variety of clinical and neuroimaging predictors from several studies that point towards possible multiple sclerosis at an initial demyelinating event have been identified. In a cohort of 116 children, 52 patients had a second attack and fulfilled the criteria for multiple sclerosis. In this study, MRI features such as lesions of the corpus callosum on the perpendicular long axis, focal lesions, well-defined lesions and more than nine lesions were suggestive of multiple sclerosis.[46] Another study included a cohort of 296 pediatric patients with acute CNS inflammatory demyelination. At the end of the 2.9 ± 3 years of follow-up, 57% of patients were diagnosed as multiple sclerosis, 29% had monophasic ADEM, and 14% had a single focal episode. The rate of a second attack was higher in patients with an age of onset ≥ 10 years, initial MRI suggestive of multiple sclerosis and optic nerve involvement. A second attack was less likely if a patient had myelitis or abnormal mental status. Of the patients with a second demyelin-ating event, 29% had an initial diagnosis of ADEM.[35] The presence of peri-ventricular lesions distinguished a first attack of multiple sclerosis from monophasic ADEM[47] (Table 2).

Table 2 Differentiating Features of Acute Disseminated Encephalomyelitis and Multiple Sclerosis

	ADEM	MS
Demographic		
Age of onset	Children (5–8 years)	Adults
M:F	1:1	1:>2
Season	Winter and spring	No specific season
Precipitating event	Infection or vaccination	No definite association
Pathological		
Pathology	Perivenous demyelination	Confluent demyelination
Clinical		
Course	Monophasic	Polyphasic
Symptoms	Poly-symptomatic	Monosymptomatic
Manifestations	Encephalopathy manifesting as altered sensorium, meningism and seizures	Encephalopathy is rare
Optic neuritis	Bilateral	Unilateral
CSF	Lymphocytic pleocytosis and increased protein	Often normal
Oligoclonal bands	Rare	Common
Neuroimaging		
MRI	Multiple ill-defined lesions	Single or few lesions with well-defined margins
	Deep white matter lesions with periventricular sparing	Periaqueductal, periventricular white matter and corpus callosum long-axis perpendicular lesions (Dawson fingers)
	Spinal cord and grey matter (brain stem, thalamus and basal ganglion) are involved	Not involved
Follow-up MRI	New lesions are rare	New lesions are frequent
Prognosis		
Outcome	Often good	Disability is common

Several groups of investigators noted that patients with ADEM whose initial brain MRI findings meet the modified McDonald criteria have a significantly higher probability of conversion to multiple sclerosis. In contrast, patients whose brain MRI findings do not meeting the modified McDonald criteria are likely to have ADEM, and they have a lesser risk of conversion to multiple sclerosis.[48] On the basis of their experience, de Seze and co-workers proposed that the presence of any two of the following three criteria could be used to differentiate patients with ADEM from those with multiple sclerosis: atypical clinical symptoms of multiple sclerosis, absence of oligoclonal bands, and grey matter involvement. On this basis they were able to classify 29 of the 35 patients (83%) in the ADEM group and 18 of the 19 patients (95%) in the multiple sclerosis group in the appropriate categories.[49]

In developing countries, the clinical and radiologic presentation of pediatric ADEM is similar to that observed in developed countries, but no conversions to multiple sclerosis have been noted.[50] Even large demyelinating lesions (tumefactive lesions) are frequently encountered; available data suggest that these patients also show an excellent response to treatment, with good functional recovery in the long term and no recurrences.[51]

12 CONCLUSION

Differentiating relapses from multiple sclerosis poses a great diagnostic challenge in patients with ADEM because of the need for long-term disease-modifying therapy. Patients with ADEM whose MRI findings meet the modified McDonald criteria have a high probability of conversion to multiple sclerosis. Although ADEM is frequently encountered in developing countries, conversion to multiple sclerosis has not been noted. Is ADEM seen in developed countries different from ADEM seen in countries poor in resources? The exact relationship between ADEM and multiple sclerosis needs further clarification.

REFERENCES

1. Tenembaum SN. Acute disseminated encephalomyelitis. *Handb Clin Neurol* 2013;**112**:1253–62. http://dx.doi.org/10.1016/B978-0-444-52910-7.00048-9.
2. Wingerchuk DM, Weinshenker BG. Acute disseminated encephalomyelitis, transverse myelitis, and neuromyelitis optica. *Continuum (Minneap Minn)* 2013;**19**:944–67.

3. Krupp LB, Banwell B, Tenembaum S, International Pediatric MS Study Group. Consensus definitions proposed for pediatric multiple sclerosis and related disorders. *Neurology* 2007;**68**(Suppl. 2):S7–S12.
4. Krupp LB, Tardieu M, Amato MP, Banwell B, Chitnis T, Dale RC, et al. International Pediatric Multiple Sclerosis Study Group criteria for pediatric multiple sclerosis and immune-mediated central nervous system demyelinating disorders: revisions to the 2007 definitions. *Mult Scler* 2013;**19**:1261–7.
5. Murthy SN, Faden HS, Cohen ME, Bakshi R. Acute disseminated encephalomyelitis in children. *Pediatrics* 2002;**110**:e21.
6. Absoud M, Lim MJ, Chong WK, De Goede CG, Foster K, Gunny R, et al. Paediatric acquired demyelinating syndromes: incidence, clinical and magnetic resonance imaging features. *Mult Scler* 2013;**19**:76–86.
7. Leake JA, Albani S, Kao AS, Senac MO, Billman GF, Nespeca MP, et al. Acute disseminated encephalomyelitis in childhood: epidemiologic, clinical and laboratory features. *Pediatr Infect Dis J* 2004;**23**:756–64.
8. Murthy JM, Yangala R, Meena AK, Jaganmohan RJ. Acute disseminated encephalomyelitis: clinical and MRI study from South India. *J Neurol Sci* 1999;**165**:133–8.
9. Murthy JM, Yangala R, Meena AK, Reddy JJ. Clinical, electrophysiological and magnetic resonance imaging study of acute disseminated encephalomyelitis. *J Assoc Physicians India* 1999;**47**(3):280–3. Erratum in J Assoc Physicians India 1999;47:412.
10. Noorbakhsh F, Johnson RT, Emery D, Power C. Acute disseminated encephalomyelitis: clinical and pathogenesis features. *Neurol Clin* 2008;**6**:759–80.
11. Mani S, Mondal SS, Guha G, Gangopadhyay S, Pani A, Das Baksi S, et al. Acute disseminated encephalomyelitis after mixed malaria infection (*Plasmodium falciparum* and *Plasmodium vivax*) with MRI closely simulating multiple sclerosis. *Neurologist* 2011;**17**:276–8.
12. Paliwal VK, Goel G, Vema R, Pradhan S, Gupta RK. Acute disseminated encephalomyelitis following filarial infection. *J Neurol Neurosurg Psychiatry* 2012;**83**:347–9.
13. Paisiou A, Goussetis E, Dimopoulou M, Kitra V, Peristeri I, Vessalas G, et al. Acute disseminated encephalomyelitis after allogeneic bone marrow transplantation for pure red cell aplasia—a case report and review of the literature. *Pediatr Transplant* 2013;**17**:E41–5.
14. Oh HH, Kwon SH, Kim CW, Choe BH, Ko CW, Jung HD, et al. Molecular analysis of HLA class II-associated susceptibility to neuroinflammatory diseases in Korean children. *J Korean Med Sci* 2004;**19**:426–30.
15. Idrissova ZhR, Boldyreva MN, Dekonenko EP, Malishev NA, Leontyeva IY, Martinenko IN, et al. Acute disseminated encephalomyelitis in children: clinical features and HLA-DR linkage. *Eur J Neurol* 2003;**10**:537–46.
16. Alves-Leon SV, Veluttini-Pimentel ML, Gouveia ME, Malfetano FR, Gaspareto EL, Alvarenga MP, et al. Acute disseminated encephalomyelitis: clinical features, HLA DRB1*1501, HLA DRB1*1503, HLA DQA1*0102, HLA DQB1*0602, and HLA DPA1*0301 allelic association study. *Arq Neuropsiquiatr* 2009;**67**:643–51.
17. Gold R, Hartung HP, Toyka KV. Animal models for autoimmune demyelinating disorders of the nervous system. *Mol Med Today* 2000;**6**:88–91.
18. Pender MP, Sears TA. The pathophysiology of acute experimental allergic encephalomyelitis in the rabbit. *Brain* 1984;**107**:699–726.
19. Pohl-Koppe A, Burchett SK, Thiele EA, Hafler DA. Myelin basic protein reactive Th2 T cells are found in acute disseminated encephalomyelitis. *J Neuroimmunol* 1998;**91**:19–27.
20. Cusick MF, Libbey JE, Fujinami RS. Molecular mimicry as a mechanism of autoimmune disease. *Clin Rev Allergy Immunol* 2012;**42**:102–11.
21. Wucherpfennig KW, Strominger JL. Molecular mimicry in T cell-mediated autoimmunity: viral peptides activate human T cell clones specific for myelin basic protein. *Cell* 1995;**80**:695–705.

22. Miller SD, Katz-Levy Y, Neville KL, Vanderlugt CL. Virus-induced autoimmunity: epitope spreading to myelin autoepitopes in Theiler's virus infection of the central nervous system. *Adv Virus Res* 2001;**56**:199–217.
23. Richards MH, Getts MT, Podojil JR, Jin YH, Kim BS, Miller SD. Virus expanded regulatory T cells control disease severity in the Theiler's virus mouse model of MS. *J Autoimmun* 2011;**36**:142–54.
24. Brilot F, Dale RC, Selter RC, Grummel V, Kalluri SR, Aslam M, et al. Antibodies to native myelin oligodendrocyte glycoprotein in children with inflammatory demyelinating central nervous system disease. *Ann Neurol* 2009;**66**:833–42.
25. Lee DH, Linker RA. The role of myelin oligodendrocyte glycoprotein in autoimmune demyelination: a target for multiple sclerosis therapy? *Expert Opin Ther Targets* 2012;**16**:451–62.
26. Van Haren K, Tomooka BH, Kidd BA, Banwell B, Bar-Or A, Chitnis T, et al. Serum autoantibodies to myelin peptides distinguish acute disseminated encephalomyelitis from relapsing- remitting multiple sclerosis. *Mult Scler* 2013;**19**(13):1726–33.
27. Pröbstel AK, Dornmair K, Bittner R, Sperl P, Jenne D, Magalhaes S, et al. Antibodies to MOG are transient in childhood acute disseminated encephalomyelitis. *Neurology* 2011;**77**:580–8.
28. Ishizu T, Minohara M, Ichiyama T, Kira R, Tanaka M, Osoegawa M, et al. CSF cytokine and chemokine profiles in acute disseminated encephalomyelitis. *J Neuroimmunol* 2006;**175**:52–8.
29. Ichiyama T, Kajimoto M, Suenaga N, Maeba S, Matsubara T, Furukawa S. Serum levels of matrix metalloproteinase-9 and its tissue inhibitor (TIMP-1) in acute disseminated encephalomyelitis. *J Neuroimmunol* 2006;**172**:182–6.
30. Habek M, Žarković K. Pathology of acute disseminated encephalomyelitis. *Transl Neurosci* 2011;**2**:252–5.
31. Young NP, Weinshenker BG, Parisi JE, Scheithauer B, Giannini C, Roemer SF, et al. Perivenous demyelination: association with clinically defined acute disseminated encephalomyelitis and comparison with pathologically confirmed multiple sclerosis. *Brain* 2010;**133**:333–48.
32. Marin SE, Callen DJ. The magnetic resonance imaging appearance of monophasic acute disseminated encephalomyelitis: an update post application of the 2007 consensus criteria. *Neuroimaging Clin N Am* 2013;**23**:245–66.
33. Garg RK. Acute disseminated encephalomyelitis. *Postgrad Med J* 2003;**79**:11–17.
34. Zhang L, Wu A, Zhang B, Chen S, Men X, Lin Y, et al. Comparison of deep gray matter lesions on magnetic resonance imaging among adults with acute disseminated encephalomyelitis, multiple sclerosis, and neuromyelitis optica. *Mult Scler* 2014;**20**(4):418–23.
35. Mikaeloff Y, Suissa S, Vallée L, Lubetzki C, Ponsot G, Confavreux C, et al. First episode of acute CNS inflammatory demyelination in childhood: prognostic factors for multiple sclerosis and disability. *J Pediatr* 2004;**144**:246–52.
36. Dale RC, Branson JA. Acute disseminated encephalomyelitis or multiple sclerosis: can the initial presentation help in establishing a correct diagnosis? *Arch Dis Child* 2005;**90**:636–9.
37. Balasubramanya KS, Kovoor JM, Jayakumar PN, Ravishankar S, Kamble RB, Panicker J, et al. Diffusion-weighted imaging and proton MR spectroscopy in the characterization of acute disseminated encephalomyelitis. *Neuroradiology* 2007;**49**:177–83.
38. Richard HT, Harrison JF, Abel TW, Maertens P, Martino AM, Sosnowski JS. Pediatric gliomatosis cerebri mimicking acute disseminated encephalomyelitis. *Pediatrics* 2010;**126**:e479–82.
39. Pace AA, Edwards S, Weatherby S. A new clinical variant of the post-malaria neurological syndrome. *J Neurol Sci* 2013;**334**(1–2):183–5.
40. Deiva K, Mahlaoui N, Beaudonnet F, de Saint Basile G, Caridade G, Moshous D, et al. CNS involvement at the onset of primary hemophagocytic lymphohistiocytosis. *Neurology* 2012;**78**:1150–6.

41. Pohl D, Tenembaum S. Treatment of acute disseminated encephalomyelitis. *Curr Treat Options Neurol* 2012;**14**:264–75.
42. Refai D, Lee MC, Goldenberg FD, Frank JI. Decompressive hemicraniectomy for acute disseminated encephalomyelitis: case report. *Neurosurgery* 2005;**56**:E872.
43. Tenembaum S, Chamoles N, Fejerman N. Acute disseminated encephalomyelitis. A long-term follow up study of 84 Pediatric patients. *Neurology* 2002;**59**:1224–31.
44. Lin CH, Jeng JS, Hsieh ST, Yip PK, Wu RM. Acute disseminated encephalomyelitis: a follow-up study in Taiwan. *J Neurol Neurosurg Psychiatry* 2007;**78**:162–7.
45. Rostásy K, Nagl A, Lütjen S, Roll K, Zotter S, Blaschek A, et al. Clinical outcome of children presenting with a severe manifestation of acute disseminated encephalomyelitis. *Neuropediatrics* 2009;**40**:211–17.
46. Mikaeloff Y, Adamsbaum C, Husson B, Vallée L, Ponsot G, Confavreux C, et al. MRI prognostic factors for relapse after acute CNS inflammatory demyelination in childhood. *Brain* 2004;**127**:1942–7.
47. Callen DJ, Shroff MM, Branson HM, Li DK, Lotze T, Stephens D, et al. Role of MRI in the differentiation of ADEM from MS in children. *Neurology* 2009;**72**:968–73.
48. Liao MF, Huang CC, Lyu RK, Chen CM, Chang HS, Chu CC, et al. Acute disseminated encephalomyelitis that meets modified McDonald criteria for dissemination in space is associated with a high probability of conversion to multiple sclerosis in Taiwanese patients. *Eur J Neurol* 2011;**18**:252–9.
49. de Seze J, Debouverie M, Zephir H, Lebrun C, Blanc F, Bourg V, et al. Acute fulminant demyelinating disease: a descriptive study of 60 patients. *Arch Neurol* 2007;**64**:1426–32.
50. Singhi PD, Ray M, Singhi S, Kumar KN. Acute disseminated encephalomyelitis in North Indian children: clinical profile and follow-up. *J Child Neurol* 2006;**21**:851–7.
51. Wattamwar PR, Baheti NN, Kesavadas C, Nair M, Radhakrishnan A. Evolution and long term outcome in patients presenting with large demyelinating lesions as their first clinical event. *J Neurol Sci* 2010;**297**:29–35.

CHAPTER 61

Narcolepsy, Infections, and Autoimmunity

María-Teresa Arango[*,†,‡,1], **Shaye Kivity**[*,§,¶], **Nancy Agmon-Levin**[*,||], **Joab Chapman**[*,#], **Gili Givaty**[*,#], **Yehuda Shoenfeld**[*,||,**]

[*]Zabludowicz Center for Autoimmune Diseases, Sheba Medical Center, Tel-Hashomer, Affiliated to Sackler Medical School, Tel Aviv University, Tel Aviv, Israel
[†]Center for Autoimmune Diseases Research, Universidad del Rosario, Bogotá, Colombia
[‡]Doctoral Program in Biomedical Sciences, Universidad del Rosario, Bogotá, Colombia
[§]Rheumatic Disease Unit, Sheba Medical Center, Tel-Hashomer, Israel
[¶]The Dr. Pinchas Borenstein Talpiot Medical Leadership Program 2013, Sheba Medical Center, Tel-Hashomer, Israel
[||]Sackler Faculty of Medicine, Tel-Aviv University, Tel-Aviv, Israel
[#]Neurology Department and Sagol Neuroscience Center, Sheba Medical Center, Tel-Hashomer, Israel
[**]Incumbent of the Laura Schwarz-Kip Chair for Research of Autoimmune Diseases, Tel Aviv University, Israel
[1]Corresponding Author: mta270686@hotmail.com

1 INTRODUCTION

Narcolepsy is a sleep disorder characterized by excessive sleepiness daytime. It is considered a rare disease, with a worldwide prevalence between 25 and 50 per 100,000 people.[1] However, it varies from one country to another. For example, in the United States it affects approximately 1 in every 3000 individuals and in Japan it has the highest reported prevalence (0.16%).[2] This range highly depends on the person's genetic background.

A consequence of the strong association with human leukocyte antigen (HLA) polymorphisms, environmental factors as well as other genetic associations related to disease onset, narcolepsy is suspected to be an autoimmune disorder. Five relevant associations support this theory.

1. Narcolepsy is highly associated with protective and risk polymorphisms in the HLA system, especially the *DQB1*06:02*, *DQA1*01:02*, and *DRB1*15:01* risk alleles. However, the strongest risk is associated with the *DQB1*06:02*: 82% to 99% of patients with narcolepsy are carriers,[3,4] whereas only 12% to 38% of healthy individuals have this allele. Indeed, homozygotic individuals for *DQB1*06:02* have an increased risk developing narcolepsy.[3,4] Other important immune-related genes have been associated with narcolepsy, such as tumor necrosis factor (*TNF*)-α,[5]

Infection and Autoimmunity
http://dx.doi.org/10.1016/B978-0-444-63269-2.00064-7

TNF (ligand) superfamily member 4 (*TNFSF4* or *OX40L*), T-cell receptor α-chain,[6] cathepsin H (*CTSH*) and DNA methyltransferase I (*DNMT1*),[7–9] among others.[10]

2. The presence of autoantibodies against Tribbles 2 (Trib2) was first described in a patient with uveitis.[11] Interestingly, 14% to 26% of narcoleptic patients also had higher anti–Trib2 titers than healthy controls.[12,13] Among the narcoleptic patients, titers were higher in proximity to disease onset.[12,13] In addition, experiments with transgenic mice demonstrated that anti–Trib2 antibodies taken from patients with narcolepsy bind directly to orexin neurons in mice brains.[12,14,15] Moreover, the passive transfer (via intraventricular injection) of total IgG from narcoleptic patients (confirmed to be anti–Trib2 positive) into mice brains induced narcoleptic-like attacks, as well as behavioral changes similar to those observed in narcoleptic patients, such as hyperactivity and long-term memory deficits.[16]

3. The importance of the environment in the pathogenesis of narcolepsy is emphasized through studies of twins, which demonstrate a concordance rate of 20-35% in monozygotic narcoleptic twins.[17] In other words, these results suggest that the development of the disease does not depend exclusively on the genetic component but also on environmental factors.

4. Interestingly, the onset of narcolepsy frequently occurs during the teenage years, suggesting that hormonal changes in puberty might trigger the disease.[2,18–21]

5. Finally, there have been numerous reports of narcolepsy appearing following the H1N1 vaccination or after H1N1 or *Streptococcus* spp. infection (see section 3).

Taken together, the interplay between these factors may serve as a trigger of an autoimmune-mediated mechanism that might allow the loss of orexin-producing neurons.

2 OREXIN AND SLEEP

It is postulated that narcolepsy is a consequence of the lack of orexin-producing neurons, which have an essential role in sleep cycle regulation. Analysis of brain autopsy of narcoleptic patients demonstrated a loss of orexin-producing neurons in the hypothalamus.[22,23] Also, orexin concentrations in the cerebrospinal fluid of human patients with narcolepsy are low or undetectable compared with healthy individuals.[5,22] As a consequence of the orexin deficiency, narcoleptic patients present abnormal sleep architecture with uncontrollable attacks of the rapid eye movement (REM) sleep stage in which the previous non-REM stage is absent. In addition, patients may present other symptoms such as cataplexy (loss of muscle tone), sleep paralysis, hallucinations, obesity, and disrupted nocturnal sleep.[5,24]

There are two different kinds of orexins, orexin A and orexin B, which are produced exclusively by orexin neurons in the hypothalamic region of the brain. Both proteins come from the same precursor: the prepro-orexin. This precursor generates two different peptides after post-translational modifications, which are very conserved among different species.[25] Furthermore, two different orexin receptors are distributed throughout the central nervous system, specifically on monoaminergic centers, which are responsible for the secretion of norepinephrine, serotonin, and histamine.[24,25] Since the orexins help mediate the production of these molecules, which are important in many different regulatory process such as feeding, cardiovascular regulation, emotions, and locomotion,[25] it is possible to understand their role in human physiology.

Regarding the sleep process, orexin is responsible for maintaining a state of wakefulness. It activates monoaminergic neurons, which in turn send inhibitory signals to the ventrolateral preoptic area (VLPO), where gamma-aminobutyric acid-producing neurons are suppressed. On the other hand, during the sleep period, the neurons in the VLPO send inhibitory signals to orexin and monoaminergic neurons, thus inducing sleep. When orexin neurons are removed from this circuit, there are mutual inhibitory signals between monoaminergic and VLPO neurons that cause the characteristic unwanted abrupt transitions between wakefulness and sleep and the rupture of the balance. This leads the previously described symptoms of the disease.[22,25–27]

3 ENVIRONMENTAL ROLE: INFECTION AND VACCINES

The current hypothesis is that a given individual with a certain genetic background may develop an autoimmune disease at some stage of life because of exposure to several environmental factors. Results from narcoleptic concordance studies suggest the importance of the environment etiology,[17] perhaps with association of the *DQB1*06:02* allele. In addition, a few studies regarding the exposure to different environmental components have been done to establish an association with narcolepsy. For instance, they demonstrated that smoking, exposure to toxics (e.g. heavy metals and fertilizers), fever and infections are related to disease onset.[21,28,29] In one case-control study, the risk for narcolepsy among carriers of the $DQB1^{*}06:02$ allele was higher among children who were passive smokers than those that were not exposed to cigarettes.[29] Another report based on questionnaires and medical records of narcoleptic $DQB1^{*}06:02$ carriers and matched controls demonstrated that those who suffered from an infectious disease, especially measles, or suffered from any unexplained fever in the past had a significantly higher risk for developing narcolepsy later. Also, they found that some stressors, such as major changes in sleeping habits or changes in living style, carried an additional risk for narcolepsy.[21] One study evaluated the effect of exposure to toxic substances on the risk for narcolepsy among 67 narcoleptic patients compared with 95 controls, both positive for the HLA $DQB1^{*}06:02$ allele. This study evaluated exposure to substances related to different activities (e.g. summer jobs) during childhood, as well as those encountered during recreational activity and other non-vocational activities. Results disclosed that exposure to heavy metals, woodwork, fertilizers, and pesticides posed a risk for acquiring narcolepsy in this population.[28] However, more studies are needed to clarify whether these exposures and stressors are important in the development of narcolepsy.

Infections are of paramount importance in triggering autoimmune diseases—and narcolepsy in particular—and they are considered the most widespread environmental factor that has been studied so far. Infections can induce autoimmunity through different mechanisms, such as molecular mimicry, epitope spreading, bystander activation and superantigens.[30–36] Most of the evidence has linked streptococcal and influenza A infections, as well as the influenza H1N1 vaccine, to narcolepsy susceptibility.[37–39]

3.1 Streptococcal Infections

The importance of streptococcal group A (SGA) infection, a gram-positive bacteria, in autoimmunity has been extensively studied. Indeed, SGA is linked to rheumatic fever, affecting susceptible individuals and leading to an immune-mediated disease that may involve the heart, joints, skin, and brain as a consequence of antigen mimicry with the M-protein.[40] SGA produces different antigens and superantigens that may stimulate auto-reactive B and T cells, leading to the production of autoantibodies.[40,41] In 2012, Cunningham summarized the relationship between specific manifestations of rheumatic fever and the relevant mimicry between streptococcal antigens and human antigens recognized by T and B cells. For instance, in carditis, cardiac myosin is recognized by anti-streptococcal antibodies directed to the bacterial carbohydrate N-acetyl-beta-D-glucosamine (GlcNAc).

SGA infections also have been related to neurological conditions such as Sydenham's chorea syndrome (the neurological manifestation of rheumatic fever), pediatric autoimmune disorders associated with streptococcal infections and different dystonias.[40,42–44] Interestingly, some reports have demonstrated the presence of autoantibodies against neuronal proteins in patients with a neurologic disorder and previous streptococcal infections.[43,44] For instance, neuronal glycolytic enzymes are human antigens recognized by anti-streptococcal antibodies. The NGE are expressed intracellularly, as well as on the neuronal cell surface, and they may have an identity between 0% and 49% similar with glycolytic streptococcal enzymes.[45] Another example is the development of movement and psychiatric disorders, which are associated with the presence of autoantibodies against neuronal structures in post-streptococcal infections.[43] Movement disorders may develop after the biding of anti-neuronal antibodies to receptors on neurons. This interaction may trigger signal cascades such as Ca2+/calmodulin-dependent protein kinase II, tyrosine hydroxylase with eventual dopamine release or the direct stimulation of dopamine receptors.[40,46–48] In the same way, the presence of anti-basal ganglia antibodies was associated with idiopathic obsessive compulsive disorder in patients with previous streptococcal infections.[49] This supports the theory of cross-reactivity as a consequence of the similarity between human and SGA molecules, leading to brain manifestations after SGA infections.

Finally, the relationship between streptococcal infections and narcolepsy was proposed after a study that detected elevated anti-streptococcal antibodies in the sera of newly diagnosed narcoleptic patients.[37] Another case-control study of *DQB1*06:02* carriers, including healthy control and narcoleptic patients, showed that childhood streptococcal throat infection was a risk factor for narcolepsy in comparison with other childhood infectious diseases such as mononucleosis, pneumonia, or hepatitis.[50] An 8-year-old child positive for DR2 (DR15) and HLA *DQB1*0602* was diagnosed with Sydenham's chorea and narcolepsy. In addition to the HLA, it was interesting that this patient had a orexin deficiency in the CSF and elevated titers of anti-streptococcal antibodies (i.e. anti-streptolysin O).[51] All this together supports the idea that streptococcal infections are associated with the onset of narcolepsy.

3.2 AH1N1 Vaccine and Influenza Infections

Perhaps the most impressive evidence that there is an environmental trigger in the development of narcolepsy is H1N1 vaccination campaigns. Following

the 2009 outbreak of pandemic influenza type AH1N1, different immunization strategies were implemented in Europe using eight different commercial
vaccines; all were designed from the A/California/7/2009 (H1N1) v-like
strain. However, the main difference between them was the adjutant used;
the ASO3-adjuvanted vaccine was the most widely used.[52,53]

After the campaign, an increase in the diagnosis of narcolepsy was
described first in Finland. In 2010, a neurologist studying children found that
the number of new cases of the disease was higher than that in the historical
records.[54,55] Afterwards, more reports and epidemiological studies contributed to proving the phenomenon. In 2010, a task force was created to determine whether there was a causal relationship between the increase in
narcolepsy cases in children from Finland and the 2009 vaccination campaign.
The task force compared the narcolepsy incidence before and after 2009 and
discovered a significant upswing after the vaccination in 2009.[56] Finally, the
analysis showed a ninefold increased risk of narcolepsy the 4- to 19-year-old
age group among those who received the ASO3-adjuvanted vaccine,[56] but
the risk of narcolepsy did not increase in the overall population with the
viral infection itself.[57] Consequently, an analysis of medical records of vaccinated individuals in Finland showed that children who had been vaccinated
had a 12.7-fold higher risk of developing narcolepsy. These results were dupli-
cated in Denmark, Sweden, France, and England[52,55,58] by retrospective studies based on information from health care databases and that evaluated the
ASO3-adjuvanted vaccine as a risk factor. It is worth mentioning that the risk
of narcolepsy associated with the AH1N1 vaccine also was related to genetic
susceptibility. For instance, studies of cases of narcolepsy/cataplexy after vaccination in Switzerland, the United States, the United Kingdom, France, and
Brazil found that all the patients were carriers of $DQB1^*06:02$,[38,55,59] and one
particular case with an additional diagnosis of multiple sclerosis was also
$DRB1^*15:01$ positive.[60]

A recent study of narcolepsy-cataplexy patients in France was performed
in a search for different sub-phenotypes between patients with and without
the H1N1 vaccine. As expected, the vaccination was associated with the disease. Nevertheless, the comparison between patients with and without the
vaccine found slight differences. Vaccinated patients in particular had a
shorter delay in diagnosis and a higher number of sleep-onset REM
periods.[61]

However, the link between H1N1 vaccination and the onset of narcolepsy
was not found in other European countries such as Italy or the United
Kingdom.[52,55] In contrast, the infection itself—and not the vaccine—was

associated with a three- to fourfold increase in the incidence of narcolepsy in China after the 2009 pandemic, where it also displayed a seasonal behavior. It is noteworthy that the incidence of narcolepsy among the Chinese population returned to baseline after this period.[19,62] Finally, functional analyses of CD4$^+$ lymphocytes from narcoleptic patients showed that these cells were able to recognize orexin peptides when they were presented by dendritic cells (homozygotic for the $DQA1^*01:02/DQB1^*06:02$ haplotype); moreover, those cells could also recognize peptides from H1N1, indicating a possible molecular mimicry between orexin and similar peptides from H1N1.[63] Therefore, these results suggest an association between the H1N1 vaccination or the infection itself and onset of narcolepsy based on geographic location and genetic background.[56]

4 DRAWING CONCLUSIONS ABOUT AUTOIMMUNE ETIOLOGY

There is no evidence of any inflammatory process in the hypothalamus; this may be because of the impossibility of analyzing the brains of patients at the time of the diagnosis.[5,23,37] The specific loss of orexin neurons found in analyses of the brains of deceased patients suggests that this precise loss is the consequence of an autoimmune-mediated process.[22,23,64] Currently, many researchers consider the association with the $DQB1^*06:02$ allele to be another strong indication of autoimmunity. However, a single polymorphic association is not enough to draw this conclusion. Indeed, there are more studies that describe associations between other genetic variants as well as environmental factors that may trigger the disease (discussed earlier).

In the past few years, Emmanuel Mignot studied the etiology of narcolepsy in animal models and human genetic studies. His group recently proposed a model that may explain how the combination of genetic and environmental factors can result in the destruction of the orexin neurons by an autoimmune process[4,65,66] (Figure 1). Briefly, almost all the genetic associations with narcolepsy are related to the immune system. Therefore, changes in antigen degradation and presentation may serve as clues to elucidate the autoimmune mechanism in narcolepsy. In addition, infections as well as pathogen (i.e. superantigens) or vaccine components may also play a crucial role in facilitating the breakdown of the blood-brain barrier[21,41] as well as the activation of autoreactive immune cells and the production of autoantibodies, which leads to the destruction of orexin neurons in the hypothalamus as collateral damage in response to infections.[4,65,66] When

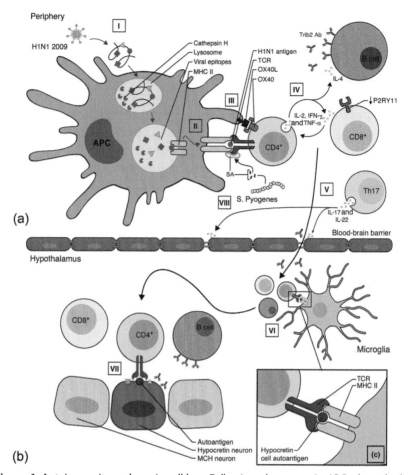

Figure 1 Autoimmunity and orexin cell loss. Following phagocytosis, APCs degrade the H1N1 influenza virus in the lysosome, a process facilitated by cathepsin H (I). Peptides from the virus are presented on the surface of APCs in the context of MHC class II (DQA1*01:02-DQB1*06:02) for cognate TCR recognition (II). Orexin-specific CD4+ T cells recognize the presented antigen and are activated. After being activated, the CD4+ T cells up-regulate the expression of OX40, which is an important co-stimulatory molecule recognized by APCs that express OX40L (III). Activated CD4+ T cells secrete IFN-γ, TNF-α and IL-2, which stimulate CD8+ T cells and drive a Th 1-mediated immune response. IL-4 from activated CD4+ T cells promotes a humoral response, leading to the production of Tribbles2 antibody by B cells (IV). Generation of superantigens as a result of *Streptococcus* infection activates Th17 cells, facilitating the breakdown of the blood-brain barrier through the secretion of IL-17 and IL-22. Increased permeability allows for the migration of activated T cells, B cells, and Tribbles-2 antibodies into the CNS (V). Migration of activated T cells and B cells through the disrupted brain-blood barrier (i.e. by fever or cytokines) is followed by interaction with CNS APCs (microglia) that present autoantigens (orexin neuron autoantigens) in the context of DQA1*01:02-DQB1*06:02 (VI). Reactivated T cells reach the hypothalamus and recognize orexin neurons, inducing effector functions such as the secretion of cytokines or cytotoxic compounds. Moreover, superantigens from streptococcus cross-link the MHC and TCR molecules independent of antigen specificity, activating the autoreactive T cell (VII and inset c). This may lead to sensitization to orexin-specific antigens and form the basis for subsequent booster reactions of cross-reactive CD4+ T cells, a process that finally ends in an autoimmune reaction against orexin neurons. MCH, melanin-concentrating hormone. *Reprinted with permission from Elsevier from Mahlios et al.[65]*

the association of the disease with infections and vaccines is considered within the context of narcolepsy, all this evidence suggests that an autoimmune-mediated process triggered by environmental factors may be the main cause of narcolepsy among genetically susceptible individuals.

Further studies are needed to clarify the actual role of the immune system in the development and autoimmune basis of narcolepsy in individuals with a specific genetic background, environmental exposures and perhaps immune disregulation. Different mechanisms such as bystander activation of autoreactive B and T cells in response to a vaccine's adjuvants or infections as well as molecular mimicry between neuronal epitopes and peptides derived from the H1N1 vaccine, H1N1 virus or *Streptococcus* spp. molecules should be explored.[4,65,66]

REFERENCES

1. Longstreth WT, Koepsell TD, Ton TG, Hendrickson AF, van Belle G. The epidemiology of narcolepsy. *Sleep* 2007;**30**(1):13–26.
2. Akintomide GS, Rickards H. Narcolepsy: a review. *Neuropsychiatr Dis Treat* 2011;**7**:507–18.
3. Mignot E, Lin L, Rogers W, Honda Y, Qiu X, Lin X, et al. Complex HLA-DR and-DQ interactions confer risk of narcolepsy-cataplexy in three ethnic groups. *Am J Hum Genet* 2001;**68**(3):686–99.
4. Kornum BR, Faraco J, Mignot E. Narcolepsy with hypocretin/orexin deficiency, infections an autoimmunity of the brain. *Curr Opin Neurobiol* 2011;**21**(6):897–903.
5. Fontana A, Gast H, Reith W, Recher M, Birchler T, Bassetti CL. Narcolepsy: autoimmunity, effector T cell activation due to infection, or T cell independent, major histocompatibility complex class II induced neuronal loss? *Brain* 2010;**133**(5):1300–11.
6. Hallmayer J, Faraco J, Lin L, Hesselson S, Winkelmann J, Kawashima M, et al. Narcolepsy is strongly associated with the T-cell receptor alpha locus. *Nat Genet* 2009;**41**(6):708–11.
7. Faraco J, Lin L, Kornum BR, Kenny EE, Trynka G, Einen M, et al. ImmunoChip study implicates antigen presentation to T cells in narcolepsy. *PLoS Genet* 2013;**9**(2):e1003270.
8. Winkelmann J, Lin L, Schormair B, Kornum BR, Faraco J, Plazzi G, et al. Mutations in DNMT1 cause autosomal dominant cerebellar ataxia, deafness and narcolepsy. *Hum Mol Genet* 2012;**21**(10):2205–10.
9. Josefowicz SZ, Wilson CB, Rudensky AY. Cutting edge: TCR stimulation is sufficient for induction of Foxp3 expression in the absence of DNA methyltransferase 1. *J Immunol* 2009;**182**(11):6648–52.
10. Han F, Lin L, Li J, Aran A, Dong SX, An P, et al. TCRA, P2RY11, and CPT1B/CHKB associations in Chinese narcolepsy. *Sleep Med* 2012;**13**(3):269–72.
11. Zhang Y, Davis JL, Li W. Identification of tribbles homolog 2 as an autoantigen in autoimmune uveitis by phage display. *Mol Immunol* 2005;**42**(11):1275–81.
12. Cvetkovic-Lopes V, Bayer L, Dorsaz S, Maret S, Pradervand S, Dauvilliers Y, et al. Elevated tribbles homolog 2-specific antibody levels in narcolepsy patients. *J Clin Invest* 2010;**120**(3):713.
13. Toyoda H, Tanaka S, Miyagawa T, Honda Y, Tokunaga K, Honda M. Anti-tribbles homolog 2 autoantibodies in Japanese patients with narcolepsy. *Sleep* 2010;**33**(7):875–8.

14. Kawashima M, Lin L, Tanaka S, Jennum P, Knudsen S, Nevsimalova S, et al. Antitribbles homolog 2 (TRIB2) autoantibodies in narcolepsy are associated with recent onset of cataplexy. *Sleep* 2010;**33**(7):869–74.
15. Lim ASP, Scammell TE. The trouble with Tribbles: do antibodies against TRIB2 cause narcolepsy? *Sleep* 2010;**33**:857.
16. Katzav A, Arango MT, Kivity S, Tanaka S, Givaty G, Agmon-Levin N, et al. Passive transfer of narcolepsy: anti-TRIB2 autoantibody positive patient IgG causes hypothalamic orexin neuron loss and sleep attacks in mice. *J Autoimmun* 2013;**45**:24–30.
17. Mignot E. Genetic and familial aspects of narcolepsy. *Neurology* 1998;**50**:S16–22.
18. Silver MH, Krahn LE, Olson EJ, Pankratz VS. The epidemiology of narcolepsy in Olmsted County, Minnesota: a population-based study. *Sleep* 2010;**25**(2):197–202.
19. Nohynek H, Jokinen J, Partinen M, Vaarala O, Kirjavainen T, Sundman J, et al. AS03 adjuvanted AH1N1 vaccine associated with an abrupt increase in the incidence of childhood narcolepsy in Finland. *PloS one* 2012;**7**(3):e33536.
20. Ohayon MM, Ferini-Strambi L, Plazzi G, Smirne S, Castronovo V. How age influences the expression of narcolepsy. *J Psychosom Res* 2005;**59**(6):399–405.
21. Picchioni D, Hope CR, Harsh JR. A case-control study of the environmental risk factors for narcolepsy. *Neuroepidemiology* 2007;**29**(3–4):185–92.
22. Rolls A, Borg JS, de Lecea L. Sleep and metabolism: role of hypothalamic neuronal circuitry. *Best Pract Res Clin Endocrinol Metab* 2010;**24**(5):817–28.
23. Thannickal TC, Nienhuis R, Siegel JM. Localized loss of hypocretin (orexin) cells in narcolepsy without cataplexy. *Sleep* 2009;**32**(8):993–8.
24. Sakurai T, Mieda M, Tsujino N. The orexin system: roles in sleep/wake regulation. *Ann N Y Acad Sci* 2010;**1200**(1):149–61.
25. Ohno K, Sakurai T. Orexin neuronal circuitry: role in the regulation of sleep and wakefulness. *Front Neuroendocrinol* 2008;**29**(1):70–87.
26. Huang W, Ramsey KM, Marcheva B, Bass J. Circadian rhythms, sleep, and metabolism. *J Clin Invest* 2011;**121**(6):2133–41.
27. Burt J, Alberto CO, Parsons MP, Hirasawa M. Local network regulation of orexin neurons in the lateral hypothalamus. *Am J Physiol Regul Integr Comp Physiol* 2011;**301**(3): R572–80.
28. Ton TGN, Longstreth WT, Koepsell TD. Environmental toxins and risk of narcolepsy among people with HLA DQB1*0602. *Environ Res* 2010;**110**(6):565–70.
29. Ton TGN, Longstreth WT, Koepsell T. Active and passive smoking and risk of narcolepsy in people with HLA DQB1*0602: a population-based case-control study. *Neuroepidemiology* 2009;**32**(2):114–21.
30. Kivity S, Agmon-Levin N, Blank M, Shoenfeld Y. Infections and autoimmunity–friends or foes? *Trends Immunol* 2009;**30**(8):409–14.
31. Sfriso P, Ghirardello A, Botsios C, Tonon M, Zen M, Bassi N, et al. Infections and autoimmunity: the multifaceted relationship. *J Leukoc Biol* 2010;**87**(3):385–95.
32. Wucherpfennig KW. Mechanisms for the induction of autoimmunity by infectious agents. *J Clin Invest* 2001;**108**(8):1097–104.
33. Samarkos M, Vaiopoulos G. The role of infections in the pathogenesis of autoimmune diseases. *Curr Drug Targets Inflamm Allergy* 2005;**4**(1):99–103.
34. Rose NR. Infection, mimics, and autoimmune disease. *J Clin Invest* 2001;**107**(8):943–4.
35. Arango M-T, Anaya J-M. Infección y enfermedad autoinmune. In: Anaya J-M, Rojas-Villarraga A, editors. *La tautología Autoinmune*. Bogotá: Editorial Univesidad del Rosario; 2012. p. 131–44.
36. Arango M-T, Shoenfeld Y, Cervera R, Anaya J-M. Infection and autoimmune diseases. In: Anaya J-M, Shoenfeld Y, Rojas-Villarraga A, Levy RA, Cervera R, editors. *Autoimmunity from bench to bedside*. Bogotá: Editorial Universidad del Rosario; 2013. p. 303–19.

37. Aran A, Lin L, Nevsimalova S, Plazzi G, Hong SC, Weiner K, et al. Elevated anti-streptococcal antibodies in patients with recent narcolepsy onset. *Sleep* 2009;**32** (8):979–83.
38. Dauvilliers Y, Montplaisir J, Cochen V, Desautels A, Einen M, Lin L, et al. Post-H1N1 narcolepsy-cataplexy. *Sleep* 2010;**33**(11):1428–30.
39. Viorritto EN, Kureshi SA, Owens JA. Narcolepsy in the pediatric population. *Curr Neurol Neurosci Rep* 2012;**12**(2):175–81.
40. Cunningham MW. Streptococcus and rheumatic fever. *Curr Opin Rheumatol* 2012;**24** (4):408–16.
41. Commons RJ, Smeesters PR, Proft T, Fraser JD, Robins-Browne R, Curtis N. Streptococcal superantigens: categorization and clinical associations. *Trends Mol Med* 2014;**20** (1):48–62.
42. Snider LA, Swedo SE. Post-streptococcal autoimmune disorders of the central nervous system. *Curr Opin Neurol* 2003;**16**(3):359–65.
43. Dale RC, Heyman I. Post-streptococcal autoimmune psychiatric and movement disorders in children. *Br J Psychiatry* 2002;**181**:188–90.
44. Dale RC. Post-streptococcal autoimmune disorders of the central nervous system. *Dev Med Child Neurol* 2005;**47**(11):785–91.
45. Dale RC, Candler PM, Church AJ, Wait R, Pocock JM, Giovannoni G. Neuronal surface glycolytic enzymes are autoantigen targets in post-streptococcal autoimmune CNS disease. *J Neuroimmunol* 2006;**172**(1–2):187–97.
46. Kirvan CA, Swedo SE, Heuser JS, Cunningham MW. Mimicry and autoantibody-mediated neuronal cell signaling in Sydenham chorea. *Nat Med* 2003;**9**(7):914–20.
47. Cox CJ, Sharma M, Leckman JF, Zuccolo J, Zuccolo A, Kovoor A, et al. Brain human monoclonal autoantibody from sydenham chorea targets dopaminergic neurons in transgenic mice and signals dopamine d2 receptor: implications in human disease. *J Immunol* 2013;**191**(11):5524–41.
48. Ben-Pazi H, Stoner JA, Cunningham MW. Dopamine receptor autoantibodies correlate with symptoms in Sydenham's chorea. *PloS one* 2013;**8**(9):e73516.
49. Dale RC, Heyman I, Giovannoni G, Church AWJ. Incidence of anti-brain antibodies in children with obsessive-compulsive disorder. *Br J Psychiatry* 2005;**187**:314–19.
50. Koepsell TD, Longstreth WT, Ton TGN. Medical exposures in youth and the frequency of narcolepsy with cataplexy: a population-based case-control study in genetically predisposed people. *J Sleep Res* 2010;**19**(1 Pt. 1):80–6.
51. Natarajan N, Jain SV, Chaudhry H, Hallinan BE, Simakajornboon N. Narcolepsy-cataplexy: is streptococcal infection a trigger? *J Clin Sleep Med* 2013;**9**(3):269–70.
52. Wijnans L, Lecomte C, de Vries C, Weibel D, Sammon C, Hviid A, et al. The incidence of narcolepsy in Europe: before, during, and after the influenza A(H1N1)pdm09 pandemic and vaccination campaigns. *Vaccine* 2013;**31**(8):1246–54.
53. O'Flanagan D, Cotter S, Mereckiene J. Pandemic A(H1N1) 2009 Influenza Vaccination Survey, Influenza season 2009/2010. Vaccine European New Integrated Collaboration Effort (VENICE). 2011
54. Käll A. The Pandemrix—narcolepsy tragedy: how it started and what we know today. *Acta Paediatr* 2013;**102**(1):2–4.
55. Zhang X, Penzel T, Han F. Increased incidense of narcolepsy following the 2009 H1N1 pandemic. *Somnologie* 2013;**17**(2):90–3.
56. THL. *National Narcolepsy Task Force Interim Report 31 January 2011*. Helsinki; 2010. p. 3–21.
57. Melén K, Partinen M, Tynell J, Sillanpää M, Himanen S-L, Saarenpää-Heikkilä O, et al. No serological evidence of influenza A H1N1pdm09 virus infection as a contributing factor in childhood narcolepsy after pandemrix vaccination campaign in Finland. *PloS One* 2013;**8**(8):e68402.

58. Miller E, Andrews N, Stellitano L, Stowe J, Winstone AM, Shneerson J, et al. Risk of narcolepsy in children and young people receiving AS03 adjuvanted pandemic A/H1N1 2009 influenza vaccine: retrospective analysis. *BMJ* 2013;**346**:f794.
59. Mendes MFSG, Valladares Neto D de C, Azevedo RA de, Caramelli P. Narcolepsy after A/H1N1 vaccination. *Clinics (Sao Paulo)* 2012;**67**(1):77–8.
60. Vrethem M, Malmgren K, Lindh J. A patient with both narcolepsy and multiple sclerosis in association with Pandemrix vaccination. *J Neurol Sci* 2012;**321**(1–2):89–91.
61. Dauvilliers Y, Arnulf I, Lecendreux M, Monaca Charley C, Franco P, Drouot X, et al. Increased risk of narcolepsy in children and adults after pandemic H1N1 vaccination in France. *Brain* 2013;**136**(Pt. 8):2486–96.
62. Han F, Lin L, Li J, Dong XS, Mignot E. Decreased incidence of childhood narcolepsy 2 years after the 2009 H1N1 winter flu pandemic. *Ann of Neurol* 2012;**73**(4):560.
63. De la Herran-Arita AK, Kornum BR, Mahlios J, Jiang W, Lin L, Hou T, et al. CD4 + T cell autoimmunity to hypocretin/orexin and cross-reactivity to a 2009 H1N1 influenza A epitope in narcolepsy. *Sci Transl Med* 2013;**5**(216):216ra176.
64. Peyron C, Faraco J, Rogers W, Ripley B, Overeem S, Charnay Y, et al. A mutation in a case of early onset narcolepsy and a generalized absence of hypocretin peptides in human narcoleptic brains. *Nat Med* 2000;**6**(9):991–7.
65. Mahlios J, De la Herrán-Arita AK, Mignot E. The autoimmune basis of narcolepsy. *Curr Opin Neurobiol* 2013;**23**(5):767–73.
66. Singh AK, Mahlios J, Mignot E. Genetic association, seasonal infections and autoimmune basis of narcolepsy. *J Autoimmun* 2013;**43**:26–31.

INDEX

Note: Page numbers followed by *b* indicate boxes, *f* indicate figures and *t* indicate tables.

I

CPI Antony Rowe
Eastbourne, UK
September 27, 2019